Cleft Lip and Palate

CLEFT LIP AND PALATE

From Origin to Treatment

Edited by
DIEGO F. WYSZYNSKI

Genetics Program
Department of Medicine
Boston University School of Medicine
and
Department of Epidemiology
Boston University School of Public Health
Boston, Massachusetts

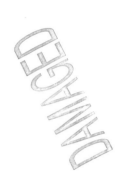

OXFORD
UNIVERSITY PRESS
2002

OXFORD
UNIVERSITY PRESS

Oxford   New York
Auckland   Bangkok   Buenos Aires   Cape Town   Chennai
Dar es Salaam   Delhi   Florence   Hong Kong   Istanbul   Karachi   Kolkata
Kuala Lumpur   Madrid   Melbourne   Mexico City   Mumbai   Nairobi
São Paulo   Shanghai   Singapore   Taipei   Tokyo   Toronto

and an associated company in Berlin

Library of Congress Cataloging-in-Publication Data
Cleft lip and palate : from origin to treatment / edited by Diego F. Wyszynski.
p. ; cm.
Includes bibliographical references and index.
ISBN 0-19-513906-2
1. Cleft lip. 2. Cleft palate. 3. Cleft lip—Surgery. 4. Cleft palate—Surgery. I.
Wyszynski, Diego F.
[DNLM: 1. Cleft lip. 2. Cleft Palate. WV 440 C62152 2002]
RD524.C525 2002
617.5′22—dc21   2001133031

2 4 6 8 9 7 5 3 1

Printed in Hong Kong
on acid-free paper

Foreword

═══════════

This book is a testament to the remarkable growth of knowledge of oral clefts in the past three-quarters of a century. In a foreword, it seems appropriate to consider the early studies of causation that were the origins of the panorama of knowledge that this volume presents. The following is a very personal view of some of the events that were milestones in oral cleft history and will undoubtedly have omissions, which are quite unintentional.

When I was in graduate school in the early 1940s, knowledge of causation had not progressed much beyond the old wive's tales that mothers would tell me about being frightened by a wolf (from *geule-de-loup*) or drawing the knife toward themselves while cutting bread.

In the late 1930s, Sheldon Read, at McGill University, began to explore the genetics of cleft lip (CL) in an ancestor of the A/Jax mouse line, and the Danish plastic surgeon Paul Fogh-Anderson, for his M.D. thesis, was collecting the monumental series of family histories of children with cleft lip and palate (CLP) and cleft palate (CP) that provided the first reliable estimates of recurrence risks for use in genetic counseling.

In the late 1940s, Ted Ingalls, a Boston pediatrician, became convinced that maternal hypoxia was teratogenic. He had seen a woman who had had a motor accident on the 52nd day of her pregnancy, had bled, and had had a child with Down syndrome. He reasoned that since all of the developmental processes that went wrong in Down syndrome happened on that day, maternal hypoxia was the cause. To his credit, he put his hypothesis to the test and showed that making pregnant mice hypoxic led to CP in the offspring, another example of the right conclusion from the wrong inference.

This, plus the recognition by the Australian ophthalmologist Norman McAlister Gregg that rubella was teratogenic and Josef Warkany's demonstration that maternal vitamin deficiencies could be teratogenic in the rat, led to a shift in attitude toward the causes of malformations. The uterus had been regarded as an invulnerable barrier, protecting the embryo from environmental harm; the causes of malformations were, by exclusion, genetic. Now the pendulum had shifted, and the causes of malformations were increasingly seen as environmental. The pendulum began to shift back to an intermediate position, not one or the other but both, when it was shown, at McGill, that the same teratogen can cause very different frequencies of a malformation on different genetic backgrounds. Genes influenced the embryo's response to teratogens, and maternal as well as embryonic genes could be involved. Cortisone and CP in mice, the first example, was soon followed by others, and from these beginnings there developed the field of teratogenics.

Studies of how the mouse palate closed and how closure was delayed by cortisone led to the concept of CP as a multifactorial/threshold trait. A continuous distribution of liability (time of shelf closure) was separated into discontinuous portions, affected and unaffected, by a threshold (the last point in time that closure was possible). Specific genetic and environmental factors were identified that altered CP frequency, by affecting either the position of the distribution or the position of the threshold.

In the meantime, the multifactorial threshold concept was being independently developed by Cedric Carter, in London. He inferred it from a peculiarity in the recurrence risks for hypertrophic pyloric stenosis. Why was the recurrence risk higher for the near relatives of affected females, when the frequency of the disorder is lower in females? The multifactorial threshold model provided a reasonable answer for this and other properties shown by the familial characteristics of pyloric stenosis. Carter and the McGill group went on to show that CL had the same characteristic properties of the model, though to a lesser extent, since the sex ratio for CLP was less distorted.

This model implied that CL usually resulted from the interaction of several genetic and environmental factors that increased susceptibility and that the particular selection of factors could be different in different individuals. Thus, identifying the specific factors in the common type of cleft would be much more difficult than it would be for those caused by genes or teratogens causing major increases in susceptibility. However, that did not discourage people from trying, as shown in Part III of this volume.

Human embryological studies were difficult because embryos could be observed only after the fact. The existence of mouse strains with a high frequency of CL and of teratogens that could produce high frequencies of CL or CP made it easier to study the embryology of oral clefts and to identify predisposing factors.

From such studies came Daphne Trasler's idea that face shape was one component of CL susceptibility, at least in the mouse. This inspired crude attempts to document, with "physioprints" or cephalograms, the relevant components of face-shape susceptibility in the parents and monozygotic twins of children with CL. These have now been happily supplanted by elegant morphometric studies (this volume, Part II). Racial differences in oral cleft frequencies were recognized early, but there have been few attempts to relate these to facial morphometrics.

Epidemiological studies are hampered by the fact that for an uncommon multifactorial trait it is virtually impossible to assemble groups large enough to allow statistically valid comparisons of potentially significant factors such as prenatal events, susceptibility genes, social class, and race. Still, with better appreciation of the problem and more sophisticated statistical approaches, things are beginning to sort out, as shown in Parts III and IV.

I cannot comment on the clinical side (Section II), except to say how dramatically treatment results have improved for the whole child, not just the cleft, at least in part because the need for a multidisciplinary approach was recognized.

Better understanding of causes often takes a long time to translate into prevention, but there is progress (Section III). Families with oral clefts can find encouragement in knowing that even though their child's cleft was not prevented, there have been great improvements in the management of clefts and their sequelae, counseling and support of the family, and social attitudes toward malformations. The very recognition of oral clefts as a public health issue augurs well for affected children and their families.

F. Clarke Fraser
Department of Human Genetics
McGill University
Montreal, Canada

Preface

Each year an estimated 150,000 babies are born with birth defects in the United States. According to a 1998 report of the National Center for Health Statistics, one in five infant deaths is due to birth defects, making them the leading cause of infant mortality. Cleft lip with or without cleft palate and isolated cleft palate, collectively termed *oral clefts*, are the second most common birth defects among newborns. It is estimated that approximately 1 out of every 1000 newborns has an oral cleft, a figure that is higher in certain ethnic groups. From these statistics it may be concluded that 4000 babies are born each year with an oral cleft in the United States. At a lifetime cost of $100,000 per case (according to the National Institute of Dental and Craniofacial Research in 1998), the expense resulting from this disorder is close to half a billion dollars per annual cohort of such children.

Among several objectives of the series *Healthy People 2010*, released by the U.S. Department of Health and Human Services in January 2000, are efforts to reduce rates of birth defects and to increase the quality and years of healthy life in the population. An understanding of the genetic and environmental factors that increase susceptibility to oral clefts is vital to their diagnosis, treatment, and, eventually, prevention. This book, therefore, is intended to provide graduate students, practitioners, and researchers with information to help them fulfill the goals of *Healthy People 2010*. The book, however, was organized with a wider readership in mind. Many of the chapters will be of interest to parents, siblings, and individuals with oral clefts.

The following chapters cover a broad range of theoretical, experimental, and clinical topics and are written by experts in the fields of craniofacial development, biomedical sciences, genetics, epidemiology, and public health. The format is that of a state-of-the-art reference text for a wide readership seeking in-depth information on oral clefts. The text is divided into three sections, Basic Principles, Treatment, and Public Health Issues, plus one appendix and a glossary.

The first section has four parts. Part I presents overarching principles of facial development, from mole-cules to tissues and organs (Chapters 1–3). These topics will be of special interest to basic scientists. Part II, Chapters 4–8, is devoted to diagnostic and morphological issues. There is still considerable debate on how to classify syndromes associated with clefts. Thus, this part will be appealing to both clinicians and researchers. Part III includes methods in oral cleft epidemiology (Chapters 9 and 10), the development and use of birth-defect surveillance systems (Chapter 11), measures of occurrence from international epidemiological studies (Chapter 12), theories on environmental exposures that may increase or decrease the risk of oral clefting (Chapters 13 and 14), and experimental (animal) models for the study of oral clefts (Chapter 15). Part IV, Chapters 16–23, covers the genetic epidemiology of oral clefts. This part, of special interest to basic researchers and health-policy analysts, describes methodological issues and recent findings. Cloning and identifying genes associated with disorders is one of the principal aims of the worldwide Human Genome Project. The consequences of these findings, however, are of importance to policy analysts and the public at large.

Section II reviews a broad set of clinical approaches to patients and families with oral clefts. Beginning with a detailed description of the craniofacial team approach (Chapter 24), it deals with pediatric and feeding issues (Chapter 25); surgery (Chapter 26); speech, language, and articulation disorders (Chapter 27); dental care and orthodontic treatment (Chapters 28 and 29); associated disorders in the ear, nose, and throat areas (Chapter 30); genetic counseling (Chapter 31); and the psychological care of children with oral clefts (Chapter 32). Due to their direct implications for treatment, this section also covers international surgical missions (Chapter 33) and evidence-based care for the individual with an oral cleft (Chapter 34).

Section III addresses emerging issues that have a direct impact on society. Chapter 35 deals with the prevention of oral clefts through multivitamin supplements. Chapter 36 describes the financial burden associated with the care of oral cleft patients, both to the family of the affected individual as well as to society. Coverage of care is discussed in Chapter 37. Parental perceptions and perspectives on having a child with a cleft and on possibilities for treatment and social interactions are the subject of Chapter 38, which includes compelling stories of parents of children with oral clefts. Numerous ethical issues involved in the care of children with craniofacial conditions are discussed in Chapter 39. "Translational" methods are presented in Chapter 40. This relatively new discipline aims at extending research findings into public health policy and action. This area is at an early stage, but as presymptomatic genetic tests become increasingly available, it is receiving much attention from the media and the public. Education of practitioners and the public is discussed in Chapter 41, and an example of international collaboration for research and treatment is presented in Chapter 42. A list of Internet resources is provided in the Appendix. Finally, a comprehensive glossary is included at the end of the volume.

Although research findings and strategies for the treatment of individuals with oral clefts will continue to evolve in the next decades, I hope that this book will be of use to all those who seek specific information in any of the areas that are covered here.

D. F. W.
Boston, Massachusetts

Acknowledgments

As the editor of this book, I wish to acknowledge with gratitude the contributors' investment of time and knowledge in the face of numerous competing demands for their attention. Drafts of each chapter were presented for formal review and comments to at least two anonymous experts in the respective field. I am grateful to the following individuals for engaging the contributors in challenging and incisive discussions and for supplying them with detailed comments about their work: Marlene Anderka, Judith A. Badner, Joan E. Bailey-Wilson, Clint Baldwin, Michael L. Begleiter, Charles D. Bluestone, Karina Boehm, Dorret Boomsma, Lorenzo Botto, Rachel Bramson, Alphonse R. Burdi, Elisa Calzolari, John Canady, Mark A. Canfield, Francesco Carinci, Suzan Carmichael, Maurizio Clementi, Alice Cusner, Muriel Davisson, Douglas S. Diekema, Virginia M. Diewert, Edward F. Donovan, David L. Duffy, Amy Feldman Lewanda, Ghali Ghali, John M. Graham, Jr., Susan Halloran Blanton, Christine Harrison, Jacqueline T. Hecht, Donald V. Huebener, Russell S. Kirby, Deborah Klein Walker, David P. Kuehn, A. Kuijpers-Jagtman, Christopher A. Kus, Edward Lammer, Don LaRossa, Susan Lieff, Ross Long, Jr., Sue Malcolm, Eden R. Martin, Michael Melnick, James Mills, Jeffrey C. Murray, Bonnie L. Padwa, Sonja Rasmussen, Paul A. Romitti, Amado Ruiz-Razura, Alan F. Scott, Melvin D. Schloss, Gary Shaw, J. C. Shirley, Robert J. Shprintzen, Keith J. Slifer, Marcy C. Speer, Kathy K. Sulik, Tsunenobu Tamura, Norman J. Waitzman, and Allen Wilcox.

My involvement in the field of craniofacial anomalies and this book are fruits of the warm support I have received from many people since I was a medical student in Argentina until the present. Some people deserve grateful recognition for inspiring me to fulfill this dream and for serving as role models: Terri Beaty, Mike Cohen, Jeff Murray, Joan Bailey-Wilson, and Laura Mitchell. As the Talmudic sage Rabbi Elazar said: "Although I learnt a tremendous amount of wisdom from my teachers, their knowledge was so vast that my learning from them could be likened to a dog that laps water from the ocean."

At Oxford University Press, I am thankful to vice president Jeffrey House, who lent his support to this project from the very beginning, and to production editor Leslie Anglin, who masterfully expedited its production. Finally, I acknowledge my lovely wife, Carolien, for her understanding and enduring belief in me, and my three children, Shoshana, Sara, and Daniel, who are my inspiration and the loves of my life.

Contents

SECTION II TREATMENT

SECTION III PUBLIC HEALTH ISSUES

Contributors

BARBARA D. ABBOTT, PH.D.
Reproductive Toxicology Division
National Health and Environmental Effects Research
    Laboratory
Environmental Protection Agency
Research Triangle Park, North Carolina

PATRICK J. ANTONELLI, M.D.
Department of Otolaryngology
University of Florida
Gainesville, Florida

TERRI H. BEATY, PH.D.
Department of Epidemiology
Johns Hopkins University Bloomberg School of
    Public Health
Baltimore, Maryland

NANCY W. BERK, PH.D.
Department of Behavioral Sciences
University of Pittsburgh School of Dental Medicine
Pittsburgh, Pennsylvania

DAVID A. BILLMIRE, M.D., F.A.C.S.
Craniofacial and Pediatric Plastic Surgery
Children's Hospital Medical Center
Cincinnati, Ohio

FELICIA S. H. CHEAH, B.S.
Department of Pediatrics
National University of Singapore
Human and Molecular Genetics Laboratory
Johns Hopkins Singapore
Science Park II, Singapore

SAMUEL S. CHONG, PH.D., F.A.C.M.G.
Departments of Pediatrics and Obstetrics
    and Gynecology
National University of Singapore
Singapore
Department of Pediatrics
Johns Hopkins School of Medicine
Baltimore, Maryland
Human and Molecular Genetics Laboratory
Johns Hopkins Singapore
Science Park II, Singapore

KAARE CHRISTENSEN, M.D., PH.D.
Center for the Prevention of Congenital Malformations
Institute of Public Health
University of Southern Denmark
Odense, Denmark

M. MICHAEL COHEN, JR., D.M.D., PH.D.,
F.C.C.M.G.
Departments of Oral and Maxillofacial Sciences,
    of Pediatrics, of Community Health and Epidemiology,
    of Health Services Administration, and of Sociology
    and Social Anthropology
Dalhousie University
Halifax, Nova Scotia, Canada

ADOLFO CORREA, M.D., PH.D.
Division of Birth Defects and Pediatric Genetics
National Center for Environmental Health
Centers for Disease Control and Prevention
Atlanta, Georgia

ANDREW E. CZEIZEL, M.D., PH.D., D.S.
Foundation for the Community Control of
    Hereditary Diseases
Budapest, Hungary

E. ROSELLEN DEDLOW, M.S.N., C.S., A.R.N.P.
Division of General Pediatrics
University of Florida
Gainesville, Florida

VIRGINIA DIXON WOOD, M.A., C.C.C.-S.L.P.
Division of General Pediatrics
University of Florida
Gainesville, Florida

LARRY D. EDMONDS, M.S.P.H.
Birth Defects and Pediatric Genetics Branch
Division of Birth Defects, Child Development,
    Disability and Health
National Center for Environmental Health
Centers for Disease Control and Prevention

FRANK FARRINGTON, D.D.S., M.S.
Department of Pediatric Dentistry
Virginia Commonwealth University School of Dentistry
Richmond, Virginia

RICHARD H. FINNELL, PH.D.
Institute of Biosciences and Technology
Texas A&M University System Health Science Center
Houston, Texas

JANEE GELINEAU-VAN WAES, D.V.M., PH.D.
Center for Human Molecular Genetics
Department of Cell Biology and Anatomy
Nebraska Medical Center
Omaha, Nebraska

JAMES K. HARTSFIELD, JR., D.M.D., PH.D.,
F.A.C.M.G.
Department of Oral Facial Development, Oral Facial
   Genetics Section, Department of Orthodontics
Indiana University School of Dentistry
Department of Medical and Molecular Genetics
Indiana University School of Medicine
Indianapolis, Indiana

CATHERINE HAYES, D.M.D., D.M.S.
Department of Oral Health Policy and Epidemiology
Harvard School of Dental Medicine
Boston, Massachusetts

NUNO V. HERMANN, D.D.S., PH.D.
Departments of Pediatric Dentistry and Clinical Genetics
   and Oral Function and Physiology
School of Dentistry, Faculty of Health Sciences
University of Copenhagen
Copenhagen, Denmark

ETHYLIN WANG JABS, M.D.
Departments of Pediatrics, Medicine, and Plastic Surgery
Center for Craniofacial Development and Disorders
Institute of Genetic Medicine
Johns Hopkins School of Medicine
Baltimore, Maryland

MARILYN C. JONES, M.D.
Department of Pediatrics
University of California, San Diego
Children's Hospital
San Diego, California

DIANA M. JURILOFF, PH.D.
Department of Medical Genetics
Faculty of Medicine
University of British Columbia
Vancouver, British Columbia, Canada

KATHLEEN A. KAPP-SIMON, PH.D.
Department of Surgery, Division of Plastic Surgery
Northwestern University Medical School
Chicago, Illinois

SVEN KREIBORG, D.D.S., D.ODONT., PH.D.
Department of Pediatric Dentistry and Clinical Genetics
School of Dentistry, Faculty of Health Sciences
University of Copenhagen
Department of Pediatrics, The Juliane Marie Center
Copenhagen University Hospital
Copenhagen, Denmark

SENG-TEIK LEE, M.B.B.S., F.R.C.S., F.A.M.S.
Department of Plastic Surgery
Singapore General Hospital
Singapore

ANDREW C. LIDRAL, D.D.S., PH.D.
Section of Orthodontics
College of Dentistry
Ohio State University
Columbus, Ohio

JULIAN LITTLE, PH.D.
Epidemiology Group
Department of Medicine and Therapeutics
University of Aberdeen
Aberdeen, Scotland

MARY L. MARAZITA, PH.D.
Division of Oral Biology
Department of Oral and Maxillofacial Surgery
School of Dental Medicine
Department of Human Genetics
Graduate School of Public Health
University of Pittsburgh
Pittsburgh, Pennsylvania

LAURA E. MITCHELL, PH.D.
Departments of Biostatistics and Epidemiology and of
   Pediatrics
Center for Clinical Epidemiology and Biostatistics
University of Pennsylvania School of Medicine
Philadelphia, Pennsylvania

CYNTHIA A. MOORE, M.D., PH.D.
National Center on Birth Defects and Developmental
   Disabilities
Centers for Disease Control and Prevention
Atlanta, Georgia

ELIZABETH S. MOORE, PH.D.
Oral Facial Genetics Section
Indiana University School of Dentistry
Indianapolis, Indiana

PETER A. MOSSEY, B.D.S., PH.D.
Dundee Dental School
Dundee, Scotland

RONALD G. MUNGER, M.P.H., PH.D.
Department of Nutrition and Food Sciences
Utah State University
Logan, Utah

JOHN A. NACKASHI, PH.D., M.D.
Division of General Pediatrics
University of Florida
Gainesville, Florida

NAGATO NATSUME, D.D.S., D.MED.SC., PH.D.
Second Department of Oral and Maxillofacial Surgery
School of Dentistry
Aichi-Gakuin University
Nagoya, Japan

KATHERINE NEISWANGER, PH.D.
Department of Oral and Maxillofacial Surgery
School of Dental Medicine
University of Pittsburgh
Pittsburgh, Pennsylvania

JANE NICHOLSON, M.D.
Division of Women's Health
University of Michigan Health System
Ann Arbor, Michigan

RICHARD S. OLNEY, M.D., M.P.H.
National Center on Birth Defects and Developmental
    Disabilities
Centers for Disease Control and Prevention
Emory University School of Medicine
Atlanta, Georgia

JEFFREY C. POSNICK, D.M.D., M.D., F.R.C.S.,
F.A.C.S.
Departments of Plastic Surgery, of Otolaryngology/Head
    and Neck Surgery, of Oral and Maxillofacial Surgery,
    and of Pediatrics
Georgetown University
Washington, D.C.
Posnick Center for Facial Plastic Surgery
Chevy Chase, Maryland

DAVID S. PRECIOUS, D.D.S., M.S.
Department of Oral and Maxillofacial Sciences
Dalhousie University
Health Sciences Centre
Halifax, Nova Scotia, Canada

JOHN E. RISKI, PH.D., F.A.S.H.A., C.C.C.-S.
Center for Craniofacial Disorders
Speech Pathology Laboratory
Children's Healthcare of Atlanta
Atlanta, Georgia

RAMON L. RUIZ, D.M.D., M.D.
Oral and Maxillofacial Surgery and Pediatrics
University of North Carolina Hospitals,
Chapel Hill, North Carolina

HOWARD M. SAAL, M.D.
Division of Human Genetics
Children's Hospital Medical Center
Department of Clinical Pediatrics
University of Cincinnati College of Medicine
Cincinnati, Ohio

GUNVOR SEMB, D.D.S., PH.D.
Orthodontic Unit
Department of Oral Health and Development
University Dental Hospital of Manchester
Manchester, England

WILLIAM C. SHAW, PH.D., M.SC.D., B.D.S., F.D.S.,
D.ORTH.R.C.S.ENG., D.D.O.R.C.P.S.GLAS.
Orthodontic Unit
Department of Oral Health and Development
University Dental Hospital of Manchester
Manchester, England

GEOFFREY H. SPERBER, B.SC., B.D.S., M.S., PH.D.,
F.I.C.D.
Faculty of Medicine and Dentistry
University of Alberta
Edmonton, Alberta, Canada

CARMELLA S. STADTER, M.S., C.G.C.
Division of Human Genetics
University of Maryland
Baltimore, Maryland

RONALD P. STRAUSS, D.M.D., PH.D.
Department of Dental Ecology
University of North Carolina School of Dentistry
Department of Social Medicine
University of North Carolina School of Medicine
Chapel Hill, North Carolina

KATHERINE W. L. VIG, B.D.S., M.S., F.D.S.,
D.ORTH.R.C.S.
Department of Orthodontics
College of Dentistry
The Ohio State University
Columbus, Ohio

RICHARD E. WARD, PH.D.
Department of Anthropology
Indiana University
Department of Oral Facial Development
Purdue University
Indianapolis, Indiana

MARTHA M. WERLER, SC.D.
Slone Epidemiology Unit
Boston University School of Public Health
Boston, Massachusetts

ERIC A. WULFSBERG, M.D.
Department of Pediatrics
University of Maryland School of Medicine
Baltimore, Maryland

DIEGO F. WYSZYNSKI, M.D., M.H.S., PH.D.
Genetics Program
Department of Medicine
Boston University School of Medicine
Department of Epidemiology
Boston University School of Public Health
Boston, Massachusetts

JOANNA S. ZEIGER, M.S., PH.D.
Department of Epidemiology
Johns Hopkins University Bloomberg School of Public
   Health
Baltimore, Maryland

I

BASIC PRINCIPLES

I

Basic Embryology of Cleft Lip and Palate

1

Formation of the primary palate

GEOFFREY H. SPERBER

To know truly is to know by causes.
Francis Bacon, De Augmentis Scientiarum

The primary palate is the keystone to the upper lip and anterior portion of the definitive palate. Its embryogenesis is fundamental to normal development of the midface, and its maldevelopment has profound clinical and sociological consequences upon breathing, suckling, swallowing, mastication, osculation, speech, and facial physiognomy.

Recent advances in molecular biology and genetics have provided significant insights into craniofacial embryology. Orofacial development in the embryo is first demarcated by the appearance of the prechordal plate at the cranial end of the embryonic disk at the 14th day postconception (Sperber, 2001). This plate designates the site of the future mouth or stomodeum. The mesenchyme that provides the facial primordia is peculiarly of ectodermal derivation, arising from neural crest cells at the apices (crests) of the neural folds prior to neural tube formation (Fig. 1.1) (La Bonne and Bronner-Fraser, 1999; Lawson et al., 2001). The neural crest cells peculiarly disrupt the ectodermal–mesodermal boundary and migrate into the subjacent tissue as ectomesenchymal cells. Their migration and proliferation are fundamental in facial development. During their migration, they interact with the extracellular matrix and adjacent epithelia, which partly determines the patterning and nature of the derivative tissues they will form. These derivatives include neural, skeletal, connective, and muscular tissues (Sarkar et al., 2001). Migration of neural crest cells into the five pharyngeal arches, which they in part create, occurs in a highly regulated manner (Graham and Smith, 2001) (Fig. 1.2).

This regulation is under the control of homeobox genes, which endow the neural crest cells and surrounding tissues with a positional identity that mediates many aspects of facial and cranial patterning (Coburne, 2000).

The stomodeal chamber that is the precursor to the future mouth, situated at the termination of the foregut, becomes a deepened central depression in the facial region as a consequence of the surrounding five primordia of the face bulging at the borders of the stomodeum (Fig. 1.3). The five primordia are the single median rostrally located frontonasal prominence and the paired bilateral maxillary and caudally located mandibular prominences (Ferguson et al., 2000). These prominences are the result of the migration and mitotic proliferation of neural crest ectomesenchyme, which originates from the caudal region of the mesencephalon and the rhombencephalon of the developing brain (Rossel and Capecchi, 1999). There is also a mesodermal contribution to the mesenchyme of the facial prominences. The destination fates of the neural crest tissue are directed by genes that control the migration, growth, differentiation, and apoptosis (cell death) of the facial primordia (Anderson, 1997; Hu and Helms, 1999; Houdayer and Bahuau, 1998; Maconochie et al., 1999; Garcia-Castro and Bronner-Fraser, 1999). The regulatory homeobox *(Hoxa-1, Hoxa-2, Hoxb-1, Hoxb-3, Hoxb-4), sonic hedgehog (SHH), OXT (orthodontical), GSC (goosecoid), DLX (distalless),* and *MSX (muscle segment)* gene families are expressed in the ectomesenchyme derived from the rhombomere neural crest. Many of these are candidate genes for orofacial clefting. Hedgehog proteins exert their effects through a highly conserved signal-transduction pathway. Proteins encoded by the homeobox genes are transcription fac-

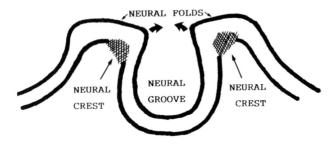

The Infolding Neural Folds (Heavy Arrows)

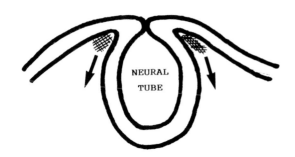

FIG. 1.1. Schematic depiction of neural crest origin and migration.

tors of RNA from the DNA (gene) template. Transcription factors can activate or repress gene expression, thereby controlling the cascade of molecular events that produce cellular patterning and morphogenesis (Thesleff, 1998). At the cellular level, control is expressed through regulatory proteins such as epidermal growth factor, the transforming growth factor family, fibroblast growth factor, and bone morphogenetic proteins (Lee et al., 2000; Lu et al., 2000). The critical timing, dosage, and combination of these factors account for the different tissues and organs and provide the key to understanding morphogenesis and dysmorphology. As an example, loss of *SHH* signaling leads to facial clefting (Hu and Helms, 1999). Many growth factors, signaling transductions, and mechanistic movements are involved in the delicate morphogenetic maneuvers of facial fabrication (Iamaroon et al., 1996; Iamaroon and Diewert, 1996). The precise and exquisite coordination of these processes creates the genetically determined characteristics of the face (Thorogood and Ferretti, 1992; Johnston and Bronsky, 1995; Morriss-Kay and Sokolova, 1996). Genetic mutations or perturbations and environmental impacts upon the complex mechanisms of craniofacial morphogenesis lead to phenotypic anomalies, of which orofacial clefting is the most common (Hibbert and Field, 1996; Dixon, 1998; Pirinen, 1998; Schutte and Murray, 1999). Further genetic defects responsible for cleft lip

and palate have been recently described (Sozen et al., 2001; Braybrook et al., 2001).

Formation of the upper lip involves an extraordinary combination of elements arising from both the frontonasal prominence and the maxillary prominence, which is a component of the first pharyngeal or mandibular arch. At the inferolateral corners of the frontonasal prominence, bilateral olfactory placodes arise. The placodes become invaginated as a consequence of the elevation of inverted horseshoe-shaped ridges, the medial and lateral nasal prominences on each side. The sinking nasal placodes form nasal pits, the precursors of the anterior nares that are initially in continuity with the stomodeum (Figs. 1.4, 1.5) (O'Rahilly, 1967). The timing and rapidity of facial formation is chronicled in Table 1.1.

The bilateral medial nasal prominences form the central tuberculum of the upper lip and provide the basis for the primary palate (Diewert and Shiota, 1990; Diewert et al., 1993a,b; Diewert and Lozanoff, 1993; Rude et al., 1994). The upper lip is completed on either side of the central tuberculum by fusion of the freely projecting medial nasal prominences with the laterally located maxillary prominences, requiring critically timed correlation of their growth, spatial location, and disintegration of their contacting surface epithelia that form the transient nasal fin (Diewert and Wang, 1992) (Fig. 1.6). Disintegration of the nasal fin by apoptosis or mesenchymal transformation allows intermingling of the underlying mesenchymal cells, providing continuity of the median and lateral com-

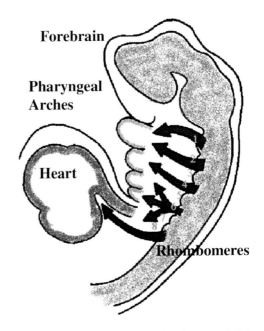

FIG. 1.2. Neural crest migration from rhombomeres 1–8 into pharyngeal arches and heart. (From Sperber, 2001, with permission.)

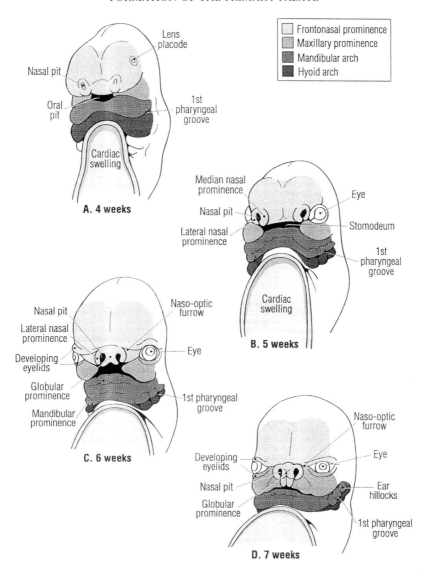

FIG. 1.3. Schematic depiction of facial formation from 4 to 7 weeks postconception. (From Sperber, 2001, with permission.)

ponents of the upper lip (Fig. 1.7) (Gui et al., 1993; Shuler, 1995). Failure of normal disintegration of the nasal fin or inadequate mesenchymal migration across the two boundaries of the maxillary and medial nasal prominences results in lip clefting, unilaterally or bilaterally, of varying degrees of severity. Bilateral clefting produces a prominent median (globular) process arising from the central tuberculum. Cleft lip (cheiloschisis) is a developmental threshold trait involving quantitative variation in the size of the embryonic maxillary and medial nasal prominences (McGonnell et al., 1998).

Clefting of the upper lip is one of the most common human malformations, with a prevalence averaging 1 in 700 live births (Tolarova and Cervenka, 1998). There is an inheritance factor in upper lip clefts, independent of the inheritability of cleft palate (Laatikainen, 1999). Genetic epidemiological studies have revealed that mutated genes involving between two and ten loci are responsible for orofacial clefting (Bender, 2000; Prescott et al., 2000; Suzuki et al., 2000; van den Boogaard et al., 2000). Lip clefting occurs twice as frequently in males as in females (Oliver-Padilla and Martinez-Gonzales, 1986), is usually unilateral, and occurs more commonly on the left side than on the right (Vanderas, 1987). Sex-dependent susceptibility to clefting is a consequence of genetic variation at the MSX1 gene locus on chromosome 4 (Blanco et al., 2001). Cleft lips can now be identified prenatally by ultrasonography (Pretorius et al., 1995; Pretorius and Nelson, 1995; Shaikh et al., 2001), allowing for parental counseling and postnatal therapeutic preparation.

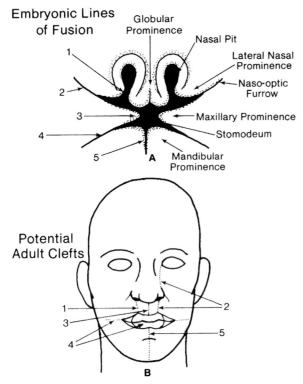

Embryonic Lines of Fusion

Globular Prominence

Nasal Pit

Lateral Nasal Prominence

Naso-optic Furrow

Maxillary Prominence

Stomodeum

Mandibular Prominence

A

Potential Adult Clefts

B

1. Uni- or bilateral cleft lip
2. Unilateral facial cleft
3. Median cleft lip (true "hare lip")
4. Micro- or macrostomia
5. Median mandibular cleft

FIG. 1.4. Schematic depiction of embryonic lip formation.

Fusion of the medial nasal and maxillary prominences not only provides continuity of the upper jaw and lip but also separates the nasal pits from the stomodeum (Fig. 1.8). The central median component of the face forms the tuberculum and philtrum of the up-

per lip, the tip of the nose, and the primary palate. The philtral ridges are formed by thickened dermis and dermal appendages (Namnoum et al., 1997). The intermaxillary segment of the upper jaw (the premaxilla), in which the four upper incisor teeth will develop, arises from the median primary palate (Mooney et al., 1991, 1992; Siegel et al., 1991). The rare absence of the primary palate is demonstrated in premaxillary agenesis, producing a median cleft lip and palate, a manifestation of holoprosencephaly (Sperber et al., 1989).

Ossification of the primary palate begins at the eighth week in the medial nasal prominence and spreads laterally across the fusion line with the maxillary prominence. The existence of a separate premaxillary ossification center from the primary ossification center of the secondary palate has been disputed and is reviewed in Chapter 2.

Development of the dentition in the primary palate and in the alveolar ridges of the maxilla and mandible is dependent on a great number of genes (*PAX9, MSX1, SHH, DLX,* and *WNT*) and growth factors (nerve growth factor, fibroblast growth factor, and bone morphogenetic protein) that are expressed in the oral ectoderm and the underlying neural crest mesenchyme. Epithelial–mesenchymal interactions are induced at specific locations to produce tooth buds from a submerged ectodermal dental lamina at 28 days postconception. Amelogenesis, dentinogenesis, and cementogenesis are programmed to form teeth (Tucker and Sharpe, 1999). Normally, four tooth buds arise in the primary palate which produce the upper incisor teeth. The location of these four teeth usually defines the limits of the primary palate, which are demarcated by incisive fissures in the fetus. The canine teeth normally arise in the secondary palate. Most commonly, clefting between the primary and secondary palates occurs at the incisive fissure sites that separate the lateral incisor

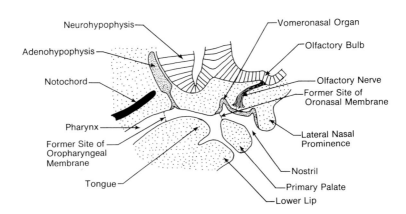

FIG. 1.5. Schematic depiction of a lateral sagittal section through the anterior facial region of an embryo at approximately 7 weeks.

TABLE 1.1. *Chronology of Key Embryonic Events*

Carnegie Stage	Postconception Age	Craniofacial Features
6	14 days	Primitive streak appears; oropharyngeal membrane forms
8	17 days	Neural plate forms
9	20 days	Cranial neural folds elevate; otic placode appears
10	21 days	Neural crest migration commences; fusion of neural folds; otic pit forms
11	24 days	Frontonasal prominence swells; first arch forms; wide stomodeum; optic vesicles form; anterior neuropore closes; olfactory placode appears
12	26 days	Second arch forms; maxillary prominences appear; lens placodes commence; posterior neuropore closes; adenohypophysial pouch appears
13	28 days	Third arch forms; dental lamina appears; fourth arch forms; oropharyngeal membrane ruptures
14	32 days	Otic and lens vesicles present; lateral nasal prominences appear
15	33 days	Medial nasal prominences appear; nasal pits form-widely separated, face laterally
16	37 days	Nasal pits face ventrally; upper lip forms on lateral aspect of stomodeum; lower lip fuses in midline; retinal pigment forms; nasolacrimal groove appears, demarcating nose; neurohypophysial evagination
17	41 days	Contact between medial nasal and maxillary prominences, separating nasal pit from stomodeum; upper lip continuity first established; vomeronasal organ appears
18	44 days	Primary palate anlagen project posteriorly into stomodeum; distinct tip of nose develops; eyelid folds form; retinal pigment; nasal pits move medially; nasal alae and septum present; mylohyoid, geniohyoid and genioglossus muscles form
19	47–48 days	Nasal fin disintegrates; (failure of disintegration predisposes to cleft lip); the rima oris of the mouth diminishes in width; mandibular ossification commences
20	50–51 days	The lidless eyes migrate medially; nasal pits approach each other; ear hillocks fuse
22	54 days	The eyelids thicken and encroach upon the eyes; the auricle forms and projects; the nostrils are in definitive position
23	56–57 days	Eyes are still wide apart but eyelid closure commences; nose tip elevates; face assumes a human fetal appearance; head elevates off the thorax; mouth opens; palatal shelves elevate; maxillary ossification commences
Fetus	60 days	Palatal shelves fuse; deciduous tooth buds form; embryo now termed a fetus

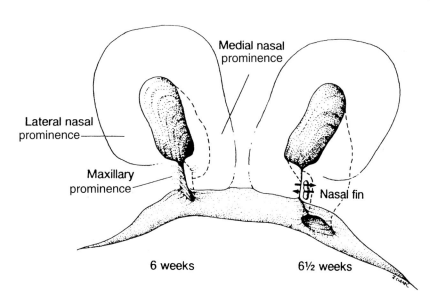

FIG. 1.6. Formation of nostril and primary palate. *Arrows* indicate disintegration of nasal fin between maxillary and medial nasal prominences. (Courtesy of Dr. J. Avery. University of Michigan and Thieme Publishing Group.)

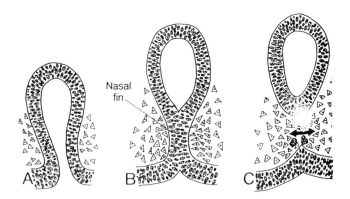

FIG. 1.7. Schematic depiction of breakdown of nasal fin. *A:* Groove between maxillary and medial nasal prominences; *B:* apposition of surface epithelia; *C: Arrows* indicate disintegration of nasal fin between maxillary and medial nasal prominences. (Courtesy of Dr. J. Avery. University of Michigan and Thieme Publishing Group.)

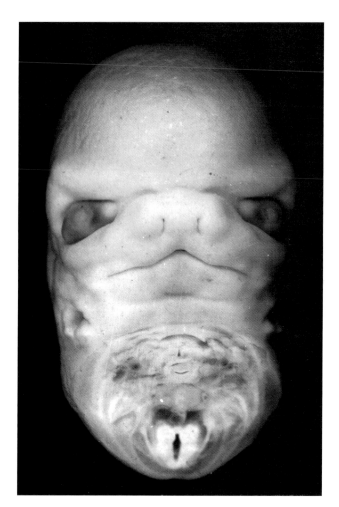

FIG. 1.8. Scanning electron micrograph of the face of a 44-day-old human embryo. The merging facial prominences have eliminated the intervening grooves. The cut surface reveals arteries, veins, the pharynx, and spinal cord. The eyelids have not yet formed. Magnification ×30. (From KV Hinrichsen, Human Embryologie. Courtesy of Springer-Verlag.)

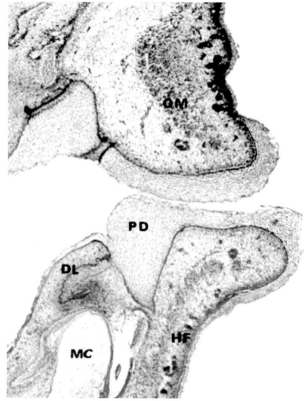

FIG. 1.9. Paramedian sagittal section of the lips of a 12-week-old fetus. Note the multilayered periderm *(PD),* the orbicularis oris muscle *(OM),* the dental lamina *(DL),* and Meckel's cartilage *(MC).* Hair follicles *(HF)* are forming in the cutaneous area. Magnification ×56. (From Sperber, 2001, with permission. Courtesy of Dr. R. R. Miethke.)

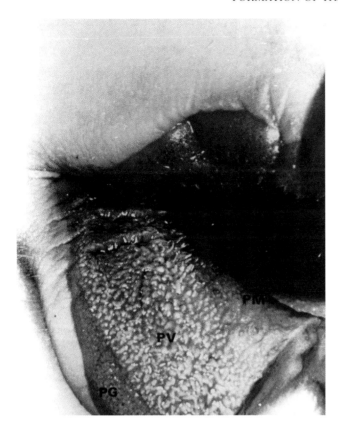

FIG. 1.10. Lips and commissure of mouth of a 39-week-old fetus. Note in the lower lip the outermost smooth pars glabra *(PG)*, which narrows toward the commissure. The central pars villosa *(PV)* is covered with fine villi. The inner vestibular zone, pars mucosa *(PM)*, is continuous with the vestibule of the mouth. Magnification ×4. (Courtesy of Dr. R. R. Miethke.)

and canine teeth. However, abnormal location or absence of these teeth may occur in variations of pre-maxillary (primary palate) hypoplasia or agenesis. The occurrence of a single median central incisor within a deficient primary palate characterizes holoprosencephaly (Wei et al., 2000; Kjaer et al., 2002). Clefts may occur within the primary palate, separating the medial and lateral incisors (Sperber et al., 1989). Distorted fetal tooth buds may be detected prenatally by ultrasonography (Ulm et al., 1999).

The lower jaw and lip are formed by midline merging of the paired mandibular prominences and are the first parts of the face to become definitively established. The future lower jaw and lower lip are essentially established by Carnegie stage 16 (37 days postconception), whereas the upper jaw and lip components will not blend until stage 19 (48 days postconception). The earlier occurrence of lower lip completion might in part account for the rarity of clefting of the lower lip in comparison to the upper lip (Oostrom et al., 1996;

Lekkas et al., 1998). The delay in upper lip formation might allow a longer period for teratogenic agents to disrupt merging of lip components, although there is undoubtedly a genetic factor accounting for the discrepancy in the incidence of upper and lower lip clefting.

The cutaneous covering of the lips of the fetus is sharply delineated from the adjacent skin and oral mucosa. The primitive epithelium of the vermilion surface of the lip forms a distinctive multilayered periderm that is shed in utero. At birth, the surface of the lips is subdivided into a central highly mobile sucking area characterized by fine villi (the pars villosa) distinct from lateral smooth zones (the pars glabra) and an inner vestibular zone (the pars mucosa) (Figs. 1.9, 1.10) (Miethke, 1977). The villous portion of the infant lip is adhesive, more so than the glabrous or vestibular portions. During suckling, the blood vessels in the villi swell, establishing an airtight seal around the nipple. This seal-

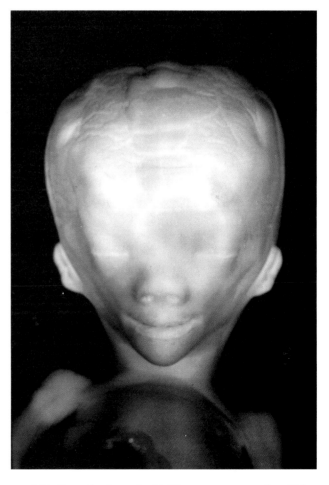

FIG. 1.11. Face of a 3-month-old (52 mm crown–rump length) human fetus depicting closed eyelids and absent philtrum. (Courtesy of Prof. Dr. E. Blechschmidt and Springer-Verlag Inc.)

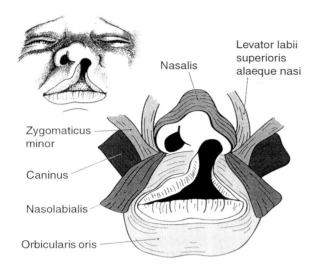

Levator labii
superioris
alaeque nasi

Nasalis

Zygomaticus
minor

Caninus

Nasolabialis

Orbicularis oris

FIG. 1.12. Depiction of the musculature surrounding a cleft lip.

ing effect is obviously not possible in clefts of the upper lip, leading to feeding difficulties. Hypertrophy of the inner pars villosa and an exaggerated boundary line demarcating it from the outer pars glabra produces a double lip (Calnan, 1952; Reddy and Roa, 1989).

The conspicuous philtrum of the neonatal upper lip is absent in fetal alcohol syndrome, which presents a characteristic flat upper lip (Fig. 1.11) (Autti-Ramo et al., 1992; Astley et al., 1999). The central depression of the philtrum normally becomes shallower during later childhood.

The lip primordia are invaded by myogenic mesenchyme derived from the sixth somitomere, which migrates into the second pharyngeal (hyoid) arch, drawing along its initially established facial nerve (VII) supply. The neural crest mesenchyme from rhombomere IV provides the epimysium, perimysium, and endomysium surrounding the myocytes of the facial muscles. The orbicularis oris muscle establishes powerful suckling movements in the neonate but is defective in cleft lips (Fig. 1.12). Defects of the orbicularis oris muscle might not be overtly visible but, nonetheless, may be part of the spectrum of the cleft lip phenotype. Detection of subclinical orbicularis oris deficiencies is now possible with ultrasonography (Martin et al., 2000; Munshi et al., 2000). The relationship of genetically determined and phenotypically expressed orofacial clefts is becoming ever more clearly defined by increasingly sophisticated mutation-detection and diagnostic techniques (Thieme et al., 2000).

I thank Anne-Marie McLean for meticulous word processing of the manuscript.

REFERENCES

Anderson, DJ (1997). Cellular and molecular biology of neural crest cell lineage determination. Trends Genet *13*: 276–280.

Astley, SJ, Magnuson, SI, Omnell, LM, Clarren, SK (1999). Fetal alcohol syndrome: changes in craniofacial form with age, cognition and timing of ethanol exposure in the macaque. Teratology *59*: 163–172.

Avery, JK (2002). *Oral Development and Histology.* 3rd ed. Stuttgart: Thieme.

Autti-Ramo, I, Gailey, E, Granstrom, ML (1992). Dysmorphic features in offspring of alcoholic mothers. Arch Dis Child *67*: 712–716.

Bender, PL (2000). Genetics of cleft lip and palate. J Pediatr Nurs *15*: 242–249.

Blanco, R, Chakraborty, R, Barton, SA et al. (2001). Evidence of a sex-dependent association between the MSX1 locus and nonsyndromic cleft lip with or without cleft palate in the Chilean population. Hum Biol *73*: 81–89.

Braybrook, C, Doudney, K, Marcano, AC et al. (2001). The T-box transcription factor gene TBX22 is marked in X-linked cleft palate and ankyloglossia. Nat Genet *29*: 179–183.

Calnan, J (1952). Congenital double lip: record of a case with a note on the embryology. J Plastic Surg *5*: 196.

Coburne, MT (2000). Construction for the modern head, current concepts in craniofacial development. J Orthod *27*: 307–314.

Diewert, VM, Shiota, K (1990). Morphological observations in normal primary palate and cleft lip embryos in the Kyoto collection. Teratology *41*: 663–677.

Diewert, VM, Lozanoff, S (1993). Growth and morphogenesis of the human embryonic midface during primary palate formation analyzed in frontal sections. J Craniofac Genet Dev Biol *13*: 162–183.

Diewert, VM, Lozanoff, S, Choy, V (1993a). Computer reconstructions of human embryonic craniofacial morphology showing changes in relations between the face and brain during primary palate formation. J Craniofac Genet Dev Biol *13*: 193–201.

Diewert, VM, Wang, KY (1992). Recent advances in primary palate and midfacial morphogenesis. Crit Rev Oral Biol Med *4*: 111–130.

Diewert, VM, Wang, KY, Tait, B (1993b). A morphometric analysis of cell densities in facial prominences of the rhesus monkey embryo during primary palate formation. J Craniofac Genet Dev Biol *13*: 236–249.

Dixon, MJ (1998). Facial growth and patterning: dysmorphology. In: *Oral Biology at the Turn of the Century,* edited by B Guggenheim and S Shapiro. Basel: Karger, pp. 79–84.

Ferguson, CA, Tucker, AS, Sharpe, PT (2000). Temporospatial cell interactions regulating mandibular and maxillary arch patterning. Development *127*: 403–412.

Garcia-Castro, M, Bronner-Fraser, M (1999). Induction and differentiation of the neural crest. Curr Opin Cell Biol *11*: 695–698.

Graham, A, Smith, A (2001). Patterning the pharyngeal arches. Bioessays *23*: 54–61.

Gui, T, Osumi-Yamashita, N, Eto, K (1993). Proliferation of nasal epithelial and mesenchymal cells during primary palate formation. J Craniofac Genet Dev Biol *13*: 250–258.

Hibbert, SA, Field, JK (1996). Molecular basis of familial cleft lip and palate. Oral Dis *2*: 238–241.

Houdayer, C, Bahuau, M (1998). Orofacial cleft defects: inference from nature and nurture. Ann Genet *41*: 89–117.

Hu, D, Helms, J (1999). The role of sonic hedgehog in normal and abnormal craniofacial morphogenesis. Development *126*: 4873–4884.

Iamaroon, A, Diewert, VM (1996). Distribution of basement membrane components in the mouse primary palate. J Craniofac Genet Dev Biol *16*: 48–51.

Iamaroon, A, Tait, B, Diewert, VM (1996). Cell proliferation and expression of EGF, TGFα and EGF receptor in the developing primary palate. J Dent Res 75: 1534–1539.

Johnston, MC, Bronsky, PT (1995). Prenatal craniofacial development: new insights on normal and abnormal mechanisms. Crit Rev Oral Biol Med 6: 368–422.

Kjaer, I, Keeling, J, Fischer Hansen, B, Becktor, KB (2002). Midline skeletodental morphology in holoprosencephaly. Cleft Palate Craniofac J 39: (in press).

Laatikainen, T (1999). Etiological aspects on craniofacial morphology in twins with cleft lip and palate. Eur J Oral Sci 107: 102–108.

LaBonne, C, Bronner-Fraser, M (1999). Molecular mechanisms of neural crest formation. Annu Rev Cell Dev Biol 15: 81–112.

Lawson, A, Anderson, H, Schoenwolf, GC (2001). Cellular mechnisms of neural fold formation and morphogenesis in the chick embryo. Anat Rec 262: 153–168.

Lee, S, Crisera, CA, Erfani, S et al. (2000). Immunolocalization of fibroblast growth factor receptors 1 and 2 in mouse palate development. Plast Reconstr Surg 107: 1776–1785.

Lekkas, C, Latief, BS, Corputty, JE (1998). Median cleft of the lower lip associated with lip pits and cleft of the lip and palate. Cleft Palate Craniofac J 35: 269–271.

Lu, H, Jin, Y, Tipoe, GL (2000). Alteration in the expression of bone morphogenetic protein-2, 3, 4, 5 mRNA during pathogenesis of cleft palate in BALB/c mice. Arch Oral Biol 45: 133–140.

Maconochie, M, Krishnamurthy, R, Nonchev, S, et al. (1999). Regulation of Hoxa2 in cranial neural crest cells involves members of the AP-2 family. Development 126: 1483–1494.

Martin, RA, Hunter, V, Neufeld-Kaiser, W, et al. (2000). Ultrasonography detection of orbicularis oris defects in first degree relatives of isolated cleft lip patients. Am J Med Genet 90: 155–161.

McGonnell, IM, Clarke, JD, Tickle, C (1998). Fate map of the developing chick face: an analysis of expansion of facial primordia and establishment of the primary palate. Dev Dyn 212: 102–118.

Miethke, RR (1977). Zur anatomie der-ober und unterlippe zwischen dem 4 intrauterinen monat und der gerburt. Gegenbaurs Morphol Jahrb 123: 424.

Mooney, MP, Siegel, MI, Kimes, KR, Todhunter, J (1991). Premaxillary development in normal and cleft lip and palate human fetuses using three-dimensional computer reconstruction. Cleft Palate Craniofac J 28: 49–53.

Mooney, MP, Siegel, MI, Kimes, KR, et al. (1992). Multivariate analysis of second trimester midfacial morphology in normal and cleft lip and palate human fetal specimens. Am J Phys Anthropol 88: 203–209.

Morris-Kay, GM, Sokolova, N (1996). Embryonic development and pattern formation. FASEB J 10: 961–968.

Munshi, AK, Hegde, AM, Srinath, SK (2000). Ultrasonographic and electromyographic evaluation of the labial musculature in children with repaired cleft lips. J Clin Pediatr Dent 24: 123–128.

Namnoum, JD, Hisley, KC, Graepel, S, et al. (1997). Three dimensional reconstruction of the human fetal philtrum. Ann Plast Surg 38: 202–208.

Oliver-Padilla, G, Martinez-Gonzales, V (1986). Cleft lip and palate in Puerto Rico: a 33 year study. Cleft Palate J 23: 48–57.

Oostrom, CA, Vermeij-Keers, C, Gilbert, PM, van der Meulen, JC (1996). Median cleft of the lower lip and mandible: case reports, a new embryologic hypothesis and subdivision. Plast Reconstr Surg 97: 313–320.

O'Rahilly, R (1967). The early development of the nasal pit in staged human embryos. Anat Rec 157: 380.

Pirinen, S (1998). Genetic craniofacial aberrations. Acta Odontol Scand 56: 356–359.

Prescott, NJ, Lees, MM, Winter, RM, Malcolm, S (2000). Identification of susceptibility loci for nonsyndromic cleft lip with or without cleft palate in a two stage genome scan of affected sib pairs. Hum Genet 106: 345–350.

Pretorius, DH, House, M, Nelson, TR, Hollenbach, KA (1995). Evaluation of normal and abnormal lips in fetuses: comparison between three- and two-dimensional sonography. AJR Am J Roentgenol 165: 1233–1237.

Pretorius, DH, Nelson, TR (1995). Fetal face visualization using three-dimensional ultrasonography. J Ultrasound Med 14: 349–356.

Reddy, KA, Roa, AK (1989). Congenital double lip: a review of seven cases. Plast Reconstr Surg 84: 420–423.

Rossel, M, Capecchi, MR (1999). Mice mutant for both Hoxa1 and Hoxb1 show extensive remodeling of the hindbrain and defects in craniofacial development. Development 126: 5027–5040.

Rude, FP, Anderson, L, Conley, D, Gasser, RF (1994). Three dimensional reconstructions of the primary palate. Anat Rec 238: 108–113.

Schutte, BC, Murray, JC (1999). The many faces and factors of orofacial clefts. Hum Mol Genet 8: 1853–1859.

Sarkar, S, Petiot, A, Copp, A et al. (2001). FGF2 promotes skeletogenic differentiation of cranial neural crest cells. Development 128: 2143–2152.

Shaikh, D, Mercer, NS, Sohan, K, Kyle, P, Soothill, P (2001). Prenatal diagnosis of cleft lip and palate. Br J Plast Surg 54: 288–289.

Shuler, CF (1995). Programmed cell death and cell transformation in craniofacial development. Crit Rev Oral Biol Med 6: 202–217.

Siegel, MI, Mooney, MP, Kimes, KR, Todhunter, J (1991). Developmental correlates of midfacial components in a normal and cleft lip and palate human fetal sample. Cleft Palate Craniofac J 28: 408–412.

Sozen, MA, Suzuki, K, Tolarova, MM, et al. (2001). Mutation of PVRL1 is associated with sporadic, non-syndromic cleft lip-palate in northern Venezuela. Nat Genet 29: 141–142.

Sperber, GH (2001). Craniofacial Development. Hamilton, Canada: B. C. Decker.

Sperber, GH, Honoré, LH, Machin, GA (1989). Microscopic study of holoprosencephalic facial anomalies in trisomy 13 fetuses. Am J Med Genet 32: 443–451.

Suzuki, K, Hu, D, Bustos, T, et al (2000). Mutations of PVRL1 encoding a cell–cell adhesion molecule/herpesvirus receptor, in cleft lip/palate-ectodermal dysplasia. Nat Genet 25: 427–430.

Thesleff, I (1998). The genetic basis of normal and abnormal craniofacial development. Acta Odontol Scand 56: 321–325.

Thieme, G, Manco-Johnson, ML, Cioffi-Ragan, D (2000). In obstetrics 3-D imaging solves clinical problems. Diagn Imaging (Suppl): 8–19.

Thorogood, P, Ferretti, P (1992). Heads and tales: recent advances in craniofacial development. Br Dent J 173: 301–306.

Tolarova, MM, Cervenka, J (1998). Classification and birth prevalence of orofacial clefts. Am J Med Genet 75: 126–137.

Tucker, AS, Sharpe, PT (1999). Molecular genetics of tooth morphogenesis and patterning: the right shape in the right place. J Dent Res 78: 826–834.

Ulm, MR, Kratochwil, A, Ulm, B, et al. (1999). 3-Dimensional ultrasonographic imaging of fetal tooth buds for characterisation of facial clefts. Early Hum Dev 55: 67–75.

Van den Boogaard, M-J, Dorland, M, Beemer, FA, van Amstel, HKP (2000). MSX1 mutation is associated with orofacial clefting and tooth agenesis in humans. Nat Genet 24: 342–343.

Vanderas, AP (1987). Incidence of cleft lip, cleft palate, and cleft lip and palate among races: a review. Cleft Palate J 24: 216–225.

Wei, X, Senders, C, Owiti, GO, et al. (2000). The origin and development of the upper lateral incisor and premaxilla in normal and cleft lip/palate monkeys induced with cyclophosphamide. Cleft Palate Craniofac J 37: 571–583.

2

Palatogenesis: closure of the secondary palate

GEOFFREY H. SPERBER

" . . . find out the cause of this effect,
or rather say, the cause of this defect,
For this effect defective comes by cause."
Shakespeare, Hamlet, act II, scene II

The secondary palate, so called because it forms after the appearance of the primary palate, constitutes both the floor of the nasal cavities and the roof of the mouth. The secondary palate is comprised of the anterior hard and the posterior soft palate and is an essential component of normal respiration, mastication, deglutition, and speech.

The very existence of the definitive secondary palate in humans characterizes a major mammalian evolutionary separation of the respiratory from the masticatory functions of the primitive stomodeal (oronasal) chamber of vertebrate antecedents. The transition of the single chamber of the embryonic stomodeum into the divided compartments of the two nasal cavities for respiration and the oral cavity for mastication represents a subdivision of this common chamber found in primitive crossopterygian fish, reptiles, birds, and early mammals. The separation of a continuous respiratory channel (the nostrils) from an intermittently required food-ingestion channel (the mouth) enabled the evolutionary development of leisurely mastication without respiratory interference. This separation occurs only anteriorly since the nasopharynx and oropharynx share a channel posteriorly, which accounts for momentary asphyxiation during swallowing. However, in the neonate and infant until 6 months of age, concomitant breathing and swallowing can occur due to the epiglottis and soft palate being in contact, forming a seal that maintains a continuous airway between the nasopharynx and laryngopharynx. Milk passes on either side of this continuous airway channel into the esophagus. An oropharynx develops only upon postnatal descent of the larynx, thereby separating the soft palate from the epiglottis. As a consequence, the risk of aspirating food may occur, protected by development of the cough reflex.

The existence of an intact palate has enabled sophisticated masticatory movements and epicurian enjoyment to evolve by virtue of the taste and texture senses embedded in the palate, accounting for the popular concept of the palate being the seat of taste (hence, *palatable*). Moreover, an intact palate is essential for the production of normal speech. Deficiencies of palatal development will result in food and salivary spillage into the nostrils and impaired articulation.

Three elements make up the secondary definitive palate: the two lateral palatal processes projecting into the stomodeum from the maxillary prominences and the primary palate derived anteriorly from the frontonasal prominence (Fig. 2.1). These three elements are initially widely separated due to the advancing edges of the palatal processes being deflected down on either side of the obtruding tongue, which initially occupies most of the stomodeal chamber (Kimes et al., 1991) (Fig. 2.2). Concomitantly, the midline cartilaginous nasal septum descends from the roof of the stomodeum as a feature of nasal capsular development (Mooney et al., 1994) (Fig. 2.3). During the 8th week postconception, a remarkable transformation of the palatal shelves occurs, when they elevate into a horizontal position as a prelude to their fusion with each other, the primary

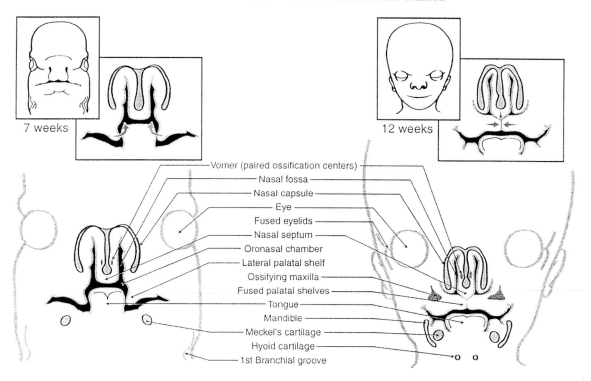

FIG. 2.1. Schematic depiction of midcoronal sections of embryonic heads at 7 and 12 weeks postconception. (From Sperber, 2001, with permission.)

palate, and the nasal septum, thereby partitioning the oronasal chamber (Fig. 2.4).

The transition from vertical to horizontal is completed within hours during the 8th week postconception. There is a sex difference in the timing of palatal closure. Shelf elevation and fusion begin a few days earlier in male than in female embryos (Burdi and Faist, 1967), the slight delay possibly accounting for the higher incidence of cleft palates in females. Several mechanisms have been proposed for the rapid elevation of the palatal shelves. They include biochemical transformations in the physical consistency of the connective tissue matrix of the shelves; variations in vasculature and blood flow to these structures (Amin et al., 1994), resulting in a sudden increase in tissue fluid turgor; rapid differential mitotic growth, muscular movements, and an intrinsic shelf force (Young et al., 1997; McGonnell et al., 1998). The intrinisic shelf elevating force is generated chiefly by the synthesis, accumulation, and hydration of hyaluronic acid and glycosaminoglycans within the extracellular matrix of the shelves (Singh et al., 1997).

The alignment of mesenchymal cells and orientation of collagen within the palatal shelves may direct the elevating forces, while palatal mesenchymal cells are themselves contractile. The withdrawal of the fetus's face from against the heart prominence by uprighting the head facilitates jaw opening (Fig. 2.5). Mouth-opening reflexes and extrinsic tongue muscle activity have been implicated in the withdrawal of the tongue from between the vertical shelves (Humphrey, 1969). Depressed fetal swallowing may delay palatal shelf elevation, precluding their conjunction, leading to clefting. Prenatal ultrasonography revealing aphagia has been correlated with cleft palate formation (Laster et al., 2001). Absence of functioning of the hyoglossus muscle, which depresses the tongue, resulting from *Hoxa* gene mutations, prevents palatal shelf lifting and consequent clefting (Barrow and Capecchi, 1999). Tongue withdrawal is further aided by movement of the lower jaw through the functioning of pharyngeal arch muscles, which in turn requires an intact neural motor system (Wragg et al., 1972; Kjaer, 1997). In this regard, the trigeminal nerve is the first motor nerve to function in the fetus and, moreover, requires a functioning incudomalleal primary jaw joint to allow opening of the mouth. The fetus must be in a floating condition in the amniotic sac to permit jaw movements; in the event of oligohydramnios,[1] deficient amniotic fluid inhibits mouth opening and tongue withdrawal, thereby precluding palatal shelf elevation, accounting for a possible source of clefting. Extracellular agents such as growth factors, hormones, and neuropeptides have been implicated in the regulation of various cellular re-

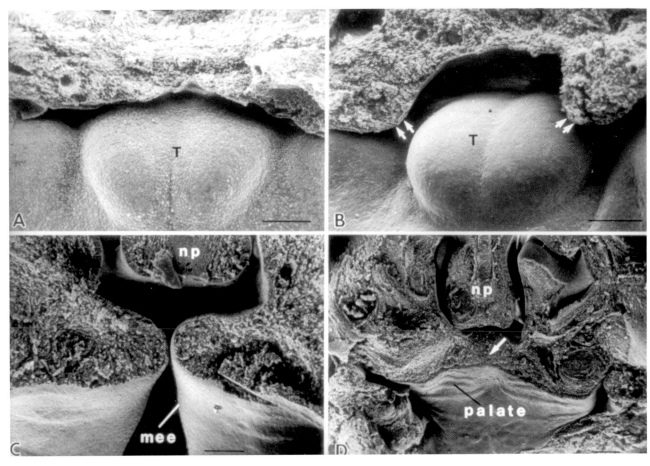

FIG. 2.2. Coronal section scanning electron micrographs of stomodeal chambers of embryos at (A) 4,
(B) 6, (C) 7, and (D) 8 weeks, revealing secondary palate development. *T*, tongue; *np*, nasal prominence
(septum); *mee*, medial edge epithelium; *double arrows*, palatal shelves; *single arrow*, midpalatal fusion
seam. (Courtesy of Dr. H. C. Slavkin. University of Southern California.)

sponses during palate development (Greene and Pratt,
1976; Morris-Wiman and Brinkley, 1992; Abbott et al.,
1998; Izadnegahdar et al., 1999; Machida et al., 1999).
Most significantly, epidermal growth factor (EGF), the
transforming growth factors (TGF-α, TGF-β1, TGF-
β3), and their receptor molecules have been identified
during all stages of palate formation (Citterio and Gaillard, 1994; Proetzel et al., 1995; Kaartinen et al., 1997;
Cui et al., 1998; Sun et al., 1998). Docking of TGF-α
with the EGF receptor results in the production of matrix metalloproteinases, a class of proteins that regulate palate closure (Miettinen et al., 1999).

During palate closure, the mandible becomes more
prognathic and the vertical dimension of the stomodeal chamber increases, though maxillary width remains
stable, allowing shelf contact to occur. Also, forward
growth of Meckel's cartilage relocates the tongue more
anteriorly, concomitant with head elevation. Mandibular growth retardation causes retrognathia that enforces

a high tongue position, preventing the shelves from fusing (Seegmiller and Fraser, 1977) to create the Pierre
Robin sequence (Lavrin, 2000).

The epithelium overlying the edges of the palatal
shelves is especially thickened, and their fusion upon
mutual contact is crucial to intact palatal development.
This fusion is dependent on targeted removal of the epithelium between the palatal shelves, which is anticipated by upregulation of keratin K5/6 and expression
of vimentin mRNA in the medial edge epithelium (Gibbins et al., 1999). Fusion also occurs between the dorsal surfaces of the fusing palatal shelves and the lower
edge of the midline nasal septum. The fusion seam initially forms anteriorly in the hard palate region, with
subsequent merging of the soft palate region (Ferguson, 1988). The mechanisms of adhesive contact, fusion, and subsequent degeneration of the epithelium are
not clearly understood. The combination of degenerat-
ing epithelial cells and a surface coat accumulation of

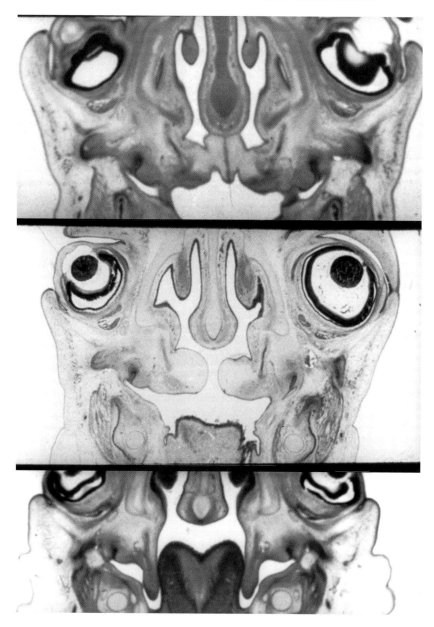

FIG. 2.3. Coronal sections of embryos at (*top*) 54, (*middle*) 57, and (*lower*) 63 days postconception, revealing elevation of lateral palatal shelves from vertical to horizontal and fusion with the nasal septum. (From the Carnegie Embryo Collection.)

glycoproteins and desmosomes facilitates epithelial adherence between contacting palatal shelves. The cell adhesion molecule syndecan is expressed as the shelves elevate, and its expression decreases during fusion (Fitchett et al., 1990). At the time of palatal shelf fusion, there is increased expression of N-cadherin. This may be instrumental in the transformation of epithelium into its different phenotypes (nasal, medial edge, and oral) and into mesenchyme. Only the medial edge epithelium of the palatal shelves (in contrast to their

oral and nasal surface epithelia) undergoes cytodifferentiation, which involves a decline of EGF receptors leading to apoptotic cell death (Greene and Pratt, 1976). The oral surface of the palatal shelves differentiates into stratified squamous epithelium, while the nasal surface becomes respiratory ciliated pseudostratified columnar epithelium (Carette et al., 1991).

Programmed cell death of the fusing medial edge epithelia is restricted to the periderm, with basal cells remaining healthy. Epithelial–mesenchymal transforma-

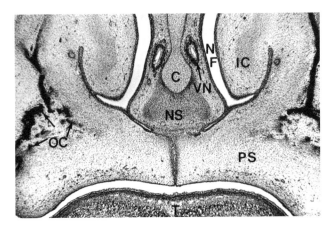

FIG. 2.4. Coronal section of the palate of an embryo immediately after midline fusion. *PS*, palatal shelves; *NS*, nasal septum; *IC*, inferior concha; *C*, cartilage of nasal septum; *VN*, vomeronasal organ; *OC*, ossification centers; *NF*, nasal fossa; *T*, tongue. (From O'Rahilly, 1975, with permission.)

tion of medial edge epithelium is essential to mesenchymal coalescence of the shelves. The surface cells lose their epithelial cell junctions and adopt a fibroblastic morphology. Cytokeratins (characteristic of epithelia), vimentin (typical of mesenchyme), and cadherins are variously expressed during this transformation (Montenegro et al., 2000). Some epithelial cells also migrate into the palatal mesenchyme, undergoing epithelial–mesenchymal transformation and contributing to seam disruption (Fitchett et al., 1990; Shuler et al., 1991, 1992; Griffith and Hay, 1992; Hay, 1995; Lavrin and Hay, 2000). The epithelium, at its leading edges, may contribute to failure of fusion by not breaking down after shelf approximation, leading to epithelial pearl formation, or by not maintaining adhesiveness beyond a critical time should palatal shelf elevation be delayed.[2] Obstructed, unfused medial palatal shelf epithelium stratifies and keratinizes before birth (Goss et al., 1970). However, the capability to fuse is retained until shortly before birth (Lavrin et al., 2001). This provides the possibility that unfused palatal shelves brought into contact by *in utero* surgical intervention could forestall clefting.

Fusion of the three palatal components initially produces a flat, unarched roof to the mouth (Fig. 2.6). The fusing lateral palatal shelves overlap the anterior primary palate, as indicated later by the sloping pathways of the junctional incisive neurovascular canals that carry the previously formed incisive nerves and blood vessels. The site of junction of the three palatal components is marked by the incisive papilla overlying the incisive canal. The line of fusion of the lateral palatal shelves is traced in the adult by the midpalatal suture[3] and on the surface by the midline raphe of the hard

palate (Fig. 2.6). This fusion seam is minimized in the soft palate by invasion of extraterritorial mesenchyme.

Ossification of the palate proceeds during the 8th week postconception from the spread of bone into the mesenchyme of the fused lateral palatal shelves and from trabeculae appearing in the primary palate as premaxillary centers, all derived from the single primary ossification centers of the maxillae (Jacobson, 1955; Wood et al., 1967; Kjaer, 1989; Nijo and Kjaer, 1993; Silau et al., 1994; Vacher et al., 1999; Vacher et al., 2001). The existence of an incisive fissure in the ossified palate at the site of fusion of the primary and secondary palates has been demonstrated in archeological material (Sejrsen et al., 1993; Maureille and Bar, 1999; Kieser et al., 1999). However, the coincidence of the incisive fissure with alveolar palatal clefts has been

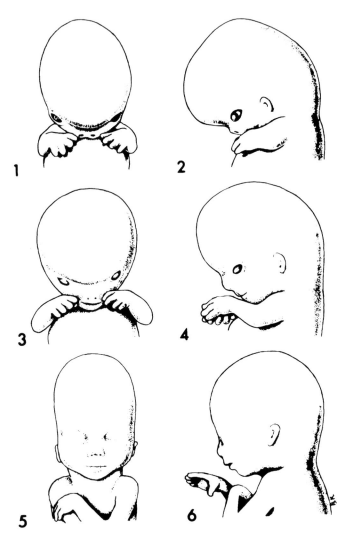

FIG. 2.5. Schematic depiction of fetal head movements from frontal (*left*) and lateral (*right*) perspectives at (*1,2*) 6, (*3,4*) 7, and (*5,6*) 8 weeks. (Courtesy of Dr. V. M. Diewert. University of British Columbia.)

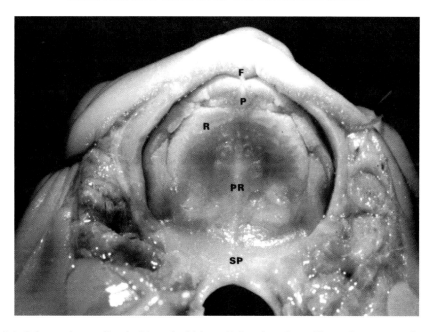

FIG. 2.6. Palate and upper lip of a 22-week-old fetus. *F*, frenulum; *P*, papilla overlying incisive foramen; PR, palatal raphe; *R*, rugae; *SP*, soft palate. (From Sperber, 2001, with permission.)

disputed (Lisson and Kjaer, 1997). Posteriorly, the hard palate is ossified by trabeculae spreading from the single primary ossification center of each of the palatine bones.

The midpalatal sutural structure is first evident at 10.5 weeks, when an upper layer of fiber bundles develops across the midline (Del Santo et al., 1998). In infancy, the midpalatal suture in coronal section has a Y shape, and it binds the vomer with the palatal shelves. In childhood, the junction between the three bones rises into a T shape, with the interpalatal section taking a serpentine course. In adolescence, the suture becomes so interdigitated that mechanical interlocking and interstitial islets of bone are formed. Cartilage may appear in islands in the suture in the neonatal period, but after 3 years the suture is exclusively fibrous (Persson, 1973). Application of expansional forces on the maxillae to widen the palate in orthodontic practice induces osteogenesis in the midpalatal suture (*distraction osteogenesis*) (Latham, 1971; Kobayashi et al., 1999). The palatine bone elements remain separated from the maxillary elements by the transverse palatomaxillary sutures into adulthood (Nijo and Kjaer, 1993).

Ossification does not occur in the most posterior part of the palate, giving rise to the soft palate. Myogenic mesenchymal tissue of the first and fourth pharyngeal arches migrates into this faucial region, supplying the musculature of the soft palate and fauces (Cohen et al., 1993, 1994). The tensor veli palatini is derived from somitomeres associated with the first pharyngeal arch; the levator palatini and uvular and faucial pillar mus-

cles are derived from somitomeres associated with the fourth pharyngeal arch, accounting for the innervation by the first arch trigeminal nerve of the tensor veli palatini muscle and by the fourth arch pharyngeal plexus and vagus nerves for all of the other muscles.

The tensor veli palatini is the earliest of the five palatal muscles to develop, forming myoblasts at 40 days postconception. It is followed by the palatopharyngeus (45 days), the levator veli palatini (8th week), the palatoglossus (9th week), and the uvular muscles (11th week). The palatoglossus, derived from the tongue musculature, attaches to the soft palate during the 11th week postconception. The hard palate grows in length, breadth, and height, becoming an arched roof for the mouth (Fig. 2.7). The fetal palate increases in length more rapidly than in width between 7 and 18 weeks postconception, after which the width increases faster than the length (Lee et al., 1992). In early prenatal life, the palate is relatively long, but from the 4th month postconception it widens as a result of midpalatal sutural growth and appositional growth along the lateral alveolar margins. At birth, the length and breadth of the hard palate are almost equal. The postnatal increase in palatal length is due to appositional growth in the maxillary tuberosity region and, to some extent, at the transverse maxillopalatine suture (Sejrsen et al., 1996).

Growth at the midpalatal suture ceases between 1 and 2 years of age, but no synostosis occurs to signify its cessation.[4] Growth in width of the midpalatal suture is larger in its posterior than in its anterior part.

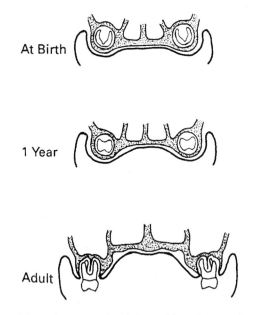

FIG. 2.7. Schematic cross-sectional views of the palate at various ages. Note the increasing depth of the palatal arch concomitant with tooth eruption. (From Sperber, 2001, with permission.)

Obliteration of the midpalatal suture may start in adolescence, but complete fusion is rarely found before 30 years of age. The timing and degree of fusion of this suture vary greatly (Wehrbein and Yildizhan, 2001).

Lateral appositional growth continues until 7 years of age, by which time the palate achieves its ultimate anterior width. Posterior appositional growth continues after lateral growth has ceased so that the palate becomes longer, rather than wider, during late childhood. During infancy and childhood, bone apposition also occurs on the entire inferior surface of the palate, accompanied by concomitant resorption from its superior (nasal) surface. This bone remodeling results in descent of the palate and enlargement of the nasal cavity. Nasal capacity must increase, to keep pace with the increasing respiratory requirements engendered by general body growth. A fundamental drive in facial growth is provision of an adequate nasal capacity; if this need is not met, the space capacity requirement is diverted to the mouth for maintenance of respiration.

The appositional growth of the alveolar processes contributes to deepening, as well as widening, of the vault of the bony palate, at the same time adding to the height and breadth of the maxillae. The lateral alveolar processes help to form an anteroposterior palatal furrow, which together with a concave floor produced by a tongue curled from side to side results in a palatal tunnel ideally suited to receive a nipple. A variable number of transverse palatal rugae develop in the mucosa covering the hard palate (Harris et al., 1990; Thomas and

Rossouw, 1991). They appear even before palatal fusion, which occurs at 56 days postconception. The rugae, which are most prominent in the infant, hold the nipple while it is being milked by the tongue. Palatal rugae are utilized as landmarks in cephalometry and orthodontics because of their stability (Hoggan and Sadowsky, 2001). The anterior palatal furrow is well marked during the first year of life (i.e., the active suckling period) and normally flattens out into the palatal arch after 3 to 4 years of age, when suckling has been discontinued. Persistence of thumb or finger sucking may retain the accentuated palatal furrow into childhood.

Anomalies of the palate occur as a consequence of disturbances of the above-mentioned developmental processes. Successful fusion of the three embryonic components of the palate involves complicated synchronization of shelf movements with growth and withdrawal of the tongue and growth of the mandible and head. Mistiming of any of these critical events, because of environmental agents or genetic predisposition, results in failure of fusion, leading to clefts of the palate. Palatal clefting is multifactorial in its etiology, and no single genetic locus has been identified as a source of its cause, despite its hereditary familial associations (Hibbert and Field, 1996). Postnatal surgical repair of cleft palate results in cicatricial formation, the scarring compromising the growth potential and final result. However, in utero repair of fetal cleft palate offers the possibility of scarless healing and is a potential future treatment (Christ, 1990; Weinzweig et al., 1999).

The entrapment of epithelial rests or pearls in the line of fusion of the palatal shelves, particularly the midline raphe of the hard palate, may give rise later to median palatal rest cysts (Arnold et al., 1998). A common superficial expression of these epithelial entrapments is development of epithelial cysts or nodules, known as *Epstein's pearls*, along the median raphe of the hard palate and at the junction of the hard and soft palates. Small mucosal gland retention cysts (*Bohn's nodules*) may occur on the buccal and lingual aspects of the alveolar ridges, and dental lamina cysts composed of epithelial remnants of this lamina may develop on the crests of the alveolar ridges. All of these superficial cysts of the palate in the newborn usually disappear by the third postnatal month. An anterior midline maxillary cyst developing in the region of the primary palate cannot be of fissural origin, but is a nasopalatine duct cyst encroaching anteriorly into the palate. Cysts are rare in the soft palate because of the mesenchymal merging of the shelves in this region, although submucous clefts may occur.

Delay in elevation of the palatal shelves from the vertical to the horizontal while the head is growing continuously results in a widening gap between the shelves

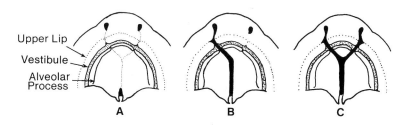

Cleft Palate Variations

A Bifid uvula

B Unilateral cleft palate and lip

C Bilateral cleft palate and lip

FIG. 2.8. Schematic depiction of cleft palate variations. (From Sperber, 2001, with permission.)

so that they cannot meet and, therefore, cannot fuse. When eventually they do become horizontal, this leads to clefting of the palate (*palatoschisis*). Other causes of cleft palate are defective shelf fusion, failure of medial edge epithelial cell death, possible postfusion rupture (Kitamura, 1991), and failure of mesenchymal consolidation and differentiation (Lavrin and Hay, 2000).

The least severe form of cleft palate is the bifid uvula, of relatively common occurrence. Increasingly severe clefts always incur posterior involvement, the cleft advancing anteriorly in contradistinction to the direction of normal fusion (Fig. 2.8). The lines of fusion of the lateral palatal shelves with the primary palate dictate the diversion from the midline of a severe palatal cleft anteriorly to either the right or left or, in rare instances, to both. If the cleft involves the alveolar arch, it usually passes between the lateral incisor and canine teeth (Lisson and Kjaer, 1997). Such severe clefting of the palate may or may not be associated with unilateral or bilateral cleft upper lip; the two conditions are deter-

mined independently. The vertical nasal septum may fuse with the left or right palatal shelf or neither in cases of severe cleft palate (Figs. 2.9, 2.10).

Clefts of the soft palate alone incur varying degrees of speech difficulty and swallowing problems because of the inability to close off the oropharynx completely from the nasopharynx during these pharyngeal functions. Clefts of the hard palate, which almost invariably include soft palate clefts, give rise to feeding problems, particularly in infants in whom the vacuum-producing sucking processes demand an intact hard palate. Spillage of food into the nasal cavity is symptomatic of feeding difficulties. The efficacy of suckling is compromised, with the necessary negative oral pressure for ingestion shifted toward the nasal cavity and pharynx. The consequent altered physiological pressures result in altered morphology of adjacent structures (Ihan-Hren et al., 2001). Such infants require early reparative surgery and/or obturator fitting to maintain good nutrition and to aid development of correct enunciation.

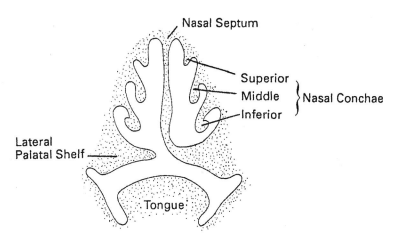

FIG. 2.9. Schematic coronal section through a unilateral cleft palate with an oral opening into one nasal cavity only. (From Sperber, 2001, with permission.)

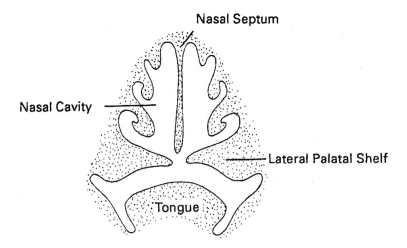

FIG. 2.10. Schematic coronal section through a bilaterally cleft palate with an oral opening into both nasal cavities. (From Sperber, 2001, with permission.)

Cleft palate is a feature of a number of congenital defect syndromes, among which are mandibulofacial dysostosis (Treacher Collins syndrome), micrognathia (Pierre Robin sequence), van der Woude syndrome, and orodigitofacial dysostosis syndrome. The palate is narrower, shorter, and lower than normal in Down syndrome (trisomy 21), although it is often described as having a high midline elevation but being horizontally flattened laterally along the alveolar ridges, creating a steeple palate (Panchón-Ruiz et al., 2000). A highly arched palate is also characteristic of Marfan syndrome, an inherited disorder manifesting skeletal and cardiovascular anomalies. Cleidocranial dysostosis, a congenital defect of intramembranous bones, also manifests a highly arched palate, with or without a cleft. Other congenital conditions displaying a highly arched palate are craniofacial dysostosis (Crouzon syndrome), acrocephalosyndactyly (Apert syndrome), progeria, Turner syndrome (XO sex chromosome complement), and oculodentodigital dysplasia. A great variety of other congenital anomalies may be associated with clefts of the lip and palate (Milerad et al., 1997; Natsume et al., 2001).

A fairly common genetic anomaly of the palate is a localized midpalatal overgrowth of bone, of varying size, known as torus palatinus. This may enlarge in adulthood, and although it does not directly influence dental occlusion, if prominent, it may interfere with the seating of a removable orthodontic appliance or upper denture.

I thank Anne-Marie McLean for meticulous word processing of the manuscript.

REFERENCES

Abbott, BD, Probst, MR, Perdew, GH, Buckalew, AR (1998). AH receptor, ARNT, glucocorticoid receptor, EGF receptor, EGF, TGFα, TGFβ₁, TGFβ₂ and TGFβ₃ expression in human embryonic palate and effects of 2, 3, 7, 8 tetrachlorodibenzo-*p*-dioxin (TCDD). Teratology *58:* 30–43.

Amin, N, Ohashi, Y, Chiba, J, et al. (1994). Alterations in vascular pattern of the developing palate in normal and spontaneous cleft palate mouse embryos. Cleft Palate Craniofac J *31:* 332–344.

Arnold, WH, Rezwani, T, Baric, I (1998). Location and distribution of epithelial pearls and tooth buds in human fetuses with cleft lip and palate. Cleft Palate Craniofac J *35:* 359–365.

Barrow, JR, Capecchi, MR (1999). Compensatory defects associated with mutations in Hoxa 1 restore normal palatogenesis to Hoxa 2 mutants. Development *126:* 5011–5026.

Burdi, AR, Faist, K (1967). Morphogenesis of the palate in normal human embryos with special emphasis on the mechanisms involved. Am J Anat *120:* 149.

Carette, MJ, Lane, EB, Ferguson, MW (1991). Differentiation of mouse embryonic palatal epithelium in culture: selective cytokeratin expression distinguishes between oral, medial edge and nasal epithelial cells. Differentiation *47:* 149–161.

Christ, JE (1990). Plastic surgery for the fetus. Plast Reconstr Surg *86:* 1238.

Citterio, HL, Gaillard, DA (1994). Expression of TGF2, EGF-R and cell proliferation during human palatogenesis: an immunohistochemical study. Int J Dev Biol *38:* 499–505.

Cohen, SR, Chen, L, Burdi, AR, et al. (1994). Patterns of abnormal myogenesis in human cleft palates. Cleft Palate Craniofac J *31:* 345.

Cohen, SR, Chen, L, Trotman, CA, et al. (1993). Soft palate myogenesis: a developmental field paradigm. Cleft Palate Craniofac J *30:* 441–446.

Cui, X-M, Warburton, D, Zhao, J, et al. (1998). Immunohistochemical localization of TGF-β type II cell receptor and TGFβ3 during palatogenesis in vivo and in vitro. Int J Dev Biol *42:* 817–820.

Del Santo, M, Jr, Minarelli, AM, Liberti, EA (1998). Morphological aspects of the mid-palatal suture in the human foetus: a light and scanning electron microscope study. Eur J Orthod *20:* 93–99.

Ferguson, MWJ (1988). Palate development. Development *103(Suppl.)*: 41–60.

Fitchett, JE, McAlmon, KR, Hay, ED, Bernfield, M (1990). Epithelial cells lose syndecans prior to epithelial–mesenchymal transformation in the developing rat palate. J Cell Biol *111*: 1459.

Gibbins, JR, Manthey, A, Tazawa, YM, et al. (1999). Midline fusion in the formation of the secondary palate anticipated by upregulation of keratin K5/6 and localized expression of vimentin mRNA in medial edge epithelium. Int J Dev Biol *43*: 237–244.

Goss, AN, Bodner, JW, Avery, JK (1970). In vitro fusion of cleft palate shelves. Cleft Palate J *7*: 737–747.

Greene, RM, Pratt, RM (1976). Developmental aspects of secondary palate formation. J Embryol Exp Morphol *36*: 225–245.

Griffith, CM, Hay, ED (1992). Epithelial–mesenchymal transformation during palatal fusion: carboxyfluorescein traces cells at light and electron microscopic levels. Development *116*: 1087–1099.

Harris, MJ, Juriloff, DM, Peters, CE (1990). Disruption of pattern formation in palatal rugae in fetal mice heterozygous for First Arch (FAR). J Craniofac Genet Dev Biol *10*: 363–371.

Hay, ED (1995). An overview of epithelio–mesenchymal transformation. Acta Anat (Basel) *154*: 8–20.

Hibbert, SA, Field, JK (1996). Molecular basis of familial cleft lip and palate. Oral Dis *2*: 238–241.

Hoggan, BR, Sadowsky, C (2001). The use of palatal rugae for the assessment of anteroposterior tooth movements. Am J Orthod Dentofac Orthoped *119*: 482–488.

Humphrey, T (1969). The relation between human fetal mouth opening reflexes and closure of the palate. Am J Anat *125*: 317–344.

Ihan-Hren, N, Oblak, P, Kozelj, V (2001). Characteristic forms of the upper part of the oral cavity in newborns with isolated cleft palate. Cleft Palate Craniofac J *38*: 164–169.

Izadnegahdar, MF, Rathanaswami, P, Shah, RM (1999). Effects of EGF and TGFβ1 on c-*myc* gene expression and DNA synthesis in embryonic hamster palate mesenchymal cells. Anat Rec *254*: 453–464.

Jacobson, A (1955). Embryological evidence for the non-existence of the premaxilla in man. J Dent Assoc S Afr *10*: 189–210.

Kaartinen, V, Cui, XM, Heisterkamp, N, et al. (1997). TGFβ3 regulates transdifferentiation of medial edge epithelium during palatal fusion and associated degradation of the basement membrane. Dev Dyn *209*: 255–260.

Kieser, JA, Dennison, KJ, Dias, GR (1999). Premaxillary suture in early Polynesians. Int J Osteoarchaeol *9*: 244–247.

Kimes, KR, Mooney, MP, Siegel, MI, Todhunter, JS (1991). Size and growth rate of the tongue in normal and cleft lip and palate human fetal specimens. Cleft Palate Craniofac J *28*: 212–216.

Kitamura, H (1991). Evidence for cleft palate as a postfusion phenomenon. Cleft Palate Craniofac J *28*: 195–210.

Kjaer, I (1989). Prenatal skeletal maturation of the human maxilla. J Craniofac Genet Dev Biol *9*: 257–264.

Kjaer, I (1997). Mandibular movements during elevation and fusion of palatal shelves evaluated from the course of Meckel's cartilage. J Craniofac Genet Dev Biol *17*: 80–85.

Kobayashi, ET, Hashimoto, F, Kobayashi, Y, et al. (1999). Force-induced rapid changes in cell fate at midpalatal suture cartilage of growing rats. J Dent Res *78*: 1495–1504.

Laster, Z, Temkin, D, Zarfin, Y, Kushnir, A (2001). Complete bony fusion of the mandible to the zygomatic complex and maxillary tuberosity: case report and review. Int J Oral Maxillofac Surg *30*: 75–79.

Latham, RA (1971). The development, structure and growth pattern of the human midpalatal suture. J Anat *108*: 31–41.

Lavrin, IG (2000). Pierre Robin sequence—a review and an animal model. In: Davidovitch, Z, Mah, J (Eds.) *The Biological Mecha-*

nisms of Tooth Movement and Craniofacial Adaptation. Harvard Society for the Advancement of Orthodontics. Boston. pp. 299–303.

Lavrin, IG, Hay, ED (2000). Epithelial–mesenchymal transformation, palatogenesis and cleft palate. Angle Orthod *70*: 181–182.

Lavrin, IG, McLean, W, Seegmiller, RE, Olsen, BR, Hay, ED (2001). The mechanism of palatal clefting in the Col11a1 mutant mouse. Arch Oral Biol *46*: 865–869.

Lee, SK, Kim, YS, Lim, CY, Chi, JG (1992). Prenatal growth pattern of the human maxilla. Acta Anat (Basel) *145*: 1–10.

Lisson, JA, Kjaer, I (1997). Location of alveolar clefts relative to the incisive fissure. Cleft Palate Craniofac J *34*: 292–296.

Machida, J, Yoshiura, K, Funkhauser, CD, et al. (1999). Transforming growth factor α: genomic structure, boundary sequences and mutation analysis in non-syndromic cleft lip/palate and cleft palate only. Genomics *61*: 237–242.

Mann, SE, Nijland, MJ, Ross, MG (1996). Mathematical modeling of human amniotic fluid dynamics. Am J Obstet Gynecol *175*: 937–944.

Maurielle, B, Bar, D (1999). The premaxilla in Neanderthal and early modern children: ontogeny and morphology. J Hum Evol *37*: 137–152.

McGonnell, IM, Clarke, JD, Tickle, C (1998). Fate map of the developing chick face: an analysis of expansion of facial primordia and establishment of the primary palate. Dev Dyn *212*: 102–118.

Miettinen, PJ, Chin, JR, Shum, L, et al. (1999). Epidermal growth factor receptor function is necessary for normal craniofacial development and palate closure. Nat Genet *22*: 69–73.

Milerad, J, Larson, O, Hagberg, C, Ideberg, M (1997). Associated malformations in infants with cleft lip and palate: a prospective, population-based study. Pediatrics *100*: 180–186.

Montenegro, MA, Rojas, M, Dominguez, S, Vergara, A (2000). Cytokeratin, vimentin and E-cadherin immunodetection in the embryonic palate in two strains of mice with different susceptibility to glucocorticoid-induced clefting. J Craniofac Genet Dev Biol *20*: 137–143.

Mooney, MP, Siegel, MI, Kimes, KR, et al. (1994). Anterior paraseptal cartilage development in normal and cleft lip and palate human fetal specimens. Cleft Palate Craniofac J *31*: 239–245.

Morris-Wiman, J, Brinkley, L (1992). An extracellular matrix infrastructure provides support for murine secondary palatal shelf remodelling. Anat Rec *234*: 575–586.

Natsume, N, Niimi, T, Furukawa, H, et al. (2001). Survey of congenital anomalies associated with cleft lip and/or palate in 701,181 Japanese people. Oral Surg Oral Med Oral Pathol Oral Radiol Endod *91*: 157–161.

Nijo, BJ, Kjaer, I (1993). The development and morphology of the incisive fissure and the transverse palatine suture in the human fetal palate. J Craniofac Genet Dev Biol *13*: 24–34.

O'Rahilly, R (1975). *A Color Atlas of Human Embryology.* Philadelphia: Saunders.

Panchón-Ruiz, A, Jornet-Carrillo, V, Sanchez del Campo, F (2000). Palate vault morphology in Down syndrome. J Craniofac Genet Dev Biol *20*: 198–200.

Persson, M (1973). Structure and growth of facial sutures. Odont Rev *24(Suppl 26)*: 1–146.

Proetzel, G, Pawlowski, SA, Wiles, MV, et al. (1995). Transforming growth factor β3 is required for secondary palate fusion. Nat Genet *11*: 409–414.

Seegmiller, RE, Fraser, FC (1977). Mandibular growth retardation as a cause of cleft palate in mice homozygous for chondrodysplasia gene. J Embryol Exp Morphol *38*: 227–238.

Sejrsen, B, Kjaer, I, Jakobsen, J (1993). The human incisal suture and premaxillary area studied on archeological material. Acta Odont Scand *51*: 143–151.

Sejrsen, B, Kjaer, I, Jakobsen, J (1996). Human palatal growth evaluated on medieval crania using nerve canal openings as references. Am J Phys Anthropol 99: 603–611.

Shuler, CF, Guo, Y, Majumder, A, Luo, R (1991). Molecular and morphological changes during the epithelial–mesenchymal transformation of palatal shelf medial edge epithelium in vitro. Int J Dev Biol 35: 463–472.

Shuler, CF, Halpern, DE, Guo, Y, Sank, AC (1992). Medial edge epithelium fate traced by lineage analysis during epithelial–mesenchymal transformation. Dev Biol 154: 318–330.

Silau, AM, Njio, B, Solow, B, Kjaer, I (1994). Prenatal sagittal growth of the osseous components of the human palate. J Craniofac Genet Dev Biol 14: 252–256.

Singh, GD, Moxham, BJ, Langley, MS, Embery, G (1997). Glycosaminoglycan biosynthesis during 5-fluro-2-deoxyuridine–induced palatal clefts in the rat. Arch Oral Biol 42: 355–363.

Sun, D, Vanderburg, CR, Odierna, GS, Hay, ED (1998). TGFβ3 promotes transformation of chicken palatal medial edge epithelium to mesenchyme in vitro. Development 125: 95–105.

Thomas, CJ, Rossouw, RJ (1991). The early development of palatal rugae in the rat. Aust Dent J 36: 342–348.

Vacher, C, Copin, H, Sakka, M (1999). Maxillary ossification in a series of six human embryos and fetuses aged from 9 to 12 weeks of amenorrhea: clinical implications. Surg Radiol Anat 21:261–266.

Vacher, C, Sakka, M, Dauge, M-C (2001). Incisive suture (fissure) in the human fetus: radiographic and histologic study. Cleft Palate Craniofac J 38: 330–336.

Wehrbein, H, Yildizhan, F (2001). The mid-palatal suture in young adults. A radiological-histological investigation. Eur J Orthod 23: 105–114.

Weinzweig, J, Panter, KE, Pantaloni, M, et al. (1999). The fetal cleft palate: II scarless healing after in utero repair of a congenital model. Plast Reconstr Surg 104: 1356–1364.

Wood, NK, Wragge, LE, Stuteville, OH (1967). The premaxilla: embryological evidence that it does not exist in man. Anat Rec 158: 485–489.

Wragg, LE, Smith, JA, Borden, CS (1972). Myoneural maturation of the foetal rat tongue at the time of secondary palate closure. Arch Oral Biol 17: 673–682.

Young, AV, Hehn, BM, Sanghera, JS, et al. (1997). The activation of MAP kinase during vertical palatal shelf development in hamster. Growth Dev Aging 61: 27–38.

NOTES

1 Oligohydramnios arises from insufficient or absent urinary output consequent to absent kidneys (renal agenesis) or ureteric defects (stenosis) inhibiting micturation. The fetus normally swallows between 200 and 600 ml of amniotic fluid per day during the last trimester of pregnancy (Mann et al., 1996).

2 In birds, the medial edge epithelium keratinizes, precluding fusion, resulting in physiological cleft palate.

3 The midpalatal suture includes the palatal portion of the intermaxillary suture and the median palatine suture between the two palatine bones.

4 Retention of a syndesmosis in the midpalatal suture into adulthood, even after growth has normally ceased at this site, permits the application of expansion. Forceful separation of the suture by an orthodontic appliance reinstitutes compensatory bone growth at this site, expanding palatal width.

APPENDIX: WORLD WIDE WEB SITE ADDRESSES FOR CL/P

http://www.nuds.nwu.edu/clphome.htm
http://www.healthanswers.com/database/ami/converted/001051.html
http://www.scottishiritechildrens.org/services/cleftwhatis/shtml
http://www.healthgate.com/hic/cleft-lip_palate/
http://www.clapa.mcmail.com/
http://www.widesmiles.org/index.html
http://www.cleft.org/index.html
http://www.cleft.com/cpf.htm

The American Cleft Palate-Craniofacial Association Web Site address is www.cleft.com, their Cleftline is www.cleftline.org, and the Cleft Palate-Craniofacial Journal is available online at http://cpcj.allenpress.com.

For genetic counseling, consult the following Web Sites:

American College of Medical Genetics

www.faseb.org/genetics/acmg/acmgmenu.htm

National Society of Genetic Counselors

www.nsgc.org

Genetic Alliance

www.geneticalliance.org

Office of Rare Disorders

http://rarediseases.info.nih.gov/ord/patient-support.html

Gene Tests

www.genetests.org/servlet/access

3

Genes implicated in lip and palate development

SAMUEL S. CHONG

FELICIA S. H. CHEAH

ETHYLIN WANG JABS

Normal development of facial structures such as the lip and palate is a dynamic, highly regulated, and complex process (Francis-West et al., 1998; Schutte and Murray, 1999). Signaling interactions control the normal outgrowth of facial primordia from undifferentiated mesenchymal cells, as well as the subsequent fusion of the frontal nasal mass and the left and right maxillary primordia to form intricate facial structures such as the lip and palate. From mouse mutant models, human syndromes, and both association and expression studies, a spectrum of gene products, such as transcription factors, growth factors, and signaling molecules, are postulated to be involved in these interactions (Table 3.1). These factors interact in a series of intra- and intercellular events that culminate in a developmentally significant pattern of gene expression. When the structure or expression of these genes is modified, a cleft of some type [cleft lip only (CL), cleft palate only (CP), or cleft lip and palate (CLP)] may occur.

TRANSCRIPTION REGULATORS

Expression of every gene is uniquely controlled, whether in its spatial or temporal pattern or in its response to extracellular signals. Transcription regulators control gene expression via activating or repressing signal-transduction pathways. These transcription regulators possess specific DNA binding domains, such as

homeodomain, basic helix-loop-helix, and basic leucine zipper. Protein–protein interactions are essential for specifying the actions of transcription regulators. Such interaction permits these regulators to distinguish relevant target sequences from many nonspecific binding sites in the genome and confers highly precise transcription-regulatory properties.

Since their discovery in 1984, homeobox genes have attracted widespread interest among molecular biologists, biochemists, geneticists, embryologists, and evolutionary biologists. These genes are defined by the presence of a homeobox, which is a characteristic 180-base pair DNA sequence coding for a relatively conserved block of 60 amino acids called the homeodomain. In mammals, there are four highly conserved homeobox-containing gene clusters (*Hox* clusters) that are closely related to the *Drosophila Antennapedia* and *Bithorax* complexes.

Extensive analysis of the gene expression pattern for the *Hox* clusters has shown that they can mediate patterning in craniofacial development (Krumlauf, 1993). Many of these homeobox-containing genes are expressed in specific regions of neural crest–derived mesenchyme of the developing facial primordia. Much interest has been focused on these genes as they may control patterning of the developing facial primordia. Expression of *Hox*-cluster genes during craniofacial development is highly conserved between mice and humans (Vieille-Grosjean et al., 1997). This supports the validity of employing the mouse as a model for understanding the role of *HOX* and other homeobox-containing genes during human craniofacial development.

MSX Genes

MSX genes are homeobox-containing genes homologous to the *Drosophila msh* (muscle segment homeobox) gene (Hill et al., 1989). The murine Msx family consists of three members, Msx1–3. Msx1 and Msx2 have been well characterized with respect to their DNA binding and transcriptional properties (Catron et al., 1995, 1996; Woloshin et al., 1995; Zhang et al., 1996), while Msx3 has been less studied (Holland, 1991; Shimeld et al., 1996). They share a highly conserved homeobox motif that encodes a DNA binding domain (the homeodomain). In addition, Msx proteins share conserved regions such as the extended homeodomain and Msx homology regions, which flank the homeodomain (Zhang et al., 1997).

Both Msx1 and Msx2 proteins function as transcriptional repressors in cellular differentiation (Catron et al., 1995, 1996; Woloshin et al., 1995; Zhang et al., 1996). Interestingly, this repressor activity occurs in-dependently of homeodomain DNA binding sites in target genes, even though the Msx proteins exhibit sequence-specific DNA binding activity. Rather, Msx proteins interact with other protein factors to modulate differentiation and/or proliferation. For example, the Msx1 homeodomain interacts directly with TATA-binding protein (Zhang et al., 1996). Additionally, Msx proteins dimerize in vitro and in vivo with other homeoproteins, such as the Dlx proteins, to modulate their own transcriptional activities (Zhang et al., 1997). This heterodimer formation results in a functional antagonism that counteracts the repressor and activator actions of Msx and Dlx, respectively, and has been proposed as a mechanism by which Msx and Dlx proteins mutually regulate their transcriptional activities in vivo.

Embryonic expression patterns of *Msx* genes are consistent with a role for Msx proteins in epithelial–mesenchymal tissue interactions during craniofacial development (Hill et al., 1989; MacKenzie et al., 1991a,b; Mina et al., 1995). *Msx* genes are differentially expressed in both migratory and postmigratory neural crest cells. The role for Msx proteins in active morphogenesis is further suggested by the lack of Msx1 ex-

TABLE 3.1. *Genes Implicated in Lip/Palate Development and Disease*

Candidate	Evidence*	Reference
Transcription regulators		
MSX genes	Mutation, animal studies	Satokata and Maas, 1994; Winograd et al., 1997; Lidral et al., 1998; van den Boogaard et al., 2000
DLX genes	Animal studies	Qiu et al., 1995, 1997
LHX genes	Animal, expression studies	Grigoriou et al., 1998; Zhao et al., 1999a
PRRX genes	Animal studies	Martin et al., 1995; ten Berge et al., 1998
Goosecoid	Animal studies	Rivera-Perez et al., 1995; Yamada et al., 1995, 1997
Growth factors		
FGF genes/receptors	Expression studies	Celli et al., 1998
TGFA gene	Expression, association studies	Ardinger et al., 1989; Dixon et al., 1991; Chenevix-Trench et al., 1992; Holder et al., 1992
TGF-β superfamily	Expression, animal studies	Brunet et al., 1995; Kaartinen et al., 1995, 1997; Proetzel et al., 1995; Feijen et al., 1994; Matzuk et al., 1995a–c
PDGF genes/receptors	Expression studies	Morrison-Graham et al., 1992; Qiu and Ferguson, 1995
EGF genes/receptor	Animal studies	Miettinen et al., 1999
Signaling molecules		
Endothelins and receptors	Animal, expression studies	Kurihara et al., 1994; Clouthier et al., 1998
Jagged and *Notch*	Animal studies	Jiang et al., 1998
Thrombospondins	Expression studies	Melnick et al., 2000
GABA and receptors	Animal, teratological studies	Wee and Zimmerman, 1983; Culiat et al., 1993, 1995; Homanics et al., 1997
RYK gene	Animal studies	Halford et al., 2000

*Type of evidence in the literature for gene being implicated in lip/palate development. *MSX,* Homologous to *Drosophila* muscle segment homeobox *(msh)* gene; *DLX,* homologous to *Drosophila* distal-less *(Dll)* gene; *LHX,* LIM (lin-11 isl-1 mec-3) homeobox; *PRRX,* paired-related homeobox; *FGF,* fibroblast growth factor; *TGFA,* transforming growth factor-α; *TGF-β,* transforming growth factor-β; *PDGF,* platelet-derived growth factor; *EGF,* epidermal growth factor; *GABA,* γ-aminobutyric acid; *RYK,* related to tyrosine kinase.

pression in cells undergoing terminal differentiation (Woloshin et al., 1995) and by restricted cellular expression of Msx1 transcript during periods of rapid cellular proliferation in tissues that are maintained in a developmentally plastic state during regeneration (Pavlova et al., 1994; Reginelli et al., 1995; Simon et al., 1995).

In mice, targeted disruption of *Msx1* leads to significant craniofacial abnormalities ranging from the loss of structures such as palatal shelves and maxillary bones to a slight shortening of the maxilla and mandible and absence of tooth development beyond the bud stage (Satokata and Maas, 1994) (Color Fig. 3.1a–c). That *MSX1* is a candidate gene for human orofacial clefting is further supported by the findings of van den Boogaard et al. (2000), who identified a Dutch family with tooth agenesis and various combinations of CP and CLP, a phenotype similar to that of *Msx1* gene knockout mice. Mutational analysis of the *MSX1* gene in affected individuals revealed heterozygosity for a nonsense mutation (S104X) in exon 1. Further evidence comes from an Iowa case-control study, which reported positive association between *MSX1* and CP (Lidral et al., 1998; Romitti et al., 1999), although a previous study in a Philippine population had shown no association (Lidral et al., 1997).

Msx2 is also involved in craniofacial development, although its role in lip and palate development is less well defined. Msx2-deficient mice show defects of skull ossification and persistent calvarial foramen (Satokata et al., 2000). These features closely resemble the defective cranial osteogenesis and enlarged parietal foraminae observed in humans with functional haploinsufficiency of *MSX2* (Wilkie et al., 2000). In contrast, a gain-of-function mutation in *MSX2* has been shown to be the cause of autosomal dominant craniosynostosis in a family with one member having a CP (Jabs et al., 1993; Ma et al., 1996). Furthermore, transgenic mice harboring either a wild-type or a mutant (P148H) human *MSX2* gene show perinatal lethality and various degrees of craniofacial malformation, including mandibular hypoplasia, cleft secondary palate, exencephaly, and median facial cleft (Winograd et al., 1997). In addition, aplasia of the interparietal bone and reduced ossification of the hyoid have been observed in these transgenic mice. These data allude to the importance of *MSX2* dosage effects during skull development.

DLX Genes

DLX genes are homeobox-containing genes homologous to the *Drosophila Distal-less* (*Dll*) gene (Price et al., 1991). They include at least six members in mice (*Dlx1, Dlx2, Dlx3, Dlx5, Dlx6*, and *Dlx7*) and encode transcription factors that are involved in the patterning of the orofacial skeleton derived from cephalic neural crest cells (Porteus et al., 1991; Price et al., 1991; Robinson et al., 1991; Robinson and Mahon, 1994; Simeone et al., 1994; Nakamura et al., 1996; Davideau et al., 1999). In mice, only Dlx1 and Dlx2 are expressed in the developing maxillary arch, while Dlx1, -2, -3, -5, and -6 are expressed in overlapping domains in the developing mandibular primordia (Dolle et al., 1992; Qiu et al., 1995, 1997).

Targeted disruption of either *Dlx1* or *Dlx2* in mice affects the development of the palatine and pterygoid bones of the palate, aside from features unique to each knockout (Qiu et al., 1995, 1997). In $Dlx1^{-/-}/Dlx2^{-/-}$ double gene knockout mice, no additional skeletal structures are affected or replaced except for the absence of maxillary molars.

LHX Genes

The *LHX* (**LIM h**omeobox) genes encode a class of transcription regulators that possess two tandemly repeated cysteine-rich double-zinc finger motifs called LIM (**lin**-11 isl-1 **mec**-3) domains, followed by a homeodomain (Freyd et al., 1990). Each LIM domain is composed of 50 to 60 amino acids with a conserved pattern of cysteine and histidine residues forming a pair of zinc fingers and separated by a linker of two amino acids.

In contrast to the DNA binding activity of the homeodomain, the LIM domains regulate the activity of the LIM protein molecules by protein–protein interaction (Sanchez-Garcia et al., 1993; Xue et al., 1993; Feuerstein et al., 1994; Taira et al., 1994; Dawid et al., 1995; Agulnick et al., 1996; Jurata et al., 1996; Bach et al., 1997; Morcillo et al., 1997; Breen et al., 1998).

Genetic studies conducted in various organisms such as *Drosophila* and mice suggest that members of the *Lhx* gene family are required for tissue patterning or specification and differentiation of different cell types during embryonic development (Cohen et al., 1992; Taira et al., 1994; Shawlot and Behringer, 1995; Sharma et al., 1998; Zhao et al., 1999b). Two of these genes, *Lhx6* and *Lhx7*, are expressed prior to initiation of tooth formation in presumptive oral and odontogenic mesenchyme of the maxillary and mandibular processes during mouse embryogenesis (Grigoriou et al., 1998). Another LIM homeobox gene, *Lhx8* (also called *L3*), is differentially expressed in the maxillary primordia, mandibular primordia, and ventral forebrain during mouse embryogenesis (Matsumoto et al., 1996). *Lhx8* has been mapped to mouse chromosome 3 syntenic segment H3-4 (Kitanaka et al., 1998), which is homologous to a human chromosomal region (4q25-q31) that has been associated with craniofacial clefting (Beiraghi et al., 1994; Mitchell et al., 1995). During different stages of palatogenesis, continuous expression of Lhx8 is observed in the mesenchyme (Zhao et al., 1999a). In mice homozygous for deletion of the *Lhx8* gene, the palatal shelves are not able to contact and fuse normally, resulting in clefting of the secondary palate (Zhao et al., 1999a) (Color Fig. 3.1d–f). The CP phenotype observed in *Lhx8*$^{-/-}$ mutant mice thus makes *Lhx8* a candidate gene for the isolated nonsyndromic form of CP in humans.

PRRX Genes

The *PRRX* (paired-related homeobox) genes encode a class of transcription regulators that have a homeodomain homologous to the *Drosophila paired* and *gooseberry* genes and to the mouse *Pax3, Pax6,* and *Pax7* genes (Nohno et al., 1993; Norris et al., 2000). The Prrx proteins have three conserved domains: the homeodomain, the aristaless domain, and the Prrx-specific domain (ten Berge et al., 1998). These proteins do not contain a paired box and have a glutamine at amino acid position 50 of the homeodomain in place of the paired-specific serine. This amino acid difference confers the DNA binding specificity of the Prrx proteins (Treisman et al., 1989).

The two best studied *Prrx* genes, *Prrx1* (also known as *Mhox, Prx1, Phox1, Pmx1,* and *K2*) and *Prrx2* (also known as *Prx2* and *S8*), are expressed in a variety of tissues, especially in the mesenchyme during embryonic development (Leussink et al., 1995, and references therein). The expression patterns of Prrx1 and Prrx2 in the developing mouse embryo overlap but differ considerably. The *Prrx1* and *Prrx2* genes have similar expression patterns in the cranium, branchial arches, body wall, and limbs; but major differences have been observed in the brain and heart. For example, Prrx1 expression is detected in most of the ectoderm, including the precursors of the brain, whereas Prrx2 expression is not detected in the developing brain.

Inactivation (loss of function) of the *Prrx1* gene in mice results in homozygous mutants with craniofacial defects such as microcephaly, low-set ears, pointed snout, clefting of the secondary palate, and mild mandibular hypoplasia (Martin et al., 1995; ten Berge et al., 1998). In contrast, inactivation of *Prrx2* does not result in any morphological abnormalities, suggesting that Prrx1 functionally compensates for the loss of Prrx2 in *Prrx2*$^{-/-}$ mice (ten Berge et al., 1998; Lu et al., 1999). *Prrx1*$^{-/-}$/*Prrx2*$^{-/-}$ double-mutant mice exhibit abnormalities similar to but more severe than *Prrx1*$^{-/-}$ mice. For example, double-mutant mice ex-

hibit absence of external ears, and 8% of them have clefting of the mandible and tongue (ten Berge et al., 1998). *Prrx1*$^{-/-}$/*Prrx2*$^{-/-}$ mice die shortly after birth, while *Prrx1*$^{-/-}$ mice survive up to 24 h after birth. These results indicate that Prrx may be essential for normal craniofacial development, including palate and mandibular formation (ten Berge et al., 1998; Lu et al., 1999).

Goosecoid

Goosecoid (GSC) is a homeodomain-containing protein that was originally isolated from a *Xenopus* dorsal blastopore lip cDNA library (Blumberg et al., 1991). Its name is derived from the fact that parts of the homeodomain are similar to the *Drosophila* genes *gooseberry* and *bicoid* (Cho et al., 1991). Highly conserved *Goosecoid* homologs have been identified in chick, zebrafish, and mouse. In addition to the homeodomain, they share a highly conserved seven–amino acid stretch known as the Goosecoid engrailed homology domain (Goriely et al., 1996; Mailhos et al., 1998).

Goosecoid acts as a transcription factor and is expressed in two distinct phases of mouse embryonic development: initially during gastrulation [embryonic day 6.4 (E6.4) to E6.7] in regions of the embryo with axial patterning activity and subsequently during organogenesis (E10.5 onward) in craniofacial regions, the ventral body wall, and limbs (Blum et al., 1992; Gaunt et al., 1993). Generally, Goosecoid appears to be involved in orchestrating the final stages of the formation of craniofacial structures such as the ear, nose, and mouth.

Homozygous disruption of the *Gsc* gene in mice results in numerous developmental defects affecting structures in which Goosecoid is expressed during the organogenesis phase of embryonic development (Rivera-Perez et al., 1995; Yamada et al., 1995). The defects predominantly involve the lower mandible and its associated musculature, including the tongue, nasal cavity, nasal pits, malleus, and external auditory meatus (Yamada et al., 1995, 1997). Rivera-Perez et al. (1995) demonstrated numerous craniofacial and rib cage abnormalities in *Gsc*$^{-/-}$ mutant mice, including reduction or absence of maxillary and frontal bones and structures of the middle ear, as well as malformation of various bones at the base of the skull, e.g., palatine. Mice chimeric for the *Gsc*$^{-/-}$ mutation display defects similar to those observed in constitutive *Gsc*$^{-/-}$ mutant mice (Rivera-Perez et al., 1999), suggesting that Goosecoid acts in a cell-autonomous manner in mesenchyme-derived tissues during craniofacial development; i.e., Goosecoid is required for the emergence, proliferation, or survival of Goosecoid-expressing cells.

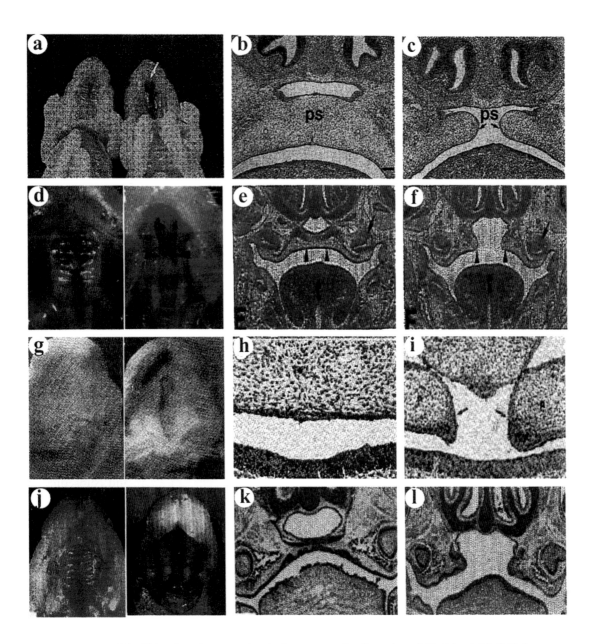

COLOR FIG. 3.1. Cleft palate phenotypes in mice homozygous for disruptions of *Msx1 (a–c)*, *Lhx8 (d–f)*, *Tgfb3 (g–i)*, and *Egfr (j–l)* genes. Gross morphology of clefts is shown in the left panels *(a, d, g, j)*, with wild-type mice on the left and –/– littermates on the right. Frontal sections through the heads of these mutant mice show failure of fusion of palatal shelves *(c, f, i, l)* compared to their wild-type sibs *(b, e, h, k)*. *ps*, palatal shelves; *t*, tongue. (From Satokata and Maas, 1994(a–c); Zhao et al., 1999a(d–f); Kaartinen et al., 1995(g–i); and Miettinen et al., 1999(j–l) with permission.)

GROWTH FACTORS

Growth factors such as fibroblast growth factor (FGF), transforming growth factor-α (TGF-α), the TGF-β superfamily, platelet-derived growth factor-α (PDGF-α), and epidermal growth factor (EGF) together with some structural extracellular matrix molecules control epithelial–mesenchymal interactions during normal palatogenesis (Ferguson, 1988; Fitzpatrick et al., 1990; Crossley and Martin, 1995; Wall and Hogan, 1995). Some of these growth factors are expressed at several stages of facial development, making it unclear which stage(s) of development is affected by mutations in any of these genes.

Fibroblast Growth Factors and Receptors

To date, at least 23 structurally similar members of the FGF family have been identified. They are associated with a wide spectrum of functions, such as angiogenesis, wound healing, embryonic development, and malignant transformation (reviewed in Basilico and Moscatelli, 1992; Yamaguchi and Rossant, 1995). They regulate cell proliferation, differentiation, and migration in many different tissues through complex signal-transduction pathways. Upon binding of FGF to its receptor, FGFR, receptor dimerization occurs, followed by kinase activation in one of the receptors. This results in the transphosphorylation of the other receptor in the dimer. The autophosphorylated FGFR can then bind and phosphorylate intracellular gene products to activate downstream signal-transduction pathways.

Although the expression patterns of many members of the Fgf gene family have not been fully characterized, at least seven members (Fgf1, Fgf2, Fgf4, Fgf5, Fgf8, Fgf9, and Fgf12) are expressed in the developing facial primordia (reviewed in Francis-West et al., 1998; Colvin et al., 1999). Some members of the Fgf family may control outgrowth of the developing facial primordia, analogous to their roles in limb bud development (Richman and Crosby, 1990; Niswander and Martin, 1992; Drucker and Goldfarb, 1993; Ohuchi et al., 1994; Crossley and Martin, 1995; Wall and Hogan, 1995; Richman et al., 1997).

The Fgfrs (Fgfr1, Fgfr2, and Fgfr3) are also expressed in the facial primordia and later associate with some regions of chondrogenesis. In a study by Celli et al. (1998), transgenic expression of a kinase-deficient mutant, Fgfr2b (a dominant-negative mutant receptor), resulted in embryonic lethality and limb and craniofacial abnormalities such as CP and reduced maxillary bone. These features are reminiscent of several human craniofacial syndromes associated with activating mutations in FGFR genes, e.g., Apert, Crouzon, Pfeiffer,

Jackson-Weiss and Beare-Stevenson syndromes (reviewed in Yamaguchi and Rossant, 1995; Passos-Bueno et al., 1999). Each of these syndromes can be associated with CP, especially Apert syndrome.

Transforming Growth Factors

The TGFs are extracellular signaling molecules that play widespread roles in regulating development in both invertebrates and vertebrates. TGF-α and TGF-β contribute to facial development, especially palate formation.

TGFA Gene. The *TGFA* gene encodes a 160–amino acid transmembrane glycoprotein called TGF-α (Derynck et al., 1984). It interacts with the EGF receptor (EGFR) and elicits downstream responses during cell-to-cell interaction (Brachmann et al., 1989). Biological relevance for *TGFA* as a candidate gene for oral clefting is supported by its expression pattern in palatal tissues, especially in the midline seam and subjacent mesenchyme of the palatal shelves at the time of shelf fusion (Dixon et al., 1991). Interestingly, however, *Tgfa* gene knockout mice have failed to demonstrate a cleft phenotype (Luetteke et al., 1993).

Some human population-based studies have yielded a positive association between *TGFA* and CL with or without CP (CL/P). Ardinger et al. (1989) first reported evidence that specific alleles of *TGFA* are associated with nonsyndromic CL/P. Subsequent results supported this association in independent Caucasian populations: Australian (Chenevix-Trench et al., 1992), British (Holder et al., 1992), French (Stoll et al., 1992), and another U.S. population, in Pennsylvania (Sassani et al., 1993). Another study, on a Chilean Caucasoid–Mongoloid population, demonstrated an association between *TGFA* and nonsyndromic CL/P (Jara et al., 1995). Conversely, two studies involving a population from the Philippines and a U.S. Caucasian population failed to replicate the earlier findings (Lidral et al., 1997, 1998).

Rather than being a necessary and sufficient determinant on its own, it has been postulated that *TGFA* acts as a modifier gene (Stoll et al., 1992; Jara et al., 1995; Murray, 1995). Nevertheless, meta-analyses of *TGFA* continue to provide strong support for a possible role in cleft etiology. Machida et al. (1999) utilized single-strand conformational polymorphism analysis to search for causal *TGFA* mutations in the coding sequence, splice junctions, and a portion of the 3′ untranslated region in 250 individuals with nonsyndromic CL/P or nonsyndromic CP. Several novel sequence substitutions were identified. Five variants were found in conserved regions of the gene and may represent rare causes of clefting in individuals.

TGF-β Superfamily. The TGF-β superfamily of polypeptides performs a wide range of regulatory functions. Members include the TGF-β family (TGF-β1, TGF-β2, TGF-β3, TGF-β4, and TGF-β5) and the more distantly related bone morphogenetic proteins, growth and differentiation factors, and the activin/inhibin family.

TGFB genes. Members of the TGF-β family, which are encoded by the *TGFB* genes, display a remarkable spectrum of effects on patterning, epithelial–mesenchymal interactions, cellular proliferation, apoptosis, and chondrogenesis during development (Kingsley, 1994). The mature and active form of TGF-β contains 110 to 140 amino acids, derived from the C-terminal region of the TGF-β precursor protein through a proteolytic process. This precursor contains an N-terminal signal peptide followed by a prodomain containing 50 to 375 amino acids and a C-terminal region. The mature domain contains six cysteine residues, which form three intrachain disulfide bonds. Each monomer has an additional N-terminal cysteine, which can form an interchain disulfide bond to generate a population of either homodimers or heterodimers, thus indirectly increasing the functional diversity of these proteins.

Tgf-β1, Tgf-β2, and Tgf-β3 are expressed in early embryogenesis and are associated later with some regions of skeletal development (Pelton et al., 1989, 1991; Millan et al., 1991). Expression of each Tgf-β is temporally and spatially regulated in the developing palate, suggesting an important role for these isoforms in this process (Fitzpatrick et al., 1990). Brunet et al. (1995) showed that depletion of Tgf-β3 using either antisense oligonucleotides or neutralizing antibodies prevents in vitro palatal fusion. In contrast, inhibition of Tgf-β1 and Tgf-β2 activities by either strategy failed to affect palate development and fusion. Studies done on *Tgfb2*$^{-/-}$ and *Tgfb3*$^{-/-}$ mutant mice have shown that both play important roles in palatogenesis (Kaartinen et al., 1995, 1997; Proetzel et al., 1995; Sanford et al., 1997). Sanford et al. (1997) demonstrated that 23% of their *Tgfb2*$^{-/-}$ mutant mice had complete anteroposterior clefting of the secondary palate extending to the soft palate, leaving the nasal septae exposed. Histological analysis of these mutants at E18.5 revealed failure of the palatal shelves to elevate into the horizontal orientation. Kaartinen et al. (1997) also demonstrated impaired basement degradation and medial edge epithelium (MEE) transdifferentiation in all *Tgfb3*$^{-/-}$ mutant mice, resulting in CP (Fig. 3.1g–i). These studies provide strong evidence for a critical role of Tgf-β2 and Tgf-β3 in the molecular control of palatal fusion.

That the *TGFB3* gene is involved in human oral clefting is supported by the findings in an Iowa case-control study, showing an association between polymorphic markers in *TGFB3* and CP (Lidral et al., 1998).

Activins, follistatin, and receptors. Activins are dimeric glycoproteins that are widely expressed during rodent development (Feijen et al., 1994; Roberts and Barth, 1994; Phillips, 2000). The first of these proteins was originally purified from ovarian follicular fluid and shown to stimulate release of follicle-stimulating hormone from the pituitary. Various other nonreproductive functions have since been attributed to the activins, such as in mesodermal and neuronal induction and in erythroid differentiation (reviewed in Phillips, 2000). The two best studied activin subunits, βA and βB, are encoded by the *INHBA* and *INHBB* genes, respectively. Activin A and activin B consist of homodimers of βA and βB, respectively, while activin AB is a heterodimer of βA and βB. Activins interact with binding proteins such as follistatin and initiate intracellular signaling by binding to serine/threonine kinase receptors, types I and II (reviewed in Phillips, 2000). The type II activin receptors (Acvr2 and Acvr2b) are constitutively active kinases. Upon binding activin, they associate with and phosphorylate a type I activin receptor (Acvr1 or Acvr1b), which then initiates intracellular signaling.

The expression patterns of the activin βA and βB subunits in the developing mouse embryo overlap but differ considerably (Feijen et al., 1994). At E10.5 to 12.5, EβA (but not βB) mRNA is abundant in mesenchymal tissues such as the developing face, body wall, heart, and precartilaginous limb condensations. The sites of type II activin receptor expression also overlap with or are adjacent to the sites of activin β subunit expression, but there are some differences between Acvr2 and Acvr2b. For example, only Acvr2 is expressed in the whisker follicles and the mandibular component of the first branchial arch.

Targeted disruption of the *Inhbb* gene, which encodes the activin βB subunit, causes defective (open) eyelids in otherwise viable homozygous mutant mice; however, females are unable to rear offspring normally (Vassalli et al., 1994). This is in contrast to mice homozygous for targeted disruption of the *Inhba* gene, which encodes the activin βA subunit. *Inhba*$^{-/-}$ mutant mice lack whiskers and incisors; have a secondary defect in the alveolar ridge of the mandible, the site of formation of the lower molars; and die within 24 h (Matzuk et al., 1995a). Significantly, approximately one-third of these mice had clefting of the secondary palate. Of the mice that did not show clefting, detailed examination revealed that one-third lacked a hard palate, while the remainder had incomplete hard palate development.

Acvr2 gene knockout mice also exhibit variable craniofacial defects (Matzuk et al., 1995b). Approximately one-fifth of *Acvr2*[-/-] mutant mice had variable mandibular hypoplasia (micrognathia) and secondary defects including CP, absence of incisors, defects in Meckel's cartilage, and open eyelids.

Matzuk et al. (1995c) also created follistatin (Fst)-deficient mice and reported that *Fst*[-/-] mutant mice were growth-retarded, had shiny skin, and died within hours of delivery. A majority of the mice either had delayed incisor development or lacked incisors altogether. Clefting of the secondary palate was observed in 6% of the null mice, while 21% (hybrid background) and 55% (inbred background) lacked a hard palate.

The incomplete penetrance of the CP phenotype in *Inhba* and *Fst* gene knockout mice is reminiscent of the complex nature of human nonsyndromic oral clefting. The malformations seen in *Acvr2* gene knockout mice, however, appear to mimic the human condition Pierre Robin syndrome, which involves defects in the development of the first branchial arch.

Platelet-Derived Growth Factors and Receptors

The PDGFs are a family of homo- and heterodimers of disulfide-bonded α- and β-polypeptide chains. The mature forms of α and β chains of PDGF are ~100 amino acids long and show ~60% amino acid sequence identity (reviewed in Heldin and Westermark, 1999). The PDGF isoforms bind to two receptors, PDGFR-α and PDGFR-β. The first has high affinity for both α and β chains of PDGF, whereas the second binds only to the β chain with high affinity. Hence, PDGF-αα can induce PDGFR-αα homodimers only, PDGF-ββ can induce all 3 dimeric combinations of α and β receptors, and PDGF-αβ can induce both PDGFR-αα homodimers and PDGFR-αβ heterodimers. Aside from their regulatory roles in central nervous and vascular system development, in the maintenance of tissue homeostasis, and in wound healing (reviewed in Heldin and Westermark, 1999), PDGFs and PDGFRs may play an important role in palate development, particularly in regulating palatal midline epithelial seam formation and degradation.

The Pdgfs and Pdgfrs are differentially expressed during development of the embryonic mouse secondary palate. For example, Pdgfr-αα is normally present during palate formation, while Pdgfr-ββ is sparse or absent (Qiu and Ferguson, 1995). Furthermore, Pdgf-α is expressed in the mandibular arch of E10.5 embryos, while Pdgfr-αα is expressed in the surface ectoderm underlying branchial arch mesenchyme (Orr-Urtreger and Lonai, 1992). The expression patterns of these genes change temporally during palatal shelf elevation and midline epithelial seam formation and degradation. At E13, before elevation of the palatal shelf, Pdgfr-αα is

expressed in the palatal mesenchyme and MEE, while only low-level expression of Pdgf-αα is detected in the palatal epithelia. During palatal midline epithelial seam formation and degradation throughout E14, intensive co-localization of Pdgf-αα and its receptor in the nasal and midline seam epithelia is observed (Qiu and Ferguson, 1995).

Homozygous knockout of the *Pdgfra* gene causes some midline defects and under-development of the face, with absence of some facial bones (Soriano, 1997). The phenotype was similar to that observed in the recessive mouse mutant *Patch* (*Ph*), which involves a deletion encompassing the *Pdgfra* gene (Morrison-Graham et al., 1992). In both mutants, neuronal derivatives of the neural crest were unaffected, suggesting that Pdgf-α affects survival of the subset of neural crest cells giving rise to nonneuronal derivatives.

Epidermal Growth Factors and Receptor

The EGF family consists of several different members, including EGF, heparin-binding EGF-like factor, amphiregulin, epiregulin, betacellulin, the neuregulins, and the neuregulin-2s (reviewed in Riese and Stern, 1998). Most of the precursor proteins are membrane-bound and can be proteolytically cleaved into soluble forms or remain as membrane-anchored hormones in signaling. They share a domain of homology of approximately 50 amino acids and together with the EGFR regulate proliferation and differentiation of various tissue types, including the palate.

Egfr gene knockout mice exhibit facial mediolateral defects such as narrow and elongated snouts, underdeveloped lower jaws, and CP (Miettinen et al., 1999) (Fig. 3.1j–l). Interestingly, palatal shelf tissues extracted from *Egfr*[-/-] mutant mice are capable of fusing but with residual epithelium in the midline frequently observed. Cultured mandibular cells from these mice exhibit diminished morphogenesis of Meckel's cartilage. Secretion of matrix metalloproteinases (MMPs) was also diminished in palatal shelf tissues of *Egfr*[-/-] mutant mice. Usually, Egf is able to increase MMP secretion; absence of Egfr prevents Egf ligand binding and downstream signal transduction, leading to decreased MMP expression. Hence, Egf/Egfr signaling is necessary for normal craniofacial development, and downstream effectors such as the MMPs mediate this role indirectly.

To further understand the respective roles of these growth factors during facial development, especially in the area of palatogenesis, functional studies are needed to determine how members of these growth factor families control the outgrowth and patterning via the different signal-transduction pathways.

SIGNALING MOLECULES

Signaling molecules are specific substances synthesized and released by signaling cells. They produce a specific response only in the target cells that have receptors for them. Endothelins, jagged proteins, and thrombospondins are some of the signaling molecules involved in normal facial development.

Endothelins and Receptors

Endothelins (ETs) were initially identified as vasoconstrictor proteins secreted by vascular endothelial cells (Yanagisawa et al., 1988). They consist of three closely related 21–amino acid polypeptides (ET1, ET2, ET3) that are capable of binding one or both ET receptors, ET_A and ET_B (Inoue et al., 1989; Arai et al., 1990; Sakurai et al., 1990). Both receptors belong to the seven-transmembrane, G protein–coupled receptor family. At physiological concentrations, only ET1 and ET2 can bind to ET_A but all three ET isoforms are able to bind to ET_B.

The ETs are first synthesized as preproendothelins of approximately 200 amino acid residues, which are then processed by a furin-like protease into biologically inactive intermediates called big ETs (Yanagisawa et al., 1998). A further cleavage at the common Trp^{21} residue by highly specific ET-converting enzymes (ECEs) yields the mature ET. Two isozymes of ECE (ECE1 and ECE2) are known, both belonging to the type II membrane-bound metalloprotease family (Xu et al., 1994; Emoto and Yanagisawa, 1995).

Recent gene knockout studies have revealed unexpected and interesting roles for Et isopeptides and their receptors. For example, mice homozygous for a null mutation of the Et_A gene demonstrate craniofacial and cardiovascular abnormalities similar to those associated with the CATCH-22 (cardiac defects, abnormal facies, thymic hypoplasia, cleft palate, hypocalcemia, associated with chromosome 22 microdeletion) syndrome (Clouthier et al., 1998). In contrast, mutant mice deficient in Et3 or Et_B gene product show developmental abnormalities of other neural crest derivatives, including melanocytes and enteric neurons, giving rise to coat-color spotting and aganglionic megacolon reminiscent of Hirschsprung disease in humans (Baynash et al., 1994; Hosoda et al., 1994). These observations suggest that two distinct Et signaling pathways likely contribute to the development of different neural crest lineages and that only some of the Et isopeptides and their receptors are essential for craniofacial development.

Endothelin 1 is expressed mainly in the epithelium of the pharyngeal arches, endothelium of the aortic arch artery, and cardiac outflow tracts; homozygous disruption of this gene results in malformations of pharyngeal arch–derived craniofacial structures, including a nonfused mandible (Kurihara et al., 1994, 1995). The zebrafish craniofacial mutant *sucker* was also shown to be caused by a mutation in the *et1* gene (Miller et al., 2000). The exact role of Et1 in neural crest development is unclear. However, one novel basic helix-loop-helix transcriptional factor, dHAND, has been shown to interact with Et1 in controlling neural crest branchial arch formation in mice (Thomas et al., 1998). Expression of dHAND is limited to the mesenchyme of the distal branchial arches, just beneath the Et1-expressing epithelium. In *dHAND* null mutant mice, lack of expression of dHAND in branchial and aortic arches results in the branchial arches becoming hypoplastic at

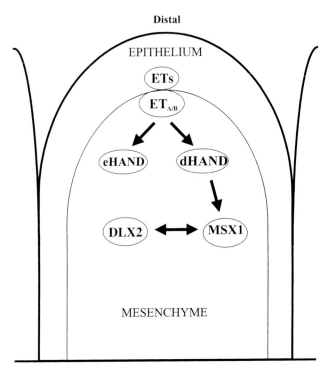

FIG. 3.2. Endothelin–HAND–MSX pathway: proposed model for regulation of branchial arch outgrowth. Endothelins (ETs) are secreted from the epithelial layer of the branchial arch into the mesenchyme. They bind to receptors ($ET_{A/B}$), which are expressed in mesenchymal and surrounding endothelial cells. This binding upregulates the expression of two basic helix-loop-helix transcription factors, dHAND and eHAND, in the distal mesenchyme. In turn dHAND upregulates expression of the homeobox protein MSX1 also in the distal mesenchyme. MSX1 interacts with another homeobox protein, DLX, and they regulate each other in an antagonistic manner. An appropriate balance between MSX1 and DLX is probably crucial in maintaining normal cell proliferation, differentiation, and death in the branchial arch, which is essential for formation of the secondary palate.

as early as E9.5, apparently secondary to the programmed cell death of the mesenchyme. Furthermore, Msx1 expression is undetectable in $dHAND^{-/-}$ mutant mice.

These data suggest a potential molecular model for the regulation of branchial arch outgrowth. In this model, Et1 is secreted from the branchial arch epithelium into the mesenchyme, while its receptor, Et_A, is expressed in mesenchymal cells and surrounding endothelial cells (Fig. 3.2). Intracellular signaling is initiated by the binding of secreted Et1 to activated Et_A receptor, which enhances the expression of dHAND in the mesenchyme. In turn, dHAND upregulates expression of Msx1 in the distal branchial arch (Thomas et al., 1998). An appropriate balance between Msx1 and its modulator Dlx2 in the distal branchial arch may be crucial for normal proliferation, differentiation, and cell death in the branchial arch, processes necessary for formation of a continuous mesenchyme in the secondary palate.

Jagged Molecules and Notch Receptors

The Notch family of receptors are important signaling molecules regulating cell fate during development. They are membrane-bound and have a large extracellular domain containing multiple tandemly arranged EGF-like repeats (Rebay et al., 1991). Jagged1 and Jagged2 (also known as Serrate1 and Serrate2) are transmembrane ligands for the Notch receptors (reviewed in Artavanis-Tsakonas et al., 1995; Robey, 1997; Francis-West et al., 1998). Their extracellular domains also contain multiple EGF-like motifs as well as a conserved motif called the DSL (delta, serrate, lag-2) domain. The DSL domain is required for interaction with their receptors.

Binding of Jagged1 and Jagged2 to the Notch receptors elicits a series of intracellular processes involving receptor proteolysis and interactions with several novel cytoplasmic and nuclear proteins (Artavanis-Tsakonas et al., 1995; Kopan et al., 1996). The Notch intercellular signaling pathway is evolutionarily conserved. It is essential for proper cell-fate specification and embryonic development in a diverse group of organisms (reviewed in Artavanis-Tsakonas et al., 1995; Gridley, 1997; Robey, 1997). In humans, mutations in the *Notch* genes have been implicated in cancer and an inherited condition causing stroke and dementia (Ellisen et al., 1991; Joutel et al., 1996).

In contrast, Jagged1 and Jagged2 proteins play a role in craniofacial and limb development. In mice, Jagged1 is expressed in both developing maxillary and mandibular primordia (Mitsiadis et al., 1997), while Jagged2 is expressed in the first to third branchial arches and the developing limb (Valsecchi et al., 1997). Haploinsuffi-

ciency of the *JAG1* gene in humans causes Alagille syndrome (Alagille et al., 1987; Li et al., 1997; Oda et al., 1997). This syndrome is characterized by a broad forehead, deep-set eyes, malformed ears, long straight nose, and pointed mandible. Some cases of Alagille syndrome result from truncation of the Jagged1 protein, which acts in a dominant-negative fashion during craniofacial development. A single–amino acid change in the Jagged2 protein is thought to be responsible for the mouse *syndactylism* (*sm*) mutant, in which the digits of the feet are fused (Sidow et al., 1997). In contrast, targeted deletion of the *Jag2* exons encoding the DSL domain results in craniofacial defects and perinatal lethality in mice (Jiang et al., 1998). $Jag2^{-/-}$ mutant mice have CP mainly due to failure of the palatal shelves to elevate and fuse. In addition, these mutant mice exhibit syndactyly of the fore- and hindlimbs. The limb defects are more severe than those seen in *sm* mutants. These studies suggest that Notch signaling mediated by Jagged2 plays an essential role during limb and craniofacial development in mice and that *sm* is a hypomorphic allele of the *Jag2* gene.

Thrombospondins

Thrombospondins (TSPs) are a family of multifunctional, extracellular matrix glycoproteins secreted by a variety of cells and consisting of five members (TSP1, TSP2, TSP3, TSP4, and COMP/TSP5) encoded by distinct genes (reviewed in Bornstein, 1992; Vacca et al., 1999). The first, TSP1, is a homotrimeric multidomain glycoprotein. Each monomer contains an amino-terminal heparin binding domain, followed by a procollagen homology domain, three TSP (properidin-like) repeats, three EGF-like repeats, seven Ca^{2+}-binding repeats, and a carboxy-terminal cell attachment domain (Bornstein and Sage, 1994). The TSPs have an affinity for cell surfaces and extracellular matrix macromolecules such as fibronectin, laminin, heparan sulfate proteoglycans, plasminogen, collagens, and histidine-rich glycoproteins (Lawler, 1986; Frazier, 1987). For example, TSP1 is involved in platelet aggregation, inflammation, and inhibition of angiogenesis, as well as cell adhesion, migration, growth, and differentiation (Bornstein and Sage, 1994).

As discussed in an earlier section, the TGF-β family is one of the numerous growth factor families involved in modulating mesenchymal proliferation of the palatal shelves. There are several pathways available for activating the TGF-βs, one of which utilizes TSPs. Expression of TSPs is prominent in head mesenchyme, including the palate. Tsp1 and Tsp2 are expressed in different but overlapping regions of cartilage and bone mesenchyme (Tooney et al., 1998; Melnick et al.,

2000). Tsp1 activates latent Tgf-β1, while Tsp2 functions as an antagonist to the function of Tsp1 by competitively binding latent Tgf-β and not activating it (Crawford et al., 1998; Melnick et al., 2000).

Although the precise roles of Tsp1 and Tsp2 in embryogenesis are poorly understood, studies based on their transcript expression and protein localization shed some light on their functions during palatogenesis. High expression of Tsp1, Tsp2, and Tgf-β mRNAs and high protein quantities are localized throughout the extracellular matrix of the palatal mesenchyme (Melnick et al., 2000). At the vertical palatal shelf stage of palatogenesis, Tsp2 protein is found throughout the extracellular matrix of the shelf mesenchyme. By the horizontal palatal shelf stage, Tsp2 protein is far less evident in the palatal shelf proper. It is principally localized in the ossification centers of the maxilla, including the palate. This is consistent with its previously purported role in craniofacial morphogenesis (Tooney et al., 1998). However, in *Thbs2* (*Tsp2*) null mutant mice, CP or other craniofacial anomalies are absent (Kyriakides et al., 1998), suggesting that Tsp2 may not be an essential participant in palatogenesis.

γ-Aminobutyric Acid and Receptors

γ-Aminobutyric acid (GABA) is a major inhibitory neurotransmitter with many critical functions as an intercellular signaling molecule in the nervous system and in a number of nonneuronal cell types (reviewed in Erdo and Wolff, 1990; Chebib and Johnston, 1999). In the GABA-utilizing neurons of the central nervous system, it is synthesized from glutamic acid by glutamic acid decarboxylase (GAD). Outside of the central nervous system, GABA is synthesized by a number of cell types, including pancreatic β cells. It binds to GABA receptors, namely GABA$_A$, GABA$_B$, and GABA$_C$. Both GABA$_A$ and GABA$_C$ belong to a superfamily of transmitter-gated ion channels that includes nicotinic acetylcholine, strychnine-sensitive glycine, and 5-hydroxytryptamine 3 receptors. The GABA$_A$ receptors are heterooligomeric Cl$^-$ channels that can be selectively blocked by the alkaloid bicuculline and modulated by steroids, barbiturates, and benzodiazepines. In contrast, GABA$_C$ receptors represent a relatively simple form of Cl$^-$ channel made up of a single type of protein subunit. The GABA$_B$ receptors are heterooligomeric receptors coupled to G proteins and can activate second-messenger systems and Ca^{2+} and K$^+$ ion channels upon binding GABA (Chebib and Johnston, 1999).

Cell culture studies have demonstrated that GABA is capable of promoting the survival, differentiation, and migration of embryonic neurons (Barbin et al., 1993; Liu et al., 1997). These observations suggest a role for GABA and its receptors in normal embryonic and fetal development. In addition, both genetic and teratological studies have suggested that GABA signaling may be involved in normal craniofacial development, including palate formation (Zimmerman and Wee, 1984; Culiat et al., 1993, 1995; Homanics et al., 1997). Teratological studies have shown that drugs such as diazepam, which can potentiate GABA action, are capable of inducing CP formation during a critical phase of mouse palate development (Miller and Becker, 1975; Wee and Zimmerman, 1983). However, the CP phenotype is observed only at high drug doses, suggesting that the effect may be nonspecific. Nonetheless, mice lacking the GABA$_A$ receptor β3 subunit (Gabrβ3) show clefting of the secondary palate (Culiat et al., 1993, 1995; Homanics et al., 1997). Furthermore, mice deficient in Gad67, one of two GAD enzymes in mice, show a similar phenotype (Condie et al., 1997), clearly demonstrating a role for GABA signaling in normal palatogenesis.

RYK

The *RYK* (related to tyrosine kinases) gene encodes a catalytically inactive member of the receptor protein tyrosine kinase (RTK) family (Hovens et al., 1992; Halford et al., 1999; Katso et al., 1999). The RTKs typically are transmembrane signal-transduction glycoproteins with an extracellular N-terminal ligand binding domain and an intracellular C-terminal tyrosine kinase domain (reviewed in van der Geer et al., 1994). They regulate diverse cellular functions, among them mitogenesis, differentiation, and morphogenesis. Because of its inability to undergo autophosphorylation or to phosphorylate substrates, RYK is unique within the RTK family. Despite this, it is able to activate downstream signaling pathways (Katso et al., 1999, and references therein).

In a study by Halford et al. (2000), most mice homozygous for targeted disruption of the *Ryk* gene failed to survive more than 24 h. In addition to some limb abnormalities, these mice have a slightly smaller and more rounded cranial vault, reflecting minor changes in size and shape of individual calvarial elements. They have a shorter snout due to shortened nasal bones, a flattened midface due to premaxillary/maxillary hypoplasia, and a reduced mandible. In addition, over 88% of the mice presented with a completely cleft secondary palate. These results indicate that Ryk is essential for normal development of craniofacial structures, including the secondary palate. These authors also provide biochemical evidence to suggest that Ryk activates downstream signaling via interaction with other members of different RTK subfamilies.

FUTURE PERSPECTIVES

The preceding list of candidate genes for lip and palate development is by no means exhaustive and underscores the concept that CL and CP are a complex, multifactorial group of disorders. The interactions of multiple genes and their polymorphisms might explain the observed variations in normal and abnormal lip and palate development. Several of these genes have been extensively characterized with respect to their roles in lip and palate development. However, evidence for the role of the other genes in lip and palate pattern formation is less conclusive, and our current understanding of the genetic factors controlling these processes remains rudimentary.

Completion of the sequencing phase of the Human Genome Project and transition to the functional genomics phase holds the promise of unraveling the complex inter- and intracellular signaling pathways controlling this developmental process. Continued utilization of targeted mutagenesis in the mouse and application of random mutagenesis methods in the mouse and other vertebrate model systems, such as the zebrafish, should accelerate the pace of gene discovery and functional analyses.

Work on this chapter was sponsored in part by National Institutes of Health grants DE 13078, DE 13939 (E. W. J.), and DE 13707 (S. S. C. and E. W. J.) and by Johns Hopkins Singapore (S. S. C., F. S. H. C., and E. W. J.).

REFERENCES

Agulnick, AD, Taira, M, Breen, JJ, et al. (1996). Interactions of the LIM-domain–binding factor Ldb1 with LIM homeodomain proteins. Nature 384: 270–272.

Alagille, D, Estrada, A, Hadchouel, M, et al. (1987). Syndromic paucity of interlobular bile ducts (Alagille syndrome or arteriohepatic dysplasia): review of 80 cases. J Pediatr 110: 195–200.

Arai, H, Hori, S, Aramori, I, et al. (1990). Cloning and expression of a cDNA encoding an endothelin receptor. Nature 348: 730–732.

Ardinger, HH, Buetow, KH, Bell, GI, et al. (1989). Association of genetic variation of the transforming growth factor-alpha gene with cleft lip and palate. Am J Hum Genet 45: 348–353.

Artavanis-Tsakonas, S, Matsuno, K, Fortini, ME (1995). Notch signaling. Science 268: 225–232.

Bach, I, Carriere, C, Ostendorff, HP, et al. (1997). A family of LIM domain–associated cofactors confer transcriptional synergism between LIM and Otx homeodomain proteins. Genes Dev 11: 1370–1380.

Barbin, G, Pollard, H, Gaiarsa, JL, Ben-Ari, Y (1993). Involvement of GABAA receptors in the outgrowth of cultured hippocampal neurons. Neurosci Lett 152: 150–154.

Basilico, C, Moscatelli, D (1992). The FGF family of growth factors and oncogenes. Adv Cancer Res 59: 115–165.

Baynash, AG, Hosoda, K, Giaid, A, et al. (1994). Interaction of endothelin-3 with endothelin-B receptor is essential for development of epidermal melanocytes and enteric neurons. Cell 79: 1277–1285.

Beiraghi, S, Foroud, T, Diouhy, S, et al. (1994). Possible localization of a major gene for cleft lip and palate to 4q. Clin Genet 46: 255–256.

Blum, M, Gaunt, SJ, Cho, KW, et al. (1992). Gastrulation in the mouse: the role of the homeobox gene goosecoid. Cell 69: 1097–1106.

Blumberg, B, Wright, CV, De Robertis, EM, Cho, KW (1991). Organizer-specific homeobox genes in Xenopus laevis embryos. Science 253: 194–196.

Bornstein, P (1992). Thrombospondins: structure and regulation of expression [published erratum appears in FASEB J (1993) 7: 237]. FASEB J 6: 3290–3299.

Bornstein, P, Sage, EH (1994). Thrombospondins. Methods Enzymol 245: 62–85.

Brachmann, R, Lindquist, PB, Nagashima, M, et al. (1989). Transmembrane TGF-α precursors activate EGF/TGF-α receptors. Cell 56: 691–700.

Breen, JJ, Agulnick, AD, Westphal, H, Dawid, IB (1998). Interactions between LIM domains and the LIM domain–binding protein Ldb1. J Biol Chem 273: 4712–4717.

Brunet, CL, Sharpe, PM, Ferguson, MW (1995). Inhibition of TGF-β3 (but not TGF-β1 or TGF-β2) activity prevents normal mouse embryonic palate fusion. Int J Dev Biol 39: 345–355.

Catron, KM, Wang, H, Hu, G, et al. (1996). Comparison of MSX-1 and MSX-2 suggests a molecular basis for functional redundancy [published erratum appears in Mech Dev (1996) 56: 223]. Mech Dev 55: 185–199.

Catron, KM, Zhang, H, Marshall, SC, et al. (1995). Transcriptional repression by Msx-1 does not require homeodomain DNA-binding sites. Mol Cell Biol 15: 861–871.

Celli, G, LaRochelle, WJ, Mackem, S, et al. (1998). Soluble dominant-negative receptor uncovers essential roles for fibroblast growth factors in multi-organ induction and patterning. EMBO J 17: 1642–1655.

Chebib, M, Johnston, GA (1999). The "ABC" of GABA receptors: a brief review. Clin Exp Pharmacol Physiol 26: 937–940.

Chenevix-Trench, G, Jones, K, Green, AC, et al. (1992). Cleft lip with or without cleft palate: associations with transforming growth factor alpha and retinoic acid receptor loci. Am J Hum Genet 51: 1377–1385.

Cho, KW, Blumberg, B, Steinbeisser, H, De Robertis, EM (1991). Molecular nature of Spemann's organizer: the role of the Xenopus homeobox gene goosecoid. Cell 67: 1111–1120.

Clouthier, DE, Hosoda, K, Richardson, JA, et al. (1998). Cranial and cardiac neural crest defects in endothelin-A receptor-deficient mice. Development 125: 813–824.

Cohen, B, McGuffin, ME, Pfeifle, C, et al. (1992). apterous, a gene required for imaginal disc development in Drosophila encodes a member of the LIM family of developmental regulatory proteins. Genes Dev 6: 715–729.

Colvin, JS, Feldman, B, Nadeau, JH, et al. (1999). Genomic organization and embryonic expression of the mouse fibroblast growth factor 9 gene. Dev Dyn 216: 72–88.

Condie, BG, Bain, G, Gottlieb, DI, Capecchi, MR (1997). Cleft palate in mice with a targeted mutation in the γ-aminobutyric acid–producing enzyme glutamic acid decarboxylase 67. Proc Natl Acad Sci USA 94: 11451–11455.

Crawford, SE, Stellmach, V, Murphy-Ullrich, JE, et al. (1998). Thrombospondin-1 is a major activator of TGF-β1 in vivo. Cell 93: 1159–1170.

Crossley, PH, Martin, GR (1995). The mouse Fgf8 gene encodes a family of polypeptides and is expressed in regions that direct outgrowth and patterning in the developing embryo. Development 121: 439–451.

Culiat, CT, Stubbs, L, Nicholls, RD, et al. (1993). Concordance between isolated cleft palate in mice and alterations within a region including the gene encoding the β3 subunit of the type A γ-aminobutyric acid receptor. Proc Natl Acad Sci USA 90: 5105–5109.

Culiat, CT, Stubbs, LJ, Woychik, RP, et al. (1995). Deficiency of the β3 subunit of the type A γ-aminobutyric acid receptor causes cleft palate in mice. Nat Genet 11: 344–346.

Davideau, JL, Demri, P, Gu, TT, et al. (1999). Expression of DLX5 during human embryonic craniofacial development. Mech Dev 81: 183–186.

Dawid, IB, Toyama, R, Taira, M (1995). LIM domain proteins. C R Acad Sci III 318: 295–306.

Derynck, R, Roberts, AB, Winkler, ME, et al. (1984). Human transforming growth factor-alpha: precursor structure and expression in E. coli. Cell 38: 287–297.

Dixon, MJ, Garner, J, Ferguson, MW (1991). Immunolocalization of epidermal growth factor (EGF), EGF receptor and transforming growth factor alpha (TGF-α) during murine palatogenesis in vivo and in vitro. Anat Embryol 184: 83–91.

Dolle, P, Price, M, Duboule, D (1992). Expression of the murine Dlx-1 homeobox gene during facial, ocular and limb development. Differentiation 49: 93–99.

Drucker, BJ, Goldfarb, M (1993). Murine FGF-4 gene expression is spatially restricted within embryonic skeletal muscle and other tissues. Mech Dev 40: 155–163.

Ellisen, LW, Bird, J, West, DC, et al. (1991). TAN-1, the human homolog of the Drosophila notch gene, is broken by chromosomal translocations in T lymphoblastic neoplasms. Cell 66: 649–661.

Emoto, N, Yanagisawa, M (1995). Endothelin-converting enzyme-2 is a membrane-bound, phosphoramidon-sensitive metalloprotease with acidic pH optimum. J Biol Chem 270: 15262–15268.

Erdo, SL, Wolff, JR (1990). γ-Aminobutyric acid outside the mammalian brain. J Neurochem 54: 363–372.

Feijen, A, Goumans, MJ, van den Eijnden-van Raaij, AJ (1994). Expression of activin subunits, activin receptors and follistatin in postimplantation mouse embryos suggests specific developmental functions for different activins. Development 120: 3621–3637.

Ferguson, MW (1988). Palate development. Development 103: 41–60.

Feuerstein, R, Wang, X, Song, D, et al. (1994). The LIM/double zinc-finger motif functions as a protein dimerization domain. Proc Natl Acad Sci USA 91: 10655–10659.

Fitzpatrick, DR, Denhez, F, Kondaiah, P, Akhurst, RJ (1990). Differential expression of TGF-β isoforms in murine palatogenesis. Development 109: 585–595.

Francis-West, P, Ladher, R, Barlow, A, Graveson, A (1998). Signalling interactions during facial development. Mech Dev 75: 3–28.

Frazier, WA (1987). Thrombospondin: a modular adhesive glycoprotein of platelets and nucleated cells. J Cell Biol 105: 625–632.

Freyd, G, Kim, SK, Horvitz, HR (1990). Novel cysteine-rich motif and homeodomain in the product of the Caenorhabditis elegans cell lineage gene lin-11. Nature 344: 876–879.

Gaunt, SJ, Blum, M, De Robertis, EM (1993). Expression of the mouse goosecoid gene during mid-embryogenesis may mark mesenchymal cell lineages in the developing head, limbs and body wall. Development 117: 769–778.

Goriely, A, Stella, M, Coffinier, C, et al. (1996). A functional homologue of goosecoid in Drosophila. Development 122: 1641–1650.

Gridley, T (1997). Notch signaling in vertebrate development and disease. Mol Cell Neurosci 9: 103–108.

Grigoriou, M, Tucker, AS, Sharpe, PT, Pachnis, V (1998). Expression and regulation of Lhx6 and Lhx7, a novel subfamily of LIM homeodomain encoding genes, suggests a role in mammalian head development. Development 125: 2063–2074.

Halford, MM, Armes, J, Buchert, M, et al. (2000). Ryk-deficient mice exhibit craniofacial defects associated with perturbed Eph receptor crosstalk. Nat Genet 25: 414–418.

Halford, MM, Oates, AC, Hibbs, ML, et al. (1999). Genomic structure and expression of the mouse growth factor receptor related to tyrosine kinases (Ryk). J Biol Chem 274: 7379–7390.

Heldin, CH, Westermark, B (1999). Mechanism of action and in vivo role of platelet-derived growth factor. Physiol Rev 79: 1283–1316.

Hill, RE, Jones, PF, Rees, AR, et al. (1989). A new family of mouse homeo box-containing genes: molecular structure, chromosomal location, and developmental expression of Hox-7.1. Genes Dev 3: 26–37.

Holder, SE, Vintiner, GM, Farren, B, et al. (1992). Confirmation of an association between RFLPs at the transforming growth factor-alpha locus and non-syndromic cleft lip and palate. J Med Genet 29: 390–392.

Holland, PW (1991). Cloning and evolutionary analysis of msh-like homeobox genes from mouse, zebrafish and ascidian. Gene 98: 253–257.

Homanics, GE, DeLorey, TM, Firestone, LL, et al. (1997). Mice devoid of γ-aminobutyrate type A receptor β3 subunit have epilepsy, cleft palate, and hypersensitive behavior. Proc Natl Acad Sci USA 94: 4143–4148.

Hosoda, K, Hammer, RE, Richardson, JA, et al. (1994). Targeted and natural (piebald-lethal) mutations of endothelin-B receptor gene produce megacolon associated with spotted coat color in mice. Cell 79: 1267–1276.

Hovens, CM, Stacker, SA, Andres, AC, et al. (1992). RYK, a receptor tyrosine kinase–related molecule with unusual kinase domain motifs. Proc Natl Acad Sci USA 89: 11818–11822.

Inoue, A, Yanagisawa, M, Kimura, S, et al. (1989). The human endothelin family: three structurally and pharmacologically distinct isopeptides predicted by three separate genes. Proc Natl Acad Sci USA 86: 2863–2867.

Jabs, EW, Muller, U, Li, X, et al. (1993). A mutation in the homeodomain of the human MSX2 gene in a family affected with autosomal dominant craniosynostosis. Cell 75: 443–450.

Jara, L, Blanco, R, Chiffelle, I, et al. (1995). Evidence for an association between RFLPs at the transforming growth factor alpha (locus) and nonsyndromic cleft lip/palate in a South American population. Am J Hum Genet 56: 339–341.

Jiang, R, Lan, Y, Chapman, HD, et al. (1998). Defects in limb, craniofacial, and thymic development in Jagged2 mutant mice. Genes Dev 12: 1046–1057.

Joutel, A, Corpechot, C, Ducros, A, et al. (1996). Notch3 mutations in CADASIL, a hereditary adult-onset condition causing stroke and dementia. Nature 383: 707–710.

Jurata, LW, Kenny, DA, Gill, GN (1996). Nuclear LIM interactor, a rhombotin and LIM homeodomain interacting protein, is expressed early in neuronal development. Proc Natl Acad Sci USA 93: 11693–11698.

Kaartinen, V, Cui, XM, Heisterkamp, N, et al. (1997). Transforming growth factor-β3 regulates transdifferentiation of medial edge epithelium during palatal fusion and associated degradation of the basement membrane. Dev Dyn 209: 255–260.

Kaartinen, V, Voncken, JW, Shuler, C, et al. (1995). Abnormal lung development and cleft palate in mice lacking TGF-β3 indicates defects of epithelial–mesenchymal interaction. Nat Genet 11: 415–421.

Katso, RM, Russell, RB, Ganesan, TS (1999). Functional analysis of H-Ryk, an atypical member of the receptor tyrosine kinase family. Mol Cell Biol 19: 6427–6440.

Kingsley, DM (1994). The TGF-β superfamily: new members, new receptors, and new genetic tests of function in different organisms. Genes Dev 8: 133–146.

Kitanaka, J, Takemura, M, Matsumoto, K, et al. (1998). Structure and chromosomal localization of a murine LIM/homeobox gene, Lhx8. Genomics 49: 307–309.

Kopan, R, Schroeter, EH, Weintraub, H, Nye, JS (1996). Signal transduction by activated mNotch: importance of proteolytic processing and its regulation by the extracellular domain. Proc Natl Acad Sci USA 93: 1683–1688.

Krumlauf, R (1993). Hox genes and pattern formation in the branchial region of the vertebrate head. Trends Genet 9: 106–112.

Kurihara, Y, Kurihara, H, Oda, H, et al. (1995). Aortic arch malformations and ventricular septal defect in mice deficient in endothelin-1. J Clin Invest 96: 293–300.

Kurihara, Y, Kurihara, H, Suzuki, H, et al. (1994). Elevated blood pressure and craniofacial abnormalities in mice deficient in endothelin-1. Nature 368: 703–710.

Kyriakides, TR, Zhu, YH, Smith, LT, et al. (1998). Mice that lack thrombospondin 2 display connective tissue abnormalities that are associated with disordered collagen fibrillogenesis, an increased vascular density, and a bleeding diathesis. J Cell Biol 140: 419–430.

Lawler, J (1986). The structural and functional properties of thrombospondin. Blood 67: 1197–1209.

Leussink, B, Brouwer, A, Khattabi, ME, et al. (1995). Expression patterns of the paired-related homeobox genes MHox/Prx1 and S8/Prx2 suggest roles in development of the heart and the forebrain. Mech Dev 52: 51–64.

Li, L, Krantz, ID, Deng, Y, et al. (1997). Alagille syndrome is caused by mutations in human Jagged1, which encodes a ligand for Notch1. Nat Genet 16: 243–251.

Lidral, AC, Murray, JC, Buetow, KH, et al. (1997). Studies of the candidate genes TGFB2, MSX1, TGFA, and TGFB3 in the etiology of cleft lip and palate in the Philippines. Cleft Palate Craniofac J 34: 1–6.

Lidral, AC, Romitti, PA, Basart, AM, et al. (1998). Association of MSX1 and TGFB3 with nonsyndromic clefting in humans. Am J Hum Genet 63: 557–568.

Liu, J, Morrow, AL, Devaud, L, et al. (1997). GABAA receptors mediate trophic effects of GABA on embryonic brainstem monoamine neurons in vitro. J Neurosci 17: 2420–2428.

Lu, MF, Cheng, HT, Kern, MJ, et al. (1999). prx-1 functions cooperatively with another paired-related homeobox gene, prx-2, to maintain cell fates within the craniofacial mesenchyme. Development 126: 495–504.

Luetteke, NC, Qiu, TH, Peiffer, RL, et al. (1993). TGF-α deficiency results in hair follicle and eye abnormalities in targeted and waved-1 mice. Cell 73: 263–278.

Ma, L, Golden, S, Wu, L, Maxson, R (1996). The molecular basis of Boston-type craniosynostosis: the Pro148 → His mutation in the N-terminal arm of the MSX2 homeodomain stabilizes DNA binding without altering nucleotide sequence preferences. Hum Mol Genet 5: 1915–1920.

Machida, J, Yoshiura, K, Funkhauser, CD, et al. (1999). Transforming growth factor-alpha (TGFA): genomic structure, boundary sequences, and mutation analysis in nonsyndromic cleft lip/palate and cleft palate only. Genomics 61: 237–242.

MacKenzie, A, Ferguson, MW, Sharpe, PT (1991a). Hox-7 expression during murine craniofacial development. Development 113: 601–611.

Mackenzie, A, Leeming, GL, Jowett, AK, et al. (1991b). The homeobox gene Hox 7.1 has specific regional and temporal expression patterns during early murine craniofacial embryogenesis, especially tooth development in vivo and in vitro. Development 111: 269–285.

Mailhos, C, Andre, S, Mollereau, B, et al. (1998). Drosophila Goosecoid requires a conserved heptapeptide for repression of paired-class homeoprotein activators. Development 125: 937–947.

Martin, JF, Bradley, A, Olson, EN (1995). The paired-like homeobox gene MHox is required for early events of skeletogenesis in multiple lineages. Genes Dev 9: 1237–1249.

Matsumoto, K, Tanaka, T, Furuyama, T, et al. (1996). L3, a novel murine LIM-homeodomain transcription factor expressed in the ventral telencephalon and the mesenchyme surrounding the oral cavity. Neurosci Lett 204: 113–116.

Matzuk, MM, Kumar, TR, Vassalli, A, et al. (1995a). Functional analysis of activins during mammalian development. Nature 374: 354–356.

Matzuk, MM, Kumar, TR, Bradley, A (1995b). Different phenotypes for mice deficient in either activins or activin receptor type II. Nature 374: 356–360.

Matzuk, MM, Lu, N, Vogel, H, et al. (1995c). Multiple defects and perinatal death in mice deficient in follistatin. Nature 374: 360–363.

Melnick, M, Chen, H, Zhou, Y, Jaskoll, T (2000). Thrombospondin-2 gene expression and protein localization during embryonic mouse palate development. Arch Oral Biol 45: 19–25.

Miettinen, PJ, Chin, JR, Shum, L, et al. (1999). Epidermal growth factor receptor function is necessary for normal craniofacial development and palate closure. Nat Genet 22: 69–73.

Millan, FA, Denhez, F, Kondaiah, P, Akhurst, RJ (1991). Embryonic gene expression patterns of TGF β1, β2 and β3 suggest different developmental functions in vivo. Development 111: 131–143.

Miller, CT, Schilling, TF, Lee, K, et al. (2000). sucker encodes a zebrafish endothelin-1 required for ventral pharyngeal arch development. Development 127: 3815–3828.

Miller, RP, Becker, BA (1975). Teratogenicity of oral diazepam and diphenylhydantoin in mice. Toxicol Appl Pharmacol 32: 53–61.

Mina, M, Gluhak, J, Upholt, WB, et al. (1995). Experimental analysis of Msx-1 and Msx-2 gene expression during chick mandibular morphogenesis. Dev Dyn 202: 195–214.

Mitchell, LE, Healey, SC, Chenevix-Trench, G (1995). Evidence for an association between nonsyndromic cleft lip with or without cleft palate and a gene located on the long arm of chromosome 4. Am J Hum Genet 57: 1130–1136.

Mitsiadis, TA, Henrique, D, Thesleff, I, Lendahl, U (1997). Mouse Serrate-1 (Jagged-1): expression in the developing tooth is regulated by epithelial–mesenchymal interactions and fibroblast growth factor-4. Development 124: 1473–1483.

Morcillo, P, Rosen, C, Baylies, MK, Dorsett, D (1997). Chip, a widely expressed chromosomal protein required for segmentation and activity of a remote wing margin enhancer in Drosophila. Genes Dev 11: 2729–2740.

Morrison-Graham, K, Schatteman, GC, Bork, T, et al. (1992). A PDGF receptor mutation in the mouse (Patch) perturbs the development of a non-neuronal subset of neural crest–derived cells. Development 115: 133–142.

Murray, JC (1995). Face facts: genes, environment, and clefts. Am J Hum Genet 57: 227–232.

Nakamura, S, Stock, DW, Wydner, KL, et al. (1996). Genomic analysis of a new mammalian distal-less gene: Dlx7. Genomics 38: 314–324.

Niswander, L, Martin, GR (1992). Fgf-4 expression during gastrulation, myogenesis, limb and tooth development in the mouse. Development 114: 755–768.

Nohno, T, Koyama, E, Myokai, F, et al. (1993). A chicken homeobox gene related to Drosophila paired is predominantly expressed in the developing limb. Dev Biol 158: 254–264.

Norris, RA, Scott, KK, Moore, CS, et al. (2000). Human PRRX1 and PRRX2 genes: cloning, expression, genomic localization, and exclusion as disease genes for Nager syndrome. Mamm Genome *11:* 1000–1005.

Oda, T, Elkahloun, AG, Pike, BL, et al. (1997). Mutations in the human *Jagged1* gene are responsible for Alagille syndrome. Nat Genet *16:* 235–242.

Ohuchi, H, Yoshioka, H, Tanaka, A, et al. (1994). Involvement of androgen-induced growth factor *(FGF-8)* gene in mouse embryogenesis and morphogenesis. Biochem Biophys Res Commun *204:* 882–888.

Orr-Urtreger, A, Lonai, P (1992). Platelet-derived growth factor-A and its receptor are expressed in separate, but adjacent cell layers of the mouse embryo. Development *115:* 1045–1058.

Passos-Bueno, MR, Wilcox, WR, Jabs, EW, et al. (1999). Clinical spectrum of fibroblast growth factor receptor mutations. Hum Mutat *14:* 115–125.

Pavlova, A, Boutin, E, Cunha, G, Sassoon, D (1994). Msx1 (Hox-7.1) in the adult mouse uterus: cellular interactions underlying regulation of expression. Development *120:* 335–345.

Pelton, RW, Nomura, S, Moses, HL, Hogan, BL (1989). Expression of transforming growth factor β2 RNA during murine embryogenesis. Development *106:* 759–767.

Pelton, RW, Saxena, B, Jones, M, et al. (1991). Immunohistochemical localization of TGF β1, TGF β2, and TGF β3 in the mouse embryo: expression patterns suggest multiple roles during embryonic development. J Cell Biol *115:* 1091–1105.

Phillips, DJ (2000). Regulation of activin's access to the cell: why is mother nature such a control freak? Bioessays *22:* 689–696.

Porteus, MH, Bulfone, A, Ciaranello, RD, Rubenstein, JL (1991). Isolation and characterization of a novel cDNA clone encoding a homeodomain that is developmentally regulated in the ventral forebrain [published erratum appears in Neuron (1992) *9:* 187]. Neuron *7:* 221–229.

Price, M, Lemaistre, M, Pischetola, M, et al. (1991). A mouse gene related to *Distal-less* shows a restricted expression in the developing forebrain. Nature *351:* 748–751.

Proetzel, G, Pawlowski, SA, Wiles, MV, et al. (1995). Transforming growth factor-β3 is required for secondary palate fusion. Nat Genet *11:* 409–414.

Qiu, CX, Ferguson, MW (1995). The distribution of PDGFs and PDGF-receptors during murine secondary palate development. J Anat *186:* 17–29.

Qiu, M, Bulfone, A, Ghattas, I, et al. (1997). Role of the *Dlx* homeobox genes in proximodistal patterning of the branchial arches: mutations of *Dlx-1, Dlx-2,* and *Dlx-1* and *-2* alter morphogenesis of proximal skeletal and soft tissue structures derived from the first and second arches. Dev Biol *185:* 165–184.

Qiu, M, Bulfone, A, Martinez, S, et al. (1995). Null mutation of *Dlx-2* results in abnormal morphogenesis of proximal first and second branchial arch derivatives and abnormal differentiation in the forebrain. Genes Dev *9:* 2523–2538.

Rebay, I, Fleming, RJ, Fehon, RG, et al. (1991). Specific EGF repeats of Notch mediate interactions with Delta and Serrate: implications for Notch as a multifunctional receptor. Cell *67:* 687–699.

Reginelli, AD, Wang, YQ, Sassoon, D, Muneoka, K (1995). Digit tip regeneration correlates with regions of Msx1 (Hox 7) expression in fetal and newborn mice. Development *121:* 1065–1076.

Richman, JM, Crosby, Z (1990). Differential growth of facial primordia in chick embryos: responses of facial mesenchyme to basic fibroblast growth factor (bFGF) and serum in micromass culture. Development *109:* 341–348.

Richman, JM, Herbert, M, Matovinovic, E, Walin, J (1997). Effect of fibroblast growth factors on outgrowth of facial mesenchyme. Dev Biol *189:* 135–147.

Riese, DJ 2nd, Stern, DF (1998). Specificity within the EGF family/ErbB receptor family signaling network. Bioessays *20:* 41–48.

Rivera-Perez, JA, Mallo, M, Gendron-Maguire, M, et al. (1995). Goosecoid is not an essential component of the mouse gastrula organizer but is required for craniofacial and rib development. Development *121:* 3005–3012.

Rivera-Perez, JA, Wakamiya, M, Behringer, RR (1999). Goosecoid acts cell autonomously in mesenchyme-derived tissues during craniofacial development. Development *126:* 3811–3821.

Roberts, VJ, Barth, SL (1994). Expression of messenger ribonucleic acids encoding the inhibin/activin system during mid- and late-gestation rat embryogenesis. Endocrinology *134:* 914–923.

Robey, E (1997). Notch in vertebrates. Curr Opin Genet Dev *7:* 551–557.

Robinson, GW, Mahon, KA (1994). Differential and overlapping expression domains of Dlx-2 and Dlx-3 suggest distinct roles for *Distal-less* homeobox genes in craniofacial development. Mech Dev *48:* 199–215.

Robinson, GW, Wray, S, Mahon, KA (1991). Spatially restricted expression of a member of a new family of murine *Distal-less* homeobox genes in the developing forebrain. New Biol *3:* 1183–1194.

Romitti, PA, Lidral, AC, Munger, RG, et al. (1999). Candidate genes for non-syndromic cleft lip and palate and maternal cigarette smoking and alcohol consumption: evaluation of genotype-environment interactions from a population based case-control study of orofacial clefts. Teratology *59:* 39–50.

Sakurai, T, Yanagisawa, M, Takuwa, Y, et al. (1990). Cloning of a cDNA encoding a non-isopeptide-selective subtype of the endothelin receptor. Nature *348:* 732–735.

Sanchez-Garcia, I, Osada, H, Forster, A, Rabbitts, TH (1993). The cysteine-rich LIM domains inhibit DNA binding by the associated homeodomain in Isl-1. EMBO J *12:* 4243–4250.

Sanford, LP, Ormsby, I, Gittenberger-de Groot, AC, et al. (1997). TGFβ2 knockout mice have multiple developmental defects that are non-overlapping with other TGFβ knockout phenotypes. Development *124:* 2659–2670.

Sassani, R, Bartlett, SP, Feng, H, et al. (1993). Association between alleles of the transforming growth factor-alpha locus and the occurrence of cleft lip. Am J Med Genet *45:* 565–569.

Satokata, I, Ma, L, Ohshima, H, et al. (2000). Msx2 deficiency in mice causes pleiotropic defects in bone growth and ectodermal organ formation. Nat Genet *24:* 391–395.

Satokata, I, Maas, R (1994). Msx1 deficient mice exhibit cleft palate and abnormalities of craniofacial and tooth development. Nat Genet *6:* 348–356.

Schutte, BC, Murray, JC (1999). The many faces and factors of orofacial clefts. Hum Mol Genet *8:* 1853–1859.

Sharma, K, Sheng, HZ, Lettieri, K, et al. (1998). LIM homeodomain factors Lhx3 and Lhx4 assign subtype identities for motor neurons. Cell *95:* 817–828.

Shawlot, W, Behringer, RR (1995). Requirement for Lim1 in head-organizer function. Nature *374:* 425–430.

Shimeld, SM, McKay, IJ, Sharpe, PT (1996). The murine homeobox gene *Msx-3* shows highly restricted expression in the developing neural tube. Mech Dev *55:* 201–210.

Sidow, A, Bulotsky, MS, Kerrebrock, AW, et al. (1997). Serrate2 is disrupted in the mouse limb-development mutant syndactylism. Nature *389:* 722–725.

Simeone, A, Acampora, D, Pannese, M, et al. (1994). Cloning and characterization of two members of the vertebrate Dlx gene family. Proc Natl Acad Sci USA *91:* 2250–2254.

Simon, HG, Nelson, C, Goff, D, et al. (1995). Differential expression of myogenic regulatory genes and *Msx-1* during dedifferentiation and redifferentiation of regenerating amphibian limbs. Dev Dyn *202:* 1–12.

Soriano, P (1997). The PDGF alpha receptor is required for neural crest cell development and for normal patterning of the somites. Development *124:* 2691–2700.

Stoll, C, Qian, JF, Feingold, J, et al. (1992). Genetic variation in transforming growth factor alpha: possible association of BamHI polymorphism with bilateral sporadic cleft lip and palate. Am J Hum Genet *50:* 870–871.

Taira, M, Otani, H, Saint-Jeannet, JP, Dawid, IB (1994). Role of the LIM class homeodomain protein Xlim-1 in neural and muscle induction by the Spemann organizer in *Xenopus* [published erratum appears in Nature (1995) *373:* 451]. Nature *372:* 677–679.

ten Berge, D, Brouwer, A, Korving, J, et al. (1998). Prx1 and Prx2 in skeletogenesis: roles in the craniofacial region, inner ear and limbs. Development *125:* 3831–3842.

Thomas, T, Kurihara, H, Yamagishi, H, et al. (1998). A signaling cascade involving endothelin-1, dHAND and msx1 regulates development of neural-crest–derived branchial arch mesenchyme. Development *125:* 3005–3014.

Tooney, PA, Sakai, T, Sakai, K, et al. (1998). Restricted localization of thrombospondin-2 protein during mouse embryogenesis: a comparison to thrombospondin-1. Matrix Biol *17:* 131–143.

Treisman, J, Gonczy, P, Vashishtha, M, et al. (1989). A single amino acid can determine the DNA binding specificity of homeodomain proteins. Cell *59:* 553–562.

Vacca, A, Di Marcotullio, L, Giannini, G, et al. (1999). Thrombospondin-1 is a mediator of the neurotypic differentiation induced by EGF in thymic epithelial cells. Exp Cell Res *248:* 79–86.

Valsecchi, C, Ghezzi, C, Ballabio, A, Rugarli, EI (1997). JAGGED2: a putative Notch ligand expressed in the apical ectodermal ridge and in sites of epithelial–mesenchymal interactions. Mech Dev *69:* 203–207.

van den Boogaard, MJ, Dorland, M, Beemer, FA, van Amstel, HK (2000). *MSX1* mutation is associated with orofacial clefting and tooth agenesis in humans [published erratum appears in Nat Genet (2000) *25:* 125]. Nat Genet *24:* 342–343.

van der Geer, P, Hunter, T, Lindberg, RA (1994). Receptor protein-tyrosine kinases and their signal transduction pathways. Annu Rev Cell Biol *10:* 251–337.

Vassalli, A, Matzuk, MM, Gardner, HA, et al. (1994). Activin/inhibin βB subunit gene disruption leads to defects in eyelid development and female reproduction. Genes Dev *8:* 414–427.

Vieille-Grosjean, I, Hunt, P, Gulisano, M, et al. (1997). Branchial *HOX* gene expression and human craniofacial development. Dev Biol *183:* 49–60.

Wall, NA, Hogan, BL (1995). Expression of bone morphogenetic protein-4 (BMP-4), bone morphogenetic protein-7 (BMP-7), fibroblast growth factor-8 (FGF-8) and sonic hedgehog (SHH) during branchial arch development in the chick. Mech Dev *53:* 383–392.

Wee, EL, Zimmerman, EF (1983). Involvement of GABA in palate morphogenesis and its relation to diazepam teratogenesis in two mouse strains. Teratology *28:* 15–22.

Wilkie, AO, Tang, Z, Elanko, N, et al. (2000). Functional haploinsufficiency of the human homeobox gene *MSX2* causes defects in skull ossification. Nat Genet *24:* 387–390.

Winograd, J, Reilly, MP, Roe, R, et al. (1997). Perinatal lethality and multiple craniofacial malformations in *MSX2* transgenic mice. Hum Mol Genet *6:* 369–379.

Woloshin, P, Song, K, Degnin, C, et al. (1995). MSX1 inhibits myoD expression in fibroblast × 10T1/2 cell hybrids. Cell *82:* 611–620.

Xu, D, Emoto, N, Giaid, A, et al. (1994). ECE-1: a membrane-bound metalloprotease that catalyzes the proteolytic activation of big endothelin-1. Cell *78:* 473–485.

Xue, D, Tu, Y, Chalfie, M (1993). Cooperative interactions between the *Caenorhabditis elegans* homeoproteins UNC-86 and MEC-3. Science *261:* 1324–1328.

Yamada, G, Mansouri, A, Torres, M, et al. (1995). Targeted mutation of the murine *goosecoid* gene results in craniofacial defects and neonatal death. Development *121:* 2917–2922.

Yamada, G, Ueno, K, Nakamura, S, et al. (1997). Nasal and pharyngeal abnormalities caused by the mouse *goosecoid* gene mutation. Biochem Biophys Res Commun *233:* 161–165.

Yamaguchi, TP, Rossant, J (1995). Fibroblast growth factors in mammalian development. Curr Opin Genet Dev *5:* 485–491.

Yanagisawa, H, Yanagisawa, M, Kapur, RP, et al. (1998). Dual genetic pathways of endothelin-mediated intercellular signaling revealed by targeted disruption of endothelin converting enzyme-1 gene. Development *125:* 825–836.

Yanagisawa, M, Kurihara, H, Kimura, S, et al. (1988). A novel potent vasoconstrictor peptide produced by vascular endothelial cells. Nature *332:* 411–415.

Zhang, H, Catron, KM, Abate-Shen, C (1996). A role for the Msx-1 homeodomain in transcriptional regulation: residues in the N-terminal arm mediate TATA binding protein interaction and transcriptional repression. Proc Natl Acad Sci USA *93:* 1764–1769.

Zhang, H, Hu, G, Wang, H, et al. (1997). Heterodimerization of Msx and Dlx homeoproteins results in functional antagonism. Mol Cell Biol *17:* 2920–2932.

Zhao, Y, Guo, YJ, Tomac, AC, et al. (1999a). Isolated cleft palate in mice with a targeted mutation of the LIM homeobox gene *Lhx8*. Proc Natl Acad Sci USA *96:* 15002–15006.

Zhao, Y, Sheng, HZ, Amini, R, et al. (1999b). Control of hippocampal morphogenesis and neuronal differentiation by the LIM homeobox gene *Lhx5*. Science *284:* 1155–1158.

Zimmerman, EF, Wee, EL (1984). Role of neurotransmitters in palate development. Curr Top Dev Biol *19:* 37–63.

II

Clinical Features of Cleft Lip and Palate

4

The orofacial examination: normal and abnormal findings

ERIC A. WULFSBERG

The discovery of an oral cleft (OC) in a baby or young child is a distressing event for the family. Parents who have been visualizing a healthy child throughout pregnancy are often shocked by the significant physical and cosmetic abnormalities that accompany an OC. Following the discovery of the OC, the parents will appropriately have many questions, which may be divided into two general categories: the first addresses the diagnosis and prognosis of the condition, involving questions such as "What is wrong?," "What can be done about it?," and "What does it mean for the future?"; the second addresses etiology and recurrence risk, typically including questions such as "Why did it happen?," "Will it happen again?," and "What are our reproductive options in the future?" These questions can be answered only after accurately determining the abnormalities that are present and establishing the etiology of the OC. When a genetic syndrome with associated mental retardation is the cause of the cleft, the developmental prognosis may be more important to the ultimate function of the individual than the specific anatomic issues surrounding the OC and its repair. Thus, this section discusses issues related to the general and orofacial evaluation of the OC patient with emphasis on clues to differentiate syndromic from nonsyndromic OCs.

While the majority of individuals with OCs have no other physical abnormalities and are developmentally normal, a significant number have associated malformations, possibly as part of a genetic or chromosomal syndrome. Most studies looking for associated abnormalities or syndromes among individuals with facial clefts have been done in craniofacial or cleft palate (CP)

clinic populations. This tends to underestimate the incidence of the most severe or lethal malformation syndromes as these children often do not survive the neonatal period. Using these populations has the advantage that craniofacial clinics often include a dysmorphologist or clinical geneticist, resulting in a more thorough morphological evaluation. A study of this type from the CP clinic in San Diego, which does not include early lethal syndromes, showed a 14% incidence of associated malformations in individuals with cleft lip (CL) with or without CP (CL/P), a 40% incidence of associated malformations among individuals with CP, and a 78% incidence of associated malformations among individuals with velopharyngeal insufficiency (Jones, 1993, 2000). For comparison, a French population-based study utilizing a birth defects registry showed a 37% incidence of associated malformations in individuals with CL/P, a 47% incidence of associated malformations among individuals with CP, and a 14% incidence of associated malformations among individuals with CL (Stoll et al., 2000). In the French study, approximately 13% of the patients with CL/P, 14% with CP, and 6% with CL had recognized multiple malformation syndromes (Stoll et al., 2000). Thus, results from these two different patient populations suggest that the type of OC can heighten or lower concerns for associated malformations or genetic syndromes. Similarly, the severity of the OC appears to be important. Bilateral CL/P is almost twice as likely to be associated with a multiple malformation syndrome than unilateral CL/P (Milerad et al., 1997).

While surgeons evaluate OC patients with reference to the best technique for good cosmetic and functional repair, the goal of the medical evaluation is to categorize the abnormality into one of three groups: *(1)* part of a multiple malformation syndrome with possible associated developmental disabilities and/or mental retardation and a recurrence risk as high as 25% to 50%, *(2)* a nonsyndromic abnormality with a presumed good developmental outcome and lower recurrence risk, or *(3)* one of a number of associated malformations not representing a known or recognized syndrome, with a guarded developmental outcome depending on the nature and severity of the associated abnormalities and an unknown recurrence risk. These distinctions are critically important for counseling but may not be immediately obvious at the initial evaluation of the OC patient. Therefore, evaluation of the OC patient is often an ongoing process that may need to be repeated over a period of time to accurately categorize the nature and etiology of an individual OC and, thus, provide important treatment, long-term prognosis, and recurrence risk counseling information. As in other areas of medicine, this clinical evaluation should include a detailed medical and family history, a careful physical examination, and appropriate diagnostic studies.

Evaluation of an individual with an OC begins by gathering medical and family history information. The pregnancy history should include the ages of the parents as chromosomal abnormalities are more frequent with advanced maternal age and new gene mutations are more frequent with advanced paternal age. Maternal health and any medications taken during the pregnancy may give clues to exposure to potential teratogens. In particular, personal habits, such as alcohol or cigarette use during the pregnancy, should be ascertained. The occupations of both parents may also suggest potential teratogen exposures. Pregnancy complications, such as maternal illnesses or premature delivery, may add important clues. Perinatal history, especially any nursery complications and feeding difficulties, is often important. While feeding difficulties may be due to the OC itself, they may also indicate associated neurodevelopmental abnormalities suggestive of a syndromic etiology. Over time, a child's growth and neurodevelopment are perhaps the two best measures of good health and normality. Abnormalities in these vital areas should raise concern of a syndromic etiology for the OC.

The family history is best done by constructing a three-generation pedigree, looking for individuals with OCs as well as other congenital and developmental abnormalities. The family history may identify other members with apparent nonsyndromic OCs, supporting a nonsyndromic etiology for the OC and altering the recurrence risk counseling. Because of the phenotypic variability of many OC syndromes, the family history may also identify individuals with other abnormalities, leading to the diagnosis of a familial OC syndrome. Updating the family history at subsequent clinic visits is important as additional information may be learned from other family members after the discovery of the individual OC and new affected individuals may be added to the family over time.

The physical examination needs to be comprehensive and thorough because extracranial as well as craniofacial abnormalities may be major components of an OC syndrome. Some dysmorphologists begin their physical examinations away from the OC and craniofacial region so as not to overlook minor abnormalities of the hands, feet, genitalia, and other body parts. The important extracranial abnormalities seen in clefting syndromes will be discussed elsewhere in this book. An important general concept to remember is that those structures with complex embryonic development, such as the brain, heart, face, and hands, are the most likely to show associated abnormalities (Stoll et al., 2000). Examination for minor abnormalities in the parents, and sometimes in other family members, is an important part of the evaluation. This may uncover features of a clefting syndrome not present in the affected individual.

When trying to understand how a structural abnormality such as an OC develops, it is important for the physician to have a thorough knowledge of the normal embryology of facial development, as described earlier in this book. The most common abnormal embryological processes that can lead to an OC include malformations and disruptions. The majority of OCs are malformations, meaning that an error in early development prevented completion of normal developmental processes, resulting in the OC (Jones, 1997). Primary malformation OCs can be nonsyndromic, part of a multiple malformation syndrome, or part of a number of associated but nonsyndromic malformations. Malformation OCs are most commonly *(1)* paramedian CL or CLP occurring at the junction of the lateral branchial arch derivatives and the frontonasal process, *(2)* isolated CP, or *(3)* medial facial clefts involving deficiency of the frontonasal process. A smaller number of OCs are the result of disruptions, meaning that the lip and palate structures were developing normally until they were interfered with by an extrinsic force such as a swallowed amniotic strand, or of a chemical teratogen such as in fetal alcohol syndrome (Jones, 1997). Clefts caused by swallowed amniotic strands are most likely to be atypical appearing oro-orbital or oroauricular clefts, but the amniotic strands can interfere with subsequent normal development and result in an oro-orbital or oroauricular cleft together with a typical appearing paramedian OC (Eppley et al., 1998).

Careful physical evaluation of the type and severity of an OC can alter the concern for associated abnormalities and syndromes. As previously discussed, CL/P, CP, median facial clefts, and velopharnygeal insufficiency are developmentally separate abnormalities showing different patterns of inheritance, recurrence risks, and syndrome associations. While typical unilateral or bilateral CL/P occurs at the boundary of the embryonic frontonasal process and lateral branchial arch derivatives, care must be taken on oral examination to recognize the occasional severe unilateral CL/P, which may mimic a less common median OC. Identification of frontonasal derivatives such as the philtral columns or prolabial segment will allow this important distinction to be made as midline structures may have been distorted and shifted to one side by a large unilateral CL/P. Identification of median OCs involving failure of formation or hypoplasia of the frontonasal process almost always signifies disturbances in underlying forebrain development with a guarded developmental prognosis and often an early lethal outcome (DeMyer, 1975). Aberrant oral frenulae are seen in a number of disorders, including Ellis-van Creveld syndrome, and are combined with midline upper lip notches in the orofaciodigital syndromes. It is likely that these disorders are embryologically different from midline OCs due to absence or hypoplasia of the frontonasal process as underlying forebrain abnormalities are not present. Paramedian lower lip pits, which contain the openings of labial mucous glands or accessory salivary glands, are found in fewer than 1% of individuals with CL/P, but are highly associated with Van der Woude's syndrome, an autosomal dominant clefting syndrome (Cervenka et al., 1967). The lip pits in Van der Woude's syndrome can occur without a CL/P so the finding of this abnormality in the parent of a child with a CL/P increases the recurrence risk for this syndrome to 50% in future offspring. In contrast to lower lip pits, upper lip pits or commissural pits, located at the angles of the mouth, have no association with CL/P or other anomalies (Lettieri, 1993). Oroauricular and oro-orbital clefts are the least common types of OC and rarely have a genetic etiology. As discussed above, oro-orbital and oroauricular clefts often result from swallowed amniotic strands, which either cause disruptions of normally formed tissues or interfere with subsequent normal lip and palate closure. Lateral oroauricular clefts, which indicate incomplete merging of the maxillary and mandibular processes, are found in Treacher Collins syndrome, the oculoauriculovertebral spectrum (including hemifacial microsomia as well as Goldenhar's syndrome), and the acrofacial dysostoses. Isolated clefts of the lower lip are exceedingly rare and presumably caused by incomplete midline merging of the two lateral mandibular processes. These most often occur as nonsyndromic abnormalities and generally have a good developmental outcome.

While there are less obvious structural differences among CPs compared to CL/Ps, the morphology of CPs may be important in separating them into broad groups with differing risks for associated abnormalities or syndromes. While a clear distinction is often not possible, most isolated nonsyndromic CPs tend to have a narrower, V-shaped appearance with relatively normal development of the mandible in relationship to the maxilla. However, CPs with a broader, more U-shaped appearance and associated hypoplasia of the mandible and glossoptosis are referred to as Robin sequence-type clefts and carry a much higher risk of being part of an associated genetic or chromosomal syndrome. Bifid uvula and submucosal CP represent mild phenotypic expression of CP and should be looked for in family members of individuals with overt CP. Thus, subtle physical distinctions on the craniofacial examination can help to raise or lower the suspicion of a syndromic association.

The history and physical examination of individuals with many of the OC syndromes characteristically show major malformations, growth and developmental delays, and minor dysmorphic features all thought to be due to a single unifying etiology (Jones, 1997). However, approximately 40% of patients with OCs have one or more associated malformations but do not have a recognizable syndrome (Jones, 1993). These individuals appear to represent a heterogeneous group, with some having a good neurodevelopmental outcome and low recurrence risk and others having a more guarded prognosis.

Future recurrence risk counseling includes not just interpretation of recurrence risk figures but also compassionate communication of those risks and reproductive options to the family and affected individual. This is an important task and should be performed by a specialized genetic counselor, clinical geneticist, or other knowledgeable professional. Therefore, the medical and family history, a detailed physical and craniofacial examination, and parental examinations are central to distinguishing those individuals with nonsyndromic OCs from those with associated malformations or an OC syndrome.

REFERENCES

Cervenka, J, Gorlin, RJ, Anderson, VE (1967). The syndrome of pits of the lower lip and cleft lip and/or palate: genetic considerations. Am J Hum Genet 19: 416–432.

DeMyer, W (1975). Median facial malformations and their implications for brain malformations. Birth Defects Original Article Series XI: 155.

Eppley, BL, David, L, Li, M, et al. (1998). Amniotic band facies. J Craniofac Surg 9: 360–365.

Jones, KL (1997). Introduction including dysmorphology approach and classification. In: *Smith's Recognizable Patterns of Human Malformation,* edited by KL Jones. Philadelphia: Saunders, pp. 1–7.

Jones, MC (1993). Facial clefting: etiology and developmental pathogenesis. Clin Plast Surg *20:* 599–606.

Jones, MC (2000). Cleft lip with or without cleft palate and cleft palate alone: a clinic based population revisited to determine the frequency of multiple malformation syndromes within the population and to define subgroups among individuals with isolated clefts. Presented at the David W. Smith Workshop on Malformation and Morphogenesis, San Diego, CA, August 2–4, 2000.

Lettieri, J (1993). Lips and oral cavity. In: *Human Malformations and Related Anomalies,* vol. 2, edited by RE Stevenson, JG Hall, and RM Goodman. New York: Oxford University Press, pp. 367–381.

Milerad, J, Larson, O, Hagberg, C, Ideberg, M (1997). Associated malformations in infants with cleft lip and palate: a prospective, population-based study. Pediatrics *100:* 180–186.

Stoll, C, Alembik, Y, Dott, B, Roth, MP (2000). Associated malformations in cases with oral clefts. Cleft Palate Craniofac J *37:* 41–47.

5

Classification and description of nonsyndromic clefts

HOWARD M. SAAL

Cleft lip (CL) with or without cleft palate (CL/P) and isolated cleft palate (CP), collectively termed *oral clefts* (OCs), are among the most common birth defects, with a prevalence that ranges between 1 case in every 500 to 1000 newborns. The prevalence of CL/P varies according to ethnicity, gender, and socioeconomic factors (Croen et al., 1998; Bender, 2000). Native Americans have the highest reported prevalence at birth, with 3.6 CL/P cases per 1000 births. Asians have the second highest prevalence at birth for CL/P, with 2.1 cases per 1000 Japanese and 1.7 cases per 1000 Chinese live births (Croen et al., 1998). Gender seems to play a role in the etiology of CL/P since males predominate by a 2:1 ratio (Tolarova, 1987). Also, population studies have shown that individuals born in more rural, lower socioeconomic conditions have a higher risk for CL/P compared to ethnically similar groups with a higher socioeconomic status (Chung et al., 1987; Cembrano et al., 1995).

The incidence of CP is much less dependent on racial and ethnic factors, being approximately 1 in 2000 live births (Vanderas, 1987; Gorlin et al., 1990). In contrast to CLP, however, there is a female predominance of CP, the ratio being approximately 3:2 females to males (Cohen, 2000).

There are many genetic and developmental conditions that can cause CL/P or CP. The Online Mendelian Inheritance in Man (www.ncbi.nlm.nih.gov/Omim/) lists over 174 Mendelian disorders associated with CL/P and 312 associated with CP. The London Dysmorphology Database, which also lists many teratogenic and other nongenetic disorders, identifies 205 disorders associated with CL/P and 441 with CP (Winter

and Baraitser, 1996). These resources do not include the substantial number of chromosomal disorders that can be associated with OCs. However, despite these figures, approximately 75% of CL/P and 50% of CP cases will be isolated, nonsyndromic OCs (Table 5.1) (Milerad et al., 1997; Saal, 1998, 2000; Tolarova and Cervenka, 1998; Jones, 2000; Stoll et al., 2000).

It is important to distinguish between syndromic and nonsyndromic CL/P and CP. This distinction has significant implications for determining management and recurrence risks for patients and families. In addition, the success of genetic studies, which search for genes that cause OCs, depends on accurate clinical diagnosis. What differentiates syndromic from nonsyndromic CL/P and CP is often subjective, differing in basic definition from one center to the next. There are no specific guidelines which define nonsyndromic OCs, although one author has specified nonsyndromic OCs as those associated with no or one major anomaly or two or fewer minor anomalies (Jones, 1988). Another study precluded consideration of a nonsyndromic cleft if there was any other major anomaly or three or more minor anomalies in addition to the OC (Tolarova and Cervenka, 1998). Major anomalies are those of functional or cosmetic significance requiring some degree of medical intervention (Spranger et al., 1982). Minor anomalies are those of minimal or no cosmetic or functional significance, which occur in less than 5% of the population (Jones, 1997; Spranger et al., 1982). If one is to equate nonsyndromic OCs with isolated OCs, it seems reasonable to include only those cases where no additional major anomaly exists. The distinctions between syndromic and nonsyndromic OCs become less clear in

TABLE 5.1. *Studies of Syndromic vs. Nonsyndromic Oral Clefts*

Study	Nonsyndromic (%)	Syndromic (%)
Tolarova and Cervenka, 1998		
CL	85.8	14.2
CLP	67.7	32.3
CP	47.5	52.5
Milerad et al., 1997		
CL/P	81	19
CP	78	22
Stoll et al., 2000		
CL/P	71.0	29.0
CP	53.2	46.7
Jones, 2000		
CL/P	87	13
CP	41	59
Saal, 1998, 2000		
CL/P	73	27
CP	45.6	54.4

CL, cleft lip; CP, cleft palate; CLP, cleft lip and palate; CL/P, cleft lip with or without cleft palate.

the presence of minor anomalies. The most helpful studies have shown that the presence of three or more minor anomalies is strongly associated with the presence of a major anomaly (Marden et al., 1964; Leppig et al., 1987, 1988). Therefore, for the purpose of definition, it is reasonable to limit nonsyndromic OC to those associated with no additional malformations and two or fewer minor anomalies. However, some syndromic OCs may be associated with two or fewer minor anomalies. For example, Van der Woude's syndrome is characterized by positive family history for OC and the presence of lower lip pits. Similarly the Robin sequence with CP and mild ear dysplasia or preauricular sinuses are found in individuals with a mild form of the branchio-oto-renal syndrome. In Stickler's syndrome, the only presenting sign may be the Robin sequence and myopia with a positive family history for CP. The diagnosis is even more challenging in the nonocular forms of Stickler's syndrome or if an affected infant has a new mutation with no family history of CP.

Oral clefts can be classified on the basis of etiology and/or pathogenesis. There have been multiple classifications of OC based on anatomic and embryological considerations (Fogh-Andersen, 1942, 1971; Millard, 1976). Fogh-Anderson (1942) divided OCs into three main groups: *(1)* CL extending to the the incisive foramen and including clefts of the alveolus (primary palate); *(2)* CL and CP (CLP), including unilateral and bilateral CLP; and *(3)* CP identified as being median and not extending beyond the incisive foramen. An-

other comprehensive approach was taken by the International Confederation for Plastic and Reconstructive Surgery, which at their 1967 congress established a classification of OC based on the embryology of the developing structures. They identified three major groups of OC (Millard, 1976).

Group 1. Clefts of the primary palate

    a. Lip
    b. Alveolus

Group 2. Clefts of the primary and secondary palate

    a. Lip
    b. Alveolus
    c. Hard palate (secondary palate)

Group 3. Clefts of the secondary palate

    a. Hard palate
    b. Soft palate

An anatomic diagnosis is clearly advantageous to the surgeon, who must decide on the best approach and timing for the surgical treatment. However, some problems with diagnosis based solely on anatomy and embryology are that it does not explain the cause of the cleft, does not allow for a comprehensive management plan of the patient for medical conditions that are not directly related to the cleft, and does not give sufficient information regarding possible recurrence risks. Classification of OCs based solely on etiology or pathogenesis supplies insufficient information regarding the severity of the cleft and the types of direct medical and surgical management required. Therefore, it is necessary to combine the two types of classification in order to optimally diagnose and treat any patient with an OC.

CLEFT LIP WITH OR WITHOUT CLEFT PALATE

Nonsyndromic CL/P accounts for between 70% and 80% of all cases (Milerad et al., 1997; Saal, 1998, 2000; Tolarova and Cervenka, 1998; Jones, 2000; Stoll et al., 2000). Affected individuals may have either CL or CLP. In nonsyndromic CL/P, the cleft is not in the midline and there is laterality to the CL. Midline CL is indicative of another underlying disorder, such as one of the oral-facial-digital syndromes or the holoprosencephaly sequence. The London Dysmorphology Database identifies at least 40 different conditions with midline clefts (Winter and Baraitser, 1996).

In nonsyndromic CL, unilateral clefts are more common than bilateral involvement (Fig. 5.1). In unilateral CL, the prevalence of left-sided CL is greater than that of right-sided CL. The left-sided:right-sided:bilateral CL/P ratio is 6:3:1 (Lettieri, 1993).

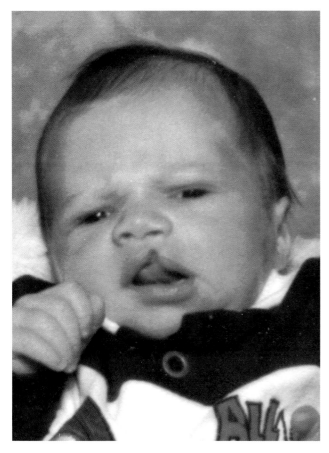

FIG. 5.1. Infant boy with isolated left-sided cleft lip.

Anatomically, the CL may be complete or incomplete. Complete CL refers to the cleft involving the entire upper lip and extending into the naris. In incomplete CL, there is a variable amount of tissue that bridges the upper lip. The connecting tissue may comprise only a narrow band, called a Simonart band (Millard, 1976).

Often, CL and CP occur concurrently. In most cases of CLP, there is a cleft of both the primary and secondary palates. Again, when there is a unilateral CLP, the cleft of the primary palate occurs on the side of the CL (Fig. 5.2). There are uncommon cases of CL with intact primary palate but clefting of the secondary palate. Such cases are often syndromic, and one must exclude associations, sequences (especially Robin sequence), and other associated anomalies. Bilateral CLP is the most severe presentation (Fig. 5.3). In this classification, there is involvement of the primary palate on the left and the right with, in most cases, clefting of the secondary palate. Although possible in patients with CLP, there is no specific pattern of expected minor anomalies. Probably, the most common minor anomaly in patients with nonsyndromic CL/P is hyper-

telorism. This also may be a sign of an underlying genetic condition, such as the Opitz G/BBB syndrome (Saal, 2000).

Recurrence risk for nonsyndromic CLP depends on several factors, including severity of the cleft, number of affected relatives, gender of the affected individual, and degree of genetic relationship to the affected individual (e.g., first-degree relatives have higher risk than second- and third-degree relatives). As noted, more severe clefts are associated with a higher recurrence risk. For example, for a child with a unilateral incomplete CL and a negative family history for clefts, the recurrence risk would be 3%. However, if the child were born with a bilateral complete CLP, the recurrence risk would be 5% (Gorlin et al., 1990; Harper, 1993; Bender, 2000).

CLEFT PALATE

Nonsyndromic CP refers to abnormal development of the secondary palate. The prevalence at birth of CP is estimated to be 1 in 2000 live births (Murray, 1995; Wyszynski et al., 1996). In contrast to CL/P, where there are obvious racial and ethnic genetic factors that

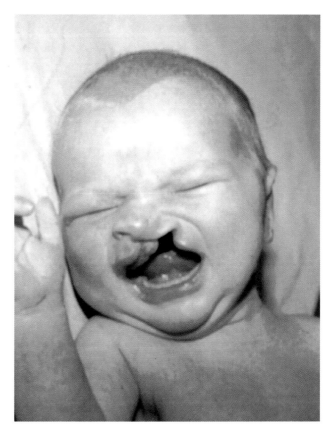

FIG. 5.2. Infant with unilateral complete cleft lip and cleft palate.

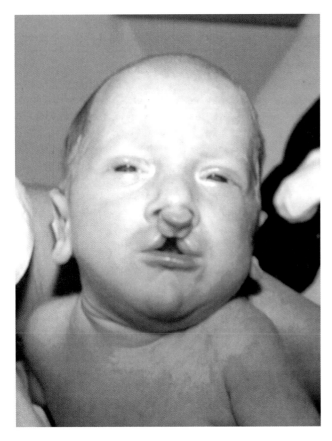

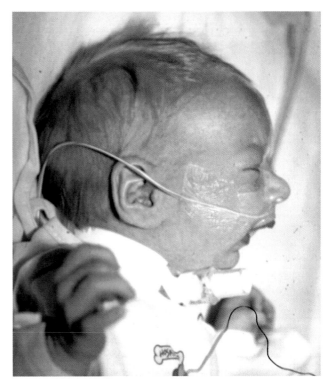

FIG. 5.4. Infant with micrognathia and Pierre Robin sequence.

FIG. 5.3. Infant with complete bilateral cleft lip and cleft palate.

contribute to the prevalence in certain populations, CP has no such population propensity. Instead, the prevalence of CP is similar in all populations studied.

CP is genetically distinct from CL/P. In families and individuals with nonsyndromic CL/P, the increased recurrence risk is for CL/P; however, the risk for having a child with CP remains at the general population level (1 in 2000). The same is true for families and individuals with nonsyndromic CP. Moreover, when individuals in the same family are born with CL/P and CP, one must look for an underlying genetic etiology, such as Van der Woude's syndrome, one of a very few syndromes where one can see both CP and CL/P (Murray, 1995).

Nonsyndromic CP is pathogenetically unrelated to the CP in patients with CLP. In CLP, the CP is a secondary phenomenon related to failure of the lip to close (Trasler and Fraser, 1977). It may be a primary malformation, reflecting abnormal palate development in one of the many critical steps including elevation, merging, and fusion of the palatal shelves. It may also be a consequence of other events, which do not primarily involve palate development, such as the Robin sequence. This condition is related to developmental fac-

tors that cause either retrognathia or micrognathia, with secondary posterior positioning of the tongue. This, in turn, may cause interference with elevation and merging of the lateral palatal shelves (Fig. 5.4) (Cohen, 1999). In the classic presentation, the CP is U-shaped,

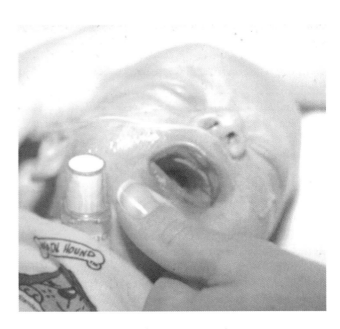

FIG. 5.5. Cleft palate secondary to Pierre Robin sequence. Note U-shaped cleft of the secondary palate.

reflecting fusion of the palatal shelves around the tongue (Fig. 5.5). Another complication of the Robin sequence is respiratory distress from pharyngeal airway obstruction from the posteriorly placed tongue *(glossoptosis).* Many cases of Robin sequence will present with a V-shaped CP, making it difficult to distinguish between CP as a malformation and as a component of the Robin sequence. Children with Robin sequence and V-shaped CP remain at high risk for glossoptosis. Therefore, it is often not possible to clinically differentiate CP as a malformation from CP as a secondary component of a sequence of events related to micrognathia or retrognathia (Cohen, 1999).

An additional difficulty in categorizing CP is classifying submucous CP and bifid uvula. Submucous CP appears to represent a microform or forme fruste of CP. As in CP, approximately 50% of cases of submucous CP are associated with underlying syndromes (Saal, 2000).

In contrast to CLP, CP is much more likely to be syndromic or associated with additional malformations (Jones, 1988, 2000; Tolarova and Cervenka, 1998; Saal, 2000; Stoll et al., 2000). In several studies, the incidence of nonsyndromic CP has ranged from 41% to to 55% (Jones, 2000; Saal, 2000; Stoll et al., 2000). The most common diagnosis is Stickler's syndrome (Saal, 2000). Stickler's syndrome has also been identified as the most common syndrome causing Robin sequence (Hanson and Smith, 1975; Cohen, 1979; Gorlin et al., 1990). It is genetically heterogeneous, with at least three genes identified (Brunner et al., 1994; Annunen et al., 1999; Martin et al., 1999; Snead and Yates, 1999). With both ocular and nonocular forms, the diagnosis may be difficult to make in infants and young children with what appear to be nonsyndromic CP. This is especially true in nonocular Stickler's syndrome, where the patient may have a mildly affected parent or a spontaneous gene mutation and absence of myopia in infancy or early childhood as a diagnostic sign.

Therefore, the diagnosis of nonsyndromic CP is challenging. In many cases, the final diagnosis of nonsyndromic CP cannot be made in infancy and must be delayed until later childhood, emphasizing the need for clinical genetics follow-up. This is especially true when there are associated developmental disabilities, including mental retardation, since these clinical signs may not become evident for several years.

CONCLUSIONS

Oral clefts are among the most common birth defects. The causes of CL/P and CP are heterogeneous and include genetic and environmental etiologies. To provide optimal long-term management and adequate genetic counseling and recurrence risks, identification of the etiology of the OC is essential. A large percentage of OC are syndromic, approximately 25% of CL/P and 50% of CP cases. Therefore, the diagnosis of isolated, nonsyndromic OC is one of exclusion of other diagnoses. This has significant implications for physicians, patients, and families since management and genetic counseling issues are often closely tied to specific diagnosis. This also has implications for those who do research in the area of OCs since much of the genetic research depends on an accurate diagnosis.

REFERENCES

Annunen, S, Korkko, J, Czarny, M, et al. (1999). Splicing mutations of 54-bp exons in the *COL11A1* gene cause Marshall syndrome, but other mutations cause overlapping Marshall/Stickler phenotypes. Am J Hum Genet 65: 974–983.

Bender, PL (2000). Genetics of cleft lip and palate. J Pediatr Nurs 15: 242–249.

Brunner, HG, van Beersum, SE, Warman, ML, et al. (1994). A Stickler syndrome gene is linked to chromosome 6 near the *COL11A2* gene. Hum Mol Genet 3: 1561–1564.

Cembrano, JRJ, Vera, JS, Joaquino, JB, et al. (1995). Familial risk of recurrence of cleft lip and palate. Philippine J Surg Surg Spec 50: 37–40.

Chung, CS, Mi, MP, Beechert, AM (1987). Genetic epidemiology of cleft lip with or without cleft palate in the population of Hawaii. Genet Epidemiol 4: 415–423.

Cohen, MM Jr (1979). Syndromology's message for craniofacial biology. J Maxillofac Surg 7: 89–109.

Cohen, MM Jr (1999). Robin sequences and complexes: causal heterogeneity and pathogenetic/phenotypic variability [editorial]. Am J Med Genet 84: 311–315.

Cohen, MM Jr (2000). Etiology and pathogenesis of orofacial clefting. Oral Maxillofac Clin North Am 12: 379–397.

Croen, LA, Shaw, GM, Wasserman, CR, Tolarova, MM (1998). Racial and ethnic variations in the prevalence of orofacial clefts in California, 1983–1992. Am J Med Genet 79: 2–7.

Fogh-Andersen, P (1942). *Inheritance of Harelip and Cleft Palate.* Copenhagen: Munksgaard.

Fogh-Andersen, P (1971). Epidemiology and etiology of clefts. In *Birth Defects: Original Article Series* (Volume VII, Part 7), edited by D. Bergsma. Baltimore: Williams and Wilkins Company, pp. 50–53.

Gorlin, R, Cohen, MJ, Levin, L (1990). *Syndromes of the Head and Neck,* 3rd ed. New York: Oxford University Press.

Hanson, JW, Smith, DW (1975). U-shaped palatal defect in the Robin anomalad: developmental and clinical relevance. J Pediatr 87: 30–33.

Harper, PS (1993). *Practical Genetic Counseling,* 4th ed. Oxford: Butterworth-Heinemann.

Jones, K (1997). *Smith's Recognizable Patterns of Human Malformation,* 5th ed. Philadelphia: Saunders.

Jones, MC (1988). Etiology of facial clefts: prospective evaluation of 428 patients. Cleft Palate J 25: 16–20.

Jones, MC (2000). Cleft lip with or without cleft palate and cleft palate alone: a clinic based population revisited to determine the frequency of multiple malformation syndromes within the population and to define subgroups among individuals with isolated clefts. Presented at the David W. Smith Workshop on Morphogenesis and Malformations, San Diego, August 9, 2000.

Leppig, KA, Werler, MM, Cann, CI, et al. (1987). Predictive value of minor anomalies. I. Association with major malformations. J Pediatr 110: 531–537.

Leppig, KA, Werler, MM, Cann, CI, et al. (1988). Minor malformations: significant or insignificant [letter]. Am J Dis Child 142: 1274.

Lettieri, J (1993). Human Malformations and Related Anomalies, edited by RE Stevenson, JG Hall, and RM Goodman. New York: Oxford University Press, pp. 367–381.

Marden, PM, Smith, DW, McDonald, MJ (1964). Congenital anomalies in the newborn infant including minor variations. J Pediatr 64: 357.

Martin, S, Richards, AJ, Yates, JR, et al. (1999). Stickler syndrome: further mutations in COL11A1 and evidence for additional locus heterogeneity. Eur J Hum Genet 7: 807–814.

Milerad, J, Larson, O, et al. (1997). Associated malformations in infants with cleft lip and palate: a prospective, population-based study. Pediatrics 100: 180–186.

Millard, DR Jr (1976). Cleft Craft, 1st ed., vol. 1. Boston: Little, Brown.

Murray, JC (1995). Face facts: genes, environment, and clefts [editorial; comment]. Am J Hum Genet 57: 227–232.

Saal, HM (1998). Syndromes and malformations associated with cleft lip with or without cleft palate. Am J Hum Genet 64: A118.

Saal, HM (2000). A prospective analysis of cleft palate: associated syndromes and malformations. Presented at the XXI David W. Smith Workshop on Morphogenesis and Malformations, San Diego, August 9, 2000.

Snead, MP, Yates, JR (1999). Clinical and molecular genetics of Stickler syndrome. J Med Genet 36: 353–359.

Spranger, J, Benirschke, K, Hall, JG, et al. (1982). Errors of morphogenesis: concepts and terms. Recommendations of an international working group. J Pediatr 100: 160–165.

Stoll, C, Alembik, Y, Dott, B, Roth, MP (2000). Associated malformations in cases with oral clefts. Cleft Palate Craniofac J 37: 41–47.

Tolarova, M (1987). Orofacial clefts in Czechoslovakia. Incidence, genetics and prevention of cleft lip and palate over a 19 year period. Scand J Plast Reconstructive Surg 21: 19–25.

Tolarova, MM, Cervenka, J (1998). Classification and birth prevalence of orofacial clefts. Am J Med Genet 75: 126–137.

Trasler, DG, Fraser, FC (1977). Time–position relationships with particular reference to cleft lip and cleft palate. In: Handbook of Teratology, Vol. 2, edited by JG Wilson and FC Fraser. New York: Plenum Press, 265–281.

Vanderas, AP (1987). Incidence of cleft lip, cleft palate, and cleft lip and palate among races: a review. Cleft Palate J 24: 216–225.

Winter, RM, Baraitser, M (1996). London Dysmorphology Database. London: Oxford University Press.

Wyszynski, DF, Beaty, TH, Maestri, NE (1996). Genetics of nonsyndromic oral clefts revisited. Cleft Palate Craniofac J 33: 16406–16417.

6

Syndromes with orofacial clefting

M. MICHAEL COHEN, JR.

Cleft lip with or without cleft palate is etiologically distinct from isolated cleft palate. In a patient with cleft lip with or without cleft palate, if another family member is affected, he or she will have either isolated cleft lip or cleft lip together with cleft palate but not isolated cleft palate alone. Similarly, if a patient has isolated cleft palate, another affected family member can have only isolated cleft palate. There are three exceptions. First, in genetic isolates that are inbred, both types may concur by chance (Cohen, 1978, 2000). Second, cleft lip and palate and cleft palate alone but not cleft lip alone have been associated with *MSX1* (J. C. Murray, personal communication, 2000). Third, in many genetic syndromes with orofacial clefting, both types may be found. For example, in the autosomal dominantly inherited Van der Woude syndrome, in which orofacial clefting is found together with lip pits, patients may have cleft lip, cleft lip and palate, or isolated cleft palate (Cohen, 1978, 2000).

When cleft data are broken down by subtype, isolated cleft palate (13%–50%) is associated more frequently with congenital malformations than cleft lip (7%–13%) or cleft lip and palate (2%–11%). Some studies have suggested that associated anomalies occur with a frequency of 44% to 64% in patients with clefts. In general, the more malformations that occur together with orofacial clefting, the lower the birth weight (Cohen, 1978, 2000; Cohen and Bankier, 1991; Hagberg et al., 1997; Källén et al., 1996).

SYNDROMES, SEQUENCES, AND ASSOCIATIONS

Syndromology is a broad and diverse field of endeavor spanning almost all areas of medicine. Approximately 1% of all newborns have multiple anomalies, or syndromes. Of these, about 40% can be diagnosed as having specific, recognized syndromes. The other 60% have unknown entities that need to be further delineated. Although many syndromes are individually rare, in the aggregate they constitute a significant portion of medicine (Cohen, 1997b). Many syndromes with orofacial clefting are known (Cohen, 1978; Cohen and Bankier, 1991).

Syndromes are composed of multiple malformations. A particular malformation can be minimally or maximally expressed. For example, bifid uvula is a minimal expression of cleft palate. More complex malformations also can be minimally or maximally expressed, as exemplified by holoprosencephaly and its attendant facial dysmorphism (Fig. 6.1).

A *syndrome* can be defined as a pattern of multiple anomalies thought to be pathogenetically related and not representing a sequence. In contrast, a *sequence* can be defined as a pattern of multiple anomalies derived from a single known or presumed prior anomaly or mechanical factor. In a syndrome, the level of understanding of a pathogenetically related set of anomalies is usually lower than in a sequence, in which the initiating event and the cascading of secondary events are frequently known. A syndrome commonly, but not always, implies a unitary etiology, e.g., del(4p) syndrome; a sequence commonly has multiple causes, e.g., oligohydramnios sequence (Cohen, 1997b; Spranger et al., 1982).

A true malformation syndrome is characterized by embryonic pleiotropy in which a pattern of developmentally *unrelated* malformation sequences occurs, i.e., the malformations that make up the syndrome occur in embryonically *noncontiguous* areas. They are not related to one another at the descriptive embryonic level; at a more basic level, the malformations have, or are

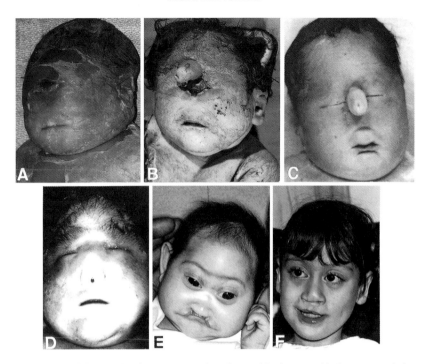

FIG. 6.1. Spectrum of dysmorphic faces associated with variable degrees of holoprosencephaly. *A:* Cyclopia without proboscis formation. Note single central eye. *B:* Cyclopia with proboscis. *C:* Ethmocephaly. *D:* Cebocephaly. Ocular hypotelorism with single-nostril nose. *E:* Median cleft lip, flat nose, and ocular hypotelorism. *F:* Ocular hypotelorism and surgically repaired cleft lip. (*A–D, F* from Cohen et al., 1971. *E* from DeMyer and Zeman, 1963. Montage from Cohen 1997b, with permission.)

presumed to have, a common cause and are thus pathogenetically related. The difference between a malformation sequence and a malformation syndrome is diagrammed in Figure 6.2. When holoprosencephaly occurs alone, it is a malformation sequence, but when it occurs with multiple noncontiguous anomalies, such as in trisomy 13 syndrome or with multiple noncontiguous anomalies in the autosomal recessively inherited Meckel syndrome, it is a malformation syndrome composed of several malformation sequences (Cohen, 1997b).

Because malformations can be relatively simple or complex, the later a defect is initiated, the simpler the malformation, and the earlier during organogenesis that a defect is initiated, the more far-reaching the consequences. The primary defect sets off a chain of secondary and tertiary events, resulting in what appear to be multiple anomalies. In holoprosencephaly, the embryonic forebrain fails to cleave sagittally into cerebral hemispheres, transversely into telencephalon and diencephalon, and horizontally into olfactory and optic bulbs. Holoprosencephaly varies in severity. At the mild end of the spectrum is simple absence of the olfactory tracts and bulbs. Holoprosencephaly is associated with facial dysmorphism, which also varies from mild to severe expression (Fig. 6.1). A single eye or closely set

eyes, proboscis formation, single-nostril nose, flattened nose, median cleft lip, or lateral cleft lip may be observed variably or in combination. All malformations encountered trace their origin developmentally to a single primary defect in morphogenesis thought to be an abnormality in the prechordal mesoderm (Cohen, 1997b).

Although median cleft lip may occur with holoprosencephaly, cases occur without holoprosencephaly (Fig. 6.3). In holoprosencephaly with median cleft lip, the head circumference is dramatically reduced,[a] but when median cleft lip occurs without holoprosencephaly, the head circumference is within two standard deviations of the mean and normotelorism is the rule. Median cleft lip, reasonable head circumference, and normotelorism predict lack of holoprosencephaly. The distinction is important clinically and surgically because survival is the rule, necessitating surgical cleft lip repair. However, some degree of mental deficiency can accompany such cases (Cohen, 2000).

An *association* can be defined as a nonrandom occurrence of several anomalies in two or more individuals. An association cannot be reduced to a sequence or syndrome. For example, orofacial clefting is associ-

[a]Except in those few cases that are accompanied by hydrocephalus.

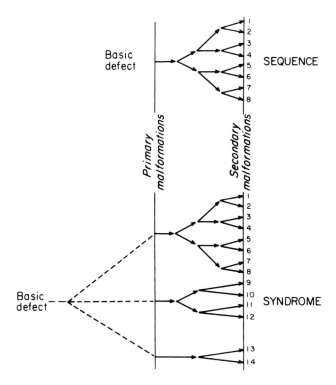

FIG. 6.2. Comparison of a malformation sequence *(top)* with a true malformation syndrome *(bottom)*. Isolated holoprosencephaly is an example of a malformation sequence. The combination of holoprosencephaly, ventricular septal defect, and polydactyly caused by trisomy 13 is a malformation syndrome. (From Cohen, 1997b, with permission.)

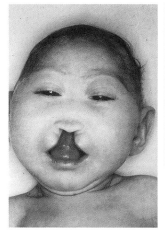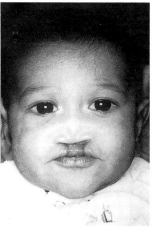

FIG. 6.3. Median cleft lip with holoprosencephaly *(left)*, note microcephaly, without holoprosencephaly *(right)*, note normal head circumference. (From Cohen, 2001, with permission.)

tion with the most learned colleagues in the field (Cohen, 1997b).

An example of a provisionally unique-pattern syndrome (Figs. 6.4–6.6) consists of a dysmorphic face with a prominent square forehead and Robin sequence,

ated with congenital heart defects more commonly than expected by chance. Cleft lip-palate is also associated with neural tube defects more commonly than expected by chance. However, when cleft palate occurs with a basilar encephalocele that herniates through the sphenoid bone, the cleft palate occurs on a mechanical basis.

SYNDROME DELINEATION

The process of syndrome delineation can be divided into the following stages: *(1)* unknown-genesis syndromes, including provisionally unique-pattern syndromes and recurrent-pattern syndromes, and *(2)* known-genesis syndromes, including pedigree syndromes, chromosomal syndromes, biochemical-defect syndromes, and environmentally induced syndromes (Cohen, 1997b).

In an unknown-genesis syndrome, the cause is simply not known. In a provisionally unique-pattern syndrome, several anomalies are observed in the same patient such that the clinician does not recognize the overall pattern of defects from his or her own experience, from searching the literature, or from consulta-

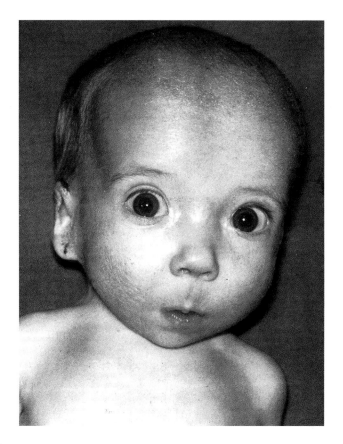

FIG. 6.4. Provisionally unique-pattern syndrome. Dysmorphic face with Robin sequence. (From Martsolf et al., 1977, with permission.)

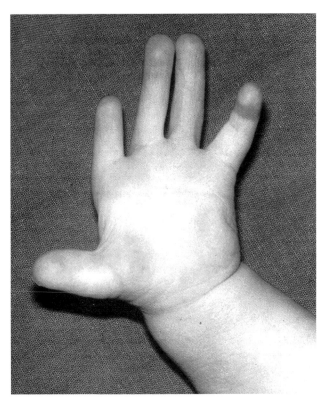

FIG. 6.5. Provisionally unique-pattern syndrome. Broad proximally placed thumb, hypoplasia of third and fifth middle phalanges, and absence of middle phalanx of index finger. (From Martsolf et al., 1977, with permission.)

broad proximally placed thumbs, hypoplasia of the third and fifth middle phalanges, absent middle phalanges in the second fingers, broad halluces, postaxial polydactyly, rhizomelic short stature, and radiographic abnormalities of the spine and pelvis (Martsolf et al., 1997).

Most likely, the anomalies in this provisionally unique-pattern syndrome have a common cause, though unknown, rather than different causes acting independently. The probability that such anomalies occur in the same patient by chance becomes less likely the more anomalies the patient has and the rarer these anomalies occur individually in the general population (Cohen, 1997b).

Obviously, if a second example of the syndrome comes to light, the condition is no longer unique. A provisionally unique-pattern syndrome is a one-of-a-kind syndrome to a particular observer at a particular point in time. There may be a nineteenth century description of a similar instance that escapes his or her attention. There may also be some instances of the syndrome in different parts of the world that remain as yet unrecognized. Thus, many syndromes appear to be unique at the time the ini-

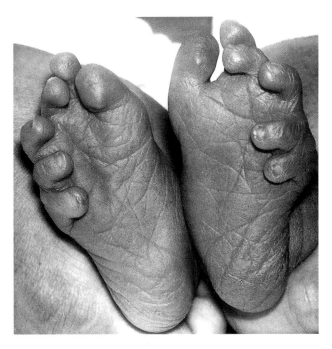

FIG. 6.6. Provisionally unique-pattern syndrome. Postaxial hexadactyly and abnormal toes. (From Martsolf et al., 1977, with permission.)

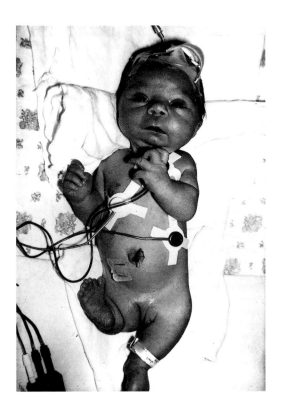

FIG. 6.7. Recurrent-pattern syndrome. Catel-Manzke syndrome with micrognathia (Robin sequence), ventricular septal defect, and talipes equinovarus.

tial patient is discovered but are no longer unique when two or more examples become known (Cohen, 1997b).

A recurrent-pattern syndrome can be defined as a similar or identical set of anomalies in two or more unrelated patients (Cohen, 1997b). An example is the Catel-Manzke syndrome, consisting of a globular cranium, Robin sequence, clinodactyly of the index finger with a supernumerary proximal phalanx in the index finger, congenital heart defects (50%), particularly ventricular septal defect, and talipes equinovarus (Gorlin et al., 1990) (Figs. 6.7–6.11).

The same abnormalities in two or more patients suggest, but do not prove, that the pathogenesis may be the same. At the recurrent-pattern stage of syndrome delineation, the etiology is still not known. In general, the validity of a recurrent-pattern syndrome increases with the more abnormalities found in the condition and the more patients recognized as having the syndrome (Cohen, 1997b). About 25 cases of Catel-Manzke syndrome have been described, mostly in males but several females have also been noted (Figs. 6.7–6.11). Although a few examples of famil-

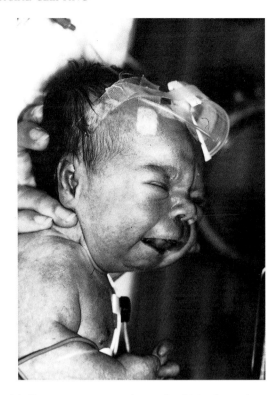

FIG. 6.9. Recurrent-pattern syndrome. Catel-Manzke syndrome. Micrognathia (Robin sequence).

ial aggregation have been reported, no pattern of inheritance has been discerned. Most cases are sporadic, and the syndrome is still of the recurrent-pattern type.

At the recurrent-pattern stage of syndrome delineation, the number of findings is usually expanded as the number of patients increases. However, because the etiology remains unknown at this time, other examples

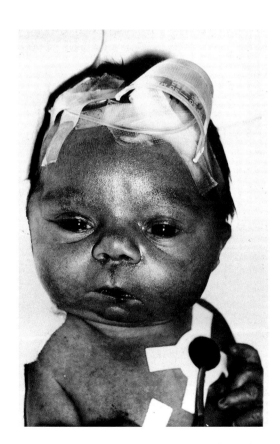

FIG. 6.8. Recurrent-pattern syndrome. Catel-Manzke syndrome. Micrognathia (Robin sequence).

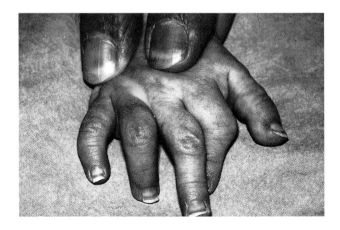

FIG. 6.10. Recurrent-pattern syndrome. Catel-Manzke syndrome. Marked clinodactyly of right index finger.

58 BASIC PRINCIPLES

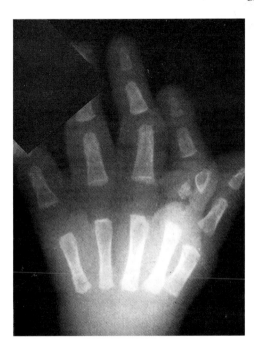

FIG. 6.11. Recurrent-pattern syndrome. Catel-Manzke syndrome. Radiograph of left hand showing extra bone at base of proximal phalanx of index finger.

of the syndrome tend to be selected because they most closely resemble the first case. This results in an artificial homogeneity of cases that emphasizes the most severe aspects of the syndrome. Thus, we should be wary of estimated frequencies given in review articles and textbooks for various anomalies that occur in a recurrent-pattern syndrome; they tend to be overestimates that can affect the prognostic risk counseling for possibly developing some features of the syndrome such as mental retardation (Cohen, 1997b).

A known-genesis syndrome can be defined as several anomalies causally related on the basis of *(1)* occurrence in the same family or, less conclusively, the same mode of inheritance in different families; *(2)* a chromosomal defect; *(3)* a specific defect in an enzyme or structural protein; or *(4)* an environmental factor. The term *pedigree syndrome* refers to known genesis on the basis of pedigree evidence alone; the basic defect itself remains undefined, although the condition is known to represent a monogenic disorder. Several examples with orofacial clefts include the autosomal recessively inherited Meckel syndrome and oral–facial–digital syndrome I, which has X-linked dominant inheritance, lethal in the male. Chromosomal syndromes, such as trisomy 13 syndrome, are cytogenetically determined. In a biochemical-defect syndrome, specific enzymatic defects are known in recessive syndromes. An example is the autosomal recessive Smith-Lemli-Opitz syn-

drome. An environmentally induced syndrome is defined in terms of the environmental factor or causative teratogen, such as diphenylhydantoin syndrome (Cohen, 1997b).

COMMENTS ON THE PROCESS OF SYNDROME DELINEATION

The process of syndrome delineation is summarized in Figure 6.12. Generally, a syndrome can be placed into one of the categories previously discussed. Occasionally, a syndrome may be delineated in one step, thus bypassing several of the stages mentioned earlier. For example, if a new chromosomal abnormality is discovered during the laboratory investigation of a patient clinically defined as having a provisionally unique-pattern syndrome, the patient represents a known-genesis syndrome of the chromosomal type in a one-step delineation. However, the variability of the clinical expression must await the discovery of more patients. In other instances, such as a large dominant pedigree with many affected individuals, a known-genesis syndrome of the pedigree type and much of its phenotypic variability can be determined in one step (Cohen, 1997b).

Provisionally unique-pattern syndromes occur with some frequency. Further delineation will often occur, given sufficient time. A truly unique-pattern syndrome may occur with a chromosomal anomaly involving two or more breaks. The condition may be sporadic or segregate within a family. Since the chance of an identical duplication-deficiency syndrome occurring in another family is very slight, the syndrome may be considered unique to an affected individual or an affected family (Cohen, 1997b).

The multiple anomalies that make up any syndrome are thought to be pathogenetically related. However, anomalies may concur either by chance or as a statistically related association in the same patient. Some associations are well-stocked pools for future syndrome delineation (Cohen, 1997b).

Syndrome delineation and the use of the delineation terms proposed should be thought of as a dynamic,

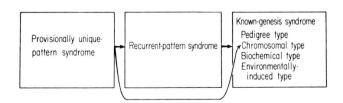

FIG. 6.12. Summary of the process of syndrome delineation. See text. (From Cohen, 1997b, with permission.)

flexible, and continually changing framework in which to view various syndromes. These categories should never be thought of as static or immutable, even at the higher stages of syndrome delineation. Etiologic and clinical heterogeneity is common and should be expected to occur even when not readily apparent. Moreover, we should not confuse syndrome delineation with understanding of the syndrome's pathogenesis, even at the higher stages of delineation. In a pedigree syndrome such as the autosomal recessively inherited Meckel syndrome, we know nothing about how the homozygous state of the Meckel gene produces such diverse features as encephalocele, orofacial clefting, polydactyly, and polycystic kidneys (Cohen, 1997b).

SIGNIFICANCE OF SYNDROME DELINEATION

The significance of syndrome delineation cannot be overestimated. As an unknown-genesis syndrome becomes delineated, its phenotypic spectrum, its natural history, and its inheritance pattern or risk of recurrence become known, allowing for better patient care and family counseling. If the phenotypic spectrum is known, the clinician can search for suspected defects that may not be immediately apparent but that may produce clinical problems at a later date, such as a hemivertebra in Goldenhar syndrome. If a certain complication can occur in a given syndrome, such as Wilms tumor in Beckwith-Wiedemann syndrome, the clinician is forewarned to monitor the patient for possible development of neoplasia. Finally, if the recurrence risk is known, the parents can be counseled properly about future pregnancies. This is particularly important if the risk is high and the disorder is severely disabling or disfiguring, has mental deficiency as one component, or has a dramatically shortened life span. For example, Stickler syndrome is an autosomal dominant disorder with a 50% recurrence risk when one parent is affected. Retinal detachment occurs in 20% of reported cases, and blindness affects 15%. Genetic counseling is important because the risk of developing serious ocular problems is high. This relatively common condition also illustrates the importance of syndrome delineation because the entity was unrecognized before 1965, although clearly it existed before then. Thus, syndrome delineation fosters good patient care. The overall treatment program gains rationality. In contrast, with a provisionally unique-pattern syndrome, the treatment program and overall management frequently leave something to be desired (Cohen, 1997b).

SYNDROME NOMENCLATURE

In general, a newly recognized syndrome can be denoted by *(1)* an eponym, *(2)* one or more striking features, *(3)* an acronym, *(4)* a numeral, *(5)* a geographic term, or *(6)* some combination of the above. None of these systems of nomenclature is without fault. Each has advantages and disadvantages. In general, nomenclature usage evolves with time. Sometimes international working groups are very helpful in standardizing nomenclature in various subfields (Cohen, 1976).

Mythical terms such as *elfin facies syndrome* and animal nomenclature such as *bird-headed dwarf* are pejorative and should be discouraged. One commonly recognized principle in the field is never to use apostrophe *s* in eponymic designations. Thus, we use Apert syndrome, not Apert's syndrome, because Apert neither had nor owned the syndrome he described (Cohen, 1976, 1997a,b).

PACE OF SYNDROME DELINEATION

Syndrome delineation is proceeding at a very rapid pace. Table 6.1 illustrates syndrome delineation through the years with respect to orofacial clefting. Toriello (1988) has estimated that newly recognized syndromes in general are being described at the rate of one or more per week and, although some represent variable expression of previously recorded conditions, many actually represent newly recognized syndromes.

Orofacial clefting is estimated for the years 1971, 1978, and 1990 in Table 6.1 (Cohen and Bankier, 1991). The 1990 estimate is based on the POSSUM

TABLE 6.1. *Syndrome Delineation Involving Orofacial Clefting*

Etiology	1971*	1978†	1990‡
Monogenic	39	79	193
Autosomal dominant	17	35	69
Autosomal recessive	18	39	104
X-linked	4	5	20
Environmentally induced	0	6	10
Chromosomal	15	29	49
Unknown cause§	18	40	90
Total	72	154	342

*Based on Gorlin et al. (1971).
†Based on Cohen (1978).
‡Based on POSSUM (1990).
§Includes distinctive syndromes of unknown genesis and associations.
Source: Cohen and Bankier (1991).

TABLE 6.2. *Genetic Aspects of Some Syndromes with Clefting*

Syndrome	Gene Map Locus	Comments
Van der Woude syndrome	1q32-q41	Autosomal dominant 17p11.1-p11.2 inheritance. Gene maps to 1q32-q41. One large Brazilian family maps to 17p11.1-p11.2. Either the syndrome is genetically heterogeneous or the gene at both loci works synergistically, 17p11.1-p11.2 increasing the risk of cleft lip with or without cleft palate.
Treacher Collins syndrome	5q32-q33.1	*Treacle* gene mutations cause premature termination of the protein.
del(22q11.2) syndrome*	22q11.2	Disruption of gene *UFD1L* alone or in combination with gene *CDC45L* and/or *HIRA* has been suggested as the most likely etiology, and the role of the dHand-UFD1L pathway has been discussed. However, many patients do not have mutations in these genes. Thus, the genetic etiology is not resolved at present.
X-linked cleft palate with or without ankyloglossia	(1) Xq21.3-q22	Genetically heterogeneous. (1) is found in German and Icelandic families.
	(2) Xq13-q21.31	(2) is found in British Columbia families.

*Formerly known as velocardiofacial syndrome, DiGeorge syndrome, or conotruncal anomalies/face syndrome. Data from Cohen (1997b, 2000), Gorlin et al. (1990), Murray (1995), Novelli et al. (1999), Saitta et al. (1999), Schutte et al. (1999), Srivastava and Yamagishi (1999), Wulfsberg et al. (1997), and Yamagishi et al. (1999).
Source: Cohen (2000).

computer based system. POSSUM (1990) is a computer program that provides an extensive catalogue of multiple anomaly syndromes, including photographs (on video disk) and references. The POSSUM estimate is compared with those of Cohen (1978) and Gorlin et al. (1971). The category "unknown cause" in Table 6.1 includes *distinctive* syndromes of unknown genesis and various simple associations.

Syndromes with orofacial clefting have been reviewed by Gorlin et al. (2001). Genetic aspects of a few syndromes are summarized in Table 6.2, and some teratogenic syndromes with occasional clefting are shown in Table 6.3.

ROBIN SEQUENCE AND ROBIN COMPLEXES

In a classic article titled "Not All Dwarfed Mandibles Are Alike," the late Samuel Pruzansky (1969) observed that "Pierre Robin syndrome" (as he and others called it in those days) was not only causally heterogeneous but also pathogenetically and phenotypically variable.

Shprintzen (1988) showed that by using different definitions of Robin sequence proposed by various authors, he could calculate different frequencies of syndromic and nonsyndromic Robin sequence in his own hospital series. Different criteria for Robin sequence are summarized in Table 6.4. Definitions I through IV are

TABLE 6.3. *Some Human Teratogenic Syndromes**

Teratogen	Use	Teratogenic Effects	Frequency of Orofacial Clefting
Ethyl alcohol	Recreational use or alcohol dependence	Growth retardation, small palpebral fissures, facial dysmorphism, microcephaly, mental deficiency, cardiovascular defects	Occasional
Diphenylhydantoin	Antiseizure drug	Growth retardation, facial dysmorphism, microcephaly, mental deficiency, hypoplastic nails	Occasional
Trimethadione	Antiseizure drug	Developmental delay, growth deficiency, V-shaped eyebrows, ear anomalies, cardiovascular defects	Occasional
Retinoids	Drugs to treat cystic acne	Abortion, craniofacial dysmorphism, various central nervous system abnormalities	Occasional
Aminopterin Methotrexate	Folic acid antagonist, has been used as an abortifacient	Abortion hydrocephalus, growth retardation, mental deficiency, craniofacial dysmorphism, limb defects	Occasional
Hyperthermia	From heat source such as fever, sauna	Neural tube defects, occasional other central nervous system abnormalities, mental deficiency	Occasional

*Data from Cohen (1997b).
Source: Cohen (2000).

TABLE 6.4. *Defining Robin Sequence Using Different Criteria*

Definition	Mandibular Deficiency	Cleft Palate*	Upper Airway Obstruction
I	+	+(U)	+
II	+	+(U or V)	+
III	+	+(U)	−
IV	+	±(U or V)	±
V (non-Robin)	−[†]	+(V)	+

*U, U-shaped cleft palate; V, V-shaped cleft palate.
[†]Mandible is normal but maybe slightly small subjectively, though it is impossible to be certain.
Source: Cohen (1997b).

clearly Robin sequence, but definition V is *non-Robin* in type. The cleft palate is V-shaped, and by polysomnography, some respiratory compromise is evident. The mandible is normal but *may be slightly small subjectively, though it is impossible to be certain.* Thus, at the interface, it is not always possible to distinguish between Robin sequence and ordinary cleft palate (Cohen, 1997b, 2000).

Shprintzen (1988) demonstrated that different mechanisms of obstruction can occur within the same syndrome and noted that glossoptosis is frequently not the cause of upper airway obstruction in some cases. Types of obstruction based on Sher (1992) are summarized in Table 6.5. Kreiborg and Cohen (1996) documented the growth pattern in Robin patients and found that catch-up growth was partial, never complete.

Because of etiologic, pathogenetic, and phenotypic differences, Robin sequence or Robin complexes of various types can occur. Table 6.6 summarizes several conditions with mandibular differences, cranial base angle changes, and different types of respiratory compromise. These changes are shown in Figure 6.13. Double lines indicate general causes: malformation, deformation, or connective tissue dysplasia. Thick arrows

indicate Robin sequence. Thin lines show possible ways that Robin complexes can occur (Cohen, 1999).

A distinction is made between micrognathia and retrognathia (Fig. 6.13). Micrognathia refers to size, retrognathia to position. In Treacher Collins syndrome, the mandible is short. In deletion 22q11.2 syndrome, the mandible is essentially normal in size but retrognathia in position because the cranial base angle is larger than normal (Table 6.6). Most Robin conditions are micrognathic or retrognathic but not both together (so-called "microretrognathia") (Cohen, 1999). Different results were found by Glander and Cisneros (1992), but their results may be questioned. These authors compared del(22q11.2) with Robin in Stickler dysplasia. No controls from the general population or from first-degree relatives were provided. Furthermore, with multiple measurements on each cephalogram, confidence intervals would have produced a more meaningful interpretation than *t*-tests of significance.

Phenotypic variability (Table 6.6) is illustrated by comparing the mandible in Treacher Collins syndrome with that found in deformational Robin sequence (Cohen, 1999). In both conditions, the mandibles are short. Catch-up growth in deformational Robin sequence is incomplete. Mandibular growth is severely affected in Treacher Collins syndrome. The two conditions differ greatly in shape; the Treacher Collins syndrome mandible is highly specific (Cohen, 1999; Kreiborg and Cohen, 1996).

Different Robin complexes are exemplified by del(22q11.2) syndrome and spondyloepiphyseal dysplasia congenita (Table 6.6). In del(22q11.2) syndrome, retrognathia, caused by an obtuse cranial base angle, and cleft palate, either submucous or true, are found. The flat cranial base angle and retrognathia do not contribute to pharyngeal obstruction, which in fact results from hypotonia (Arvystas and Shprintzen, 1984). Robin sequence does not occur. Rather, in this form of Robin complex, all of the manifestations are causally, but not sequentially, related (Cohen, 1999).

TABLE 6.5. *Types of Obstruction in Robin Sequence/Complex (n = 52)*

	True Glossoptosis	Tongue Retracts Posteriorly with Velum Interposed between Tongue and Posterior Pharyngeal Wall	Medial Movement of Lateral Pharyngeal Wall	Pharynx Constricts in Sphincteric Manner
Stickler syndrome	15	6	1	0
22q11 syndrome	4	0	1	1
Treacher Collins syndrome	3	0	1	1
Isolated Robin	5	1	0	0
Other	4	4	2	3

Source: Sher (1992).

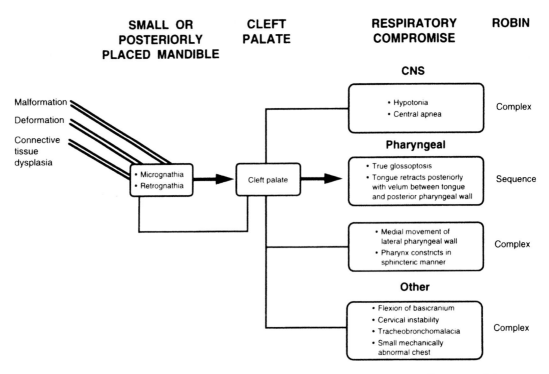

FIG. 6.13. Robin sequence and complexes. *Double lines* indicate general causes: malformation, deformation, or connective tissue dysplasia. *Thick arrows* indicate Robin sequence. *Thin lines* show all possible ways that Robin sequence can occur. (From Cohen, 1999, with permission.)

TABLE 6.6. *Robin Sequences and Complexes*

Condition (Sequence or Complex)	Cause	Mandible	Cranial Base Angle	Respiratory Compromise
Malformation				
Treacher Collins syndrome (mandibulo-facial dysostosis) (sequence)	Mutations in *TCOF1* (gene map location: 5q32-q33.1)	Short body, short ramus, characteristic shape, growth severely affected	Decreased	Pharyngeal
del(22q11.2) syndrome* (complex)	del(22q11.2)	Retrognathia, essentially normal in shape	Increased	Hypotonia
Deformation (sequence)	Intrauterine constraint	Short body, short ramus, increased gonial angle, incomplete catch-up growth	Decreased	Pharyngeal
Connective tissue dysplasia				
Stickler dysplasia (complex)	Heterogeneous; mutations in *COL2A1* (gene map location: 12q13.1-q13.3) (protein: type II collagen)	Short ramus, antegonial notching	Decreased	Pharyngeal
	Mutations in *COL11A1* (gene map location: 6p21.3) (protein: type XI collagen)			
Spondyloepiphyseal dysplasia congenita (complex)	Mutations in *COL2A1* (gene map location: 12q13.1-q13.3)	Short body	—	Small mechanically abnormal chest and/or tracheobronchomalacia and/or cervical instability (resulting in central apnea)

*Formerly known as "velocardiofacial syndrome," "DiGeorge syndrome," or "conotruncal anomalies/face syndrome."
Source: Cohen (1999).

An example of multiple mechanisms of respiratory compromise can be found in spondyloepiphyseal dysplasia congenita (Table 6.6): small mechanically abnormal chest, tracheobronchomalacia, and/or central apnea due to cervical or medullary compression caused by cervical instability (Harding et al., 1990) in addition to the possibility of upper respiratory obstruction based on Robin sequence.

UNUSUAL CRANIOFACIAL CLEFTS AND THE TESSIER CLASSIFICATION

Tessier (1976) outlined an anatomic and descriptive classificatory system in which the various types of bony and soft tissue defects, which he called clefts, are situated along definite axes with numbers assigned to the sites of clefting, depending on their relationships to the sagittal midline (Fig. 6.14). Clefting may involve bone and/or soft tissue but rarely to the same extent. From the sagittal midline to the infraorbital foramen, abnormalities of soft tissue predominate. From the infraorbital foramen to the temporal bone, however, osseous defects are more severe than those of soft tissue, a notable exception being the ear. Clefts through the orbit use the lower eyelid as an equator. Cleft numbered lines may be either northbound (cranial) or southbound (facial). Cranial numbered lines have facial numbered counterparts, yet these numbers are different to avoid the implication that they necessarily have the same etiopathogenesis. Thus, the Tessier classification permits description of both the location and the extent of unusual facial clefts. Several different types of Tessier clefts may occur in the same patient (Fig. 6.15).

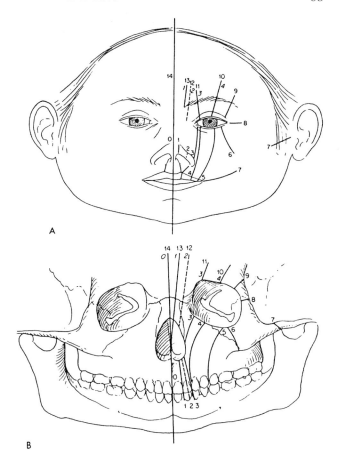

FIG. 6.14. Tessier craniofacial clefting system. *A:* Soft tissue clefts. *B:* Bony clefts. *Dotted lines* represent uncertain localization or uncertain clefting. Note that northbound cranial line has a different number from southbound facial line. Thus, system is descriptive and anatomic and avoids etiologic or pathogenetic speculation. For example, the cause of a number 10 cleft may be different from the cause of a number 4 cleft. (From Cohen, 1999, with permission.)

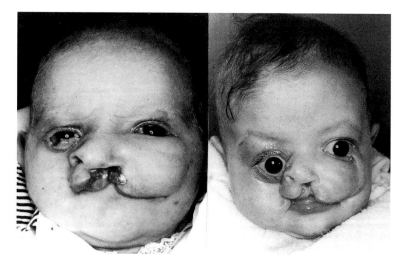

FIG. 6.15. Multiple clefts. *Left:* Cleft lip with Tessier number 7 cleft on left side and cleft numbers 5 and 6 on right. *Right:* Cleft lip and palate with Tessier number 6 cleft on left side and number 4 cleft on right. Courtesy of A. Richieri-Costa (Bauru, Brazil).

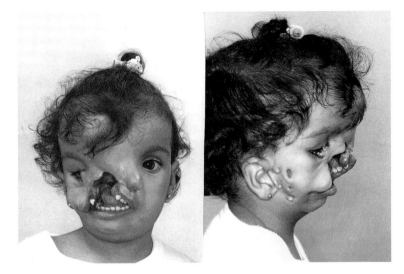

FIG. 6.16. Complex clefting. Hairline indicator points to cleft area. Computed tomographic scan showed anterior cranium bifidum occultum and gap in sphenoid bone. Note ear tags. Courtesy of A. Richieri-Costa (Bauru, Brazil).

In some instances, overlying soft tissue defects predict the possibility of underlying bony clefts. Elsewhere I have referred to such features (e.g., colobomatous notching of the upper or lower eyelids or the nostrils or interruption of the eyelashes or the eyebrows) as Tessier signs (Cohen, 1997b). Also included in this category are hairline indicators that may point to the cleft (Moore et al., 1988) (Fig. 6.16).

The causes of most Tessier clefts are unknown. The overwhelming majority occur sporadically. One exception is Treacher Collins syndrome, which is autosomal dominantly inherited. Some Tessier clefts are malformations that can be explained by faulty embryogenesis. However, others represent disruptions, such as those associated with amniotic bands (Cohen, 1997b).

REFERENCES

Arvystas, M, Shprintzen, RJ (1984). Craniofacial morphology in the velocardiofacial syndrome. J Craniofac Genet Dev Biol 4: 39–45.
Cohen, MM, Jr (1976). Syndrome designations. J Med Genet 13: 266–270.
Cohen, MM, Jr (1978). Syndromes with cleft lip and palate. Cleft Palate J 15: 306–328.
Cohen, MM, Jr (1997a). Apert syndrome, not Apert's syndrome: Apert neither had nor owned the syndrome that bears his name. Plast Reconstr Surg 100: 532–533.
Cohen, MM, Jr (1997b). The Child with Multiple Birth Defects. New York: Oxford University Press.
Cohen, MM, Jr (1999). Robin sequences and complexes: causal heterogeneity and pathogenetic variability. Am J Med Genet 84: 311–315.
Cohen, MM, Jr (2000). Etiology and pathogenesis of orofacial clefting. In: Cleft Lip and Palate: A Physiological Approach, Oral and Maxillofacial Surgery Clinics of North America vol. 12. pp. 379–397.
Cohen, MM, Jr (2001). Perspectives on craniofacial anomalies, syndromes, and other disorders. In: Craniofacial Surgery: A Multi-Disciplinary Approach to Craniofacial Anomalies, edited by K. Y. Lin, R. C. Ogle, and J. A. Jane, 2002, Chapter 1, pp. 1–38.
Cohen, MM, Jr, Bankier, A (1991). Syndrome delineation involving orofacial clefting. Cleft Palate-Craniofac J 28: 119–120.
Cohen, MM, Jr, Jirasek, JE, Guzman, RT, Gorlin, RJ, Peterson, MQ (1971). Holoprosencephaly and facial dysmorphia: nosology, etiology and pathogenesis. Birth Defects 7(7): 125–135.
DeMyer, WE, Zeman, W (1963). Alobar holoprosencephaly (arhinencephaly) with median cleft lip and palate: clinical, electroencephalographic and nosologic considerations. Confin Neurol 23: 1–36.
Glander, K II, Cisneros, GJ (1992). Comparison of the craniofacial characteristics of two syndromes associated with the Pierre-Robin sequence. Cleft Palate Craniofac J 29: 210–219.
Gorlin, RJ, Cervenka, J, Pruzansky, S (1971). Facial clefting and its syndromes. Birth Defects 7(7): 3–49.
Gorlin, RJ, Cohen, MM, Jr, Hennekam, RCM (2001). Syndromes of the Head and Neck, 4th ed. New York: Oxford University Press.
Gorlin, RJ, Cohen, MM, Jr, Levin, LS (1990). Syndromes of the Head and Neck, 3rd ed. New York: Oxford University Press.
Hagberg, C, Larson, O, Milerad, J (1997). Incidence of cleft lip and palate and risks of additional malformations. Cleft Palate-Craniofac J 35: 40–45.
Harding, CO, Green, CG, Perloff, WH (1990). Respiratory complications in children with spondyloepiphyseal dysplasia congenita. Pediatr Pulmonol 9: 49–54.
Källén, B, Harris, J, Robert, E (1996). The epidemiology of orofacial clefts: 2. Associated malformations. J Craniofac Genet Dev Biol 16: 242–248.
Kreiborg, S, Cohen, MM, Jr (1996). Syndrome delineation and growth in orofacial clefting and craniosynostosis. In: Facial Clefts and Craniosynostosis Principles and Management, edited by TA Turvey, KWL Vig, and RJ Fonseca. Philadelphia: WB Saunders, Chapter 3, pp. 57–75.
Martsolf, JT, Reed, MH, Hunter, AGW (1977). Case report 56. Skeletal dysplasia, Robin anomalad, and polydactyly. Syndrome Ident 5(1): 14–18.
Moore, MH, David, DJ, Cooter, RD (1988). Hairline indicators of craniofacial clefts. Plast Reconstr Surg 82: 589–593.

Murray, JC (1995). Face facts: genes, environment, and clefts. Am J Hum Genet 57: 227–232.

Novelli, G, Amati, F, Dallapiccola, G (1999). UFDIL and CDC45L: a role in DiGeorge syndrome and related phenotypes? Trends Genet 15: 251–253.

POSSUM (1990). Computer software system. Melbourne, Australia: Murdoch Institute for Research into Birth Defects.

Pruzansky, S (1969). Not all dwarfed mandibles are alike. Birth Defects 5(2): 120–129.

Saitta, SC, McGrath, JM, Mensch, H, et al. (1999) A 22q11.2 deletion that excludes UFDIL and CDC45L in a patient with conotruncal and craniofacial defects. Am J Hum Genet 65: 562–566.

Schutte, BC, Basart, AM, Watanabe, Y (1999). Microdeletions at chromosome bands 1q32-q41 as a cause of Van der Woude syndrome. Am J Med Genet 84: 145–150.

Sher, AE (1992). Mechanisms of airway obstruction in Robin sequence: implications for treatment. Cleft Palate-Craniofac J 29: 224–231.

Shprintzen, RJ (1988). Pierre Robin, micrognathia, and airway obstruction: the dependency of treatment on accurate diagnosis. Int Anesthesiol Clin 26: 64–71.

Spranger, JW, Benirschke, K, Hall, JG, Lenz, W, Lowry, RB, Opitz, JM, Pinsky, L, Schwarzacher, HG, Smith, DW (1982). Errors of morphogenesis: concepts and terms. J Pediatr 100: 160–165.

Srivastava, D, Yamagishi, H (1999). Role of the dHAND-UFDIL pathway. Trends Genet 15: 253–254.

Tessier, P (1976). Anatomical classifications of facial, craniofacial and laterofacial clefts. J Maxillofac Surg 4: 69–92.

Toriello, HV (1988). New syndromes from old: the role of heterogeneity and variability in syndrome delineation. Am J Med Genet Suppl 1: 50–70.

Wulfsberg, EA, Leana-Cox, J, Neri, C (1997). Reply to "What's in a name? The 22q11.2 deletion" (letter to the editor). Am J Med Genet 72: 248–249.

Yamagishi, H, Garg, V, Matsuoka, R (1999). A molecular pathway revealing a genetic basis for human cardiac and craniofacial defects. Science 283: 1158–1161.

7

Morphometric characteristics of subjects with oral facial clefts and their relatives

RICHARD E. WARD

ELIZABETH S. MOORE

JAMES K. HARTSFIELD, JR.

The relationship between cleft lip and palate (CLP) and facial form is widely recognized, frequently studied, and poorly understood. Thus, after nearly a century of research, it remains uncertain which aspects of facial form are related to the primary underlying cause of the cleft and which aspects are secondary to the effects of the cleft or of its repair. Clearly, complete CLP will distort normal facial growth but so may its later surgical repair. It is also suspected that certain facial shapes are more predisposed to developing CLP than others.

To address these issues, facial form has been evaluated in three distinct groups of subjects: untreated individuals with oral facial clefts, affected individuals with repaired clefts, and unaffected relatives of individuals with clefts. An astonishing number of studies over the last 50 years have examined one or more of these populations and have generated considerable, frequently conflicting information. Variations in methodology, sample composition, and the degree to which the studies have controlled for differences in cleft type and etiology have made it difficult to generalize from this information. We make no pretense of comprehensively reviewing every one of the several hundred articles written on these topics. Instead, in this chapter, we summarize a select group of key publications and extract from them common themes that represent what is known at the start of a new century of research.

More specifically, we review the morphometric methods that have been used to assess facial form in clefts, summarize what is known about facial form in untreated persons as well as individuals who have had their clefts repaired, and finally discuss the current understanding of facial form in unaffected relatives of individuals with clefts. There can be little doubt that we stand on the threshold of a new era of understanding as emerging technologies and a revolution in our knowledge of the interplay between genes and the "environment of development" promise to resolve many of the questions that remain unanswered. Nevertheless, this progress must grow from a foundation established by the work of dentists, physicians, anatomists, anthropologists, and other "morphometricians" who have attempted to penetrate the complexities of this most frequently encountered form of craniofacial anomaly.

MORPHOMETRICS

Morphometrics describes a variety of methods used to measure and assess form. Since its introduction by Broadbent in 1931, the two-dimensional lateral cephalometric radiograph has been the morphometric medium of choice for assessing cranial facial form. Less often, facial measurements have been taken directly *(anthropometrics)* (Farkas and Lindsay, 1971, 1972a,b; Šmahel and Brejcha, 1983; Šmahel, 1984a,b,d; Farkas et al., 1993) or derived from photographs *(photogrammetrics)* (Vegter et al., 1997). More recently, computerized tomography and other forms of three-dimensional radiography (Baumrind et al., 1983;

Cheverud et al., 1983; Grayson et al., 1983, 1985; Savara et al., 1985; Ras et al., 1994a,b) have augmented these methods.

Data derived from any of these methods must be adjusted mathematically so that individuals of different ages, sizes, and sexes can be compared. To create equations that control for size, age, and sex differences, investigators convert original data to standard deviation units (z-scores) or perform regression analysis. However, such adjustments are seldom completely effective. For example, regression equations are sensitive to the variation within the samples from which they are generated, and z-scores must be calculated against some normative or control population that may or may not be well matched to the study population. Therefore, even adjusted data are likely to retain some variation due to age, sex, and size, an often overlooked fact that can confound comparisons of results from different studies.

There is also considerable debate over the efficacy of morphometric techniques derived from fixed but often arbitrarily defined landmarks. For example, Moyers and Bookstein (1979) noted that traditional cephalometrics provides limited or even misleading information regarding the true shape and size of craniofacial structures. Compressing a complex three-dimensional structure into two dimensions distorts form, occludes anatomy, and creates artifacts. Furthermore, two-dimensional measurements cannot reveal differences clearly visible in three dimensions. Analyzing lines and angles to measure the shape and size of such a distorted image compounds the problem. Moyers and Bookstein (1979) noted that the standard measure of mandibular length (gonion to menton) is likely to be highly inaccurate because it uses a straight line to measure a complex, curved surface. Finally, they argue that classic serial cephalometric studies are inadequate because there is little relationship between the superimposed points moving in apparent succession and the actual geometry of growth.

In response to these challenges, new technologies and analytical techniques have been proposed to extract more accurate information from radiographic images. Geometric analytical techniques originally proposed by Thompson (1917) have come of age with the development of computer-assisted programs that are able to carry out the necessary complex equations (Bookstein, 1982; Grayson et al., 1987; Trotman and Ross, 1993; Lestrel et al., 1999). These techniques use geometric forms to assess change in shape over time or to compare form between individuals.

Despite the availability of new technologies and analytical techniques most studies of facial form in clefting continue to rely on traditional cephalometric approaches. It is likely that this reflects less a resistance to innovation and precision than the reality that most investigators do not have ready access to the technology, software, or training necessary to carry out the more sophisticated analyses. Moreover, while the more advanced imaging techniques generate stunningly detailed images, they cost more, increase radiation exposure, and generally lack adequate control or reference data. In addition, many investigators find that traditional analyses continue to yield useful results. Nevertheless, there appears to be little reason to doubt that our understanding of oral facial clefting will improve as we find more effective means to employ these more refined approaches and to couple them with the exploding technologies in developmental and molecular genetics (McAlarney and Chiu, 1997; Mossey et al., 1997; Peltonen and McKusick, 2001).

FACIAL FORM IN INDIVIDUALS WITH ORAL FACIAL CLEFTS

As noted above, inconsistencies in study design, including method of evaluation (judgment vs. measurement), demographics of the patient population, selection of cephalometric or anthropometric landmarks, and methods of statistical analysis, make it difficult to compare results. In addition, as Bishara et al. (1985) and Gaggl et al. (1999) have pointed out, many studies have limitations such as small sample size; inconsistent age distribution; unspecified combinations of untreated, partially treated, and late treated individuals; as well as a mixture of individuals with different types of cleft. Despite the difficulties, we summarize in the following sections relevant morphometric literature and distill common findings regarding the craniofacial phenotype of the various forms of cleft both pre- and posttreatment. The discussion on cleft lip with or without cleft palate (CL/P) and cleft palate (CP) is separated because these are best regarded as etiologically and developmentally distinct anomalies. The review of the CL/P phenotype is divided into sections based on degree of facial disruption, beginning with the most severe (untreated bilateral complete CLP) and proceeding through the least severe (repaired CL without cleft alveolus). Where possible, facial form in untreated individuals is contrasted to that in individuals whose clefts have been repaired. The often confusing use of anatomical landmarks as descriptors has been avoided. Instead, we discuss anatomical areas and what individual measurements reveal about these structures.

Cleft Lip with or without Cleft Palate

Untreated Bilateral Cleft Lip and Palate. The most dramatic effects on facial structures occur in individuals with untreated complete bilateral CLP. Most structural abnormalities are obvious at birth (Huddart, 1970), and some, unless treated, worsen with age. In addition to the anterior facial areas directly affected by the cleft, adjacent and posterior areas (including the neurocranium and cranial base) often deviate from normal morphology.

Neurocranium and cranial base. Smaller craniofacial dimensions have been found in many different cleft types (Dahl, 1970; Ross and Johnston, 1972; Semb, 1991a,b; da Silva Filho et al., 1992; Capelozza Filho et al., 1993), including untreated bilateral cleft patients (da Silva Filho, 1998). In the latter study (da Silva Filho, 1998), there were generally no differences in the cranial base angle compared to controls, in spite of the finding that cranial base linear (sagittal) dimensions were smaller in the untreated CLP group. However, Šmahel et al. (1985) reported that maximum head width was significantly increased in untreated bilateral CLP patients relative to controls (without a cleft).

da Silva Filho et al. (1998) studied a sample of adult (Caucasian) Brazilians with untreated, complete bilateral CLP (20 males and 8 females) and compared these to a matched control, noncleft population. There was a general reduction in cranial and facial size in the untreated group with the means for most linear dimensions significantly reduced compared to controls.

Facial widths. da Silva Filho et al. (1998) reported significantly greater cranial and facial widths, including maximum head width, and bizygomatic, interorbital, and nasal widths. There was a significant sex effect, with males showing greater average mandibular retrognathia and females showing greater average facial convexity. Farkas et al. (1993) found that most untreated bilateral CLP patients had borderline-large to abnormally large facial widths and all had abnormally large nasal widths.

Craniofacial heights and profiles. An extremely prominent premaxilla combined with a smaller mandible results in marked facial convexity and an extreme imbalance between the jaws (Šmahel et al., 1985; da Silva Filho et al., 1998). da Silva Filho et al. (1998) also found significantly greater facial convexity in the untreated group. The bilateral group had a combination of a smaller nasomaxillary–pharyngeal complex and reduced upper posterior facial height (Brader, 1957; Levin, 1963; Dahl, 1970).

Maxillary, palatal, and mandibular structures. In infancy prior to surgery, the overall maxillary size tends to be larger and the maxilla retrognathic (Huddart, 1970). Infants with unrepaired bilateral CLP also appear to have a surprising degree of asymmetry in left and right maxillary arch size (Huddart, 1970). In addition, the premaxilla is rotated and protrusive (Huddart, 1970). The projection of the premaxilla continues if left untreated (Handelman and Pruzansky, 1968; Friede and Pruzansky, 1972; Bishara et al., 1978; da Silva Filho et al., 1998), contributing to the extreme premaxillary prominence that is the most striking feature in adult untreated bilateral CLP patients (da Silva Filho et al., 1998).

The mandible tends to be small and retruded in unrepaired bilateral CLP individuals (Bishara et al., 1985; Dahl et al., 1989; da Silva et al., 1998), a characteristic found in untreated adult patients with other types of cleft (Mars and Houston, 1990; da Silva Filho et al., 1992, 1993). In addition, there is a tendency for the mandibular plane to be steep (Bishara et al., 1985). Most studies have also found that untreated individuals with bilateral CLP have significantly more obtuse gonial angles (Brader, 1957; Levin, 1963; Dahl, 1970; Horowitz et al., 1976, 1980; da Silva Filho et al., 1998).

Dental arches and relationships. Incisors in both jaws tend to be retroclined (da Silva Filho et al., 1998), and the two maxillary segments rotate medially, causing various degrees of arch collapse. Decreased maxillary intercanine width and increased incidence of crossbite in the canine region are found (Bishara et al., 1985). Patients with unoperated CLP tend to have greater maxillary alveolar widths than operated cleft subjects (Motohashi et al., 1994; Trotman et al., 1997).

Untreated Unilateral Cleft Lip and Palate. Individuals with unrepaired unilateral CLP exhibit many of the same features seen in bilateral CLP, such as a tendency for wide nasal cavities (Atherton, 1967a; Farkas et al., 1993), midface retrusion, acute nasaolabial angle, and relatively excessive lower facial height (Dahl, 1970; Bishara et al., 1985, 1986; Šmahel et al., 1985; Mars and Houston, 1990). In addition, individuals with unrepaired unilateral CLP tend to have significantly more obtuse gonial angles as well as a smaller nasomaxillary–pharyngeal complex and reduced upper posterior facial height, as reported in bilateral cases (Brader, 1957; Levin, 1963; Dahl, 1970; Horowitz et al., 1976, 1980).

In general, the cranial base of subjects with unrepaired unilateral CLP is similar to that of controls with the exception of reduced cranial base length (Bishara et al., 1976; Mars and Houston, 1990; Capelozza Filho et al., 1993). In individuals with unilateral CLP, the unoperated maxilla usually maintains a normal relationship to the cranial base, while the premaxilla tends to rotate forward on the noncleft side. In contrast, the mandible is generally rotated backward (retruded), which some researchers have suggested is secondary to the biomechanical effect of the cleft on the mandible (Atherton, 1967b; Dahl, 1970; Chierici et al., 1973; Bishara et al., 1985;

Mars and Houston, 1990; Capelozza Filho et al., 1993). Capelozza Filho et al. (1993) also reported a smaller mandibular body and ramus height in subjects with untreated unilateral CLP. Several researchers have concluded that these subjects also had significant increases in the angle of the mandibular plane (Ortiz-Monasterio et al., 1966; Bishara et al., 1976; Mars and Houston, 1990; Capelozza Filho et al., 1993).

Ortiz-Monasterio et al. (1959) and Mestre et al. (1960) reported that the size of the maxilla in patients with unoperated clefts was within normal limits, while Capelozza Filho et al. (1993) found that the maxilla was smaller and protruded at the alveolar level. Capelozza Filho et al. (1993) employed posterior–anterior cephalograms in their study, while other researchers used lateral cephalograms. This may account for the variability in results. In the maxillary arch, the relationship of the cleft segment to the noncleft segment varied from normal to degrees of medial collapse, particularly in the canine area. This resulted in an increased incidence of crossbite (Atherton, 1967a; Bishara et al., 1976, 1985). There was also an increased incidence of buccal overjet of the maxillary premolars (Bishara et al., 1985). The side of the cleft was not found to cause significant differences in craniofacial morphology in either pre- or postsurgery individuals (Jain and Krogman, 1983a; Hermann et al., 1999, 2000). However, there appeared to be a greater incidence of lingual crossbite on the cleft side compared to individuals with unilateral CL and alveolus but not CP (Bishara et al., 1985). Tang and So (1992) noted that the majority of individuals with unilateral CLP had severe malocclusion at an early age. In two samples of unoperated adults with unilateral CLP, the upper incisors were found to be similar to those of noncleft subjects in one study (Mars and Houston, 1990) and proclined in another (Capelozza Filho et al., 1993).

Repaired Bilateral Cleft Lip and Palate Compared to Repaired Unilateral Cleft Lip and Palate and Noncleft Individuals. Most morphometric studies of bilateral CLP have reported that with treatment the severe facial dysmorphology was greatly improved, although some residual effects remained (Trotman and Ross, 1993). However, several cephalometric studies have reported only minimal differences between subjects who had surgically repaired bilateral clefts and their nonrepaired counterparts (Dahl, 1970; Narula and Ross, 1970; Hanada and Krogman, 1975; Wepner and Hollman, 1975). In general, the facial differences found in the treated bilateral CLP group were similar to those found in treated unilateral CLP (Dahl, 1970; Ishiguro et al., 1976; Šmahel and Brejcha, 1983; Farkas et al., 1993).

Neurocranium, and cranial base. Šmahel (1984b) compared lateral cephalograms of surgically repaired adult males with complete bilateral CLP to unaffected controls as well as surgically repaired adult males with unilateral CLP. In the bilateral CLP group, the height of the neurocranium was reduced, the supraorbital frontal width was increased, and the posterior cranial base was significantly shorter compared to noncleft controls. In comparison to subjects with unilateral CLP, the cranial base was slightly but significantly flatter and the clivus significantly shorter. In a related study on the same group of treated adult males using anthropometrics, Šmahel (1984c) noted that head circumference, head length, head width, and bizygomatic and bitragal (cranial base) widths were not significantly different compared to controls.

There has been less agreement regarding the cranial base in studies of repaired CLP. Aduss (1971) reported that there were no significant differences in the cranial base of patients with unilateral CLP compared with noncleft patients, while Krogman et al. (1975), in a longitudinal study of infants and children, found that all linear cranial base measurements were significantly longer and the cranial base angle was smaller in the unilateral CLP group compared to a noncleft control group. In contrast to both of these studies, Hayashi et al. (1976) reported no significant differences in the length of the anterior cranial base but noted that the cranial base angle was more obtuse in their unilateral CLP group compared to the noncleft group. Horswell and Gallup (1992) found that the age at which the linear dimensions became significantly reduced varied but that, in general, both anterior and posterior dimensions became significantly reduced between ages 8 and 9 (and remained so thereafter). No significant differences were found in the cranial base angle of either the unilateral or bilateral CLP individuals. In contrast, Semb (1991a) noted that cranial base angulation was greater in unilateral CLP subjects when compared to noncleft controls but also found a sex effect, with the angle being significantly greater for affected females compared to affected males. Failure to consider variations due to age and sex may help to explain the lack of agreement in previous studies, as may the use of inappropriate control samples and other variations in methodology (Horswell and Gallup, 1992).

Facial widths. As was the case for untreated individuals, most studies of treated subjects with CLP have described excessive widths across the midface. For example, Šmahel and Brejcha (1983) and Šmahel (1984b) reported a widening of the nasal cavity and the interocular distance in both unilateral and bilateral subjects. In a longitudinal study comparing three different cleft types (bilateral CLP, unilateral CLP, and CP),

Ishiguro et al. (1976) found that, in general, the repaired bilateral CLP group had significantly greater facial breadths than the other two cleft groups or the noncleft group. Athanasiou et al. (1990) found that individuals with repaired bilateral CLP also exhibited increases in nasal and intergonial widths compared to noncleft controls. However, Farkas et al. (1993) suggested that this might not be universal among affected individuals. Using direct anthropometry, they reported that 71% of patients with repaired unilateral CLP had normal soft tissue nasal width, while only 48% of repaired patients with bilateral CLP had normal soft tissue nasal width. Surprisingly, the mean values for these variables did not differ significantly between the two groups. They also noted that individuals with surgically repaired CLP tended to have normal or, in some cases, abnormally narrow bizygomatic width. Part of the difference between the outcomes of the radiographic and direct methods may be that the direct method measures the soft tissue, which may not absolutely correlate with the underlying skeletal structures. On the other hand, an uncritical reliance on group mean values can obscure meaningful differences between study populations.

Craniofacial heights and profiles. Both bilateral and unilateral surgically repaired groups had a combination of a smaller nasomaxillary–pharyngeal complex and reduced upper posterior facial height (Brader, 1957; Levin, 1963; Dahl, 1970; Friede and Johanson, 1974, 1977; Horowitz et al., 1976, 1980; Semb, 1991a,b). In contrast, both groups tended to exhibit relatively excessive anterior lower facial height (Dahl, 1970; Farkas and Lindsay, 1971; Krogman et al., 1975; Ross, 1987; Enemark et al., 1990; Semb, 1991a,b). Krogman et al. (1975) reported that both upper and lower anterior facial heights were increased in unilateral CLP children compared to controls, while Hayashi and colleagues (1976) found that the upper anterior facial height was reduced and the lower anterior facial height was increased, resulting in normal total facial height. Šmahel and Brejcha (1983) supported these findings. In comparison to individuals with unilateral CLP, individuals with bilateral CLP tended to have an increased length of the face as a whole but normal upper facial measurements (Šmahel, 1984b). A midfacial deficit was reported in the sagittal plane in patients with repaired bilateral CLP, as was a moderate reduction in height of the midface in favor of the lower face (Gaggl et al., 1999).

In contrasting repaired unilateral and bilateral CLP groups, the relatively greater increase in facial height in the bilateral cleft group was associated with an even more noticeable posterior growth rotation of the face, retroclination of the palatal plane, and greater retru-sion of the mandible. This was reflected by the significant difference between the angulation of the midface relative to the cranial base in these two series (Šmahel, 1984b). The configuration of the soft tissue profile tended to correspond to its skeletal framework (Šmahel and Brejcha, 1983). Again, however, Farkas and colleagues (1993) demonstrated considerable individual variability in the expression of facial height deviations. They reported that in both unilateral and bilateral CLP groups the anthropometric height of the upper face was normal in two-thirds of individuals, in spite of the differences in mean values for facial height between the CLP and control groups.

Maxillary, palatal, and mandibular structures. In patients with repaired complete bilateral CLP, Narula and Ross (1970) found severe protrusion of the premaxilla at 6 years of age that reduced to almost normal by 16 years of age. They also found superior and posterior positioning of the lateral maxillary segments, although the length of the segments was normal. Similarly, Šmahel and Brejcha, (1983) found that in repaired bilateral cases there was displacement of the premaxilla forward and more marked displacement of the maxilla backward. This caused retrusion of the upper face similar to that found in cases with complete unilateral CLP, although the retrusion of lateral dentoalveolar segments and maxilla was even greater than in individuals with unilateral clefts. In addition, there was posterior displacement of the zygomatic bones and orbits in the repaired bilateral cases that reflected the more posterior positioning of the maxilla (Šmahel and Brejcha 1983; Schultes et al., 2000). Midfacial growth deficiencies and posterior displacement of the upper jaw have been reported in both unilateral and bilateral groups (Ross, 1987; Mars and Houston, 1990; Chen and So, 1997). Several studies have found that the palatal plane was rotated in a clockwise direction in treated CLP subjects (Dahl, 1970; Friede and Johanson, 1974, 1977; Horowitz et al., 1980).

Trotman and Ross (1993) concluded that the greatest effects of growth and treatment on the face of individuals with CLP were in the area of the maxilla. This region was consistently smaller and all its landmarks were located closer to the cranial base, implying a less developed midface and oropharynx. As noted, the premaxilla began in a grossly protruded position in the treated bilateral cases but gradually resolved until the relative protrusion was decreased in the adult. The nasal bones were longer and more protruded relative to the cranial base, and the posterior segments of the maxilla were hypoplastic, as evidenced by their posterior displacement and deficiency (Trotman and Ross, 1993). Gaggl et al. (1999) used cephalometric and model analyses to assess the long-term growth effects of surgical repair and orthodontic treatment in adults with complete bilateral CLP. Compared with standard values, all patients in their study retained a small extent of maxillary retrognathia and retroposition of the midface with a retrognathic type of face.

Schultes et al. (2000) used the same methods to assess the surgical and orthodontic treatment of adults with unilateral CLP or isolated CP. They found that, similar to the bilateral CLP group, the unilateral group had maxillary growth disturbances. On average, the unilateral CLP group had no growth disturbances in the higher midface region.

The maxillary deficiencies associated with surgical repair of CLP are associated with skeletal discrepancies between the upper and lower jaws (Pruzansky and Aduss, 1967; Ross and Johnston, 1972; Nordén et al., 1973; Bergland and Sidhu, 1974; Dahl and Hanusardottir, 1979; Šmahel and Müllerová, 1986). However, Friede and Pruzansky (1972) suggested that it was the palatoplasty and not the lip repair that most affected midfacial development. In their patients with bilateral CLP who had surgical closure of the lip without a premaxillary setback, facial profile measurements in early adolescence approximated those of the averages of noncleft individuals. Other morphometric studies have suggested that surgically induced scar tissue was a major contributing factor to the facial growth problems seen in patients with clefts (Graber 1949, 1954; Ortiz-Monasterio et al., 1959, 1966; Mestre et al., 1960; Glass, 1970; Narula and Ross, 1970; Boo-Chai, 1971; Friede and Pruzansky, 1972).

Trotman and Ross (1993), in their study of individuals with repaired bilateral CLP, suggested that, compared to controls, the main shape differences in the mandible were concentrated at the gonial angle. They found, as had many others, that patients with treated bilateral CLP tended to have a significantly more obtuse gonial angle than noncleft controls (Narula and Ross, 1970; Horowitz et al., 1980; Šmahel, 1984b). Trotman and Ross (1993) also found that the mandibular length was smaller in surgically repaired patients at 6 years of age but not different in adults. In contrast, Narula and Ross (1970) found normal mandibular length in children with bilateral CLP, and Šmahel (1984b) reported that the mandibular length in an adult male study population was significantly shorter than in noncleft controls. Šmahel and Brejcha (1983) found that a higher degree of posterior growth rotation of the mandible was accompanied by an even more marked compensatory increase of the anterior height compared to individuals with unilateral clefts. They also found that subjects with unilateral CLP exhibited deficient mandibular growth, which was associated with changes in its shape, specifically a decrease in gonial angle and

shortening of the mandibular body. Finally, several studies have reported that individuals with repaired complete unilateral CLP tend to have persistent facial asymmetries and nasal deformities (Harvold, 1954; Aduss and Pruzansky, 1967; Dahl, 1970; Mars and Houston, 1990; Molsted and Dahl, 1990; Molsted et al., 1992; Sandham and Murray, 1993; Trotman et al., 1993; Motohashi et al., 1994; Ras et al., 1994b; Kyrkanides et al., 1995).

Dental arches and relationships. Handelman and Pruzansky (1968) noted the presence of a significant overjet by the age of 4 in individuals with complete repaired bilateral CLP; however, Ross and Johnston (1972) found that significant overjet was rare but that 38% of their CLP sample exhibited incisor crossbite. According to Trotman and Ross (1993), the differences reported in the aforementioned studies were likely the result of differences in the surgical management of the two samples. Other differences in dental and arch relationships between individuals with repaired bilateral and unilateral clefts included a more pronounced retroclination of the upper incisors and of the alveolar process in the bilateral group (Šmahel and Brejcha, 1983; Trotman and Ross, 1993). In contrast, Šmahel and Brejcha (1983) noted a tendency toward overeruption of the posterior teeth in individuals with repaired unilateral CLP. They suggested that this could occur as compensatory growth due to the vertical posterior maxillary hypoplasia.

The occlusal plane in surgically repaired CLP appeared not to differ significantly from that of controls (Narula and Ross, 1970; Trotman and Ross, 1993). However, Gaggl et al. (1999) employed model analysis to show that for most patients with repaired CLP either the maxillary or the mandibular arch was too wide and that all had transverse space deficits as well as a reduction in sagittal measurements, even after termination of orthodontic treatment. Interestingly, patients with bilateral CLP tended to possess a better-formed anterior dental arch compared to patients with unilateral CLP or CP. According to Gaggl et al. (1999), sagittal and transverse space deficits in bilateral CLP patients were consistent with the earlier observations reported by Steinhäuser and Rudzki-Janson (1994). A sagittal space deficit was observed in half of the bilateral CLP group studied by Gaggl and colleagues (1999), but positional abnormalities of the upper incisors were rare. The majority of patients with bilateral CLP also had alveolar midline displacement of the maxilla and mandible (Gaggl et al., 1999).

In a similar study of individuals with repaired unilateral CLP, Schultes et al. (2000) noted that an even higher percentage of patients had a negative sagittal space available compared to individuals with bilateral

CLP (88% vs. 50%, respectively). In most cases with unilateral CLP, there was a reduction in sagittal length, implying a sagittal space deficit. This may reflect the reduction of maxillary growth in an anteroposterior direction that has been reported in other CLP types (Bishara et al., 1979; da Silva Filho et al., 1998; Mars and Houston, 1990). Schultes et al. (2000) also found a unilateral persistent transverse space deficit in the premolar and molar regions (also reported by Bishara et al., 1985).

Cleft Lip with or without Cleft Alveolus

Most researchers agree that the craniofacial morphology of individuals with cleft lip with or without cleft alveolus (CL/A) is very similar to that found in noncleft controls (Dahl, 1970; Nakamura et al., 1972; Hirschfeld and Aduss, 1974; Cronin and Hunter, 1980; Šmahel, 1984d; Friede et al., 1986; Horswell and Gallup, 1992). However, Šmahel et al. (1985) noted several small but significant differences between individuals with unrepaired CL/A and normal controls. Specifically, head width, bizygomatic width, interocular width, nasal width, mouth width, total facial height and upper facial height, were significantly increased in the untreated CL group (although the degree of difference was generally less than that seen in CL/P). Several studies have agreed that the effects in this group seemed to center around the cleft area (Innes, 1962; Dahl, 1970; Bishara et al., 1976, 1985), although this does not account for the greater interocular and cranial widths often reported in this group.

Morphometric analysis of the craniofacial complex of individuals with CL/A after surgery showed little residual effect from lip and alveolar repair and suggested that the skeletal craniofacial relationship of CL/A patients posttreatment is similar to that in noncleft faces (Dahl, 1970; Bishara et al., 1985). However, only a few investigators have examined the craniofacial morphology of individuals with CLA (but not palate) independently from individuals with CL only (Bishara et al., 1976, 1985; Friede et al., 1986). Friede et al. (1986) argued that there were important distinctions between these two groups that accounted for some of the variability in results reported in the literature and suggested further that using CL/A individuals as normal controls (Dahl, 1970; Dahl et al., 1982; Nakamura et al., 1972) would be imprudent given the small but notable differences consistently described in these populations. In the following sections, the term CL/A is used only for those studies where it is clear that such distinctions have been noted.

Cranial base and facial widths. Dahl et al. (1982) found that adults with unrepaired CL had a (lateral)

widening of the cranial base and increased interocular distance. This finding has been documented by numerous investigators in both pre- and postoperative CL/A patients (Ross and Coupe, 1965; Dahl, 1970; Aduss, 1971; Farkas and Lindsay, 1972a; Nakamura et al., 1972; Hirschfeld and Aduss, 1974; Šmahel, 1984d; Friede et al., 1986; Šmahel et al., 1985).

Craniofacial heights and profiles. In addition to the increase in anterior facial heights previously reported by Šmahel et al. (1985), Casal et al. (1997) reported an increase in facial convexity in treated CL/A, which was secondary to mandible retrognathism, and a decrease in mandibular body length together with a degree of mandibular rotation. Cronin and Hunter (1980) also noted a slight clockwise rotation of the mandible in individuals with repaired CL.

Maxillary, palatal, and mandibular structures. In their study of individuals with repaired CL/A, Nakamura et al. (1972) found a greater transverse maxillary dimension. The following features were also reported: decreased inclination of the nasal bones (Dahl, 1970; Nakamura et al., 1972), more superiorly placed anterior nasal spine (Ross and Coupe, 1965; Dahl, 1970; Nakamura et al., 1972), and increased length of the maxilla and mandible (Dahl et al., 1982). However, there has been some disagreement among investigators in regard to maxillary width. Dahl (1970) found a decreased maxillary width, while Friede et al. (1986) reported that the maxillary width of CL patients closely approximated noncleft values. The latter study also did not find the clockwise rotation of the mandible described by Cronin and Hunter (1980). It is possible that the differences were secondary to age discrepancies, treatment differences, and differential inclusion of alveolar clefts. Thus, Friede et al. (1986) employed a mixed longitudinal study of CL patients (excluding CLA patients) from infancy to 6 years of age, while most of the other studies were conducted on adult CL (possibly including CLA), in which most had undergone some type of orthodontic treatment.

Casal et al. (1997) found that in a small sample ($n = 6$) of young children with repaired isolated CL, mandibular body length was significantly shorter and mandibular position significantly more retruded than in the control population, leading to greater convexity. These findings were similar to those reported for CLP, but other investigators did not find these features in their generally older populations (Dahl et al., 1982). Thus, Casal et al. (1997) may have described a transient manifestation of CL that disappeared as the more normal growth trajectory of this group occurred or as orthodontic treatment proceeded.

Dental arches and relationships. Individuals with unrepaired CLA tended to have an increased overjet and canines that were edge-to-edge and sometimes in crossbite. The teeth on either side of the cleft tended to roll superiorly, resulting in infraocclusion, with a localized open bite tendency. Bishara et al. (1985) used lateral cephalometric analysis to compare unoperated CLA individuals to unoperated CLP individuals. They found that the mandibular incisors were significantly more lingually inclined in the CLP group and more labially inclined in the CLA group. This appeared to be different from what was seen in individuals with repaired CL alone. Casal et al. (1997) reported that such children had lingual inclination of the upper and lower teeth, which resulted in widening of the interincisal angle and a reduction in the incisor overjet prior to orthodontic treatment.

Isolated Cleft Palate

Debate persists about the degree to which isolated CP and/or its surgical repair affect facial form. Some researchers have reported significant craniofacial differences in children with unrepaired CP compared to controls (Šmahel et al., 1987) and to children with unilateral CL (Dahl et al., 1982). Significant differences were described in adult females with CP (both pre- and postpalatoplasty combined) compared to a noncleft control sample (Bishara, 1973a; Bishara and Iverson, 1974). However, Mestre et al. (1960) found no significant differences in facial morphology in adult Puerto Ricans with unoperated CP compared to a noncleft group. Bishara (1973a) suggested that the disagreement in results might be due to differences in the populations studied and to differences in the methods of study. Bishara (1973b) also found that sex and the extent of the cleft were not correlated with significant changes in the craniofacial complex. However, Dahl (1970) found a "systematic tendency for the morphological changes to be most marked in extensive clefts."

In regard to the effects of surgical repair, several investigators have found that the craniofacial morphology of patients with surgically repaired CP differed significantly from that of noncleft patients (Shibaski and Ross, 1969; Dahl, 1970; Farkas and Lindsay, 1972b; Bishara, 1973a; Bishara and Iverson, 1974; Krogman et al., 1975). However, Bishara (1973a,b) and Bishara and Iverson (1974) found no significant differences in the craniofacial morphology of unrepaired and repaired (but obturated) CP adult females, which suggested that the morphometric features were not the result of surgical repair. However, Šmahel et al. (1987) argued that surgical repair did affect later growth, particularly in the restraint of further widening of the palate and surrounding structures. They also suggested that the relative maxillary shortening was progressive after palato-

plasty. Finally, some deviations which occurred in adults, including changes in mandibular shape, were mostly insignificant before palatal surgery, as documented by Dahl et al. (1982) as well as Šmahel et al. (1987).

The phenotypic differences between individuals with untreated CP and individuals with untreated CLP reinforce the point that CP differs both etiologically and morphologically and, in general, is believed to result in less overall facial abnormality. Nevertheless, many phenotypic similarities between individuals with isolated CP and other forms of oral facial cleft occur.

Neurocranium and cranial base. Dahl et al. (1982) used lateral, anteroposterior, and axial cephalometry to demonstrate that infants with untreated CP compared to untreated CL infants (used as a "normal" control) had shorter anterior cranial bases. Šmahel et al. (1987) also found evidence for shortening of the cranial base in children before their palates were repaired.

Facial widths. Widening of the nasal cavity and of neighboring structures in all types of cleft with involvement of the palate prior to palatoplasty was demonstrated early by Subtelny (1955) and Coupe and Subtelny (1960). The finding of widening of the nasal cavity was also in agreement with the observations of Dahl et al. (1982). However, Šmahel et al. (1987) could not demonstrate a significant difference in interocular dimensions in their unrepaired CP subjects compared to controls. Šmahel (1984a) also reported that the increased nasal cavity width almost disappeared in adulthood, probably as a result of growth modifications caused by the repair. Farkas and Lindsay (1972b) used direct anthropometry to assess facial morphology in adult males and females with CP who underwent palate surgery in childhood. They found that both male and female CP patients had on average a significantly narrower bizygomatic diameter than noncleft age- and sex-matched controls. The soft tissue width of the nose was also significantly smaller in adults with repaired CP. Similarly, Jain and Krogman (1983b) could not demonstrate an increase in facial widths in their treated CP subjects, at least compared to their CLP groups. These findings contrast with those for CLP (and in some cases CL), where increased orbital and nasal widths were commonly reported in both untreated and treated subjects.

Craniofacial height and profile. Šmahel et al. (1987) found a reduction of the posterior height of the upper face in pretreated children but not in adults with surgically repaired palates. Individuals with unrepaired palatal clefts also failed to exhibit the shortening of the anterior height of the upper face or the elongation of the lower face typical of the CLP group. Farkas and Lindsay (1972b), however, found the total height of the face to be greater in adults with repaired CP than in controls, but the difference was significant in males only. The difference could be attributed almost entirely to an increase in anterior mandibular height, which was significantly greater in both male and female adults with repaired CP compared to controls. The anterior heights of the upper and middle parts of the face were similar in both groups (Farkas and Lindsay, 1972a).

Maxillary, palatal, and mandibular structures. Dahl et al. (1982) demonstrated that children with CP prior to surgical repair exhibited a short maxilla and reduced posterior maxillary height in addition to reduced dimensions of the mandible (especially mandibular length), narrow naso- and pharyngeal airways, and retrognathia. They noted shortening of both jaws as early as age 2 to 3 months in infants with isolated CP compared to infants with incomplete CL. Dahl (1970) found that in adult males with CP, untreated and treated combined, there was a tendency for the maxilla to be smaller in length and retrognathic. The maxilla was retruded in relation to the cranial base and to the mandible compared to a noncleft control group. In a study that combined untreated and treated adult females with CP, Bishara (1973a) reported similar results. There was a tendency toward posterior positioning of the maxilla and mandible in relation to the cranial base, while the maxillary–mandibular relation was not significantly different from that of noncleft controls. However, Šmahel et al. (1987) found no evidence of a posterior positioning of the maxilla in their study of 60 children prior to palatal repair.

Several studies have found serious aberrations in the craniofacial morphology of CP patients with repaired clefts, although it is unclear whether these are due to the repair or to the cleft. For example, two groups of investigators reported a relatively posterior position of the maxilla and mandible in relation to the cranial base in operated patients with CP compared to controls (Shibaski and Ross, 1969; Dahl, 1970). Reduction in the size of the mandible of children with repaired CP was reported by Nakamura et al. (1972). Šmahel et al. (1987) noted shortening of both jaws in adults who had undergone palatal repair as children, although Dahl et al. (1982) also found this feature in children prior to palatal repair. Šmahel et al. (1987) did not find retrognathia, commonly associated with CLP, or significant differences in other areas of the face except a reduction in the mandibular plane inclination in their sample of individuals with repaired CP. Casal et al. (1997) found no evidence of retrognathia in their study of young children with repaired CP but suggested that this may be secondary to the early age at reconstructive surgery.

Dental arches and relationships. Shortening of the dentoalveolar arch prior to palatoplasty was demonstrated by Peterka (1979). Shibasaki and Ross (1969), in a cross-sectional growth study of children with operated isolated CP, found that the maxillary underdevelopment progressed with age but that an acceptable facial balance was achieved because of the positional changes of the mandible. In addition, both Bishara (1973a) and Casal et al. (1997) found that, despite the posterior positioning of the maxilla and mandible, the maxillary–mandibular relationship was normal and similar to the noncleft group.

Discussion

Given the diversity of research designs, sample composition, treatment protocols, and analytical approaches evident in studies of facial form associated with oral clefts, disagreement is not surprising. Nevertheless, some common findings can be discerned (Table 7.1). Investigators have demonstrated consistently that the facial morphology of infants, children, adolescents, and adults with various types of cleft and various stages of treatment deviated from normal (or control) populations (Ross and Coupe, 1965; Dahl, 1970; Aduss, 1971; Friede and Johanson, 1977; Dahl et al., 1982, 1989; Friede et al., 1987; Molsted et al., 1987; Kilpeläinen and Laine-Alava, 1996; Kilpeläinen et al., 1996; Hermann et al., 1999). There is greater facial disruption in bilateral than in unilateral CLP and in

TABLE 7.1. *What We Know about Facial Shape in Cleft Lip with or without Cleft Palate and in Cleft Palate Alone*

1. Facial morphology in infants, children, adolescents, and adults with various types of cleft and various stages of treatment deviates from normal.

2. There is a large range of variation within each cleft type in the expression of associated morphological patterns.

3. This variation is associated with the severity of the defect: individuals with complete clefts deviate more severely than those with incomplete clefts and individuals with isolated cleft lip have fairly normal facial development but a similar morphometric pattern in key ways to more severe forms of cleft lip.

4. There is a tendency among individuals with clefts involving the lip, alveolus, and/or palate to demonstrate increased mandibular rotation, increased anterior mandibular height, and total facial height, as well as reduced facial convexity.

5. Residual deformities are often observed in cleft individuals, even following corrective surgery and/or orthodontic treatment.

6. Growth deficiencies of the midface region following surgery have also been reported as a problem in patients with cleft lip and palate or cleft palate alone.

7. Widening of the nasal cavity and of interorbital dimensions has been a persistent feature in studies of all forms of cleft lip with cleft palate, but this feature is infrequently reported in untreated or treated cleft palate.

unilateral CLP than in isolated CP or CL, in that order. Researchers have shown consistently that individuals with isolated CL have fairly normal facial development in comparison to subjects with some form of CLP or isolated CP (Dahl, 1970). However, even these CL individuals have been shown to differ, on average, from control values and in a fashion consistent with other forms of CLP.

Šmahel (1984a) concluded that the configuration of the face in complete unilateral and bilateral CLP was characterized by essentially identical patterns. This pattern included retroclination of the dentoalveolar component of the upper jaw, retroposition of the mandible and of the maxilla per se, and posterior growth rotation of the face. There was impairment of vertical growth within the lateral parts of the upper face in both groups. Šmahel (1984a) further suggested that increased intraorbital widths might be an intrinsic characteristic that predisposed the individual to develop the cleft.

Among the many unresolved questions is the effect of surgery on the growth and development of the face in individuals with oral facial clefts. In a recent series of studies that compared infants with early surgical repair of complete unilateral CLP with a group who had repaired incomplete unilateral CL, Hermann et al. (1999, 2000) argued that bimaxillary retrognathia, short posterior height of the maxilla, and short mandible were intrinsic in the CLP population and not the consequence of surgery. However, the maxillary–mandibular discrepancies reported in operated unilateral CLP patients were not frequently observed in the unrepaired faces of individuals with unilateral CLP, indicating that these features may be secondary to the treatment (Bishara, 1973a,b; Bishara et al., 1976, 1985).

In regard to isolated CP, debate centers around the merits of early palatoplasty, which increases the likelihood of normal speech, vs. later closure, which may maximize maxillary growth potential (and hence reduce the impact of surgery on growth). Rohrich and Byrd (1990) suggested that four key variables determine the outcome of cleft surgery: cleft type, surgeon's expertise, operative technique, and timing of the repair. They concluded from a careful review of the literature that the type of surgery and the skill with which it was carried out predicted outcome better than the timing of the palatal closure. Šmahel et al. (1999) argued in a similar vein, noting that surgical impact on growth was greater in their sample of 187 adult men with CLP, CP, and CL, all of whom had their surgical repairs before the "contemporary state of treatment," which includes both alveolar repair and treatment with fixed orthodontic appliances. They found no difference in the basic bony facial characteristics of CP vs. CLP, a fact that

underscores the overriding impact of the palatal repair in these two otherwise distinct populations.

Finally, there is great phenotypic variation within any group of individuals with oral facial clefts, even those who would be grouped together on the basis of cleft location or severity (Farkas et al., 1993; Ishikawa et al., 2000). This fact is seldom discussed but readily evident in studies where standard deviations are reported. Consistently, these measures of variation within the sample are larger in the cleft groups than in the controls. This is significant because nearly every study of facial morphometrics among individuals with oral clefts utilizes mean values to characterize cleft types (e.g., bilateral vs. unilateral.) However, these mean phenotypes are probably a poor representation of the individual cases comprising the category.

FACIAL FORM IN RELATIVES OF AFFECTED INDIVIDUALS

Family Members of Individuals with Cleft Lip or Cleft Lip and Palate

The interest in a possible relationship between facial shape and increased risk for CL/P can be traced to studies on differences in the susceptibility of various strains of mice to CL/P. Trasler (1968) suggested that variations in embryonic facial shape and growth dynamics were factors in the increased susceptibility to CL in the A/J mouse compared to the C57BL strain. Specifically, she proposed that the more prominent and centrally placed medial nasal process characteristic of the A/J strain led to greater rates of failure in the fusion of medial and lateral nasal processes and in subsequent breakdown of the isthmus of tissue connecting medial, lateral, and maxillary processes. In effect, these mice had a heritable facial shape that led to a lower threshold (and hence a greater incidence) for CL.

As a result of Trasler's work, Fraser and Pashayan (1970) suggested the following: "if the shape of the embryonic face is related to the shape of the postnatal face, and if the face shape is at least in part genetically determined, and if face shape is indeed related to the predisposition to cleft lip, it follows that the parents of children with cleft lip should have faces that are, on the average, of a different shape than those of the general population." These authors tested their hypothesis by examining 50 parents of children with CL/P (25 males and 25 females) and contrasting this sample with normal controls drawn from other clinical (noncleft) populations and hospital staff. Using direct measurements, measurements from photographs, and "physioprints" (after Sassouni, 1962), they concluded that the parental group tended to have, on average, longer facial heights (intraocular to chin dimensions), narrower bizygomatic widths, underdeveloped maxilla, thin upper lips, and more rectangular or trapezoidal facial shapes than ovoid (Fraser and Pashayan, 1970). Moreover, they argued that these deviations were more pronounced in parents who had more than one affected child. Finally, they suggested the following: "Though the genetic basis for the quantitative differences demonstrated in this study is [sic] likely to be complex, it is possible that specific traits showing simple Mendelian inheritance can be distinguished. Their identification would help to clarify the biological basis for the genetically determined susceptibility to cleft lip."

Subsequent research can be divided into three categories, based on research design and theoretical assumptions. In the majority of studies, researchers have followed the basic design and assumptions first outlined by Fraser and Pashayan (1970). Thus, a multifactorial model was assumed and a population of parents was contrasted *en masse* to a population of controls. Differences were then documented using straightforward statistical tests of means. A second category of research design reflects the growing awareness of the etiological and genetic variability present within and between CLP and CP populations. This approach requires more sophisticated statistical models and the acceptance of the possibility that risk factors are not evenly distributed among or between parental pairs. The third category of research has emerged in the last several years as investigators have attempted to link suspected genetic markers associated with oral facial clefts to specific morphological patterns seen in the parents. This approach combines our greatly increased understanding of craniofacial morphogenetics with our knowledge of craniofacial morphometrics.

Multifactorial Models. Coccaro et al. (1972) built on the results of Fraser and Pashayan (1970), comparing cephalometric radiographs from a group of 40 parents (20 males and 20 females) of children with CL/P to a group of 40 control individuals. Their experimental group consistently displayed a more acute cranial base angle, smaller upper facial heights, shorter palatal lengths, shorter anterior lengths of the palate, and shorter noses. Mandibular length was greater in the experimental group than in the controls. They speculated that it was the "unfavorable variation" or disharmony between the upper and lower facial sizes that was passed on to their children, disrupting normal development and leading to increased frequency of clefting. Their research again supported the idea that parents of children with CL/P demonstrate a facial form that distinguishes them from the general population, implying a heritable predisposition to the condition.

Erickson (1974), citing Trasler (1968) and Fraser and Pashayan (1970), examined siblings of affected children and showed that they too had distinctive facial features. They compared palatal form, dental arch shape, and facial profile in siblings of children with CL/P and siblings from families with no immediate history (first- or second-degree relatives) of CL/P. While only one of the three traits (palatal form) differed significantly between the study siblings and controls, consistent differences were found that tended in the direction of those previously reported in parents. Thus, the facial profile in the sibs of cleft children tended to be less convex than in controls and palatal form was tapered and highly arched. As in previous studies (and most of those that have followed), the presumptive genetic model being tested was the multifactorial threshold (MFT) model. Therefore, when calculating values for sibs, Erickson (1974) used the mean value derived from combining the scores of each (unaffected) child in the sibship for each variable. The "midsib" values were then compared between treatment and control groups. If another model is presumed (major gene) or if, as Fraser and Pashayan (1970) suggested, some pertinent aspects of facial form exhibit Mendelian patterns of inheritance, then it might be expected that the associated phenotype would not be equally distributed between members of a sibship. Therefore, any attempt to combine or average their values would weaken the ability to define the relevant phenotypic pattern.

Nakasima and Ichinose (1983) demonstrated that the unique facial phenotype transcended ethnicity. They examined lateral and posterior–anterior cephalometric head plates from parents of 251 children in Japan with oral facial clefts and an equal number of control pairs. These investigators included parents of children with CP as well as CLP and broke the latter sample into subgroups based on severity (CL/P and CL). They utilized a total of 53 cephalometric variables as well as multivariate statistical procedures (analysis of variance and discriminant function analysis) to further explore the data. As in all previous studies, an MFT mode of inheritance was presumed. Thus, the investigators averaged the values for both parents for each variable and compared the group means of these midparental scores to the means derived from the averaged scores of randomly selected pairs of male and female controls.

Their findings were largely consistent with those reported by previous researchers. Parents of CL/P children had on average significantly shorter heads and maxillary lengths as well as shorter anterior middle or upper facial heights coupled with a more open, rotated mandible (greater mandibular angle) and a significantly less convex face than controls. The midparental average for head width in the CL/P parent group was significantly smaller than in the control group. However, outer orbital width was significantly greater, as were forehead and nasal widths. The researchers also examined left–right asymmetry from the frontal radiographs and found that, for the most part, this was not increased in any of the study groups (the exceptions were alveolar width asymmetry and nasal floor height asymmetry among parents of children with CLP).

Given the smaller cranial dimensions in the study group, it would be reasonable to ask to what extent the facial measurements were affected by this general reduction in size. Nakasima and Ichinose (1983) addressed this question by examining proportional relationships between cranial dimensions (maximum head width) and five midfacial widths (outer orbital width, forehead width, nasal width, zygomatic width, and maxillary width). With the exception of the cranial index, the proportions were always larger in the study groups, indicating that the facial measurements were not simply reflections of a generalized reduction in body or head size. Nakasima and Ichinose (1984) investigated this question further in a study that compared cranial area in four groups: children with oral facial clefts, their parents, a control sample of children without clefts, and their parents. Cranial area (brain case) was significantly smaller in both the affected group and their parents (again expressed as a midparental average) compared to the control children and their parents (midparental average). They also found higher correlation coefficients between the control children and their parents for cranial area than between the affected children and their parents and suggested that this might reflect varied disruptions to normal growth caused by the cleft and its subsequent surgical repair. They argued as well that the small brain case appeared to be an inherited factor passed from the parents to the children with clefts and suggested that it may be related to susceptibility to oral facial clefting (Nakasima and Ichinose, 1983).

In the same study, the authors found a correlation between cleft severity in the child and facial form in the parents. Hence, they demonstrated that parents of children with CL alone consistently displayed less pronounced deviations from control values than did parents of children with CLP. This was noted both in mean values of the various measurements and in the number of these values that differed significantly from control values. However, these differences were minor compared to the differences with controls, as indicated by discriminant function analysis. This multivariate technique was unable to successfully separate the three study groups (CL, CL/P, and CP) from one another, but each could be separated from the controls, as could the study group as a whole. The authors proposed that

these differences were great enough to serve as a possible mechanism for identifying parents at greater risk for having an affected child (Nakasima and Ichinose, 1983).

Raghavan et al. (1994) analyzed a set of 38 parents of children with CL/P from India and compared these individuals to a control set of 24 parents of healthy children from the same area. They utilized both lateral and posterior–anterior cephalograms to assess mean differences between the experimental group and the control group for 30 variables. Midparental values were used to generate mean values for each group, once again reflecting the assumption of a multifactorial mode of inheritance. Seven of the 22 means derived from the lateral films were significantly different between the two samples, with the experimental group demonstrating on average a significantly more obtuse cranial base angle, a more acute articular angle, shorter upper facial height, shorter posterior facial height, a greater palatal length, a more projecting midface, and a more obtuse mandibular angle. In contrast, seven of the eight width dimensions differed significantly between the control and experimental groups, with maximum head width, bizygomaticofrontal suture width, zygomatic width, alveolar width, gonial width, and total facial height being smaller in the experimental group. Only nasal cavity width was greater in the experimental group. These results are somewhat at odds with those reported by previous researchers. Examination of their published data, however, offers a possible explanation for this apparent discrepancy: head size appears to be reduced on average in the experimental group. Had these investigators followed Nakasima and Ichinose (1983) and used ratios to explore the possibility that the experimental group might exhibit facial widths that were broad compared to head size, a different set of conclusions would have resulted. Ratios can be calculated from the mean values in their tables, and these indicate that for inner orbital width, frontal width, and bigonial width (in addition to nasal width) the values from the experimental group ranged from 3% to 16% larger than those for the controls, a finding that is much more in keeping with those reported earlier.

Investigating Phenotypic Heterogeneity. Kurisu et al. (1974) expanded on all previous studies in a landmark work that still stands as a model of methodological rigor. Their study used a greatly increased sample size and included parents of children with isolated CP as well as CL/P. In addition, they utilized two independent control samples, one from Lancaster, Pennsylvania, and the other from Ann Arbor, Michigan. They also utilized posterior–anterior cephalograms, in addition to the more traditional lateral head films, to obtain a set of 20 linear and angular variables. Theirs was the first study to analyze fathers separately from mothers. Their methods included both factor analysis to generate a better understanding of the underlying biological (anatomical) differences between the groups and a form of cluster analysis (Q-mode correlations in conjunction with principal components analysis) to study the multivariate or global differences between the study and control groups.

In general, Kurisu et al. (1974) found the same phenotypic associations reported by Coccaro et al. (1972). Thus, parents of children with CL/P tended to have more concave facial profiles, more relative mandibular prognathism, and shorter vertical and wider horizontal dimensions in the upper face. However, fathers demonstrated these features more dramatically than mothers in regard to both individual variables and factor scores. (Their results relative to parents of children with CP are discussed in a later section of this chapter, Parental Facial Form in Isolated Cleft Palate.) The researchers found no correlation between cleft severity and degree of facial abnormality in either parent and called into question the MFT model of inheritance, which would predict such a correlation. Interestingly, they also found significant differences between the two normal control populations and cautioned that such variation is likely to account for some of the discrepancies reported between studies using different control populations.

Ward et al. (1989, 1994) criticized previous studies, including that of Kurisu et al. (1974), because parental samples were treated as uniform entities. They argued that in any large sample, whether parents of sporadic or of familial CLP children, a variety of etiologies would likely be represented. For example, among the sporadic cases, some would have a greater familial or genetic component than others (it is well known that a percentage of sporadic cases become familial cases after a subsequent affected child is born). Even in those cases with a stronger familial component, there were likely to be multiple genetic loci associated with increased risk for clefting, not all associated with the same or any effect on facial form in the parents. Furthermore, Ward et al. (1989) noted that in most previous studies the MFT model had been assumed, in which both parents contributed to the risk of an affected child. Hence, parental phenotypes were considered *en masse* even when values were separated by sex. There is nothing in the MFT model that requires the parental contributions to be equal, and moreover, there is ample evidence that the MFT model is inadequate for explaining the inheritance of many cases of oral facial clefting. Finally, when relying on mean values

alone, little attention is paid to variation within samples.

To overcome these methodological shortcomings, these investigators sorted their parental sample (lateral cephalograms from 82 parents of children with sporadic CL/P) using multivariate cluster analysis. This technique generated multivariate distance or similarity measures to identify individuals with similar phenotypes. A dendrogram, or tree diagram, was produced from these results, which displayed the pattern of similarity between groups of individuals. Resulting clusters were compared to one another using linear regression analysis, which measures the correlation, or similarity in the pattern of variation, between two clusters (with a value of 1 representing pattern identity).

The results of this analysis supported the contention that there was considerable variability in phenotypes among parents of children with CL/P. While half of the parents sorted into a large group ($n = 39$) with mean values that differed only in being consistently (but insignificantly) a little larger than the published norms, the remaining 43 parents sorted into a series of smaller groupings that had major deviations from the published norms. All clusters were compared (using regression analysis) to an independent and unrelated sample of 16 individuals with repaired CLP. Interestingly, the largest two phenotypically unusual groupings ($n = 17$ and $n = 12$) exhibited patterns of variation that were surprisingly similar to the phenotype seen in individuals with CLP. Correlations between the facial pattern of these two clusters and that of the group with overt clefts were ($r = 0.88$) and ($r = 0.68$), respectively. In contrast, there was little correlation between the pattern in the cleft group and the largest (nominally normal) cluster of parents ($r = 0.37$).

Another outcome of Ward et al.'s (1989) different methodological approach was the documentation that, at least in this sample, it was rare for both parents to be in one of the "phenotypically unusual" groups. Thus, in only 15% of the pairs were both parents unusual. In over half of the pairs (54%), only one member showed an unusual facial phenotype, and in 31% of the pairs neither parent was unusual. These findings suggest that some sporadic cases have a genetic or familial component while others do not.

Mossey et al. (1998b) examined 40 fathers and 43 mothers of children with CL, CLP, and isolated CP. They analyzed fathers and mothers separately, echoing the concerns of Ward et al. (1989) that combining parents in a single group ignored the likelihood that parental contributions to risk in children are unequal. The parents were compared to a carefully selected group of 100 control individuals from the same general population (Glasgow). Thirty-seven measurements of the head and face were derived from lateral cephalograms and included area measurements as well as angles and linear measures. Univariate analysis revealed that both fathers and mothers differed significantly from controls but displayed little concordance in the specific traits that were significantly different. In fathers, the mean mandibular area measurement was significantly smaller than in controls, as was the mean palatal length. The mean cranial base angle was significantly more acute and the mean cross-sectional area of the cranium significantly smaller than those derived from control males. Only the mean area of occipital subtenuce was larger in fathers than control males. In contrast, means for mothers exhibited significant increases in mandibular length, total facial height, anterior cranial base, and clivus length. Mothers resembled fathers in having significantly reduced means for cranial area.

AlEmran et al. (1999) also found differences in fathers and mothers of children with clefts. Specifically, utilizing frontal cephalograms, they reported that fathers tended to exhibit significantly greater nasal widths and narrower maxillary widths compared to controls. Mothers tended to display significantly smaller head, bizygomatic, alveolar, and bigonial widths (although these differences were not apparent when considered as ratios to head width). Both mothers and fathers had significantly increased facial asymmetry in orbital and alveolar measurements to a constructed midline compared to controls. However, these results are difficult to interpret because the investigators apparently did not separate parents of children with CP from those with other types of cleft.

Some investigators have examined populations with familial forms of isolated CLP on the assumption that these may be more likely to display a heritable facial phenotype associated with the risk for oral facial clefts. Thus, Ward et al. (1994) studied a single multiplex family using lateral and posterior–anterior cephalograms to assess seven craniofacial variables. They demonstrated that the four individuals in this family who would be classified as likely gene carriers by pedigree analysis (i.e., they had an affected parent or a sib and an affected child but were not cleft themselves) exhibited a distinct craniofacial phenotype, similar in some ways to that reported in previous studies (Fraser and Pashayan, 1970; Cocarro et al., 1972; Nakasima and Ichinose, 1983). Thus, these individuals had significantly larger means for (outer) orbital widths and nasal cavity widths. However, in contrast to previous studies, the carriers had significantly shorter lower faces than either the affected or the obligate normal group. Carriers also did not show the decreased facial convexity or increased lower facial heights frequently de-

scribed in previous studies. Multivariate discriminant function analysis showed that two functions comprised of four variables (nasal cavity width, facial profile angle, palatal length, and lower facial height) correctly classified 89% of the affected, carrier, and obligate normal family members (no carriers were misclassified, one affected individual was misclassified as obligate normal, and one obligate normal was classified as an obligate carrier). The fact that carriers had even greater mean values for nasal cavity width and outer orbital width than affected (though treated) individuals suggests that these phenotypic characteristics do not simply result from the oral cleft (since the carriers have no cleft).

Suzuki et al. (1999) examined 65 individuals (25 fathers and 40 mothers) who were parents of children with CL/P but who also had at least one (blood) relative with CL/P within the last three generations. These familial cases were compared to an unspecified control sample of 413 parental pairs using 19 ratios (to adjust for the effects of sex) derived from lateral and posterior–anterior cephalograms. Their results indicated that on average the adjusted measurements for interorbital width, bicoronoid width, nasal cavity width, and anterior cranial base length were significantly increased in the parental sample compared to the controls. Discriminant function analysis indicated that parents and controls could be correctly classified 68% of the time. This value is considerably less than that reported by Ward et al. (1994), but Suzuki et al. (1999) used a sample that was nearly 45 times larger.

Linking Morphometrics and Morphogenetics. Mossey et al. (1998a) combined molecular and morphometric techniques. Specifically, they examined polymorphisms in the *transforming growth factor alpha* (TGF-α) locus in 83 parents (the same sample reported in Mossey et al., 1998b). They found that one polymorphism (the C2 allele of the *TGF-α* Taq1 polymorphism), although rare in general, had a significantly higher occurrence in the parents of both CL/P and CP children than in controls. Also, by combining these genotypic predictors of risk status with cephalometric predictors, discriminant function classification improved. They correctly classified 76% of the CP and 94% of the CL/P parents (compared to controls). The authors acknowledged that it is unlikely that the *TGF-α* gene plays a major role in the susceptibility to oral facial clefts but speculated that it might be a modifying factor. Beiraghi et al. (1994), who linked the risk of CL/P to the 4p− region of chromosome 4, examined the same family as Ward et al. (1994). In an unpublished study, Ward and Beiraghi (personal communication) found that there was 100% correspondence between the individuals identified as carriers by genetic marker analysis and morphometric analysis.

Parental Facial Form in Isolated Cleft Palate

Craniofacial form in parents of children with isolated CP has not been as extensively studied, and the few studies that can be found exhibit many of the same deficiencies in research design described in the previous section. Nevertheless, the same tendency for parents of affected children to exhibit unusual patterns of facial form has been reported in each of these studies. The nature of this pattern differed in significant ways from that described in parents of children with CLP. Thus, Kurisu et al. (1974) and Nakasima and Ichinose (1983) found that the parents of children with CP evidenced fewer deviations from normal compared to the parents of children with CL/P; however, the general direction for the differences was similar. Kurisu et al. (1974) also noted that while fathers and mothers tended to have the same pattern of deviation from normal, the specific list of variables that differed significantly from controls varied by sex. For example, both fathers and mothers had, on average, larger maxillary widths and shorter anterior mid-facial measurements, but the former reached a value that was significant in the mothers while the latter reached significance in the fathers. In general, fathers differed more than mothers compared to control values. Prochazkova and Tolarová (1986) also examined mothers and fathers of CP children separately (20 mothers and 20 fathers). These subjects were compared to a control sample of 75 university students for a series of 34 characteristics taken from lateral cephalograms and dental casts. They reported that parents on average had a significantly longer anterior cranial base, longer palate, and shorter mandibular body. Soft tissue lower facial heights were greater in parents compared to controls. Again, there were a few minor differences in significance levels for variables between mothers and fathers, and, in general, the fathers showed greater deviation from normal in most measurements. In a later study, Prochazkova and Vinsova (1995) found that males tended to have significantly larger mandibles compared to controls, but this feature was not characteristic of females. Both males and females however, differed from controls in a number of other cephalometric and anthropometric variables.

Mossey et al. (1997) examined 35 parents of children with CP as well as 12 with CL children and 36 with children who had CL/P derived from a population in western Scotland. Using 37 linear, angular, and area measurements from lateral cephalograms, they concluded that were no significant differences between parents of children with CL and CL/P but a few significant differences between parents of children with CP and CL/P. However, these differences were apparent only if the sample was first subdivided by sex. In this case, means for mothers of children with CP were consistently greater for mandibular length, mandibular ramus length, mandibular area, and cranial area when compared to the means for mothers of children with CL/P. Stepwise discriminant function analysis could correctly classify 80% of the CL/P mothers and 75% of the CP mothers using just mandibular ramus length and cranial height. Mandibular ramus length alone could correctly classify 71% of the CP parents and 63% of the CL/P parents regardless of sex.

All of these research efforts suffered from the same methodological assumption of a multifactorial mode of inheritance seen in most of the studies of relatives of CLP cases. In an ongoing research effort in our lab, we are using a different approach but observing similar sex specific morphometric differences in parents of children with CP. More specifically, Sammons (1999) examined 15 parental pairs who had a child with isolated CP. Seventeen variables from lateral cephalograms and 25 posterior–anterior variables were analyzed and compared to published data derived from the same geographic region (Saksena et al., 1987, 1990). Twenty of the 42 variables differed significantly from the reference means. Most values were smaller in the parental group (14/20), although mean values for inner orbital width, nasal shelf width, mandibular angle, mandibular protrusion, lower facial height, and palatal length were larger in the parental group. However, Sammons (1999) went the additional step of using cluster analysis to determine if distinct groups could be identified with in this parental sample. Two groupings could be defined, one comprised largely of females and the other of males. The predominantly female group (9/12 or 75%) was characterized by relatively greater reductions in facial height, shorter palates, longer mandibular bodies, and greater mandibular prognathism compared to the cluster that was predominantly male (12/18 or 67%). While these findings do not correspond directly with those reported by Mossey et al. (1998b), they do support the contention that sex has an important influence on the expression of facial features that differentiate parents of CP children from the general population.

Discussion

What has been learned in the 30 years since Fraser and Pashayan (1970) first suggested that facial form in parents might relate to the risk of oral facial clefts in their offspring? The answer to this question is complex. As

Mossey and coworkers (1998a,b) have demonstrated in their reviews of this subject, there is a lack of agreement on the specific craniofacial features that distinguish parents with such risk factors from the general population. However, we can make some generalizations (Table 7.2).

In spite of the differences in study design, variables assessed, and ethnic origin of the populations under study, investigators have consistently found that, taken as a group, parents of children with isolated CL/P and CP display morphometric features that distinguish them from the general population (as represented by control subjects). This in and of itself would not be surprising because, as Kurisu et al. (1974) demonstrated, even two reference normal populations can exhibit an alarming number of statistically significant differences if they are drawn from different regions of the country and/or are measured by different investigators. However, the differences exhibited by the parents of children with oral clefts are quite similar to those shown by individuals with oral facial clefts (as demonstrated by Ward et al., 1989). Two classes of shared traits stand out. First, the repeated finding of excess intraorbital widths in both

TABLE 7.2. *What We Have Learned about Facial Shape in Relatives of Individuals with Orofacial Clefts*

1. Every study has found significant craniofacial differences between parents of children with clefts and the general population.

2. These differences exist for parents of both sporadic cases of cleft and cases within multiplex families.

3. Many features that distinguish parents from controls also distinguish affected (pretreated and treated) individuals from controls.

4. Common findings in affected individuals with cleft lip with or without cleft palate and their unaffected relatives include greater lower facial height, increased interorbital distances, and rotated mandibular position.

5. In studies where the methodology has been appropriate, it has been demonstrated that these facial features are not uniformly distributed within the parental sample, within parental pairs, or between sexes.

6. The pattern of expression of unusual facial features within parental samples supports the contention that cleft lip with or without cleft palate and cleft palate are separate entities but that both represent common phenotypic outcomes of a heterogeneous complex of genetic and environmental causes.

7. This heterogeneity further supports the probability of the inheritance of major genes in some cases of clefting, a multifactorial threshold inheritance in others, and a more purely environmental cause in others.

8. At least in some cases, it has been demonstrated that the unusual cleft phenotype in the parental sample correlates with the inheritance of genetic markers potentially associated with the inheritance of cleft lip and/or palate.

affected individuals and noncleft parents of children with CL/P reinforces the original observations of Fraser and Pashayan (1970) and suggests that increased facial width may be a heritable trait that predisposes one to an oral cleft by reducing the threshold for its occurrence. Second, the excessive width through the orbits (and in some cases other regions of the midface) may indicate a general disturbance in growth, perhaps caused by a major gene operating in the craniofacial developmental pathway. In this case, altered facial form could be seen as a forme fruste of the full-blown cleft.

One possible developmental anomaly that may explain the peculiar set of features shared by parents and affected individuals, at least for CLP, is the size and shape of the cartilaginous cranial base. In studies using axial projection instead of standard cephalometrics, Molsted and colleagues (1993) found that there were significant differences in the width of the spheno-occipital synchondrosis and cranial base dimensions between a group of infants with untreated CLP and a group of infants with untreated CL with minor incomplete clefts (used as a normal control). They also found that the CLP group exhibited significantly greater widths in the superior as well as the inferior part of the spheno-occipital synchondrosis. No difference between the groups was found in the cranial base length. However, the distance from the synchondrosis to the sella point was significantly shorter in the CLP group (Molsted et al., 1993). In their 1995 study, Molsted et al. reported that the CLP group had an increased width of the cranial base and that the angle between the right and left ala major of the sphenoid bone and the angle between the petrous part on the right and left side was also increased. Also, the posterior width of the maxilla was greater. Others have found that anterior–posterior cranial base dimensions are reduced in individuals with oral clefts (Bishara and Iversen, 1974; Horswell and Gallup, 1992). Dahl et al. (1982) suggested that the reduced anterior–posterior dimensions of the cranial base might be an intrinsic (predisposing) factor in CP. We do not know whether such specific morphometric features are heritable, but if so, the primary defect in some forms of CLP could be an abnormally wide but short cranial base. This would account for the greater facial widths in both a parent and the affected child, as well as abnormal midfacial depths (retruded maxilla, etc.), and could, following Trasler's (1968) original suggestion, lower the threshold for expression of the cleft.

The second area where common morphometric abnormalities can be seen is the mandible, which tends to be posteriorly rotated both in people with CL/P and in (some) otherwise normal parents of these individuals. This rotation also gives rise to either an increased total facial height or lower facial height and often an associated decrease in facial convexity. Mossey and coworkers (1997) suggested that in parents expressing some primary defect in maxillary growth (a finding in many studies of parents of children with CL/P) the mandibular abnormalities may reflect functional adaptation to the deficiency in the midface. They further suggested, as did Cocarro et al. (1972), that these differences in mandibular growth might interact with embryonic tongue positioning in a susceptible offspring and subsequently interfere with lip and/or palatal closure. However, the fact that an increased intraorbital width *and* a posterior rotation of the mandible occur together in otherwise normal parents of children with CL/P argues for a more generalized disturbance in craniofacial growth.

The suggestion that variations in the shape of the cranial base or in any other region of the face correlate with morphological changes in structures far removed from the primary defect is a logical consequence of the functional matrix theory, especially in its most recent incarnations (Moss, 1997a,b). It also may indicate that many cases of oral facial clefts are best seen as part of larger malformation sequences, as suggested by Shprintzen et al. (1985) and Horswell and Gallup (1992).

It is interesting that in most studies of parents of children with CP the morphometric differences with the control population are less pronounced and seldom include significant differences in facial width or cranial size. However, variations in mandibular morphology may be more common in some relatives of individuals with CP. There also appears to be a stronger correlation between facial morphology and sex in parents of CP children. These differences suggest that heritable differences in facial form may be less important in producing a child with CP than some as yet unspecified influence of sex or imprinting coming from the parents.

CONCLUSIONS

Facial form associated with CL/P reflects a complex mix of primary and secondary factors. Thus, in both noncleft relatives and individuals with CL/P prior to treatment, excessive width through the midface (orbits and nasal cavity) and posterior rotation of the mandible suggest that facial form itself may be a causal factor or a minimal expression of the cleft. It is equally clear that an untreated cleft, whether of an isolated palate, lip and palate, or primary palate, interferes with facial growth and distorts facial form. Finally, treatment and surgical repair can also disrupt the normal pattern of facial growth. However, one of the great remaining difficulties faced by morphometricians, developmental biolo-

gists, and clinicians is that presented by the variability of expression within the population of individuals with oral clefts (and their families). The standard approach to studying facial form as it relates to CL/P has always been to compare groups of individuals with a certain cleft phenotype to groups lacking this trait. This of course ignores the likelihood of genetic and etiological heterogeneity within the cleft population (Shprintzen et al., 1985). This intrinsic variability is further obscured by the practice of summarizing the phenotype through the use of mean values for the traits in question. The consequent tendency to rely on phenotypic typologies that may poorly reflect underlying etiological typologies remains the biggest hindrance to a meaningful linkage between morphometrics and morphogenetics. Finally, Moss (1997a,b) suggested that variant genes in the developmental pathway interact in an as yet unrecognized but undoubtedly complex fashion with epigenetic (environmental) factors to produce a given phenotype. From this perspective, variability is an inevitable expression of developmental complexity, and it is unlikely that we will ever understand the morphometrics of individuals with oral clefts without equal attention to both genetic and epigenetic factors that can influence facial form. This problem is underscored by research in the last two decades that has identified a number of genetic loci that may be linked to the expression of oral clefts in different individuals (Mossey et al., 1998a).

It appears that, as Fraser and Pashayan (1972) first predicted, facial shape may be an important aid in sorting out the genetic contributions to oral facial clefts. Specific morphometric patterns may serve as a marker for identifying individuals or families in which there may be a greater risk for inheriting this condition. The possibility of utilizing this information in combination with emerging technologies of genetic linkage analysis has not gone unnoticed (Ward et al., 1989, 1994; Mossey et al., 1998a). However, future morphometric research must recognize the lessons already learned, and a more sophisticated research design must be used than has generally been employed in the past. First, morphometric research must allow for variable expression of the key features in individuals affected by oral clefts and their otherwise unaffected relatives. Indeed, it is likely that there are multiple rather than singular characteristic phenotypes within the traditional cleft typologies of bilateral, unilateral, complete, and incomplete CL/P. For example, individuals with CLP caused primarily by intrauterine exposure to a teratogen may have a different phenotypic pattern than those who inherited a cleft-susceptible facial form. Research has shown that among parents of affected individuals, significant phenotypic differences exist within and between parental pairs as well as by sex. Second, future research must be guided by our increasing understanding of the complex developmental pathways that can lead to an oral cleft. Mossey and colleagues (1998a) were the first to utilize such a combined approach, but it may be expected that more productive lines of inquiry will emerge as our understanding of the genetics of craniofacial development improves; i.e., it may be possible to associate specific genetic variants with different patterns of facial form as well as with the probability of the appearance of CL/P in one's offspring. Third, whether we are studying facial form as it relates to the effects of the oral facial clefts, their surgical repair, or subtle differences among family members, the new three-dimensional technologies and geometrically based analyses of form must be harnessed to create a more precise understanding of facial morphology and its inheritance. If these new techniques become as readily accessible as the two-dimensional head plate and associated cephalometric analysis have been, the new century can expect to see a resolution of those questions that escaped the last.

REFERENCES

Aduss, H (1971). Craniofacial growth in complete unilateral cleft lip and palate. Angle Orthod 41: 202–213.

Aduss, H, Pruzansky, S (1967). The nasal cavity in complete unilateral cleft lip and palate. Arch Otolaryngol 85: 53–61.

AlEmran, SE, Fatani, E, Hassanain, JE (1999). Craniofacial variability in parents of children with cleft lip and cleft palate. J Clin Pediatr Dent 23: 337–341.

Athanasiou, AE, Tseng, CY, Zarrinnia, K, Mazaheri, M (1990). Frontal cephalometric study of dentofacial morphology in children with bilateral clefts of lip, alveolus and palate. J Craniomaxillofac Surg 18: 49–54.

Atherton, JD (1967a). Morphology of facial bones in skulls with unoperated unilateral cleft palate. Cleft Palate J 4: 18–30.

Atherton, JD (1967b). A descriptive anatomy of the face in human fetuses with unilateral cleft lip and palate. Cleft Palate J 4: 104–114.

Baumrind, S, Moffit, F, Curry, S (1983). Three-dimensional x-ray stereometry from paired coplanar images. A progress report. Am J Orthod 84: 313.

Beiraghi, S, Foroud, T, Diouhy, S, et al. (1994). Possible localization of a major gene for cleft lip and palate to 4q. Clin Genet 46: 255–256.

Bergland, O, Sidhu, SS (1974). Occlusal changes from the deciduous to the early mixed dentition in unilateral complete clefts. Cleft Palate J 11: 317–326.

Bishara, SE (1973a). Cephalometric evaluation of facial growth in operated and non-operated individuals with isolated clefts of the palate. Cleft Palate J 10: 239–246.

Bishara, SE (1973b). The influence of palatoplasty and cleft length on facial development. Cleft Palate J 10: 390–398.

Bishara, SE, de Arrendondo, RS, Vales, HP, Jakobsen, JR (1985). Dentofacial relationships in persons with unoperated clefts: comparisons between three cleft types. Am J Orthod 87: 481–507.

Bishara, SE, Iversen, WW (1974). Cephalometric comparisons on the cranial base and face in individuals with isolated clefts of the palate. Cleft Palate J 11: 162–175.

Bishara, SE, Jakobsen, JR, Krause, JC, Sosa-Martinez, R (1986). Cephalometric comparisons of individuals from India and Mexico with unoperated cleft lip and palate. Cleft Palate J 23: 116–25.

Bishara, SE, Krause, CJ, Olin, WH, et al. (1976). Facial and dental relationships of individuals with unoperated clefts of the lip and/or palate. Cleft Palate J 13: 238–252.

Bishara, SE, Olin, WH, Krause, CJ (1978). Cephalometric findings in two cases with unrepaired bilateral cleft lip and palate. Cleft Palate J 15: 233–238.

Bishara, SE, Sierk, DL, Huang, KS (1979). A longitudinal cephalometric study on unilateral cleft lip and palate subjects. Cleft Palate J 16: 59–71.

Boo-Chai, K (1971). The unoperated adult bilateral cleft of the lip and palate. Br J Plast Surg 24: 250–257.

Bookstein, FL (1982). On the cephalometrics of skeletal change. Am J Orthod 82: 177–198.

Brader, AC (1957). A cephalometric x-ray appraisal of morphological variations in cranial base and associated pharyngeal structures: implications in cleft palate therapy. Angle Orthod 27: 179–194.

Broadbent, BH (1931). A new x-ray technique and its application to orthodontia. Angle Orthod 1: 45–66.

Capelozza Filho, L, Taniguchi, SM, da Silva Filho, OG (1993). Craniofacial morphology of adult unoperated complete unilateral cleft lip and palate patients. Cleft Palate Craniofac J 30: 376–381.

Casal, C, Rivera, A, Rubio, G, et al. (1997). Examination of craniofacial morphology in 10-month to 5-year-old children with cleft lip and palate. Cleft Palate Craniofac J 34: 490–497.

Chen, KF, So, LL (1997). Soft tissue profile changes of reverse headgear treatment in Chinese boys with complete unilateral cleft lip and palate. Angle Orthod 67: 31–38.

Cheverud, J, Lewis, JL, Bachrach, W, Lew, WD (1983). The measurement of form and variation in form: an application of three-dimensional quantitative morphology by finite-element methods. Am J Phys Anthropol 62: 151–165.

Chierici, G, Harvold, EP, Vargervik, K (1973). Morphogenetic experiments in cleft palate: mandibular response. Cleft Palate J 10: 51–61.

Coccaro, PJ, D'Amico, R, Chavoor, A (1972). Craniofacial morphology of parents with and without cleft lip and palate children. Cleft Palate J 9: 28–38.

Coupe, TB, Subtelny, JD (1960). Cleft palate—deficiency or displacement of tissue. Plast Reconstr Surg 26: 600–612.

Cronin, DG, Hunter, WS (1980). Craniofacial morphology in twins discordant for cleft lip and/or palate. Cleft Palate J 17: 116–126.

Dahl, E (1970). Craniofacial morphology in congenital clefts of the lip and palate. An x-ray cephalometric study of young adult males. Acta Odontol Scand 28: 11–164.

Dahl, E, Hanusardottir, B (1979). Prevalence of malocclusion in the primary and early mixed dentition in Danish children with complete cleft lip and palate. Eur J Orthod 1: 81–88.

Dahl, E, Kreiborg, S, Jensen, BL (1989). Roentgen-cephalometric studies of infants with untreated cleft lip and palate. In: What Is a Cleft Lip and Palate? A Multidisciplinary Update, edited by O Kriens. Stuttgart: Georg Thieme Verlag, pp. 113–115.

Dahl, E, Kreiborg, S, Jensen, BL, Fogh-Andersen, P (1982). Comparison of craniofacial morphology in infants with incomplete cleft lip and infants with isolated cleft palate. Cleft Palate J 19: 258–266.

da Silva Filho, OG, Carvalho Lauris, RC, Capelozza Filho, L, Semb, G (1998). Craniofacial morphology in adult patients with unoperated complete bilateral cleft lip and palate. Cleft Palate Craniofac J 35: 111–119.

da Silva Filho, OG, Normando, AD, Capelozza Filho, L (1992). Mandibular morphology and spatial position in patients with clefts: intrinsic or iatrogenic? Cleft Palate Craniofac J 29: 369–375.

da Silva Filho, OG, Normando, AD, Capelozza Filho, L (1993). Mandibular growth in patients with cleft lip and/or cleft palate—the influence of cleft type. Am J Orthod Dentofacial Orthop 104: 269–275.

Enemark, H, Bolund, S, Jorgensen, I (1990). Evaluation of unilateral cleft lip and palate treatment: long term results. Cleft Palate J 27: 354–361.

Erickson, JD (1974). Facial and oral form in sibs of children with cleft lip with or without cleft palate. Ann Hum Genet 38: 77–88.

Farkas, LG, Hajnis, K, Posnick, JC (1993). Anthropometric and anthroposcopic findings of the nasal and facial region in cleft patients before and after primary lip and palate repair. Cleft Palate Craniofac J 30: 1–12.

Farkas, LG, Lindsay, WK (1971). Morphology of the adult face following repair of bilateral cleft lip and palate in childhood. Plast Reconstr Surg 47: 25–32.

Farkas, LG, Lindsay, WK (1972a). Morphology of the orbital region in adults following the cleft lip-palate repair in childhood. Am J Phys Anthropol 37: 65–73.

Farkas, LG, Lindsay, WK (1972b). Morphology of adult face after repair of isolated cleft palate in childhood. Cleft Palate J 9: 132–142.

Fraser, FC, Pashayan, H (1970). Relation of face shape to susceptibility to congenital cleft lip. A preliminary report. J Med Genet 7: 112–117.

Friede, H, Johanson, B (1974). A follow-up study of cleft children treated with primary bone grafting. 1. Orthodontic aspects. Scand J Plast Reconstr Surg 8: 88–103.

Friede, H, Johanson, B (1977). A follow-up study of cleft children treated with vomer flap as part of a three-stage soft tissue surgical procedure. Facial morphology and dental occlusion. Scand J Plast Reconstr Surg 11: 45–57.

Friede, H, Figueroa, AA, Naegele, ML, et al. (1986). Craniofacial growth data for cleft lip patients infancy to 6 years of age: potential applications. Am J Orthod Dentofacial Orthop 90: 388–409.

Friede, H, Moller, M, Lilja, J, et al. (1987). Facial morphology and occlusion at the stage of early mixed dentition in cleft lip and palate patients treated with delayed closure of the hard palate. Scand J Plast Reconstr Surg Hand Surg 21: 65–71.

Friede, H, Pruzansky, S (1972). Longitudinal study of growth in bilateral cleft lip and palate, from infancy to adolescence. Plast Reconstr Surg 49: 392–403.

Gaggl, A, Schultes, G, Karcher, H (1999). Aesthetic and functional outcome of surgical and orthodontic correction of bilateral clefts of lip, palate, and alveolus. Cleft Palate Craniofac J 36: 407–412.

Glass, D (1970). The early management of bilateral cleft of lip and palate. Br J Plast Surg 23: 130–141.

Graber, TM (1949). A cephalometric analysis of the developmental pattern and facial morphology in cleft palate. Angle Orthod 19: 91–100.

Graber, TM (1954). The congenital cleft palate deformity. J Am Dent Assoc 48: 375–395.

Grayson, BH, Bookstein, FL, McCarthy, JG, Mueeddin, T (1987). Mean tensor cephalometric analysis of a patient population with clefts of the palate and lip. Cleft Palate J 24: 267–277.

Grayson, BH, McCarthy, JG, Bookstein, F (1983). Analysis of craniofacial asymmetry by multiplane cephalometry. Am J Orthod 84: 217–224.

Grayson, BH, Weintraub, N, Bookstein, FL, McCarthy, JG (1985). A comparative cephalometric study of the cranial base in craniofacial anomalies. Part I: Tensor analysis. Cleft Palate J 22: 75–87.

Hanada, K, Krogman, WM (1975). A longitudinal study of postoperative changes in the soft-tissue profile in bilateral cleft lip and palate from birth to 6 years. Am J Orthod 67: 363–376.

Handelman, CS, Pruzansky, S (1968). Occlusion and dental profile with complete bilateral cleft lip and palate. Angle Orthod 38: 185–198.

Harvold, E (1954). Cleft lip and palate. Am J Orthod 40: 493–506.

Hayashi, I, Sakuda, M, Takimoto, K, Miyazaki, T (1976). Craniofacial growth in complete unilateral cleft lip and palate: a roentgeno-cephalometric study. Cleft Palate J 13: 215–237.

Hermann, NV, Jensen, BL, Dahl, E, et al. (1999). Craniofacial growth in subjects with unilateral complete cleft lip and palate, and unilateral incomplete cleft lip, from 2 to 22 months of age. J Craniofac Genet Dev Biol 19: 135–147.

Hermann, NV, Jensen, BL, Dahl, E, et al. (2000). Craniofacial comparisons in 22-month-old lip-operated children with unilateral complete cleft lip and palate and unilateral incomplete cleft lip. Cleft Palate Craniofac J 37: 303–317.

Hirschfeld, WJ, Aduss, H (1974). Interorbital distance in cleft lip and palate: significant differences found by sign test. J Dent Res 53: 947.

Horowitz, SL, Graf, B, Bettex, M, et al. (1980). Factor analysis of craniofacial morphology in complete bilateral cleft lip and palate. Cleft Palate J 17: 234–244.

Horowitz, SL, Graf-Pinthus, B, Bettex, M, et al. (1976). Factor analysis of craniofacial morphology in cleft lip and palate in man. Arch Oral Biol 21: 465–472.

Horswell, BB, Gallup, BV (1992). Cranial base morphology in cleft lip and palate: a cephalometric study from 7 to 18 years of age. J Oral Maxillofac Surg 50: 681–686.

Huddart, AG (1970). Maxillary arch dimensions in bilateral cleft lip and palate subjects. Cleft Palate J 7: 139–155.

Innes, CO (1962). Some observations on unrepaired hare-lips and cleft palates in adult members of the Dusan tribes of north Borneo. Br J Plast Surg 15: 173–181.

Ishiguro, K, Krogman, WM, Mazaheri, M, Harding, RL (1976). A longitudinal study of morphological craniofacial patterns via P-A x-ray headfilms in cleft patients from birth to six years of age. Cleft Palate J 13: 104–126.

Ishikawa, H, Kitazawa, S, Iwasaki, H, Nakamura, S (2000). Effects of maxillary protraction combined with chin-cap therapy in unilateral cleft lip and palate patients. Cleft Palate Craniofac J 37: 92–97.

Jain, RB, Krogman, WM (1983a). Cleft type and sex differences in craniofacial growth in clefting from one month to ten years. Cleft Palate J 20: 238–245.

Jain, RB, Krogman, WM (1983b). Craniofacial growth in clefting from one month to ten years as studied by P-A headfilms. Cleft Palate J 20: 314–326.

Kilpeläinen, PV, Laine-Alava, MT (1996). Palatal asymmetry in cleft palate subjects. Cleft Palate Craniofac J 33: 483–488.

Kilpeläinen, PV, Laine-Alava, MT, Lammi, S (1996). Palatal morphology and type of clefting. Cleft Palate Craniofac J 33: 477–482.

Krogman, WM, Mazaheri, M, Harding, RL, et al (1975). A longitudinal study of the craniofacial growth pattern in children with clefts as compared to normal, birth to six years. Cleft Palate J 12: 59–84.

Kurisu, K, Niswander, JD, Johnston, MC, Mazaheri, M (1974). Facial morphology as an indicator of genetic predisposition to cleft lip and palate. Am J Hum Genet 26: 702–714.

Kyrkanides, S, Bellohusen, R, Subtelny, JD (1995). Skeletal asymmetries of the nasomaxillary complex in noncleft and postsurgical unilateral cleft lip and palate individuals. Cleft Palate Craniofac J 32: 428–433.

Lestrel, PE, Berkowitz, S, Takahashi, O (1999). Shape changes in the cleft palate maxilla: a longitudinal study. Cleft Palate Craniofac J 36: 292–303.

Levin, HS (1963). A cephalometric analysis of cleft palate deficiencies in the middle third of the face. Angle Orthod 33: 186–194.

Mars, M, Houston, WJ (1990). A preliminary study of facial growth and morphology in unoperated male unilateral cleft lip and palate subjects over 13 years of age. Cleft Palate J 27: 7–10.

McAlarney, ME, Chiu, WK (1997). Comparison of numeric techniques in the analysis of cleft palate dental arch form change. Cleft Palate Craniofac J 34: 281–291.

Mestre, J, DeJesus, J, Subtelny, JD (1960). Unoperated oral clefts at maturation. Angle Orthod 30: 78–85.

Molsted, K, Dahl, E (1990). Asymmetry of the maxilla in children with complete unilateral cleft lip and palate [published erratum appears in Cleft Palate J 1990;27: 444]. Cleft Palate J 27: 184–192.

Molsted, K, Asher-McDade, C, Brattstrom, V, et al. (1992). A six-center international study of treatment outcome in patients with clefts of the lip and palate: Part 2. Craniofacial form and soft tissue profile. Cleft Palate Craniofac J 29: 398–404.

Molsted, K, Kjaer, I, Dahl, E (1993). Spheno-occipital synchondrosis in three-month-old children with clefts of the lip and palate: a radiographic study. Cleft Palate Craniofac J 30: 569–573.

Molsted, K, Kjaer, I, Dahl, E (1995). Cranial base in newborns with complete cleft lip and palate: radiographic study. Cleft Palate Craniofac J 32: 199–205.

Molsted, K, Palmberg, A, Dahl, E, Fogh-Andersen, P (1987). Malocclusion in complete unilateral and bilateral cleft lip and palate. The results of a change in the surgical procedure. Scand J Plast Reconstr Surg Hand Surg 21: 81–85.

Moss, ML (1997a). The functional matrix hypothesis revisited. 3. The genomic thesis. Am J Orthod Dentofacial Orthop 112: 338–342.

Moss, ML (1997b). The functional matrix hypothesis revisited. 4. The epigenetic antithesis and the resolving synthesis. Am J Orthod Dentofacial Orthop 112: 410–417.

Mossey, PA, Arngrimsson, R, McColl, J, et al. (1998a). Prediction of liability to orofacial clefting using genetic and craniofacial data from parents. J Med Genet 35: 371–378.

Mossey, PA, McColl, J, O'Hara, M (1998b). Cephalometric features in the parents of children with orofacial clefting. Br J Oral Maxillofac Surg 36: 202–212.

Mossey, PA, McColl, JH, Stirrups, DR (1997). Differentiation between cleft lip with or without cleft palate and isolated cleft palate using parental cephalometric parameters. Cleft Palate Craniofac J 34: 27–35.

Motohashi, N, Kuroda, T, Capelozza Filho, L, Freitas, JA (1994). P-A cephalometric analysis of nonoperated adult cleft lip and palate. Cleft Palate Craniofac J 31: 193–200.

Moyers, RE, Bookstein, FL (1979). The inappropriateness of conventional cephalometrics. Am J Orthod 75: 599–617.

Nakamura, S, Savara, BS, Thomas, DR (1972). Facial growth of children with cleft lip and/or palate. Cleft Palate J 9: 119–131.

Nakasima, A, Ichinose, M (1983). Characteristics of craniofacial structures of parents of children with cleft lip and/or palate. Am J Orthod 84: 140–146.

Nakasima, A, Ichinose, M (1984). Size of the cranium in parents and their children with cleft lip. Cleft Palate J 21: 193–203.

Narula, JK, Ross, RB (1970). Facial growth in children with complete bilateral cleft lip and palate. Cleft Palate J 7: 239–248.

Nordén, E, Linder-Aronson, S, Stenberg, T (1973). The deciduous dentition after only primary surgical operations for clefts of the lip, jaw, and palate. Am J Orthod 63: 229–236.

Ortiz-Monasterio, F, Afonso Serrano, R, Gustavo Barrera, P, et al. (1966). A study of untreated adult cleft palate patients. Plast Reconstr Surg 38: 36–41.

Ortiz-Monasterio, F, Rebiel, A, Valderrama, M, Crux, R (1959). Cephalometric measurements in adult patients with non-operated cleft palate. Plast Reconstr Surg 24: 53–61.

Peltonen, L, McKusick, V (2001). Dissecting human diseases in the postgenomic era. Science 291: 1224–1229.

Peterka, M (1979). Prenatal Growth and Damage of the Orofacial Complex [in Czech]. Prague: Czechoslovak Academy of Sciences. Dissertation.

Prochazkova, J, Tolarová, M (1986). Craniofacial morphological features in parents of children with isolated cleft palate. Acta Chir Plast 28: 194–204.

Prochazkova, J, Vinsova, J (1995). Craniofacial morphology as a marker of predisposition to isolated cleft palate. J Craniofac Genet Dev Biol 15: 162–168.

Pruzansky, S, Aduss, H (1967). Prevalence of arch collapse and malocclusion in complete unilateral cleft lip and palate. Rep Congr Eur Orthod Soc 365–382.

Raghavan, R, Sidhu, SS, Kharbanda, OP (1994). Craniofacial pattern of parents of children having cleft lip and/or cleft palate anomaly. Angle Orthod 64: 137–144.

Ras, F, Habets, LL, van Ginkel, FC, Prahl-Andersen, B (1994a). Three-dimensional evaluation of facial asymmetry in cleft lip and palate. Cleft Palate Craniofac J 31: 116–21.

Ras, F, Habets, LL, van Ginkel, FC, Prahl-Andersen, B (1994b). Facial left–right dominance in cleft lip and palate: three-dimension evaluation. Cleft Palate Craniofac J 31: 461–465.

Rohrich, RJ, Byrd, HS (1990). Optimal timing of cleft palate closure. Speech, facial growth, and hearing considerations. Clin Plast Surg 17: 27–36.

Ross, RB (1987). Treatment variables affecting facial growth in complete unilateral cleft lip and palate. Cleft Palate J 24: 3–89.

Ross, RB, Coupe, TB (1965). Craniofacial morphology in six pairs of monozygotic twins discordant for cleft lip and palate. J Can Dent Assoc 31: 149–157.

Ross, RB, Johnston, MC (1972). Cleft Lip and Palate. Baltimore: Williams & Wilkins.

Saksena, SS, Bixler, D, Yu, P (1990). A Clinical Atlas of Roentgencephalometry in Norma Frontalis. New York: Alan R. Liss.

Saksena, SS, Walker, GF, Bixler, D, Yu, P (1987). A Clinical Atlas of Roentgencephalometry in Norma Lateralis. New York: Alan R. Liss.

Sammons, E (1999). Cephalometric Similarity among Parents of Individuals with Sporadic Isolated Cleft Palate: Is There Evidence for an Inherited Predisposition? Indianapolis: Indiana University School of Dentistry. Dissertation.

Sandham, A, Murray, JA (1993). Nasal septal deformity in unilateral cleft lip and palate. Cleft Palate Craniofac J 30: 222–226.

Sassouni, V (1962). The Face in Five Dimensions, 2nd ed. Morgantown: West Virginia University Press.

Savara, BS, Miller, SH, Demuth, RJ, Kawamoto, HK (1985). Biostereometrics and computer graphics for patients with craniofacial malformation: diagnosis and treatment planning. Plast Reconstr Surg 75: 495.

Schultes, G, Gaggl, A, Karcher, H (2000). A comparison of growth impairment and orthodontic results in adult patients with clefts of palate and unilateral clefts of lip, palate and alveolus. Br J Oral Maxillofac Surg 38: 26–32.

Semb, G (1991a). A study of facial growth in patients with unilateral cleft lip and palate treated by the Oslo CLP Team. Cleft Palate Craniofac J 28: 1–21.

Semb, G (1991b). A study of facial growth in patients with bilateral cleft lip and palate treated by the Oslo CLP Team. Cleft Palate Craniofac J 28: 22–39.

Shibasaki, Y, Ross, RB (1969). Facial growth in children with isolated cleft palate. Cleft Palate J 6: 290–302.

Shprintzen, RJ, Siegel-Sadewitz, VL, Amato, J, Goldberg, RB (1985). Anomalies associated with cleft lip, cleft palate, or both. Am J Med Genet 20: 585–595.

Šmahel, Z (1984a). Variations in craniofacial morphology with severity of isolated cleft palate. Cleft Palate J 21: 140–158.

Šmahel, Z (1984b). Craniofacial morphology in adults with bilateral complete cleft lip and palate. Cleft Palate J 21: 159–169.

Šmahel, Z (1984c). Cephalometric and morphologic facial changes in adults with complete bilateral cleft lip and palate. Acta Chir Plast 26: 200–215.

Šmahel, Z (1984d). Craniofacial changes in unilateral cleft lip in adults. Acta Chir Plast 26: 129–149.

Šmahel, Z, Brejcha, M (1983). Differences in craniofacial morphology between complete and incomplete unilateral cleft lip and palate in adults. Cleft Palate J 20: 113–127.

Šmahel, Z, Brousilova, M, Müllerová, Z (1987). Craniofacial morphology in isolated cleft palate prior to palatoplasty. Cleft Palate J 24: 200–208.

Šmahel, Z, Hradisky, D, Müllerová, Z (1999). Multivariate comparison of craniofacial morphology in different types of facial clefts. Acta Chir Plast 41: 59–65.

Šmahel, Z, Müllerová, Z (1986). Craniofacial morphology in unilateral cleft lip and palate prior to palatoplasty. Cleft Palate J 23: 225–232.

Šmahel, Z, Pobisova, Z, Figalova, P (1985). Basic cephalometric facial characteristics in cleft lip and/or cleft palate prior to the first surgical repair. Acta Chir Plast 27: 131–144.

Steinhäuser, EW, Rudzki-Janson, JM (1994). Kieferorthopädische Chirurgie: Eine interdisziplinäre Aufgabe. Berlin: Quintessenz Verlag.

Subtelny, JD (1955). Width of the nasopharynx and related anatomic structures in normal and unoperated cleft palate children. Am J Orthod 41: 889–909.

Suzuki, A, Takenoshita, Y, Honda, Y, Matsuura, C (1999). Dentocraniofacial morphology in parents of children with cleft lip and/or palate. Cleft Palate Craniofac J 36: 131–138.

Tang, EL, So, LL (1992). Prevalence and severity of malocclusion in children with cleft lip and/or palate in Hong Kong. Cleft Palate Craniofac J 29: 287–291.

Thompson, DW (1917). On Growth and Form. Cambridge: Cambridge University Press.

Trasler, DG (1968). Pathogenesis of cleft lip and its relation to embryonic face shape in A-J and C57BL mice. Teratology 1: 33–49.

Trotman, CA, Collett, AR, McNamara, JA, Jr, Cohen, SR (1993). Analyses of craniofacial and dental morphology in monozygotic twins discordant for cleft lip and unilateral cleft lip and palate. Angle Orthod 63: 135–139.

Trotman, CA, Papillon, F, Ross, RB, et al. (1997). A retrospective comparison of frontal facial dimensions in alveolar bone-grafted and nongrafted unilateral cleft lip and palate patients. Angle Orthod 67: 389–394.

Trotman, CA, Ross, RB (1993). Craniofacial growth in bilateral cleft lip and palate: ages six years to adulthood. Cleft Palate Craniofac J 30: 261–273.

Vegter, F, Mulder, JW, Hage, JJ (1997). Major residual deformities in cleft patients: a new anthropometric approach. Cleft Palate Craniofac J 34: 106–110.

Ward, RE, Bixler, D, Jamison, PL (1994). Cephalometric evidence for a dominantly inherited predisposition to cleft lip–cleft palate in a single large kindred. Am J Med Genet 50: 57–63.

Ward, RE, Bixler, D, Raywood, ER (1989). A study of cephalometric features in cleft lip–cleft palate families. I: Phenotypic heterogeneity and genetic predisposition in parents of sporadic cases. Cleft Palate J 26: 318–326.

Wepner, F, Hollmann, K (1975). Mid-face anthropometry on the cephalometric radiograph in cleft lip and palate cases. J Maxillofac Surg 3: 188–197.

8

Craniofacial morphology and growth in infants and young children with cleft lip and palate

SVEN KREIBORG

NUNO V. HERMANN

Cleft lip and palate (CLP) may have severe consequences for affected individuals because oral clefts interfere with two of the most important means of communication: facial expression and speech. Individuals with either unoperated or operated clefts usually have a face which differs from that of unaffected individuals. Studies including both unoperated and operated individuals have shown that some deviations are directly caused by the primary anomaly, while others are caused by the surgical interventions and the subsequent dysplastic and compensatory growth of the facial bones (Dahl, 1970; Ehmann, 1989; Mars and Houston, 1990; Dahl and Kreiborg, 1995; Sandham and Foong, 1997).

Semb and Shaw (1996) suggested several factors that may be potential sources of interference with the normal craniofacial growth pattern in individuals with clefts:

1. Variations intrinsically associated with the cleft malformation
2. Other variations intrinsically associated with the cleft
3. Functional adaptations
4. Surgical iatrogenesis.

Severe surgical iatrogenesis to maxillary development in individuals with clefts has been documented repeatedly (Graber, 1949, 1954; Slaughter and Brodie, 1949; Bishara and Olin, 1972; Friede and Pruzansky, 1972a,b; Friede and Johanson, 1974; Tomanova and Müllerova, 1994). Attention has been drawn to the harmful interference with the maxillary growth zones (Friede, 1998), including the premaxillary–vomerine complex (Pruzansky, 1971; Friede and Morgan, 1976; Friede, 1977, 1978). As a consequence of these studies, certain surgical procedures, such as premaxillary setback and primary bone grafting, have been largely abandoned because they were shown to lead to disturbed maxillary growth and facial concavity. However, even more cautious surgical procedures are claimed to interfere with maxillary growth. Maxillary retrognathia is a good example. Some authors believe that in subjects with CLP, maxillary retrognathia is intrinsically associated with the primary cleft malformation. Others, however, claim it to be caused by surgical iatrogenesis (Bishara et al., 1976; Dahl et al., 1982, 1989; Semb and Shaw, 1996; Hermann et al., 1999a). The major reason for this disagreement is the scarcity of data based on large, consecutive, well-controlled samples on the craniofacial morphogenesis of infants with oral clefts before surgery. This lack of information is not surprising. In many institutions, cleft lip (CL) is surgically treated within the first couple of months after birth. Thus, the available period to examine the unoperated state is short.

Comprehensive quantitative analysis of the infant's craniofacial morphology requires the use of infant roentgencephalometry (Pruzansky and Lis, 1958), including several projections, combined with study models of the maxilla. Although infant cephalometry was introduced more than 50 years ago and has been shown to be useful in the study of congenital craniofacial anomalies (Pruzansky and Lis, 1958; Kreiborg, 1985), few investigators have adopted these techniques in the evaluation of patients with CLP (Mazaheri and Sahni, 1969; Pruzansky, 1971, 1973; Robertson and Hilton, 1971; Friede and Pruzansky, 1972a,b; Dahan, 1974; Krogman et al., 1975, 1982a,b; Ishiguru et al., 1976; Friede, 1977; Kreiborg et al., 1977, 1985; Dahl et al., 1982, 1989; Long et al., 1982; Jain and Krogman, 1983a,b; Friede et al., 1986; Berkowitz, 1995; Han et al., 1995; Mølsted et al., 1995; Kreiborg and Cohen, 1996; Hermann et al., 1999a,b; 2000, 2001b). Furthermore, most of the relatively few cephalometric studies of unoperated infants with CLP have been limited to the lateral projection, a few have included the frontal projection, and only a handful have included the lateral, frontal, and axial projections (Dahan, 1974; Dahl et al., 1982; Mølsted et al., 1995; Hermann et al., 1999a,b, 2000). All but one of the latter studies come from our group in Copenhagen, and these studies form the basis of this chapter.

Additional information about the primary anomaly can be obtained from studies of older children, adolescents, and adults with unoperated clefts. A number of such roentgencephalometric studies have been published on subjects from Brazil, Cameroon, Czekoslovakia, Denmark, India, Mexico, and Sri Lanka, among others (Ortiz-Monasterio et al., 1959, 1966; Bishara, 1973; Bishara et al., 1976, 1985, 1986; Dahl, 1970; Smahel et al., 1987; Ehmann, 1989; Mars and Houston, 1990; da Silva Filho et al., 1992a,b, 1998; Capelozza et al., 1993; Capelozza Filho et al., 1996). However, most of these studies are limited by small sample sizes and the mixture of unoperated, partially operated, and late operated individuals. Cephalometric findings are also limited since often they only include the lateral projection or perform simplistic cephalometric analyses, typically based on 15 to 20 reference points, or measure maxillary prognathism as the nasion-sella-point A angle or similar measurements to the premaxilla.

The aim of this chapter is to summarize the available information on the intrinsic craniofacial morphology in individuals with oral clefts. The data presented here come primarily from our own studies but are supplemented with findings from the literature, especially regarding unoperated older children, adolescents, and adults.

MATERIAL AND METHODS

Inspired by Dr. Samuel Pruzansky, we designed a three-projection cephalometer in the mid-1970s (Kreiborg et al., 1977) (Figs. 8.1, 8.2). From 1976 to 1981, we examined nearly all infants born with a cleft in Denmark (Jensen et al., 1988). Almost all children were examined at both 2 months (prior to any surgery) and 22 months of age by three-projection cephalometry and impressions of the palate. More than 600 consecutive cases were examined. A comprehensive set of cephalometric landmarks ($n = 279$), defining all craniofacial regions, was built into a digitizing system (Kreiborg, 1981, 1989; Heller et al., 1995; Hermann et al., 2001a) (Color Figs. 8.3, 8.4, Fig. 8.5).

The total sample of nonsyndromic oral cleft individuals comprised more than 600. Patients were divided into four groups: CL (cleft of the primary palate only); CP (cleft of the secondary palate only); Robin sequence (RS) (CP, glossoptosis, and micrognathia); and CLP (cleft of both the primary and secondary palate). Cases with CLP were subsequently classified according to severity (Jensen et al., 1988) (Fig. 8.6).

By the time this chapter was submitted for publication, the following groups had been analyzed:

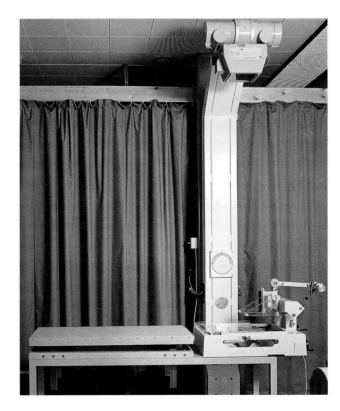

FIG. 8.1. Roentgencephalometric unit with two high-kilovoltage x-ray tubes for infants. (From Kreiborg et al., 1977, with permission.)

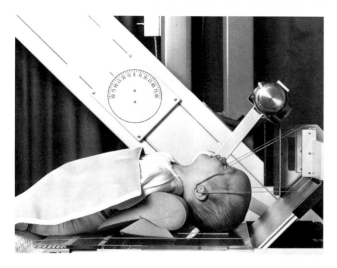

FIG. 8.2. The x-ray tube above the cephalostat is tilted 45 degrees for the axial projection. The center of rotation is located at the axial ray of the x-ray tube for the lateral projection. The correct orientation of the head is secured by the ear rods and a light cross projected on the face. Note that the casette holder for this projection has an angulation of 45 degrees to the vertical plane. (From Kreiborg et al., 1977, with permission.)

1. Unilateral incomplete CL (UICL) at 2 and 22 months of age (Hermann et al., 1999a,b, 2000, 2001b; Darvann et al., 2001)
2. Isolated CP at 2 and 22 months of age (Dahl et al., 1982, 1989; Kreiborg et al., 1985; Kreiborg and Cohen, 1996; Hermann et al., 2001b)
3. RS at 2 and 22 months of age (Kreiborg et al., 1985; Kreiborg and Cohen, 1996; Hermann et al., 2001b)
4. Unilateral complete CLP (UCCLP) at 2 and 22 months of age (Hermann et al., 1999a,b, 2000, 2001b; Darvann et al., 2001)
5. Bilateral complete CLP (BCCLP) at 2 months of age (Dahl et al., 1989)

Cleft Lip

Isolated CL involves only structures of the embryonic primary palate. The craniofacial morphology in subjects with CL is fairly normal, except for the small region of the cleft including the premaxilla and the incisors. In unoperated bilateral complete CL, the premaxilla may protrude markedly. In unilateral complete CL, the protrusion is less pronounced but asymmetric. In subjects with UICL, the protrusion of the premaxilla is negligible (Hermann et al., 1999a). The interorbital distance in subjects with CL appears to be slightly increased. The basal part of the maxilla has normal prognathism in relation to the anterior cranial base, and the mandible is of normal size, shape, and

inclination (Dahl, 1970; Hermann et al., 1999a). Following lip surgery, the premaxilla is molded into a normal position by pressure from the soft tissue and maxillary prognathism measured to point A or ss (subspinale) is normal (Dahl, 1970; Han et al., 1995; Hermann et al., 1999a,b, 2000) (Fig. 8.7). Consequently, for the purpose of this chapter, the group of patients with UICL was used as a control.

Cleft Palate

Isolated CP involves only structures of the embryonic secondary palate. Dahl et al. (1982, 1989) reported on 30 unoperated 2-month-old cases with CP from our sample. In Figure 8.8, the mean facial diagram of the CP group is superimposed on the mean facial diagram of a group of age-matched infants with CL (control group). The major deviations in the CP group were bimaxillary retrognathia, reduced length and posterior height of the maxilla, and reduced length of the mandible with mandibular retrognathia. The sagittal jaw relationship was normal. In the CP group, the upper airway dimensions were reduced. Hermann et al. (2001b) found similar deviations in infants with CP. They also observed increased width of the maxilla and nasal cavity. The mean facial growth pattern in the CP group from 2 to 22 months of age, before palatal surgery, was reported by Kreiborg and Cohen (1996) (Fig. 8.9). The facial growth pattern seemed harmonious. The bimaxillary retrognathia, with a normal sagittal jaw relationship, persisted. The cranial base angle decreased somewhat. The direction of facial growth was, however, more vertical than in the control group.

Bimaxillary retrognathia has been documented in unoperated older children (Smahel et al., 1987) and adults (Dahl, 1970; Bishara, 1972) with CP and must be considered as a variation intrinsically associated with the cleft malfornation. Dahl (1970) found an increased vertical dimension of the face in adult CP subjects (Fig. 8.10).

Robin Sequence

Robin sequence is defined by the presence of the following three cardinal signs: isolated CP, micrognathia, and glossoptosis (Gorlin et al., 1990). It may be part of several syndromes, e.g., Treacher Collins syndrome (Kreiborg and Cohen, 1996; Cohen, 1997). In this chapter, only nonsyndromic cases of RS will be discussed. We consider this to be a subgroup of the larger CP group.

Kreiborg et al. (1985) and Kreiborg and Cohen (1996) have described the unoperated infant facial

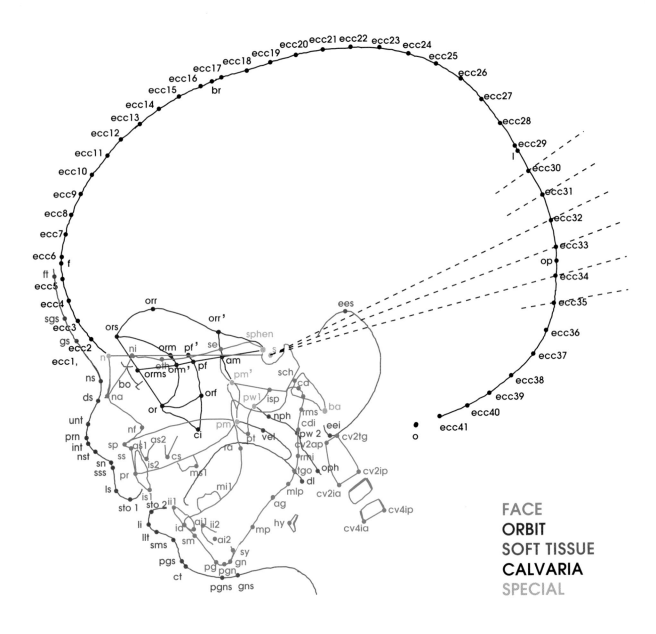

COLOR FIG. 8.3. Landmarks and their names in the lateral x-ray. Landmarks denoted *ecc1–42* are defined by radii drawn from a center point (sella) 5 degrees apart. All landmarks are defined as belonging to a certain layer *(Face, Orbit, Soft tissue, Calvaria)*, indicated by a color code, or to the group denoted *Special*, which indicates that they exist in all four layers. (From Hermann et al., 1999a, with permission.)

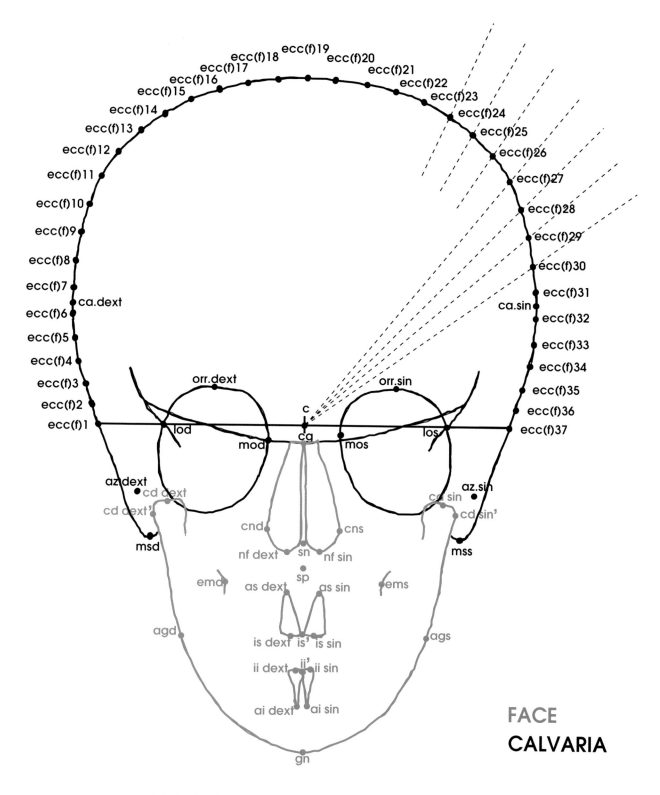

COLOR FIG. 8.4. Landmarks and their names in the frontal x-ray. Landmarks denoted *ecc(f)37* are defined by radii drawn from a center point (sella) 5 degrees apart. All landmarks are defined as belonging to one of the two layers *Face* or *Calvaria*. (From Hermann et al., 1999a, with permission.)

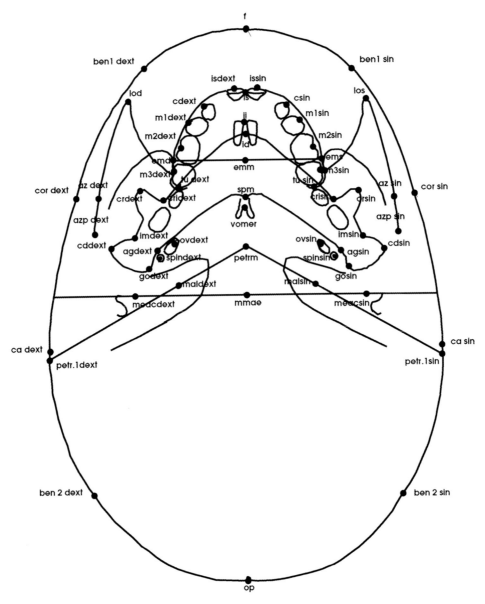

FIG. 8.5. Landmarks and their names in the axial x-ray. All landmarks belong to one single layer. (From Hermann et al., 1999a, with permission.)

morphology and early facial growth in eight consecutive cases from our sample. In Figure 8.11, the mean facial diagram of the RS group at 2 months of age is superimposed on the mean facial diagram of an age-matched CP group (Kreiborg and Cohen, 1996). The RS infants had a significantly smaller cranial base angle (nasion-sella-basion), shorter mandible with more marked mandibular retrognathia, and smaller depth of the bony nasopharynx than the CP infants. The degree of maxillary retrognathia was similar in the RS and the CP groups compared to infants with UICL. The marked mandibular retrognathia in the RS group was confirmed by Hermann et al. (2001b), documenting

significant mandibular retrognathia in the CP group and even more marked retrognathia in RS subjects. Both studies concluded that RS subjects probably represent the extreme part of the CP population in terms of mandibular retrognathia and upper airway constriction.

The facial growth pattern in the RS group from 2 to 22 months of age, before palatal surgery, is illustrated in Figure 8.12 (Kreiborg and Cohen, 1996). Facial growth seemed harmonious. At 22 months of age, the maxilla was still retrognathic and the mandible was also still markedly retrognathic compared to the CP group (Fig. 8.13). However, all patients with RS had

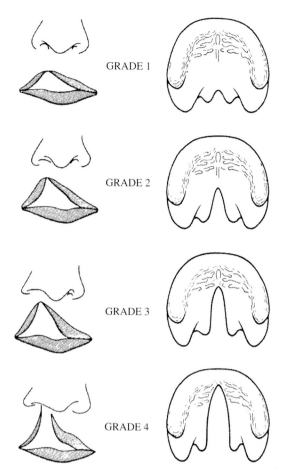

GRADE 1

GRADE 2

GRADE 3

GRADE 4

FIG. 8.6. The principle of catagorizing cleft lip and palate (Jensen et al., 1988). The extent of the cleft lip and the cleft palate was divided into four grades. Cleft lip: grade 1, up to one-third of lip height; grade 2, greater than one-third to two-thirds of lip height; grade 3, greater than two-thirds to subtotal; grade 4, total. Cleft palate: grade 1, soft palate; grade 2, one-third of hard palate; grade 3, greater than one-third up to subtotal; grade 4, total.

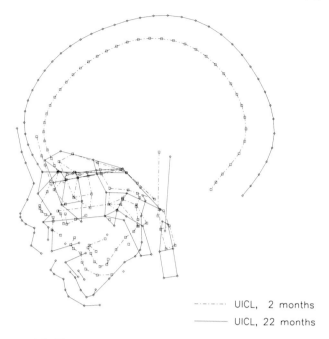

------- UICL, 2 months
——— UICL, 22 months

FIG. 8.7. The average craniofacial growth from 2 to 22 months of age in the unilateral incomplete cleft lip *(UICL)* group *(n = 45)* in the lateral projection. (From Hermann et al., 1999b, with permission.)

outgrown their airway problems because of the increase in facial and airway dimensions.

As mentioned above, the RS group is considered a special subgroup of the CP group. Accordingly, it is believed that the bimaxillary retrognathia is intrinsically associated with clefting of the secondary palate.

Cleft Lip and Palate

Combined clefts of the lip, alveolous, and palate involve structures of both the embryonic primary palate and secondary palate. In Figure 8.14, the mean cranio-facial morphology in 2-month-old unoperated infants with UCCLP is compared to a control group consisting of individuals with UICL (Hermann et al., 1999a). No marked differences were observed in the calvaria or cranial base. A number of significant differences were

found, however, in the facial structures. In the UCCLP group, the most pronounced deviations were observed in the maxillary complex and the mandible. The most striking findings were the markedly increased width of the maxilla and nasal cavity, a short mandible, and bimaxillary retrognathia except for the premaxillary area, which was relatively protruding and asymmetric. Facial retrognathia was also suggested to be part of the primary anomalies associated with the cleft deformity in

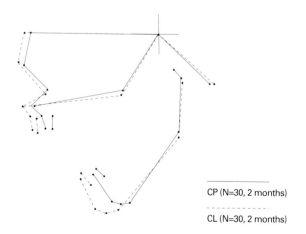

CP (N=30, 2 months)

CL (N=30, 2 months)

FIG. 8.8. Mean drawings of the 2-month-old unoperated cleft palate *(CP)* and cleft lip *(CL)* groups *(n = 30* in both groups) superimposed on the nasion-sella line and registered on the sella. (Modified from Dahl et al., 1989.)

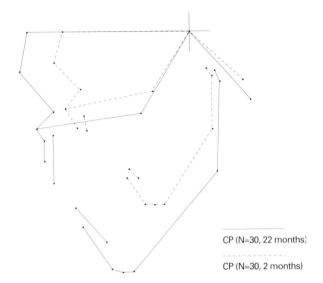

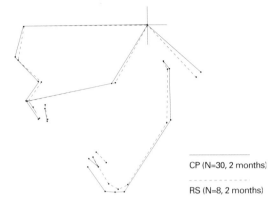

FIG. 8.11. Mean drawings of 2-month-old unoperated cleft palate *(CP*, n = 30) and Robin sequence *(RS, n* = 8) groups superimposed on the nasion-sella line and registered on the sella. (Modified from Kreiborg and Cohen, 1996.)

FIG. 8.9. Average facial growth in the cleft palate *(CP)* group *(n* = 30) from 2 to 22 months of age. Mean drawings are superimposed on the nasion-sella line and registered on the sella. (Modified from Kreiborg and Cohen, 1996.)

unilateral CLP by Sandham and Foong (1997). Increased width of the midface and nasal cavity has been reported in unoperated UCCLP infants (Han et al., 1995) and in unoperated adults with UCCLP (Motohashi et al., 1994). Relative protrusion and asymmetry of the premaxilla have also been reported in unoperated UCCLP

children, adolescents, and adults (Ortiz-Monasterio et al., 1959, 1966; Bishara et al., 1976, 1985, 1986; Capelozza et al., 1993), probably due to overgrowth in the premaxillary–vomerine complex (Pruzansky, 1971; Friede and Morgan, 1976; Friede, 1978). The overgrowth is probably an effect of the lack of structural integrety in the region. The relative protrusion of the premaxilla explains why the measurements *s-n-ans* (sella-nasion-anterior nasal spine) and *s-n-ss* (S-N-A) in the infant UCCLP group are comparable to the values in the control group, despite the fact that the UCCLP group showed significant maxillary retrognathia measured to the lateral segments. Also, several studies of older unoperated UCCLP children and adults have found

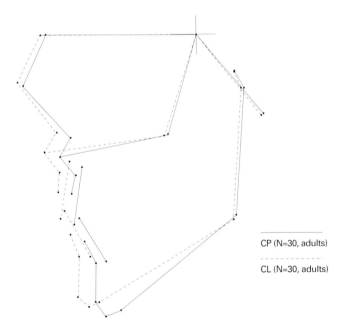

FIG. 8.10. Mean drawings of adult cleft palate *(CP)* and cleft lip *(CL)* groups *(n* = 30 in both groups) superimposed on the nasion-sella line and registered on the sella. (Modified from Dahl et al., 1989.)

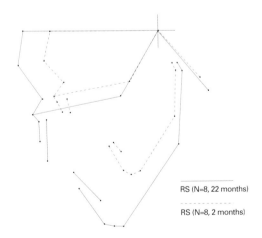

FIG. 8.12. Average growth in the Robin sequence *(RS)* group *(n* = 8) from 2 to 22 months of age. Mean drawings are superimposed on the nasion-sella line and registered on the sella. (Modified from Kreiborg and Cohen, 1996.)

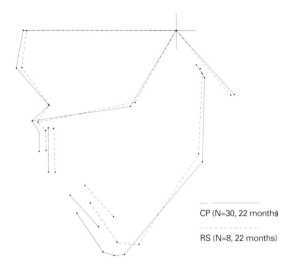

CP (N=30, 22 months)

RS (N=8, 22 months)

FIG. 8.13. Mean drawings of 22-month-old unoperated cleft palate (*CP*, *n* = 30) and Robin sequence (*RS*, *n* = 8) groups superimposed on the nasion-sella line and registered on the sella. (Modified from Kreiborg and Cohen, 1996.)

the maxillary prognathism to be within normal limits or even increased compared to normative data (Ortiz-Monasterio et al., 1959, 1966; Mars and Houston, 1990; Capelozza et al., 1993). All of these studies, however, measured prognathism only to the *A point* or to the point *ANS*, both located in the relatively protruding premaxilla. Ortiz-Monasterio et al. (1959) concluded the following, based on their findings in unoperated adults with UCCLP: "The embryonic factor responsible for the facial cleft does not interfere with maxillary growth. This evidence leads us to believe that growth defects of the middle third of the face so frequently seen are caused by early or repeated and agressive surgery." We disagree somewhat with this conclusion. Based on our studies of infants with UCCLP, the maxillary retrognathia in this group appears to be part of the intrinsic variations associated with the cleft malformation of the secondary palate. In the unoperated infant and the unoperated adult, the maxillary retrognathia is, however, partly masked by relative protrusion of the premaxilla, secondary to overgrowth in the premaxillary–vomerine suture. Surgical closure of the lip at 2 months of age molds the premaxilla back into place, unmasking the maxillary retrognathia (Figs. 8.15, 8.16). Thus, we believe that the bimaxillary retrognathia shown in Figure 8.15 illustrates the facial type characteristic of the 22-month-old lip-operated UCCLP group. The maxillary retrognathia observed at 22 months of age, therefore, should not be considered the result of surgical iatrogenesis. Rather, it represents a normalization of the "intrinsic facial type" characteristic of subjects with UCCLP. By the time this

chapter went to press, the sample had not yet been re-examined at older ages. Therefore, it is not possible to comment on facial growth and signs of further surgical iatrogenesis after the age of 2 years.

Dahl et al. (1982) analyzed facial morphology in 2-month-old infants with unoperated BCCLP (*n* = 22) from our sample. Figure 8.17 illustrates the mean facial diagram of the BCCLP group superimposed on the mean facial diagram of an age-matched group with UICL (*n* = 30). The most obvious features in the BC-CLP group were protrusion of the premaxilla, increased width of the maxilla and nasal cavity, reduced posterior maxillary height, and a short and retrognathic mandible. The body of the maxilla was, however, retrognathic when measured to both its anterior and posterior aspects. Thus, the protruding premaxilla was situated in a totally retrognathic face. The protruding premaxilla is probably the result of overgrowth in the premaxillary–vomerine complex secondary to lack of structural integrity in the region, as discussed above.

For comparison, Mars and Houston (1990) and da Silva Filho et al. (1998) described groups of adult unoperated patients with BCCLP and found extreme protrusion of the premaxilla and a very convex profile measured as the ANB angle. No measurements were performed to describe the position of the body of the maxilla.

The retrognathia of the body of the maxilla and the short and retrognathic mandible found in the present sample are, in our opinion, variations intrinsically associated with the cleft of the secondary palate (as discussed above). The facial growth pattern, from the time of lip surgery at 2 months of age to the time of palatal closure at 22 months of age, was characterized by a normal amount of jaw growth but an increased vertical growth direction (Hermann et al., 1999b) (Color Fig. 8.18).

DISCUSSION AND CONCLUSIONS

The findings discussed in this chapter support the suggestion of Dahl (1970) and others that facial clefts should be classified based on embryonic facial development, i.e., into clefts involving the primary palate only (CL), clefts involving the secondary palate only (CP), and clefts involving structures of both the primary and secondary palate (CLP). The postnatal facial morphology and growth in these groups differ greatly.

It has been the aim of this chapter to summarize the available information about the intrinsic variations in facial morphology associated with the different types of cleft malformation, to form a basis for valid esti-

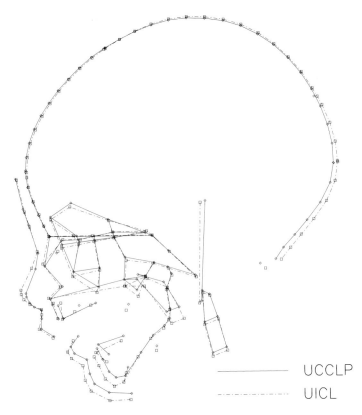

FIG. 8.14. Craniofacial mean drawings of 2-month-old unoperated unilateral complete cleft lip and palate (*UCCLP, n = 82*) and unilateral incomplete cleft lip (*UICL, n = 75*) groups superimposed on the nasion-sella line and registered on the sella. (From Hermann et al., 1999a, with permission.)

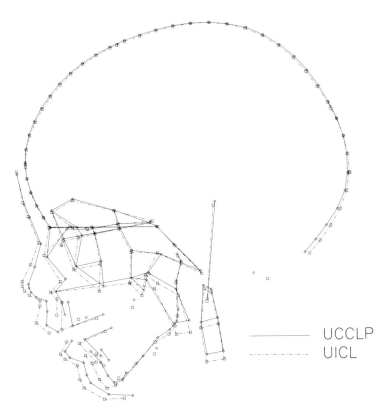

FIG. 8.15. Craniofacial mean drawings of 22-month-old lip-operated unilateral complete cleft lip and palate (*UCCLP, n = 82*) and unilateral incomplete cleft lip (*UICL, n = 75*) groups superimposed on the nasion-sella line and registered on the sella. (From Hermann et al., 2000, with permission.)

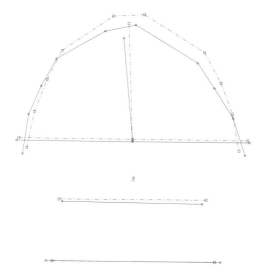

FIG. 8.16. Axial maxillary mean drawings of 22-month-old lip-operated unilateral complete cleft lip and palate (solid line) (*n* = 82) and unilateral incomplete cleft lip (dashed line) (*n* = 75) groups superimposed on the line between the left and right foramen ovale and registered on the midpoint of this line. (From Hermann et al., 2000, with permission.)

mations of the amount of surgical iatrogenesis, especially to the maxillary development, introduced by different surgical procedures and regimes, including the timing of treatment.

Cleft Lip

Several studies indicate that clefts involving structures of the primary palate only are associated with minor variations in facial morphogenesis except for the area of the primary malformation. In general, unilateral and in-

complete clefts show the mildest deviations (Dahl, 1970). Surgical closure of the CL, does not lead to disturbed maxillary growth (Dahl, 1970; Hermann et al., 2000). The development of the cranial base and mandible is unremarkable. However, a slight increase in interorbital distance has been reported (Dahl, 1970; Ishiguru et al., 1975; Dahl et al., 1982; Motohashi et al., 1994).

Cleft Palate

Isolated CP appears to be associated with bimaxillary retrognathia, reduced length and posterior height of the maxilla, increased width of the maxilla and nasal cavity, reduced mandibular length, and reduced dimensions of the upper airway (Dahl, 1970; Dahl et al., 1982, 1989; Hermann et al., 2001b). The sagittal jaw relationship is normal and early facial growth in unoperated patients revealed no change in the facial pattern up to 22 months of age (Kreiborg and Cohen, 1996). This lack of change in facial pattern may be observed even into adulthood, except for a relative increase in anterior facial height, which can probably be explained by a more vertical growth pattern, most likely related to altered function, e.g., change in head posture (Sandham and Foong, 1997).

Robin Sequence

Subjects with RS represent the extreme part of the CP population in terms of mandibular retrognathia and upper airway constriction. In our study, patients with RS outgrew their breathing problems even without closure of the CP, simply through the growth in facial dimensions. However, at 22 months of age, the mandible was still significantly shorter and more retrognathic than in the CP group (Kreiborg and Cohen, 1996).

Cleft Lip and Palate

Complete clefts of the lip and palate (unilateral or bilateral) appear to be associated with the following intrinsic variations in the newborn:

1. Protrusion (or relative protrusion) of the premaxilla
2. Retrognathia of the body of the maxilla
3. Increased maxillary width
4. Increased width of the nasal cavity
5. Reduced posterior height of the maxilla
6. Short and retrognathic mandible
7. Reduced dimensions of the upper airway

Secondary to surgical closure of the lip at 2 months of age in UCCLP, we found that the premaxilla was molded into place, unmasking the intrinsic maxillary retrognathia and leading to a normal sagittal jaw rela-

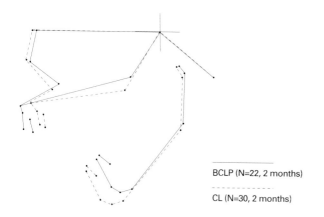

BCLP (N=22, 2 months)

CL (N=30, 2 months)

FIG. 8.17. Mean drawings of 2-month-old unoperated bilateral cleft lip and palate (*BCLP*, *n* = 22) and cleft lip (*CL*, *n* = 30) groups superimposed on the nasion-sella line and registered on the sella. (Modified from Dahl et al., 1989.)

A

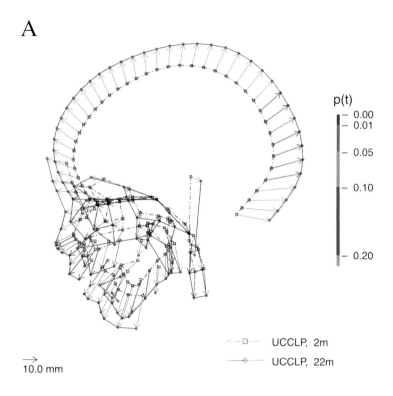

p(t)
— 0.00
— 0.01

— 0.05

— 0.10

— 0.20

---□--- UCCLP, 2m
——◇—— UCCLP, 22m

→
10.0 mm

B

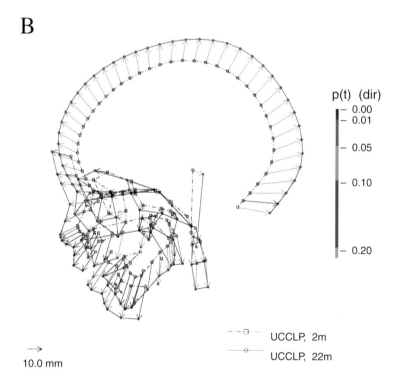

p(t) (dir)
— 0.00
— 0.01

— 0.05

— 0.10

— 0.20

---□--- UCCLP, 2m
——◇—— UCCLP, 22m

→
10.0 mm

COLOR FIG. 8.18. Facial growth pattern from 2 to 22 months of age in unilateral complete cleft lip and palate *(UCCLP)*. Growth vectors have been color-coded according to the significance of the differences between the growth in the UCCLP group relative to the unilateral incomplete cleft lip *(UICL)* group (control group). Red, significant difference at the 1% level; yellow, 5%; green, 10%; blue, >10%. *A:* Differences in the total amount of growth (length of growth vectors) between the two groups. *B:* Differences in the direction of growth (angle of growth vectors in relation to the nasion-sella line) between the two groups, the UCCLP group showing a significantly more vertical growth pattern than the control group.

tionship at 22 months of age. The amount of jaw growth was similar, except for the premaxillary molding, in both the UCCLP and the UICL (control) groups. The direction of growth, however, was more vertical in the UCCLP group.

Based on this concept, we found that surgery to the lip and anterior part of the hard palate at 2 months of age in UCCLP subjects appeared to influence the development of the maxillary complex, as observed at 22 months of age, in two beneficial ways: *(1)* the premaxilla was no longer relatively protruding and *(2)* it was less asymmetric. The nasal septum deviated less toward the noncleft side. The width of the nasal cavity and the posterior part of the maxilla had become relatively more normal, and the transverse position of the lateral maxillary segment on the noncleft side was closer to normal. The posterior height of the maxilla was still reduced to the same degree, the mandible was still short and retrognathic to the same degree, and bimaxillary retrognathia was still present. The only iatrogenic effect observed was that the lateral maxillary segment on the cleft side had become displaced toward the midsagittal plane anteriorly, resulting in a very narrow dental arch at the level of the deciduous canine (Hermann et al., 2000).

In conclusion, our findings suggest that subjects with cleft of the secondary palate have a special "intrinsic" facial type, primarily characterized by bimaxillary retrognathia and increased maxillary width. This facial type could be a "liability factor," increasing the probability of CP or CLP (Hermann et al., 1999a,b). Finally, when evaluating the outcome of cleft surgery in subjects with CLP at adolescence or adulthood, comparisons should not be made to normal standards but rather to the adolescent and adult morphology seen in subjects with CP.

REFERENCES

Berkowitz, S (1995). The value of longitudinal facial and palatal records in clinical research. *Cleft Lip and Palate. Perspectives in Management.* San Diego: Singular Publishing Group, pp. 7–12.

Bishara, SE (1973). Cephalometric evaluation of facial growth in operated and non-operated individuals with isolated clefts of the palate. Cleft Palate J 10: 239–246.

Bishara, SE, de Arrendondo, RSM, Vales, HP, Jakobsen, JR (1985). Dentofacial relationships in persons with unoperated clefts: comparison between three cleft types. Am J Orthod 87: 481–507.

Bishara, SE, Jakobsen, JR, Krause, JC, Sosa-Martinez, R (1986). Cephalometric comparisons of individuals from India and Mexico with unoperated cleft lip and palate. Cleft Palate J 23: 116–125.

Bishara, SE, Krause, CJ, Olin, WH, et al. (1976). Facial and dental relationships of individuals with unoperated clefts of the lip and/or palate. Cleft Palate J 13: 238–252.

Bishara, SE, Olin, WH (1972). Surgical repositioning of the premaxilla in complete bilateral cleft lip and palate. Angle Orthod 42: 139–147.

Capelozza, L, Jr, Taniguchi, SM, da Silva Filho, OG, Jr (1993). Craniofacial morphology of adult unoperated complete unilateral cleft lip and palate patients. Cleft Palate Craniofac J 30: 376–381.

Capelozza Filho, L, Jr, Normando, ADC, da Silva Filho, OG, Jr (1996). Isolated influences of lip and palate surgery on facial growth: comparison of operated and unoperated male adults with UCLP. Cleft Palate Craniofac J 33: 51–56.

Cohen, MM, Jr (1997). Etiologic and pathogenetic heterogeneity. In: *The Child with Multiple Birth Defects.* New York: Oxford University Press, pp. 164–196.

Dahan, J (1974). Die dreidimensionale röntgenkephalometrische Untersuchung von Fällen mit Pierre-Robin-Syndrom. Fortschr Kieferorthop 35: 240–255.

Dahl, E (1970). Craniofacial morphology in congenital clefts of the lip and palate. Acta Odontol Scand 28 (Suppl 57): 1–167.

Dahl, E, Kreiborg, S (1995). Craniofacial malformations. In: *Introduction to Orthodontics,* 2nd ed, edited by B Thilander and O Rönning. Stockholm: Gothia, pp. 239–254.

Dahl, E, Kreiborg, S, Jensen, BL (1989). Roentgencephalometric studies of infants with untreated cleft lip and palate. In: *What is a cleft lip and palate? A multidisciplinary update,* edited by O Kriens. Stuttgart: Georg Thieme Verlag, pp. 113–115.

Dahl, E, Kreiborg, S, Jensen, BL, Fogh-Andersen, P (1982). Comparison of craniofacial morphology in infants with incomplete cleft lip and infants with isolated cleft palate. Cleft Palate J 19: 258–266.

Darvann, TA, Hermann, NV, Huebener, DV, et al. (2001). The CT-scan method of 3D form description of the maxillary arch. Validation and an application. Transactions of the 9th International Congress on Cleft Palate and Related Craniofacial Anomalies, Göteborg, Sweden, 25–29 June, edited by J Lilja, pp. 223–233.

da Silva Filho, OG, Carvalho Lauris, RC, Capelozza Filho, L, Semb, G (1998). Craniofacial morphology in adult patients with unoperated complete bilateral cleft lip and palate. Cleft Palate Craniofac J 35: 111–119.

da Silva Filho, OG, Jr, Normando, ADC, Capelozza, L, Jr (1992a). Mandibular morphology and spatial position in patients with clefts: intrinsic or iatrogeneic? Cleft Palate Craniofac J 29: 369–375.

da Silva Filho, OG, Jr, Ramos, AL, Abdo, RCC (1992b). Influence of surgery on maxillary growth in cleft lip and/or palate patients. J Craniomaxillofac Surg 20: 111–118.

Ehmann, G (1989). Cephalometric findings in normal and unoperated CLAP Fulbe-tribe adults of northern Cameroon. In: *What is a cleft lip and palate? A multidisciplinary update,* edited by O Kriens. Stuttgart: Georg Thieme Verlag, pp. 121–122.

Friede, H (1977). Studies on Facial Morphology and Growth in Bilateral Cleft Lip and Palate. Göteborg: Univ. of Göteborg. Dissertation.

Friede, H (1978). The vomero-premaxillary suture—a neglected growth site in mid-facial development of unilateral cleft lip and palate patients. Cleft Palate J 15: 398–404.

Friede, H (1998). Growth sites and growth mechanisms at risk in cleft lip and palate. Acta Odontol Scand 56: 346–351.

Friede, H, Figueroa, AA, Naegele, ML, et al. (1986). Craniofacial growth data for cleft lip patients from infancy to 6 years of age: potential applications. Am J Orthod 90: 388–409.

Friede, H, Johanson, B (1974). A follow-up study of cleft children treated with primary bone grafting. Scand J Plast Reconstr Surg 8: 88–103.

Friede, H, Morgan, P (1976). Growth of the vomero-premaxillary suture in children with bilateral cleft lip and palate. Scand J Plast Reconstr Surg 10: 45–55.

Friede, H, Pruzansky, S (1972a). Longitudinal study of growth in bilateral cleft lip and palate, from infancy to adolescence. Plast Reconstr Surg 49: 392–403.

Friede, H, Pruzansky, S (1972b). Changes in profile in complete bilateral cleft lip and palate from infancy to adolescence. Trans Eur Orthod Soc 147–157.

Gorlin, RJ, Cohen, MM, Jr, Levin, LS (1990). *Syndromes of the Head and Neck*, 3rd ed. New York: Oxford University Press, pp. 693–783.

Graber, TM (1949). A cephalometric analysis of the developmental pattern and facial morphology in cleft palate. Angle Orthod 19: 91–100.

Graber, TM (1954). The congenital cleft palate deformity. J Am Dent Assoc 48: 375–395.

Han, B-J, Suzuki, A, Tashiro, H (1995). Longitudinal study of craniofacial growth in subjects with cleft lip and palate: from cheiloplasty to 8 years of age. Cleft Palate Craniofac J 32: 156–166.

Heller, A, Kreiborg, S, Dahl, E, Jensen, BL (1995). X-ray: cephalometric analysis system for lateral, frontal, and axial projections. Presented at the 5th European Craniofacial Congress, Copenhagen, Denmark, June 15–17. Abstract nr. 61: 33.

Hermann, NV, Jensen, BL, Dahl, E, et al. (1999a). A comparison of the craniofacial morphology in 2 months old unoperated infants with unilateral complete cleft lip and palate, and unilateral incomplete cleft lip. J Craniofac Genet Dev Biol 19: 80–93.

Hermann, NV, Jensen, BL, Dahl, E, et al. (1999b). Craniofacial growth in subjects with unilateral complete cleft lip and palate, and unilateral incomplete cleft lip, from 2 to 22 months of age. J Craniofac Genet Dev Biol 19: 135–147.

Hermann, NV, Jensen, BL, Dahl, E, et al. (2000). Craniofacial comparisons in 22-month-old lip-operated children with unilateral complete cleft lip and palate and unilateral incomplete cleft lip. Cleft Palate Craniofac J 37: 303–317.

Hermann, NV, Jensen, BL, Dahl, E, et al. (2001a). A method for three-projection infant cephalometry. Cleft Palate Craniofac J 38: 300–316.

Hermann, NV, Kreiborg, S, Darvann, TA, et al. (2001b). Mandibular retrognathia in infants with cleft of the secondary palate. Transactions of the 9th International Congress on Cleft Palate and Related Craniofacial Anomalies, Göteborg, Sweden, 25–29 June, edited by J Lilja, pp. 151–154.

Ishiguro, K, Krogman, WM, Mazaheri, M, Harding, RL (1976). A longitudinal study of morphological craniofacial patterns via P-A x-ray headfilms in cleft patients from birth to six years of age. Cleft Palate J 13: 104–126.

Jain, RB, Krogman, WM (1983a). Cleft type and sex differences in craniofacial growth in clefting from one month to ten years. Cleft Palate J 20: 238–245.

Jain, RB, Krogman, WM (1983b). Craniofacial growth in clefting from one month to ten years as studied by P-A headfilms. Cleft Palate J 20: 314–326.

Jensen, BL, Kreiborg, S, Dahl, E, Fogh-Andersen, P (1988). Cleft lip and palate in Denmark 1976–1981. Epidemiology, variability, and early somatic development. Cleft Palate J 25: 1–12.

Kreiborg, S (1981). Crouzon syndrome. A clinical and roentgencephalometric study. Scand J Plast Reconstr Surg Suppl 18: 1–198.

Kreiborg, S (1985). The application of roentgencephalometry to the study of craniofacial anomalies. J Craniofac Genet Dev Biol (Suppl 1): 31–41.

Kreiborg, S (1989). Quantitative methods in the study of abnormal cranio-facial growth. In: *What is a cleft lip and palate? A multidisciplinary update*, edited by O Kriens. Stuttgart: Georg Thieme Verlag, pp. 123–125.

Kreiborg, S, Cohen, MM, Jr (1996). Syndrome delineation and growth in orofacial clefting and craniosynostosis. In: *Facial clefts and craniosynostosis. Principles and management*, edited by TA Turvey, KWL Vig, and RJ Fonseca. Philadelphia: WB Saunders, pp. 57–75.

Kreiborg, S, Dahl, E, Prydsø, U (1977). A unit for infant roentgencephalometry. Dentomaxillofac Radiol 6: 29–33.

Kreiborg, S, Jensen, BL, Dahl, E, Fogh-Andersen, P (1985). Pierre Robin syndrome. Early facial development. Presented at the 5th International Congress on Cleft Palate and Related Craniofacial Anomalies, Monte Carlo. 2–7 September. Abstract nr. 303.

Krogman, WM, Jain, RB, Long, RE, Jr (1982a). Sex differences in craniofacial growth from one month to ten years of cleft lip and palate. Cleft Palate J 19: 62–71.

Krogman, WM, Jain, RB, Oka, SW (1982b). Craniofacial growth in different cleft types from one month to ten years. Cleft Palate J 19: 206–211.

Krogman, WM, Mazaheri, M, Harding, RL, et al. (1975). A longitudinal study of the craniofacial growth pattern in children with clefts as compared to normal, birth to six years. Cleft Palate J 12: 59–84.

Long, RE, Jr, Jain, RB, Krogman, WM (1982). Possible sex-discriminant variables in craniofacial growth in clefting. Am J Orthod 82: 392–402.

Mars, M, Houston, WJB (1990). A preliminary study of facial growth and morphology in unoperated male unilateral cleft lip and palate subjects over 13 years of age. Cleft Palate J 27: 7–10.

Mazaheri, M, Sahni, PP (1969). Techniques of cephalometry, photography and oral impressions of infants. J Prosthet Dent 21: 315–323.

Mølsted, K, Kjær, I, Dahl, E (1995). Cranial base in newborns with complete cleft lip and palate: radiographic study. Cleft Palate J 32: 199–205.

Motohashi, N, Kuroda, T, Capelozza Filho, L, Jr, de Souza Freitas, JA (1994). P-A cephalometric analysis of nonoperated adult cleft lip and palate. Cleft Palate Craniofac J 31: 193–200.

Ortiz-Monasterio, F, Rebeil, AS, Valderrama, M, Cruz, R (1959). Cephalometric measurements on adult patients with nonoperated cleft palates. Plast Reconstr Surg 24: 53–61.

Ortiz-Monasterio, F, Serrano, A, Barrera, G, et al. (1966). A study of untreated adult cleft palate patients. Plast Reconstr Surg 38: 36–41.

Pruzansky, S (1971). The growth of the premaxillary–vomerine complex in complete bilateral cleft lip and palate. Tandlaegebladet 75: 1157–1169.

Pruzansky, S (1973). Monitoring growth of the infant with cleft lip and palate. Trans Eur Orthod Soc 539–546.

Pruzansky, S, Lis, EF (1958). Cephalometric roentgenography of infants: sedation, instrumentation and research. Am J Orthod 44: 159–186.

Robertson, NRE, Hilton, R (1971). The changes produced by presurgical orthopaedics. Br J Plast Surg 24: 57–68.

Sandham, A, Foong, K (1997). The effect of cleft deformity, surgical repair and altered function in unilateral cleft lip and palate. In: Transactions of the 8th International Congress on Cleft Palate and Related Craniofacial Anomalies, edited by ST Lee. Academy of Medicine, Singapore, pp. 673–678.

Semb, G, Shaw, WC (1996). Facial growth in orofacial clefting disorders. In: *Facial clefts and craniosynostosis. Principles and management*, edited by TA Turvey, KWL Vig, and RJ Fonseca. Philadelphia: WB Saunders, pp. 28–56.

Slaughter, WB, Brodie, AG (1949). Facial clefts and their surgical management in view of recent research. Plast Reconstr Surg 4: 203–224.

Smahel, Z, Brousilova, M, Müllerova, Z (1987). Craniofacial morphology in isolated cleft palate prior to palatoplasty. Cleft Palate J 24: 200–208.

Tomanova, M, Müllerova, Z (1994). Effects of primary bone grafting on facial development in patients with unilateral complete cleft lip and palate. Acta Chir Plast 36: 38–41.

III

Epidemiology of Cleft Lip and Palate

9

Methodological issues in epidemiological studies of oral clefts

KAARE CHRISTENSEN

At a first glance, oral clefts (OCs) seem an ideal group of congenital malformations to be studied. They are among the most common congenital malformations and, compared to most other anomalies, easily diagnosed and described. However, even such a seemingly straightforward task as estimating the frequency of OC imposes its own problems. The first part of this chapter addresses methodological issues in the assessment of OC frequency, including frequency measurements and the completeness and biases in various ascertainment sources. The second part covers some methodological issues in connection with the two major design options for assessing environmental risk factors for OC: case-control studies and follow-up studies.

ASSESSING THE FREQUENCY OF ORAL CLEFTS

Although OCs are among the most frequent congenital malformations and relatively easily assessed, the statistical power of most etiological studies is low, especially because most studies subdivide OCs into cleft lip (CL) with or without cleft palate (CL/P) and isolated cleft palate (CP) and, furthermore, into syndromic and nonsyndromic cases. These subdivisions are based on observations that nonsyndromic CL/P and CP rarely segregate in the same family (Fogh-Andersen, 1942) and that a substantial number of syndromic cases have a strong association with specific genetic mutations. Additionally, it may be of interest to study OCs stratified by familial occurrence and severity [bilateral vs. unilateral CL/P, cleft lip and palate (CLP) vs. CL] (Mitchell, 1997). Finally, some studies have suggested that the nonsyndromic CP group may consist of two etiologically different subtypes: CP affecting the soft palate only and CP affecting both the hard and soft palate (Christensen and Fogh-Andersen, 1994; Clementi et al., 1997). A number of etiological factors are likely shared by these subgroups, while other factors may be unique to a subgroup. Therefore, the emerging international collaborative efforts are essential to obtain reasonable statistical power in analyses of the subgroups.

Incidence or Prevalence?

In epidemiology, the three major measures of disease frequency are incidence, prevalence, and risk. *Incidence* is the number of disease onsets per risk time (observation time), *prevalence* is the proportion of a population that has a disease at a specific point in time, and *risk* is a cumulative incidence proportion, i.e., the proportion of a given population that becomes cases within a given time period (Rothman, 1986). The frequency of OCs is one usually reported as 1 to 2/1000 births. There has been a long semantic and conceptual discussion about this frequency measurement: is it a measure of incidence, prevalence, or risk?

The primary palate and the palatine shelves fuse at the end of the first trimester of gestation. Hence, the population at risk includes all conceptions surviving to the time of normal fusion. Since it is not possible to ascertain all conceptions that occur and survive until this point and not feasible to assess whether fusion has occurred in all cases, neither the incidence nor the risk measure of disease frequency is obtainable. What could be measured is the proportion of OCs among newborns, stillborns, and abortions occurring after the first trimester. Therefore, only OC prevalence may be measured (Rothman and Greenland, 1998).

Prevalence data have severe limitations when used for etiological research because prevalence depends on both the incidence of new cases and the survival of cases. If first-trimester exposure to an environmental risk factor increases OC risk when the exposure intensity is moderate and the same exposure leads to spontaneous abortion when the exposure is intense (the so-called two-threshold model), then paradoxical results may occur (Dronamraju et al., 1982; Rothman and Greenland, 1998). A reduction in the exposure could lead to a reduction in the number of spontaneous abortions and an increase in OC prevalence. Therefore, in principle, it would not be possible to know whether an association between an exposure (environmental or genetic) and OC occurrence is due either to better survival of an exposed OC fetus compared to nonexposed OC fetuses or to an increased susceptibility of OC formation in exposed fetuses. Formally, additional evidence is needed to disentangle these effects, e.g., through studies of spontaneous abortion. In reality, however, estimating prevalence is the basis of OC epidemiology research; therefore, high-quality methods of collecting prevalence data are essential.

Change in Oral Cleft Frequency over Time

Most countries have undergone dramatic changes during the last century in terms of living conditions, work environment, health care, and lifestyle. Therefore, it is of considerable interest to test whether the frequency of OCs is associated with both gradual changes, such as improved living conditions, and more delimited exposures, such as war, changes in legislation, and new health programs. Such studies, however, rely heavily on the assumption of the same level of completeness of registration. False results may be obtained, e.g., if registration is less complete during war or a famine. However, spurious results may also occur even in settings with very good registration systems. The following example will illustrate this point.

A uniform and standardized registration system has been used in Denmark since the 1930s. These data have been entered into the Danish Facial Cleft Register, which includes 7290 oral cleft cases born between 1936 and 1987. Figure 9.1 is based on the Danish Facial Cleft Register and summarizes the estimated yearly prevalence of CL/P and CP in the period 1936–1987. From Figure 9.1, it is clear that in the second half of the period (1962–1987) the prevalence at birth was fairly constant for both CL/P (around 1.4 to 1.5/1000) and CP (around

0.7 to 0.9/1000). In contrast, there was apparently a steady increase in the prevalence of both CL/P and CP during the first half of the period (1936–1961).

However, the most likely explanation of this increase in the middle of the century is an improvement in the survival of newborn CL/P cases (especially those with associated anomalies) and a better ascertainment during these 26 years (especially of milder CP forms and OC cases with associated anomalies). Figure 9.1 shows that a substantial part of the increase in prevalence in that period was due to an increased proportion of cases with associated anomalies and milder forms of OC. The nearly constant prevalence of the most severe OC forms (nonsyndromic bilateral CL/P and CP including the hard palate) suggests that no major changes in the prevalence of OC have occurred in the 52-year period. If the overall figures were taken at face value, it might be concluded that OCs became increasingly common during the middle of the twentieth century. Detailed description of the cases, however, suggests the presence of ascertainment bias.

Change in Oral Cleft Frequency with Season

Another example of why trends in rates should be interpreted with caution is seasonal variation in the dates of birth of children with congenital malformations. Seasonality has been studied to gain insight into the possible role of diet, infections, and other factors that may vary with season. Seasonal variation in the dates of birth of children with nonsyndromic CL/P has been studied in nearly 600 cases born in Montreal between 1950 and 1996 (Fraser and Gwyn, 1998). A significant tendency for children with CL/P to be born more often in the summer than in the winter was found. In another report, which used the Danish CL/P data set from Fogh-Andersen's (1942) thesis, no variation was found in month of birth among females, but a peak in April–May was observed for males. These analyses were based on the distribution of month of birth for CL/P cases. Applying this method to the entire Danish 1936–1987 cohort yielded a small seasonal variation similar to that observed in the data from Canada for both nonsyndromic CL/P and CP.

A critical point to take into account when studying OC seasonality is that pregnancy-timing preferences (i.e., when parents prefer to have their children) may vary between settings and time periods. For example, in the Scandinavian countries, the frequency of births is 10% to 20% higher in spring and summer compared to winter (NOMESKO, 1993). Hence, the Danish CL/P and CP seasonality pattern can be explained by the variation in the overall seasonality pattern of births;

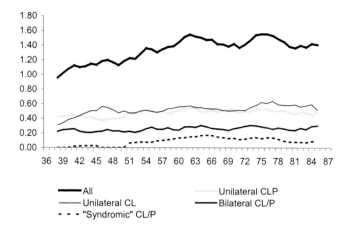

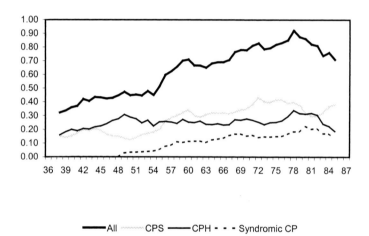

FIG. 9.1. Change in the frequency of oral clefts over time. Smoothed prevalence (5-year moving average) of subgroups of cleft lip with or without cleft palate *(CL/P)* and cleft palate *(CP)* per 1000 live births in Denmark in the period 1936–1987. *CL,* cleft lip; *CLP,* cleft lip and palate; *CPS,* nonsyndromic CP including only the soft palate (submucous CP included here); *CPH,* nonsyndromic CP including the hard palate. (Modified from Christensen, 1999, with permission.)

i.e., the larger number of OC births in the spring and summer can simply be explained by the larger number of total births at that time of year.

Oral Clefts and Associated Anomalies

A longstanding debate in OC research is whether cases with associated anomalies should be excluded ("splitting") or included ("lumping") in etiological studies. The rationale for splitting is to reduce etiological heterogeneity, i.e., to eliminate all OC cases with known etiology (e.g., monogenic diseases such as Van der Woude's syndrome and chromosomal abnormalities such as trisomy 18). The rationale for lumping is that there may be common etiological factors in nonsyndromic and syndromic OC cases. For example, although OC occurs frequently in trisomy 18, far from all trisomy 18 cases have OC.

The factors that might increase susceptibility to OC in trisomy 18 may be the same as those that increase risk in chromosomally normal individuals.

The splitting vs. lumping problem also applies to minor and more subtle associated anomalies, for which it is considerably harder to make a uniform ascertainment and classification. The wide range in the reported frequency of associated anomalies for OC (CL/P 2%–15%, CP 10%–50%) is partially due to differences in the definition of associated anomalies, how long after birth and how carefully the individuals are examined, and the selection of patients.

The 22q11 deletion syndrome illustrates this problem. Patients with this syndrome often display only CP and a minor heart defect and/or learning disability, and many such cases are undiagnosed (Goldberg et al., 1993; Brøndum-Nielsen and Christensen, 1996). The inclusion of cases with 22q11 deletion syndrome in a study of nonsyndromic CP could reduce the power of the study if the risk factors for CP in this syndrome are different from the risk factors for nonsyndromic CP.

As mentioned above, the rationale behind splitting is to reduce etiological heterogeneity. However, splitting may introduce bias. If the definition of minor anomalies includes conditions that occur at a rather high frequency in the general population (e.g., learning disabilities), OC cases without any such conditions might represent an otherwise very healthy group. Furthermore, as mentioned above, a number of environmental and genetic factors likely affect both syndromic and nonsyndromic OC cases; i.e., syndromic and nonsyndromic cases may have some common etiological factors.

Therefore, as long as the delineation of strictly nonsyndromic OC cases depends strongly on definitions of associated anomalies as well as the length and intensity of follow-up, the most reasonable approach is to obtain as much information on associated anomalies as possible and, later, to perform analyses with and without the OC cases with associated anomalies.

Sources of Ascertainment

The baseline epidemiological characteristics of OC are important both for scientific purposes and for public health planning. These data are usually obtained through population-based clinical records, cleft treatment centers, surveillance systems, or birth certificates. The completeness of such files highly depends on the practice and organization of the country, state, or facility providing them.

Population-Based Clinical Records. Population-based records of treated or hospitalized cases introduce a bias in favor of surviving cleft cases, which leads to underreporting of OC (Aabyholm, 1978). Surgical files have played a major role in OC research; e.g., the Danish surgical files have been the basis of numerous, often quoted studies (Fogh-Andersen, 1942, 1971; Bixler et al., 1971; Shields et al., 1979, 1981; Melnick et al., 1980; Marazita et al., 1984; Chung et al., 1986).

The completeness of various ascertainment sources was studied in Denmark for the period 1983–1987 using three nationwide ascertainment sources and an autopsy study in a 10% sample of the Danish population. The nationwide ascertainment sources were (1) a centralized surgical facility, which had treated all OC cases since the 1930s; (2) the National Institute for Defects of Speech, which has coordinated the registration and follow-up treatment of all OC cases, also since the 1930s; and (3) the National Register of Congenital Malformations, which was based on doctors' notifications and reports (Christensen et al., 1992).

Based on these comparisons, it was estimated that more than 95% ascertainment was obtained by means of surgical files for CL/P without associated malformations/syndromes. However, the comparison showed that surgical files should not be used for studying CP. Surgical files included only 60% of these cases. Surgical files were found to be unsuitable for studying the prevalence of associated malformations or syndromes in cases with OC. Figure 9.2 illustrates the completeness of the centralized surgical files in Denmark and the reasons for nonregistration.

Cleft Treatment Centers. Cleft treatment centers often have high-quality information on OC cases in terms of associated malformations and other characteristics. However, these cases often cannot be used for estimat-

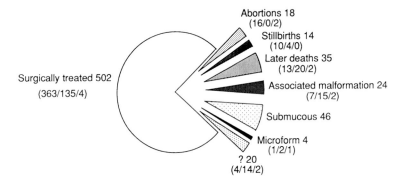

FIG. 9.2. Sources of ascertainment of oral cleft cases. Classification of 663 known facial cleft cases born in Denmark during 1983–1987, identified through three nationwide ascertainment sources. *Small slices* represent nonoperated cases. When a nonoperated case could be classified as belonging to more than one slice, the vertically uppermost was chosen. Parentheses show the number of cases with cleft lip with or without cleft palate, isolated cleft palate, and atypical facial clefts within each slice. (From Christensen et al., 1992, with permission.)

ing the prevalence of OC or other epidemiological characteristics because the population from which they come is not well defined. Furthermore, cleft treatment centers often have a very high frequency of associated anomalies among OC cases. This is partially due to differences in the definition of associated anomalies, how long after birth and how carefully the individuals are examined, as well as the referral practice. A bias in ascertainment arises in highly specialized centers that attract severe or complicated cases (Fraser, 1970; Shprintzen et al., 1985).

Surveillance Systems. Registries of congenital malformations were established in various countries after the thalidomide epidemic. The primary aim of these registries was surveillance to avoid similar epidemics. While some of the registries are limited to surveillance, others include etiological substudies within the register (Dolk et al., 1998). A number of these registries have also been used in OC research. The efficiency of these record systems is highly dependent on the local practice and organization, but even the most well-established registries may have significant underreporting of cases with OC, particularly CP, which showed an under-reporting of 12% in one study (Ericson et al., 1977).

Birth Certificates. Birth certificates are a poor source for OC data, particularly for milder forms of CL/P and CP. Green et al. (1979) found that only 65% of known OC cases in a register of congenital malformation in Arkansas were recorded as having a cleft on the birth certificate and that only 48% were correctly classified regarding cleft type. The same pattern was observed in Denmark by Olsen (1982a,b), who found that only approximately 75% of OC cases had any indication of OC on the birth certificate.

Death Certificates and Autopsy Series. Death certificates and autopsies of fetuses can supplement other ascertainment sources. However, OCs might not be recorded on death certificates when multiple defects coexist because other, more severe malformations are most likely to be registered as the causes of death. Underreporting in autopsies of fetuses is also likely because of the difficulty of recognizing and diagnosing OCs in them (Kraus et al., 1963; Christensen et al., 1992).

DESIGN OPTIONS FOR ASSESSING ENVIRONMENTAL RISK FACTORS FOR ORAL CLEFTS: METHODOLOGICAL ISSUES

As pointed out in Chapter 17, there is convincing evidence that both genetic and environmental factors play a role in the etiology of OCs. However, what environmental and genetic factors these are is still largely an enigma. A number of design options for assessing OC risk factors are available. This section covers some methodological issues in connection with the two major design options for assessing environmental risk factors for OC: case-control studies and follow-up studies.

Case-Control Studies

The case-control study design is by far the most commonly used to evaluate environmental risk factors for OC. During the last decade, case-control studies have been used increasingly for genetic association studies as well. The basic concept is to compare the first-trimester exposures of mothers of OC cases with those of mothers of controls. Ideally, a case-control study uses incident cases from a well-defined population and has four to five controls, who would have been cases in the study if they had had OC, for each case (Rothman and Greenland, 1998). As mentioned above, it is not possible to obtain incident cases in studies of OC; the best available option is to include cases and controls in the study as shortly after birth (or abortion) as possible.

If one uses older cases with OC, the window of exposure of interest (the first trimester) will be further back in time, increasing the likelihood of recall bias (Werler et al., 1989). This bias would arise if case mothers reported differently from control mothers (e.g., if case mothers were more inclined to remember all exposures during the first trimester). Therefore, a study would be substantially strengthened if exposure information were obtained during pregnancy (e.g., from general practitioners' records), before the mother knew whether the fetus had OC or not. For self-reported exposures, it is often useful to collect the date of recognition of the pregnancy as well as the exposure information before and after this date. This is because many women change their lifestyle to some degree when they recognize that they are pregnant. For example, in a Danish case-control study of OC, both case mothers and control mothers reported changes in their lifestyle after recognition of pregnancy: cigarette consumption decreased by one-third and alcohol consumption decreased by 60% among all mothers (who were interviewed on average 1–2 weeks after birth). If the date of recognition of the pregnancy is known as well as the exposure before and after the recognition, a first-trimester dose can be calculated for each mother (Christensen et al., 1999).

The number of controls necessary for each case is a compromise between statistical power and costs. However, it can be shown that including more than four or five controls per case increases the statistical power only slightly (Rothman, 1986). Selection of controls needs special attention. Matching on time and place of birth is a commonly used method that is logistically appealing. However, a disadvantage is that it does not allow the study of time and place of birth as potential risk factors. It has been argued that the control group should be selected among newborns with congenital malformations other than OC. The rationale for this is to avoid recall bias since both cases and controls would be equally motivated to recall exposures. However, this approach presents several disadvantages. First, risk factors will be overlooked if they are associated with both OCs and the congenital malformations in the control group. Second, it might be difficult to obtain a large control group if it consists of children with other congenital malformations. Third, it may be difficult to inform the parents of children with congenital malformations in the control group that the study is aimed at identifying causes of OC but not of the problem their children have. If the inclusion criterion in the case group is isolated OC, then the control group should have an isolated anomaly as well. If, however, OC cases with associated anomalies/syndromes are included, then controls with other anomalies/syndromes should not be excluded.

A special situation arises when genetic factors are included in case-control studies of ethnically heterogeneous populations. If the ethnic composition is different in the case and control groups, then any genetic factor which is unequally distributed among ethnic groups might show an association with OC (without having any etiological role); this is called *population stratification*. This potential bias can be reduced by matching on ethnic background or by conducting studies in ethnically homogeneous populations. Recent developments in methodology extend the case-control design to overcome such and other problems embedded in case-control studies of genetic factors. One option is to sample *case triads* (i.e., an OC case and his or her parents) and similar control-triads in the study. The use of such triads makes it possible to assess or avoid bias, such as population stratification (Umbach and Weinberg, 2000).

Follow-Up Studies (Cohort Studies)

From a strictly methodological point of view, a prospective follow-up or cohort study is preferable over a case-control study. If pregnant women are followed-up from recognition of pregnancy, exposure information can be obtained with no recall bias. This is because these pregnant women do not yet know who will eventually be a case mother or a control mother. Despite OCs being among the most common congenital malformations, the drawback of this approach is that 1000 women would have to be followed in order to identify two cases. Such studies are enormous undertakings. In the period 1959–1966, such a study was conducted in the United States, the Collaborative Perinatal Project. In this study, about 56,000 pregnant women were followed from the first prenatal visit through labor and delivery, and their offspring were later followed-up to assess, among other things, the frequency of congenital malformations (Myrianthopoulos and Chung, 1974).

An even larger study is emerging from Denmark. During the years 1998–2002, approximately 100,000 pregnant women and their offspring will be included in a longitudinal study through a large collaborative effort. Women are typically enrolled in the study at the first visit to their general practitioner (usually in the first trimester). At this time, women who decide to participate, provide a blood sample and are interviewed about a broad range of health-related issues, including potential fetal risk factors and lifestyle information. Around the beginning of the third trimester, women who wish to participate again provide a blood sample and are interviewed. At birth, an umbilical blood sample is drawn, and later, punches are obtained from the newborn's screening card. Finally, 6 and 18 months after delivery, mothers participate in an interview. At this time, data including information on hospitalizations and surgeries are obtained from national health registries. This study allows for the assessment of risk factors even before the woman knows the outcome of her pregnancy, thereby avoiding recall bias. Also, it makes it feasible to include both maternal and infant genotypes in the analysis and to measure changes in maternal plasma antibodies during pregnancy. The latter will allow evaluation of the influence of various maternal infections in the etiology of OC. It should be emphasized, however, that even such a large study will not be able to obtain incident data since women experiencing spontaneous abortions prior to their first prenatal visit will not be included.

SUMMARY

Oral clefts are among the most common congenital malformations and, compared to most other anomalies, relatively easily diagnosed and described. Delineation of nonsyndromic OC cases depends on the definition of associated anomalies as well as on the length and intensity of follow-up. The most reasonable approach in epidemiological studies is to collect as much information as possible on associated anomalies and to perform analyses with and without OC cases with associated anomalies. A fundamental problem of all studies is that they use only cases with OC who have survived at least two trimesters. Hence, it is not possible to distinguish factors which increase the risk of OC in fetuses and factors which enhance the survival chances of OC fetuses. In reality, however, prevalence measures of OC are the basis of OC epidemiology research; therefore, high-quality methods of collecting prevalence data are essential.

The validity of comparing OC frequency between settings and at different time periods depends heavily on the degree of ascertainment. Many different ascertainment sources are used, and all have limitations. Population-based clinical records (surgical files) can provide high ascertainment of cases of CL/P without associated malformations/syndromes. However, they are not useful for CP cases or cases with associated malformations or syndromes. For assessing environmental risk factors, the case-control study is logistically the most appealing design. Ideally, a case-control study uses cases ascertained shortly after birth from a well-defined population and has four or five controls for each case. However, the case-control study is subject to recall bias and selection of appropriate controls might be difficult. Follow-up studies of pregnant women and their offspring yield excellent exposure information, but such studies are logistically enormous.

This work was supported by the Egmont Foundation and the National Institute of Dental and Craniofacial Research (grant R01 DE 11948).

REFERENCES

Aabyholm, FR (1978). Cleft lip and palate in Norway I. Registration, incidence and early mortality of infants with CLP. Scand J Plast Reconstr Surg 12: 29–34.

Bixler, D, Fogh-Andersen, P, Conneally, PM (1971). Incidence of cleft lip and palate in the offspring of cleft parents. Clin Genet 2: 155–159.

Brøndum-Nielsen, K, Christensen, K (1996). Chromosome 22q11 deletion and other chromosome aberrations in cases with cleft palate, congenital heart defects and/or mental disabilities. A survey based on the Danish facial cleft register. Clin Genet 50: 116–120.

Christensen, K (1999) The 20th century Danish facial cleft population—epidemiological and genetic–epidemiological studies. Cleft Palate Craniofac J 36: 96–104.

Christensen, K, Fogh-Andersen, P (1994). Etiological subgroups in non-syndromic isolated cleft palate? A genetic–epidemiological study of 52 Danish birth cohorts. Clin Genet 46: 329–335.

Christensen, K, Holm, NV, Olsen, J, et al. (1992). Selection bias in genetic-epidemiological studies of cleft lip and palate. Am J Hum Genet 51: 654–659.

Christensen, K, Olsen, J, Nørgaard-Pedersen, B, et al. (1999). Oral clefts, transforming-growth-factor-alpha gene variants, and maternal smoking. A population based case-control study in Denmark 1991–1994. Am J Epidemiol 149: 248–255.

Chung, CS, Bixler, D, Watanabe, T, et al. (1986). Segregation analysis of cleft lip with or without cleft palate: a comparison of Danish and Japanese data. Am J Hum Genet 39: 603–611.

Clementi, M, Tenconi, R, Forabosco, P, et al. (1997). Inheritance of cleft palate in Italy. Evidence for a major autosomal recessive locus. Hum Genet 100: 204–207.

Dolk, H, Vrijheid, M, Armstrong, B, et al. (1998). Risk of congenital anomalies near hazardous-waste landfill sites in Europe: the EUROHAZCON study. Lancet 352: 423–427.

Dronamraju, KR, Bixler, D, Majumder, PP (1982). Fetal mortality associated with cleft lip and cleft palate. Johns Hopkins Med J 151: 287–289.

Ericson, A, Källén, B, Winberg, J (1977). Surveillance of malformations at birth: a comparison of two record systems run in parallel. Int J Epidemiol 6: 35–41.

Fogh-Andersen, P (1942). Inheritance of Harelip and Cleft Palate. Copenhagen: Arnold Busck.

Fogh-Andersen, P (1971) Epidemiology and etiology of clefts. Birth Defects 7: 51–53.

Fraser, FC (1970). Counseling in genetics: its intent and scope. Birth Defects 6: 7–12.

Fraser, FC, Gwyn, A (1998). Seasonal variation in birth date of children with cleft lip. Teratology 57: 93–95.

Goldberg, R, Motzkin, B, Marion, R, et al. (1993). Velo-cardio-facial syndrome: a review of 120 patients. Am J Med Genet 45: 313–319.

Green, HG, Nelson, CJ, Gaylor, DW, Holson, JF (1979). Accuracy of birth certificate data for detecting facial cleft defects in Arkansas children. Cleft Palate J 16(2): 167–170.

Kraus, BS, Kitamura, H, Ooe, T (1963). Malformations associated with cleft lip and palate in human embryos and fetuses. Am J Obstet Gynecol 86: 321–328.

Marazita, ML, Spence, MA, Melnick, M (1984). Genetic analysis of cleft lip with or without cleft palate in Danish kindreds. Am J Med Genet 19: 9–18.

Melnick, M, Bixler, D, Fogh-Andersen, P, Conneally, PM (1980). Cleft lip +/− cleft palate: an overview of the literature and an analysis of Danish cases born between 1941 and 1968. Am J Med Genet 6: 83–97.

Mitchell, LE, Christensen, K (1997). Evaluation of family history data for Danish twins with nonsyndromic cleft lip with or without cleft palate. Am J Med Genet 72: 120–121.

Myrianthopoulos, NC, Chung, CS (1974). Congenital malformations in singletons: epidemiologic survey. Report from the Collaborative Perinatal project. Birth Defects 10: 1–58.

NOMESKO (1993). Birth and infant mortality in the Nordic countries. Copenhagen: Nordic Medico-Statistical Committee.

Olsen, J (1982a). The register of congenital anomalies in Funen County. I. The number of notifications and their sources [in Danish]. Ugeskr Laeger 144: 1333–1337.

Olsen, JH (1982b). Forplantning, miljø og kemiske stoffer. Copenhagen: Miljøstyrelsen.

Rothman, KJ (1986). Modern Epidemiology. Boston: Little, Brown.

Rothman, KJ, Greenland, S (1998). Modern Epidemiology, 2nd ed. Philadelphia: Lippincott-Raven.

Shields, ED, Bixler, D, Fogh-Andersen, P (1979). Facial clefts in Danish twins. Cleft Palate J 16: 1–6.

Shields, ED, Bixler, D, Fogh-Andersen, P (1981). Cleft palate: a genetic and epidemiological investigation. Clin Genet 20: 13–24.

Shprintzen, RJ, Siegel-Sadewitz, VL, Armato, J, Goldberg, RB (1985). Anomalies associated with cleft lip, cleft palate or both. Am J Med Genet 20: 585–595.

Umbach, DM, Weinberg, CR (2000). The use of case–parent triads to study joint effects of genotype and exposure. Am J Hum Genet 66: 251–261.

Werler, MM, Pober, BR, Nelson, K, Holmes, LB (1989). Reporting accuracy among mothers of malformed and non-malformed infants. Am J Epidemiol 129: 415–421.

10

Exposure assessment in studies of oral clefts

MARTHA M. WERLER

One challenge in studying environmental exposures related to oral cleft risks is assessment of exposure. This chapter provides a general discussion of study design issues and how they relate to the assessment of exposures. There is a brief description of the consequences of inaccurate assessment and approaches to measuring it. Then, several sources of exposure information are described. Following is a section describing the methods of assessing specific exposures that are relevant to the study of oral clefts.

STUDY DESIGNS

Accurate assessment of exposures depends, to a large extent, on the study design. As described in Chapter 9, the cohort and case-control observational designs are the most widely used, in addition to the cross-sectional method. Cohort studies typically measure exposure status prospectively before the outcome is known. Prospective studies are considered optimal for assessment of exposures. In the case of oral clefts, prospective studies involve identifying a cohort of pregnant women, measuring exposure status, and following the women to the end of pregnancy to determine the presence or absence of oral clefts in their offspring. Case-control studies identify cases with the outcome of interest and a control group, then measure exposure status, typically, retrospectively for the etiologically relevant time period. Accurate retrospective assessment is a major challenge in case-control studies, but certain steps can be taken to maximize accuracy. Cross-sectional studies identify cases and controls in similar fashion to that in a retrospective study, but exposure status is measured at the time of case/control identification or later. Unless maternal exposure status after delivery reflects the status early in pregnancy, inferences made from cross-sectional findings are severely limited.

Although oral clefts are one of the most common birth defects, their occurrence at birth (1.7/1000) is rare enough to complicate their study. Since it is most appropriate to separate cleft lip with or without cleft palate from cleft palate alone (see Chapters 1, 2, and 5), prevalence rates are further reduced to 1.1/1000 births and 0.6/1000 births, respectively. Hence, prospective studies must follow approximately 50,000 pregnant women to identify 85 infants with cleft lip with or without cleft palate and 30 infants with cleft palate alone. The greater efficiency of the case-control design explains why the majority of oral cleft studies are retrospective. However, the gain in efficiency of retrospective studies is countered by difficulties in accurate exposure assessment.

EXPOSURE ASSESSMENT

Misclassification

The main goal of conducting studies of environmental exposures in relation to oral clefts is to estimate risk. As exposure is more accurately assessed, so the risk measure is more accurately estimated. When exposure status is poorly ascertained across all study subjects and large portions of subjects are misclassified, the net result is usually underestimation of risk. In other words, in the presence of random misclassification, risk measures (e.g., odds ratios or relative risks) are biased toward the null value. When exposure status is poorly ascertained for one of the study groups compared to the other, known as differential misclassification, the effect on risk measures may be great but the direction (under- or overestimation) is more difficult to predict. Both random and differential misclassification can be present in any of the three previously described study designs. However, there is particular concern over differential misclassification in retrospective studies based on self-reported exposure information, referred to as *recall bias*.

Recall Bias

Concern about recall bias stems from the intuitive idea that a mother who gives birth to a child with an oral cleft may reflect back on her pregnancy, searching for a reason to explain why her baby is affected. Indeed, many a clinician can relay stories of concerned mothers asking whether one exposure or another in pregnancy could be 'the reason'. Under this scenario, case mothers would be more accurate reporters than mothers of 'normal' children. Conversely, the reverse situation can be invoked, where mothers of cases might deny exposures that women are warned to avoid in pregnancy (e.g., alcohol) and reporting accuracy would be greater for controls than cases. There is little empirical evidence of recall bias in studies of oral clefts, not because there is evidence that it does not exist but, rather, because it is difficult to measure. To measure recall bias, a gold standard must be available against which exposure status is compared. For example, retrospective maternal reports might be compared to some other source of exposure information such as stored biologic samples or documentation in medical records. However, such sources are often not available. Further, medical records may provide an inaccurate assessment of exposure and, thus, a poor gold standard (Drews et al., 1990; Werler et al., 1989). Prospective studies in which information was collected from women both during and after pregnancy (MacKenzie and Lippman, 1989; Klemetti and Saxén, 1967) have been important in measuring accuracy of recall, but they offer less in terms of assessing recall bias. This is due to the rarity of oral clefts and other malformations. The gold standard (whether prospective interview data or some other source) would need to be available on hundreds of thousands of pregnant women to compare postpartum recall accuracy between mothers of oral cleft cases and mothers of normal infants for exposures that are rare (<10%). Further, it is likely that the accuracy of recall and the potential for recall bias would vary across ex-

posures, depending on the respondent's attitude, society's view, or whether the media had recently cast any negative attention on it. Also, increased length of time between interview and early pregnancy is thought to negatively affect recall. Due to concerns of recall bias, some retrospective studies have used a control group comprised of infants with other major structural malformations, assuming that accuracy of recall would be similar between mothers of oral cleft cases and mothers of infants with other major malformations. Such a study design requires that the exposure(s) under study not be associated with the malformations in the control group (Swan et al., 1992), to avoid introducing a selection bias. Since retrospective studies are often launched with the intent of gathering information on a wide variety of exposures, it may be difficult to predict which exposures are vulnerable to recall bias and which are associated with non-oral cleft malformations. If resources allow, both non-malformed and malformed control groups may be utilized, to address concerns of potential recall and selection biases. Studies have shown that risk estimates for various exposures do not vary when malformed and non-malformed controls are used (Werler et al., 1996, 1999; Khoury et al., 1994). In any event, the best approach is to obtain the most accurate exposure information possible for all study subjects, to reduce the likelihood of either random or differential misclassification.

Validity Assessment

Despite the difficulties described above in determining the presence of recall bias or differential misclassification, there is considerable merit in determining the validity of measuring exposures in both prospective and retrospective studies (Drews and Greenland, 1990). Validity assessment involves comparing the exposure measure of interest to a gold standard. One measure of validity is *sensitivity*, or the probability of being classified as exposed if truly exposed. Conversely, *specificity* is the probability of being classified as not exposed if truly unexposed. Using the data presented in Table 10.1 as an example, smoking measured by interview is com-

TABLE 10.1. *Validity Assessment of Cigarette Smoking*

Maternal Report	Cotinine		
	Exposed	Unexposed	Total
Exposed	25	1	26
Unexposed	5	69	74
Total	30	70	100

pared to cotinine levels in first-trimester urine samples (as the gold standard). Sensitivity would be the proportion of cotinine identified-smokers who were classified by interview as smokers (25/30 = 83%); specificity would be the proportion of women identified by cotinine levels as nonsmokers who were also classified by interview as nonsmokers (69/70 = 99%).

Exposure information may be available from two separate sources or measures, but one may not necessarily be considered a gold standard. In this instance, the amount of agreement or correlation between the two exposure measures can be assessed. Simple percent agreement can be misleading because a certain amount of agreement occurs by chance. For dichotomous factors, the Kappa statistic corrects for the amount of agreement that is expected to occur by chance (Thompson and Walter, 1988; Fleiss, 1973). The Kappa statistic is considered to represent excellent agreement when greater than 0.75, fair to good agreement in the range of 0.4 to 0.75, and poor agreement when less than 0.4. However, it is particularly dependent on the prevalence of exposure, tending to approach low values when prevalence rates are low, regardless of sensitivity and specificity.

It has been recommended that sensitivity analyses be employed to assess the likelihood that an observed association between exposure and disease might be due to measurement error. This is a theoretical exercise where effect estimates (e.g., odds ratios) are calculated after assuming certain amounts of error in exposure measurement (i.e., a particular sensitivity value). For example, a study of cigarette smoking in pregnancy, based on birth certificate data, observed 35% of cases exposed and 20% of controls exposed and produced an odds ratio of 2.2 (Table 10.2).

If the sensitivity of the observed cigarette smoking data was assumed to be higher for cases than controls (80% vs. 60%, as might occur in the presence of re-

call bias), the odds ratio would decrease to 1.6. If the sensitivity disparity were greater, say 70% vs. 40%, the odds ratio would decrease to 1.0. However, in the former scenario, the prevalence of smoking among controls would be 50%, which is unreasonably high based on reported smoking and cotinine measures in pregnant women (Kendrick and Merritt, 1996; Haddow et al., 1987). Hence, it would be reasonable to assume that extreme differential recording of cigarette smoking would not completely account for the increased risk in the example.

Gestational Timing

As described in detail in Chapter 1, fusion of the upper lip and palate occurs within the first 10 weeks of gestation. Thus, epidemiologic studies should aim at capturing exposure status early in pregnancy. To do so, it is necessary to establish gestational timing of pregnancy. The usual approach is based on the last menstrual period. However, approximately 5% of women have unreliable dates due to irregular cycles or missed menstrual periods. Sonograms in the first half of pregnancy accurately assess gestational timing, with a general rule being that the earlier in gestation the sonogram is performed, the more accurate the dating (Mongelli et al., 1996; Hall, 1990). Other methods of gestational dating, such as fundal height of the mother and Dubowitz exam of the infant, are considered less reliable (Hall, 1990).

SOURCES OF INFORMATION

Biologic Specimens

There is a range of possible biologic specimens that can serve as potential markers of exposure, including amniotic fluid; placenta; maternal serum, urine, hair, and nails; and infant serum and urine. Each tissue has its own set of advantages and disadvantages. For example, maternal hair or nail samples have the advantage of representing cumulative exposure levels in previous months, thus allowing the time of sampling to follow the etiologically relevant time period; however, only limited exposures can reliably be measured from hair, such as trace elements and cocaine, and contamination is not uncommon (Hunter, 1990). Maternal cumulative exposure may not be the best indicator of fetal exposure. For example, maternal blood measurements of compounds that are stored in fat or bone represent circulating levels and may more closely represent fetal exposure than measurements of storage tissues, which would represent maternal cumulative exposure. How-

TABLE 10.2. *Sensitivity Analysis*

Outcome	Sensitivity Cases/Controls	Smoking Exposed	Unexposed	Odds Ratio
	1.00/1.00			
Cases		35	65	2.2
Controls		20	80	Reference
	0.80/0.60			
Cases		44	56	1.6
Controls		33	67	Reference
	0.70/0.40			
Cases		50	50	1.0
Controls		50	50	Reference

ever, blood samples would need to be collected during early pregnancy, which is not always feasible. When the exposure of interest is a one-time event, such as acute exposure to a toxin resulting from an environmental disaster, then compounds with long half-lives can be measured in biologic tissues years later, allowing identification of exposed and unexposed subjects retrospectively. Exposures that are likely to change during pregnancy (e.g., diet, cigarette smoking, coffee consumption, and alcoholic beverage drinking) can be more difficult to accurately measure in biologic samples from a feasibility standpoint in that the timing of measurement should coincide with the etiologically relevant time period, i.e., early gestation.

Biologic measures may reflect intake amount or levels in tissues but not always both. In other words, intake amounts may not correlate with tissue levels because other factors (e.g., genetic factors, bioavailability, other exposures) may play a role. Both intake amounts and tissue levels are of interest; the former is potentially modifiable, and the latter is more closely related to risk (Hunter, 1990).

Environmental or Occupational Sampling

Testing of exposures in the environment can be done to measure air pollutants, water contaminants, or soil contaminants. These measures may not represent individual exposure levels; thus, they are indirect or ecologic measures. Occupational records are sometimes available as either indirect or direct measures of exposure. An example of an indirect measure of occupational exposure would be employment in an industry or building known to use solvents, thereby indicating the potential for exposure. Direct measurement would indicate exposure status per individual rather than per residence, employment category, or site. Because direct measurement of environmental exposures can be difficult, requiring personal monitoring devices, indirect measures are more often used. However, the accuracy of indirect measures can be improved by collecting information on individual behaviors that may influence the likelihood of exposure. For example, the number of days of employment in a particular occupation as an indirect measure of an occupational exposure could be enhanced by asking employees if they wore protective devices. Another example is that individual residences linked to water distribution records (as an indirect measure of exposure to contaminated water) could be enhanced by asking individuals about consumption of tap vs. bottled water. Environmental databases on air pollution dispersion, pesticide use patterns, water pollution, and toxic waste sites can be accessed for geographic information systems studies (Rodenbeck

et al., 2000; Moore and Carpenter, 1999). Also, more involved dosimetric models can be implemented which incorporate environmental, individual, and biologic data (Hatch and Thomas, 1993). Use of these sophisticated models can help to characterize potential exposure, but without information on individual exposure factors, they are likely to fall short of accurate assessment.

Records

Medical records can be an excellent source for exposures or procedures that are accurately and routinely documented in a standardized manner. For example, infertility procedures or anesthetic exposures are usually well documented in medical records. Other exposures, such as vitamin use, over-the-counter medication use, or infectious diseases, may not be well documented. For prescription medications, pharmacy records are a reasonable source, assuming the woman was compliant in her use.

Vital records are sometimes used as a source of information. Birth certificates include demographic information, such as maternal age, race, and birth order. In most U.S. states, information is also available on maternal exposures such as cigarette smoking, alcohol consumption, and illicit drug use during pregnancy. However, this source is considered inaccurate for such exposures, and details on level and timing of exposure are typically not recorded (Dietz et al., 1998).

Maternal Report

Finally, maternal report is a common source of exposure information. Reported exposures rely on maternal recall and, therefore, are subject to error. Studies have shown that such errors and the resulting random and differential misclassification can be reduced by asking standardized and detailed questions (Mitchell et al., 1986; Klungel et al., 2000; Eskenazi and Pearson, 1988). Questions that are open-ended or that lead the respondent should be avoided. In addition, if questions on a particular exposure or set of exposures can be asked in several ways, it has been shown that reporting increases. For example, information on medication use can be elicited by indication ("Did you take anything for headache?"), type of drugs ("Did you take any pain- or fever-reducing medications?"), and specific drugs ("Did you take any aspirin, acetaminophen, or ibuprofen?"). In addition, questions can be tailored to elicit details on the most relevant information, i.e., exposure timing (onset and duration), dose, frequency, changes in use, gestational timing, and potential confounders.

The method of administering a questionnaire is related to the quality of information. Self-administered questionnaires depend on the literacy and sometimes intellect of the respondent. Further, questions may be unintentionally skipped or left incomplete (O'Toole et al., 1986). Both telephone and in-person interviews can overcome these limitations, with higher-quality information obtained in person (Patterson et al., 1998; Hermann, 1985; Weeks et al., 1983; Einarson et al., 1999). In addition, participation rates tend to be higher when study subjects are verbally asked to participate (Weeks et al., 1983).

SPECIFIC EXPOSURES

Cigarette Smoking

There are several biomarkers of exposure to cigarette smoke; but cotinine, the main nicotine metabolite, is at present the most stable, sensitive, and specific marker for either individual exposure or passive exposure (Benowitz, 1999; Jauniaux et al., 1999). Cotinine can be measured in blood, saliva, urine, and amniotic fluid. Findings on cigarette smoking in relation to oral cleft risk appear to be dose-dependent (number of cigarettes smoked per day); hence, details on quantity of smoking should be collected. However, quantity and timing of smoking in pregnancy are not well documented on birth certificates in the United States, with approximately 30% underreporting compared to urinary cotinine measures (Kendrick et al., 1995). Documentation in prenatal medical records is generally better than on birth certificates; but underreporting remains, and information on quantity and timing is often missing. The quality of questionnaire data on smoking depends on the way questions are asked. Kharrazi et al. (1999) compared four questions on smoking in pregnancy to cotinine levels determined from second-trimester blood samples. Timing-specific questions on cigarette smoking by telephone interview were estimated to be 87% sensitive, whereas a simple yes/no question during a prenatal care visit was only 47% sensitive. Data suggest that pregnant smokers under-report that they smoke at all and that, among those who report smoking, the amount smoked is underreported (Ford et al., 1997).

Alcohol

Maternal alcohol consumption is difficult to accurately measure in early pregnancy. Various biologic markers of alcohol consumption have been examined, including mean red cell volume, γ-glutamyl transpeptidase, acetaldehyde in whole blood, and carbohydrate-deficient transferrin, each with different sensitivities and specificities. Stoler et al. (1998) used all four markers as a screen for alcohol abuse in pregnant women and found greater sensitivity than with each marker alone, using abnormal phenotype in offspring as the gold standard. Several different screens, such as TWEAK, T-ACE, Michigan Alcohol Screening Test or MAST, and CAGE (Russell et al., 1996), have been developed to identify heavy alcohol consumers with reasonably high sensitivity and specificity (>75%). However, moderate and occasional binge alcohol drinking are more common behaviors and may carry risks for oral clefts (Werler et al., 1991; Munger et al., 1996). To measure these more casual or intermittent patterns of use, separate questions on average and binge frequency (how often), timing (when), dose (drinks per day), and type (beer, wine, liquor) should be asked in detail. One pitfall in collecting alcohol information is asking separately about the frequency and dose of beer, wine, and liquor intake. Data collected in this manner cannot accurately assess the total frequency and dose without assuming that only one type of beverage is consumed on any given day. For example, a woman may report drinking two glasses of wine per drinking day 3 days per week and two liquor drinks per drinking day 3 days per week. If the woman drank only 3 days per week, her daily dose would be four drinks; if she drank 6 days per week, her average daily dose would be two drinks. Sensitivity and specificity values have not been estimated for various questions on patterns of use, but presumably sensitivity is not high and specificity is not low.

Medications and Illnesses

Various medications and illnesses, such as antiepileptics (Abrishamchian et al., 1994) and the common cold (Zhang and Cai, 1993), have been suggested to affect oral cleft risk; and other such exposures deserve to be studied. Information on prescription medications can be obtained from medical records, but one must assume that the woman followed her clinician's orders in a timely and otherwise compliant fashion. Pharmacy records are one step closer in that they indicate that the prescription was filled, but one must assume that the woman took the medication as prescribed. Also, a woman may have taken a medication that was not documented in her medical record or was filled at a different pharmacy. Medical records and pharmacy sources are most useful for cohorts of pregnant health maintenance organization members, where different medical and pharmacy services are documented within one system. These sources have the added benefit of being documented during pregnancy and are not subject to recall bias. However, most medications taken in pregnancy are not prescribed (Werler and Mitchell, 2000) and are more difficult to ascertain because they tend not to be documented in medical records. The most common approach to assessing exposure to over-the-counter medications is by interview. Questions must be detailed on specific product, frequency, dose, timing, and indication for use. To assess confounding by underlying illness in drug analyses, it is necessary to obtain information on the illness(es) among unmedicated women as well. Also, depending on the drug, route of administration may be important; e.g., corticosteroid exposure includes oral, inhaled, and topical routes. For over-the-counter drugs, particularly cough/cold/analgesic products, it is important to identify the product name, type (capsule, packet, liquid), and packaging because product lines are often labeled according to the symptoms they treat and vary in the components they contain. For example, Tylenol® contains acetaminophen and Tylenol Flu® contains acetaminophen, dextromethorphan, and pseudoephedrine. Over-the-counter medications are usually taken intermittently and on a more casual basis, which complicates accurate assessment, presumably reducing both sensitivity and specificity.

Issues surrounding the assessment of illnesses in pregnancy parallel those of medication use in pregnancy. Chronic or severe illnesses are more likely to be reliably documented in medical records than those that are acute or less severe. Infectious illnesses can be extremely difficult to accurately assess in observational studies because it is prohibitive to conduct sequential serology tests in early pregnancy to identify true exposure to any given specific agent. Thus, studies usually rely on reported illness events, such as colds or flu. Assessment of fever is subject to many of the same limitations. In interview studies on illnesses, the quality of information can be improved by asking details on timing, whether the illness was diagnosed by a clinician, what symptoms were experienced, whether medication was taken and what type, and whether fever accompanied the illness (and, if so, fever duration and highest temperature).

Vitamins and Diet

For biologic measurement of various nutrients, serum and plasma are commonly used. However, red blood cells may provide a better indication of nutrient status due to greater stability compared to serum and plasma levels. One potentially useful source of second-trimester blood samples, for which measurements might correlate with early gestation levels, is banked maternal serum following prenatal screening. Long-term storage

may result in degradation of nutrients, but such degradation should not be differential for cases and controls. Detailed discussion of sampling and measurement issues can be found elsewhere (Hunter, 1990). Hair and nail samples provide stable measures of heavy metals but are subject to contamination from cleansing and polishing products.

Many studies rely on reported supplement and dietary intakes to assess nutrient status. For supplements, questions must be asked about specific products because there are hundreds of multivitamin products with varying amounts of different vitamin and mineral components. Most women begin use of prenatal multivitamin preparations after pregnancy is clinically recognized (Werler et al., 1999), regardless of whether or not they were routine vitamin takers before pregnancy. Therefore, it is important to ascertain the timing of use of each supplement and to determine exposure status during the developmentally relevant time period.

Approaches to assessing dietary intake include 24 h dietary recalls, food diaries, and food-frequency questionnaires (Witschi, 1990). The first two methods are effective for measuring dietary intake but reflect intake at the time of data collection. Since dietary patterns often change during early pregnancy due to nausea and then change again once nausea has passed, intake at the time of measurement may not reflect the developmentally relevant time period. One advantage of food-frequency questionnaires is that they can refer to a specific time, e.g., pre-pregnancy or early pregnancy. Indeed, food-frequency questions can identify changes in diet during pregnancy (Brown et al., 1996) and have been validated among pregnant women (Wei et al., 1999). However, if there is a long delay between early pregnancy and when dietary intake is measured, recall of dietary patterns may be difficult for the relatively short period of organogenesis (approximately 8 weeks). If there is an interval of several months or more between early gestation and the time that dietary information is collected, food-frequency questions targeted to average diet during the months preceding pregnancy may be better recalled and may better reflect nutrient status of very early gestation.

The validity of food-frequency data collected retrospectively has been examined in several non-pregnant populations (Sobell et al., 1989; Block et al., 1990; Mares-Perlman et al., 1993) but to date has not been reported in postpartum populations as a reflection of early or prepregnancy diet. Among nonpregnant women, correlation coefficients for retrospective measurement of diet compared to 24 h recalls vary across the range of foods from low to high but, on average, are in the moderate range (0.52) (Salvini et al., 1989); for specific nutrients, correlation coefficients ranged from 0.36 for vitamin A without supplementation to 0.75 for vitamin C with supplements (Willett et al., 1985). A detailed discussion of assessment of diet can be found elsewhere (Willett, 1990).

Solvents and Pesticides

Because exposure to solvents and pesticides can come from more than one source, it is important to be as comprehensive as possible in assessments. For example, occupational studies should include assessment of exposure away from the workplace. This requires contact with study individuals, which in some occupational or environmental studies may not be feasible; but if at all possible, the gain in accuracy of exposure assessment may be worth the extra expense. Further, in occupational, environmental, and home settings, exposure to a single product may involve several different chemical agents. Every attempt should be made to determine the exact chemicals of exposure. In occupational settings, records of chemicals used can be assessed. There is an Environmental Protection Agency number (EPA Reg. No.) on all pesticide products sold in the United States. This unique identifier can be easily ascertained from products that are still on hand and then linked to its chemical contents. The typical research goal is to identify whether risks are confined to a particular chemical or group of chemicals, but often there is so much overlap in exposure to individual chemicals that it prohibits estimating independent effects. Nevertheless, there is value in identifying risks associated with mixes of chemicals because public health interventions may occur for an overall exposure scenario rather than for a specific chemical (Hertz-Picciotto, 1998). A detailed discussion of pesticide and solvent exposure measurement can be found elsewhere (Armstrong et al., 1992).

Confounding Factors

While accurate assessment of exposure is important in epidemiologic studies, potential confounding factors also deserve careful attention. In studies of oral clefts, factors that are known to be associated with their occurrence are obvious candidates as confounders. For oral clefts, information should be collected on infant's race; ethnicity; sex; maternal and paternal ages; maternal epilepsy; maternal use of anticonvulsants, corticosteroids, high-dose vitamin A, or trimethoprim; maternal occupation; maternal smoking; and maternal use of alcohol. However, other factors which have not previously been identified may be related to both oral clefts and the exposure under study. It is important to collect accurate information on potential confounders, to

reduce the likelihood of spurious estimation of adjusted risks (Greenland, 1980).

Likewise, factors that may act as effect modifiers should be accurately measured. Positive family history of oral clefts is one such potential effect modifier. Accurate assessment is best accomplished by contacting family members individually for medical information. One study has documented that family history of birth defects was more accurately obtained by this method as opposed to maternal report (Romitti et al., 1997). Inaccurate measurement can result in an apparent lack of effect modification when in fact it exists or in an apparent interaction when none exists (Greenland, 1980).

Data Collection

It is important to record data in a way that allows clear understanding of exposure status. Because most sources of exposure information are not perfect, allowance must be made for incomplete or missing information. For example, no notation on alcohol consumption in a medical record may represent truly missing information (the question was never asked of the patient) or a negative response (only positive responses were recorded). Likewise, medical records or maternal report may indicate use of cough medication, but the specific agent is missing. In addition, recall of details of illnesses and medication use that occurred several months earlier can be difficult. Data collection instruments should include options such as "missing," "not otherwise specified," and "don't know" to accommodate these situations. In maternal interviews, there is a natural tendency to try to force a study participant into an exposed or unexposed category; however, random misclassification will be reduced if truly unclear information is recorded and analyzed as such.

CONCLUSION

Accurate assessment of exposures is essential for valid study of risk factors for oral clefts. Prospective studies may reduce exposure misclassification by collecting information closer to the etiologically relevant time period (the first trimester), but they are less efficient than retrospective studies. Therefore, the majority of studies of environmental risk factors for oral clefts are retrospective in design and thereby present further challenges in accurate exposure assessment. It is important that efforts be made to collect detailed exposure information in as complete and accurate a fashion as possible, to reduce the likelihood of misclassification. While such efforts can be laborious during the data collection phase of studies, there is a gain in the validity of risk estimation that justifies the added effort.

I thank Allen Mitchell for his helpful comments.

REFERENCES

Abrishamchian, AR, Khoury, MJ, Calle, EE (1994). The contribution of maternal epilepsy and its treatment to the etiology of oral clefts: a population based case-control study. Genet Epidemiol 11: 343–351.

Armstrong, BK, White, E, Saracci, R (1992). Principles of Exposure Measurement in Epidemiology. Monographs in Epidemiology and Biostatistics, Vol. 21. Oxford: Oxford University Press.

Benowitz, NL (1999). Biomarkers of environmental tobacco smoke exposure. Environ Health Perspect 107(Suppl 2): 349–355.

Block, G, Woods, M, Potosky, A, Clifford, C (1990). Validation of a self-administered diet history questionnaire using multiple diet records. J Clin Epidemiol 43: 1327–1335.

Brown, JE, Buzzard, IM, Jacobs, DR, Jr, et al. (1996). A food frequency questionnaire can detect pregnancy-related changes in diet. J Am Diet Assoc 96: 262–266.

Dietz, PM, Adams, MM, Kendrick, JS, et al. (1998). Completeness of ascertainment of prenatal smoking using birth certificates and confidential questionnaires: variations by maternal attributes and infant birth weight. Am J Epidemiol 148: 1048–1054.

Drews, CD, Greenland, S (1990). The impact of differential recall on the results of case-control studies. Int J Epidemiol 19: 1107–1112.

Drews, CD, Kraus, JF, Greenland, S (1990). Recall bias in a case-control study of sudden infant death syndrome. Int J Epidemiol 19: 405–411.

Einarson, A, Ahmed, SF, Gallo, M, et al. (1999). Reproducibility of medical information obtained via the telephone vs personal interview. Vet Hum Toxicol 41: 397–400.

Eskenazi, B, Pearson, K (1988). Validation of a self-administered questionnaire for assessing occupational and environmental exposures of pregnant women. Am J Epidemiol 128: 1117–1129.

Fleiss, JL (1973). Statistical Methods for Rates and Proportions. New York: John Wiley & Sons.

Ford, RP, Tappin, DM, Schluter, PJ, Wild, CJ (1997). Smoking during pregnancy: how reliable are maternal self reports in New Zealand? J Epidemiol Community Health 51: 246–251.

Greenland, S (1980). The effect of misclassification in the presence of covariates. Am J Epidemiol 112: 564–569.

Haddow, JE, Knight, GJ, Palomaki, GE, et al. (1987). Cigarette consumption and serum cotinine in relation to birthweight. Br J Obstet Gynaecol 94: 678–681.

Hall, MH (1990). Definitions used in relation to gestational age. Paediatr Perinat Epidemiol 4: 123–128.

Hatch, M, Thomas, D (1993). Measurement issues in environmental epidemiology. Environ Health Perspect 101(Suppl 4): 49–57.

Herrmann, N (1985). Retrospective information from questionnaires. II. Intrarater reliability and comparison of questionnaire types. Am J Epidemiol 121: 948–953.

Hertz-Picciotto, I (1998). Environmental epidemiology. Domain of environmental epidemiology. In: Modern epidemiology, 2nd ed., edited by KJ Rothman and S Greenland. Philadelphia: Lippincott-Raven, pp. 555–583.

Hunter, D (1990). Biochemical indicators of dietary intake. In: Nutritional epidemiology. Monographs in epidemiology and biostatistics, Vol. 15, edited by W Willett. New York: Oxford University Press, pp. 143–216.

Jauniaux, E, Gulbis, B, Acharya, G, et al. (1999). Maternal tobacco exposure and cotinine levels in fetal fluids in the first half of pregnancy. Obstet Gynecol 93: 25–29.

Kendrick, JS, Merritt, RK (1996). Women and smoking: an update for the 1990s. Am J Obstet Gynecol 175: 528–535.

Kendrick, JS, Zahniser, SC, Miller, N, et al. (1995). Integrating smoking cessation into routine public prenatal care: the Smoking Cessation in Pregnancy project. Am J Public Health 85: 217–222.

Kharrazi, M, Epstein, D, Hopkins, B, et al. (1999). Evaluation of four maternal smoking questions. Public Health Rep 114: 60–70.

Khoury, MJ, James, LM, Erickson, JD (1994). On the use of affected controls to address recall bias in case-control studies of birth defects. Teratology 49: 273–281.

Klemetti, A, Saxén, L (1967). Prospective versus retrospective approach in the search for environmental causes of malformations. Am J Public Health 57: 2071–2075.

Klungel, OH, de Boer, A, Paes, AHP, et al. (2000). Influence of question structure on the recall of self-reported drug use. J Clin Epidemiol 53: 273–277.

Mackenzie, SG, Lippman, A (1989). An investigation of report bias in a case-control study of pregnancy outcome. Am J Epidemiol 129: 65–75.

Mares-Perlman, JA, Klein, BE, Klein, R, et al. (1993). A diet history questionnaire ranks nutrient intakes in middle-aged and older men and women similarly to multiple food records. J Nutr 123: 489–501.

Mitchell, AA, Cottler, LB, Shapiro, S (1986). Effect of questionnaire design on recall of drug exposure in pregnancy. Am J Epidemiol 123: 670–676.

Mongelli, M, Wilcox, M, Gardosi, J (1996). Estimating the date of confinement: ultrasonographic biometry versus certain menstrual dates. Am J Obstet Gynecol 174: 278–281.

Moore, DA, Carpenter, TE (1999). Spatial analytical methods and geographic information systems: use in health research and epidemiology. Epidemiol Rev 21: 143–161.

Munger, RG, Romitti, PA, Daack-Hirsch, S, et al. (1996). Maternal alcohol use and risk of orofacial cleft birth defects. Teratology 54: 27–33.

O'Toole, BI, Battistutta, D, Long, A, Crouch, K (1986). A comparison of costs and data quality of three health survey methods: mail, telephone and personal home interview. Am J Epidemiol 124: 317–328.

Patterson, RE, Kristal, AR, Levy, L, et al. (1998). Validity of methods used to assess vitamin and mineral supplement use. Am J Epidemiol 148: 643–649.

Rodenbeck, SE, Sanderson, LM, Rene, A (2000). Maternal exposure to trichloroethylene in drinking water and birth-weight outcomes. Arch Environ Health 55: 188–194.

Romitti, PA, Burns, TL, Murray, JC (1997). Maternal interview reports of family history of birth defects: evaluation from a population-based case-control study of orofacial clefts. Am J Med Genet 72: 422–429.

Russell, M, Martier, SS, Sokol, RJ, et al. (1996). Detecting risk drinking during pregnancy: a comparison of four screening questionnaires. Am J Public Health 86: 1435–1439.

Salvini, S, Hunter, DJ, Sampson, L, et al. (1989). Food-based validation of a dietary questionnaire: the effects of week-to-week variation in food consumption. Int J Epidemiol 18: 858–867.

Sobell, J, Block, G, Koslowe, P, et al. (1989). Validation of a retrospective questionnaire assessing diet 10–15 years ago. Am J Epidemiol 130: 173–187.

Stoler, JM, Huntington, KS, Peterson, CM, et al. (1998). The prenatal detection of significant alcohol exposure with maternal blood markers. J Pediatr 133: 346–352.

Swan, SH, Shaw, GM, Schulman, J (1992). Reporting and selection bias in case-control studies of congenital malformations. Epidemiology 3: 356–363.

Thompson, WD, Walter, SD (1988). A reappraisal of the kappa coefficient. J Clin Epidemiol 41: 949–958.

Weeks, MF, Kulka, RA, Lessler, JT, Whitmore, RW (1983). Personal versus telephone surveys for collecting household health data at the local level. Am J Public Health 73: 1389–1394.

Wei, EK, Gardner, J, Field, AE, et al. (1999). Validity of a food frequency questionnaire in assessing nutrient intakes of low-income pregnant women. Matern Child Health J 3: 241–246.

Werler, MM, Hayes, C, Louik, C, et al. (1999). Multivitamin supplementation and risk of birth defects. Am J Epidemiol 150: 675–682.

Werler, MM, Lammer, EJ, Rosenberg, L, Mitchell, AA (1991). Maternal alcohol use in relation to selected birth defects. Am J Epidemiol 134: 691–698.

Werler, MM, Louik, C, Shapiro, S, Mitchell, AA (1996). Prepregnant weight in relation to risk of neural tube defects. JAMA 275: 1089–1092.

Werler, MM, Mitchell, AA (2000). Medication use in pregnancy in the U.S. [Abstract]. Teratology 62: 363.

Werler, MM, Pober, BR, Nelson, K, Holmes, LB (1989). Reporting accuracy among mothers of malformed and nonmalformed infants. Am J Epidemiol 129: 415–421.

Willett, W (1990). Nutritional Epidemiology. Monographs in Epidemiology and Biostatistics, Vol. 15. New York: Oxford University Press.

Willett, WC, Sampson, L, Stampfer, MJ, et al. (1985). Reproducibility and validity of a semiquantitative food frequency questionnaire. Am J Epidemiol 122: 51–65.

Witschi, JC (1990). Short-term dietary recall and recording methods. In: Nutritional epidemiology. Monographs in epidemiology and biostatistics, Vol. 15, edited by W Willett. New York: Oxford University Press, pp. 52–68.

Zhang, J, Cai, WW (1993). Association of the common cold in the first trimester of pregnancy with birth defects. Pediatrics 92: 559–563.

11

Birth defects surveillance systems and oral clefts

ADOLFO CORREA

LARRY EDMONDS

Oral clefts are among the more frequent and readily diagnosed major congenital anomalies. Accordingly, they have been the subject of many studies that have increased our knowledge of their epidemiology. For instance, studies of the variation in prevalence by race/ethnicity have shown a high rate of oral clefts in Asians, followed by whites and African-Americans (Vanderas, 1987). Etiologic studies have identified possible increases in the risk of oral clefts with a number of factors, including maternal smoking (Khoury et al., 1989; Kallen 1997; Lieff et al., 1999), alcohol consumption (Shaw et al., 1999), use of corticosteroids (Carmichael and Shaw, 1999), and occupational factors (Bianchi et al., 1997; Lorente et al., 2000) (see Chapters 16 and 17). Data for these studies have come from population-based surveillance systems for birth defects. This chapter examines the methods of population-based birth defects surveillance systems, reviews recent prevalence data on oral clefts from state and international monitoring programs, and offers some recommendations for enhancing the use of birth defects surveillance programs for studies of oral clefts.

METHODS OF BIRTH DEFECTS SURVEILLANCE

Population-based birth defects surveillance programs aim at having a relatively complete or representative sample of affected infants in the population and, as such, can provide more accurate and reliable estimates of rates and risk factors for birth defects than birth defects registries based on a selected sample of hospitals. Therefore, after the epidemic of limb reduction defects associated with thalidomide use in the 1960s, interest was extensive in population-based surveillance systems for identifying increases in the frequency of birth defects possibly associated with maternal exposure to teratogens in the general population. As methodologic issues of this approach became apparent (Khoury and Holtzman, 1987), birth defects surveillance programs expanded their functions; and interest in birth defect surveillance has grown, with population-based programs currently monitoring the occurrence of birth defects in 31 U.S. states and internationally (Centers for Disease Control and Prevention, 2000; International Clearinghouse for Birth Defects Monitoring Systems, 2000).

The fundamental objective in population-based surveillance for birth defects, including oral clefts, is the description of their frequency in the population and how this frequency varies with time, place, and personal characteristics of infants with birth defects and their mothers (e.g., child's sex, maternal age). Accordingly, the general methods in surveillance for birth defects, including oral clefts, are as follows: *(1)* specification of the population covered; *(2)* definition and ascertainment of affected infants and children (i.e., cases) in the population; *(3)* collection of clinical and descriptive data; *(4)* coding and classification of cases; and *(5)* data analysis and dissemination. The methods used (e.g., case criteria, case classification) need to be related to the specific objectives of the surveillance program.

Population Covered

The population covered by the surveillance system needs to be specified in terms of the geographic area, number of yearly live births and stillbirths to area residents, and hospitals in the study area where births are delivered and children undergo medical evaluations. Given the variation in the race/ethnicity characteristics in the population of the United States and the known variation in prevalence of oral clefts by race/ethnicity, surveillance systems in the United States collect information on the race/ethnicity characteristics of the yearly births. For example, the population covered by the Metropolitan Atlanta Congenital Defects Program (MACDP), a population-based surveillance system for birth defects in operation since 1967, included about 47,000 births in 1999 in 22 area hospitals, occurring among residents of five counties in metropolitan Atlanta. The percent of nonwhite births has increased over time from about 27% in 1967 to 46% in 1999.

Case Definition

The definition of a case specifies the inclusion criteria, such as (1) births with any major defect (i.e., a defect that can cause death or a major disability in the absence of treatment), infants with any one of a select subgroup of major defects, infants with major or minor defects, or infants with other groups of birth defects; (2) period of detection of birth defects; (3) age by which cases should be ascertained; and (4) inclusion of live-born infants and stillbirths, 20 weeks of gestation or more, or 500 g or more. For example, within MACDP the case definition includes all infants born to residents of five counties in metropolitan Atlanta and who have at least one major birth defect diagnosed in their first year and identified by MACDP within their first 5 years of life.

Case Ascertainment

Affected children can be identified from a variety of routine data sources: (1) vital records (birth certificates, fetal death certificates, and infant death certificates), where health professionals are asked report the presence of structural defects at birth or as a cause of death; (2) newborn hospital discharge summaries and obstetric and nursery logs; (3) hospital records of subsequent hospitalizations; and (4) data from other sources, including specialty clinics (such as medical genetics for syndrome diagnosis), pathology reports for terminations, abortion records, autopsy records, and cytogenetic laboratories. Each of these sources of information affects the quality of the data.

Vital records have several strengths: (1) the complete coverage of the population since they are population-based, (2) availability of some information on the type of defect, (3) availability of some information on characteristics of the parents, (4) availability of data for previous years, (5) low cost, and (6) potential for linkage with other data for the conduct of follow-up studies of children with birth defects. The weaknesses of vital records include (1) underreporting of several birth defects because of diagnostic difficulties (e.g., limited evaluations for defects), (2) inaccurate diagnoses because of limited evaluations, (3) lack of specificity of the diagnosis for most birth defects, (4) possible exclusion of case infants born outside of the state, and (5) lack of timeliness of the death certificates. That underascertainment of oral clefts may result from the use of birth certificates as the only source of cases is well documented. In a study in Norway, a 14.5% underreporting error was noted for cleft lip and palate patients' birth records when compared to subsequent surgery records (Åbyholm, 1978). Sixteen percent of orofacial clefts and other anomalies were underreported in Pennsylvania's birth certificates (Ivy, 1957), and 35% of facial cleft anomalies were not recorded as such in the birth certificates of affected infants in Arkansas (Green et al., 1979). Furthermore, many cases of oral clefts that are reported on the birth certificates are misclassified (Meskin and Pruzansky, 1967). For instance, 52% of all facial clefts in Arkansas were reported incorrectly (Green et al, 1979).

Newborn hospital discharge summaries have several strengths: (1) more complete recording of birth defects than in the birth certificate, (2) more readily available data (usually within 6 months of discharge), (3) data that may be already computerized and in digital form in many hospitals. The weaknesses of newborn hospital discharge summaries include (1) incomplete recording of information on birth defects, (2) possible incomplete or incorrect preliminary diagnosis in the newborn period, (3) lack of access to personal identifiers (making follow-up difficult), (4) difficulties in defining the population base because many infants born at home are not included, (5) difficulties in establishing the representativeness of the case data, and (6) lack of information about maternal characteristics. The potential problem of relying solely on newborn discharge summaries was highlighted by a study of hospital newborn records as the sole source for oral facial clefts in King County, Washington, for the years 1956–1965 (Emanuel et al., 1973). This study showed that hospital newborn records ascertained 98.5% of the total cases of oral clefts found through all sources combined but that only 68.4% of them had been coded correctly on the discharge abstract.

Records from subsequent hospitalizations, specialty clinics, pathology reports, abortion reports, and cytogenetic laboratories are potentially very useful in that they can provide clinical and laboratory data that may help clarify questions about possible diagnoses. However, such records may be collected and maintained only on a select sample of cases, and practical or legal considerations may limit their availability. Consequently, population-based birth defects surveillance programs do not rely on such records as sole sources for case ascertainment. In 1999, none of the 31 operational birth defects surveillance programs in the United States relied solely on medical records for case ascertainment (Centers for Disease Control and Prevention, 2000). Twenty-two of these programs reported use of medical records as one of several sources for case ascertainment.

Use of multiple sources for case ascertainment offers the best potential for complete case finding and for obtaining the best quality data on affected children. The strengths of multiple-source case ascertainment include *(1)* relative completeness of the recording of cases, *(2)* more precise and accurate diagnoses, *(3)* availability of maternal and infant data, and *(4)* relative ease for researchers to conduct follow-up studies of children with birth defects. The weaknesses of multiple-source case ascertainment include *(1)* more time and effort required to collect data from multiple sources, *(2)* higher costs (often limiting the use of this method to small populations), *(3)* more time and effort to prepare the database, and *(4)* more time needed to establish the baseline rates. Of the 31 operational birth defects surveillance systems in the United States in 1999, 29 used two or more sources

for case ascertainment and two relied on vital records alone (Centers for Disease Control and Prevention, 2000).

Case ascertainment can be characterized also by the intensiveness of the efforts involved. Case ascertainment may be limited to identification of cases from vital records or from reports submitted to the surveillance program by staff from hospitals, clinics, or other facilities. Such reports may be submitted voluntarily or through reporting systems established by law or regulation. More intensive surveillance methods entail the identification of cases by trained staff who actively seek cases in hospitals, clinics, or other facilities by systematically reviewing medical and other records. They may also query personnel who know about the newly diagnosed cases. Program staff record the case information on standard forms designed for the program.

Figure 11.1 shows the geographic distribution birth defects surveillance systems that were operational or in the planning phase in the United States in August of 2000. Among the 31 operational systems, 28 were statewide and 3 were limited to specific counties within a state. Among the operational systems, 10 (Alabama, Arizona, California, Georgia, Hawaii, Iowa, Massachusetts, Oklahoma, South Carolina, and Texas) had intensive surveillance, 7 (Colorado, Illinois, New Mexico, New Jersey, New York, North Carolina, and Utah) had mandatory reporting with follow-up and quality-control procedures, 11 (Arkansas, Connecticut, Delaware, Florida, Kentucky, Maryland, Mississippi, Missouri, Nebraska, Virginia, and West Virginia) had mandatory hospital reporting but no follow-up or quality-control procedures, and 9 (Louisiana, Montana, New

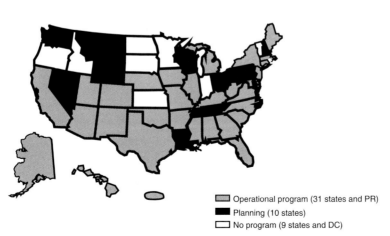

50 States, Washington DC and Puerto Rico

Operational program (31 states and PR)
Planning (10 states)
No program (9 states and DC)

FIG. 11.1. State birth defects surveillance systems in the United States, 2000. (From Centers for Disease Control and Prevention, 2000, with permission.)

Hampshire, Ohio, Pennsylvania, Tennessee, Washington, Wisconsin, and Wyoming) were planning or developing a registry.

Data Collection

Information collected on infants that meet the case definition may include *(1)* identifying information on infant and parents, *(2)* demographic information (such as maternal age, race/ethnicity), *(3)* pregnancy history and birth outcomes, *(4)* information on the index pregnancy and outcome, *(5)* diagnostic information on the types of birth defect, *(6)* cytogenetic and laboratory data, and *(7)* information on the hospital and physician to facilitate follow-up procedures. To evaluate the completeness and accuracy of the data, surveillance systems may set up quality-control procedures.

Coding and Classification of Birth Defects

Information may be collected on several defects for each affected infant. These defects may then be reviewed by a clinician/dysmorphologist and coded according to established procedures. For instance, MACDP uses a modified British Paediatric Association (BPA) six-digit code (British Paediatric Association, 1979) that is more detailed than the *International Classification of Diseases, Ninth Revision, Clinical Modification* (ICD-9-CM codes) (World Health Organization, 1979). These modified BPA codes for orofacial clefts are as follows: cleft palate without cleft lip, 749.000–749.099; and cleft lip with and without cleft palate, 749.100–749.299. Based on the clinical reviews, cases can be further classified into patterns of associated defects (isolated, sequences, syndromes with recognized cause, and "multiples") (Spranger et al., 1982; Stevenson and Hall, 1993).

Data Analysis and Dissemination

Data on major defects are analyzed to monitor the frequency of birth defects and to detect variations by calendar time or any unusual patterns. The frequency of birth defects is usually measured as prevalence at birth, expressed as the number of affected infants per 1000 or 10,000 births. Some systems include late fetal deaths (stillbirths) in the prevalence estimates. In addition, the gestational age at which delivery must occur for a classification of fetal death as late varies, being 20 weeks in some systems and 28 weeks in others. Prevalence data are monitored by statistical evaluation of the difference between observed and expected numbers of specific defects or defect combinations for a specified time in a specified area. Expected numbers are obtained from baseline prevalence data. Such comparisons may lead to the identification of clusters of birth defects and to epidemiologic studies to identify possible risk factors.

STATE AND INTERNATIONAL MONITORING PROGRAMS

The objectives of birth defects monitoring programs are to describe the magnitude of the problem by quantifying its prevalence, to serve as a source of cases for studies of risk factors, and to enable follow-up studies of the impact of these conditions on children's health and development and of the need of health and social services. This section describes recent prevalence rates for oral clefts and the extent to which birth defects surveillance systems are being used to address these objectives.

Prevalence Rates

Estimates of the birth prevalence of oral clefts have been published recently for selected state surveillance systems in the United States and for the International Clearinghouse for Birth Defects Monitoring Systems (ICBDMS).

State Birth Defects Surveillance Systems in the United States. Prevalence data are available for cleft lip with or without cleft palate and for cleft palate without cleft lip from 26 state surveillance systems in the United States for calendar year 1996 (except for a few states where data are available only for 1991, 1993, 1994, or 1995) by race (white and other) (National Birth Defects Prevention Network, 2000). The state birth defects surveillance programs that provided data on oral clefts vary in several respects: *(1)* case ascertainment methods, *(2)* definition of birth defects, *(3)* coding systems, *(4)* inclusion of stillbirths and pregnancy terminations in counts of birth defects occurrences, and *(5)* population coverage. In addition, some states do not include conditions noted in the medical chart as possible birth defects and in need of definitive confirmation or exclusion, while other states do. Because of these differences, state surveillance data on the prevalence of oral clefts cannot be combined to give a reliable overall national rate for the United States or be used to make meaningful comparisons between states. However, it is possible to examine the variation in prevalence of oral clefts by subgroup of oral clefts and race within each state as methods of case ascertainment are likely to vary less within than between states.

For cleft lip with or without cleft palate (Table 11.1), overall prevalence varied from 6 to 16 cases per 10,000 births (median 10/10,000), with rates generally higher for white than for nonwhite infants. Among white infants, the prevalence of cleft lip with or without cleft palate varied from 6 to 26 per 10,000 births (median 13/10,000); among infants of other races, it varied from 1 to 15 per 10,000 births (median 7/10,000).

For cleft palate without cleft lip (Table 11.2), the overall prevalence varied from 1 to 14 cases per 10,000 births (median 6/10,000) with some (but less pronounced) variation by race. Among white infants, the prevalence of cleft palate without cleft lip varied from 2 to 19 per 10,000 births (median 6/10,000); among infants of other races, it varied from 0 to 15 per 10,000 births (median 4/10,000).

Within each surveillance system, the prevalence for cleft lip with or without palate tended to be higher than that for cleft palate without cleft lip. In addition, the

TABLE 11.1. *Prevalence Rates for Cleft Lip with and without Cleft Palate per 10,000 Live Births and Stillbirths by Surveillance System, Reporting Year, and Race*

State	Year	White	Other	Total
Alaska	1996	7.47	2.29	5.98
Arizona	1991	10.61	13.55	11.02
Arkansas	1996	12.91	13.70	13.10
California	1995	9.45	10.23	10.00
Colorado	1996	12.02	5.31	10.33
Connecticut*	1994	8.00	3.32	6.77
Georgia*	1996	13.06	5.89	9.78
Hawaii	1996	12.55	15.29	14.44
Illinois	1996	6.16	4.40	5.75
Iowa†	1996	11.18	12.49	11.52
Maryland	1996	5.77	5.23	5.58
Massachusetts	1996	6.75	10.27	7.22
Missouri*	1996	12.96	10.35	12.48
Nebraska	1996	11.72	4.80	11.10
Nevada	1996	9.32	7.11	8.90
New Jersey*	1996	7.52	7.30	7.43
New Mexico	1996	10.93	30.16	14.36
New York*	1996	7.50	3.87	6.60
North Carolina	1996	10.77	7.39	9.77
Oklahoma	1996	11.20	19.83	12.92
South Carolina	1996	10.77	5.23	8.72
Tennessee	1993	8.77	4.31	7.64
Texas	1995	25.36	1.53	9.23
Utah	1996	12.29	40.54	13.71
Virginia†	1996			9.00
Wisconsin	1996	15.81	15.13	15.69

*Total births include live births only.
†Total births include live births, stillbirths, and terminations.
Source: National Birth Defect Prevention Network (2000).

TABLE 11.2. *Prevalence Rates for Cleft Palate without Cleft Lip per 10,000 Live Births and Stillbirths by Surveillance System, Reporting Year, and Race*

State	Year	White	Other	Total
Alaska	1996	4.48	8.96	5.98
Arizona	1991	4.45	3.13	4.26
Arkansas	1996	6.46	3.42	5.73
California	1995	8.00	7.07	7.28
Colorado	1996	9.20	7.67	8.73
Connecticut*	1994	6.52	0.83	5.02
Georgia*	1996	5.40	6.96	6.11
Hawaii	1996	2.09	8.34	6.71
Illinois	1996	4.32	3.24	4.07
Iowa†	1996	4.59	4.16	4.82
Maryland	1996	4.85	2.01	3.82
Massachusetts	1996	4.60	14.94	5.98
Missouri*	1996	4.76	1.59	4.20
Nebraska	1996	7.97	0.00	7.26
New Jersey*	1996	8.49	3.48	7.17
New Mexico	1995			1.08
New York*	1996	5.49	4.28	5.20
North Carolina	1996	6.33	7.39	6.64
Ohio	1996	9.73	3.34	8.40
Oklahoma	1996	7.10	7.31	7.32
Tennessee	1993	3.11	2.69	3.00
Texas	1995	19.24	0.77	6.75
Utah	1996	6.02	13.51	6.38
Virginia†	1996			4.22
Wisconsin	1996	14.36	12.74	14.06

*Total births include live births only.
†Total births include live births, stillbirths, and terminations.
Source: National Birth Defect Prevention Network (2000).

prevalence of oral clefts tended to be higher among white than among nonwhite infants. These observations have been noted before (Edmonds, 1997; Tolarova and Cervenka, 1998; Amidei et al., 1994; Croen et al., 1998; Robert et al., 1996).

International Clearinghouse for Birth Defects Monitoring Systems. The ICBDMS, an organization of birth defects monitoring programs around the world, recently published its *Annual Report 2000*, which includes prevalence data for several birth defects (International Clearinghouse for Birth Defects Monitoring Systems, 2000). These data include prevalence rates for cleft lip with or without cleft palate and for cleft palate without cleft lip for 1974–1998 for 25 systems: Australia, USA Atlanta, Canada National, New Zealand, Canada Alberta, England and Wales, Norway, North Netherlands, Finland, Ireland Dublin, Italy Birth Defects Registry of Campania (BDRCAM), Italy North East, Italy Tuscany, Italy Emilia-Romagna Registry of

Congenital Malformations (IMER), Italy Sicilian Registry of Congenital Malformations (ISMAC), France Strasbourg, France Central East, France Paris, Mexico Registry and Epidemiological Surveillance of External Congenital Malformations (RYVEMCE), Spanish Collaborative Study of Congenital Malformations (ECEMC), South America Latin American Collaborative Study of Congenital Malformations (ECLAMC), Czech Republic, Hungary, Israel Birth Defects Monitoring System (IBDMS), and Japan Association of Obstetricians and Gynecologists (JAOG). The clearinghouse programs

differ in their methods, so meaningful between-program comparisons are not possible. However, the clearinghouse data do allow for monitoring of temporal trends within each program.

In 1998, the prevalence rate for cleft lip with or without cleft palate varied from 4 to 17 cases per 10,000 live births and stillbirths among the 25 reporting systems (Fig. 11.2). Between 1974 and 1998, the prevalence of cleft lip with or without cleft palate showed a consistent decline in six systems (USA Atlanta, New Zealand, England and Wales, North Netherlands, Italy

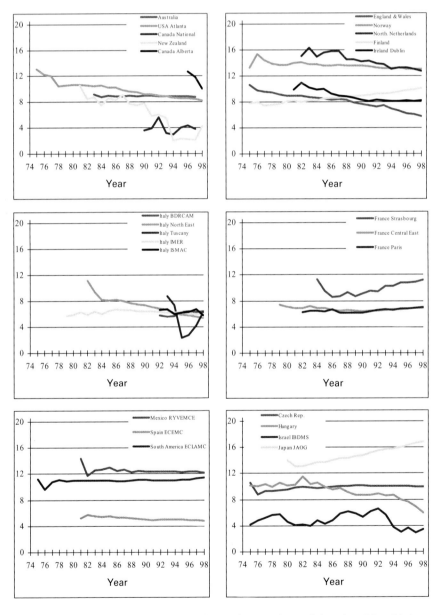

FIG. 11.2. Time trends in prevalence of cleft lip with or without cleft palate [(live births + stillbirths)/10,000] in programs participating in the International Clearinghouse for Birth Defects Monitoring Systems 1974–1998. (From International Clearinghouse for Birth Defects Monitoring Systems, 2000, with permission.)

Northeast, and Hungary), a consistent increase in three systems (Finland, France Strasbourg, and Japan JAOG), and no consistent change for the rest.

In 1998, the prevalence rate for cleft palate without cleft lip varied from 3 to 15 cases per 10,000 live births and stillbirths among the 25 reporting systems (Fig. 11.3). Between 1974 and 1998, the prevalence for cleft palate without cleft lip showed a consistent decline in six systems (USA Atlanta, England and Wales, North Netherlands, Italy Northeast, France Strasbourg, and Japan JAOG), a consistent increase in five systems

(Australia, Finland, Norway, France Central East, and France Paris), and no appreciable change for the rest.

Within each ICBDMS surveillance system, the prevalence of cleft lip with or without palate tended to be higher than that for cleft palate without cleft lip, consistent with data from state surveillance systems in the United States. Temporal trends for both subgroups of oral clefts showed no consistent patterns. The reasons for these temporal trends are unclear. Possibilities include changes in methods or changes in risk factors in the population over time. Without additional informa-

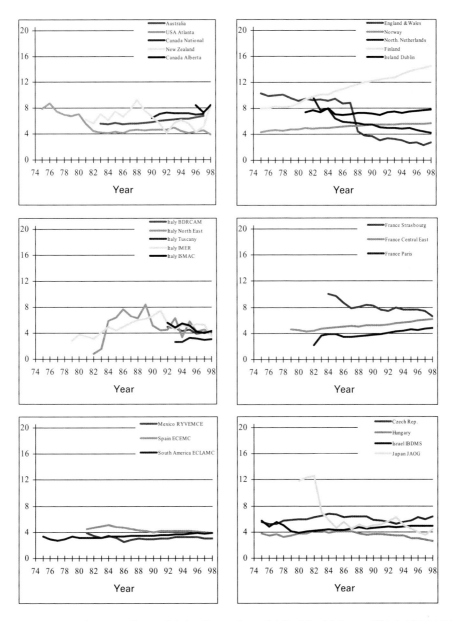

FIG. 11.3. Time trends in prevalence of cleft palate without cleft lip [(live births + stillbirths)/10,000] in programs participating in the International Clearinghouse for Birth Defects Monitoring Systems 1974–1998. (From International Clearinghouse for Birth Defects Monitoring Systems, 2000, with permission.)

tion on possible changes in case ascertainment, methods of diagnosis, and patterns of prenatal detection and pregnancy termination, interpreting these temporal changes in prevalence of oral clefts is difficult.

Source of Cases for Etiologic and Follow-Up Studies

In addition to monitoring trends in prevalence, population-based surveillance programs have become an important source of cases for etiologic studies. Cases of oral clefts ascertained by population-based surveillance programs have been included in case-control studies of a wide range of risk factors (see Chapters 13 and 14). Examples of such etiologic studies include studies of cigarette smoking (Khoury et al., 1989; Lieff et al., 1999; Kallen, 1997), alcohol consumption (Shaw and Lammer, 1999), corticosteroid use (Rodriguez-Pinilla and Martinez-Frias, 1998; Carmichael and Shaw, 1999), occupational factors (Bianchi et al., 1997; Lorente et al., 2000), use of multivitamins and folic acid (Shaw et al., 1995; Czeizel et al., 1999), and interactions between genetic factors and cigarette smoking (Hwang et al., 1995; Beaty et al., 1997). Currently, eight population-based birth defects surveillance programs in the United States serve as sources of cases for the National Birth Defects Prevention Study, a multicenter case-control study of birth defects that is evaluating the role of genetic and environmental factors and gene–environment interactions in the risk of oral clefts.

Children with oral clefts are at increased risk for several disorders that can impair normal development, including dental problems (Ranta, 1986; Bokhout et al., 1997), hearing disorders (Koempel and Kumar, 1997), speech and hearing problems (Broen et al., 1998), and cognitive and psychomotor deficits (Speltz et al., 2000; Kapp-Simon and Krueckeberg, 2000). Much of this knowledge has been derived from studies of children with oral clefts referred to evaluation or treatment facilities. Studies of children referred for treatment may select for the more severe surviving cleft cases or for the group of cases in the segment of the population served by the treating facility (Oka, 1979). Consequently, such a select group of cases may not reflect the wide spectrum of oral clefts in the population and may result in biased assessment of the natural history, morbidity, and developmental deficits associated with oral clefts.

CONCLUDING REMARKS

Many genetic and epidemiologic studies have focused on oral clefts, resulting in increased knowledge about the different types of oral cleft and their differences in genetic and epidemiologic characteristics. However, meaningful characterization of the spatial variation of the prevalence of oral clefts through comparisons of rates across regions, a basic goal of descriptive epidemiology and a useful source of etiologic hypotheses, has not been possible because of differences in methods between surveillance systems. One approach to address this issue is to compare prevalence rates among surveillance programs that use similar methods. With the continued development of birth defects surveillance systems in the United States and efforts to standardize the methods used, analyses of spatial variations will be more feasible.

In recent years, use of sophisticated diagnostic procedures to detect and diagnose birth defects in utero has increased, resulting in a corresponding increase in elective terminations of affected pregnancies. Such practices can result in underestimation of the prevalence of birth defects at birth. A recent study in Hawaii (Forrester et al., 1998) found that the proportion of oral cleft cases diagnosed prenatally was 14% for cleft lip with or without cleft palate and 0% for cleft palate without cleft lip and that the resulting underestimation of the prevalence rates was not substantial. Whether this limited impact of prenatal diagnosis on the prevalence of oral clefts at birth is similar for other geographic areas and likely to remain in future years is unclear. Further monitoring of the impact of prenatal diagnoses on the prevalence of oral clefts at birth may become increasingly important, particularly in interpreting temporal trends in relation to changes in risk or preventive factors in the population.

Oral clefts represent a heterogeneous group of defects, including cleft lip only, cleft lip and palate, and cleft palate only. Cleft lip with or without palate and cleft palate without cleft lip are different entities that can occur as isolated defects, as part of a sequence of primary defects, or as a multiple congenital anomaly (Fogh-Andersen, 1942; Lettieri, 1993). In addition, oral clefts can be part of a known monogenetic syndrome, part of a chromosomal aberration, part of an association, or part of a complex of multiple defects of unknown etiology (Cohen, 1991). Because these different types of oral cleft may have different etiologies, surveillance systems may need to invest more resources in classifying infants with oral clefts into subgroups to account for such heterogeneity in descriptive and risk factor studies.

Because the causes of oral clefts remain unknown, population-based surveillance systems will continue to serve as sources of cases for studies of etiologic hypotheses. Such studies will be instrumental in identifying primary prevention strategies for population-based interventions for oral clefts, as was done for neural tube defects with folic acid interventions. If and when such interventions become available, surveillance systems for birth defects are likely to play a key role in the evaluation of their effectiveness. In addition, population-based surveillance systems of birth defects are likely to play an important role in population-based studies of the long-term effects of oral clefts on children's health and development and of prognostic and risk factors for developmental delays and morbidity associated with oral clefts. These efforts may ultimately help to further control and prevent the morbidity associated with oral clefts and thereby to improve the quality of life of affected children and their families.

The authors thank the International Clearinghouse of Birth Defects for permission to print the figures on temporal trends for oral clefts, and Ms. Cara Mai for valuable technical assistance with formatting of the illustrations.

REFERENCES

Åbyholm, FE (1978). Cleft lip and palate in Norway: II. A numerical study of 1555 CLP-patients admitted for surgical treatment 1954–75. Scand Plast Reconstr Surg *12:* 35–43.

Amidei, RL, Hamman, RF, Kassebaum, DK, Marshall, JA (1994). Birth prevalence of cleft lip and palate in Colorado by sex distribution, seasonality, race/ethnicity, and geographic variation. Special Care Dent *14:* 233–240.

Beaty, TH, Maestri, NE, Hetmanski, JB, et al. (1997). Testing for interaction between maternal smoking and *TGFA* genotype among oral cleft cases born in Maryland 1992–1996. Cleft Palate Craniofac J *34:* 447–454.

Bianchi, F, Cianciulli, D, Pierini, A, Seniori Constantini, A (1997). Congenital malformations and maternal occupation: a registry-based study. Occup Environ Med *54:* 223–228.

Bokhout, B, Hofman, FX, van Limbeck, J, et al. (1997). Incidence of dental caries in the primary dentition in children with a cleft lip and/or palate. Caries Res *31:* 8–12.

British Paediatric Association (1979). British Paediatric Association Classification of Diseases: Codes Designed for Use in the Classification of Paediatric and Perinatal Disorders. London: British Paediatric Association, vol. 2.

Broen, PA, Devers, MC, Doyle, SS, et al. (1998). Acquisition of linguistic and cognitive skills by children with cleft palate. J Speech Lang Hear Res *41:* 676–687.

Carmichael, SL, Shaw, GM (1999). Maternal corticosteroid use and risk of selected congenital anomalies. Am J Med Genet *86:* 242–244.

Centers for Disease Control and Prevention (2000). State birth defects surveillance programs directory. Teratology *61:* 33–85.

Cohen, MM (1991). Syndrome delineation involving orofacial clefting. Cleft Palate J *28:* 119–120.

Croen, LA, Shaw, GM, Wasserman, CR, Tolarova, MM (1998). Racial and ethnic variations in the prevalence of orofacial clefts in California, 1983–1992. Am J Med Genet *79:* 42–47.

Czeizel, AE, Timar, L, Sakozi, A (1999). Dose-dependent effect of folic acid on the prevention of orofacial clefts. Pediatrics *104:* e66.

Edmonds, LD (1997). Birth defects surveillance data from selected states. Teratology *56:* 115–175.

Emanuel, I, Culver, BH, Erickson, JD, et al. (1973). The further epidemiological differentiation of cleft lip and palate: a population study of clefts in King County, Washington, 1956–1965. Teratology *7:* 271–282.

Fogh-Andersen, P (1942). *Inheritance of Harelip and Cleft Palate.* Copenhagen: Arnold Busck.

Forrester, MB, Mertz, RD, Yoon, PW (1998). Impact of prenatal diagnosis and elective termination on the prevalence of selected birth defects in Hawaii. Am J Epidemiol *148:* 1206–1211.

Green, HG, Nelson, CJ, Gaylor, DW, Holson, JF (1979). Accuracy of birth certificate data for detecting facial clefts in Arkansas children. Cleft Palate J *16:* 167–170.

Hwang, SH, Beaty, TH, Panny, SR, et al. (1995). Association study of transforming growth factors alpha (TGFα) Taq1 polymorphism and oral clefts: indication of gene–environment interaction in a population-based sample of infants with birth defects. Am J Epidemiol *141:* 629–636.

International Clearinghouse for Birth Defects Monitoring Systems (2000). *Annual Report 2000.* Rome: International Centre for Birth Defects, pp. 115–116.

Ivy, RH (1957). Congenital anomalies. As recorded on birth certificates in the Division of Health Statistics of Pennsylvania Department of Health, for the period 1951–1955, inclusive. Plast Reconstr Surg *41:* 50–53.

Kallen, K (1997). Maternal smoking and orofacial clefts. Cleft Palate-Craniofacial J *34:* 11–16.

Kapp-Simon, KA, Krueckeberg, S (2000). Mental development in infants with cleft lip and/or palate. Cleft Palate Craniofac J *37:* 65–70.

Khoury, MJ, Gomez-Farias, M, Mulinare, J (1989). Does maternal cigarette smoking during pregnancy cause cleft lip and palate in offspring? Am J Dis Child *143:* 333–337.

Khoury, MJ, Holtzman, NA (1987). On the ability of birth defects monitoring to detect new teratogens. Am J Epidemiol *126:* 136–143.

Koempel, JA, Kumar, A (1997). Long-term otologic status of older cleft palate patients. Indian J Pediatr *64:* 793–800.

Lettieri, J (1993). Lips and oral cavity. In: *Human Malformations and Related Anomalies.* Vol. II. *Oxford Monographs on Medical Genetics 27,* edited by RE Stevenson, JG Hall, and RM Goodman. New York: Oxford University Press, pp. 367–380.

Lieff, S, Olshan, AF, Werler, M, et al. (1999). Maternal cigarette smoking during pregnancy and risk of oral clefts in newborns. Am J Epidemiol *150:* 683–694.

Lorente, C, Cordier, S, Bergeret, A, et al. (2000). maternal occupational risk factors for oral clefts. Occupational Exposure and Congenital Malformation Working Group. Scand J Work Environ Health *26:* 137–145.

Meskin, LH, Pruzanski, S (1967). Validity of the birth certificate in the epidemiologic assessment of facial clefts. J Dent Res *46:* 1456–1459.

National Birth Defect Prevention Network (2000). Congenital malformations surveillance report. Teratology *61:* 87–158.

Oka, SW (1979). Epidemiology and genetics of clefting: with implications for etiology. In: *Cleft Palate and Cleft Lip: A Team Approach to Clinical Management and Rehabilitation of the Patient,* edited by HK Cooper, RL Harding, WM Krogman, et al. Philadelphia: WB Saunders, pp. 108–143.

Ranta, R (1986). A review of tooth formation in children with cleft lip/palate. Am J Orthod Denofacial Orthop *90:* 11–18.

Robert, E, Kallen, B, Harris, J (1996). The epidemiology of orofacial clefts. 1. Some general epidemiological characteristics. J Craniofac Genet Dev Biol *16:* 2343–241.

Rodriguez-Pinilla, E, Martinez-Fria, SML (1998). Corticosteroids during pregnancy and oral clefts: a case-control study. Teratology 58: 2–5.

Shaw, GM, Lammer, EJ (1999). Maternal periconceptional alcohol consumption and risk for orofacial clefts. J Pediatr 134: 298–303.

Shaw, GM, Lammer, EJ, Wasserman, CR, et al. (1995). Risks of orofacial clefts in children born to women using multivitamins containing folic acid periconceptionally. Lancet 346: 393–396.

Speltz, ML, Endriga, MC, Hill, S, et al. (2000). Cognitive and psychomotor development of infants with orofacial clefts. J Pediatr Psychol 25: 185–190.

Spranger, J, Benirscke, K, Hall, JG, et al. (1982). Errors of morphogenesis: concepts and terms. Recommendations of an international working group. J Pediatr 100: 160–165.

Stevenson, RE, Hall, JG (1993). Terminology. In: Human malformations and related anomalies. Vol. I. Oxford Monographs on Medical Genetics 27, edited by RE Stevenson, JG Hall, and RM Goodman. New York: Oxford University Press, pp. 21–30.

Tolarova, MM, Cervenka, J (1998). Classification and birth prevalence of orofacial clefts. Am J Med Genet 75: 126–137.

Vanderas, AP (1987). Incidence of cleft lip, cleft palate and cleft lip and palate among races: a review. Cleft Palate J 24: 216–225.

World Health Organization. (1979). International Classification of Diseases, 9th rev. Geneva: World Health Organization.

12

Epidemiology of oral clefts: an international perspective

PETER A. MOSSEY

JULIAN LITTLE

Cleft lip with or without cleft palate (CL/P) and isolated cleft palate (CP) are serious birth defects, which on a worldwide level affect approximately 1 in every 600 newborn babies. This means that assuming a global birth rate of 15,000 children per hour (United States Bureau of the Census, www.census.gov/ipc/www/ibd-new.html, 2001), a child with a cleft is born somewhere in the world every 2.5 min. From birth to maturity, children with oral clefts (OCs) undergo multidisciplinary surgical and nonsurgical treatment with considerable disruption to their lives and often adverse psychological consequences to themselves and their families.

Efforts over the years have been made to record the frequency of birth defects, and accurate data on epidemiology are important for documenting the burden in relation to the planning of public health services. They also form the basis for research into causes. The eventual objective must be, from both scientific and humanitarian viewpoints, to advance the knowledge and understanding of causative factors and to institute primary preventive measures. Among the barriers to achieving this objective are *(1)* the heterogeneity of OCs, *(2)* the lack of standard criteria for the collection of data, and *(3)* the lack of and/or failure to apply an internationally comparable OC classification.

SEARCH STRATEGY FOR IDENTIFICATION OF RELEVANT STUDIES

The search strategy began with a free text search of Medline (from 1966, www.ncbi.nlm.nih.gov/PubMed/)

and EMBASE (from 1989, www.silverplatter.com/catalog/embx.htm) and OVID (www.ovid.com/sales/medical.cfm), which incorporates Medline, BIDS and a number of university medical databases. The PubMed database was searched with the key words *cleft, lip, palate,* and *incidence,* producing 377 records ranked by date. EMBASE was searched using *cleft lip* or *cleft palate* combined with *prevalence* or *incidence,* yielding a total of 239 references. OVID was searched using *cleft lip, cleft palate,* and *incidence* or *prevalence,* producing a total of 755 references dating back to 1965. In addition, selected literature was hand-searched, including the *Cleft Palate Journal* dating back to 1960, and references were identified in earlier work on neural tube defects (Elwood et al., 1992). Where available, the following information was also noted: gender distribution, ethnic origin of the parents, and whether the figures included stillbirths and induced abortions. This hand search concentrated on reports from more obscure journals and from various parts of the world, for which the above data sets may not contain complete records. This included the Indian subcontinent, Africa, Asia, and the Middle East. In all searches, there was no restriction on language and original papers were sought. For a small percentage of the literature, only abstracts were reviewed. Bibliographies and review articles from the literature obtained in the hand search enabled identification of any missed articles. The searches are supplemented by EUROCAT (www.iph.fgov.be/eurocat/eurocat.htm) and ICBDMS (www.icbd.org) reports, in particular for examining time trends.

Among the minimum data required for eligibility were the following:

- Year of publication, reference population, and sample size
- Subdivision into cleft subgroups
- Type of pregnancy outcome included, e.g., live births, stillbirths, induced abortions

Other issues affecting comparison of studies, e.g., ascertainment methods, association of abnormalities or syndromes, family history, were noted but not used as criteria for exclusion.

METHODOLOGICAL ISSUES RELEVANT TO THE DATA PRESENTED

Descriptive Epidemiology

The completeness of ascertainment may differ between countries, depending on the number and type of sources of ascertainment, the type of pregnancy outcome (live births, terminations, stillbirths), and the recognition of syndromic individuals. These issues can considerably affect the comparability of such data (McMahon and Pugh, 1970; Leck, 1983). Epidemiological data were derived from OC registries or surgical records, which may be different from the actual number of affected OC individuals. Temporal trends in the prevalence at birth of OCs exist, which can in part be explained by the differing levels of ascertainment within countries as they develop.

Another critical requirement is that the observer defines precisely the population in which the frequency of malformation is measured. A major issue is whether one reports or estimates rates in all recognized conceptuses, all births, or all live births. The term *births* is somewhat ambiguous because it (usually) included stillbirths, which does not have a uniform definition. In summarizing the data, we have considered issues such as *(1)* live births vs. stillbirths, *(2)* associated malformations, and *(3)* particular factors contributing to the prevalence of isolated CP.

Live Births vs. Stillbirths. The proportion of serious malformations is higher in stillbirths than in live births, so the inclusion of stillbirths tends to elevate the birth prevalence or incidence rates over those derived if only live births are considered. Similarly, inclusion of data on miscarriages and abortions, i.e., losses earlier in gestation, may increase rates over those found if only live births and stillbirths are analyzed.

Vanderas (1987) examined the problem of inclusion or exclusion of stillbirths in the ascertainment of OCs in a number of international studies, some of which included live births, stillbirths, and abortions in their evaluation of prevalence at birth. The OC rates were 6.43/1000 stillbirths vs. 2.16/1000 live births in a study of the white population of Iowa (Hay, 1971). In a study on live births in the pooled data from black, Mexican, and white populations (Lutz and Moor, 1955), rates were 2.72/1000 stillbirths vs. 0.91/1000 live births. The risk of developing clefts in stillbirths and abortions appears therefore to be about three times as frequent as in live births. Also, clefts with associated malformations behaved differently epidemiologically in comparison to clefts without associated malformations.

A further study, in Hungary (Czeizel, 1984), reported that the proportion of CP without cleft lip (CL) was about sevenfold greater in stillbirths (primary fetal deaths 28 weeks or older) than in live births (2.38/1000 vs. 0.36/1000). In comparison, for CL/P, the ratio was a little less than threefold (3.17/1000 vs. 1.15/1000). As may be expected, this differential between live births and stillbirths is greater for individuals with additional malformations elsewhere than for those with only CL, CP, or both (CLP).

Krause et al. (1963), examined human embryos and fetuses and reported that the frequency of clefts with associated malformations was 11.61/1000 and that the frequency of clefts without associated malformations was 7.22/1000. Nishimura et al. (1966) reported the frequency of CL/P in 1213 voluntarily aborted human embryos to be 14.7/1000. In a separate study of 5117 voluntarily aborted human embryos, Iizuka (1973) found that the prevalence at birth of CL was 4.3/1000, that of CLP was 8.10/1000, and that of isolated CP was 3.2/1000. Thus, the lumping of figures that include not only live births but also stillbirths and/or induced abortions will not be comparable to figures for live births only. If fetal deaths or earlier losses are included in summary rates, then this should be noted specifically and rates should be presented separately for live births and for embryonic and fetal deaths.

Associated Malformations. It is generally accepted that associated malformations occur less frequently in infants who have CLP than in those who have CP and even less still in those with isolated CL. For example, a 17-year study in north-eastern France reported rates of associated malformations to be 46.7% in CP, 36.8% in CLP, and 13.6% in CL (Kallen et al., 1996). Cornel et al. (1992) reported associated abnormalities in 23% of CL/P cases and in 52% of cases with isolated CP. Numerous other studies also found congenital anomalies to be much more commonly associated with CP than with CL/P (Ingalls et al., 1964; Drillien et al., 1966; Moller, 1972; Emanuel et al., 1973). In the Finnish population, however, CL/P was as often associated with other malformations as was CP (Saxen and Lath, 1974). Familial background was also more often reported in association with CP than with CL/P in Finland, which contrasts with the findings of others, e.g., Fogh-Andersen (1942) in Denmark.

Some studies also subdivide CL/P into unilateral and bilateral groups when examining additional malformations and report an increase in additional malformations in the bilateral subgroup (Hagberg et al., 1997). Some reports do not define what is meant by *associated abnormalities,* while others give ambiguous descriptions. Conway and Wagner (1966) recorded only the "ten most common" associated abnormalities listed on birth certificates over an 11-year period. This may explain some of the variation observed in the reporting of the frequency of other abnormalities accompanying OCs (see tables in Appendix I).

Prevalence of Isolated Cleft Palate. There is considerable heterogeneity in what is described as isolated CP. Many figures for isolated CP are provided without an adequate explanation of inclusion/exclusion criteria. For instance, the most common syndrome with isolated CP as a feature is the Pierre Robin syndrome, and inclusion or exclusion may make a substantial difference to the figures. This subgroup is also more susceptible to ascertainment bias as the prevalence of submucous clefting within the general population is thought to be as common as overt isolated CP. In a detailed study of isolated CP in Denmark, Christensen and Fogh-Andersen (1994) noted a marked difference in sex ratios for nonsyndromic overt CP including the hard palate and non-syndromic overt CP of the soft palate only. This, combined with the tendency for hard palate and soft palate clefts not to occur within the same families indicates that they may be two etiologically distinct subgroups of CP. Therefore, the authors recommended that future studies on isolated CP distinguish between hard palate, soft palate, and submucous hard palate in an attempt to disclose etiological heterogeneity within secondary palatal clefting.

Inclusion of the Robin sequence is also complicated by the fact that its etiology is heterogeneous and its diagnosis inconsistent. Some authorities state that respiratory distress is an essential part of the anomaly (Shprintzen and Singer, 1992), while others make a diagnosis on the basis of glossoptosis and micrognathia with the cleft, whether or not there is respiratory distress (Caouette-Laberge et al., 1994). The Pierre Robin anomaly also occurs in association with other monogenic disorders, e.g., Stickler's syndrome.

Further complications in the consideration of isolated CP are two recognized genetic phenomena: *(1)* the association of CP with 22q11.2 deletion in the velocardiofacial syndrome and *(2)* X-linked clefting. The prevalence at birth of velocardiofacial syndrome in many populations is unknown, and diagnosis may be delayed, thus affecting the birth prevalence figures. X-linked clefting has been reported in some populations, e.g., the Icelandic population (Moore et al., 1987), but has not been investigated in many others. Also, Lowry and Renwick (1969) reported X-linked submucous CP as part of an X-linked recessive trait, which might complicate the picture regarding CP birth prevalence and sex ratio figures.

GEOGRAPHICAL VARIATION IN THE EPIDEMIOLOGY OF ORAL CLEFTS

Epidemiological data for OCs from the three different sources outlined above are presented as follows:

- Peer-reviewed publications, Table 12.1 (complete data shown in Appendix 12.I)
- Data from the European Registry of Congenital Anomalies and Twins (EUROCAT) registration system, Appendix 12.II
- Data collected through the National Birth Defects Prevention Network (NBDPN) in the United States, Appendix 12.III
- A series of maps (Figs. 12.1–12.6) are included to illustrate some of the birth prevalence data for isolated CP and cleft lip and palate (CL/P). The data used for the maps were taken from individual reports or from registries that are mentioned in the text of the chapter (Appendix 12.I).
- There is insufficient detail in the maps (Figs. 12.1–12.6) to reflect regional differences within countries. These maps are intended merely to illustrate general trends in the population distribution of CP and CL/P. They also indicate that there is a dearth of published information available for some countries and geographical areas of the world.

The commentary relates mainly to the peer-reviewed literature, with occasional reference to the other registration systems, and deals with CL/P and CP separately.

Prevalence of Cleft Lip with or without Cleft Palate

United States and Canada. One of the fundamental differences between the OC epidemiology data in Europe and North America is the ethnic heterogeneity that characterizes most of the North American population. It was therefore important to examine the North American data in the light of ethnic origin. The highest prevalence of CL/P was found in British Columbia among Native Americans, 2.73/1000 live births (Lowry and Renwick, 1969). The next highest, 1.99/1000 births, is

TABLE 12.1A. *Extremes of Cleft Lip with or without Cleft Palate Prevalence: Highest and Lowest Figures*

Continent/Country	Total Births	Prevalence (per 1000 births)	Reference
Europe			
N. Netherlands	60,584	1.46	Cornel et al. (1992)
France (Rhone-Alpes-Auvergne)	813,513	0.67	Long et al. (1992)
United States and Canada			
USA California	13,545	1.99	Croen et al. (1998)
USA New York (*Native American*)	344,929	0.29	Conway and Wagner (1966)
Central and South America			
Bolivia	79,296	2.28	Castilla et al. (1999)
Caribbean (Santo Domingo)	704,410	0.42	Garcia-Godoy (1980)
Oceania			
Australia (*Aborigines*)	9,695	2.27	Bower et al. (1989)
New Zealand (*Maoris*)	178,240	0.39	Chapman (1983)
Far East			
Japan (Hiroshima, Nagasaki)	63,806	2.13	Neel (1958)
Japan	55,103	0.97	Kondo (1987)
Middle East			
Saudi Arabia	62,557	1.89	Borkar et al. (1993)
Israel (*Jews*)	47,768	0.37	Azaz and Koyoumdjisky-Kaye (1967)
Indian Subcontinent			
India (Maharashtra)	3014	2.32	Chaturvedi and Banerjee (1989)
India (Madurai)	11,619	0.77	Kamala et al. (1978)
Africa			
Kenya (Nairobi)	3061	1.63	Khan (1965)
South Africa (Johannesburg, *blacks*)	29,633	0.20	Kromberg and Jenkins (1982)

TABLE 12.1B. *Extremes of Cleft Palate Prevalence: Highest and Lowest Figures*

Continent/Country	Total Births	Prevalence	Reference
Europe			
Finland	2,258,850	0.97	Rintala (1986)
Denmark	1,631,376	0.36	Fogh-Andersen (1961)
United States and Canada			
USA Native Americans	13,545	1.11	Croen et al. (1998)
New York (*nonwhite*)	344,929	0.22	Conway and Wagner (1966)
Central and South America			
Chile	297,583	0.46	Castilla et al. (1999)
Peru	72,864	0.06	Castilla et al. (1999)
Oceania			
Australia (*Whites*)	170,760	0.67	Bower et al. (1989)
New Zealand (*Maoris*)	178,240	0.39	Chapman (1983)
Far East			
Japan (Tokyo)	49,645	0.73	Mitani (1954)
China	1,243,284	0.15	Xiao (1989)
Middle East			
Kuwait	53,786	0.42	Srivastava and Bang (1990)
Israel (*Jews*)	47,768	0.17	Azaz and Koyoumdjisky-Kaye (1967)
Indian Subcontinent			
Kanpur	4150	0.48	Mital and Grewal (1969)
New Delhi	7590	0.32	Singh and Sharma (1980)
Africa			
Tunisia	10,000	0.40	Khrouf et al. (1986)
Zaire	56,637	0.02	Ogle (1993)

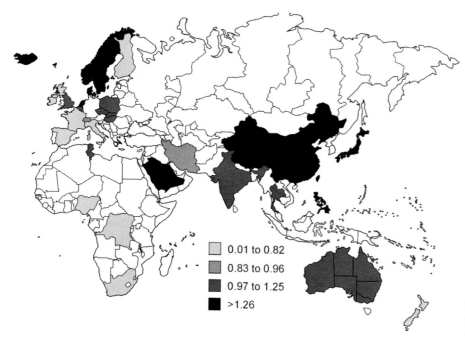

FIG. 12.1. Distribution of cleft lip with or without cleft palate for Europe, Africa, Asia, and Australia.

from the Californian registry in the period 1983–1992 (Croen et al., 1998), representing Native Americans only. The lowest figures are from nonwhite populations in New York [0.29 reported by Conway and Wagner (1966)] and Mississippi [0.30 as reported by Das et al. (1995)].

The NBDPN examined OC prevalence by U.S. state. The highest recorded is for New Mexico at 1.73/1000 live births in the 1995–1996 cohort, which included stillbirths as well as live births and is a relatively small

sample. In Wisconsin 1989–1995, prevalence was 1.56/1000 with live births and stillbirths combined. The lowest recorded prevalence rate for CL/P was 0.59 in Alaska and Illinois; the Alaskan sample was for 1996 only, while the Illinois sample was a 7-year sample (1989–1996) and included stillbirths.

Central and South America. Most of the registers in South America report through the Latin American Collaborative Study of Congenital Malformations

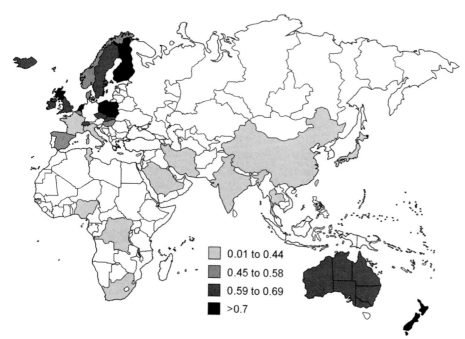

FIG. 12.2. Distribution of cleft palate for Europe, Africa, Asia, and Australia.

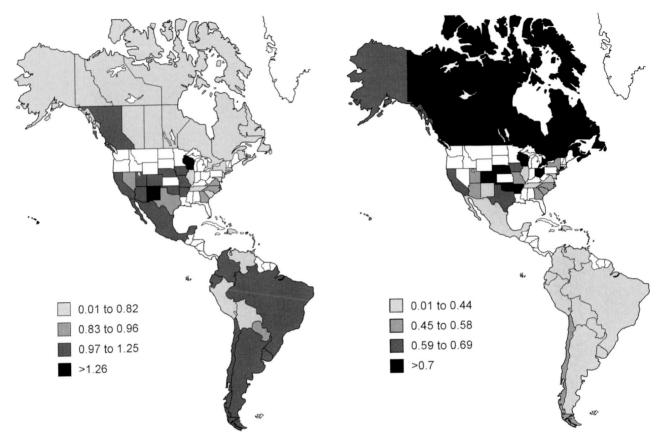

0.01 to 0.82
0.83 to 0.96
0.97 to 1.25
>1.26

0.01 to 0.44
0.45 to 0.58
0.59 to 0.69
>0.7

FIG. 12.3. Distribution of cleft lip with or without cleft palate for North and South America.

FIG. 12.4. Distribution of cleft palate for North and South America.

(ECLAMC; Appendix I, Table 12.IC), and the OC figures include associated abnormalities. The highest CL/P prevalence figure is from Bolivia (2.28/1000), with Argentina (1.16/1000) and Chile (1.13/1000) next. These are geographically in the southern, and generally less developed, parts of South America. At the lowest end of the scale is the geographically and genetically different population in Central America and the Caribbean, with Das et al. (1995) reporting a prevalence of 0.42/1000, the next lowest rate is for Venezuela (on the northern coast), with a prevalence of 0.77/1000.

Australia and New Zealand. The figures for Australia and New Zealand recognize the different ethnic origins of the indigenous people of these islands and the settlers. Prevalence figures range from remarkable extremes for nonsyndromic clefts of 2.27 in Aborigines in a study between 1980 and 1987 (Bower et al., 1989) to the lowest recorded figure outside of Africa of 0.39 in New Zealand Maoris between 1960 and 1976. In

the same study, New Zealand whites occupied an intermediate position (1.19) (Chapman, 1983).

Europe. The highest birth prevalence of CL/P from all European countries was 1.46 (Cornel et al., 1992). Overall, the areas of highest prevalence within Europe are Norway, Denmark, Sweden, Iceland, and the northern Netherlands. Intermediate levels occur in Central Europe, and the lowest are in southern Europe. In the British Isles, the frequency varies between 0.6 and 1.04, which is nearer to the southern European figures.

Middle East. In the Middle East, the highest record for CL/P prevalence is 1.89/1000 in a Saudi Arabian hospital-based study (Borkar et al., 1993). The next highest is considerably lower (1.06/1000 live births) for nonsyndromic OCs, reported in Kuwait between 1985 and 1987 (Srivastava and Bang, 1990). Taher (1992) reported what he regarded as a cluster in one hospital in Tehran with a prevalence of 3.12/1000. Chemical

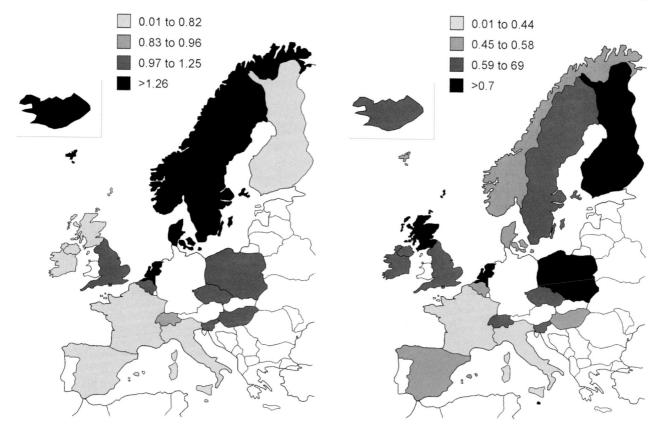

FIG. 12.5. Distribution of cleft lip with or without cleft palate for Europe.

FIG. 12.6. Distribution of cleft palate for Europe.

sulfur mustard gas was implicated in the etiology during this 4-year period, 1983–1988. The lowest prevalence (0.37/1000 live births) was recorded by Azaz and Koyoumdjisky-Kaye (1967) in a hospital-based study of Israeli Jews between 1960 and 1962. The next lowest recorded prevalence was 0.85/1000 live births in Iran (Rajabian and Sherkat, 2000).

Far East. Data on CL/P prevalence from the Far East are often quoted as single figures with all clefts combined rather than separate figures for CP and CL/P. The highest rate reported is from Japanese data, a hospital-based sample in Hiroshima between 1948 and 1954, revealing a prevalence of 2.13/1000 live births (Neel, 1958). In the Philippines, Murray et al. (1997) reported a prevalence of 1.94/1000 live births in a 7-year survey of hospital records between 1989 and 1996, with this figure including syndromic clefts (21%). The lowest quoted figure is also from a hospital-based study

of live births in Japan between 1979 and 1982 (Kondo, 1987), 0.97/1000; the next lowest was reported by Natsume et al. (1987), 1.02/1000 live births, in Haichi, Japan. These studies are not strictly comparable because of differences in ascertainment criteria; they also reveal the difficulty of comparing hospital- vs. population-based studies.

Indian Subcontinent. On the Indian subcontinent, highest CL/P prevalences were recorded in Maharashtra (2.32/1000) in a hospital-based study that included live births and stillbirths (Chaturvedi and Banerjee, 1989). This is followed by a rate of 1.61/1000 in Calcutta in a 29-month hospital-based study (Nair and Mathai, 1964). The lowest prevalences were seen in Madurai (0.77/1000 live births) in a hospital-based study (Kamala et al., 1978) and in a small 2-year hospital-based study in New Delhi (0.41/1000 live births) (Kulshrestha et al., 1983).

Africa. In Africa, the highest figure of 1.63 comes from a relatively small 6-month hospital-based study in Nairobi reported by Khan (1965), which is out of step with other African studies; selection bias is suspected. The next highest rate is from Tunisia in northern Africa, where live births and stillbirths were recorded in a 9-month study, with a prevalence of 1/1000 births (Khrouf et al., 1986). Many of the studies reveal figures less than half of that; e.g., the next highest is from Nigeria (0.47/1000) (Gupta, 1969) and the lowest (0.2, 0.21, and 0.3/1000 live births) were recorded in hospital-based studies in Johannesburg (Kromberg and Jenkins, 1982) and Nigeria (Iregbulem, 1982; Ogle, 1993). All three of these were small studies that may be suspected of underascertainment.

Prevalence of Isolated Cleft Palate

United States and Canada. In North America, the highest reported prevalence for CP is 1.11 for Native Americans in the Californian registry between 1983 and 1992 (Croen et al., 1998). This is followed closely by the East Indian ethnic subgroup in California in the same study (1.06/1000). The lowest figures reported are 0.22 for nonwhites in New York City (Conway and Wagner, 1966) and 0.24/1000 for nonwhites in Mississippi in 1980–1989 (Das et al., 1995). In the NBDPN, which compared the frequency of clefts in various states, the highest reports come from Wisconsin (1.45) and Connecticut (0.95), with the lowest in New Mexico (0.18) and Tennessee (0.29).

Central and South America. The prevalence of CP in South America shows remarkably little variation, with eight out of the 10 South American countries contributing to the ECLAMC Registry; prevalence rates are between 0.2 and 0.4/1000 births. The lowest is 0.06/1000 in Peru, while the highest prevalence was recorded in Chile, 0.46/1000. The figures from Central America for prevalence of isolated CP were 0.2/1000 in a hospital-based study in the Caribbean (Garcia-Godoy, 1980) and 0.27/1000 in a hospital-based register in Mexico (Perez-Molina et al., 1993).

Australia and New Zealand. In Oceania, a remarkably high figure for isolated CP was reported for the Maoris in New Zealand, with a prevalence of 1.87/1000 between 1960 and 1976 (Chapman, 1983); figures of 0.64 and 0.67 were reported for whites in New Zealand (Chapman, 1983) and Australia (Bower et al., 1989), respectively.

Europe. The prevalence of isolated CP is highest in Finland, with a rate of 0.97/1000 from in a study be-

tween 1948 and 1975 (Rintala, 1986); in a later study, between 1974 and 1988, Tolarova and Cervenka (1995) reported a birth prevalence of 1.01. The next highest rate in Europe was reported by Womersley and Stone (1987) in the west of Scotland, 0.81, between 1974 and 1985. The lowest reported European figures come from Denmark (0.36/1000) in a study between 1938 and 1957 (Fogh-Andersen, 1961) and central and eastern France (0.42/1000) (Kallen et al., 1996). In the EUROCAT regional registry (which does not include Finland), the highest figure is from Glasgow (western Scotland) (0.94) and the lowest (0.25/1000) is from Northern Ireland in the same time period (1990 and 1994). In general, the figures from Europe are characterized by significant variation, not only between countries but also within. For instance, the Paris registry reveals a relatively low frequency of CP (0.47/1000), while the figure for Strasbourg is 0.88/1000 (ICBDMS, 2000).

Middle East. From the relatively few studies from the Middle East, the extremes in CP birth prevalence range from a low of 0.17/1000 in a hospital-based study of Israeli Jews (Azaz and Koyoumdjisky-Kaye, 1967) to a high of 0.42/1000 for nonsyndromic clefts (Srivastava and Bang, 1990) in a population-based study in Kuwait. Taher (1992) reported what he regarded as a cluster in one hospital in Tehran with a birth prevalence of 0.62/1000 for CP (and a remarkably high figure of 3.12/1000 for CL/P). Chemical sulfur mustard gas was implicated in the etiology during this 4-year period (1983–1988).

Far East. The highest recorded figure for isolated CP comes from an 18-year hospital-based study in Tokyo, in which Mitani (1954) reported 0.73/1000 births. The lowest figure, 0.15/1000 live births, was recorded by Xiao (1989) in a large cross-sectional study of 945 hospitals in China in a 12-month period between October 1986 and September 1987. The next lowest figure comes from a report by Emanuel et al. (1972), who recorded a figure of 0.16/1000 in a hospital-based study in Taipei (Taiwan).

Indian Subcontinent. Much of the data from India come from relatively small local hospital-based studies recording the prevalence of birth defects including OCs. While the majority of these studies record figures for CL/P, many do no record isolated CP. Of those that do, the lowest figure, 0.32/1000, comes from a study by Singh and Sharma (1980) in New Delhi. The highest figure, 0.48/1000, comes from a small study in Kanpur by Mital and Grewal (1969). While a meta-analysis was carried out by Verma and Mathews (1983), this was methodologically flawed and included various prospective and retrospective studies of live births and stillbirths throughout India. However, the figures of 1.20/1000 for CL/P and 0.44/1000 for CP appear to be the best available estimates for OC prevalence in the Indian subcontinent.

Africa. The lowest recorded birth prevalence for OC comes from Africa, and the lowest rate of any study in the world is that from the hospital live births series reported by Ogle (1993) between October 1977 and June 1979 in a hospital-based study in Nigeria. The prevalence at birth was 0.02/1000 in a study of over 56,000 live births. The next lowest, 0.07/1000, was recorded by Iregbulem (1982) in another hospital series, in Enugu, Nigeria. The highest prevalence rates come from Tunisia on the north coast, where Khrouf et al. (1986) recorded 0.4/1000 in a hospital-based study that included the recording of abnormalities in stillbirths. The next highest, 0.33/1000, comes from a hospital-based study in Nairobi reported by Khan (1965).

DISCUSSION

Ethnic Origin, Migration, and Population Admixture Studies

While only a few studies have been carried out in Africa to examine cleft prevalence, they suggest a low prevalence of both CP and CL/P. African-Americans have lower rates for both CP and CLP than whites in the United States, and a study in Birmingham (UK) showed that those originating from the Caribbean have low OC rates (Leck and Lancashire, 1995) (Table 12.2). Studies from Asia reveal high rates of CL/P but not CP in mainly hospital-based series, and similarly higher rates on the Indian subcontinent. Studies in North America also reveal high rates of CL/P in persons of Japanese or Chinese origin (Croen et al., 1998; Tolarova and Cervenka, 1998).

Ching and Chung (1974) have shown that the racial differences in CL/P birth prevalence are likely to have a genetic basis. In an extensive study from Hawaii, they showed that Japanese immigrants continue to have increased birth prevalence of CL/P and, by studying interracial crosses, that Caucasian–Japanese matings have intermediate birth prevalence, suggesting that the racial differences are independent of environment. Support for this theory is provided by Leck (1972), who showed that the variation in the birth prevalence of CL/P between different ethnic groups living in the same areas is eight times greater that that among geographically scattered populations of the same ethnic origin.

Among Filipinos, prevalence data for CL/P revealed a difference by country, with the highest prevalence observed in the Philippines, an intermediate prevalence in Hawaii, and the lowest prevalence in California (Croen et al., 1998). Such variations in cleft prevalence according to maternal country of birth may reflect changes in nongenetic risk factors, such as maternal diet, that may occur following migration. Variations in prevalence may also be related to racial and ethnic differences in nongenetic factors associated with clefting risk, and this assists with the formulation of future hypotheses in OC research.

In the United States, Croen et al. (1998) recognized that the considerable population admixture requires investigation of variation of OC prevalence according to parental race, ethnicity, and maternal country of birth. This issue is particularly relevant in OC with the known ethnic variations; it is therefore important to pursue clues as to the relative contribution of genetics and environmental factors to the etiology. Croen and colleagues (1998) subdivided patients in the Californian birth defects monitoring program into 13 ethnic subsets. They also recorded OC risk according to whether mother and father were of the same race or ethnicity.

A further study in the United States examined rates of CL/P by state (Table 12.3) and Hispanic ethnicity by subdividing the data into three subgroups: Hispanics, non-Hispanic whites, and non-Hispanic blacks (Kirby et al., 2000). They concluded that CL/P prevalence was greatest among whites (1.03/1000) and lowest among blacks (0.54/1000), with Hispanics having an intermediate prevalence (0.97/1000).

Relative Proportions of Different Cleft Types

When considering OC frequency, the proportion of different types of cleft has important implications for the clinical workload but is also of interest in providing clues about the underlying etiology. The relative pro-

TABLE 12.2. *Prevalence at Birth of Oral Clefts by Ethnic Group of Parents (Birmingham 1960–1984)*

Ethnic Group	Prevalence at birth (per 10,000)	
	Cleft Lip with or without Cleft Palate	Cleft Palate
Both parents originating from		
Europe	10.9	6.6
Indian subcontinent	12.1	7.4
Caribbean	5.2*	2.2*
Mother European, father Caribbean	1.5†	6.1
Mother Caribbean, father European	0.0	0.0

*p < 0.05.
†p < 0.01.

TABLE 12.3. *Number and Rates of Cleft Lip with or without Cleft Palate by State and Hispanic Ethnicity (USA National Center for Health Services 1993–1995)*

	Hispanic all			Non-Hispanic white			Non-Hispanic black		
	Cases	Rate*	95% CI	Cases	Rate*	95% CI	Cases	Rate*	95% CI
Arizona	78	13.5	10.7–16.9	126	10.8	9.1–13.0	7	9.4	4.1–20.3
California	564	10.4	9.5–11.3	217	10.0	8.8–11.5	5 2	7.8	5.9–10.3
Colorado	48	14.8	11.–19.8	136	11.7	9.9–13.9	3	3.7	1.0–11.9
New Jersey	8	4.3	1.9–8.5	40	6.1	4.4–8.4	7	3.7	1.6–7.9
New York	91	5.8	4.7–7.1	367	10.9	9.9–12.1	63	4.3	3.4–5.6
Texas	52	8.6	6.5–11.3	26	7.6	5.1–11.4	8	5. 9	2.7–12.1
Totals	841	9.7	9.0–10.3	912	10.3	9.7–11.0	140	5.4	4.5–6.4

*Rate is quoted per 10,000 births. 95% CI, confidence interval.
Source: Kirby et al. (2000).

portions of syndromic clefts and associated abnormalities are also important in determining etiological factors. European and U.S. studies on nonsyndromic cleft prevalence in general suggest that unilateral CLP is the most frequent single type of cleft, accounting for about 30% to 35% of cases. Isolated CL and CP each account for between 20% to 25%, and bilateral CLP is the most rare (about 10%), with submucous and other clefts accounting for the rest (Hagberg et al., 1997).

Furthermore, of all CLP cases, 80% are unilateral and 20% are bilateral. Overall, 15% of all OCs are syndromic (12% of CL/P and 25% of CP). Over 300 syndromes are recognized (involving the oral, cardiac, skeletal, and other body areas), and of the remaining 85% of OC individuals, 50% have other less well-defined anomalies (OMIM, 2000; www3.ncbi.nlm.nih.gov/omim/).

Fogh-Andersen (1942), using data from Denmark, reported a CL:CLP:CP ratio of 1:2:1, which is often quoted as the normal ratio for the different types of cleft, especially for European or Caucasian populations. This has on occasion been used as a guide [e.g., Woolf et al. (1963), who felt that, because of underascertainment of isolated CP in their hospital-based sample in Utah, the figure should be adjusted in line with this ratio]. It may, however, be erroneous to assume this as a universal figure, as other studies indicate. A number of Japanese studies (Natsume and Kawai, 1986; Natsume et al., 1987) reveal a much lower prevalence at birth of CP, with a CL:CP ratio of 8:3. Similarly, in Africa, CP is a much lower proportion of the overall prevalence at birth of clefting, being 4% in a newborn Zairian sample (Ogle, 1993) and 19% in a large Nigerian study (Iregbulem, 1982). In the latter study, CL was much more common than CLP, the ratios being 49% for CL, 32% for CLP, and 19% for CP.

Closer inspection of the figures in studies that provide a breakdown of clefts into different subgroups is interesting. Table 12.4 was compiled from a selection of studies that provide this information and presents in particular the relative frequency of CL and CLP, as well as the overall prevalence of CL/P. The general trend is that in those regions of the world where cleft prevalence is highest, the ratio of CLP to CL is highest, and in regions of lowest cleft prevalence, the proportion of the more severe forms of clefting is correspondingly low. This provides indirect support for the multifactorial threshold model and for the notion of OC being a threshold characteristic with genetic predisposition.

The data in Table 12.4, however, need to be interpreted with caution because of the heterogeneity associated with the ascertainment methods from which the figures were derived. The data are from a range of studies of varying sizes, some looking at nonsyndromic cases only, and some including associated malformations; also, some included stillbirths as well as livebirths and some did not. Since other studies have revealed a greater proportion of associated malformations with the more severe clefts and the milder clefts may not be as easily ascertained in areas with a higher proportion of severe cases, these factors must be accounted for before firm conclusions can be drawn.

Gender Ratios in Various Types of Cleft

Among the accepted epidemiological differences between CL/P and isolated CP is the now widely accepted male predilection for CL/P and female tendency toward CP. Therefore, to quote a sex ratio for OC as a whole, in view of the acknowledged differences in sex ratios for the subgroups, is meaningless.

The differences in sex ratios within the OC groups have proven to be more complicated, varying with severity of the cleft, number of affected siblings in a family, and ethnic origin. In all studies of white populations, CL/P occurs more frequently in males than fe-

TABLE 12.4. *Relative Proportions of Cleft Lip Subtypes in a Sample of Studies*

Country	Relative proportions of cleft types (%)				Reference
	Prevalence CL/P	CL	CLP	Ratio CLP:CL	
New York City (nonwhites)	0.29	27.0	31.0	1.15	Conway and Wagner (1966)
Africa (Nigeria)	0.34	49.0	32.0	0.65	Iregbulem (1982)
Israeli Jews	0.37	31.0	38.0	1.23	Azaz and Koyoumdjisky-Kaye (1967)
Caribbean (Santo Domingo)	0.42	36.4	31.4	0.86	Garcia-Godoy (1980)
Africa (Zaire)	0.44	50.0	46.0	0.92	Ogle (1993)
New York City (whites)	0.60	33.0	37.0	1.12	Conway and Wagner (1966)
Iran	0.85	35.0	48.0	1.37	Rajabian and Sherkat (2000)
USA Wisconsin	0.86	26.0	44.0	1.69	Gilmore and Hofman (1966)
Denmark	1.08	33.5	41.7	1.27	Fogh-Andersen (1961)
Bohemia	1.21	24.3	42.5	1.75	Tolarova (1987)
Thailand	1.22	26.0	48.0	1.84	Chuangsuwanich et al. (1998)
British Columbia	1.23	23.0	39.0	1.70	Lowry et al. (1989)
Australia (non-Aboriginal)	1.24	21.0	44.0	2.09	Bower et al. (1989)
Iceland	1.33	25.0	43.8	1.75	Moller (1965)
Japan	1.43	41.3	46.0	1.11	Natsume and Kawai (1986)
Australia (Aboriginal)	2.27	17.0	59.0	3.47	Bower et al. (1989)
Canadian Native Americans	2.73	8.0	78.0	9.75	Lowry et al. (1969)

CL, cleft lip; CP, cleft palate; CLP, cleft lip and palate; CL/P, cleft lip with or without cleft palate.

males, with an average male to female ratio of 2:1 (Wyszynski et al., 1996). In Japanese populations, there is a significant male excess in the CLP group but not in the CL only group (Fujino et al., 1963). In the white population, the male excess in the CL/P group becomes more apparent with increasing severity of cleft (Fogh-Andersen, 1942) and less apparent when more than one sibling is affected in the family (Niswander et al., 1972). In both races, there appears to be a slight excess of affected females in the CP group (Fraser, 1970; Wyszynski et al., 1996), although there remains some uncertainty and variation in the gender distribution of isolated CL. No generally accepted explanation for these gender differences exists, although sex differences in the timing of critical developmental stages in craniofacial development are thought to have an as yet undefined role in their etiology (Burdi and Silvey, 1969).

It is generally considered that clefts with associated malformations are different epidemiologically from clefts without associated malformations (Vanderas, 1987). However, the subdivision of primary palatal clefting into CL and CLP is somewhat controversial. Some argue that they are embryologically the same structure and the pathogenesis is presumably chronologically the same, with clefting of the hard palate being a secondary phenomenon occurring because of the disturbance surrounding the primary palate cleft (Fogh-

Andersen, 1942). It is, however, possible to have a CL and/or primary palate and a separate cleft of the soft palate with an intact hard palate between the two clefts, suggesting that they may be separate events (Hook and Porter, 1982; Vanderas, 1987; Sayetta et al., 1989).

A review of the literature reveals that only a subset of the epidemiological reports sub-divide the primary palatal clefting into CL and CLP. For those that do, there is considerable variation in the gender ratio for CL. There also tends to be less variation in CLP, and by virtue of the fact that CLP is much more common than isolated CL, the gender ratios for CL/P invariably reveal a male predilection. This may, however, mask an important underlying trend in CL gender ratios with considerable variation between ethnic groups. Womersley and Stone, (1987) reported a CL male to female ratio of 3:1 in the west of Scotland, which is considerably higher than other U.K. and European figures. For example, in Czechoslovakia, the CL male to female ratio was 1.5 (Tolarova, 1987) and in Denmark, 1.73 (Melnick et al., 1980). Precisely the same value (1.73) was reported by Woolf et al. (1963) in Utah. Similar gender ratios have been reported in other U.S. studies, such as Gilmore and Hofman (1966) in Wisconsin and Shaw et al. (1991) in California. However, the ratio is much lower in other countries, such as Nigeria (1.1 to 1; Iregbulem, 1982). In China, Yi et al. (1999) reported a male to female ratio of 0.85 to 1. In a 15-year sample of clefts in Iran (Rajabian and Sherkat, 2000) and in a small sample of clefts in the Jewish population in Israel (Azaz and Koyoumdjisky-Kaye, 1967), CL was also more common in females.

Unilateral Clefts and Laterality

The tendency for unilateral CL to be left-sided has proved to be a consistent finding. Of unilateral CL (80%–85% of all CL cases), approximately two-thirds have left-sided defects regardless of sex, ethnic group, and severity of defect (Fogh-Andersen, 1942; Fraser and Calnan, 1961). Since then, this predilection for the left side in unilateral clefts has been a recurrent finding in the OC literature (Bonaiti et al., 1982; Tolarova, 1987; Jensen et al., 1988), and this seems to be a feature in all ethnic groups.

No convincing explanation for these differences has been advanced, but a proposed explanation is that blood vessels, supplying the right side of the fetal head, leave the aortic arch closer to the heart and are perhaps better perfused by blood than those going to the left side (Johnston and Brown, 1980). Therefore, this left-sided characteristic would equally affect males and females, and this was confirmed for both unilateral CL and unilateral CL/P in a study of the Metropolitan Atlanta Congenital Defects Program (Paulozzi and Lary, 1999). An earlier report from the Netherlands by Cornel et al. (1992), however, examined laterality according to gender in an 8-year study and found that the predilection to left-sided clefting was seen only in boys.

Time Trends

The best data on which to base judgments on time trends for OC prevalence at birth are provided by the registries, where the criteria and infrastructure for the collection of data over a time period in a defined geographical area are relatively consistent. Data from the EUROCAT registry Report 6 (1980–1992) and Report 7 (1990–1994) provide a reasonable estimate of time trends in prevalence during these two time periods for CP and CL/P subgroups. While interesting variations during these time periods can be observed in various registries, there is no overall consistent trend to suggest that OC is significantly increasing or reducing in prevalence.

The ICBDMS, like EUROCAT, does not reveal any remarkable time trends in the period 1974–1998, with the occasional exception, such as the Finnish data. In Finland, the prevalence of CP has steadily increased over this period and, for CL/P, there is a similar, though lesser, trend. In contrast, many of the other countries that contribute data to ICBDMS, e.g., the United States and most of the European countries such as England and Wales, Ireland, northern Netherlands, Italy, and Hungary, reveal a tendency to reduction in frequency of CL/P. Apart from the aforementioned trend in Finland, the birth prevalence of CP remains remarkably consistent throughout this time period.

One of the most comprehensive data sets comes from Denmark, where there is a mandatory reporting system and a rigorous ascertainment procedure. The reported birth prevalence of OC in Denmark has risen from 1/667 live-born infants in 1942 to 1/529 in 1981 (Jensen et al., 1988). This increase may be due to better reporting and recording, decreased neonatal mortality, increasing environmental teratogens (e.g., drugs), and increased frequency of marriage among cleft patients because of better care.

The decline in OC in England and Wales apparent in notification data does not appear in the EUROCAT Registry data from Liverpool or Glasgow (EUROCAT Reports, 1995, 1996). However, EUROCAT data from Northern Ireland show a consistent decline in birth prevalence for CP. In parallel with the increased prevalence in Denmark over time between the 1940s and 1970s, increases were also noted in Finland during the same period. Seasonal patterns are little studied, but where they have been (Saxen and Lathi, 1974), no consistency has been noted.

Genetics and Environmental Factors

The overall variation in craniofacial morphology worldwide is related to ethnicity, and heritable characteristics (parental craniofacial characteristics being an example) are associated with ethnicity. The myriad of identifiable environmental causes are not uniform worldwide, individual countries and regions of countries being subjected to considerably differing lifestyle factors and environmental conditions. Maternal cigarette smoking and alcohol consumption remain the most plausible environmental factors in the cause of OC, but the evidence is not entirely consistent and may differ for CP and CL/P. Gene–environment interactions may also play a role, and in two studies smoking has been shown to be a more potent risk factor when present in conjunction with the transforming growth factor-alpha TaqI C2 allele (Hwang et al., 1995; Shaw et al., 1996). Specific environmental etiologies were implicated in OC in the Tehran study (Taher, 1992), and Zieglowski and Hemprich (1999) showed a dramatic increase (9.4%) in CLP 1 year after the Chernobyl nuclear accident, though there may be an element of selection bias in this figure.

Variations in genotype are associated with ethnicity, and thus it is possible that the effects of gene–environment interactions may vary considerably between ethnic groups. This may also account for some of the ethnic and geographic variation in the epidemiology of OC.

Socioeconomic Status

A number of studies have speculated on socioeconomic status, but in general, little attempt has been made to record it accurately or to analyze the correlation with CP or CLP. Croen et al. (1998) examined variation in the prevalence of CP and CL/P among Filipinos in California, Hawaii, and the Philippines and demonstrated a gradient, with the highest prevalence observed in the Philippines, an intermediate prevalence in Hawaii, and the lowest prevalence in California. They speculated that this variation may reflect differences in environmental risk factors, such as lack of maternal periconceptional vitamin supplementation.

Womersley and Stone (1987) examined the prevalence of facial clefting within Greater Glasgow according to housing and social characteristics. The highest rates were observed in areas of high unemployment, poor housing, and unskilled workers, whereas the lowest rates were found in affluent areas with large owner-occupied housing and professional or non-manual workers. The majority of cases examined were CP, and there appeared to be less variation in CL/P cases. The authors concluded that a deprived environment enhances the susceptibility to CP and that interaction between low socioeconomic status or a poor environment with a teratogen might explain Glasgow's high prevalence of CP. Diet, infection, and drugs were suggested.

Sivaloganathan (1972) examined social class and OC in a hospital-based sample in Kuala Lumpur, Malaysia, between September 1969 and May 1971. They found that 65% of clefts were from the lower class, 28% from the middle class, and 7% from the upper class, indicating either that clefting is associated with poor socioeconomic status and environmental factors or that there is a genetic predisposition. In a similar hospital-based study in Thailand, Chuangsuwanich et al. (1998) reported that low socio-economic status is also a significant etiological factor for OC.

It might be expected that if low socioeconomic status were a significant factor, time trend data would reflect this in areas where there have been improvements in living standards. Some trends are detectable from the available data in Europe (of which the EUROCAT data are regarded as being the most reliable), and these show that globally there was no reduction in the birth prevalence of OC between 1980 and 1996. This is despite considerable improvements in living conditions and nutrition during this same time period. This might well be due to a concomitant increase in exposure to other environmental teratogens, or it may be a genetic phenomenon. In the context of gene–environment interaction, Khoury and James (1993) state that if genetic susceptibility is not accounted for in the study of environmental factors, the results may be misleading.

It may be that the factors associated with low socioeconomic status can account for some of the worldwide variation in the prevalence of OC. The overall conclusion is that socio-economic status in OC is not well studied. One of the barriers to investigation of the role of socioeconomic status in OC is that common criteria for the description of low socioeconomic status do not exist. Also, in those studies where socioeconomic status or social class have been examined, different criteria have been used, making valid intercenter comparisons impossible.

RECOMMENDATIONS FOR PRODUCING BETTER DESCRIPTIVE STATISTICS IN ORAL CLEFTS EPIDEMIOLOGY

Oral clefting is a heterogeneous group of defects with a considerable range of severity; therefore, there will inevitably be variability in ascertainment rates. Many earlier publications were less discriminating on the differences in frequency between CP and CL/P, often quoting a combined figure. Many of the more recent papers do differentiate and some subdivide CL and CLP.

For example, the overall data from Europe show a fivefold variation in CL/P and a threefold variation in CP. The explanation for such variation may, at least partly, be due to the variable quality of data. It is therefore important that methods of ascertainment are specified, as well as whether studies were population-based or hospital-based. Accurate data require a recording system using multiple sources of ascertainment.

Population-Based vs. Hospital-Based Registries

In much of the older literature and in current work in less developed countries, data are often available only on births delivered in hospital. Unless almost all births occur in hospital, such data may be biased. However, if hospital confinement is more available to women from the upper socio-economic groups, hospital-derived rates may underestimate those for the community as a whole.

Interpretation of hospital series, therefore, is not straightforward unless the proportion of births in the community delivered in hospital approaches 100%.

Even so, when hospital records alone are searched, the number of cases expressed as a percentage of all known cases found using multiple sources of ascertainment may be low, as indicated by the Hungarian figure of 52.5% based on this one source of ascertainment (Czeizel and Revesz, 1970).

While complete ascertainment is almost impossible to achieve, we can come close to this by pooling data from several overlapping sources. The quality of a population-based perinatal register will depend on how many sources are used and how thorough the ascertainment process is; also, cleft registers or hospital-based registers tend to be a subset, excluding stillbirths, early deaths, minor anomalies not requiring surgery, patients who move away, miscoding, etc. As well as being less complete, a hospital-based registry will tend to have fewer cases with associated abnormalities because of stillbirths and perinatal deaths and because another feature may be more important than the cleft.

Multiple Sources of Ascertainment

Multiple sources of ascertainment from population-based samples should be used for incidence statistics, and complete censuses or representative samples should be employed for prevalence statistics. These constitute the best approaches available for preparing accurate estimates of rates because no single data source has sufficient reliability (Czeizel and Tusnadi, 1971).

In preparing incidence data to support genetic and other etiological studies, all abortions and stillbirths should be included or appropriate adjustments made. Whether terminations and fetal deaths are included, the inclusion criteria, and the methods used should be clarified. Similarly, the effects of differential prenatal and postnatal death rates on the apparent sex ratios for clefts should be documented. All degrees of cleft expression should be diagnosed to prevent underascertainment.

Cleft Type and Associated Malformations

All epidemiological and genetic data should be presented by specific cleft type whenever possible (Fogh-Andersen, 1942; Fraser, 1970). Each cleft type should be subdivided by the presence or absence of associated congenital malformations (Emanuel et al., 1973). Where possible, syndromic cleft cases should be separated from nonsyndromic ones and the classification used and how this was done should be explained, e.g., by a dysmorphologist. Birth prevalence statistics for clefts will further benefit risk factor studies if they are tallied separately for familial and sporadic cases (Melnick et al., 1980; Bixler, 1981), in which the genetic

and environmental risk factors may differ, and then for syndromic vs. nonsyndromic status within these categories. Since the major cleft phenotypes are actually heterogeneous entities, disaggregating them for statistical purposes may aid the investigation of unitary disease categories.

Ethnic Grouping

Where possible, data within countries should be presented by ethnic group, although it must be recognized that grouping by ethnic origin is not entirely objective. Also, in light of some emerging evidence, it may be useful to have a record of socioeconomic status. Ideally, data sets containing core information agreed by consensus should be collected, while additional information should be collected for studies in suspected high-risk population subgroups: specific parental genotypes or phenotypes, older parents, medicated mothers, mothers with certain chronic diseases, and parents with unique dietary or other environmental exposures.

CONCLUSIONS

The overall conclusions to be drawn from the data presented in this chapter are as follows:

- There is ample evidence of the distinctly different nature of CL/P and CP and emerging evidence of distinct differences in subgroups within these overall conditions.
- There is a great deal of geographical variation, which is more apparent for CL/P than CP.
- There is considerable variation in the proportion of OC cases with additional congenital anomalies and syndromes.
- The limited available data suggest that migrant groups retain rates of CL/P similar to those of their area of origin.
- There is no consistent evidence of time trends, nor is there consistent variation by socioeconomic status or seasonality, but these areas have not been adequately studied. There is a need to investigate such parameters within as well as between different populations.
- There is considerable international variation in the frequency of OCs, but validity and comparability of data are adversely affected by numerous factors: source population of births considered (hospital vs. population), time period, method of ascertainment, inclusion/exclusion criteria, and sampling fluctuation.
- There are many parts of the world for which we have little or no information on the frequency of OCs, in particular parts of Africa, Asia, and Eastern Europe.

REFERENCES

Abyholm, FE (1978). Cleft lip and palate in Norway. I. Registration, incidence and early mortality of infants with CLP. Scand J Plast Reconstr Surg 12: 29–34.

Altemus, LA (1966). The incidence of cleft lip and palate among North American Negroes. Cleft Palate J 3: 357–361.

Antoszewski, B, Kruk-Jeromin, J (1997). The incidence of cleft lip and (or) palate in children of Lodz in the years 1982–1991. Pol Merkuriusz Lek 3: 10–12.

Azaz, B, Koyoumdjisky-Kaye, E (1967). Incidence of clefts in Israel. Cleft Palate Craniofac J 4: 227–233.

Beckman, L, Myrberg, N (1972). The incidence of cleft lip and palate in northern Sweden. Hum Hered 22: 417–422.

Bellis, TH, Wohlgemuth, B (1999). The incidence of cleft lip and palate deformities in the south-east of Scotland (1971–1990). Br J Orthod 26: 121–125.

Bixler, D (1981). Genetics and clefting. Cleft Palate J 18: 10–18.

Bonaiti, C, Briard, ML, Feingold, J, et al. (1982). An epidemiological and genetic study of facial clefting in France: epidemiology and frequency in relatives. J Med Genet 19: 8–15.

Borkar, AS, Mathur, AK, Mahaluxmivala, S (1993). Epidemiology of facial clefts in the central province of Saudi Arabia. Br J Plast Surg 46: 673–675.

Bower, C, Forbes, R, Seward, M, Stanley, F (1989). Congenital malformations in Aborigines and non-Aborigines in Western Australia, 1980–1987. Med J Aust 151: 245–248.

Brogan, WF, Woodings, JL (1974). A decline in the incidence of cleft lip and palate in Western Australia, 1963 to 1972. Med J Aust 2: 8–11.

Burdi, AR, Silvey, RG (1969). Sexual differences in closure of the human palatal shelves. Cleft Palate J 6: 1–7.

Calzolari, E, Milan, M, Cavazzuti, GB, et al. (1988). Epidemiological and genetic study of 200 cases of oral cleft in the Emilia Romagna region of northern Italy. Teratology 38: 559–564.

Caouette-Laberge, L, Bayet, B, Larocque, Y (1994). The Pierre Robin sequence: review of 125 cases and evolution of treatment modalities. Plast Reconstr Surg 93: 934–942.

Castilla, EE, Lopez-Camelo, JS, Campaña, H (1999). The Altitude as a Risk Factor for Congenital Anomalies. Am J Med Genet 86: 9–14.

Chandra, P, Harilal, KT (1977). Congenital malformation in Madras—a study of 24,192 consecutive births. Med Genet India 1: 47–52.

Chapman, CJ (1983). Ethnic differences in the incidence of cleft lip and/or cleft palate in Auckland, 1960–1976. N Z Med J 96: 327–329.

Chaturvedi, P, Banerjee, KS (1989). Spectrum of congenital malformations in the newborns from rural Maharashtra. Indian J Pediatr 56: 501–507.

Chi, S, Godfrey, K (1970). Cleft lip and palate in New South Wales. Med J Aust 2: 1172.

Ching, GHS, Chung, CS (1974). A genetic study of cleft lip and palate in Hawaii. 1. Interracial crosses. Am J Hum Genet 26: 162–172.

Choudhury, AR, Mukherjee, M, Sharma, A, et al. (1989). Study of 126,266 consecutive births for major congenital defects. Indian J Pediatr 56: 493–499.

Choudhury, AR, Talukder, G, Sharma, A (1984). Neonatal congenital malformations in Calcutta. Indian J Pediatr 21: 399–405.

Christensen, K, Fogh-Andersen, P (1994). Etiological subgroups in non-syndromic isolated cleft palate. A genetic epidemiological study of 52 Danish birth cohorts. Clin Genet 46: 329–335.

Chuangsuwanich, A, Aojanepong, C, Muangsombut, S, Tongpiew, P (1998). Epidemiology of cleft lip and palate in Thailand. Ann Plast Surg 41: 7–10.

Chung, CS, Myrianthopoulos, NC (1968). Racial and prenatal factors in major congenital malformations. Am J Hum Genet 20: 44.

Conway, H, Wagner, KJ (1966). Incidence of clefts in New York City. Cleft Palate J 3: 284–290.

Cooper, ME, Stone, RA, Liu, Y, et al. (2000). Descriptive epidemiology of nonsyndromic cleft lip with or without cleft palate in Shanghai, China from 1980 to 1989. Cleft Palate Craniofac J 37: 274–280.

Cornel, MC, et al. (1992). Some epidemiological data on oral clefts in the northern Netherlands 1981–1988. J Craniomaxillofac Surg 20: 147–152.

Coupland, MA, Coupland, AI (1988). Seasonality, birth prevalence and sex distribution of cleft lip and palate births in the Trent region. Cleft Palate J 25: 33–37.

Croen, LA, Shaw, GM, Wasserman, CR, Tolarova, MM (1998). Racial and ethnic variations in the prevalence of orofacial clefts in California, 1983–1992. Am J Med Genet 79: 42–47.

Czeizel, A (1984). Incidence and prevalence as measures of the frequency of birth defects. Am J Epidemiol 119: 141–142.

Czeizel, A, Revesz, C (1970). Major malformations of the central nervous system in Hungary. Br J Prev Soc Med 24: 205–222.

Czeizel, A, Tusnadi, G (1971). An epidemiologic study of cleft lip with or without cleft palate and posterior cleft palate in Hungary. Hum Hered 21: 17–38.

Czeizel, AE (1997). First 25 years of the Hungarian Congenital Abnormality Registry. Teratology 55: 299–305.

Das, SK, Runnels, RSJ, Smith, JC, Cohly, HH (1995). Epidemiology of cleft lip and cleft palate in Mississippi. South Med J 88: 437–442.

Davis, JS (1924). The incidence of congenital clefts of the lip and palate. Ann Surg 80: 363.

Drillien, CM, Ingram, TTS, Wilkinson, EM (1966). *The Causes and Natural History of Cleft Lip and Palate*. Edinburgh.

Elwood, JM, Little, J, Elwood, JH (1992). *Epidemiology and Control of Neural Tube Defects*. Oxford: Oxford University Press, pp. 96–101.

Emanuel, I, Culver, BH, Erickson, JD, et al. (1973). The further epidemiological differentiation of cleft lip and palate: a population study of clefts in King County, Washington, 1956–1965. Teratology 7: 271–281.

Emanuel, I, Huang, SW, Gutman, LT, et al. (1972). The incidence of congenital malformations in a Chinese population: the Taipei collaborative study. Teratology 5: 159.

Fitzpatrick, DR, Raine, PA, Boorman, JG (1994). Facial clefts in the west of Scotland in the period 1980–1984: epidemiology and genetic diagnoses. J Med Genet 31: 126–129.

Fogh-Andersen, P (1942). *Inheritance of Harelip and Cleft Palate*. Copenhagen: Arnold Busck.

Fogh-Andersen, P (1961). Incidence of cleft lip and palate: constant or increasing? Acta Chir Scand 122: 106–111.

Fraser, FC (1970). The genetics of cleft lip and cleft palate. Am J Hum Genet 22: 336–352.

Fraser, GR, Calnan, JS (1961). Cleft lip and palate: seasonal incidence, birth weight, birth rank, sex, site, associated malformations and parental age. Arch Dis Child 36: 420–423.

Garcia-Godoy, F (1980). Cleft lip and cleft palate in Santo Domingo. Community Dent Oral Epidemiol 8: 89–91.

Ghosh, S, Santosh, K, Butani, B, Butani, R (1985). Congenital malformations in a longitudinally studied birth cohort in an urban community. Indian J Med Res 82: 427–433.

Gilmore, SI, Hofman, SM (1966). Clefts in Wisconsin: incidence and related factors. Cleft Palate J 3: 186–199.

Goravalingappa, JP, Nashi, HK (1979). Congenital malformations in a study of 2398 consecutive births. Indian J Med Res 69: 140–146.

Goulet, O, Hochez, J, Berchel, C, et al. (1986). Incidence des malformations congenitales à la naissance dans une maternité guadeloupéenne. Arch Fr Pediatr 43: 507–511.

Grace, GL (1943). Frequency of occurrence of cleft palates and harelips. J Dent Res 22: 495.

Gregg, T, Boyd, D, Richardson, A (1994). The birth prevalence of cleft lip and palate in Northern Ireland from 1980–1990. Br J Orthod 21: 387–392.

Gupta, B (1969). Incidence of congenital malformation in Nigerian children. West Afr Med J 18: 22–27.

Gupta, BM, Mathur, HC, Sharda, DC (1971). A study of congenital malformations in central Rajasthan. Arch Child Health 13: 30–36.

Harrison, KA, Rossiter, CE, Ekanem, AD, Chong, H (1985). Childbearing, health and social priorities: a survey of 22,774 consecutive hospital births in Zana, northern Nigeria. Br J Obstet Gynaecol 5: 81–85.

Hay, S (1971). Incidence of selected congenital malformation in Iowa. Am J Epidemiol 94: 572–584.

Hikita, Y (1953). Incidence of harelip and cleft palate in Nagasaki [in Japanese]. Nagasaki Med J 28: 1371.

Hixon, EH (1951). A study of the incidence of cleft lip and cleft palate in Ontario. Can J Public Health 4: 508.

Hook, EB, Porter, IH (1982). Incidence and prevalence as measures of the frequency of birth defects. Am J Epidemiol 116: 743–747.

Hwang, SJ, Beaty, TH, Panny, SR, et al. (1995). Association study of transforming growth factor alpha (TGFα) TaqI polymorphism and oral clefts: indication of gene–environment interaction in a population-based sample of infants with birth defects. Am J Epidemiol 141: 629–636.

Iizuka, T (1973). High incidence of cleft lip and cleft palate in the human embryos and early fetuses. Okajimas Folia Anat Jpn 50: 259–271.

Ingalls, TH, Taube, IE, Kilingberg, MA (1964). Cleft lip and cleft palate: epidemiological considerations. Plast Reconstr Surg 1–10.

Iregbulem, LM (1982). The incidence of cleft lip and palate in Nigeria. Cleft Palate J 19: 201–205.

Ivy, RH (1962). The influence of race on the incidence of certain congenital anomalies, notably cleft lip–cleft palate. Plast Reconstr Surg 30: 581.

Jensen, BL, Kreiborg, S, Dahl, E, Fogh-Andersen, P (1988). Cleft lip and palate in Denmark 1976–1981: epidemiology variability and early somatic development. Cleft Palate J 25: 258–269.

Kallen, B, Harris, J, Robert, E (1996). The epidemiology of orofacial clefts. 2. Associated malformations. J Craniofac Genet Dev Biol 16: 242–248.

Kamala, KG, Raghavendran, VD, Krishnamurthy, KA (1978). Congenital malformations in the newborn in Madurai. Med Genet India 2: 53–59.

Khan, AA (1965). Congenital malformation in African neonates in Nairobi. J Trop Med Hyg 68: 272.

Khanna, KK, Prasad, LSN (1967). Congenital malformations in the newborn. Indian J Pediatr 34: 63–72.

Khoury, MJ, James, LM (1993). Population and familial relative risks of disease associated with environmental factors in the presence of gene/environment interaction. Am J Epidemiol 137: 1241–1250.

Khrouf, N, Spang, R, Podgorna, T, et al. (1986). Malformations in 10,000 consecutive births in Tunis. Acta Paediatr Scand 75: 534–539.

Kirby, R, Petrini, J, Alter, C (2000). Collecting and interpreting birth defects surveillance data by Hispanic ethnicity: a comparative study. The Hispanic Ethnicity Birth Defects Workgroup. Teratology 61: 21–27.

Kjaskova, B (1973). An epidemiology study of cleft lip in Bohemia. Acta Chir Plast 15: 258–262.

Knox, G, Braithwaite, F (1962). Cleft lips and palates in Northumberland and Durham. Arch Dis Child 38: 66–70.

Kobayasi, Y (1958). A genetic study on harelip and cleft palate [in Japanese with English summary]. Jpn J Hum Genet 3: 73.

Kondo, K (1987). Seasonal patterns of birth defects in Japan. Seasonal Effects Reprod Psychoses Prog Biometeorol 5: 133–138.

Kozelj, V (1996). Epidemiology of orofacial clefts in Slovenia, 1973–1993: comparison of the incidence in six European countries. J Craniomaxillofac Surg 24: 378–382.

Krause, BS, Kitamure, H, Ooe, T (1963). Malformations with cleft lip and palate in human embryos and foetuses. Am J Obstet Gynecol 86: 321.

Kromberg, JGR, Jenkins, T (1982). Common birth defects in South African blacks. S Afr Med J 62:

Kulshrestha, R, Nath, LM, Upadhyaya, P (1983). Congenital malformations in liveborn infants in a rural community. Indian Pediatr 20: 45–49.

Kurozumi, S (1963). A genetic study of harelip and cleft palate [in Japanese with English summary]. Jpn J Hum Genet 8: 120.

Leck, I (1969). Ethnic differences in the incidence of malformations following migration. Br J Prev Soc Med 23: 166.

Leck, I (1972). The etiology of human malformations: insights from epidemiology. Teratology 5: 303–314.

Leck, I (1983). Fetal malformations. In: Obstetrical Epidemiology. London: Academic Press.

Leck, I, Lancashire, RJ (1995). Birth prevalence of malformations in members of different ethnic groups and in the offspring of matings between them, in Birmingham, England. J Epidemiol Community Health 49: 171–179.

Lesi, FEA (1969). The significance of congenital defects in developing countries. Med Today 4: 347–353.

Ligutic, I, Barisic, I, Kapitanovic, H, et al. (1997). Eleven years of registration of congenital anomalies in Croatia associated with the EUROCAT international project. Lijec Vjesn 119: 47–53.

Long, S, Robert, E, Laumon, B, et al. (1992). Epidemiologie des fentes labiales et palatines dans la region Rhone-Alpes/Auvergne/Jura. A propos de 903 cas enregistres entre 1978 et 1987. Pediatrie 47: 133–140.

Lowry, RB, Renwick, DH (1969). Incidence of cleft lip and palate in British Columbia Indians. J Med Genet 6: 67–69.

Lowry, RB, Trimble, BK (1977). Incidence rates for cleft lip and palate in British Columbia 1952–71 for North American Indian, Japanese, Chinese and total populations: secular trends over twenty years. Teratology 16: 277–283.

Lowry, RB, Thunem, NY, Uh, SH (1989). Birth prevalence of cleft lip and palate in British Columbia between 1952 and 1986: stability of rates. CMAJ 140: 1167–1170.

Lutz, KR, Moor, FB (1955). A study of factors in the occurrence of cleft palate. J Speech Hear Dis 20: 271.

Master-Notani, P, Kolah, PJ, Sanghvi, LD (1968). Congenital malformations in the new born in Bombay part II. Acta Genet (Basel) 18: 193–205.

Mathur, BC, Karan, S, Vijaya Devi, KK (1975). Congenital malformation in the newborn. Indian Pediatr 12: 179–183.

McMahon, B, McKeown, T (1953). The birth prevalence of harelip and palate related to birth rank and maternal age. Am J Hum Genet 5: 176–183.

McMahon, B, Pugh, TF (1970). Epidemiology: Principles and Methods. Boston: Little, Brown.

Melnick, M, Shields, ED, Bixler, D (1980). Studies of cleft lip and cleft palate in the population of Denmark. Prog Clin Biol Res 46: 225–248.

Menegotto, BG, Salzano, FM (1991). Epidemiology of oral clefts in a large South American sample. Cleft Palate Craniofac J 28: 373–377.

Milan, M, Astolfi, G, Volpato, S, et al. (1994). 766 cases of oral cleft in Italy. Eur J Epidemiol 10: 317–324.

Mital, VK, Grewal, RS (1969). Congenital anomalies in neonates. Indian J Pediatr 36: 356–365.

Mitani, S (1954). Malformations of the newborn infants. J Jpn Obstet Gynecol Soc 1: 301.

Moller, P (1965). Cleft lip and cleft palate in Iceland. Arch Oral Biol 10: 407–420.

Moller, P (1972). Epidemiological and genetic study of cleft lip and palate in Iceland. Ala J Med Sci 119–136.

Moore, GE, Ivens, A, Chambers, J, et al. (1987). Linkage of an X-chromosome cleft palate gene. Nature 326: 91–92.

Murray, JC, Daack-Hirsch, S, Buetow, KH, et al. (1997). Clinical and epidemiological studies of cleft lip and palate in the Philippines. Cleft Palate Craniofac J 34: 7–10.

Myrianthopoulos, NC, Chung, CS (1974). Congenital malformations in singletons: epidemiologic survey (report from the Collaborative Perinatal Project). Birth Defects 10: 11.

Nair, NS, Mathai, NM (1964). Congenital malformation in the newborn at Calicut—a preliminary report. Antiseptic 61: 823–829.

National Birth Defects Prevention Network (2000). Teratology 61: 86–158.

Natsume, N, Kawai, T (1986). Incidence of cleft lip and cleft palate in 39,696 Japanese babies born during 1983. Int J Oral Maxillofac Surg 15: 565–568.

Natsume, N, Suzuki, T, Kawai, T (1987). Maternal reactions to the birth of a child with cleft lip and/or palate. Plast Reconstr Surg 79: 1003–1004.

Neel, IV (1958). A study of major congenital defects in Japanese infants. Am J Hum Genet 10: 398.

Nishimura, H, Takano, K, Tanimura, T, Yasuda, M (1968). Normal and abnormal development of human embryos: first report of the analysis of 1,213 intact embryos. Teratology 1: 281–290.

Niswander, JD, Adams, MS (1967). Oral clefts in the American Indians. Public Health Rep 82: 807–812.

Niswander, JD, MacLean, CJ, Chung, CS, Dronamraju, K (1972). Sex ratio and cleft lip with or without cleft palate. Lancet 2: 858–860.

Ogle, OE (1993). Incidence of cleft lip and palate in a newborn Zairian sample. Cleft Palate Craniofac J 30: 250–251.

Owens, JR, Jones, JW, Harris, F (1985). Epidemiology of facial clefting. Arch Dis Child 60: 521–524.

Paulozzi, LJ, Lary, JM (1999). Laterality patterns in infants with external birth defects. Teratology 60: 265–271.

Perez-Molina, JJ, Alfaro-Alfaro, N, Angulo-Castellanos, E, Nario-Castellanos, JG (1993). The prevalence and risk factors of cleft lip and cleft palate in 2 hospitals in the city of Guadalajara, Jalisco, Mexico. Bol Med Hosp Infant Mex 50: 110–113.

Rajabian, MH, Sherkat, M (2000). An epidemiologic study of oral clefts in Iran: analysis of 1669 cases. Cleft Palate Craniofac J 37: 191–196.

Rank, BK, Thomson, JA (1960). Cleft lip and palate in Tasmania. Med J Aust 10: 683.

Rintala, AE (1986). Epidemiology of orofacial clefts in Finland: a review. Ann Plast Surg 17: 456–459.

Sato, M (1966). Statistical study on the congenital malformations in Japan. J Jpn Obstet Gynecol Soc 18: 74.

Saxen, I (1975). Epidemiology of cleft lip and palate: an attempt to rule out chance correlations. Br J Prev Soc Med 29: 103–110.

Saxen, I, Lathi, A (1974). Cleft lip and palate in Finland: incidence, secular, seasonal geographical variations. Teratology 9: 217–224.

Sayetta, RB, Weinrich, MC, Coston, GN (1989). Incidence and prevalence of cleft lip and palate: what we think we know. Cleft Palate J 26: 242–248.

Sharma, B, Bajpai, PC, Sharma, NL (1972). Some observations on congenital malformations. Indian J Pediatr 39: 286–292.

Shaw, GM, Croen, LA, Curry, CJ (1991). Isolated cleft malformations in the families of South American oral cleft neonates. J Med Genet 28: 110–113.

Shaw, GM, Wasserman, CR, Lammer, EJ, et al. (1996). Orofacial clefts, parental cigarette smoking, and transforming growth factor-alpha gene variants. Am J Hum Genet. 58: 551–561.

Shija, JK, Kingo, ARM (1985). A prospective clinical study of congenital anomalies seen at Harare Central Hospital, Zimbabwe. Cent Afr J Med 31: 145–149.

Shprintzen, RJ, Singer, L (1992). Upper airway obstruction and the Robin sequence. Int Anesthesiol Clin 30: 109–114.

Singh, M, Sharma, NK (1980). Spectrum of congenital malformations in the newborn. Indian J Pediatr 47: 239–244.

Sivaloganathan, V (1972). Cleft lips in Malaysians. Plast Reconstr Surg 49: 176–179.

Spry, CC, Nugent, MAC (1975). Some epidemiological aspects of clefts of the primary and secondary palate in South Australia, 1949–1968. Aust Dent J 20: 250–256.

Srivastava, A, Bang, RL (1990). Facial clefting in Kuwait and England: a comparative study. Br J Plast Surg 43: 457–462.

Stevenson, AC, Johnston, HA, Stewart, MIP, Golding, DR (1966). A report of a study of series of consecutive births in 24 centers. Bull WHO 34: 1–127.

Stoll, C, Alembik, Y, Dott, B, Roth, MP (2000). Associated malformations in cases with oral clefts. Cleft Palate Craniofac J 37: 41–47.

Stoll, C, Alembik, Y, Dott, B, Roth, MP (1992). Epidemiological and genetic study in 207 cases of oral clefts in Alsace, north-eastern France. J Med Genet 28: 325–329.

Taher, AA (1992). Cleft lip and palate in Tehran. Cleft Palate Craniofac J 29: 15–16.

Tal, Y, Dar, H, Winter, ST, Bar-Joseph, G (1974). Frequency of cleft lip and palate in northern Israel. Israel J Med Sci 10: 515.

Tan, KL (1988). Incidence and epidemiology of cleft lip/palate in Singapore. Ann Acad Med Singapore 17: 311–314.

Tanaka, T (1972). A clinical, genetic and epidemiological study on cleft lip and/or cleft palate. Jpn J Hum Genet 16: 278.

Tandu-Umba, NF, Ntabona, B, Mputu, L (1984). Etude epidemiologique des malformations congenitales visibles en milieu zairois. Gynecol Obstet 79: 131–135.

Tolarova, MM (1987). Orofacial clefts in Czechoslovakia: incidence, genetics and prevention of cleft lip and palate over a 19 year period. Scand J Plast Reconstr Surg 21: 19–25.

Tolarova, MM, Cervenka, J (1998). Classification and birth prevalence of orofacial clefts. Am J Med Genet 75: 126–137.

Tsukamoto, S (1956). In discussion on the malformations [in Japanese]. World Obstet Gynecol 8: 843.

Tsutsui, H (1951). Study on the etiology of clefts of the lip and the palate I. Clinico-statistical observation [in Japanese]. J Dent (Japan) 8: 3.

Tyan, ML (1982). Differences in the reported frequencies of cleft lip plus cleft lip and palate in Asians born in Hawaii and the continental United States (41,474). Proc Soc Exp Biol Med 171: 41–45.

United States Bureau of the Census. International Data Base. 2001. www.census.giv/ipc/www/ibdnew.html

Vanderas, AP (1987). Social and Biological Effects on Perinatal Mortality. Budapest: WHO.

Verma, IC, Mathews, AR (1983). Congenital malformations in India. (Reprinted from Peoples of India, edited by GV Satyavati. New Delhi: Indian Council of Medical Research, 1983).

Wayne Loretz, MPH, et al. (1961). The study of cleft lip and cleft palate births in California. Am J Public Health 51: 873–877.

Wei, PY, Chen, YP (1965). Congenital malformations, especially anencephalus, in Taiwan. Am J Obstet Gynecol 91: 870.

Womersley, J, Stone, DH (1987). Epidemiology of facial clefts. Arch Dis Child 62: 717–720.

Woolf, CM, et al. (1963). A genetic study of cleft lip and palate in Utah. Am J Hum Genet 15: 209–215.

Wyszynski, DF, Beaty, TH, Maestri, N (1996) Genetics of Non-Syndromic Cleft Lip with or without Cleft Palate Revisited. Cleft Pal Craniof J 33: 406–417.

Xiao, KZ (1989). Epidemiology of cleft lip and cleft palate in China. Chung Hua I Hsueh Tsa Chih 69: 192–194.

Yi, NN, Yeow, VK, Lee, ST (1999). Epidemiology of cleft lip and palate in Singapore—a 10 year hospital-based study. Ann Acad Med Singapore 28: 655–659.

Zieglowski, V, Hemprich, A (1999). Facial cleft birth rate in former East Germany before and after the reactor accident in Chernobyl. Mund Kiefer Gesichtschir 3: 195–199.

APPENDIX 12.I. INTERNATIONAL PREVALENCE FIGURES FOR ORAL CLEFTS

TABLE 12.IA. *International Epidemiology of Oral Clefts—Europe** *

Population	Time Period	Sources of Ascertainment	No. of Births	Birth prevalence CL/P	Birth prevalence CP	Birth prevalence All Clefts	Associated Abnormalities	Reference
Czech Republic (Bohemia)	1964–1971	Population-based registry	1,831,036	1.21	0.60	1.81	Nonsyndromic	Tolarova (1987)
	1964–1982	Registry (multiple sources)	689,967	1.28	0.63	1.95	2.1% Syndromic	Kjaskova (1973)
Croatia	1983–1993	Zagreb Registry EUROCAT	65,100	—†	—	1.10		Ligutic et al. (1997)
Denmark	1936–1961	Population-based	2,031,559	—	0.47	—	Included submucous	Christensen and Fogh-Andersen (1994)
	1938–1957	Surgical records	1,631,376	1.08	0.36	1.44	Syndromes included	Fogh-Andersen (1961)
	1941–1968	Population-based	2,066,153	1.30	No data	No data	Nonsyndromic	Melnick et al. (1980)
	1942	Population-based		1.25	0.38	1.62	Nonsyndromic	Fogh-Andersen (1942)
	1962–1987	Population-based	1,761,504	n.d.	0.77	—	Nonsyndromic (including submucous)	Christensen and Fogh-Andersen (1994)
England	1976–1981	Population-based	359,027	1.37	0.52	1.89	Included	Jensen et al. (1988)
	1940–1950	Multiple sources	218,693	—	—	1.30		McMahon and McKeown (1953)
Birmingham	1949–1958	Multiple sources	404,124	0.95	0.47	1.42		Knox and Braithwaite (1962)
Liverpool	1950–1959	Multiple sources	186,046	—	—	1.90		Leck (1969)
	1960–1982	Multiple sources	325,727	—	—	1.40		Owens et al. (1985)
Birmingham	1960–1984	Population-based registry LB + SB	432,778	1.04	0.62	1.66	Included	Leck and Lancashire (1995)
Trent	1973–1982	Hospital activity analysis	617,940	—	—	1.51		Coupland and Coupland (1988)
Finland	1948–1975	Population-based registry	2,258,850	0.77	0.97	1.74	—	Rintala (1986)
	1962–1967	Multiple sources	110,299	—	—	1.30		Saxen and Lathi (1974)
	1967–1971	Registry	347,316	0.83	0.86	1.72	20% CL/P 22% CP	Saxen and Lathi (1974)
		Multiple sources						
	1972–1973	Multiple sources	116,407	0.73	0.90	1.63	25% CL/P 30% CP	Saxen (1975)
France	1974–1988			0.81	1.01	1.82	Nonsyndromic	Tolarova and Cervenka (1995)
Rhone-Alpes/Auvergne	1978–1987	Registry	813,513	0.67	0.44	1.11	Nonsyndromic	Long et al. (1992)
Alsace	1979–1987	Registry	118,286	0.98	0.77	1.75	Included	Stoll et al. (1991)
Strasbourg	1979–1996	Population based	238,942	1.08	0.85	1.93	36.7%	Stoll et al. (2000)

(continued)

TABLE 12.IA. *International Epidemiology of Oral Clefts—Europe* (continued)*

Population	Time Period	Sources of Ascertainment	No. of Births	Birth prevalence			Associated Abnormalities	Reference
				CL/P	CP	All Clefts		
East Central	n.d.	Registry	1,460,000	0.56	0.42	0.98	Chromosomal anomalies 4.3% CL/P 4.5% CP	Kallen et al. (1996)
Hungary (Budapest)	1962–1967	Registry		1.03	0.27	1.30	—	Czeizel (1997)
	1970–1976	Registry		1.16	0.48	1.64	Included	Czeizel (1997)
Iceland	1956–1962	Multiple sources LB only	32,979	1.33	0.61	1.94	6.3%	Moller (1965)
Italy								
Emilia Romagna	1978–1986	Population-based	150,168	0.75	0.58	1.33	32%	Calzolari et al. (1988)
Emilia Romagna and northeast Italy)	1981–1989	Hospital and population-based data LB + SB	561,539	0.82	0.61	1.43	23% CL/P 43% CP	Milan et al. (1994)
Northern Ireland	1980–1990	Regional database	310,838	0.60	0.68	1.28	Nonsyndromic	Gregg et al. (1994)
Netherlands	1981–1988	Multiple sources LB + SB	73,879	1.46	0.81	2.27	Syndromic (453 SB) 23% CL/P 52% CP	Cornel et al. (1992)
Norway	1967–1988	Registry	516,657	1.43	0.65	2.08	Included	Abyholm (1978)
	1974–1988			1.42	0.50	1.92	—	Tolarova and Cervenka (1995)
Poland	1981–1995	Hospital (surgical cases)	132,783	1.16	0.84	2.00	Nonsyndromic	Antoszewski and Kruk-Jeromin (1997)
Scotland	1971–1990	Regional database	356,922	0.77	0.63	1.40	Nonsyndromic	Bellis and Wohlegemuth (1999)
Southeast and Highlands								
West	1974–1985	Registry	158,333	0.75	0.81	1:56	Nonsyndromic	Wormsley and Stone (1987)
West	1980–1984			0.74	0.79	1.53	Included 26% CL/P 39.5% CP	Fitzpatrick et al. (1994)
Slovenia	1973–1993	Cleft registry	179,268	0.98	0.66	1.64	LB Nonsyndromic	Kozelj (1996)
Sweden (Stockholm)	1958–1970	Cleft registry	253,468	1.17	0.55	1.72	Nonsyndromic	Beckman and Myrberg (1972)
	1973–1983	Cleft registry		1.00	0.47	1.47	Nonsyndromic	McWilliam (1997)
	1984–1994	Cleft registry		0.95	0.53	1.48	Nonsyndromic	McWilliam (1997)
	1991–1995	Population-based LB only	122,148	1.35	0.65	2.00	17%	Hagberg et al. (1997)
	n.d.	Registry	2.07 million	1.27	0.65 (includes PR)	1.92	Chromosomal anomalies 2.1% CL/P 2.2% CP	Kallen et al. (1996)

*CL/P, cleft lip with or without cleft palate; CP, cleft palate; LB, live births; SB, stillbirths; PR, Pierre Robin; n.d., not defined.
†Data not available.

TABLE 12.IB. *International Epidemiology of Oral Clefts—USA and Canada**

Population	Time Period	Sources of Ascertainment	No. of Births	Birth prevalence			Associated Abnormalities	Reference
				CL/P	CP	All Clefts		
Canada								
Ontario	1943–1949	Surgical records	655,322	—†	—	1.06		Hixon (1951)
British Columbia	1952–1986	Registry	1,299,495	1.23	0.75	1.98	Nonsyndromic	Lowry et al. (1989)
Chinese	1952–1971	Multiple sources	12,5000	—	—	1.76		Lowry and Trimble (1977)
White	1952–1971	Multiple sources	713,316	—	—	1.97		Lowry and Trimble (1977)
Japanese	1952–1971	Multiple sources	3571	—	—	3.36		Lowry and Trimble (1977)
	1952–1964	Registry LB + SB	452,147	1.09	0.54	1.63	Included	Lowry and Renwick (1969)
Native Americans	1952–1964	Registry LB + SB	20,819	2.73	0.44	3.17	Included	Lowry and Renwick (1969)
Canada	1997	Registry (ICBD)	262,741	0.33	0.74	1.07		ICBDMS (2000)
USA	n.d.	Deliveries	15,565	—	0.74	1.09		Davis (1924)
Baltimore *White*								
Black	n.d.	Deliveries	12,500	—	—	0.56		Davis (1924)
Los Angeles *White*	1936–1951	Hospital records LB + SB	29,000	—	—	1.00		Lutz and Moor (1955)
Black	1936–1951	Hospital records LB + SB	16,901	—	—	0.71		Lutz and Moor (1955)
California	1955	Birth certificates, population-based	313,164	0.82	0.36	1.18	Included 18.2%	Wayne Loretz et al. (1961)
White	1955	Birth certificates	282,812	—	—	1.20		Wayne Loretz et al. (1961)
Black	1955	Birth records	21,532	—	—	0.60		Wayne Loretz et al. (1961)
California	1983–1986	Registry	452,287	0.74	0.38	1.12	Included	Shaw et al. (1991)
California	1983–1993	Registry	2,509,881	0.77	0.31	1.08	Nonsyndromic	Tolarova and Cervenka (1998)
California	n.d.	Registry	1.62 million	1.00	0.57* (includes PR)	1.57 / 7	Chromosomal anomalies .4% CL/P 8.4% CP	Kallen et al. (1996)
Hawaii *Japanese*	1948–1966	Multiple sources	67,170	—	—	2.65		Ching and Chung (1974)
White	1948–1986	Multiple sources	77,013	—	—	1.55		Ching and Chung (1974)
Japanese	1974–1977	Birth records	2905	—	—	2.41		Tyan (1982)
White	1963	Multiple sources	58,686	1.60	0.61	2.21	Included	Hay (1971)

(continued)

TABLE 12.IB. International Epidemiology of Oral Clefts—USA and Canada* (continued)

Population	Time Period	Sources of Ascertainment	No. of Births	Birth prevalence CL/P	Birth prevalence CP	Birth prevalence All Clefts	Associated Abnormalities	Reference
Mississippi								
White	1980–1989	Birth certificates	228,156	0.93	0.43	1.36	Nonsyndromic	Das et al. (1995)
Nonwhite	1980–1989	Birth certificates	211,198	0.30	0.24	0.54		Das et al. (1995)
New York City	Jan 1952–Dec 1962	Birth certificates	1,478,315	0.60	0.26	0.86	Included	Conway and Wagner (1966)
White							13% CL/P	
Nonwhite	Jan 1952–Dec 1962	Birth certificates	344,929	0.29	0.22	0.51	27% CP	Conway and Wagner (1966)
Pennsylvania	1942	Birth records	191,161	—	—	1.26		Grace (1943)
White								
Black	1942	Birth records	39,130	—	—	0.23		Grace (1943)
White	1961	Birth certificates	213,778	—	—	1.32		Ivy (1962)
Black	1961	Birth certificates	26,086	—	—	0.23		Ivy (1962)
Black	1961	Birth certificates	28,350	—	—	0.95		Ivy (1962)
(Utah) (white)	Jan 1951–Jan 1961	Nursery records	59,650	1.24	0.27	1.51	Included	Woolf et al. (1963)
Washington D.C.	1952–1961	Hospital records	79,842	0.49	0.49	0.98	Included	Altemus (1966)
Black								
White	1956–1965	Multiple sources	189,096	—	—	1.75		Emanuel et al. (1973)
Black	1956–1965	Multiple sources	8730	—	—	1.26		Emanuel et al. (1973)
Chinese	1956–1965	Multiple sources	1,237	—	—	4.04		Emanuel et al. (1973)
Japanese	1956–1965	Multiple sources	2,538	—	—	1.97		Emanuel et al. (1973)
Wisconsin (white)	1943–1962	Multiple sources	1,756,409	0.86	0.37	1.23	Included	Gilmore and Hofman (1966)
USA	1983–1992	Registry	2,221,755	1.07	0.68	1.75	Nonsyndromic	Croen et al. (1998)
White	1983–1992	Registry	1,005,727	1.05	0.72	1.77	Nonsyndromic	Croen et al. (1998)
African-American	1983–1992	Registry	172,557	0.62	0.54	1.16	Nonsyndromic	Croen et al. (1998)
Japanese	1983–1992	Registry	14,314	1.05	0.77	1.82	Nonsyndromic	Croen et al. (1998)
Chinese	1983–1992	Registry	53,113	0.96	0.60	1.50	Nonsyndromic	Croen et al. (1998)
Hispanic	1983–1992	Registry	769,866	1.01	0.56	1.57	Nonsyndromic	Croen et al. (1998)
Filipino	1983–1992	Registry	61,012	1.00	0.92	1.92	Nonsyndromic	Croen et al. (1998)
Native	1983–1992	Registry	13,545	1.99	1.11	3.10	Nonsyndromic	Croen et al. (1998)

East Indian	1983–1992	Registry	1.14	1.06	2.20	Nonsyndromic	Croen et al. (1998)
Pacific	1983–1992	Registry	0.83	0.83	1.66	Nonsyndromic	Croen et al. (1998)
Korean	1983–1992	Registry	0.65	0.26	0.91	Nonsyndromic	Croen et al. (1998)
Laotian	1983–1992	Registry	1.46	0.67	2.13	Nonsyndromic	Croen et al. (1998)
Vietnamese	1983–1992	Registry	1.23	0.45	1.68	Nonsyndromic	Croen et al. (1998)
Cambodian	1983–1992	Registry	0.97	0.32	1.29	Nonsyndromic	Croen et al. (1998)
14 Institutions *Whites*	n.d.	Follow-up pregnancies	—	—	1.82		Chung and Myrianthopoulos (1967)
Blacks	n.d.	Follow-up pregnancies	—	0.82	—		Chung and Myrianthopoulos (1967)
12 Institutions *Whites*	1973–1974	Follow-up pregnancies	—	—	2.69		Myrianthopoulos and Chung (1974)
Blacks	1973–1974	Follow-up pregnancies	—	1.67	—		Myrianthopoulos and Chung (1974)
Native Americans	1963–1966	Population-based	1.38	0.59	1.97	—	Niswander and Adams (1967)

*CL/P, cleft lip with or without cleft palate; CP, cleft palate; LB, live births; SB, stillbirths; PR, Pierre Robin; ICBD, International Clearinghouse for Birth Defects; n.d., not defined.
†Data not available.

TABLE 12.IC. *International Epidemiology of Oral Clefts—Central and South America**

| Population | Time Period | Sources of Ascertainment | No. of Births | Birth prevalence | | | Asscoiated Abnormalities | Reference |
				CL/P	CP	All Clefts		
Caribbean (Santo Domingo)	1973–1976	Hospital records	704,410	0.42	0.20	0.62	Nonsyndromic	Garcia-Godoy (1980)
Mexico (Guadalajara)	Nov 1988–June 1991	Hospital registry (4 hospitals)	33,461	1.05	0.27	1.32	Included	Perez-Molina et al. (1993)
South America	1967–1981	56 hospitals	849,381	0.87	0.13	1.00	Nonsyndromic	Menegotto and Salzano (1991)
South America								
Argentina	1982–1998	Registry	2,982,893	1.09	0.36	1.45	Included	ECLAMC (2000)
Bolivia	1982–1998	Registry	1,122,870	1.16	0.36	1.52	Included	ECLAMC (2000)
Brazil	1982–1998	Registry	79,296	2.28	0.21	2.50	Included	ECLAMC (2000)
Chile	1982–1998	Registry	754,657	1.01	0.39	1.40	Included	ECLAMC (2000)
Colombia	1982–1998	Registry	297,583	1.13	0.46	1.59	Included	ECLAMC (2000)
Ecuador	1982–1998	Registry	68,089	1.03	0.30	1.28	Included	ECLAMC (2000)
Paraguay	1982–1998	Registry	56,199	1.05	0.37	1.42	Included	ECLAMC (2000)
Peru	1982–1998	Registry	94,433	1.19	0.36	1.55	Included	ECLAMC (2000)
Uruguay	1982–1998	Registry	72,864	0.81	0.06	0.87	Included	ECLAMC (2000)
Venezuela	1982–1998	Registry	181,275	0.85	0.37	1.22	Included	ECLAMC (2000)
West Indies (Guadeloupe)	1982–1998	Registry	255,627	0.77	0.33	1.10	Included	ECLAMC (2000)
	July 1979–Feb 1983	Population-based LB only	8,142	—[†]	—	2.08	29% + 41% SB	Goulet et al. (1986)

*CL/P, cleft lip with or without cleft palate; CP, cleft palate; LB, live births; SB, stillbirths; ECLAMC, Latin American Collaborative Study of Congenital Malformations.
[†]Data not available.

TABLE 12.ID. *International Epidemiology of Oral Clefts—Australia and New Zealand**

Population	Time Period	Sources of Ascertainment	No. of Births	Birth prevalence			Associated Abnormalities	Reference
				CL/P	CP	All Clefts		
Australia								
Aboriginal	1980–1987	Registry	9695	2.27	0.72	2.99	Nonsyndromic	Bower et al. (1989)
Non-Aboriginal	1980–1987	Registry	170,760	1.24	0.67	1.91	Nonsyndromic	Bower et al. (1989)
Tasmania (*whites*)	1945–1957	Multiple sources	96,510	—†	—	1.66		Rank and Thomson (1960)
New South Wales (*Whites*)	1964–1966	Hospital records	143,948	—	—	1.21		Chi and Godfrey (1970)
New South Wales (*Whites*)	1963–1972	Multiple sources	193,520	0.54	0.68	1.22		Brogan and Woodings (1974)
South Australia (*whites*)	1949–1968	Multiple sources	392,228	—	—	1.41		Spry and Nugent (1975)
New Zealand (Auckland)	1960–1976	Urban population	178,240	0.39	1.87	2.26	Nonsyndromic	Chapman (1983)
Maoris								
Whites	1960–1976	Urban population	26,460	1.19	0.64	1.83	Nonsyndromic	Chapman (1983)

*CL/P, cleft lip with or without cleft palate; CP, cleft palate.
†Data not available.

TABLE 12.IE. *International Epidemiology of Oral Clefts—Far East**

Population	Time Period	Sources of Ascertainment	No. of Births	Birth prevalence				Associated Abnormalities	Reference
				CLP	CP	All Clefts			
China									
Hong Kong	n.d.	Hospital births	9876	—[†]	—	1.62			Stevenson et al. (1966)
	Oct 1986–Sept 1987	945 hospitals	1,243,284	1.67	0.15	1.82		Nonsyndromic	Xiao (1989)
Shanghai	1980–1989	Population-based cohort	541,504	1.2	—	—		Nonsyndromic	Cooper et al. (2000)
Japan									
Osaka	n.d.	Hospital birth records	16,373	—	—	2.41			Tsutsui (1951)
Tokyo	1922–1940	Hospital	49,645	1.17	0.73	1.90		Included	Mitani (1954)
	1922–1952	Hospital birth records	80,423	—	—	1.89			Mitani (1954)
	1922–1955	Questionnaire to hospitals	114,815	—	—	2.05			Tsukamoto (1956)
	1940–1956	Hospital birth records	46,635	—	—	2.08			Kobayasi (1958)
Nagasaki	1948–1952	Survey of ABCC	27,016	—	—	2.48			Hikita (1953)
Hiroshima, Nagasaki	1948–1954	Survey of ABCC	63,976 (excluding multiple births)	2.13	0.55	2.68		Included	Neel (1958)
Okayama	1953–1960	Hospital birth records	35,366	—	—	1.64			Kurozumi (1963)
	1957–1961	Questionnaire to hospitals	280,000	—	—	1.65			Sato (1966)
Hokkaido	1965–1967	Questionnaire to hospitals	105,586	—	—	1.79			Tanaka (1972)
	1979–1982	Hospital LB only	55,103	0.97	0.29	1.26		Nonsyndromic	Kondo (1987)
Aichi	1982	293 hospitals	40,304	1.02	0.27	1.29			Natsume et al. (1987)
	1983	Hospital	39,696	1.43	0.21	1.64		Nonsyndromic	Natsume and Kawai (1986)

Population	Years	Source	Sample size				Comment	Reference
Malaysia (Kuala Lumpur, *Chinese*)	n.d.	Hospital births	16,026	—	—	1.56	Included 21% at birth	Stevenson et al. (1966)
Philippines	1989–1996	Medical records	47,969	1.94	No data	No data		Murray et al. (1997)
Singapore	1985–1994	Hospital LB only	474,542	1.59	0.48	2.07	All-inclusive 1.5% of clefts	Yi et al. (1999)
Chinese	n.d.	Hospital births	39,655	—	—	1.74		Stevenson et al. (1966)
	1986–1987	Hospital	33,672	1.04	0.53	1.57	Nonsyndromic	Tan (1988)
	1986–1987	Hospital	30,411	1.15	0.59	1.74		Tan (1988)
Taiwan *Chinese*	1955–1962	Hospital births	14,583	—	—	1.92		Wei and Chen (1965)
Chinese	1965–1968	Hospital births	25,517	—	—	1.45		Emanuel et al. (1972)
Taipei	Jan 1965–Jan 1968	6 hospitals LB + SB >28 weeks	25,814	1.29	0.16	1.45	35%	Emanuel et al. (1972)
Thailand (Sirirai Hospital)	1990–1996	Hospital records	130,236	1.22	0.40	1.62	Included 4.38%	Chuangsuwanich et al. (1998)

*CL/P, cleft lip with or without cleft palate; CP, cleft palate; LB, live births; SB, stillbirths; ABCC, Atomic Bomb Casualty Committee; n.d., not defined.
†Data not available.

TABLE 12.IF. *International Epidemiology of Oral Clefts—Middle East**

Population	Time Period	Sources of Ascertainment	No. of Births	Birth prevalence			Associated Abnormalities	Reference
				CL/P	CP	All Clefts		
Iran								
Tehran	Aug 1976–Sept 1991	Hospital (surgical cases)	19,369 LB only	0.85	0.18	1.03	7.73%	Rajabian and Sherkat (2000)
Tehran	1983–1988	One hospital	21,138	3.12	0.62	3.74	Chemical sulfur mustard gas implicated in CL/P	Taher (1992)
Israel								
Jews	1960–1962	6 hospitals	47,768	0.37	0.17	0.54	27%	Azaz and Koyoumdjisky-Kaye (1967)
Whites	1961–1971	Multiple sources	218,750	—†	—	0.80		Tal et al. (1974)
Kuwait	1985–1987	Population	53,786	1.06	0.42	1.48	Nonsyndromic	Srivastava and Bang (1990)
Saudi Arabia	1989–1992	Hospital-based	62,577	1.89	0.30	2.19	CP 21.5% CL/P	Borkar et al. (1993)
United Arab Emirates	1998	Hospital-based LB + SB	7500	0.40	0.27	0.67	Included	ICBDMS (2000)

*CL/P, cleft lip with or without cleft palate; CP, cleft palate; LB, live births; SB, stillbirths.
†Data not available.

TABLE 12.IG. *International Epidemiology of Oral Clefts—Indian Subcontinent**

Population	Time Period	Sources of Ascertainment	No. of Births	Birth prevalence CL/P	CP	All Clefts	Associated Abnormalities	Reference
India	Various prospective and retrospective studies	Hospital-based LB+ SB (meta-analysis)	224,341	1.20	0.44	1.64		Verma and Mathews (1983)
Bombay	June 1960–Dec 1963	Pregnancy terminations	24,248	1.59	—[†]	—		Master-Notani et al. (1968)
Calicut	Jan 1962–May 1964	Hospital	3721	1.61	—	1.61 (6 clefts)	Included	Nair and Mathai (1964)
Lucknow	Sept 1963–Oct 1964	Hospital LB + SB	2851	—	—	1.40 (4 clefts)	Included	Sharma et al. (1972)
Patna	1 March 1964–30 Nov 1964	Hospital-based	5376	1.50	—	—		Khanna and Prasad (1967)
Jaipur	Jan 1965–Dec 1969	Hospital LB only	28,511	—	—	0.70	Included	Hemrajani et al. (1971)
Kanpur	Feb 1967–April 1968	Hospital LB + SB	4150	0.96	0.48	1.44 (6 clefts)	Included	Mital and Grewal (1969)
Rajastan	1969	Hospital LB + SB	2145	0.93 (2 clefts)	—	—		Gupta et al. (1971)
New Delhi	Dec 1969–March 1973	Hospital LB only	7590	1.05	—	—		Ghosh et al. (1985)
New Delhi	1975–1978	Hospital LB only	6274	1.43 (9 clefts)	0.32 (2 clefts)	1.75	Included	Singh and Sharma (1980)
Hyderabad	April–July 1970	Hospital LB + SB	1060	1.75	0.9	2.65 (4 clefts)	Included 2 SB	Mathur et al. (1975)
Madras	1975–1976	Hospital LB + SB	24,192	—	—	1.71 (28 clefts)	Included	Chandra and Harilal (1977)
Haryana	Jan 1976–Dec 1977	Population LB only	2409	0.41	0.41	0.82 (2 clefts)	Included	Kulshrestha et al. (1983)
Madurai	Jan 1976–July 1977	Hospital-based	11,619	0.77	—	—		Kamala et al. (1978)
Hubli	1 July 1976–30 Sept 1977	Hospital LB + SB	2398	1.25 (3 clefts)	—	—		Goravalingappa and Nashi (1979)
Calcutta	1976–1980	Hospital LB + SB + terminations	21,016	—	—	0.62		Choudhury et al. (1984)
Malda	1976–1987	6 hospitals LB + SB	126,266	—	—	0.74		Choudhury et al. (1989)
Maharashtra	April 1985–March 1986	Hospital LB + SB	3014	2.32	—	2.32	Nonsyndromic	Chaturvedi and Banerjee (1989)

*CL/P, cleft lip with or without cleft palate; CP, cleft palate; LB, live births; SB, stillbirths.
[†]Data not available.

TABLE 12.IH. *International Epidemiology of Oral Clefts—Africa**

Population	Time Period	Sources of Ascertainment	No. of Births	Birth prevalence			Associated Abnormalities	Reference
				CL/P	CP	All Clefts		
Nairobi	1 Nov 1963–30 April 1964	Hospital-based	3061	1.63	0.33	1.96		Khan (1965)
Nigeria	1 Feb–31 July 1964	Adeoyo Hospital	4220	0.47	0.24	0.71		Gupta (1969)
Lagos	1966–1967	Hospital LB + SB	16,720	0.36	—†	0.36 (5 clefts)	Included	Lesi (1969)
	1976–1980	Clinical exam at birth	21,624	0.30	0.07	0.37	18%	Iregbulem (1982)
	1976–1980	Hospital records	973,236	0.3	0.07	0.37	Included	Iregbulem (1982)
Zaria	1976–1980	Hospital	23,512	0.21	0.08	0.29	Included	Harrison et al. (1985)
South Africa (Johannesburg, *blacks*)	Jan 1976–Dec 1977	Hospital-based	29,633	0.20	0.10	0.30	22%	Kromberg and Jenkins (1982)
Tunisia	4 Oct 1983–16 July 1984	Hospital LB + SB	10,000	1.00	0.40	1.40		Khrouf et al. (1986)
Zaire	Jan 1970–Dec 1980	Hospital	64,777	—	—	1.20	Nonsyndromic	Tandu-Umba et al. (1984)
	Oct 1977–June 1979	Hospital LB only	56,637	0.44	0.02	0.46	Nonsyndromic	Ogle (1993)
Zimbabwe	March–July 1984	Hospital	18,033	—	—	0.16	Included	Shija and Kingo (1985)

*CL/P, cleft lip with or without cleft palate; CP, cleft palate; LB, live births; SB, stillbirths.
†Data not available.

APPENDIX 12.II. TIME TRENDS FOR ORAL CLEFT PREVALENCE IN EUROPE

TABLE 12.II. *Time Trends in Birth Prevalence of Cleft Palate (CP) and Cleft Lip with or without Cleft Palate (CL/P) from Overlapping Time Periods in Consecutive EUROCAT Reports (EUROCAT 1995 = 1980–1992, EUROCAT 1996 = 1990–1994)*

Population	Time Period	Birth prevalence		
		CL/P	CP	All Clefts
Belgium				
Antwerp	1980–1992/1990–1994	0.97/1.00	0.35/0.30	1.32/1.30
Hainaut-Namur	1980–1992/1990–1994	1.19/1.26	0.61/0.75	1.80/2.01
Denmark (Odense)	1980–1992/1990–1994	1.59/1.29	0.75/0.78	2.34/2.07
France				
Bouches-du-Rhone	1980–1992/1990–1994	0.87/0.74	0.85/0.86	1.72/1.60
Paris	1980–1992/1990–1994	0.78/0.97	0.47/0.62	1.25/1.59
Strasbourg	1980–1992/1990–1994	1.01/1.25	0.86/0.88	1.87/2.13
Northern Ireland (Belfast)	1980–1992/1990–1994	0.72/0.33	0.61/0.25	1.33/0.58
Ireland				
Dublin	1980–1992/1990–1994	0.88/0.88	0.70/0.75	1.58/1.63
Galway	1980–1992/1990–1994	0.78/0.62	0.47/0.54	1.25/1.16
Italy (Tuscany)	1980–1992/1990–1994	0.75/0.82	0.58/0.43	1.33/1.25
Malta	1980–1992/1990–1994	0.45/0.65	0.53/0.84	0.98/1.49
Northern Netherlands	1980–1992/1990–1994	1.52/1.53	0.66/0.72	2.18/2.25
Spain				
Asturias	1980–1992/1990–1994	0.65/0.82	0.61/0.63	1.26/1.45
Basque Country	1980–1992/1990–1994	0.57/0.55	0.43/0.49	1.00/1.04
Switzerland	1980–1992/1990–1994	0.86/0.87	0.66/0.65	1.52/1.43
United Kingdom				
Glasgow	1980–1992/1990–1994	0.65/0.87	0.84/0.94	1. 49/1.93

Sources of ascertainment, regional population-based registry. Associated anomalies: live births, stillbirths, and induced abortions.

APPENDIX 12.III. BIRTH PREVALENCE OF ORAL CLEFTS IN SELECTED U.S. STATES

TABLE 12.III. *Birth Defect Surveillance Data from Selected U.S. States, 1989–1996**

| | | | | Birth prevalence | | | | |
| | | | | White | | Other | | |
Population	Time Period	Sources of Ascertainment	No. of Births	CL/P	CP	CL/P	CP	All Clefts
Alaska	1996	NBDP LB only	10,041	0.75	0.45	0.30	0.90	1.18
Arizona	1989–1991	NBDP LB only	203,982	1.12	0.49	1.79	0.62	1.73
Arkansas	1993–1996	NBDP LB + SB	141,666	1.26	0.78	1.12	0.56	1.96
California	1989–1995	NBDP LB + SB	2,021,110	1.00	0.75	1.08	0.66	1.73
Colorado	1989–1995	NBDP LB + SB	435,615	1.15	0.80	0.88	0.82	1.98
Connecticut	1993–1994	NBDP LB only	92,453	0.80	1.00	0.46	0.83	1.66
Georgia	1989–1996	NBDP LB only	313,404	1.19	0.58	0.67	0.57	1.51
Hawaii	1989–1996	NBDP LB + SB	167,354	0.79	0.73	1.03	1.18	2.01
Illinois	1989–1996	NBDP LB + SB	1,530,996	0.65	0.41	0.42	0.26	0.96
Iowa	1989–1995	NBDP LB, SB, + terminations	306,265	1.20	0.62	1.10	0.62	1.89
Maryland	1989–1995	NBDP LB + SB	564,152	0.66	0.43	0.53	0.22	0.97
Massachusetts	1994–1996	NBDP LB + SB	246,538	0.65	0.48	1.51	1.33	1.35
Missouri	1989–1996	NBDP LB only	606,325	1.18	0.58	0.76	0.36	1.64
Nebraska	1989–1996	NBDP LB + SB	189,863	1.12	0.82	1.30	0.42	1.90
Nevada	1989–1996	NBDP LB + SB	182,744	0.97		0.67		0.91
New Jersey	1989–1996	NBDP LB only	951,117	0.72	0.69	0.72	0.52	1.39
New Mexico	1995–1996	NBDP LB + SB	55,464	1.57	0.14	0.29		1.91
New York	1989–1996	NBDP LB only	2,263,026	0.75	0.58	0.46	0.40	1.21
North Carolina	1989–1996	NBDP LB + SB	726,358	0.96	0.52	0.62	0.58	1.38
Ohio	1989–1996	NBDP LB + SB	1,488,493	1.00		0.34		—†
Oklahoma	1994–1996	NBDP LB + SB	138,100	1.21	0.71	1.50	0.77	1.99
South Carolina	1989–1996	NBDP LB + SB	441,488	0.96		0.43		—
Tennessee	1991–1993	NBDP LB + SB	222,073	0.80	0.31	0.48	0.21	1.05
Texas	1995	NBDP LB + SB	112,620	1.27	0.96	0.07	0.03	1.59
Utah	1994–1996	NBDP LB + SB	120,554	0.97	0.45	2.39	0.80	1.51
Virginia	1989–1996	NBDP LB, SB, + terminations	1,053,667	—	—	—	—	1.30
Wisconsin	1989–1995	NBDP LB + SB	563,141	1.62	1.51	1.31	1.56	3.01

*CL/P, cleft lip with or without cleft palate; CP, cleft palate; LB, live births; SB, stillbirths; NBDP, National Birth Defects Prevention Network.

†Data not available.

Source: National Birth Defects Prevention Network (2000).

13

Environmental risk factors and oral clefts

CATHERINE HAYES

Although the literature regarding the etiology of oral clefts is extensive, unique causal factors remain unknown. The widely held belief is that oral clefts are of multifactorial etiology, with both genetic predisposition and environmental influence playing a role. In this chapter, the term *environmental* is used in its broadest sense to include characteristics of the individual, such as age, sex, and race; behaviors, such as smoking and alcohol use; as well as other exposures, such as occupational or environmental ones. While no strong risk factors for oral clefts have been identified, several potential environmental risk factors have been investigated, including smoking, alcohol, caffeine, benzodiazepines, and corticosteroids. In evaluating the role of specific risk factors or a category of risk factors in epidemiology, several criteria are examined for causality. These include consistency, strength of association, biologic plausibility, temporal sequence, and dose-response relationship. Often, there is a remarkable lack of consistency for several of the risk factors discussed in this chapter. Also, many of the measures of association are not strong. In addition, usually there is little information regarding the temporal sequence between exposure and outcome. A dose–response relationship can seldom be demonstrated. Therefore, making inferences about the causality of oral clefts is largely an inconclusive task. In this chapter, the current evidence regarding the role of environmental risk factors in the etiology of oral clefts is discussed.

MATERNAL CIGARETTE SMOKING

Several studies examining the association between maternal cigarette smoking and oral clefts have found con-

flicting results. While some have concluded that smokers are more likely to have a child with an oral cleft (Ericson et al., 1979; Khoury et al., 1987, 1989; Shaw et al., 1996), others have not demonstrated a positive, statistically significant association (Saxen, 1975; Seidman et al., 1990; Kelsey et al., 1978; Evans, 1979; Werler et al., 1990; Lieff et al., 1999). A meta-analysis of these studies concluded that the overall odds ratio (OR) for cleft lip with or without cleft palate (CL/P) was 1.29 [95% confidence interval (CI) 1.18–1.42] and that for CP was 1.32 (95% CI 1.10–1.62), indicating a weak association between maternal smoking and oral clefts (Wyszynski et al., 1997).

In some of these studies, positive associations were found for some, but not all, oral cleft groups. This is not unexpected as it is often seen in studies of oral clefting; i.e., a risk factor may be associated with one type of cleft (e.g., CL/P) but not another [e.g., cleft palate (CP)]. This inconsistency is most likely related to the fact that oral clefts represent a heterogeneous group of anomalies. Therefore, specific environmental factors may not have the same effect on the various subgroups. Also, the sample sizes in the subgroups are typically unequal, resulting in a difference in the statistical power to detect an effect, if one exists.

A gene–environment interaction has been proposed in the occurrence of oral clefts in children with the rare allele C2 of the transforming growth factor α *(TGF-α)* gene born to women who smoked during pregnancy (Hwang et al., 1995; Shaw et al., 1996; Beaty et al., 1997; Romitti et al., 1999). This provided the first empirical evidence for the multifactorial etiology of oral clefts. More details on this may be found in Chapter 23.

In a study conducted in Sweden, infants with CL/P born between 1983 and 1992 (*n* = 1834) were identified from the Swedish Registry of Congenital Malformations and the Medical Birth Registry. Smoking was recorded as none, <10 cigarettes/day, or ≥10 cigarettes/day. Four groups of oral clefts were evaluated: cleft lip (CL), CL/P, CP, and the Robin sequence. A statistically significant increased risk was observed for isolated CP with an OR of 1.35 and a 95% CI of 1.12–1.63 (Kallen, 1997).

Khoury et al. (1987, 1989) consistently reported an increased risk for oral clefts among smokers in two reports using data from the Maryland Birth Defects Reporting and Information System. In both studies, cases were ascertained at birth and reported by hospitals on a special form that included demographic information, obstetric variables, and prenatal illnesses and exposures. Smoking history was obtained by an obstetric nurse directly from the mother by asking (1) "Did you smoke at any time during pregnancy?" and (2) "If yes, how many cigarettes a day (1–5, 6–10, 11–20, >20)." Statistically significant increased risks were obtained for both CL/P (OR = 1.55, 95% CI 1.10–2.18) and CP (OR = 1.96, 95% CI 1.10–3.50) in the latter study and for CL/P (OR = 3.33, 95% CI 1.3–8.4) in the former.

In another case-control study, mothers were interviewed within 6 months of delivery. This study included 400 cases with CL/P and 215 cases with CP compared to 2710 controls with other malformations (Werler et al., 1990). Smokers were categorized into the following groups: 1–14, 15–24, or ≥25 cigarettes/day. No statistically significant increased ORs were observed for any cleft category after adjustment for age, education, race, maternal alcohol use, vitamin A supplementation, and medical and reproductive histories. Adjusted ORs were 0.70 (95% CI 0.3–1.6) for CL/P and 0.80 (95% CI 0.3–2.2) for CP. In a later extension of this study (Lieff et al., 1999), no significant increased risk for oral clefts were seen among cases in the highest smoking level. Adjusted ORs were 0.91 (95% CI 0.63–1.32) for CL/P and 0.99 (95% CI 0.54–1.91) for CP.

A large prospective cohort study resulted in no statistically significant increase in risk for smoking in either subcategory of clefts (Shiono et al., 1986). In this study, information was obtained from the Kaiser-Permanente Birth Defects Study and the Collaborative Perinatal Project. Smoking status was ascertained by self-report when women were seen for routine prenatal care. In the Kaiser-Permanente Birth Defects study, women were categorized as to smoking status and information regarding congenital malformations was ascertained from medical charts, discharge diagnoses, neonatologists' notes, and autopsy reports. In the Collaborative Perinatal Project, pregnancy outcomes were ascertained by physician examination conducted at birth, 4 months, and 1 year, as well as from medical

and autopsy reports. A total of 54 congenital anomalies were evaluated in the pregnancy outcomes of 86,946 live births. The OR for CL/P was 1.1 (95% CI 0.5–2.4) based on 22 cases and that for 0.7 CP was (95% CI 0.3–1.8) based on 19 cases. These results may be due to insufficient power in both study groups.

In a population-based case-control study from the Washington State Birth Registry, no statistically significant increased risk for oral clefts was observed (Van den Eeden et al., 1990). Smoking information was collected from birth certificate data and categorized as "yes/no," which likely resulted in misclassification bias. This information was available for 96% of controls and 97% of cases. One hundred five isolated CL/P and 37 CP cases were included in the analysis. Adjusted ORs were 1.5 (95% CI 1.0–2.3) for CL/P and 1.2 (95% CI 0.6–2.5) for CP.

In a multicenter case-control study (Lorente et al., 2000b), the ORs for first-trimester maternal smoking were 1.79 (95% CI 1.07–3.04) for CL/P and 0.86 (95% CI 0.40–1.87) for CP. Smoking was categorized as regular smokers, never smokers, and ex-smokers; however, modest information was provided on how smoking history was ascertained. In addition, only 63% of eligible cases were interviewed, thereby limiting the interpretation and generalizability of the results.

Data from the U.S. Natality database of 1996 were evaluated in a case-control study (Chung et al., 2000). Information was available for 3,891,494 births, including 2207 cases with oral clefts. Controls (n = 4414) were randomly selected from newborns without congenital anomalies. The database included maternal demographic information, maternal health risk factors, and infant health characteristics. Smoking history, as well as the number of cigarettes smoked per day during pregnancy, was recorded in the database. The smoking categories were none, 1–10, 11–20, and >21 cigarettes/day. The overall adjusted OR for CL/P was 1.34 (95% CI 1.16–1.54), with dose-response rates reported for the three smoking categories of 1.50 (95% CI 1.28–1.76), 1.55 (95% CI 1.23–1.95), and 1.78 (95% CI 1.22–2.59), respectively. Unfortunately, birth certificates from the U.S. Natality database do not discriminate between CL/P and CP. This represents the largest study to date examining the association between smoking and oral clefts.

Overall, the results of the studies described above are inconsistent (Table 13.1). These inconsistencies are likely due to different study designs, case definitions, exposure assessments, and timing of exposure. The evidence to date suggests that maternal cigarette smoking during the first trimester of gestation may be weakly associated with risk of oral clefting in the offspring. However, considering the number of women who

TABLE 13.1. *Adjusted Odds Ratios (95% CIs) for Highest Smoking Category and Isolated Oral Clefts*

Reference	CL/P	CP
Saxen (1974)	1.81 (0.89–3.78)	1.59 (0.75–3.45)
Ericson et al. (1979)	2.73 (1.21–6.32)	2.29 (0.43–15.63)
Shiono et al. (1986)	1.1 (0.5–2.4)	0.7 (0.3–1.8)
Khoury et al. (1987)	3.33 (1.3–8.4)	1.82 (.67–4.9)
Khoury et al. (1989)	1.55 (1.10–2.18)	1.96 (1.10–3.50)
Van den Eeden et al. (1990)	1.5 (1.0–2.3)	1.2 (0.6–2.5)
Werler et al. (1990)	0.7 (0.3–1.6)	0.8 (0.3–2.2)
Beaty et al. (1997)	1.96 (0.84–4.59)	1.76 (0.73–4.26)
Kallen (1997)	1.13 (0.99–1.29)	1.35 (1.12–1.63)
Romitti et al. (1999)	1.3 (0.7–2.3)	2.3 (1.1–4.6)
Christensen et al. (1999)	1.4 (0.99–2.00)	0.87 (0.5–1.52)
Lieff et al. (1999)	0.91 (0.63–1.32)	0.99 (0.54–1.81)

*CL/P, cleft lip with or without cleft palate; CP, cleft palate; CI, confidence interval.

smoke during pregnancy, even a weak association would have a significant public health impact.

ALCOHOL

Several studies have examined the association between maternal alcohol intake and oral clefts in the offspring. For example, Werler and colleagues (1990) explored the association between maternal alcohol use and defects in neural crest–derived structures/tissues of the ear, face, anterior neck, and heart. The number of drinking days per week, as well as the average number of drinks in a drinking day, were recorded separately for beer, wine, and liquor during the first 4 lunar months of pregnancy. Data were collected between 1983 and 1987. Cases were defined as infants with defects of neural crest–derived structures/tissues such as the face, ear, mouth, anterior neck, thymus, thyroid, parathyroid, branchial arch arteries, ventricular septum, and truncus. Cases associated with known Mendelian disorders were excluded. A total of 1464 cases were available for analysis. Controls were infants with malformations of non-neural crest–derived tissues. Three measures of alcohol exposure were used: *(1)* maximum number of drinks in any 1 day (maximum intensity), *(2)* number of drinking days per week (average frequency), and *(3)* number of drinks per drinking day (average intensity). Mothers who consumed at least one drink were compared to mothers who drank less than one drink. The reference category included mothers who reported no intake or a fraction of a drink. Logistic regression analysis was used to estimate

relative risks, adjusting for mother's age, smoking history, race, religion, seizure history, diabetes, stillbirth, pregnancy history of rubella or measles, and family history of malformation in first-degree relatives. Consumption of alcohol at the highest level, defined as an average of 5 or more drinks per day on five or more drinking days, was more frequent among cases than controls. The only statistically significant increased risk was seen among CL/P cases in the highest intake category, five or more drinks per drinking day (OR = 3.0, 95% CI 1.1–8.5). Although no significant increase in risk for CP was demonstrated, there were almost twice as many CL/P cases ($n = 333$) as CP cases ($n = 188$). Statistical power might have been too modest in the latter group.

In a population-based case-control study conducted in Iowa between 1987 and 1991, cases were obtained from the Iowa Birth Defects registry. The registry includes data on birth defects diagnosed during the first year of life among infants born to Iowa residents (Munger et al., 1996). Ascertainment sources for cases included medical records of all Iowa hospitals, hospitals of neighboring states serving Iowa residents, and prenatal clinics. Diagnoses were confirmed by a medical record specialist, nurse geneticist, and two board-certified geneticists. Cases were selected from all live births, stillbirths, and aborted fetuses. Controls were randomly selected from all Iowa-resident live births listed with the Iowa Department of Public Health. Alcohol use was obtained via telephone interview and reported as number of drinks per month. Mothers were questioned as to alcohol use during the period of 3 months before pregnancy until the end of pregnancy.

Alcohol intake was categorized as 1–3, 4–10, or >10 drinks per month. Participation rates were 74% for cases and 54.6% for controls. More mothers with lower levels of education were non-participants, potentially introducing bias if they had higher levels of alcohol intake. The only statistically significant increased risk was observed in the highest alcohol consumption group (>10 drinks/month) for isolated CL/P ($n = 118$), with an OR of 4.0 (95% CI 1.1–15.1). In the CL/P group, no significant ORs were recorded for the lower consumption groups (4–10 drinks/month, OR = 3.5, 95% CI 0.8–15.4; 1–3 drinks/month, OR = 1.5, 95% CI 0.9–2.4). No significant increased risk for isolated CP ($n = 56$) was demonstrated for any of the alcohol intake levels. The models were adjusted for household income, maternal education, maternal smoking, maternal vitamin use, and gender of the child. However, for CL/P the χ^2 test for trend was statistically significant, indicating increased risk with increasing alcohol exposure.

In a population-based case-control study of California births from 1987 to 1989, cases were ascertained by review of hospital and genetic center records (Shaw and Lammer, 1999). Cases were diagnosed within 1 year after birth, and controls were randomly selected from all live-born infants from the same geographic area as the cases born during the same time period. Telephone interviews were completed with 734 case mothers (84.7%) and 732 controls (78.2%). Women were asked to report information regarding exposures during the period of 1 month before pregnancy until 3 months after conception. They were asked how often during this period they had any alcoholic beverage, including wine, beer, whiskey, or any other alcoholic drink. Responses were categorized as never, 1–3 during the 4-month critical window period, 1–3/month, 1–4/week, or every day. Those who reported any drink were further asked how often they had five or more drinks at one sitting. No increased risk for oral clefts was found among those categorized as having low alcohol consumption (less than weekly, weekly, daily). However, for those who reported consuming five or more drinks per drinking occasion, the ORs were significantly elevated for isolated CL/P ($n = 348$, OR = 3.4, 95% CI 1.1–9.7), for CL/P associated with other malformations ($n = 99$, OR = 4.6, 95% CI 1.2–18.8), and for oral clefts occurring with known syndromes ($n = 69$, OR = 6.9, 95% CI 1.9–28.6). There was no significant increased risk for isolated CP (OR = 1.0, 95% CI 0.23–8.5). There were no infants with CP associated with other malformations in the highest intake category.

Another population-based case-control study in Iowa (Romitti et al., 1999) showed a significant increase in risk of CL/P among women reporting ≥4 drinks/month during the periconceptional period. Alcohol exposure was ascertained for the period of 3 months before conception to 9 months following conception. Information regarding the number of days per month and the typical number of drinks consumed on those days was used to calculate the maximum number of drinks consumed in a 24 h period. Cases were ascertained through the Iowa Birth Defects registry from 1987 to 1994. Controls were selected from all eligible Iowa live births during the same time period. Information on alcohol intake was assessed for the 1-month period prior to pregnancy through the 9-month period following conception. Women were asked to detail the number of days per month that they consumed alcohol, the typical number of drinks per day, and the maximum number of drinks consumed in a 24 h interval. The average number of drinks per month was then determined for each subject. Response rates were 64% ($n = 142$) for cases and 60.6% ($n = 230$) for controls. For CL/P, the ORs for women who reported one to three drinks/month were 1.3 (95% CI 0.9–2.0) and for those who reported four or more drinks per month 2.8 (95% CI 1.2–6.6). For CP, the ORs were 1.1 (95% CI 0.6–1.9) and 1.7 (95% CI 0.5–6.4), respectively.

In a multicenter case-control study in four European countries (France, United Kingdom, Italy, and The Netherlands), cases were defined as any live-born or stillborn child or fetus with a major congenital malformation diagnosed prenatally or during the perinatal period (birth to 6 days) (Lorente et al., 2000b). Controls were born immediately after cases and identified in maternity wards or from birth records. Sixty-three percent of eligible case mothers were interviewed. Alcohol intake was assessed via personal interview in the hospital after birth. Alcohol consumption was dichotomized as <70 g or ≥70 g per week. Ex-drinkers included those who reported drinking one drink per day up until a few weeks before pregnancy and who reported stopping at the beginning of pregnancy. The only statistically significant increased risk was for CP (OR = 2.28, 95% CI 1.02–5.09). This increase was significant for isolated CP as well as for CP associated with other anomalies. This finding was not consistent with the studies discussed above, which showed no increased risk for CP.

Each of the above studies used different definitions for highest alcohol intake, ranging from ≥4 drinks/month to ≥5 drinks/drinking occasion (Table 13.2). Despite these differences, these studies consistently demonstrated, with one exception (Lorente et al., 2000b), an increased risk for CL/P with high alcohol intake, with significant point estimates ranging from 2.8 to 4.0. The fact that there was no increased risk

TABLE 13.2. *Adjusted Odds Ratios (95% CIs) for Highest Alcohol Intake Category and Isolated Oral Clefts**

Reference	Level of Alcohol Intake	CL/P (95% CI)	CP (95% CI)
Werler et al. (1991)	≥5 drinks/drinking day	3.0 (1.1–8.5)	0.9 (0.1–7.2)
Munger et al. (1996)	>10 drinks/month	4.0 (1.1–15.1)	1.8 (0.3–12.1)
Shaw and Lammer (1999)	≥5 drinks ≥once/week	3.4 (1.1–9.7)	1.0 (0.23–8.5)
Romitti et al. (1999)	≥4 drinks per month	2.8 (1.2–6.6)	1.7 (0.5–6.4)

*CL/P, cleft lip with or without cleft palate; CP, cleft palate; CI, confidence interval.

demonstrated for CP in all but one study may be explained by inadequate statistical power to detect an increased risk.

CAFFEINE

Only one case-control study has examined the association between caffeine and oral clefts (Rosenberg et al., 1982). In this study, information on beverage consumption was obtained by asking mothers about their daily consumption of decaffeinated coffee, coffee containing caffeine, tea, cola, and other soft drinks during pregnancy. Those who drank between one and four cups during their entire pregnancy were classified as "occasional drinkers," and those who drank between five and six cups per week were considered "daily drinkers." A total of 2030 mothers of malformed infants were interviewed between March 1976 and December 1980. Caffeine consumption was estimated by summing the intake from tea (35 mg), caffeinated coffee (100 mg), and cola (45 mg). There were 299 cases of CL/P and 120 of CP, which were compared to 712 controls with other malformations. Caffeine consumption, examined separately for cola, tea, and coffee, was categorized as none, 1–2, or ≥3 beverages/day or occasional use. Overall daily caffeine consumption was categorized as none, 1–199 mg, 200–399 mg, or ≥400 mg. None of the ORs were significantly greater than 1.0, indicating that caffeine use is not associated with oral clefts. However, no definitive conclusion should be made based on a single study.

EPILEPSY

Epileptic women are at increased risk of having a child with an oral cleft (Niswander and Wertelecki, 1973; Dronamraju et al., 1970; Speidel and Meadow, 1972; Monson et al., 1973; Friis, 1979; Hecht et al., 1989; Abrishamchian et al., 1994). It is unclear if it is the epilepsy per se, the drug therapy used to treat the epilepsy, or an underlying genetic link between epilepsy and clefting that accounts for this increased prevalence of clefting disorders among children of epileptic women. Use of anticonvulsants, several of which are known folic acid antagonists, may affect the developing fetus, resulting in congenital malformations, most notably oral clefts (Meadow et al., 1970; Millar and Nevin, 1973; Monson et al., 1973; Kelly et al., 1984; Dansky et al., 1992). Although some authors have pointed out that it may be the mother's epilepsy and not the use of anticonvulsants that leads to the formation of oral clefts, this has not been adequately demonstrated (Dronamraju, 1970; Monson et al., 1973; Friis, 1979; Friis et al., 1981; Kelly et al., 1984). Further, there may be a genetic relationship between epilepsy and oral clefts (Durner et al., 1992).

A review of studies investigating clefts among families with a history of epilepsy found that there was no familial occurrence of clefts in individuals with epilepsy (Hecht and Annegers, 1990). A case-control study by Abrishamchian et al. (1994) demonstrated an increased risk for CL/P among women with epilepsy (OR = 3.78, 95% CI 1.65–7.88). A statistically significant increased risk for CP, however, was not demonstrated.

An increased risk associated with drug therapy for epilepsy during pregnancy was demonstrated, especially for polytherapy, with a 10-fold increased risk for CL/P (OR = 10.5, 95% CI 1.52–59.9). These results come from a population-based study and might represent the most convincing evidence to date of an association between epilepsy, its treatment, and oral clefts. The authors pointed out, however, that the attributable risks for clefts associated with epilepsy and its treatment are very low (3.3% for CL/P and 0.9% for CP). The association between antiepileptic drugs and oral clefts may be related to the fact that many antiepileptic drugs reduce plasma folate levels (Schwaninger et al., 1999).

Although the underlying mechanism for the development of oral clefts in the offspring of women with seizure disorders is not well understood, the risk of having a child with an oral cleft among women with seizures has been reported to be four to 11 times that of women with no seizure disorders (Dansky and Finnell, 1991). The conflicting reports, however, make it difficult to draw any strong conclusions as to whether it is the use of anticonvulsants by epileptic women during early pregnancy that increases the risk of having a child with an oral cleft. The lack of evidence for a strong familial occurrence may lead to the conclusion that an environmental influence plays a significant role in the association between epilepsy and oral clefts. In summary, the data suggest a strong association between seizure disorders in the mother, and perhaps the use of medications to treat them, and the occurrence of oral clefts in the offspring.

BENZODIAZEPINES

Use of benzodiazepines during pregnancy and oral clefts in the offspring has been the subject of several reports. Benzodiazepines are prescribed to decrease anxiety, induce sedation, and treat eclampsia and pre-eclampsia (Bergman et al., 1992). In one of the first analytical epidemiologic studies, information was obtained from the Metropolitan Atlanta Birth Defects Program (Safra and Oakley, 1975). Drug use information was collected through open-ended questionnaires with specific questions regarding the use of "tranquilizers." Mothers were also shown a card with samples of several tranquilizers, e.g., chlordiazepoxide (Librium), diazepam (Valium), prochlorperazine (Compazine), amitriptyline (Elavil), and haloperidol (Haldol). All interviews were completed within 4 months after delivery. Cases were mothers of infants with CL/P, and controls were mothers of infants with other congenital anomalies. Increased risks for first-trimester use of diazepam were demonstrated for all CL/P cases (OR = 4.1, 95% CI 1.5–11.5) as well as isolated CL/P (OR = 4.9, 95% CI 1.6–14.7).

In another case-control study (Rosenberg et al., 1983), no association was demonstrated between use of diazepam during pregnancy and oral clefts. Due to the timing of oral cleft development, the authors did not include first exposure to diazepam after the fourth lunar month in their exposed category. In this study, there were 445 CL/P cases, 166 CP cases, and 2498 controls. The control group consisted of mothers of infants with other malformations. Reported exposure to diazepam during the first 4 lunar months of pregnancy was compared between case subgroups and controls. No statistically significant increased risk was observed for any oral cleft subgroup. All relative risks approximated 1.0.

A study conducted in Hungary from 1980 to 1984 did not demonstrate an increased risk for oral clefts among women exposed to benzodiazepines during pregnancy (Czeizel, 1987). In this study, 630 cases with CL/P and 179 cases with CP were compared to matched controls with no significant increase in risk for any oral cleft demonstrated regardless of timing of diazepam use during pregnancy.

A prospective study reported no increase in risk of oral clefts for first-trimester diazepam use for any oral cleft (OR = 1.22, 95% CI 0.17–8.95) (Shiono and Mills, 1984). In a case-control study (Laegreid et al.,1990), benzodiazepine use was assessed by serum analysis from blood samples taken in early pregnancy (prior to 12 weeks). Eighteen cases of congenital malformation were compared to 60 controls. Of these, six cases were classified as CLP. The OR for exposure to benzodiazepines during early pregnancy was 14.5 (p = 0.04). A subgroup analysis was not presented, nor was it clearly stated whether these were isolated clefts or clefts associated with other anomalies.

A meta-analysis of case-control and cohort studies concluded that cohort studies did not demonstrate an association between benzodiazepines and oral clefts, with a summary OR of 1.19 (95% CI 0.34–4.15), while case-control studies did demonstrate a slightly increased risk for oral clefts, with a summary OR of 1.79 (95% CI 1.13–2.82) (Dolovich et al., 1998). These results were not broken down for cleft subgroups, thereby limiting their interpretation. Attaining a large sample size by "lumping" all types of cleft might increase the statistical power to detect an association. However, due to the heterogeneity of oral cleft subgroups, this "lumping" might not be a good idea. Furthermore, the lack of agreement between case-control and cohort studies in the combined analysis was most likely due to the lower number of cases in cohort studies.

If an association between use of benzodiazepines and oral clefts does exist, the increase in risk is likely weak and perhaps modified by other factors. A possible mechanism has been proposed based on the theory that these drugs may disrupt the neurotransmitter mechanisms that regulate embryonic development. There is evidence from mouse models that γ-aminobutyric acid inhibits palatal shelf orientation. It is theorized that diazepam may mimic γ-aminobutyric acid, leading to the development of oral clefts (Zimmerman, 1984). Although this theory is plausible, the evidence to date from human studies does not indicate a strong association between diazepam use and risk for oral clefts.

CORTICOSTEROIDS

Corticosteroids, which are administered topically, systemically, or via inhalation, are mainly used to treat asthma, lupus, and rheumatoid disorders; and it has been proposed that they may promote fetal maturation (Czeizel and Rockenbauer, l997). The potential association between oral clefts and corticosteroid use during pregnancy was first proposed from animal studies (Baxter and Fraser, 1950). A case-control study demonstrated an increased risk of oral clefts in infants of women who used corticosteroids during pregnancy (Carmichael and Shaw, 1999). In this study, mothers were interviewed by telephone and asked about various exposures, illnesses, and medication use during the period of 1 month prior to conception to the third month of gestation. The average interval between interview and delivery was similar for cases (3.7 years) and controls (3.8 years). A statistically significant increased risk was demonstrated for CL/P (OR = 4.3, 95% CI 1.1–17.2) as well as for CP (OR = 5.3, 95% CI 1.1–26.5). Similar increased risks were not observed for other congenital anomalies, such as neural tube defects and conotruncal defects, indicating that the effect of corticosteroid may be specific to oral cleft malformations.

In a case-control study in Spain, Rodriguez-Pinilla and Martinez-Frias (1998) demonstrated an increased risk of oral clefting in the offspring of mothers exposed to corticosteroids during pregnancy. This hospital-based case-control study reported the results of the Spanish Collaborative Study on Congenital Malformations, in which 1184 cases of nonsyndromic oral clefts were examined by physicians and the diagnoses were made within 3 days after birth. There were three sets of controls: (1) the next nonmalformed infant born in the same hospital, (2) infants born at the same hospital as the case infant within 45 days (before or after) of the date of birth of the case infant, and (3) remaining malformed infants without oral clefts. Medication use was ascertained via physician interview and included month or week of intake, duration of treatment, and daily and total dosages. During the period April 1976 through December 1995, a total of 1,287,345 live-born infants were surveyed. There were a total of 24,038 (1.9%) malformed infants, 1184 oral clefts, and 23,517 controls. Exposure to any systemic corticosteroid during the first trimester was analyzed. Logistic regression was used to estimate ORs, with CL/P as the outcome and exposure to any systemic corticosteroid as the main exposure variable. The model was adjusted for smoking during the first trimester; first-degree relative with CL/P; maternal treatment with corticosteroids during the first trimester; and exposure to antiepileptic drugs, benzodiazepines, metronidazole, or sex hormones. Point estimates were similar when comparing all oral clefts to paired controls or controls born within 45 days of cases, 5.0 and 5.2, respectively. The increased risk was significant only for the second control group (95% CI 1.53–17.06). When the one CP case was excluded, the ORs for CL/P when compared to the second control group as well as to the malformed control group remained statistically significantly increased. No conclusion can be made regarding the risk for CP.

In a case-control study conducted in Hungary (Czeizel and Rockenbauer, 1997), cases were identified using the Hungarian Congenital Abnormality Registry. Controls were selected from the national birth registry and matched to cases according to sex, week of birth, and parents' residential district. A questionnaire was mailed to all eligible cases and controls. In addition, the prenatal care logbook (which included information on prescribed drugs and diseases during pregnancy recorded by the physician) and medical documents were requested of parents. Response rates were 82% for cases (n = 20,830) and 65% for controls (n = 35,727). No significant increase in risk for CP was observed for topical or systemic corticosteroid use. An increase in risk for CL/P with topical steroid use was observed for use during the entire pregnancy (OR = 2.21, 95% CI 1.11–4.39) and use in the first month of gestation (OR = 4.19, 95% CI 1.47–11.97). However, the risk was not significant for use during the second or third month of gestation.

Possible mechanisms for the association between corticosteroid intake and oral clefts have been proposed. One theory is that the steroid acts directly on the fetus, resulting in disruption of glycosaminoglycan or collagen synthesis or both, weakened midline fusion, and loss of amniotic fluid (Greene and Kochhar, 1975). Further, receptors for glucocorticoids have been demonstrated to be more common in palatal mesenchymal cells, which may explain why palatal tissues are affected by this drug (Goldman et al., 1978; Pratt, 1985). Regardless of the underlying mechanism, the data suggest that there is an increased risk (ranging from threefold to ninefold) for CL/P associated with use of corticosteroids during pregnancy. The information regarding the risk for CP is less convincing.

ORGANIC SOLVENTS/PESTICIDES

Several investigators have examined the relationship between exposure to organic solvents and pesticides and risk of oral clefts. In one study, which investigated the association between organic solvents and oral clefts (Laumon et al., 1996), cases were live-born infants born between 1985 and 1989 in the Rhone-Alpes region of France with an oral cleft, ascertained through any of six maxillofacial surgery clinics. For each case, two controls were selected among newborns without congenital anomalies born in the same delivery unit and whose mothers had the same obstetrician as the case mother. Case mothers were interviewed at the time of their first visit to the surgeon. Controls were interviewed in the maternity unit a few days after birth. The interviewer and questionnaires were the same for cases and controls. Exposures were described by brand names of paints, dyes, glues, or other solvent-containing products. An occupational physician who translated them into trace or significant exposure categories blindly reviewed trade names. Solvents were divided into nine groups: halogenated aromatics, other aromatics, halogenated aliphatics, other aliphatics, alcohols, glycols, ketones, aldehydes, and esters. There were 200 cases of oral clefts and 400 controls. A significant increased risk was demonstrated only for halogenated aliphatic solutions and all oral clefts (OR = 4.4, 95% CI 1.41–16.15) and for CL/P (OR = 4.0, 95% CI 1.25–14.91). Since there was only one case with CP, the results are not clearly interpretable.

A cohort of men who were members of three printer's unions in Norway were studied and categorized into four exposure groups: lead only, solvents only, lead plus solvents, other exposure (Kristensen et al., 1993). Information on children was ascertained by linking parents' union membership files with the birth registry in Norway, which is a record of all live births and stillbirths of ≥16 weeks' gestation. The standardized morbidity ratio for CL/P was 1.6 (95% CI 0.97–2.5).

In a study in Finland, 388 mothers of infants with oral clefts born between December 1977 and May 1980 were identified from the Finnish Registry of Congenital Malformations (Holmberg et al., 1982). Mothers were questioned as to occupational and in-home exposures to organic solvents via personal interview. Nine cases of CP were born to exposed mothers compared to two cases in the nonexposed group; five CL/P cases were observed among exposed mothers compared to two cases in the nonexposed group. The total numbers of exposed and nonexposed subjects were not included; therefore, an OR could not be calculated. The authors reported a McNemar's test with $p < 0.05$. There are several limitations of this study, most notably, random and nonrandom misclassification bias.

A study conducted in France, Italy, the United Kingdom, and The Netherlands using European Registration of Congenital Anomalies registries, included livebirths, stillbirths (fetal death after 20 weeks' gestation), and induced abortions with a confirmed congenital anomaly diagnosed prenatally, at birth, or within the first week of life (Cordier et al., 1997). Oral clefts were divided into CL/P ($n = 109$) and CP ($n = 52$). Controls, which were the first infant born with no anomaly after the case, were selected from the same hospital as cases. A standardized questionnaire was used in all centers to obtain information regarding socioeconomic status, mother's medical and obstetric history, and occupational exposures. Occupational exposures were obtained by questioning the mother as to occupations before and during pregnancy. Occupations were coded following the International Standard Industrial Classification of all Economic Activities and the International Standard Classification of Occupations. Exposures were further categorized as to (1) route (inhalation, cutaneous, or both), (2) level (low, medium, or high), (3) frequency (<5% of work time or 5%–50% of work time), and (4) reliability of assessment (possible, probable, or certain exposure). Only mothers who worked during pregnancy were included. Potential exposure to glycol ethers was assessed by experts for a variety of occupations. The OR for CP was 1.68 (95% CI 0.75–3.76) and that for CL/P was 2.03 (95% CI 1.11–3.73). Several limitations hamper the interpretability of the results of this study, including small numbers, misclassification bias, and recall bias.

A study conducted in the United States evaluated fetuses exposed to agricultural chemicals in Iowa and Michigan. Data were obtained from the National Center for Health Statistics and county and city data book computerized files based on the 1970 U.S. Census, the 1974 U.S. Census of Agriculture, and the 1976 update of Area Health Education Centers (Gordon and Shy, 1981). Iowa and Michigan were selected because they best met the criteria for this study, which included good birth defect monitoring programs, adequate numbers of births per year, participation in a community pesticide study, and being agricultural states. The study population included live-born singletons and controls, which were selected randomly by sampling two per center of live births in each state with a 5:1 control:case ratio. Exposures were classified as crops only, all pesticidal chemicals and fertilizers, and suspect chemicals. Each county was rated as "high" or "low," using midpoints of each of the three categories. A score was calculated for each exposure category within each county. Results revealed an increased risk of oral clefts for males and females in Iowa, with ORs of 4.25 (95% CI 1.08–16.67) and 7.13 (95% CI 1.20–42.49), respectively. In Michigan, the ORs for oral clefts were not statistically significantly increased (for males, OR = 1.46, 95% CI 0.59–3.62; for females, OR = 1.00, 95% CI 0.33–2.99). Subgroup analyses were not included; thus, the interpretation of the results is limited. Caution must be used in drawing conclusions based on this study because of the likelihood of bias due to misclassification of exposure, as well as the lumping of heterogeneous cases of oral clefts.

In another multicenter case-control study (Lorente et al., 2000a), data were obtained from the EUROCAT study and included live births, still births, and therapeutic abortions with a major congenital malformation diagnosed prior to birth or during the perinatal period. Controls were recruited for each case. A standardized questionnaire was used to obtain information from cases and controls for the periods before conception and during each trimester of pregnancy regarding socioeconomic status, age, residence, country of origin, mother's medical and obstetric history, alcohol use, tobacco use, drug use, occupation, and hobbies. Information on occupations before and during pregnancy was collected, including a description of tasks, products handled, frequency and timing of use (1 month before conception and first, second, and third trimesters), and typical job categories. Of eligible cases with oral clefts, 63% were interviewed. Controls were matched to oral cleft or to other cases in the parent study. Analysis of occupational exposures was conducted for those women who worked during pregnancy. The ORs were adjusted for center, mother's socio-economic status, urbanization, and country of origin. The ORs for oral clefts were estimated for each type of cleft and each type of occupation. The only statistically significant ORs were reported for CP among housekeepers (OR = 2.8, 95% CI 1.08–7.24) and hairdressers (OR = 5.1, 95% CI 1.10–25.9). The two most likely limitations of this study include misclassification of exposure and the substantial likelihood of spurious associations due to the high number of analyses. Chance is a likely explanation for the findings for CP.

In a case-control study in 15 maternity hospitals in France (Cordier et al., 1992), cases included all products of conception with major congenital malformations born to mothers attending one of the study hospitals, including all live births, still births, and therapeutic abortions with major defects detected prenatally or during prenatal period. For each case, one control who was normal at birth and born immediately after the case in the same maternity ward was selected. Mothers of cases and controls were interviewed in the hospital regarding age; place of residence; family, medical, and obstetric history; use of alcohol or drugs during pregnancy; and specific occupations. Occupational histories of mothers were reviewed blindly by an industrial hygienist, who assessed the presence of any chemical exposure for each work period and estimated frequency of exposure for 10% of the work time, 10% to 50% of the work time, and >50% of the work time. Twenty-nine cases of oral clefts were included. A statistically significant increased risk for all oral clefts was demonstrated for solvents with high frequency (OR = 7.9, 95% CI 1.8–44.9). These results are difficult to interpret since all oral clefts were evaluated as one case group. The limitations of misclassification bias and spurious associations cannot be ruled out as possible explanations for the findings of these studies.

A population-based case-control study (Shaw et al., 1991) included all live-born infants and fetal deaths (≥20 weeks' gestation) diagnosed with orofacial clefts, neural tube defects, conotruncal heart defects, and limb anomalies from most California counties between January 1987 and December 1988 (n = 344,214). Orofacial clefts were ascertained by the California Birth Defects Monitoring Program staff, reviewed by medical geneticists, confirmed by surgical or autopsy report. Controls (n = 972) were randomly selected from all infants born alive (n = 548,844) in the same geographic region and time period who had no major congenital anomaly diagnosed before the first birthday. Telephone interviews were conducted, and the information collected included pesticide exposure and other covariates. The periconceptional window was defined as 1 month prior to and 3 months following conception. Of cases with oral clefts, 85% completed interviews, as did 78% of controls. Pesticide information was collected from the following sources: (1) occupation (reviewed by an industrial hygienist); (2) home use, including weed killer treatments for insects, tree diseases, treatment of pests inside and outside of the home, and treatment of fleas; and (3) residential proximity to agricultural crops. The majority of exposed women were employed in agriculture, in housekeeping, as florists, or as animal handlers. The covariates included in the analysis were periconceptional vitamin use, cigarette smoking, education level, race, and ethnicity. The only statistically significant increased risk was found for CP associated with multiple anomalies and use of insect fogger (OR = 2.0, 95% CI 1.0–4.4). The limitations of this study include misclassification of exposure, the likelihood of spurious associations due to multiple testing, and low power for stratified analysis.

OTHER POTENTIAL RISK FACTORS

In addition to the studies discussed above, there have been numerous investigations regarding other potential risk factors for oral clefts (Wyszynski and Beaty, 1996). Reports have been published on chemical combustion (ten Tusscher et al., 2000), bed-heating devices (Shaw et al., 1999b; Dlugosz et al., 1992), proximity to hazardous waste sites (Croen et al., 1997), and stress (Carmichael and Shaw, 2000). The findings from these studies are variable, and most are limited by significant methodologic challenges encountered in capturing these exposures accurately. Little information is available to draw any conclusions on the role of these exposures and the risk of oral cleft formation.

SUMMARY

In summary, some of the exposures discussed in this chapter have demonstrated associations with increased risk of oral clefts, most notably use of alcohol, corticosteroids, or anticonvulsant medications and seizure disorders. For the most part, these association are weak or modest for CL/P but not for CP. Perhaps this indicates that CL/P has a stronger environmental component to its etiology than CP. None of the environmental risk factors studied to date stands out as a strong and consistent risk factor for oral clefts. There is a tremendous amount of heterogeneity in the study designs and assessment of exposures. It is likely that the mystery surrounding the etiology of oral clefts will be unlocked as technology advances and the ability to examine gene–environment interactions increases.

REFERENCES

Abrishamchian, AR, Khoury, MJ, Calle, EE (1994). The contribution of maternal epilepsy and its treatment to the etiology of oral clefts: a population based case-control study. Genet Epidemiol 11: 343–351.

Baxter, HD, Fraser, FC (1950). Production of congenital defects in the offspring of female mice treated with cortisone. McGill Med J 19: 245–249.

Beaty, TH, Maestri, NE, Hetmanski, JB, et al. (1997). Testing for interaction between maternal smoking and TGFA genotype among oral cleft cases born in Maryland 1992–1996. Cleft Palate Craniofac J 34: 447–454.

Bergman, U, Roas, FW, Baum, C, et al. (1992). Effects of exposure to benzodiazepine during fetal life. Lancet 340: 694–696.

Carmichael, SL, Shaw, GM (1999). Maternal corticosteroid use and risk of selected congenital anomalies. Am J Med Genet 86: 242–244.

Carmichael, SL, Shaw, GM (2000). Maternal life event stress and congenital anomalies. Epidemiology 11: 30–35.

Christensen, K, Olsen, J, Norgaard-Pedersem, B, et al. (1999). Oral clefts: transforming growth factor alpha gene variants, and maternal smoking: a population-based case-control study in Denmark, 1991–1994. Am J Epidemiol 149: 248–255.

Chung, KC, Kowalski, CP, Kim, HM, Buchman, SR (2000). Maternal cigarette smoking during pregnancy and the risk of having a child with cleft lip/palate. Plast Reconstr Surg 105: 485–491

Cordier, S, Bergeret, A, Goujard, J, et al. (1997). Congenital malformations and maternal occupational exposure to glycol ethers. Epidemiology 8: 355–363.

Cordier, S, Ha, MC, Ayme, S, Goujard, J (1992). Maternal occupational exposure and congenital malformations. Scand J Work Environ Health 18: 11–17.

Croen, LA, Shaw, GM, Sanbonmatsu, L, et al. (1997). Maternal residential proximity to hazardous waste sites and risk for selected congenital malformations. Epidemiology 8: 347–354

Czeizel, A. (1987). Lack of evidence of teratogenicity of benzodiazepine drugs in Hungary. Reprod Toxicol 1: 183–188.

Czeizel, AE, Rockenbauer, M (1997). Population based case control study of teratogenic potential of corticosteroids. Teratology 56: 335–340.

Dansky, LV, Finnell, RH (1991). Parental epilepsy, anticonvulsant drugs, and reproductive outcome: epidemiologic and experimental findings spanning three decades. 2: Human studies. Reprod Toxicol 5: 301–355.

Dansky, LV, Rosenblatt, DS, Andermann, E (1992). Mechanisms of teratogenesis. Neurology 42(Suppl 5): 32–42.

Dlugosz, L, Vena, J, Byers, T, et al. (1992). Congenital defects and electric bed heating in New York state: a register-based case control study. Am J Epidemiol 135: 1000–1011.

Dolovich, LR, Addis, A, Vaillancourt, JMR, et al. (1998). Benzodiazepine use in pregnancy and major malformations or oral cleft: meta-analysis of case control and cohort studies. BMJ 317: 839–843.

Dronamraju, KR (1970). Epilepsy and cleft lip and palate. Lancet 2: 876–877.

Durner, M, Greenberg, DA, Delgado-Escueta, V (1992). Is there a genetic relationship between epilepsy and birth defects. Neurology 42(Suppl 5): 63–67.

Ericson, A, Kallen, B, Welesterholm, P (1979). Cigarette smoking as an etiologic factor in cleft lip and palate. Am J Obstet Gynecol 135: 348–351.

Evans, DR, Newcombe, RG, Campbell, H (1979). Maternal smoking habits and congenital malformations: a population study. BMJ 2: 171–173.

Friis, ML (1979). Epilepsy among parents of children with facial clefts. Epilepsia 20: 69–76.

Friis, ML, Broeng-Nielsen, B, Sindrup, EH, et al. (1981). Facial clefts among epileptic patients. Arch Neurol 38: 227–229.

Goldman, AS, Shapiro, BH, Katsumata, M (1978). Human foetal palatal corticoid receptors and teratogens for cleft palate. Nature 272: 464–466.

Gordon, JE, Shy, CM (1981). Agricultural chemical use and congenital cleft lip and/or palate. Arch Environ Health 36: 213–221.

Greene, RM, Kochhar, DM (1975). Some aspects of corticosteroid-induced cleft palate: a review. Teratology 11: 47–56.

Hecht, JT, Annegers, JF (1990). Familial aggregation of epilepsy and clefting disorders: a review of the literature. Epilepsia 31: 574–577.

Hecht, JT, Annegers, JT, Kutland, LT (1989). Epilepsy and clefting disorders: lack of evidence of familial association. Am J Med Genet 33: 244–247.

Holmberg, PC, Hernberg, S, Kurppa, K, et al. (1982). Oral clefts and organic solvent exposure during pregnancy. Int Arch Occup Environ Health 50: 371–376.

Hwang, SJ, Beaty, TH, Panny, SR, et al. (1995). Association study of transforming growth factor alpha (TGFA) Taq1 polymorphism and oral clefts: indication of gene–environment interaction in a population-based sample of infants with birth defects. Am J Epidemiol 141: 629–636.

Kallen, K (1997). Maternal smoking and orofacial clefts. Cleft Palate Craniofac J 34: 11–16.

Kelly, TE, Rein, M, Edwards, P (1984). Teratogenicity of anticonvulsant drugs: the association of clefting and epilepsy. Am J Med Genet 19: 451–458.

Kelsey, JL, Dwyer, T, Holford, TR, Bracken, MB (1978). Maternal smoking and congenital malformations: an epidemiological study. J Epidemiol Community Health 32: 102–107.

Khoury, MJ, Gomez-Frias, M, Mulinare, J (1989). Does maternal cigarette smoking during pregnancy cause cleft lip and palate in offspring? Am J Dis Child 143: 333–337.

Kristensen, P, Irgens, LM, Daltveit, AK, Andersen, A (1993). Perinatal outcome among children or men exposed to lead and organic solvents in the printing industry. Am J Epidemiol 137: 134–144.

Laegreid, L, Olegard, R, Conradi, N, et al. (1990). Congenital malformations and maternal consumption of benzodiazepines: a case control study. Dev Med Child Neurol 32: 432–441.

Laumon, B, Martin, JL, Bertucat, I, et al. (1996). Exposure to organic solvents during pregnancy and oral clefts: a case control study. Reprod Toxicol 10: 15–19.

Lieff, S, Olshan, AF, Werler, MM, et al. (1999). Maternal cigarette smoking during pregnancy and risk of oral clefts in newborns. Am J Epidemiol 150: 683–94.

Lorente, C, Cordier, S, Bergeret, A, et al. (2000a). Maternal occupational risk factors for oral clefts. Scand J Work Environ Health 26: 137–145.

Lorente, C, Cordier, S, Goujard, J, et al. (2000b). Tobacco and alcohol use during pregnancy and risk of oral clefts. Am J Public Health 90: 415–419.

Meadow, SR (1970). Congenital abnormalities and anticonvulsant drugs. Proc R Soc Med 63: 48–49.

Millar, JHD, Nevin, NC (1973). Congenital malformations and anticonvulsant drugs. Lancet 10: 328.

Monson, R, Rosenberg, L, Hartz, SC, et al. (1973). Diphenylhydantoin and selected congenital malformations. N Engl J Med 289: 1049–1052.

Munger, RG, Romitti, PA, Daack-Hirsch, S, et al. (1996). Maternal alcohol use and risk of orofacial cleft birth defects. Teratology 54: 27–33.

Niswander, JD, Wertelecki, W (1973). Congenital malformation among offspring of epileptic women. Lancet 1: 1062.

Pratt, RM (1985). Receptor-dependent mechanism of glucocorticoid and dioxin-induced cleft palate. Environ Health Perspect 61: 35–40.

Rodriguez-Pinilla, E, Martinez-Frias, ML (1998). Corticosteroids during pregnancy and oral clefts: a case control study. Teratology 58: 2–5.

Romitti, PA, Lidral, AC, Munger, RG, et al. (1999). Candidate genes for nonsyndromic cleft lip and palate and maternal cigarette smoking and alcohol consumption: evaluation of genotype–environment interactions from a population-based case-control study of orofacial clefts. Teratology 59: 39–50.

Rosenberg, L, Mitchell, A, Parsells, JL, et al. (1983). Lack of relation of oral clefts to diazepam use during pregnancy. N Engl J Med 309: 1282–1285.

Rosenberg, L, Mitchell, A, Shapiro, S, Slone, D (1982). Selected birth defects in relation to caffeine-containing beverages. JAMA 247: 1429–1432.

Safra, MJ, Oakley, GP (1975). Association between cleft lip with or without cleft palate and prenatal exposure to diazepam. Lancet 13: 478–480.

Saxen, I (1974). Cleft lip and palate in Finland: parental histories, course of pregnancy and selected environmental factors. Int J Epidemiol 3: 263–270.

Schwaninger, M, Ringleb, P, Winter, R, et al. (1999). Elevated plasma concentrations of homocysteine in antiepileptic drug treatment. Epilepsia 40: 345–350.

Seidman, DS, Ever Hadani, P, Gale, R (1990). Effect of maternal smoking and age on congenital anomalies. Obstet Gynecol 76: 1046–1050.

Shaw, GM, Lammer, EJ (1999). Maternal periconceptional alcohol consumption and risk for orofacial clefts. J Pediatr 134: 298–303.

Shaw, GM, Nelson, V, Todoroff, K, et al. (1999b). Maternal periconceptional use of electric bed-heating devices and risk for neural tube defects and orofacial clefts. Teratology 60: 124–129.

Shaw, GM, Wasserman, CR, Lammer, EJ, et al. (1996). Orofacial clefts, parental cigarette smoking, and transforming growth factor alpha gene variants. Am J Hum Genet 58: 551–561.

Shaw, GM, Wasserman, CR, O'Malley, CD, et al. (1999a) Maternal pesticide exposure from multiple sources and selected congenital anomalies. Epidemiology 10: 60–66.

Shiono, P, Mills, J (1984). Oral clefts and diazepam use during pregnancy. N Engl J Med 311: 919–920.

Shiono, PH, Klebanoff, MA, Berendes, HW (1986). Congenital malformations and maternal smoking during pregnancy. Teratology 34: 65–71.

Speidel BD, Meadow SR (1972). Maternal epilepsy and abnormalities of the fetus and newborn. Lancet 2: 839–843.

ten Tusscher, GW, Stam, G, Koppe, J (2000). Open chemical combustions resulting in a local increased incidence of orofacial clefts. Chemosphere 40: 1263-1270.

Van den Eeden, SK, Karagas, MR, Daling, JR, Vaughan, TL (1990). A case-control study of maternal smoking and congenital malformations. Paediatr Perinat Epidemiol 4: 147–155.

Werler, MM, Lammer, EJ, Rosenberg, L, Mitchell, AA (1990). Maternal cigarette smoking during pregnancy in relation to oral clefts. Am J Epidemiol 132: 926–932.

Werler, MM, Lammer, EJ, Rosenberg, L, Mitchell, AA (1991). Maternal alcohol use in relation to selected birth defects. Am J Epidemiol 134: 691–697.

Wyszynski, DF, Beaty, TH (1996). The role of potential teratogens in the origin of human non-syndromic oral clefts. Teratology 53: 309–317.

Wyszynski, DF, Duffy, DL, Beaty, TH (1997). Maternal cigarette smoking and oral clefts: a meta-analysis. Cleft Palate Craniofac J 34: 206–210.

Zimmerman, EF (1984). Neuropharmacologic teratogenesis and neurotransmitter regulation of palate development. Am J Ment Defic 88: 548–558.

14

Maternal nutrition and oral clefts

RONALD G. MUNGER

Inadequate maternal nutrition during pregnancy has been suspected as a possible cause of oral clefts in humans since at least the early 1900s (Strauss, 1914). Evidence for this view has accumulated from several areas of research, including animal experiments, observational studies of human populations, and in some limited cases human experimental studies, yet many gaps remain in our understanding of the etiology of oral clefts. Each of these areas of research will be reviewed in this chapter.

Oral clefts comprise one of the most common groups of birth defects in the world (World Health Organization, 1998), and there is considerable geographic variation in occurrence. Asian populations in Asia and Native Americans (of Asian genetic ancestry) have higher rates of oral clefts than other major groups (Chung and Kau, 1985; Croen et al., 1998). The burden of oral cleft birth defects is great because affected children require substantial medical care and speech training. In areas of the developing world where corrective surgery is not available, affected children face having a serious disability for their entire lives and are often shunned by others. Hence, there is a strong public health imperative for a better understanding of the causes and prevention of oral clefts in all populations, and these insights may provide clues to the etiology of other birth defects.

Poverty has been linked to the occurrence of oral clefts. In Glasgow, oral clefts were found to be more common in socioeconomically deprived areas than elsewhere in the city (Womersley and Stone, 1987). Studies in metropolitan Manila found evidence of a social class gradient in oral cleft risk: the prevalence was higher among births in a hospital serving a more im-

poverished group of patients at the Philippine General Hospital than among births to wealthier patients in the Makati financial district a few kilometers away (Lasa and Manalo, 1989). Social class may be a determinant of maternal nutritional status, but it may also be related to other environmental exposures that have a bearing on the risk of oral clefts.

Several environmentally induced causes of clefting have been identified. Maternal cigarette smoking is perhaps the best-studied environmental risk factor for oral clefts. In a meta-analysis of 11 published studies, smoking was associated with an increased risk for both cleft lip with or without cleft palate (CL/P) and cleft palate alone (CP) (Wyszynski and Beaty, 1996). The association between maternal smoking and risk of clefting may be due in part to confounding in studies that do not account for maternal diet or nutritional status. Maternal alcohol use has been associated with an increased risk of oral clefts in some studies (Werler et al., 1991; Munger et al., 1996; Romitti et al., 1998; Shaw and Lammer, 1999; Lorente et al., 2000) but not all (Natsume et al., 2000). Examination of the social and dietary context in which alcohol consumption takes place may help to clarify its relation to risk of oral clefts. For example, the risk from alcohol consumed while drinking beer at a pub is not likely to be equivalent to that from the same amount of alcohol consumed while drinking wine with a nutritious meal. Other environmental exposures linked to increased risks for oral clefts include agricultural chemicals, solvents, and medications (reviewed in detail in Chapter 13).

Genetic and developmental studies have provided evidence that the etiology of cleft lip (CL) with or without cleft of the primary (hard) palate is different compared to clefts affecting only the secondary (soft) palate (Fraser, 1955). Oral clefts are often classified into four groups: isolated CL/P, isolated CP, CL/P in association with other major birth defects, and CP in association with other major birth defects. In isolated cases, affected individuals have no other physical or developmental anomalies (Murray, 1995). Most studies suggest that about 60% to 70% of cases are isolated and, thus, not associated with any syndrome of malformations (Jones, 1988). Most of the remaining 30% to 40% of cases occur with a pattern of multiple malformations and either are classified as recognized syndromes related to chromosomal abnormalities, one of several hundred known Mendelian disorders, or known teratogen exposures (e.g., phenytoin or alcohol) or become candidates for newly defined syndromes. Some studies of maternal nutrition and oral clefts have used subgroups of clefts in their analyses, and this approach is clearly needed in all future studies. More information on the clinical classification of oral clefts may be found in Chapters 5 and 6 of this volume.

NEURAL TUBE DEFECTS AND MATERNAL NUTRITION: RELEVANCE FOR ORAL CLEFTS

The literature on nutritional causes of neural tube defects (NTDs) is extensive and relevant to oral clefts because some structures of the craniofacial region are derived from cephalic neural crest cells; thus, these two conditions may share some developmental origins (Been and Lieuw Kie Song, 1978; Lammer et al., 1985). Malnutrition was suspected as a cause of NTDs as early as the 1960s, when it was noted that women in the United Kingdom from the poorer social classes had an elevated risk of NTDs in their pregnancies (Hibbard, 1964; Hibbard and Smithells, 1965). Attention was later focused on the role of folic acid, but early attempts at supplementation trials provoked controversy because they were not fully controlled by randomization and there was no masking of the treatment status (Smithells et al., 1976; Wald and Polani, 1984). The Medical Research Council Vitamin Study was a randomized, controlled trial of folic acid and multivitamin supplementation that provided strong evidence of the role of folic acid supplementation in reducing the risk of NTDs in the pregnancies of women who had previously had a pregnancy with an NTD (MRC Vitamin Study Research Group, 1991). Folic acid supplementation has also been shown to reduce the primary occurrence of NTDs in Hungary (Czeizel and Hirschberg, 1997) and China (Berry et al., 1999).

The mechanism for the protective effect of folic acid against NTDs remains unknown, and several features of folate–homocysteine metabolic pathways have been under investigation (Daly et al., 1997). Red cell folate is a more accurate indicator of long-term folate status compared to plasma folate (Herbert, 1989). Research has focused on understanding the shape of the dose-response curve between the maternal red cell folate level, the risk of NTDs, and the levels of folate intake required to result in a desired red cell folate level (Daly et al., 1997; Wald et al., 1998). The risk of NTDs decreases in a continuous dose-response relationship with increasing maternal level of red cell folate. A high level of plasma total homocysteine is an indicator of impaired folate and vitamin B_{12} metabolism and has been observed in mothers of children with NTDs compared to unaffected controls (Steegers-Theunissen et al., 1994; Mills et al., 1995). The major catabolic pathway for homocysteine involves cystathione β-synthase with vitamin B_6 as a co-factor. Low levels of vitamin B_{12} have also been implicated as a cause of NTDs and, thus, may be relevant for the discussion of oral clefts (Kirke et al., 1993)

An irony of the folic acid–NTD success story is that other nutrients, including those identified years ago in the animal experiments described below, have been largely overlooked in recent epidemiologic studies of human populations.

EXPERIMENTAL ANIMAL STUDIES ON MATERNAL NUTRITION AND ORAL CLEFTS

The role of maternal nutrition in the formation of oral clefts has been studied extensively in experimental animal models over the past 70 years (Table 14.1). A surprising number of specific nutritional deficiencies have been found to cause oral clefts, and in most cases multiple birth defects and excessive fetal loss also have been observed. In light of the history of animal experimentation, it is remarkable that recent investigations in human populations have been so narrowly focused, neglecting many nutrients that may be important causes of oral clefts.

The first reported observations from animal studies were anecdotal, yet with scant evidence authors were eager to promote nutritional interventions for the prevention of oral clefts in humans. As early as 1914, maternal diet was thought to influence the occurrence of CP among lions at the London Zoological Gardens (Pickerill, 1914). Cleft palate was reported among nearly all of the lion cubs born during a period when the lionesses were fed a diet of meat alone. When the diet was changed to whole small animals, which were consumed entirely, the occurrence of oral clefts among subsequent births dropped immediately and consider-

TABLE 14.1. *Nutritional Factors Found to Cause Oral Clefts in Experimental Animal Models*

Nutritional Factor	Type of Exposure	Animal Model	Reference
Vitamin A	Dietary deficiency	Pig	Hale (1935)
		Mouse	Kochhar (1967)
		Primate	Fantel et al. (1977)
	Retinoic acid	Mouse	Abbott et al. (1988), Abbott and Pratt (1988a, b)
		Mouse	Tyan and Tyan (1993)
		Rat	Whitby et al. (1994)
		Mouse	Soprano and Soprano (1995)
		Rabbit	Ross (1999)
Riboflavin (Vitamin B$_2$)	Dietary deficiency	Rat	Warkany and Nelson (1940)
		Rat	Noback and Kupperman (1944)
		Rat	Giroud and Boisselot (1947)
		Rat	Leimbach (1949)
		Rat	Piccioni and Bologna (1949)
		Rat	Giroud and Boisselot (1951)
		Mouse	Kalter and Warkany (1957)
Folate	Dietary deficiency + folate antagonist	Mouse	Nelson and Evans (1947)
	Folate antagonist	Chicken	Karnofsky et al. (1949)
	Folate antagonist	Chicken	Sunde et al. (1950)
	Dietary deficiency	Rat	Giroud and Boisselot (1951), Giroud and Lefebvres (1951), Giroud et al. (1951)
	Folate antagonist	Rat	Thiersch and Philips (1950)
	Folate antagonist	Rat	Evans et al. (1951)
	Folate antagonist	Rat	Nelson et al. (1952)
	Folic acid supplementation	Dog	Elwood and Colquhoun (1997)
Pyridoxine (Vitamin B$_6$)	B$_6$ + corticosteroid-induced cleft model	Mouse	Peer et al. (1958a)
		Mouse	Peer et al. (1958b)
	B$_6$ + vitamin A–induced cleft model	Rat	Yamaguchi (1968)
	Dietary deficiency	Mouse	Davis et al. (1970)
	B$_6$ antagonist + corticosteroid-induced cleft model	Mouse	Miller (1972)
	B$_6$ + corticosteroid-induced cleft model	Mouse	Yoneda and Pratt (1982a,b)
	B$_6$ + cyclophosphamide-induced cleft model	Mouse	Dostal and Schubert (1990)
	B$_6$ + β-aminonitrile–induced cleft model	Rat	Jacobsson and Granstrom (1997)
Plant-derived alkaloids	Feeding experiments with native plants and isolated alkaloids	Sheep, cattle	James (1999)

ably. Pickerell attributed the reduction to the added consumption of bones and suggested that women with a family history of frequent oral clefts should be given a diet during early pregnancy with added powdered fresh bone or lime phosphate. In the same year, experiments with cats in the United States were reported, in which oral clefts were easily induced by unspecified manipulations of diet and environmental conditions (Strauss, 1914). Strauss noted that in humans the occurrence of clefts seemed to be more frequent among the poor and suggested that a "hypoplastic condition of the blood" due to "faulty metabolism" was respon-

sible even if the mother generally seemed to be well-nourished and that these nutritional factors acted in concert with "hereditary tendencies" to result in oral clefts. Nearly 100 years later, the interaction between maternal nutritional status and genes is still invoked as a cause of oral clefts, yet the specific components remain unclear.

The identification and isolation of vitamins led to animal experiments with great specificity, and the first vitamins characterized were included in the earliest teratologic studies. Hale, of the Texas Agricultural Experiment Station, reported in 1933 that sows raised on rations deficient in vitamin A gave birth to pigs without eyes and in 1935 that cleft lip and palate (CLP) and ear and kidney malformations also occurred in these animals. Hale cited further breeding experiments as evidence against genetic causes of the defects in his experimental animals. When control animals were bred on the same rations but with added cod-liver oil or were allowed to graze on green pastures, no birth defects were produced. Impressed with the protective effect of green pastures, Hale (1935) wrote that "perhaps we have been forcing our spinach on the wrong victims; it ought to be administered to the mothers instead of the children."

Warkany and the Development of Animal Models of Teratogenesis

Josef Warkany began his pioneering work on nutrition and birth defects in 1938 after immigrating to Cincinnati from Vienna (Kalter 1993). Warkany was inspired by Hale's previous work and set out to challenge the prevailing view that nearly all congenital malformations were hereditary (Warkany, 1954). At that time, it was commonly asserted that maternal nutrition could not have an important effect on the development of the embryo, which was viewed as a small parasite that could easily extract the small amount of needed nutrients from the unlimited stores of the mother.

Warkany had developed a broad view of nutrition and health from his early childhood experiences. As a boy foraging for food for his family during wartime in the Austrian countryside, Warkany was struck by the sight of physically and mentally disabled *cretins* and developed a lifelong interest in the role of maternal iodine nutrition in this condition. Likewise, he became interested in the role of nutrition in rickets, then common in the European mountain villages he frequented (Kalter, 1993). Warkany often cited these as examples of evidence of important nutritional causes of birth defects.

Warkany and his first co-worker in the United States, Rose Nelson, developed techniques for breeding Sprague-Dawley rats in states of nutritional deficiency. Female rats fed on rations made from cornmeal, wheat gluten, calcium carbonate, and sodium chloride gave birth to young with multiple skeletal and craniofacial anomalies, including CP. The addition of 2% dried pig liver to the rations completely prevented the anomalies, and these investigators set out to discover the specific vitamins responsible. B-complex vitamins, including thiamine, riboflavin, niacin, pyridoxine, and pantothenic acid, had recently become available in crystalline form, and Warkany found that riboflavin alone prevented oral clefts and all of the other malformations

among offspring of female rats bred while on the deficient diet. In further studies of the timing of deficiencies during gestation, Warkany found that riboflavin supplementation before day 13 prevented the malformations but that later supplementation did not. Other investigators confirmed that riboflavin deficiency caused malformations in rats (Noback and Kupperman, 1944; Giroud and Boisselot, 1947, 1951; Leimbach, 1949; Piccioni and Bologna, 1949) and fowl (Lepkovsky et al., 1938; Romanoff and Bauernfeind, 1942). The mechanism by which riboflavin deficiency caused oral clefts and other malformations was not clear, and subsequent studies in the late 1940s of riboflavin deficiency in mice did not replicate the cleft findings in the rat studies (Fraser and Fainstat 1951a). A subsequent study by Kalter and Warkany (1957) reported malformations in mice caused by riboflavin deficiency, but little if any work has been done on the teratogenic effects of riboflavin deficiency since then.

Vitamin A

The role of vitamin A deficiency in the growth and reproduction of rats was further studied by Warkany, who reported patterns of malformations including defects of the skeleton, eyes, kidney, urogenital tract, and aortic arch; no oral clefts were mentioned however (Warkany and Shraffenberger, 1944). The possible role of vitamin A in craniofacial abnormalities did not appear in the literature until many years later, when reports on the role of excess exposure to vitamin A and related compounds in oral clefts and other birth defects in animal studies were published. Retinoic acid and other retinoids were discovered to cause oral clefts and other malformations in several animal species, including mice, rats, rabbits, and primates; and the specific effects were found to be dependent on the precise timing of exposure during early fetal development (Kochhar, 1967, 1973; Fantel et al., 1977; Kochhar et al., 1984; Soprano and Soprano, 1995). After gestational day 10 in the mouse, retinoic acid–induced oral clefts result from abnormally small palatal shelves that do not contact one another and medial epithelial cells of the shelves differentiate into oral-like epithelial tissue; after day 12, shelves of normal size form but fail to fuse and medial cells proliferate and abnormally differentiate into nasal-like epithelium (Abbott et al., 1988a,b; Abbott and Pratt, 1988a,b). Abbott and Birnbaum (1990) found that RA exposure disrupts the specific expression pattern of growth factors, including transforming growth factors α, $\beta 1$, and $\beta 2$, during this period of development and suggested that the timing of this disruption determines whether the cleft is due to the formation of small palatal shelves that never con-

tact one another or to abnormal differentiation of medial epithelial cells and failure of fusion of the palatal
shelves. Other important variables found to influence
the expression of oral clefts after retinoid exposure in
animal experiments include form of retinoid, dose,
species studied, rate of metabolism (Ross, 1999), interaction with ethanol and other exposures including
vitamin A (Whitby et al., 1994), and genetic susceptibility (Tyan and Tyan, 1993).

Folate

The role of folate in malformations began to be studied in the late 1940s by several groups of investigators
using folate antagonists in animal experiments. By this
time, Nelson had moved to Berkeley from Cincinnati,
further developed the experimental methods she had
established earlier with Warkany, and in 1947 demonstrated that folic acid deficiency caused the resorption of 26% of rat fetuses using a purified diet with
the addition of succinyl-sulfathiazole (Nelson and
Evans, 1947). Folic acid deficiency induced by folate
antagonists was shown to cause beak malformations in
chickens (Karnofsky et al., 1949). Oral clefts and other
malformations were produced in rats by folic acid deficiency in combination with sulfonamide treatment to
suppress folic acid production by maternal intestinal
bacteria (Giroud and Boisselot, 1951; Giroud and
Lefebvres, 1951). The folate antagonist 4-aminofolic
acid was shown to be sufficient to cause resorption of
embryos (Thiersch and Philips, 1950), and Nelson
found that addition of the folic acid antagonist X-
methyl-pteroylglutamic acid to her previous protocol
further increased adverse reproductive effects in rats
and that the timing of the induced folate deficiency was
more important than the dose of folate antagonist in
producing malformations and fetal deaths (Evans et al.,
1951; Nelson et al., 1952). Folate deficiency induced
between days 1 and 9 of gestation resulted in 100%
fetal resorptions and that induced between days 10 and
11 resulted in 100% stillbirths, in which 94% had CP;
when the induction of folate deficiency was delayed until day 15, only 6% were stillborn and none had cleft
palates. Nelson et al. (1952) noted that the malformations induced by folic acid deficiency were similar to
but more severe than those produced by deficiencies of
riboflavin (Warkany and Nelson, 1941), vitamin A
(Wilson and Warkany, 1948), pantothenic acid (Boisselot, 1949, 1951), and vitamin B_{12} (O'Dell et al.,
1951) and concluded that similar patterns of malformations result from interference with any one of a number of metabolic pathways during critical developmental periods.

Folate antagonists were subsequently found to be
highly toxic to human embryos (Meltzer, 1956;

Thiersch, 1956; Warkany et al., 1959; Emerson, 1962;
Goetsch, 1962; Milunsky et al., 1968; Shaw and Steinbach, 1968; Powell and Ekert, 1971). Methotrexate, a
folate antagonist used in cancer therapy, was found to
cause oral clefts, craniofacial anomalies, and other malformations in rats and rabbits, although rabbits required a dose level 60 times greater than rats to produce similar effects (Jordan et al., 1977). The A/WySn
strain of mice is genetically predisposed to oral clefts
and has been used to examine the interaction of genetic
susceptibility to oral clefts with folate status. The occurrence of oral clefts in the offspring of A/WySn dams
was increased after they had been fed a low-folate diet
(Lidral et al., 1991) and reduced when dams were
treated with folinic acid, the most stable intermediate
of folic acid metabolism, via continuous delivery by
way of an osmotic minipump (Paros and Beck, 1999).

A high incidence of CP was observed over a 30-year
period in a breeding line of Boston Terrier dogs, and
in 1982 animals from this group were supplemented
with a daily dose of 5 mg folic acid for the purpose of
reducing aggressiveness in the mother toward the pups
after birth. Cleft prevention was apparently not the
original reason for the supplementation (Elwood and
Colquhoun, 1997). The occurrence of oral clefts in the
period after supplementation began (1982–1997) was
significantly less than in the presupplementation period
(1974–1981) [4.2% of 191 pups from supplemented
pregnancies were affected vs. 17.6% of 51 unsupplemented pups; odds ratio (OR) = 0.20, 95% confidence
interval (CI) 0.07–0.62]. Studies in several animal models have thus shown that folic acid plays an important
role in fetal viability and normal development of the
craniofacial region and other structures. The mechanisms by which folate deficiency causes oral clefts and
other malformations remain unclear.

Vitamin B_6

Vitamin B_6 has been shown to protect against teratogen-induced oral clefts in many animal studies. Vitamin B_6 is the generic term for 3-hydroxy-2-methylpyri-
dine derivatives that have the biologic activity of
pyridoxine. Vitamin B_6 plays many vital roles in amino
acid metabolism, including transamination and decar-
boxylation reactions, acting as the coenzyme of glycogen phosphorylase, steroid hormone action, and acting
as a coenzyme in the degradation of homocysteine;
thus, there are many potential pathways in which vitamin B_6 protects against oral clefts. Corticosteroid exposure has been used as a model for teratogen-induced
oral clefts in mice since the 1950s (Fraser and Fainstat,
1951a,b; Kalter, 1957; Bonner and Slavkin, 1975; Melnick et al., 1981), and Peer et al. (1958a,b) demonstrated that vitamin B_6 supplementation reduced the

occurrence of corticosteroid-induced oral clefts in mice. Vitamin B_6 deficiency alone was demonstrated to cause CP and other birth defects in mice (Davis et al., 1970). Miller (1972) demonstrated that dietary vitamin B_6 deprivation in mice resulted in isolated oral clefts in 20% of the offspring, and the prevalence increased to 61% to 100% when deoxypyridine, a vitamin B_6 antagonist, or cortisone was administered to the pyridoxine-deficient mothers. Later studies demonstrated that vitamin B_6 also prevented the induction of oral clefts by vitamin A excess (Yamaguchi, 1968), cyclophosphamide (Dostal and Schubert, 1990), and β-aminoproprionitrile (Jacobsson and Granstrom, 1997); hence, the role of vitamin B_6 in cleft prevention may be complex and involve several different mechanisms.

The susceptibility to corticosteroid-induced oral clefts in mice is strain-dependent, raising the possibility that the protective effects of vitamin B_6 may depend on genotype (Marazita et al., 1988). Vitamin B_6 appears to regulate the activity of hormones, including androgens, estrogens, progesterone, retinol, retinoic acid, thyroid hormones, calcitriol, and glucocorticoids, by binding to nuclear receptor proteins and influencing transcription and gene expression (Jacobsson and Granstrom, 1997). Cytoplasmic levels of glucocorticoid receptors in the developing secondary palate of mice are associated with the susceptibility to glucocorticoid-induced oral clefts (Salomon et al., 1979; Salomon and Pratt, 1979). These authors suggested that glucocorticoids inhibit the growth of palatal mesenchyme cells at a critical point in palatal formation. Yoneda and Pratt (1982a,b) found that vitamin B_6 inhibited the specific binding of labeled glucocorticoid to cytosolic receptors from cultured mouse palatal mesenchyme and suggested that it reduces the occurrence of cortisone-induced oral clefts by altering the binding of glucocorticoids to their cytoplasmic receptors and, consequently, nuclear acceptors.

Plant Toxins

Naturally occurring toxins in plants cause malformations, including oral clefts in sheep, cattle, and other grazing animals. Extensive studies of the role of plant toxins have been conducted since the 1950s in the arid mountainous regions of the western United States, where many poisonous plant species have caused epidemics of birth defects with significant morbidity and mortality in livestock. The production and sequestering of toxins by plants appear to have evolved as defense mechanisms against herbivores, especially in arid regions where plant growth is quite limited. Many of the plants with potent toxins are in the legume family of flowering plants, and alkaloids are often found to be the active compound. Exposure of pregnant ewes to

Veratrum californicum (false hellebore) on day 14 of gestation resulted in cyclopic craniofacial anomalies and CLP in the lambs (James, 1999). The teratogens isolated from *V. californicum* include the steroidal alkaloids cyclopamine, jervine, and cycloposine (Keeler, 1968, 1990). A potential mechanism for the teratogenic action of the *Veratrum* alkaloids includes disruption of signal transduction mediated by Sonic hedgehog proteins, responsible for developmental patterning of the mammalian craniofacial region (Cooper et al., 1998; Incardona et al., 1998). Oral clefts and skeletal defects are also caused in cattle that graze on *Lupine* species (James, 1999). Humans are exposed to alkaloids from a variety of plant sources, including *Nicotiana* (tobacco), *Lobelia* (medications), *Punica* (pomegranate), *Duboisia* (medications), *Carica* (papaya), and *Prosopis* (mesquite); but the relevance of these alkaloid exposures to human birth defects is largely unexplored.

HUMAN OBSERVATIONAL STUDIES OF MATERNAL NUTRITION AND ORAL CLEFTS

Peer et al. (1958b) were among the first to publish data on a series of mothers of cleft patients that included vitamin use. The subtitle of their 1958 paper on the results of 400 human pregnancies is "protective effect of folic acid and vitamin B_6 therapy," yet no evidence from human studies was presented to support these conclusions. Recognizing that existing medical records were inadequate, the authors sent questionnaires to 1000 mothers of cleft-affected children who were surgical patients at St. Barnabus Medical Center in Newark, New Jersey. Four hundred mothers responded. The racial composition of the sample was not reported, although it was the impression of the authors that oral clefts were less common among African-Americans than in other groups. Because 77% of the oral clefts occurred in families without a previous history, the authors believed that environmental causes were important. Five pairs of identical twins with oral clefts were described, three of whom had one affected and one unaffected twin. Douglas (1958) had cited similar discordant sets of identical twins in which the cleft-affected twin had a lower birth weight and length than the unaffected twin as evidence that differences in the fetal environment, perhaps related to unequal maternal blood supply between twins, may give rise to a cleft in the more compromised fetus. Peer et al. (1958b) noted that 90% of the mothers in their series either had not used vitamin supplements or had used them late in pregnancy or irregularly; no data from a control group were cited, making the significance of this observation uncertain.

Montreal Case-Control Study

Fraser and Warburton (1964) collected family history and medical information from mothers of 187 children with CL/P and 59 with CP in the Montreal area and compared these data to reports from 90 mothers of children with genetically determined diseases that did not include oral clefts. This study thus represents the first of a growing list of case-control studies of oral clefts (Table 14.2). The authors were primarily interested in whether stressful life events were associated with the risk of oral clefts via excessive adrenal gland secretion of glucocorticoids. Both case and control mothers reported more stressful events during the pregnancy of their affected children than during the pregnancies of their other unaffected children, and the authors attributed this finding to maternal recall bias. Prescribed nutritional supplements were taken during pregnancy by 67% of the CL/P mothers, 77% of the CP mothers, and 71% of the control mothers; the authors concluded that use of prescribed dietary supplements was not associated with the occurrence of CL/P or CP. The strengths of this early case-control study include collection of data from a structured questionnaire, use of a control group with children affected with known genetic diseases, and consideration of the role of maternal recall bias by comparing the results of reports from affected pregnancies to those of unaffected pregnancies from the same mothers. No information was provided on the demographic characteristics of the sample, type of nutritional supplements, or diets of the mothers.

Finland Case-Control Study

The Finnish Register of Congenital Malformations was used by Saxen (1975) in a study of medication and vitamin supplement use during pregnancy in relation to oral clefts. The register covered 98% of Finnish births in 1967; thus, this report was the most representative population-based sample at that time. Mothers of 232 CL/P children, 232 CP children, and 232 control children were contacted by midwives after their deliveries while working with the Maternity Welfare Centres and interviewed with a standard questionnaire. Controls were unaffected children born in the same district just prior to a case child; thus, they were matched on place of residence and time of pregnancy. Use of iron, vitamin supplements, or both was tabulated by trimester of pregnancy; during the first trimester, use was greater for CL/P case mothers compared to controls (63.8% vs. 54.4%) and similar for CP case mothers and controls (46.6% vs. 47.8%). Use of supplements increased to 82% for all mothers in the third trimester, with no significant differences between groups. Several medications were used more often among cases vs. controls in the first trimester, including salicylates, other antipyretic analgesics, opiates, tetracyclines, chloramphenicol, and antineurotics. The strengths of the Finnish study included being among the first population-based case-control studies of nutritional supplements and cleft risk, an adequate sample size, and assessment of exposure by trimester of pregnancy. The limitations of the study include the simple exposure variable of all supplement use combined (most of which may have been iron alone), lack of dietary data, possible overmatching of cases and controls by place of residence, and lack of information on possible confounding factors. The medication data indicated that case mothers had more illnesses during pregnancy than controls; thus, it is possible that these illnesses compromised the nutritional status of case mothers more often than controls.

Baltimore Case-Control Study of Maternal Metabolic Factors

Maternal metabolic factors were studied in a case-control study by Niebyl et al. (1985). Cases were 59 mothers of children with CL/P recruited through surgical clinics and advertisements in the Baltimore area. Controls were a convenience sample of 56 mothers of unaffected children drawn from the authors' private patients or hospital employees. The sample size was thus small, was not population-based, and yielded controls of higher socioeconomic status (40% college graduates vs. 24% among cases); thus, the results may be confounded by these differences. No information on diet or supplement use was presented. The authors collected blood specimens and conducted a broad spectrum of biochemical studies, including folate status and phenytoin pharmacokinetics. In cases compared to controls, mean red cell folate was higher (143 vs. 138 ng/ml) and serum folate was lower (6.0 vs. 6.3 ng/ml), but these differences were not statistically significant. In a more detailed substudy of 10 cases and 10 controls, the mean baseline red cell folate was higher in cases vs. controls (150 vs. 118 ng/ml) but the mean peak serum folate after a 1.0 mg dose of pteroylmonoglutamate was lower in cases vs. controls (63.5 vs. 83.3 ng/ml); these differences were not statistically significant, but this approach may be useful in characterizing differences in folate metabolism in larger samples of cleft case mothers vs. controls. After a 1-week period of phenytoin treatment (300 mg/day), the mean peak serum folate values of cases and controls were similar (56.4 vs. 52.9 ng/ml), as were the phenytoin elimination kinetics.

TABLE 14.2. *Case-Control Studies of Maternal Nutritional Status in Pregnancy and Risk of Oral Clefts*[a]

References	Population	Sample of mothers		Assessment of Maternal Nutritional Status	Findings[b]
		Cases	Controls		
Fraser and Warburton (1964)	Montreal Canada	187 CL/P 59 CP	90 AC	Self-reported MV use	MV use in pregnancy: CTL 71%, CL/P 67% ($p = 0.49$), CP 77% ($p = 0.57$)
Saxen (1975)	Finland	232 CL/P 232 CP	232 UC-CL/P[c] 232 UC-Cp[d]	Self-reported MV use	MV use in first trimester: CL/P 63.8% vs. CTL 54.4% ($p = 0.047$), CP 46.6% vs. CTL 47.8% ($p = 0.85$)
Niebyl et al. (1985)	Baltimore, MD	59 CL/P	56 UC	Biochemical measures after delivery	No significant differences in serum or red cell folate between CL/P and CTL
Hill et al. (1988)	England	676 OC	676 UC	Medical record review of MV use	MV use in pregnancy: OC 1.9%, CTL 1.3% ($p = 0.52$); FA use in pregnancy: OC 1.2%, 0.9% CTL ($p = 0.79$)
Khoury et al. (1989)	Atlanta, GA	238 CL/P 107 CP	2809 UC	Self-reported MV use	MV use in periconceptional[e] period: CL/P vs. CTL: OR = 0.74 (0.56–0.97); CP vs. CTL: OR = 0.93 (0.62–1.40)
Bower and Stanley (1992)	Western	13 OC	115 UC	Self-reported diet and MV use	No significant differences in folate intake between OC and CTL
Shaw et al. (1995)	California	448 CL/P 215 CP	734 UC	Self-reported MV + FA use	MV + FA use in periconceptional period: CL/P-ISO vs. CTL: OR = 0.50 (0.36–0.68); CL/P-M vs. CTL: OR = 0.61 (0.35–1.1); CP-ISO vs. CTL: OR = 0.73 (0.46–1.2); CP-M vs. CTL: OR = 0.64 (0.35–1.2)
Czeizel et al. (1996)	Hungary	1246 CL/P 537 CP	1246 UC-CL/P[c] 537 UC-CP[d]	Medical record review and self-reported FA use	FA use in critical period[e] of cleft development: CL/P vs. CTL: OR = 0.72 (0.55–0.92); CP vs. CTL: OR = 0.86 (0.66–1.13)
Hayes et al. (1996)	Boston, Toronto, Philadelphia	195 CL/P 108 CP	1167 AC	Self-reported MV + FA use	MV + FA use in periconceptional period: CL/P vs. CTL: OR = 1.2 (0.7–2.0); CP vs. CTL: OR = 0.9 (0.5–1.7)
Werler et al. (1999)	Boston, Toronto, Philadelphia	114 CL/P 46 CP	521 UC 442 AC	Self reported MV use	MV use in critical period of cleft development: CL/P vs. CTL (UC): OR = 0.8 (0.5–1.3); CP vs. CTL (UC): OR = 0.4 (0.2–0.8)
Stoll et al. (1999)	Strasbourg, France	14 CL/P	340 UC	Biochemical measures in previously stored samples	No significant CL/P–CTL differences in trace elements, serum folate, vitamin A, vitamin B_{12}
Wong et al. (1999)	Nijmegen, Netherlands	35 CL/P	56 UC	Biochemical measures 1–6 years after delivery	Serum hyperhomocysteinemia:[e] CL/P (15.6%) vs. CTL (3.6%), OR = 5.3 (1.1-24.2). Higher mean serum and red cell folate and poorer vitamin B_6 status in CL/P vs. CTL

[a]OC, unspecified oral cleft; CL/P, cleft lip with or without cleft palate; CP, cleft palate; ISO, isolated cleft; M, cleft with multiple birth defects; UC, unaffected control child; AC, affected control child with noncleft birth defect or genetic disease; CTL, control; MV, multivitamin and mineral supplement; FA, folic acid; OR, odds ratio (95% confidence interval).
[b]p values from two-sided Fisher's exact test.
[c]UC-CL/P, separate control group for comparison to CL/P group.
[d]UC-CP, separate control group for comparison to CP group.
[e]See text for definition.

Hill's Case-Control Study in England

Medication use during pregnancy was the focus of a study of 676 mothers of cleft-affected children and an equal number of mothers of unaffected children born during 1983–1984 in England (Hill et al., 1988). Cases were ascertained by the congenital malformation surveillance system of the Office of Population Censuses and Surveys. Data were not presented by type of cleft. Each case child was matched with the next unaffected child born in the same general medical practice. The family medical practitioners of case and control children were identified from the District Health Authorities and visited by a medical officer of the study, who abstracted information on maternal medical and family history from the written records of the medical practice. No demographic data were presented for cases or controls, and no data were collected directly from mothers. Medical records provided very limited information on supplement use during the 3-month period before the last menstrual period: vitamin use was indicated in only 1.9% of cases and 1.3% of controls, and folic acid supplementation was indicated in only 1.2% of cases and 0.9% of controls. More case than control mothers reported use of one or more of 13 categories of medications. Thus, this study design was useful for evaluation of exposure to medications but inadequate to capture data on use of nutritional supplements. Prescription of nutritional supplements by physicians for mothers in this study seemed nearly nonexistent, and no data were provided on the use of supplements obtained outside of the medical system.

Metropolitan Atlanta Congenital Defects Program

The Atlanta Birth Defect Case-Control Study investigated a wide variety of risks for birth defects, including oral clefts, in the Atlanta metropolitan area (Khoury et al., 1989). Cleft cases were ascertained during 1968–1980 via multiple sources as part of the routine surveillance of the Metropolitan Atlanta Congenital Defects Program and included 238 with CL/P and 107 with CP; data were reported on these separate groups, but each group included isolated, multiple, and syndromic birth defects. Controls were mothers selected among 323,421 live births to women in the same population and frequency-matched to cases by birth period, race, and hospital of birth The focus of the report was on maternal cigarette smoking, but data on vitamin use were presented, although not controlled for potential confounding factors. Mothers were interviewed by telephone, and the participation rate was 70%. Mothers were asked whether they used vitamins during the periconceptional period, defined as 3 months prior to conception through 3 months after pregnancy began. No further information was provided regarding what constituted vitamin use, i.e., frequency, regularity, and type of vitamins used; and no information was provided on maternal diet. The percent of mothers reporting vitamin use was 53.3% for CL/P, 58.9% for CP, and 60.7% for controls; the OR for risk of oral clefts associated with vitamin use was 0.74 for CL/P (95% CI 0.56–0.98) and 0.93 for CP (95% CI 0.62–1.40).

Western Australia

A case-control study in Western Australia, in which an inverse association was found between maternal dietary intake of folate and risk of NTDs (Bower and Stanley, 1989), was extended to examine midline birth defects, some of which included oral clefts. (Bower and Stanley, 1992). In the original study, all cases of NTDs in infants born during mid-1982 through 1984 and ascertained via the Western Australia Birth Defects Registry were eligible. Two control groups were drawn from the same population, one with major malformations other than NTDs and the other including unaffected live-born infants. Midline defects were identified in 59 infants of the malformed control group in the original study, and these were designated as cases in the study of midline defects. Infants with chromosomal anomalies or known Mendelian syndromes were excluded. The controls used in the midline study were 115 unaffected infants used as controls in the original study of NTDs. Mothers were interviewed by telephone and completed a self-administered food-frequency questionnaire regarding their diet for the period 3 months before to 9 months after their last menstrual period before pregnancy. The questionnaire was limited to food items that contained substantial amounts of folate and included questions on cooking methods, dietary changes, and use of vitamin supplements. Intake of free folic acid and total folate was calculated using food-composition tables and adjusted for cooking practices (Paul and Southgate, 1979; Truesdale, 1984). Folate intake was divided into quartiles, and the risk of midline defects was evaluated with the lowest quartile as the reference level in multivariate models that included several potential confounding factors. No consistent relationship was observed between risk of midline defects and either free folic acid or total folate intake. The power of this study was limited by the small sample size, and the heterogeneity of the sample further compounded this problem. Only 13 of the 59 cases with midline defects had oral clefts. While there remains a strong and plausible argument for shared causes in this diverse group of birth defects, the most promising approach in identifying these causes is to focus on cleft defects per se and to use homogeneous subgroups such as isolated CL/P and CP in case-control analyses.

California Birth Defects Monitoring Program

The California Birth Defects Monitoring Program provided a large population-based sample of oral clefts for the case-control study reported by Shaw et al. (1995). Cases were infant births or fetal deaths during 1987–1989 with oral clefts ascertained via multiple sources throughout California. All cases were reviewed by a medical geneticist and classified as isolated CL/P or CP either in isolation or with multiple birth defects. Known monogenic syndromes were excluded. Controls were randomly sampled from all unaffected infants born during the same period and matched to cases by county of residence. Mothers of 731 cases and 734 controls were interviewed by telephone and asked about use of vitamin and mineral supplements, intake of cold breakfast cereals, and other traits and demographic factors. The periconceptional exposure period of interest for vitamin use was defined as 1 month before conception through 2 months afterward, and mothers who started vitamin use in the third month after conception were excluded from the analyses. Doses of folic acid were imputed as 0.8 mg for reports of prenatal vitamin use and 0.4 mg for all other vitamin supplements that contained folic acid. Fewer case than control mothers reported any use of multivitamins containing folic acid during the periconceptional period (57.2% vs. 69.1%) and during the 1-month period before conception (14.3% vs. 18.9%). The ORs indicating risk of specific types of oral cleft with any use of multivitamins with folic acid in the periconceptional period were 0.50 for isolated CL/P, 0.61 for CL/P with multiple birth defects, 0.73 for isolated CP, and 0.64 for CP with multiple birth defects. The 95% CI for isolated CL/P excluded 1.0 and was narrow (95% CI 0.36–0.68), based on the substantial sample size of 348 cases in this subgroup; the CIs for the other subgroups included 1.0 but were based on much smaller sample sizes. The risk of oral clefts by subgroup was evaluated over four levels of average daily intake of folic acid from multivitamins, with the lowest (none) as the reference level. The highest level of intake (≥ 1.0 mg/day) was uninformative because only four cases of isolated CL/P, one case of multiple CL/P, and no CP cases were in this level and the number of controls in this level was not presented. The ORs for isolated CL/P were 0.47 (95% CI 0.33–0.67) for 0.4 mg or less folic acid per day and 0.52 (95% CI 0.36-0.76) for 0.4 to 0.9 mg/day, indicating that the risk of this type of cleft was reduced by half with any use of multivitamins containing folic acid, and no dose-response relationship was discernible. The results appeared similar for the

other subgroups of oral clefts but more variable, perhaps because of smaller sample sizes in each. Vitamin use may be associated with other healthy lifestyle characteristics, so Shaw et al. (1995) rigorously controlled for potential confounding factors, including race and ethnicity, education, age, gravidity, smoking, alcohol use, family history of oral clefts, maternal medical history, and use of folate-antagonist medications; the reduced risk with multivitamin use was not influenced by these factors. Throughout this report, the relevant exposure was described as use of "multivitamins containing folic acid," yet this placed an artificial emphasis on folic acid because most of the multivitamin preparations contained folic acid and a large number of other vitamins and minerals. The authors noted that of the 954 case and control mothers using vitamins, only two reported using a supplement with folic acid only and only 27 used a multivitamin supplement without folic acid. Shaw et al. (1995) extended their analyses by examining the risk of oral clefts in mothers who consumed cold cereals, an unspecified proportion of which were fortified with vitamins and minerals. Among the mothers who used no multivitamins in the periconceptional period, the risk of clefting was reduced among those with daily cereal consumption (OR = 0.41, 95% CI 0.17–0.98) for isolated CL/P and suggestive for other cleft types, although the small number of case mothers with these characteristics (22 case and 32 control mothers) limited the analyses. The Californian study, one of the most exhaustive to date, provides compelling evidence that maternal multivitamin use in the periconceptional period is associated with a reduced risk of oral clefts, but the specific role of folic acid remains uncertain.

Hungarian Case-Control Surveillance of Congenital Abnormalities

The Hungarian Case-Control Surveillance of Congenital Abnormalities has collected data since 1980 on cases of birth defects identified among infants in the first 3 months of life and in fetal deaths ascertained by the Hungarian Congenital Abnormality Registry. Controls were selected from unaffected births via the national birth registry and matched to cases by sex, birth week, and district of parental residence. Data on cleft cases were reported by Czeizel et al. (1996) and later updated (Czeizel et al., 1999); the latest analyses were based on 1246 matched pairs of CL/P cases and controls and 537 matched pairs of CP cases and controls. Data were collected from mothers on use of vitamin supplements, use of medications, and medical and pregnancy history by mailed questionnaire, review of antenatal logbooks and medical records, and (for nonresponding cases) interviews by visiting nurses. Folic acid supplementation was evaluated from these records, and according to the authors, the commonly available form during the period of study was a 3.0 mg tablet prescribed by obstetricians in the amount of 1 to 3 tablets/day; the usual dose was assumed to be 6.0 mg/day. Use of folic acid alone was uncommon (14% of controls and 13% of cases) and not further evaluated; among the remaining majority of participants, other vitamins, minerals, and medicines were taken; but these details were not reported. The onset of folic acid supplement use was reported by month of pregnancy for cases and controls, and the critical period of exposure was defined as months 1 to 2 for CL/P and 1 to 3 for CP. The ORs describing risk of oral clefts for mothers using folic acid supplements in the critical period vs. all others were 0.72 (95% CI 0.55–0.92) for CL/P and 0.86 (95% CI 0.66–1.13) for CP. Shaw et al. (1995) excluded from their analyses mothers in California who began use of supplements after 3 months; thus, the remaining comparison was mothers using supplements in the periconceptional period vs. nonusers. Applying this approach to the 1999 Hungarian data yields an OR of 0.62 (95% CI 0.46–0.83) for the risk of CL/P among mothers using folic acid supplements in the critical period vs. nonusers. When late users (beyond the second month of pregnancy) were compared to nonusers, the OR for risk of CL/P was 0.77 (95% CI 0.62–0.96); because this exposure period is after cleft formation, these results indicate that the association between supplement use and reduced risk of oral clefts may be confounded by other personal characteristics associated with supplement use and risk of oral clefts. A similar analysis of the CP data yields an OR of 0.71 (95% CI 0.52–0.98) for use in the critical period (months 1–3) vs. nonuse, and the contrast of late supplement users (beyond the third month) and nonusers yields an OR of 0.79 (95% CI 0.54–1.15). The Hungarian findings, like the Californian findings, reveal associations between the use of nutritional supplements and reduced risk of clefting, but the independent role of folic acid per se also remains uncertain. Some of the reduced risk associated with maternal vitamin use appears to be due to confounding factors because mothers who initiated supplement use after the period of cleft formation also appeared to have a reduced risk of clefting compared to mothers who did not use supplements.

Strasbourg Case-Control Study

Plasma samples were routinely collected during the first antenatal visit of women in the Strasbourg area for subsequent case-control comparisons of mothers of children affected and unaffected with malformations (Stoll et al., 1999). The bank of samples represented births occurring between 1985 and 1994, and each was stored at −20°C until the assays were completed. Biochemical studies of maternal plasma trace elements and vitamin B_{12}, vitamin A, and folic acid were evaluated in a nested case-control study. Mothers of 170 children with congenital malformations ascertained by the local registry of congenital malformations were included as cases, and two controls per case were matched for sex, age of mother, hospital of delivery, obstetric history, and social class. The sample included only 14 cases of CL/P. The other major groups and numbers of malformations included heart ($n = 72$), vesicorenal reflux ($n = 8$), limb reduction defects ($n = 12$), spina bifida ($n = 6$), and hydrocephaly ($n = 6$). There were no significant differences between all malformations and controls or between specific subgroups of defects in mean plasma zinc, copper, magnesium, manganese, folate, vitamin B_{12}, or vitamin A. The sample size was adequate to detect a 1.0 standard deviation difference in mean trace elements at $\alpha = 0.05$ and $\beta = 0.10$ between the congenital heart defects ($n = 72$) and controls but lacked power for comparisons with the other subgroups including oral clefts. The close matching of cases and controls on a number of characteristics including social class and hospital of delivery may have resulted in an artificial similarity between cases and controls.

Boston–Philadelphia–Toronto Case-Control Studies

The Slone Epidemiology Unit has combined surveillance of birth defects and medication use with case-control studies since 1976 in participating hospitals in the Boston, Philadelphia, and Toronto metropolitan areas. Hayes et al. (1996) reported results of a case-control study of oral clefts that, like the Western Australia Study, was derived from a previous investigation of NTDs. Cases included mothers of infants live- or stillborn during 1988–1991 with CL/P ($n = 195$) or CP ($n = 108$). Mendelian conditions were excluded. Controls were 1167 mothers of live-born children with congenital anomalies other than NTDs or midline defects, and the larger groups were renal anomalies ($n = 177$), gastrointestinal anomalies ($n = 156$), limb defects ($n = 139$), craniosynostosis ($n = 115$), and chromosomal anomalies ($n = 90$). Case and control mothers were interviewed by a trained nurse within 6 months of birth regarding demographic background, medical and family history, dietary practices, and use of nutritional supplements and medications. Dates of initiation and cessation of supplement use were determined with the aid of a calendar, highlighting the exposure periods of interest. The relevant period of periconceptional exposure was defined as 1 month prior to the last menstrual period though the fourth month of pregnancy (16 weeks after last menstrual period). Medication and supplement bottles were examined for content and dose information. Supplementation was defined as use of a folic acid–containing multivitamin or a folic acid supplement alone; 95% of the folic acid supplementation, however, was in the form of a multivitamin, so the effects of folic acid could not be separated from those of other nutrients as in the Californian and Hungarian studies. Reported use of supplements at any time during the periconceptional period was 68% among controls, 70% among CL/P cases, and 62% among CP cases. When mothers using supplements daily throughout the periconceptional period were compared with mothers not using them in the same period, the OR estimate of risk was 1.2 (95% CI 0.7–2.0) for CL/P and 0.9 (95% CI 0.5–1.7) for CP; thus, no evidence was found of a protective association between maternal use of multivitamin and mineral supplements and risk of oral clefts.

A second study of maternal nutrition and oral clefts in the same populations was reported from the Slone group by Werler et al. (1999), in which case and control mothers for birth years 1993–1996 were recruited using similar procedures. A second control group was included of mothers of children without birth defects selected from the same birth hospitals in the surveillance program. The 822 case mothers represented eight major categories of birth defects, and of these, 114 were CL/P and 46 were CP. Data-collection procedures were the same as in the earlier study, and participation rates were nearly the same in cases, malformed controls, and normal controls (66% overall). Multivitamin supplementation was defined more broadly than in the earlier study and included daily use of a supplement with two or more water-soluble vitamins and two or more fat-soluble vitamins. Reported use of supplements at any time during months 1 through 4 was 76% among both malformed and non-malformed control mothers, 75% among CL/P case mothers, and 64% among CP case mothers; each represented slight increases over the previous study. Supplementation was categorized by the month of pregnancy of first use, and use in the 1-month period before the last menstrual period was not a criterion for exposure as in the earlier study. The critical exposure period was defined as months 1 through 3 for CL/P and 1 through 4 for CP because of the later period of palatal closure. The reference group included mothers with no supplement use or use that began after the critical period. Maternal characteristics associated with supplement use included age, education, race, planned pregnancy, nausea and vomiting in first month, and geographic center; these were included as covariates in multivariate models. Using the non-malformed control group, the OR indicating risk of CL/P with any use of supplements in the critical period was 0.8 (95% CI 0.5–1.3); the CL/P results using the malformed control group were similar (OR = 0.7, 95% CI 0.4–1.1). A reduced risk of CP was significantly associated with supplement use in the comparisons using non-malformed controls (OR = 0.4, 95% CI 0.2–0.8) and malformed controls (OR = 0.4, 95% CI 0.2–0.9). Both studies used similar methods of ascertainment and the same rigorous data-collection methods; supplement use increased only slightly between the earlier and later periods of study. The data from these studies do not provide evidence for a protective effect of multivitamin supplements against CL/P. The difference between the null association for CP in the earlier study and the positive association in the later study may be partially explained by the use in the earlier study of some groups of malformed controls excluded in the later one, i.e., groups including limb defects and urinary tracts defects. The parallel use of malformed and non-malformed controls and the similarity of results provide strong evidence that maternal recall of supplement use is not biased between mothers of affected and unaffected children. The possibility remains, despite the best efforts of investigators, that residual confounding factors related to maternal vitamin use and risk of oral clefts may affect the findings of the Slone studies as in other case-control studies.

The Netherlands Case-Control Study of Maternal Metabolic Factors

The University of Nijmegen in The Netherlands has been a center of innovative studies of homocysteine metabolism in relation to NTDs (Steegers-Theunissen et al., 1991, 1994, 1995; Wong, 1999). Exposure to high levels of homocysteine alters the migration of neural crest cells and causes malformations in experimental avian models (Rosenquist et al., 1996). Wong et al. (1999) demonstrated the usefulness of investigating biochemical markers of maternal nutritional status in case-control studies of oral clefts. Cases of nonsyndromic oral clefts, both CL/P and CP, were ascertained by the Nijmegen Cleft Palate Team from patients treated between 1992 and 1997, and 71 eligible mothers of case children between ages 1 and 5 years were identified. Of these, three could not be contacted, 17 declined participation, and others were excluded because of current vitamin use ($n = 6$) or pregnancy ($n = 10$); 35 case mothers completed the study. Control mothers were selected from the nearby population (methods not specified), and 56 completed the study; 1 was excluded because of recent vitamin use. Mean ages of mothers were 32.0 years for cases and 34.8 years for controls. Venous blood samples were collected for measurement of serum and red cell folate, plasma homocysteine, serum vitamin B_{12}, and vitamin B_6 (as pyridoxal-5-phosphate) in whole blood. Oral methionine-loading tests (Steegers-Theunissen et al., 1992) were then performed, and plasma homocysteine was measured again after 6 h. Case mothers had higher mean plasma homocysteine levels than controls for both the fasting (12 vs. 9 μmol/l, $p < 0.01$) and methionine afterload (35 vs. 31 μmol/l, $p < 0.05$) samples. Hyperhomocysteinemia, defined as fasting or afterload values above the 97.5 percentile, was found in 15.6% of case mothers and 3.6% of control mothers (OR = 5.5, 95% CI 1.1–24.2). Unexpectedly, case mothers compared to controls had higher mean levels of serum folate (16 vs. 13 nmol/l, $p < 0.01$) and red cell folate (550 vs. 490 nmol/l, $p < 0.05$). Vitamin B_{12} levels were not significantly different between groups, but case mothers had lower levels of whole-blood pyridoxal-5-phosphate compared to controls (41 vs. 52 nmol/l, $p < 0.05$). The mild hyperhomocysteinemia of case mothers thus was not explained by low folate values but may have been related to the poorer vitamin B_6 status of case mothers compared to controls. The advent of biochemical studies of maternal nutritional status, even years after the affected pregnancies, appears to be a significant methodologic advance in case-control studies of oral clefts. This method, however, is still subject to many of the pitfalls of case-control studies, including biased selection of participants. The Nijmegen results are based on a small number of case mothers from a single clinical center and had different rates of participation and exclusion between cases and controls. These studies should be extended to a larger sample in The Netherlands and other populations.

HUMAN EXPERIMENTAL TRIALS OF VITAMIN SUPPLEMENTATION FOR THE PREVENTION OF ORAL CLEFTS

Soon after the demonstration that vitamin deficiencies produced oral clefts in animal models in the 1940s, physicians became interested in whether vitamin supplementation could prevent the recurrence of oral clefts. The prevailing view at that time was that gene mutations were the most important cause of birth defects. In contrast, Douglas (1958) presented clinical observations of identical twins that were discordant for clefting in which the affected twin weighed less than the normal twin as evidence that variations in maternal blood supply between twins may adversely affect fetal nutritional status and risk of clefting. After the report

by Warkany (1942) that riboflavin deficiency induced skeletal abnormalities in rats, Douglas began adding riboflavin to the diets of pregnant women in Tennessee who had previously given birth to a child with a cleft. Douglas (1958) justified the intervention with the statement that "riboflavin and other vitamins in proper amounts as a supplement could not possibly harm the mother or the fetus in any way; further when one considers that it could only improve the mother's general welfare and might lower the risk of her having a second deformed child." Douglas reported no further details of efforts to reduce the recurrence of oral clefts other than the fact that not a single treated mother had another affected child; she acknowledged that the expected prevalence of oral clefts at birth in the area at that time was 0.6 to 1.0/1000 births and that the number of patients in the study was too small to be significant.

The next reported experimental trial to prevent the recurrence of oral clefts in humans was described by Conway (1958) just months after the report by Douglas appeared. Aspects and results of the trial by Conway (1958) and subsequent ones are listed in Table 14.3. Conway (1958) cited the work of Fogh-Andersen (1942) on the genetic determination of oral clefts in humans and the induction of oral clefts in animal models and concluded that "the occurrence of induced deformities is influenced by the genetic background of the experimental animals and that alteration of environmental factors is important in bringing out the deformities." Conway (1958) was also influenced by the work of Warkany and Kalter (1957) and cited their admonition that "it would be premature and dangerous to infer that parallels exist between the etiologies of the experimental and human abnormalities." Conway, working at the Cornell Medical College during 1946–1957, provided vitamin supplements for mothers of cleft-affected children during the periconceptional period of their subsequent pregnancies. Multivitamin capsules were given daily and included vitamin A (12,500 USP units), vitamin D (1000 USP units), vitamin C (100 mg), vitamin B_1 (5 mg), vitamin B_2 (5mg), vitamin B_6 (2 mg), vitamin B_{12} (4 μg), calcium pantothenate (10 mg), nicotinamide (30 mg), and folic acid (0.5 mg). In addition, an intramuscular injection of vitamins was given every other day, including vitamin B_1 (5 mg), vitamin B_2 (2 mg), vitamin B_6 (5 mg), vitamin B_{12} (2.5 μg), nicotinamide (75 mg), and sodium pantothenate (2.5 mg). No details were provided on the method of assignment of treatment; thus, it is unclear what selective factors and possible biases were involved. Participants included private, semiprivate, and "pavillion" (presumably indigent) patients; but the distributions of these patient types in the treated and un-

TABLE 14.3. *Trials of Maternal Vitamin Supplementation for the Prevention of Recurrence of Oral Clefts in the Pregnancies of High-Risk Women*

References	Population	Treatment Group*	Control Group	Design of Trial	Results†
Conway (1958)	New York	Vitamins A, B₁, B₂, B₆, B₁₂, C, D, FA, PT, N	No supplements	Method of treatment assignment not specified	0 clefts in 59 treated pregnancies, 4 clefts in 78 control pregnancies (p = 0.13)
Peer et al. (1958b, 1963, 1964), Briggs (1976)	New Jersey	Vitamins B₁, B₂, B₆, B₁₂, C, FA, P, N	No supplements	Method of treatment assignment not specified	7 clefts in 228 treated pregnancies, 20 clefts in 417 control pregnancies (p = 0.41)
Tolarova (1982), Tolarova and Harris (1995)	Czech Republic	Vitamins A, B₁, B₂, B₆, C, D, E, FA, PT, N	No supplements	Treatment group included mothers accepting supplements; controls were mothers who refused supplements or failed to comply; additional interventions encouraged for treatment group but not for control group	3 clefts in 211 treated pregnancies, 77 clefts in 1824 control pregnancies (p = 0.058)
Czeizel and Dudas (1992) Czeizel (1993a,b, 1998), Czeizel and Hirschberg (1997)	Hungary	Vitamins A, B₁, B₂, B₆, B₁₂, C, D, E, FA, PT, N, BT Minerals: Ca, P, Mg, Fe Trace elements: Cu, Mn, Zn	Cu, Mn, Zn vitamin C; lactose	Randomized, double-blind, intention-to-treat analysis	4 clefts in 2471 treated pregnancies, 6 clefts in 2391 control pregnancies (p = 0.57)

*BT, biotin; FA, folic acid; N, nicotinamide; P, phosphorus; PT, pantothenate. See text for doses.
†p values from two-sided Fisher's exact test.

treated groups was not reported. Of the 196 mothers under observation, 87 subsequently become pregnant; of these, 39 were given vitamin therapy and 48 received no vitamin therapy. The 39 mothers receiving vitamin therapy had a total of 59 subsequent pregnancies, and none of the infants had an oral cleft. Among the 48 mothers receiving no vitamin therapy, there were 78 subsequent pregnancies and four infants with oral clefts, including one with congenital heart defects. No statistical analyses were reported; application of Fisher's exact test to these data revealed that the difference between groups was not statistically significant ($p = 0.13$).

Peer et al. (1958a) reported that because animal studies showed protective effects of vitamin B_6 and folic acid against cleft induction in cortisone-treated mice, he routinely provided these vitamins to mothers of children with oral clefts during the early weeks of their subsequent pregnancy. Appeals were made to other plastic surgeons to do the same with their patients and contribute their data on pregnancy outcome to a pooled analysis. Peer et al. (1963, 1964) reported on patients in Newark, New Jersey, and 51 patients referred by colleagues at other locations. No details of the patient population were provided other than that each mother had a previous child with a cleft. Treatment consisted of prenatal vitamin capsules and an additional 5 mg folic acid and 10 mg vitamin B_6, each taken daily during the first trimester. The prenatal vitamin capsule also contained vitamin B_6 (2 mg); thus, the total daily dose of vitamin B_6 was 12 mg. Other vitamins in the prenatal capsule included vitamin B_1 (10 mg), vitamin B_2 (10 mg), vitamin B_{12} (4 μg), vitamin C (300 mg), niacinamide (100 mg), and calcium pantothenate (20 mg). Briggs (1976) provided an updated account of Peer's work and reported on the results of births to 228 treated mothers and 417 untreated control mothers. No details were provided on the methods of assigning women to the treatment or control group. Among the 228 subsequent births of the treated mothers, seven had oral clefts (3.1%); among the 417 subsequent births to the untreated women, 20 had oral clefts (4.8%). No statistical analyses were provided in the original publication; the difference between groups was not statistically significant (Fisher's exact $p = 0.41$). Briggs (1976) further stratified the data according to the type of cleft of the index child of each mother. Among mothers of children with CL/P, recurrence was 1.9% among the 161 pregnancies of treated mothers and 5.5% among the 275 pregnancies of untreated mothers ($p = 0.08$). Among mothers of index children with CP, recurrence was 6.0% in the treated group and 3.5% in the untreated group ($p = 0.47$). Briggs (1976) concluded, without statistical support for his claim, that

the supplementation was most helpful for mothers of CL/P index children and that supplementation might be "specifically detrimental when evaluating the incidence of cleft palate alone." He attempted to extend the sample size by including additional births of treated mothers who had already delivered one child while in the trial, but no comparable mothers in the untreated group were included; this may have introduced confounding related to differences in parity and social class between treated and untreated mothers.

Additional studies of the effect of vitamin supplementation on the reduction of the recurrence of oral clefts were reported by von Krebig and Stoeckenius (1978), Gabka (1981), and Schubert et al. (1990). These authors claimed success in reducing the risk of oral clefts with vitamin supplements, yet each of these studies either was too small or had insufficient data to allow a detailed evaluation of the results.

Czech Cleft Prevention Trial

A collection of pedigrees of 8250 cleft patients born between 1886 and 1982 in Bohemia provided an opportunity for Tolarova (1986, 1987a,b) at the Czechoslovak Academy of Sciences in Prague to explore the occurrence, genetics, and prevention of oral clefts. The Bohemian data include careful clinical classification of cleft type and genetic studies of the more recent patients and their families. In 1976, Tolorova began providing vitamin supplements to mothers deemed at high risk of cleft recurrence because they had either a cleft themselves or a child with a cleft. Mothers were instructed to take three tablets of the "Spofavit" multivitamin preparation each day beginning 3 months before conception and continuing until the end of the first trimester of pregnancy. Each tablet included vitamin A (2000 IU), vitamin B_1 (1 mg), vitamin B_2 (1 mg), vitamin B_6 (1 mg), vitamin C (50 mg), vitamin D (100 IU), vitamin E (2 mg), nicotinamide (10 mg), and calcium pantothenate (1 mg); in addition, mothers were given 10 mg of folic acid per day. The treatment group consisted of mothers who accepted the vitamin supplements when offered, and controls were mothers who declined the vitamin supplements or failed to comply with the treatment regimen. Tolarova (1982) reported that 1 of 85 supplemented pregnancies and 10 of 212 unsupplemented pregnancies were affected with oral clefts. The results were updated in 1987 (Tolarova, 1987a,b) and 1995 (Tolarova and Harris, 1995), and the most recent results revealed that 3 of 211 supplemented pregnancies and 77 of 1824 unsupplemented pregnancies were affected with oral clefts. A Fisher exact p value of 0.03 from a one-sided test was provided; the p value for the two-sided test was 0.058.

The exclusion of noncompliant participants in a clinical trial may seriously bias the results, even if the trial began with random assignment of treatments; this is the basis for "intention-to-treat" analyses in the design of modern clinical trials (Meinert, 1986). A serious limitation of the Czech study was the lack of random assignment of mothers to treatment or no treatment. Mothers in the treatment group were acceptors of the offer of supplementation and compliant, while the control group consisted of mothers who rejected the offer of supplementation or failed to adequately comply with the treatment regimen. This may have resulted in important confounding differences between groups related to lifestyle factors and risk of clefting. The authors noted that mothers in the supplemented group received additional interventions, including advice to conceive in the late spring and summer months because of the greater availability of fresh fruit and green vegetables and a lesser risk of respiratory tract infections; this advice was not given to the control group. Because the Czech trial did not include randomization, was a comparison of compliers and noncompliers by design, included additional lifestyle interventions for the supplemented group but not for the control group, and included an intervention with multiple vitamins, the results are uninterpretable with regard to the role of any specific nutrient in the prevention of oral clefts.

Hungarian Birth Defects Prevention Trial

The Hungarian Family Planning Program (HFPP) is a comprehensive program of medical care and social services devoted to improving reproductive health. This setting was used for a clinical trial of the efficacy of periconceptional multivitamin supplementation in the prevention of birth defects and other complications of pregnancy (Meinert, 1986; Czeizel and Dudas, 1992; Czeizel 1993a,b; Czeizel et al., 1994; Czeizel and Hirschberg, 1997; Czeizel, 1998; Czeizel et al., 1999). The HFPP included 26 centers coordinated by the Department of Human Genetics and Teratology at the Hungarian National Institute of Hygiene and is a World Health Organization Collaborating Center for the Community Control of Hereditary Diseases. Participants were offered extensive medical examinations, genetic counseling, and health education, including recommendations on diet and the avoidance of tobacco, alcohol, and other hazardous substances. Women attending the HFPP were recruited for a multivitamin supplementation trial and randomly assigned to take either a multivitamin or a trace-element tablet daily for the period 1 month before conception until the third month of gestation. The trial was double-blind. The multivitamin (Elevit Pronatal; Hoffman-La Roche,

Nutley, NJ) contained vitamin A (6000 IU until 1989 and 4000 IU thereafter); vitamin B_1 (1.6 mg); vitamin B_2 (1.8 mg); vitamin B_6 (2.6 mg); vitamin B_{12} (4 μg); vitamin C (100 mg); vitamin D (500 IU); vitamin E (15 mg); folic acid (15 mg); nicotinamide (19 mg); calcium pantothenate (10 mg); biotin (0.2 mg); four minerals including calcium (125 mg), phosphorus (125 mg), magnesium (100 mg), and iron (60 mg); and three trace elements including copper (1 mg), manganese (1 mg), and zinc (7.5 mg). The trace-element control group took a tablet with the same amounts of copper, manganese, and zinc with the addition of vitamin C (7.3 mg) and lactose (736 mg). All live births and other pregnancy outcomes were evaluated for the presence of congenital abnormalities through participating obstetrical clinics. The compliance of participants in pill taking was carefully assessed, and participants in 29% of the multivitamin group and 27% in the trace-element group were classified as taking no supplements or only a partial course. The outcome of pregnancy was assessed in 99% of participants, and the final results (Czeizel, 1998; Czeizel et al., 1999), based on an intention-to-treat analysis of all participants, revealed a significant reduction in NTDs (0 in 2471 vitamin-supplemented pregnancies vs. 6 in 2391 trace element–treated pregnancies; $p = 0.02$), but no significant differences were observed in the occurrence of a small number of oral clefts between treatment groups (4 among the vitamin-supplemented and 5 in the trace element–supplemented pregnancies; $p = 0.57$). The multivitamin group had higher rates of conception (71.3% vs. 67.9%), multiple births (3.7% vs 2.7%), and fetal deaths (13.4% vs. 11.4%) compared to the trace-element group.

NUTRIENT–GENE INTERACTIONS IN ORAL CLEFTS

A major role for genes in the development of normal craniofacial structures is evident from the common observation that monozygotic twins are nearly identical in appearance. Patterns of genetic inheritance of clefting were first described by Fogh-Andersen (1942) and confirmed by segregation analysis (Marazita et al., 1986; Mitchell and Risch, 1992; Mitchell and Christensen, 1996). The processes involved in the construction of the face have begun to be established through studies of animal models, human mutations, and recognized teratogens. Facial development is a complex process dependent on a broad spectrum of signaling molecules, homeobox genes, and growth factors (Murray, 1995). Development is initiated by migrating neural crest cells, which combine with mesodermal cells to establish the facial primordia.

A variation in the methylenetetrahydrofolate reductase gene (*MTHFR*, C677T allele) is the first known genetic risk factor for NTDs and may be relevant to oral clefts. Persons homozygous for the *MTHFR* T allele have a more thermolabile form of the *MTHFR* enzyme with reduced activity, which in the presence of low plasma folate (presumably low folate intake) results in higher plasma homocysteine levels (Jacques et al., 1996; Christensen et al., 1997). Not all studies, however, have shown a significant increase in risk of NTDs associated with the *MTHFR* T allele (Mornet et al., 1997). Shaw et al. (1998b) found a modest association between the *MTHFR* genotype of infants and risk of NTDs but no evidence of interaction between infant *MTHFR* genotype and maternal intake of folic acid–containing supplements.

The *MTHFR*–NTD association is an example of a possible nutrient–gene interaction in which the combination of these factors explains more than genotype or nutritional status alone. Christensen et al. (1999) extended the analysis of nutrient–gene interactions to include the genotype of both mother and child. The combination of the *MTHFR* TT genotype for mother and child yields an OR estimate of NTD risk of 6.0 (95% CI 1.26–28.53). The OR for mothers alone with the TT genotype was 1.29, and that for TT children alone was 2.0 (neither was statistically significant). When the combination of mother's TT genotype and low red cell folate was considered, the OR was 3.28 (95% CI 0.84–12.85). The combination of child's TT genotype and low maternal red cell folate yielded an OR of 13.43 (95% CI 2.49–72.33). This example illustrates both the potentials and the pitfalls of analyses of nutrient–gene interactions: uncovering strong interactions yields far more insight than studying single genotypes or nutrients alone, yet large sample sizes are needed to accurately estimate the effect because the combination of relatively uncommon genotypes with the probability of being in the lowest part of the distribution of an indicator of nutritional status results in a comparison group that is a small fraction of the total original sample. This is presumably why Christensen et al. (1999) were unable to report on the risk of NTDs among mother–child pairs in which both mother and child had the TT genotype and the mother had low red cell folate. Substantially larger sample sizes will be necessary to probe the extent of this and other complex interactions. As more data become available on multiple genes related to vitamin B_6 and folate metabolism, there will be more opportunities to explore the interaction between genes. Botto and Mastroiacovo (1998) analyzed the risk of NTDs in the presence of variations in both *MTHFR*

and cystathionine β-synthase and found an OR for gene–gene interaction of 5.2 (95% CI 0.8–2.1); this represents the estimate of the factor by which the OR for persons with both mutations is different from the multiplied effect of each mutation alone.

The *MTHFR*–NTD associations provide an interesting model, which at first glance may seem useful in understanding the causes of oral clefts. Early evidence, however, indicates that the association between *MTHFR* genotype and cleft risk may be different from that of NTDs. In a California study of isolated CL/P, Shaw and colleagues (1998a) found no increase in cleft risk among infants with the C677T allele (T); in the largest ethnic subgroup, non-Hispanic whites, the T allele was associated with a reduced risk of CL/P. In a follow-up report on isolated CP in the same study, a reduced risk of clefting was also found; the risk of CP, relative to infants with the CC genotype, was 0.6 (95% CI 0.3–1.3) for TT infants and 0.8 (95% CI 0.5–1.2) for CT infants (Shaw et al., 1999).

Further understanding of the role of *MTHFR* polymorphisms and cleft risk will require determinations of biochemical markers of folate and other nutrients, and insights might be gained from study of other *MTHFR*–disease associations. The C677T allele has also been associated with a reduced risk of colon cancer in the Health Professionals Follow-up Study (Chen et al., 1999), the Physicians' Health Study (Ma et al., 1997), and a case-control study conducted in Utah and Minnesota (Slattery et al., 1999). The mechanism by which the C677T allele contributes to the reduction in colon cancer risk has been hypothesized to include either imbalanced DNA methylation or altered synthesis of nucleic acids (Ma et al., 1996, 1997, 1999; Bagley and Selhub, 1998; Chen et al., 1998; Chen et al., 1998). Presence of the C677T allele was shown by Bagley and Selhub (1998) to be associated with an accumulation of formylated folates in red blood cells relative to the CC genotype; this shift in the distribution of folate forms may favor DNA synthesis and repair because of the dependence of these pathways on nonmethylated forms of folate.

DISCUSSION

Maternal nutrition is likely an important environmental factor responsible for the occurrence of oral clefts in humans. Evidence for this view has accumulated from studies over most of the past century from experimental animals, observational studies of human populations, and some limited human experimental studies. The history of experimental studies of oral clefts in experimental animals reveals several nutrients that might be used to prevent oral clefts in susceptible populations. The leading candidate nutrients include folic acid, vitamin B_6, and vitamin A. A lesser body of evidence implicates riboflavin, vitamin B_{12}, zinc, pantothenic acid, and biotin.

Josef Warkany was a pioneer in the early experimental studies of teratogenesis but remained cautious about the relevance of animal studies for congenital anomalies in humans: "experimental cleft palate has been going on for 40 years . . . to my knowledge the brilliant studies on mechanisms involved in cleft palate formation have not led to the prevention of human palate defects" (Kalter, 1993). Warkany died at the age of 90 about the time that the results from the MRC trial (MRC Vitamin Study Research Group, 1991) provided proof that maternal supplementation with folic acid substantially reduced the recurrence of NTDs and a source of optimism that improved maternal nutritional status might reduce the burden of other birth defects.

The relevance of folic acid supplementation for the prevention of human oral clefts remains unclear despite a number of studies that have addressed this hypothesis. Folate was an early focus in animal experiments on oral clefts, long before it was implicated in NTDs. Warkany's colleague Rose Nelson established methods for inducing dietary folate deficiency and exacerbating it with folate antagonists to produce fetal deaths, oral clefts, and other malformations. This work was replicated by Giroud and Boisselot (1951) in Paris, and a detailed description of the importance of the timing of folate deficiency during gestation emerged. Folate deficiency may even have relevance in dogs: a daily dose of 5 mg folic acid prevented oral clefts in a line of Boston Terriers with a genetic predisposition to this disorder.

Case-control studies of folate nutrition and oral clefts in humans have been limited by the facts that folate intake is difficult to estimate, folates have a wide range of bioavailability, and folic acid supplements are usually taken with other vitamins, minerals, and trace elements that may also have protective effects against oral clefts. Studies of medications that disrupt folate metabolism may shed more light on the role of folate nutrition in human oral clefts. Another useful approach is the study of biochemical indicators of maternal folate status (and other nutrients) even long after the fact of the affected pregnancy. The approach of examining biochemical markers of maternal nutritional status has rarely been employed in case-control studies but makes sense because mothers tend to resume their prepregnancy dietary habits and each mother, of course, has the same genotype at each time point in the study, which is important in determining tissue levels of nu-

trients. Maternal red cell folate levels were determined 1 year after delivery in a study in north London and found to be reasonably correlated with values determined early in pregnancy (Leck et al., 1983).

Studies of nutrient–genotype interactions may clarify the role of folate and other nutrients in oral clefts. The early indications from *MTHFR* studies are that the oral cleft results are quite different from expectations based on studies of NTDs. These findings underscore the importance of developing new methods for folate analyses that will characterize the distribution of various forms of folate so that the metabolic consequences of genetic variation may be examined in large-scale epidemiologic studies.

The human experimental trials conducted to date have done little to clarify the causal role of maternal folate nutrition in human oral clefts. These trials either have had an inadequate number of participants to provide sufficient statistical power, have not included study of folic acid apart from other nutrients, have not randomly assigned participants to treatment or control groups, or have failed to use intention-to-treat analyses.

Despite the extensive investigation of the role of vitamin B_6 in animal models of oral clefts since the 1950s, there is little information on the relevance of vitamin B_6 to oral clefts in humans, and this remains an important gap in our present knowledge. The use of antinausea medications was associated with a reduced risk of congenital heart defects in the Atlanta Birth Defects Case-Control Study (Erickson, 1991), and vitamin B_6 may have a role in this story. Further analyses of these findings revealed that maternal nausea during the first 2 months of pregnancy and use of the antinausea combination of doxylamine, dicyclomine and vitamin B_6 (Bendectin) (Merrell Dow Pharmaceuticals, Midland, MI) was significantly associated with a reduced risk of congenital heart defects (Boneva et al., 1999). The authors pointed out that Bendectin was composed of doxylamine succinate (10 mg), dicyclomine (10 mg, dropped from the formulation in 1976), and vitamin B_6 (pyridoxine, 10 mg) and that vitamin B_6 was often used alone for treatment of nausea in pregnancy. Portions of the developing heart are linked to cellular migration from the cranial neural crest; thus, it is plausible that vitamin B_6 may be related to several types of birth defect, including oral clefts, with common developmental origins in the neural tube and neural crest.

Biochemical analyses of maternal vitamin B_6 status in case-control studies also hold great promise, as shown in the Nijmegen study in The Netherlands (Wong et al., 1999). Adequate maternal vitamin B_6 nutrition may be important in lowering the risk of oral clefts by reducing plasma homocysteine levels. Animal experiments have provided evidence of other mechanisms for the protective effects, including a role for vitamin B_6 in glucocorticoid metabolism. The prevalence of vitamin B_6 deficiency is not well described worldwide, and little attention has been given to vitamin B_6 in public health nutrition policy in the United States and elsewhere. There are no regulations mandating the fortification of food with vitamin B_6 in the United States as there are with thiamine (vitamin B_1), riboflavin (vitamin B_2), niacin, and folic acid. Vitamin B_6 deficiency results from the use of medications including isoniazid treatment of tuberculosis and oral contraceptives (Sauberlich et al., 1972); thus, these factors should be considered in future studies of vitamin B_6 status.

Both abnormally low and high levels of vitamin A intake by mothers early in pregnancy may increase the risk of oral clefts and other malformations in their offspring. Despite Hale's early discovery that vitamin A deficiency caused ocular defects, oral clefts, and other malformations in pigs (Hale, 1933, 1935), little research has been subsequently conducted on the role of inadequate dietary vitamin A intake in experimental animal or human oral clefts. One recent exception has been the work of Natsume and colleagues (1999) in Japan, who found that intake of vegetables rich in β-carotene (and folate) was associated with a reduced risk of CL/P. Vitamin A deficiency is widespread, especially in developing countries around the world (West et al., 1999). Much work has been done on the effects of vitamin A deficiency on maternal and child health, especially related to morbidity and mortality due to increased susceptibility to infectious diseases, impaired vision, blindness, and other eye problems. Congenital anomalies may occur in the setting of vitamin A deficiency but may go unnoticed because of the larger burden of other health problems.

In a prospective study of over 22,000 pregnancies of American women, Rothman et al. (1995) found that malformations of structures derived from the embryonic cranial neural crest were more common among women who consumed more than 10,000 IU of vitamin A in the periconceptional period. Humans and other primates are thought to be more susceptible to retinoid-induced birth defects than rodents and rabbits, although the types of malformation are similar between species and include the craniofacial and other malformations mentioned above. The greater susceptibility to retinoid exposure among humans compared to other animals may be due to a higher rate of placental transfer, longer plasma half-life, and differences in metabolite formation (Ross, 1999).

Our understanding of the mechanisms involved in teratogenesis requires narrowly focused experiments in human and nonhuman animal studies and well-targeted hypotheses in observational epidemiologic studies. The flip side of this coin is that reductionism may obscure our recognition of other nutrients that may play important roles in the prevention of birth defects. Many researchers and public health advocates seem to have lost sight of the fact that a balanced diet based on wholesome foods is critical for providing the vitamins, minerals, macronutrients, and energy needed to sustain a healthy pregnancy.

A new generation of epidemiologic studies may help to establish a broader and more balanced view of the role of maternal nutrition in oral clefts. A good starting point would be studies of the co-occurrence of NTDs and oral clefts (or the lack of it). While it is possible that NTDs and clefts share developmental origins, it may be useful to try to understand how the nutritional and other causes of NTDs and oral clefts are different. Well-designed case-control studies with detailed assessment of biochemical markers of maternal nutritional status are needed to fill the gaps in our understanding of the role of maternal nutrition in oral clefts. Genetic studies of the underlying susceptibility to nutritional deficiency will clarify our understanding further. International collaboration will be essential to uncover nutrition-related and other important causes of oral clefts and to discover feasible public health interventions, to reduce their occurrence. Studies in diverse populations around the globe will likely uncover multiple nutritional, environmental, and genetic causes of oral clefts. Consistency of research methods across studies is highly desirable, and considerable efforts are now under way to organize a global network of cleft researchers with common case-control study protocols that will enhance the comparison and combination of the results of individual studies (Wyszynski and Mitchell, 1999). As the results from the next wave of enhanced case-control studies become available, rigorously designed intervention trials of vitamin supplementation will be the next logical step toward the prevention of oral clefts.

Supported by grant RO1-HD39061 from the U.S. National Institute of Child Health and Human Development and the National Institute for Dental and Craniofacial Research.

REFERENCES

Abbott, BD, Adamson, ED, Pratt, RM (1988). Retinoic acid alters EGF receptor expression during palatogenesis. Development 102: 853–867.

Abbott, BD, Birnbaum, LS (1990). Retinoic acid–induced alterations in the expression of growth factors in embryonic mouse palatal shelves. Teratology 42: 597–610.

Abbott, BD, Harris, MW, Birnbaum, LS (1988b). Etiology of retinoic acid–induced cleft palate varies with the embryonic stage. Teratology 40: 533–553.

Abbott, BD, Pratt, RM (1988a). EGF receptor expression in the developing tooth is altered by exogenous retinoic acid and EGF. Dev Biol 128: 300–304.

Abbott, BD, Pratt, RM (1988b). Influence of retinoids and EGF on growth of embryonic mouse palatal epithelia in culture. In Vitro Cell Dev Biol 24: 343–352.

Bagley, PJ, Selhub, J (1998). A common mutation in the methylenetetrahydrofolate reductase gene is associated with an accumulation of formylated tetrahydrofolates in red blood cells. Proc Natl Acad Sci USA 95: 13217–13220.

Been, W, Lieuw Kie Song, SH (1978). Harelip and cleft palate conditions in chick embryos following local destruction of the cephalic neural crest. A preliminary note. Acta Morphol Neerl Scand 16: 245–255.

Berry, RJ, Li, Z, Erickson, JD (1999). Prevention of neural-tube defects with folic acid in China. China–U.S. Collaborative Project for Neural Tube Defect Prevention. N Engl J Med 341: 1485–1490.

Boisselot, J (1949). Malformations foetales par insuffisance en acide pantothenique. Arch Pediatr 6: 1.

Boisselot, J (1951). Role tertogene de la deficience en acide pantothenique chez le rat. Ann Med 52: 225.

Boneva, RS, Moore, CA, Botto, L, et al. (1999). Nausea during pregnancy and congenital heart defects: a population-based case-control study. Am J Epidemiology 149: 717–725.

Bonner, J, Slavkin, H (1975). Cleft palate susceptibility linked to histocompatibility-2 (H-2) in the mouse. Immunogenetics 2: 213–218.

Botto, LD, Mastroiacovo, P (1998). Exploring gene–gene interactions in the etiology of neural tube defects. Clin Genet 53: 456–459.

Bower, C, Stanley, FJ (1989). Dietary folate as a risk factor for neural-tube defects: evidence from a case-control study in Western Australia. Med J Aust 150: 613–619.

Bower, C, Stanley, FJ (1992). Dietary folate and nonneural midline birth defects: no evidence of an association from a case-control study in Western Australia [see comments]. Am J Med Genet 44: 647–650.

Briggs, RM (1976). Vitamin supplementation as a possible factor in the incidence of cleft lip/palate deformities in humans. Clin Plast Surg 3: 647–652.

Chen, B, Wang, X, Yu, J, et al. (1998). Relationship between methylenetetrahydrofolate reductase gene polymorphism and coronary heart disease [in Chinese]. Chung Hua I Hsueh I Chuan Hsueh Tsa Chih 15: 300–302.

Chen, J, Giovannucci, E, Hankinson, SE, et al. (1998). A prospective study of methylenetetrahydrofolate reductase and methionine synthase gene polymorphisms, and risk of colorectal adenoma. Carcinogenesis 19: 2129–2132.

Chen, J, Giovannucci, EL, Hunter, DJ (1999). MTHFR polymorphism, methyl-replete diets and the risk of colorectal carcinoma and adenoma among U.S. men and women: an example of gene–environment interactions in colorectal tumorigenesis. J Nutr 129(Suppl 2): 560S–564S.

Christensen, B, Arbour, L, Tran, P, et al. (1999). Genetic polymorphisms in methylenetetrahydrofolate reductase and methionine synthase, folate levels in red blood cells, and risk of neural tube defects. Am J Med Genet 84: 151–157.

Christensen, B, Frosst, P, Lussier-Cacan, S, et al. (1997). Correlation of a common mutation in the methylenetetrahydrofolate reductase gene with plasma homocysteine in patients with premature coronary artery disease. Arterioscler Thromb Vasc Biol 17: 569–573.

Chung, CS, Kau, MC (1985). Racial differences in cephalometric measurements and incidence of cleft lip with or without cleft palate. J Craniofac Genet Dev Biol 5: 341–349.

Conway, H (1958). Effect of supplemental vitamin therapy on the limitation of incidence of cleft lip and cleft palate in humans. Plast Reconstr Surg 22: 450–453.

Cooper, MK, Porter, JA, Young, KE, et al. (1998). Teratogen-mediated inhibition of target tissue response to Shh signaling [see comments]. Science 280: 1603–1607.

Croen, LA, Shaw, GM, Wasserman, CR, et al. (1998). Racial and ethnic variations in the prevalence of orofacial clefts in California, 1983–1992. Am J Med Genet 79: 42–47.

Czeizel, AE (1993a). Controlled studies of multivitamin supplementation on pregnancy outcomes. Ann N Y Acad Sci 678: 266–275.

Czeizel, AE (1993b). Prevention of congenital abnormalities by periconceptional multivitamin supplementation. BMJ 306: 1645–1648.

Czeizel, AE (1998). Periconceptional folic acid containing multivitamin supplementation. Eur J Obstet Gynecol Reprod Biol 78: 151–161.

Czeizel, AE, Dudas, I (1992). Prevention of the first occurrence of neural-tube defects by periconceptional vitamin supplementation [see comments]. N Engl J Med 327: 1832–1835.

Czeizel, AE, Dudas, I, Metneki, J, et al. (1994). Pregnancy outcomes in a randomised controlled trial of periconceptional multivitamin supplementation. Final report. Arch Gynecol Obstet 255: 131–139.

Czeizel, AE, Hirschberg, J (1997). Orofacial clefts in Hungary. Epidemiological and genetic data, primary prevention. Folia Phoniatr Logop 49: 111–116.

Czeizel, AE, Timar, L, Sarkozi, A, et al. (1999). Dose-dependent effect of folic acid on the prevention of orofacial clefts. Pediatrics 104: e66.

Czeizel, AE, Toth, M, Rockenbauer, M, et al. (1996). Population-based case control study of folic acid supplementation during pregnancy. Teratology 53: 345–351.

Daly, S, Mills, JL, et al. (1997). Minimum effective dose of folic acid for food fortification to prevent neural-tube defects [see comments]. Lancet 350: 1666–1669.

Davis, SD, Nelson, T, Shepard, T, et al. (1970). Teratogenicity of vitamin B$_6$ deficiency: omphalocele, skeletal and neural defects, and splenic hypoplasia. Science 169: 1329–1330.

Dostal, M, Schubert, J (1990). Further studies on protective effects of vitamins in cyclophosphamide-induced cleft palate. Int J Oral Maxillofac Surg 19: 308–311.

Douglas, B (1958). The role of environmental factors in the etiology of so-called congenital malformations. I. Deductions from the presence of cleft lip and palate in one of identical twins, from embryology and from animal experiments. Plast Reconstr Surg 22: 94–108.

Elwood, JM, Colquhoun, TA (1997). Observations on the prevention of cleft palate in dogs by folic acid and potential relevance to humans. N Z V J 45: 254–256.

Emerson, DJ (1962). Congenital malformation due to attempted abortion with aminopterin. Am J Obstet Gynecol 84: 356–357.

Erickson, JD (1991). Risk factors for birth defects: data from the Atlanta Birth Defects Case-Control Study. Teratology 43: 41–51.

Evans, HM, Nelson, MM, Asling, CW (1951). Multiple congenital abnormalities resulting from folic acid deficiency during gestation. Science 114: 479.

Fantel, AG, Shepard, TH, Newell-Morris L, Moffett, BC (1977). Teratogenic effects of retinoic acid in pigtail monkeys (Macaca nemestrina). I. General features. Teratology 15: 65–71.

Fogh-Andersen, P (1942). Inheritance of Harelip and Cleft Palate. Copenhagen: Arnold Busck.

Fraser, FC (1955). Thoughts on the etiology of clefts of the palate and lip. Acta Genet 5: 358–369.

Fraser, FC, Fainstat, TD (1951a). Causes of congenital defects. Am Med Assoc J Dis Child 32: 593–603.

Fraser, FC, Fainstat, TD (1951b). Production of congenital defects in the offspring of pregnant mice treated with cortisone. Pediatrics 8: 527–533.

Fraser, FC, Warburton, D (1964). No association of emotional stress or vitamin supplement during pregnancy to cleft lip or palate in man. Plast Reconstr Surg 33: 395–399.

Gabbka, J (1981). Verhutung von lippen-kiefer-gaumenspalten: klinisch erfahrungen. Munch Med Wschr 123: 1139–1141.

Giroud, A, Boisselot, J (1947). Repercussions de l'avitaminose B₂ sur l'embryon du rat. Arch Pediatr 4(4): 317–327.

Giroud, A, Boisselot, J (1951). Influence teratogene de la carence en acide folique. C R Soc Biol 145: 526–527.

Giroud, A, Lefebvres, J (1951). Anomalies provoquées chez le foetus en l'absence d'acide folique. Arch Pediatr 8: 648–656.

Giroud, A, Levy, G, Lefebvres, J, et al. (1951). Variations du taux de la riboflavine chez la mére et le foetus, et leurs repercussions. Bull Soc Chim Biol 33(9): 1214–1222.

Goetsch, C (1962). An evaluation of aminopterin as an abortifacient. Am J Obstet Gynecol 83: 1474–1477.

Hale, F (1933). Pigs born without eyeballs. J Hered 24: 105–106.

Hale, F (1935). The relation of vitamin A to anophthalmos in pigs. Am J Opthalmol 18: 1087–1092.

Hayes, C, Werler, MM, Willett WC, Mitchell AA (1996). Case-control study of periconceptional folic acid supplementation and oral clefts. Am J Epidemiol 143: 1229–1234.

Herbert, V (1989). Development of human folate deficiency. In: Folic Acid Metabolism in Health and Disease, edited by MF Picciano, ELR Stokstad, and JFI Gregory. New York: Wiley-Liss, pp. 195–200.

Hibbard, B (1964). The role of folic acid in pregnancy with particular reference to anaemia, abruption and abortion. J Obstet Gynaecol Br Commonw 71: 529–542.

Hibbard, B, Smithells, R (1965). Folic acid metabolism and human embryopathy. Lancet i: 1254.

Hill, L, Murphy, M, McDowall M, Paul AH (1988). Maternal drug histories and congenital malformations: limb reduction defects and oral clefts. J Epidemiol Community Health 42: 1–7.

Incardona, JP, Gaffield, W, Kapur RP, Roelink H (1998). The teratogenic Veratrum alkaloid cyclopamine inhibits sonic hedgehog signal transduction. Development 125: 3553–3562.

Jacobsson, C, Granstrom, G (1997). Effects of vitamin B₆ on beta-aminoproprionitrile-induced palatal cleft formation in the rat. Cleft Palate Craniofac J 34: 95–100.

Jacques, PF, Bostom, AG, Williams, RR, et al. (1996). Relation between folate status, a common mutation in methylenetetrahydrofolate reductase, and plasma homocysteine concentrations [see comments]. Circulation 93: 7–9.

James, LF (1999). Teratological research at the USDA-ARS poisonous plant research laboratory. J Nat Toxins 8: 63–80.

Jones, MC (1988). Etiology of facial clefts: prospective evaluation of 428 patients. Cleft Palate J 25: 16–20.

Jordan, RL, Wilson, JG, Schumacher HJ, et al. (1977). Embryotoxicity of the folate antagonist methotrexate in rats and rabbits. Teratology 15: 73–80.

Kalter, H (1957). Factors influencing the frequency of cortisone-induced cleft palate in mice. J Exp Zool 134: 449–467.

Kalter, H (1993). Josef Warkany, 1902–1992. Teratology 48: 1–3.

Kalter, H, Warkany, J (1957). Congenital malformations in inbred strains of mice induced by riboflavin-deficient, galactoflavin-containing diets. J Exp Zool 136: 531–536.

Karnofsky, DA, Patterson, PA, Ridgway, LR, et al. (1949). Effect of folic acid, "4-amino"-folic acids, and related substances on growth of chick embryo. Proc Soc Exp Biol Med 71: 447.

Keeler, RF (1968). Teratogenic compounds of Veratrum californicum (Durand). IV, First isolation of veratramine and alkaloid Q and a reliable method for isolation of cyclopamine. Phytochemistry 7: 303–306.

Keeler, RF (1990). Early embryonic death in lambs induced by Veratrum californicum. Cornell Vet. 80: 203–207.

Khoury, MJ, Gomez-Farias, M, Mulinare, J, et al. (1989). Does maternal cigarette smoking during pregnancy cause cleft lip and palate in offspring? Am J Dis Child 143: 333–337.

Kirke, PN, Molloy, AM, Daly, LE, et al. (1993). Maternal plasma folate and vitamin B₁₂ are independent risk factors for neural tube defects. Q J Med 86: 703–708.

Kochhar, DM (1967). Teratogenic activity of retinoic acid. Acta Pathol Microbiol Scand 70: 398–404.

Kochhar, DM (1973). Limb development in mouse embryos. I. Analysis of teratogenic effects of retinoic acid. Teratology 7: 289–298.

Kochhar, DM, Penner, JD, Tellone, CI (1984). Comparative teratogenic activities of two retinoids: effects on palate and limb development. Teratog Carcinog Mutagen 4: 377–387.

Lammer, EJ, Chen, DT, Hoar, RM, et al. (1985). Retinoic acid embryopathy. N Engl J Med 313: 837–841.

Lasa, C, Manalo, P (1989). Update on the occurrence rate of cleft lip and palate. Philippine Journal of Surgery and Surgical Specialities 44: 109–111.

Leck, I, Iles, CA, Sharman, IM, et al. (1983). Maternal diet and nutrition during early pregnancy and after delivery in north London. In: Prevention of Spina Bifida and Other Neural Tube Defects, edited by J Dobbin. London: Academic Press. Appendix I. pages 197–218.

Leimbach, DG (1949). Rev Int Vitaminol 21: 222.

Lepkovsky, S, Taylor, LW, Jukes, TH, Almquist, HJ (1938). Hilgardia 11: 559–591.

Lidral, AC, Johnston, MC, Switzer, R (1991). The relationship between vitamins and the prevalence of cleft lip in mice. J Dent Res 68(Suppl): 524.

Lorente, C, Cordier, S, Goujard, J, et al. (2000). Tobacco and alcohol use during pregnancy and risk of oral clefts. Occupational Exposure and Congenital Malformation Working Group. Am J Public Health 90: 415–419.

Ma, J, Stampfer, MJ, Christensen, B, et al. (1999). A polymorphism of the methionine synthase gene: association with plasma folate, vitamin B₁₂, homocyst(e)ine, and colorectal cancer risk. Cancer Epidemiol Biomarkers Prev 8: 825–829.

Ma, J, Stampfer, MJ, Giovannucci, E, et al. (1997). Methylenetetrahydrofolate reductase polymorphism, dietary interactions, and risk of colorectal cancer. Cancer Res 57: 1098–1102.

Ma, J, Stampfer, MJ, Hennekens, CH, et al. (1996). Methylenetetrahydrofolate reductase polymorphism, plasma folate, homocysteine, and risk of myocardial infarction in US physicians [see comments]. Circulation 94: 2410–2416.

Marazita, ML, Goldstein, AM, Smalley, SL, Spence, MA (1986). Cleft lip with or without cleft palate: reanalysis of a three-generation family study from England. Genet Epidemiol 3: 335–342.

Marazita, ML, Jaskoll, T, Melnick, M (1988). Corticosteroid-induced cleft in short-ear mice. J Craniofac Genet Dev Biol 8: 47–51.

Meinert, CL (1986). Clinical Trials. Design, Conduct, and Analysis. New York: Oxford University Press.

Melnick, M, Jaskoll, T, Slavkin, HC (1981). Corticosteroid-induced cleft palate in mice and H-2 haplotype: maternal and embryonic effects. Immunogenetics 13: 443–450.

Meltzer, HJ (1956). Congenital anomalies due to attempted abortion with 4-amino-pteroylglutamic acid. JAMA 161: 1253.

Miller, TJ (1972). Cleft palate formation: a role for pyridoxine in the closure of the secondary palate in mice. Teratology 6: 351–356.

Mills, JL, McPartlin, JM, Kirke, PN, et al. (1995). Homocysteine metabolism in pregnancies complicated by neural-tube defects [see comments]. Lancet 345: 149–151.

Milunsky, A, Graef, JW, Gaynor, MF (1968). Methotrexate-induced congenital malformations. J Pediatr 72: 790–795.

Mitchell, LE, Christensen, K (1996). Analysis of the recurrence patterns for nonsyndromic cleft lip with or without cleft palate in the families of 3,073 Danish probands. Am J Med Genet 61: 371–376.

Mitchell, LE, Risch, N (1992). Mode of inheritance of nonsyndromic cleft lip with or without cleft palate: a reanalysis. Am J Hum Genet 51: 323–332.

Mornet, E, Muller, F, Lenvoise-Furet A, et al. (1997). Screening of the C677T mutation on the methylenetetrahydrofolate reductase gene in French patients with neural tube defects. Hum Genet 100: 512–514.

MRC Vitamin Study Research Group (1991). Prevention of neural tube defects: results of the Medical Research Council Vitamin Study. MRC Vitamin Study Research Group [see comments]. Lancet 338: 131–137.

Munger, RG, Romitti, PA, Daack-Hirsch, S, et al. (1996). Maternal alcohol use and risk of orofacial cleft birth defects. Teratology 54: 27–33.

Murray, JC (1995). Face facts: genes, environment, and clefts [editorial; comment]. Am J Hum Genet 57: 227–232.

Natsume, N, Kawai, T, Ogi, N, et al. (2000). Maternal risk factors in cleft lip and palate: case control study. Br J Oral Maxillofac Surg 38: 23–25.

Natsume, N, Sugimoto, S, Yoshida, K (1999). Influence of maternal anaemia during early pregnancy on the development of cleft palate [letter; comment]. Br J Oral Maxillofac Surg 37: 330–331.

Nelson, M, Asling, C, Evans, HM (1952). Production of multiple congenital abnormalities in young by maternal pteroylglutamic acid deficiency during gestation. J Nutr 48: 61–66.

Nelson, MM, Evans, HM (1947). Reproduction in the rat on purified diets containing succinylsulfathiazole. Proc Soc Exp Biol Med 66: 289.

Niebyl, JR, Blake, DA, Rocco, LE, et al. (1985). Lack of maternal metabolic, endocrine, and environmental influences in the etiology of cleft lip with or without cleft palate. Cleft Palate J 22: 20–28.

Noback, CR, Kupperman, HS (1944). Proc Soc Exp Biol Med 57: 183.

O'Dell, BL, Whitley, JR, Hogan, AG (1951). Vitamin B$_{12}$, a factor in prevention of hydrocephalus in infant rats. Proc Soc Exp Biol Med 76: 349.

Paros, A, Beck, SL (1999). Folinic acid reduces cleft lip [CL(P)] in A/WySn mice. Teratology 60: 344–347.

Paul, AA, Southgate, DA (1979). McCance and Widdowson's "The composition of foods": dietary fibre in egg, meat and fish dishes. J Hum Nutr 33: 335–336.

Peer, L, Bryan, W, Strean, LP, et al. (1958a). Induction of cleft palate in mice by cortisone and its reduction by vitamins. J Int Coll Surg 30: 249–254.

Peer, L, Gordon, H, Bernhard, WG (1964). Effect of vitamins on human teratology. Plast Reconstr Surg 34: 358–363.

Peer, L, Strean, L, Walker, JC, et al. (1958b). Study of 400 pregnancies with birth of cleft lip–palate infants: protective effect of folic acid and vitamin B$_6$ therapy. Plast Reconstr Surg 22: 442–449.

Peer, LA, Gordon, HW, Bernhard, WG (1963). Experimental production of congenital deformities and their possible prevention in man. J Int Coll Surg 39:

Piccioni, V, Bologna, U (1949). Clin Obstet 51: 173.

Pickerill, HP (1914). The anatomy and physiology of cleft palate and a new method of treatment. In: Transactions of the Sixth International Dental Congress, London. pp. 453–469.

Powell, HR, Ekert, H (1971). Methotrexate induced congenital malformations. Med J Aust 58: 1076–1077.

Romanoff, AL, Bauernfeind, JC (1942). Anat Rec 82: 11.

Romitti, PA, Munger, RG, Murray, JC, et al. (1998). The effect of follow-up on limiting non-participation bias in genetic epidemiologic investigations. Eur J Epidemiol 14: 129–138.

Rosenquist, TH, Ratashak, SA, Selhub, J (1996). Homocysteine induces congenital defects of the heart and neural tube: effect of folic acid. Proc Natl Acad Sci USA 93: 15227–15232.

Ross, CA (1999). Vitamin A and retinoids. In: Modern Nutrition in Health and Disease, edited by ME Shils, JA Olson, M Shike and AC Ross. Baltimore: Williams and Wilkins.

Rothman, KJ, Moore, LL, Singer, MR, et al. (1995). Teratogenicity of high vitamin A intake [see comments]. N Engl J Med 333: 1369–1373.

Salomon, DS, Gift, VD, Pratt, RM (1979). Corticosterone levels during midgestation in the maternal plasma and fetus of cleft palate-sensitive and -resistant mice. Endocrinology 104: 154–156.

Salomon, DS, Pratt, RM (1979). Involvement of glucocorticoids in the development of the secondary palate. Differentiation 13: 141–154.

Sauberlich, HE, Canham, JE, Baker, EM, et al. (1972). Biochemical assessment of the nutritional status of vitamin B$_6$ in the human. Am J Clin Nutr 25: 629–642.

Saxen, I (1975). Associations between oral clefts and drugs taken during pregnancy. Int J Epidemiol 4: 37–44.

Schubert, J, Schmidt, R, Raupach, HW (1990). New findings explaining the mode of action in prevention of facial clefting and first clinical experience. J Craniomaxillofac Surg 18: 343–347.

Shaw, EB, Steinbach, HL (1968). Aminopterin-induced fetal malformations. Am J Dis Child 115: 477–482.

Shaw, GM, Lammer, EJ (1999). Maternal periconceptional alcohol consumption and risk for orofacial clefts. J Pediatr 134: 298–303.

Shaw, GM, Lammer, EJ, Wasserman, CR, et al. (1995). Risks of orofacial clefts in children born to women using multivitamins containing folic acid periconceptionally [see comments]. Lancet 346: 393–396.

Shaw, GM, Rozen, R, Finnell, RH, et al. (1998). Infant C677T mutation in MTHFR, maternal periconceptional vitamin use, and cleft lip [see comments]. Am J Med Genet 80: 196–198.

Shaw GM, Rozen, R, Finnell, RH, et al. (1998b). Maternal vitamin use, genetic variation of infant methylenetetrahydrofolate reductase, and risk for spina bifida [see comments]. Am J Epidemiol 148: 30–37.

Shaw, GM, Todoroff, K, Finnell, RH, et al. (1999). Maternal vitamin use, infant C677T mutation in MTHFR, and isolated cleft palate risk [letter]. Am J Med Genet 85: 84–85.

Slattery, ML, Potter, JD, Samowitz, W, et al. (1999). Methylenetetrahydrofolate reductase, diet, and risk of colon cancer. Cancer Epidemiol Biomarkers Prev 8: 513–518.

Smithells, RW, Sheppard, S, Schorah, CJ (1976). Vitamin dificiencies and neural tube defects. Arch Dis Child 51: 944–950.

Soprano, DR, Soprano, KJ (1995). Retinoids as teratogens. Annu Rev Nutr 15: 111–132.

Steegers-Theunissen, RP, Boers, GH, Blom, HJ, et al. (1995). Neural tube defects and elevated homocysteine levels in amniotic fluid. Am J Obstet Gynecol 172: 1436–1441.

Steegers-Theunissen, RP, Boers, GH, Steegers, EA, et al. (1992). Effects of sub-50 oral contraceptives on homocysteine metabolism: a preliminary study. Contraception 45: 129–139.

Steegers-Theunissen, RP, Boers, GH, Trijbels, FJ, Eskes, TK, (1991). Neural-tube defects and derangement of homocysteine metabolism [letter]. N Engl J Med 324: 199–200.

Steegers-Theunissen, RP, Boers, GH, Trijbels, FJ, et al. (1994). Maternal hyperhomocysteinemia: a risk factor for neural-tube defects? Metabolism 43: 1475–1480.

Stoll, C, Dott, B, Alembik, Y, et al. (1999). Maternal trace elements, vitamin B$_{12}$, vitamin A, folic acid, and fetal malformations. Reprod Toxicol 13: 53–57.

Strauss, OA (1914). Predisposing causes of cleft palate and harelip. In: Transactions of the Sixth International Dental Congress, London. pp. 470–471.

Sunde, ML, Cravens, WW, Elvehjem, CA, et al. (1950). The effect of folic acid on embryonic development of the domestic fowl. Poultry Sci 29: 696.

Thiersch, JB (1956). The control of reproduction in rats with the aid of antimetabolites, and early experiments with antimetabolites as abortifacient agents in man. Acta Endocr 28(Suppl): 37–45.

Thiersch, JB, Philips, FS (1950). Effect of 4-amino-pteroylglutamic acid (aminopterin) on early pregnancy. Proc Soc Exp Biol Med 74: 204–208.

Tolarova, M (1982). Periconceptional supplementation with vitamins and folic acid to prevent recurrence of cleft lip [letter]. Lancet 2: 217.

Tolarova, M (1986). Incidence of orofacial clefts in Bohemia 1975–1982 [in Czech]. Cesk Pediatr 41: 131–135.

Tolarova, M (1987a). Orofacial clefts in Czechoslovakia. Incidence, genetics and prevention of cleft lip and palate over a 19-year period. Scand J Plast Reconstr Surg Hand Surg 21: 19–25.

Tolarova, M (1987b). A study of the incidence, sex-ratio, laterality and clinical severity in 3,660 probands with facial clefts in Czechoslovakia. Acta Chir Plast 29: 77–87.

Tolarova, M, Harris, J (1995). Reduced recurrence of orofacial clefts after periconceptional supplementation with high-dose folic acid and multivitamins. Teratology 51: 71–78.

Truesdale, K (1984). Nutrition to meet the needs of the elderly. Can Dent Hyg 18: 40–41.

Tyan, ML, Tyan, DB (1993). Vitamin A–enhanced cleft palate susceptibility gene maps between C4 and B144 within the H-2 complex. Proc Soc Exp Biol Med 202: 482–486.

von Krebig, VT, Stoeckenius, M (1978). Fehlbildungen beim menschen: lippen-kiefer-gaumenspalten. Med Monatsschr Pharm 1: 243–249.

Wald, NJ, Law, M, Jordan, R (1998). Folic acid food fortification to prevent neural tube defects [letter; comment]. Lancet 351: 834–835.

Wald, NJ, Polani, PE (1984). Neural-tube defects and vitamins: the need for a randomized clinical trial. Br J Obstet Gynaecol 91: 516–523.

Warkany, J (1954). Congenital malformations induced by maternal dietary deficiency: experiments and their interpretation. In: The Harvey Lectures. 1952–1953. New York: Academic Press. pp. 89–109.

Warkany, J, Beaudry, PJ, Hornstein, S (1959). Attempted abortion with aminopterin (4-amino-pteroylglutamic acid). Am J Dis Child 97: 274–281.

Warkany, J, Kalter, H (1957). Experimental cleft palate: interpretations and misinterpretations. Bull Am Assoc Cleft Palate Rehabil 7: 9.

Warkany, J, Nelson, RC (1940). Appearance of skeletal abnormalities in the offspring of rats reared on a deficient diet. Science 92: 383–384.

Warkany, J, Nelson, RC (1941). Skeletal abnormalities in the offspring of rats reared on deficient diets. Anat Rec 79: 83.

Warkany, J, Nelson, RC, Schraffenberger, E (1942). Congenital malformations induced in rats by maternal nutritional deficiency. II. Use of varied diets and of different strains of rats. Am J Dis Child 64: 860.

Warkany, J, Shraffenberger, E (1944). J Nutr 27: 477.

Werler, MM, Hayes, C, Louik, C, et al. (1999). Multivitamin supplementation and risk of birth defects. Am J Epidemiol 150: 675–682.

Werler, MM, Lammer, EJ, Rosenberg, L, Mitchell, AA (1991). Maternal alcohol use in relation to selected birth defects. Am J Epidemiol 134: 691–698.

West, KP, Jr, Katz, J, Khatry, SK, et al. (1999). Double blind, cluster randomised trial of low dose supplementation with vitamin A or beta carotene on mortality related to pregnancy in Nepal. The NNIPS-2 Study Group [see comments]. BMJ 318: 570–575.

Whitby, KE, Collins, TF, Welsh, JJ, et al. (1994). Developmental effects of combined exposure to ethanol and vitamin A. Food Chem Toxicol 32: 305–320.

Wilson, JG, Warkany, J (1948). Malformations in the genito-urinary tract induced by maternal vitamin A deficiency in the rat. Am J Anat 83: 357.

Womersley, J, Stone, DH (1987). Epidemiology of facial clefts. Arch Dis Child 62: 717–720.

Wong, WY, Eskes, TK, Kuijpers-Jagtman, AM (1999). Nonsyndromic orofacial clefts: association with maternal hyperhomocysteinemia. Teratology 60: 253–257.

World Health Organization (1998). World Atlas of Birth Defects. Geneva: World Health Organization.

Wyszynski, DF, Beaty, TH (1996). Review of the role of potential teratogens in the origin of human nonsyndromic oral clefts. Teratology 53: 309–317.

Wyszynski, DF, Mitchell, LE (1999). Report of the newly formed International Consortium for Oral Clefts Genetics. Cleft Palate Craniofac J 36: 174–178.

Yamaguchi, T (1968). Effects of riboflavin, pridoxine, and folic acid on the incidence of malformations in the rat caused by hypervitaminosis A. Congenit Anom 8: 175–182.

Yoneda, T, Pratt, RM (1982a). Vitamin B$_6$ reduces cortisone-induced cleft palate in the mouse. Teratology 26: 255–258.

Yoneda, T, Pratt, RM (1982b). Glucocorticoid receptors in palatal mesenchymal cells from the human embryo: relevance to human cleft palate formation. J Craniofac Genet Dev Biol 1: 411–423.

15

Experimental models for the study of oral clefts

BARBARA D. ABBOTT

Toxicology and teratology studies routinely utilize animal models to determine the potential for chemical and physical agents to produce reproductive and developmental toxicity, including birth defects such as cleft palate (CP). The standardized teratology screen typically tests compounds in two species, one of which is a nonrodent. The laboratory rat and rabbit are often the species of choice for such screens. However, research examining the mechanisms through which agents induce their teratogenic effects has been conducted in a variety of mammalian species, including mice, rats, and hamsters, as well as in nonmammalian species, including birds, fish, and frogs. A variety of in vitro models are also available to researchers interested in the study of palatogenesis. The literature presenting palatal research is extensive, and many outstanding studies could be cited in which a wide range of models were developed and applied; however, it is beyond the scope of this chapter to present more than a brief overview of some of these models and an example of their application in the study of environmental contaminants. An overview of in vivo and in vitro models is presented and the specialized requirements for research addressing the etiology of clefting are discussed. The final section of the chapter provides examples of these models, testing the environmental contaminant 2,3,7,8-tetrachlorodibenzo-p-dioxin (TCDD).

IN VIVO MODELS

Teratology and Developmental Toxicology Studies

The teratology or developmental toxicology screen typically examines near-term fetuses following exposure in utero throughout the period of organogenesis. These studies are important for evaluating the potential of a chemical or physical agent to disrupt development and produce major morphological malformations. Typically, this test is preceded by a dose-response pilot study to define the toxic range of the chemical. Although a compound can be identified as teratogenic with the standardized testing approach, an understanding of the cellular and molecular mechanisms through which the chemical produces its effects requires additional studies with specific design requirements.

For molecular and cellular mechanistic studies, it is desirable to identify, if possible, a dose regimen that produces a high incidence of CP in the exposed litters, while producing minimal or no toxicity in the maternal animal. It is especially helpful in mechanistic studies to identify a single day and dose that induce a high response rate. This window of sensitivity has to be determined for each chemical under study as it will depend on the mechanism through which the agent acts (e.g., one agent may retard palatal shelf elevation and thus be most effective prior to or during that event, while another may block processes involved in the fusion of shelves after elevation).

Traditionally, dose-response studies relate the amount of compound administered to the pregnant dam to the incidence of some toxicological or teratological outcome. Greater detail regarding the absorption, distribution, metabolism and elimination of the chemical is important for comparison between species and for applying laboratory animal data to human health risk assessment. The teratogenic agent may be a metabolite of the administered compound, and the specifics related to metabolism can influence the selection of species and/or the use of culture models. These data can be difficult to acquire, in part because of the very limited amounts of tissue during early stages of embryonic development. Determining the levels of the compound that reach an embryonic target tissue (such as the palatal shelf) and characterizing the time course of that distribution present unique challenges, but the effort is justified by the impact such data can have for interspecies extrapolations of response and for risk assessment determinations. Also, recent advances in the development and application of physiologically based pharmacokinetic and biologically based dose-response models support the importance of characterizing the concentrations of teratogen within the target tissue.

Studies that initiate the exposure with a single dose at specific developmental stages provide valuable insight into the mechanism(s) of action of the chemical. Examination of these embryos at critical stages of morphogenesis following the exposure may allow initial hypotheses to be formed regarding the molecular and cellular etiology. For example, morphological observations may identify the clefting as primarily due to one of the following: failure of secondary palatal shelves to form, reduction in growth of the shelves, failure of the shelves to elevate above the tongue (in rodents the shelf is initially vertical beside the tongue) or to elevate at the required time, inadequate expansion/growth of shelves after elevation, contact but failure to adhere, and failure of opposing shelves to fuse. These possibilities can generally be distinguished when observations are made at close intervals during palatogenesis, but conversely it is unlikely that observations of the near-term rodent fetus can identify a specific morphological basis for the clefting. For example, even shelves that were in contact at the appropriate time but failed to fuse for other reasons will be widely separated in the near-term fetus due to further cranial growth during the late fetal period. Once an initial morphological basis can be identified, cellular and molecular events that may be involved in such a response can be postulated and tested. Mechanisms could involve disruption of cell proliferation, migration, differentiation, interaction between cells or between cells and the extracellular matrix, cell migration, programmed cell death *(apoptosis)*, and production and/or remodeling of the extracellular matrix. Each of these processes could potentially be linked with pathways (e.g., gene expression, receptor binding and signal transduction, enzymatic activities) known to regulate such events during development.

In summary, to study the effects of a teratogen on developmental gene expression, it may be necessary to collect the embryonic tissues soon after the dose is given and subsequently at close time intervals. Ideally, such a dosing regimen would previously have been demonstrated to produce a high incidence of CP in the term fetus. Advances in molecular biological methods and in sequencing the genome of the rat, mouse, and human have provided valuable tools to the developmental biologist and toxicologist; and studies can be designed to examine gene expression, protein and mRNA localization, functionality of enzymes, and potential modification of other biological processes critical to palatogenesis.

Transgenic Mice

The development of transgenic animal models has stimulated rapid gains in basic biological research, and palatal research has also benefitted from these efforts. There are numerous examples of targeted inactivation of a specific gene which resulted in a transgenic phenotype that included CP. Some of these were unanticipated, while other studies specifically targeted genes believed to be involved in the etiology of clefting. A few examples will be presented, although there are many other reports and undoubtedly more to come in the future. The transforming growth factor-β3 *(TGF-β3)* gene was knocked out (genotype of the transgenic is denoted as −/−, inactive genes on both chromosomes), and the pups with no growth factor expression had cleft secondary palate, which was attributed to failure of the medial epithelia to adhere on contact and fuse (Proetzel et al., 1995). Transgenic −/− palates were put in organ culture to test the hypothesis that TGF-β3 is required for fusion. This was shown by supplementing the medium with TGF-β3 and observing that the opposing shelves fused. These studies further defined the defect in −/− animals as a failure of the basement membrane under the epithelium to degrade and permit transdifferentiation of cells to the mesenchyme (Chai et al., 1997; Kaartinen et al., 1997; Taya et al., 1999). Another transgenic knockout exhibiting CP is the mouse in which function was eliminated for *MSX-1* (Nugent and Greene, 1998). Allelic variants of this gene and *TGF-β3* appear to be associated with increased risk for non-syndromic cleft lip and palate (CLP) in cases where there was maternal cigarette smoking and alcohol consumption (Romitti et al., 1999). Thyroid dysgenesis and CP have been reported for mice lacking function of TTF-2, a forkhead domain–containing transcription factor (De Felice et al., 1998). Transgenic inactivation of the genes *Pax9*, *Hoxa1*, *endothelin-1*, and β-3 $GABA_A$ (neurotransmitter γ-aminobutyric acid) receptor also results in fetuses with CP, and further evidence has been provided for the roles of each gene in normal palatogenesis. Additional discussion of the genetic regulation of palatal development is presented in other chapters of this volume.

IN VITRO

There are several in vitro approaches for the study of CP, and these can be valuable supplements to the in vivo studies. Several of the culture models described in this section have proven useful in mechanistic studies and for comparison of the sensitivity and response to a teratogenic agent across species. The models discussed include palatal organ culture, cell culture, whole embryo culture, and a few utilizing non-mammalian species.

Palatal Organ Culture

Palatal organ culture models have been developed for mouse, rat, hamster, chick, and human secondary palates. The secondary palatal shelves can be cultured by being either supported on grids or a gel slab above the medium (Trowel's type cultures) or submerged in medium; both approaches have advantages. Each of these methods can be useful in addressing specific hypotheses regarding palatal fusion and in evaluating the responses to exogenous chemical agents. These experiments can also test the responses to excess endogenous regulatory factors [growth factors, vitamins, and essential minerals, such as epidermal growth factor (EGF), retinol, or selenium] and to reductions in the activity or abundance of specific proteins, mRNAs, or enzymes (e.g., with neutralizing antibodies, antisense RNA, or inhibitory compounds, respectively).

Culture of palates on a supporting platform requires placement of isolated secondary palatal shelves with the opposing medial edges in contact on the support, to evaluate the potential to fuse along the midline. Suspension cultures typically submerge the dissected midfacial region of the embryo (maxillary arch and associated tissues of primary and emerging secondary palate with removal of hindbrain, mandible, and tongue) under the medium. In this system, early-stage palatal shelves develop in situ, allowing outgrowth, elevation, contact, and fusion to occur as the tissue floats freely under the medium. Several variations of the suspension models for mice and rats have been published (Shiota et al., 1990; Abbott and Buckalew, 1992; Al-Obaidi et al., 1995), and a detailed laboratory protocol for a serum-free palatal organ culture model is presented in *Methods in Molecular Biology* (Abbott, 1999). Palatal organ culture models have a number of advantages and permit manipulations that are not possible with in vivo studies. The progress of palatal development can be followed for individual embryonic tissues, and experimental exposures or other manipulations can be initiated or terminated at specific stages/times. Serum-free conditions are useful for evaluation of growth factor influences on the critical stages of palatogenesis and fu-

sion of the palates. Culture methods are similar for mouse and rat studies; however, successful fusion of the rat palate in suspension culture varies with different strains of rat and usually requires modifications in the supplementation of the medium, relative volume of medium per tissue explant, and oxygenation of medium for later stages of the culture period . Palatal organ culture models include species other than rat and mouse, such as chick, hamster, or alligator; and some of these investigations have incorporated combinations of palatal shelves from different species and even recombinations of epithelia and mesenchyme from different species (Ferguson et al., 1984; Shah et al., 1985; Sun et al., 1998). Applications of palatal culture models are numerous, but only a few examples are included here.

The chemotherapeutic agent 5-fluorouracil (5-FU) is teratogenic and produces CP. This agent was used as a model compound to develop biologically based dose-response models, and a component of that effort involved characterization of the inhibition of the enzyme thymidylate synthetase (TS) and evaluation of cell proliferation. Palatal organ culture was included in this study, and it provided a unique data set in which palatal morphometric analysis, palatal fusion, cell cycle analysis, quantitative measures of ^{3}H-thymidine uptake, as well as autoradiographic localization, DNA and protein content, and biochemical data (TS enzyme inhibition) were correlated for multiple doses across a time course (Abbott et al., 1993). This study illustrated the range of end points available in such a model and provided an example of the correlation of end points in an experimental design that might not be possible in vivo. Also in this study, a variation of the model was used in which embryos were exposed in utero and subsequently removed at specific intervals for culture in serum-free control medium. This allowed the exposure to be limited, as well as retention of the initial distribution and/or metabolism of an in vivo exposure scenario. This experimental design made it possible to determine that brief exposure to 5-FU in utero was sufficient to produce palatal growth retardation and dysmorphogenesis (Shuey et al., 1994).

The palatal organ culture model has proven effective in defining the influences and roles of various growth factors in palatogenesis. A good example of this is a study examining the importance of TGF-β3 in palatal fusion. This endogenous growth factor was inactivated at specific developmental stages by inclusion of antibody and/or antisense RNA. Addition of these agents to the medium blocked the normal production and function of TGF-β3 and allowed investigators to conclude that this growth factor is essential for palatal fusion (Brunet et al., 1995). Similarly, the roles of EGF, platelet-derived growth factor, TGF-α, and other members of the TGF-β family have been evaluated using the culture system (Dixon and Ferguson, 1992).

Human embryonic palatal tissues have been cultured using the supported and submerged models. Palatogenesis in the human spans approximately gestational days (GDs) 48 to 59, and generally the outgrowth of the secondary palate can be detected around 49 days, with fusion in most cases by gestational day 54 to 55 (Abbott et al., 1999a). (This is based on specimens obtained from the Central Laboratory for Human Embryology, University of Washington, Seattle. The determination of gestational age was based on an extensive database correlating foot length, morphological features, and gestational age.) Craniofacial tissues that were placed in a serum-free suspension culture at GD 50 to 52 and cultured for 4 to 5 days achieved secondary palatal growth and fusion in vitro (Abbott and Buckalew, 1992). Culture models for human tissue are nearly identical to those for other species and appear to reasonably model human palatogenesis and, thus, provide a unique opportunity for linking animal models of palatogenesis with human embryonic developmental responses to challenge. However, there are difficulties which limit application of the human model. Tissues suitable for use in culture are typically available only from voluntary terminations of pregnancy in the seventh to eighth week. The availability of such early developmental stages is limited, as are research centers or programs that collect and distribute such tissues to researchers. Also, research with human tissues requires protocols approved by an institutional review board, and the collection and use of the materials occurs under National Institutes of Health standard guidelines for research involving human subjects. In general, during the previous decade, basic research requiring human embryonic/fetal tissue, but not involving clinical applications, was allowed in institutions receiving federal research funding. However, regulations and guidelines regarding research utilizing human embryonic/fetal tissues are under ongoing review, and updates regarding bans on specific research can be issued at any time. Even with potential restrictions and limited availability of specimens, human palatal cultures have the potential to provide unique information on normal palatogenesis and to allow interspecies comparison of responses to teratogens. In an example which will be presented in more detail later in this chapter, human palatal organ cultures were used to assess the potential for the environmental contaminant TCDD to induce clefting in the developing human embryo.

Cultured Cells

Palatal culture models also include isolated cultured cells, epithelial sheets, as well as primary mesenchymal cell cultures of mouse (MEPM) or human (HEPM) origin. The epithelial sheet of cells covering the palatal shelf can be dissociated from the underlying mesenchyme and cultured as an intact sheet on a extracellular matrix–coated plastic substrate. There are some examples of these cultures in which the responses to growth factor and/or retinoic acid were examined (Tyler and Pratt, 1980; Abbott and Pratt, 1988). The ability to dissociate the epithelial and mesenchymal components permits investigation of the contribution of each in regulating the events of palatogenesis or in the response to an experimental treatment. Investigators have even recombined dissociated epithelia and mesenchyme from different species (Ferguson et al., 1984). Though not widely applied due to the technical challenges presented by these approaches, the availability of such options can be intriguing.

The MEPM and HEPM cultures are based on enzymatic digestion of the palatal shelf with subsequent culture under conditions favoring survival and proliferation of isolated mesenchymal cells. Both of these models have been used to evaluate mechanisms of palatogenesis and teratogenic responses. The MEPM cultures have been used to study the responses to regulators of growth and differentiation (Greene and Lloyd, 1985; Sharpe et al., 1992; Gehris et al., 1994; Potchinsky et al., 1997) and to examine the interactions of growth factors with retinoic acid (Nugent and Greene, 1995; Nugent et al., 1995). The HEPM applications include evaluation of the ability of teratogenic compounds to interfere with intercellular communication (Welsch et al., 1985) and to inhibit cell growth (Pratt and Willis, 1985). Isolated HEPM cells, which were developed as a cell line, may not accurately model the responses of mesenchymal cells in situ, as all cultured cells have the potential to change during the culture period as well as with increasing passage (or generations) of the cultures. Even with primary cultures, removing the cells from the normal milieu of the extracellular matrix, as well as elimination of potentially critical interactions between different cell types, can modify the responses of cells, affect the interpretation of experimental data, and render inaccurate any attempt to extrapolate from the culture model to an in vivo situation. Applications of in vitro models should always be interpreted with consideration of the potential of that model to deviate from a normal developmental scenario.

Whole Embryo Culture

Although not a model for secondary palate formation, the whole embryo culture (WEC) system has been used to study the early embryonic morphogenetic events preceding and essential to normal formation of maxillary arch derivatives. The WEC system encompasses a period of neural crest cell migration and formation of the branchial or visceral arches. This model detects problems with early craniofacial morphogenesis and can be applied to post-implantation rat or mouse embryos. Applications to developmental biology and teratology have been reviewed (Sadler, 1985; Sadler et al., 1985; Flynn, 1987). Briefly, this model requires dissection of presomite or early somite embryonic stages, which are then cultured in serum or serum-containing culture medium for 24 to 48 h (typically, GD 9–11 for the rat and GD 8–10 for the mouse). The WEC system can include co-culture with cells to metabolically activate the test compound, and in some cases serum from treated animals is used as the exposure paradigm. With some modifications to the standard protocol, the later-stage mouse embryo can be cultured from GD 10 to 12 (Pratt et al., 1987). A detailed anatomical scoring system developed by Brown and Fabro (1981) is commonly used to evaluate the development of cultured embryos and biochemical measures, as well as DNA, RNA, and protein analyses. There is an extensive literature reporting teratogenic responses in WEC, and this model has also been extensively used in developmental biology research.

NONMAMMALIAN MODELS

Nonmammalian models may also be used in the laboratory to study craniofacial morphogenesis; these may include the chick, quail, fish, and frog. A variety of fish species are studied in the laboratory, including lake trout, Japanese medaka, zebra fish, and flathead minnow (Henry et al., 1997, 1998; Hornung et al., 1999). Generally, these models detect major malformations and defects in morphogenesis of the cranial region, and their application to teratological research was reviewed by Collins (1987). Basic research addressing the fundamental mechanisms of developmental biology utilizes many of these models, and there is an extensive literature reporting such applications.

APPLICATION OF PALATAL MODELS TO STUDY AN ENVIRONMENTAL CONTAMINANT

Dioxins, furans, and polychlorinated biphenyls are structurally related members of a class of compounds found in the environment. Many of the members of this class are poorly metabolized and do not readily degrade in the environment; thus, they persist and bioaccumulate in ecological and biological systems. Several reviews of the literature have provided information regarding the sources, bioaccumulation, and biological effects (Birnbaum, 1994b; Schecter, 1995). The most

toxic member of this class is TCDD, which is found throughout the environment. Sources of release include incineration of waste (municipal, medical, and rural domestic waste), automobile exhaust, industrial chlorine bleaching, and in the past production of herbicides. It is associated with a wide range of biological responses in wildlife, laboratory animals, and humans exposed through food contamination, industrial accidents, or herbicide spraying. In laboratory animals, the biological effects include carcinogenesis, immunotoxicity, reproductive toxicity, cancer, and teratogenesis. In humans, high exposure can produce chloracne and has been associated with cancer and neurological and hormonal effects (Peterson et al., 1993; Holladay and Luster, 1994; Birnbaum and Abbott, 1996; Abbott, 1997; Abbott and Birnbaum, 1998). Dioxin produces developmental toxicity in every species that has been examined, and the responses include fetal mortality, decreased fetal weight, edema, thymic atrophy, hemorrhaging, structural and functional defects in reproductive organs, and immunological deficiencies (Couture et al., 1990; Peterson et al., 1993; Birnbaum, 1995). Cleft palate is produced in the mouse, rat, and guinea pig; however, in the latter two species, this response is observed at fetotoxic levels. The C57BL/6N strain of mice is especially sensitive to the induction of CP by TCDD, and the response occurs at doses that are not overtly toxic to either the pregnant dam or the fetus. The only other teratogenic effect is hydronephrosis in the pups. The sensitivity of this strain correlates with expression of a high-affinity aryl hydrocarbon receptor (AhR). A considerable research effort has characterized the molecular pathways of response to this class of chemicals using TCDD as the prototypic compound (Nebert et al., 1993; Birnbaum, 1994a; Okey et al., 1994). Basically, the dioxin and dioxin-like compounds, which are very lipid-soluble, diffuse into the cell and bind to the AhR, which then interacts with the aryl hydrocarbon nuclear translocator (ARNT) protein and moves into the nucleus of the cell, where it binds to specific sequences of DNA (referred to as dioxin response elements). The bound complex then regulates expression of the gene associated with the dioxin response element. In this way, TCDD regulates expression of specific genes that have the potential to alter development in the embryo or normal cell function in the adult.

To assess the potential for TCDD to affect palatogenesis in the human, it was necessary to identify the mechanisms through which TCDD induces CP and to compare the morphological, cellular, and molecular responses in the mouse to those occurring in cultured human palatal shelves. It was important to establish that the molecular mechanisms for response are present in palates of both species (i.e., AhR and ARNT proteins were expressed), to determine that the in vitro model accurately reflects the in vivo responses for the mouse, and that these responses occur at comparable tissue burdens of the chemical and then to compare the morphological, cellular, and molecular responses in the mouse palates after exposure in vivo or in culture with those of the cultured human palates. It was also important to examine gene expression in human palates that were not cultured for comparison with cultured tissues.

Formation of the secondary palate in the mouse or human requires that complex developmental processes are regulated to produce shelves that expand across the oral cavity, make contact, and fuse along the medial edge. In the mouse, after exposure to TCDD palatal shelves form and expand to establish contact along the medial edge; however, these shelves fail to fuse (Pratt et al., 1984). This is associated with hyperplasia of the medial epithelium, which is attributed to excessive proliferation and formation of a stratified, squamous epithelial phenotype (Abbott and Birnbaum, 1989; Abbott et al., 1989). These responses are correlated with effects on expression of growth factors that regulate proliferation and differentiation (EGF, TGF-α, TGF-

β1, TGF-β2, and TGF-β3) (Abbott and Birnbaum, 1990). These responses are observed after exposure in vivo or in Trowell's or submerged cultures (Abbott et al., 1989). Human palates responded to TCDD in Trowell's and suspension cultures with responses similar to those observed in the mouse (Abbott and Birnbaum, 1991; Abbott and Buckalew, 1992; Abbott et al., 1998).

Human embryonic palates had similar, although not identical, patterns of growth factor mRNA and protein expression compared to comparable stages of mouse palatogenesis (GD 49–59 human compared with GD 12–16 mouse palates). A comparison of growth factor expression in human and mouse palates is shown in Table 15.1A. Human and mouse palates were dissimilar in particular spatiotemporal patterns of expression of these genes. Human tissues differed from mouse tissues in the expression of EGF at early palatal stages, the expression of EGF receptor and TGF-α throughout fusion events, and the uniform expression of TGF-β3 in all epithelial regions without specifically higher levels in the medial cells. The effects of TCDD on growth factor expression also differed somewhat between mice and humans (Table 15.1B). Responses to TCDD were

TABLE 15.1A. *Summary of Human and Mouse Embryonic Gene Expression in Palatogenesis**

	Mouse	Human
EGF receptor	Decreased in medial epithelial cells prior to fusion	Increased in mesenchyme, expressed in medial epithelium through fusion events
TGF-α	Decreases with age, expression in epithelium and mesenchyme similar	Expressed through palatogenesis, increases with age
EGF	Increases with age, greater expression in epithelium than mesenchyme.	No change with age, greater expression in epithelium than mesenchyme
TGF-β1	No change with age, epithelium and mesenchyme similar	No change with age for epithelium, increase in mesenchyme with age, greater in mesenchyme than epithelium.
TGF-β2	High in early stages, becomes regional, decreases in mesenchyme	Expression varies between individuals, no trend detected
TGF-β3	Higher in medial epithelium at contact and fusion	Not higher in medial cells, greater in epithelium than mesenchyme

TABLE 15.1B. *Summary of Human and Mouse Palatal Response to TCDD*[†]

	AhR	ARNT	GR	EGFR	EGF	TGF-α	TGF-β1	TGF-β2	TGF-β3
	Human in culture at 1×10^{-8} M TCDD								
Protein	▲	▲	▲	▲	▲	▲	▼	▲	▲
mRNA	▼	▲	▲	◆	▲	▲	▲	◆	▼
	Mouse in vivo								
Protein	▼	na	▲	▲	▼	◆	▼	◆	na
mRNA	▼	na	▲	na	na	na	na	na	na

*EGF, epidermal growth factor; TGF, transforming growth factor.

[†]AhR, aryl hydrocarbon receptor; ARNT, aryl hydrocarbon nuclear translocation; GR, glucocorticoid receptor; EGFR, epidermal growth factor receptor; TCDD, 2,3,7,8-tetrachloro-dibenzo-p-dioxin.

Relative to control: ▲, increase; ▼, decrease; ◆, unchanged; na, data not available.

Source: Abbott et al. (1998).

compared after exposures in culture (human, $EC_{100} = 1 \times 10^{-8}$ M) or in vivo (mouse $ED_{100} = 24$ μg/kg on GD 12) that altered the morphology and proliferation of the medial epithelium. In human palates, EGF, TGF-α, and TGF-β2 proteins increased after TCDD; but mouse palates showed decreased expression of EGF and no change in TGF-α and TGF-β2. The variation in growth factor expression during normal palatogenesis may have some role in the differential responsiveness of humans and mice to the disruptive effects of TCDD. In the mouse, the coordinated regulation of growth factors may be more easily disturbed by the exposure. For example, in the mouse palate, stage-dependent shifts in TGF-α in the absence of EGF are apparently important in early stages of palate formation; but in the human palate. both growth factors are detected at that stage

of palatogenesis. Also, TCDD increased expression of both growth factors in the human palate but in mice TGF-α appeared to be unaffected while EGF expression decreased at a time when expression of this growth factor normally increases (Abbott et al., 1998, 1999a). Thus, interspecies differences in growth factor expression may influence the response to a teratogen that affects those regulatory peptides.

Although mouse and human palates showed slightly different growth factor responses to TCDD, the morphological outcomes (medial epithelial hyperplasia and proliferation) were similar. However, the level of TCDD required to produce these responses in humans was 1×10^{-8} M, which is about 200 times higher than the effective concentration for mice, 5×10^{-11} M (Table 15.2). Comparing the responses in culture with

TABLE 15.2. *Interspecies Comparison of Embryonic Responsiveness to TCDD*

EC$_{100}$ for Morphological and Cellular Responses[a–c]			
	Mouse in vivo[a] 24 μg/kg	Mouse in vitro[b] 5×10^{-11} M	Human in vitro[c] 1×10^{-8} M

Distribution of TCDD In Vivo and In Vitro[d–g]				
TCDD (ppt) pg/g wet weight pg/g protein	Mouse in vivo[d] 24 μg/kg 440 7800	Mouse in vitro[e] 5×10^{-11} M (1636)[f] 29,000	Human in vitro 1×10^{-8} (3×10^5)[f] 5.3×10^6	Human fetal TCDD burden[g] (8–14 weeks, $n = 10$) 1.4 (lipid-adjusted, 0.647% lipid) and TEQ = 5.3 ng/kg lipid

CYP1A1 Induction in Molecules/100 fg Total RNA[h]			
Time after exposure 6 h	Mouse in vivo[h] 14,545	Mouse in vitro 14,234	Human in vitro 9.2	TCDD concentration in medium 1×10^{-9} M

AhR and ARNT Expression in Molecules/100 fg Total RNA[h,i]					
	AhR			*ARNT*		
	Range	Median	Mean	Range	Median	Mean
Human in vitro	0.2–26	2	4	0.03–6	0.98	1.18
Mouse in vivo[h]	93–1979	692	765	16–445	133	130

Relative expression of AhR:ARNT
  Mouse = 6.8:1
  Human = 3.9:1

[a]EC$_{100}$ = concentration or dose of TCDD that produced responses in 100% of exposed palates (Abbott and Birnbaum, 1989, 1990).
[b]Abbott et al. (1989).
[c]Abbott and Birnbaum (1991), Abbott and Buckalew (1992).
[d]Data from Abbott et al. (1989).
[e]Abbott et al. (1996).
[f]Values for culture extrapolated from mouse in vivo (pg/g wet weight) using the distribution relationship between in vitro and in vivo determined for protein (pg/g).
[g]Schecter (1995), Schecter et al. (1996).
[h]Abbott et al. (1998).
[i]Mouse in vivo data from Abbott et al. (1998). Mouse and human ratio, mean, median, and range include mRNA expression across all times for control and TCDD-treated palates.
TCDD, 2,3,7,8-tetrachlorodibenzo-p-dioxin; AhR, aryl hydrocarbon receptor; ARNT, aryl hydrocarbon nuclear translocator; TEQ, toxic equivalent.

those of the mouse embryo exposed in vivo requires knowing more than just the concentration in the medium. It is impossible to compare the dose administered orally to the pregnant mouse with the concentration present in the culture medium. These comparisons require knowledge of the TCDD concentration in the palatal tissues. Knowing the tissue concentrations is critical for comparing the cellular and molecular responses of mouse and human palates. To achieve this goal, distribution studies were performed in which radiolabeled TCDD was used for in vivo dosing of mice and in the submerged palatal organ culture model (Abbott et al., 1989, 1996). After oral dosing of the pregnant female mouse, TCDD reached the embryos rapidly and remained at a constant level in the palatal tissue for up to 3 days. With this distribution profile, the culture model represents a reasonable exposure scenario as the compound rapidly diffused throughout the cultured organs and levels were maintained throughout the duration of culture. The tissue burden or concentration was expressed in each experiment as a ratio of picograms of TCDD per gram of protein and picograms of TCDD per gram of wet tissue weight (Table 15.2). These units made it possible to compare tissue levels from the vitro and vivo experiments and to discuss the cellular, morphological, and molecular end points at various time points and after different exposures relative to the tissue concentrations.

As shown in Table 15.2, the differences between mouse and human sensitivity to TCDD are apparent in comparisons of the amount of TCDD required to produce cellular and morphological responses. At 24 h after oral dosing (24 μg/kg on GD 12), 440 pg TCDD were localized per gram palatal wet weight (also expressed as 7800 pg TCDD/g total protein). Palates exposed to 5×10^{-11} M TCDD in medium for 24 h retain 29,000 pg TCDD/g total protein. This is approximately 3.7 times the amount detected following in vivo exposure at 24 h. Human embryonic palates of similar developmental stages to the mouse require 200 times more TCDD to alter differentiation, proliferation, and growth factor expression. The difference is apparent in both the concentration in medium that is required to produce effects (1×10^{-8} M TCDD) and the tissue burdens (5.3×10^6 pg TCDD/g total protein) after 24 h exposure. Limited data are available regarding tissue levels in human embryos; however, in a sample of 10 embryos aged 8 to 14 weeks, approximately 1.4 pg TCDD/g tissue (ppt) was detected (lipid-adjusted, assuming 0.65% lipid) (Schecter et al., 1996). This average tissue burden for human embryos is considerably below that required to produce morphological, cellular, or molecular responses in cultures palates. As shown in Table 15.2, the EC$_{100}$ of 3×10^5 ppt in cultured palates is approximately 2000 times higher than the average embryonic tissue burden determined by Schecter et al. (1996).

Both human and mouse secondary palates express AhR and ARNT, the requisite transcriptional regulators of the response to TCDD, and there are similar patterns of localization for these proteins and their mRNAs (determined immunohistochemically and by in situ hybridization, respectively). Quantitation of AhR and ARNT mRNA by reverse-transcription polymerase chain reaction showed that the expression of both was considerably lower in human palates (based on median values AhR was 346 times lower and ARNT 135-fold lower in humans, Table 15.2). In both species, AhR is expressed at higher levels relative to ARNT; however, AhR:ARNT ratios are approximately 7:1 for humans and 4:1 for mice. In cultured human palates, TCDD did not alter expression of either AhR or ARNT in either a dose- or a time-related manner (Abbott et al., 1998, 1999a,b).

Expression of some of the members of the cytochrome P-450 family of metabolic phase I enzymes is induced by exposure to TCDD, and CYP1A1 mRNA is considered a biomarker of response to compounds that act by binding to the AhR. Expression of that gene is directly regulated through binding of the AhR:TCDD:ARNT complex to its dioxin response element. In the palate, expression of AhR and ARNT correlated with induction of CYP1A1 mRNA. In the mouse palate, where expression of both AhR and ARNT is higher compared to humans, induction of CYP1A1 mRNA was 435 times higher that that observed in human palates (Table 15.2). Comparisons of this induction response were made 6 h after exposure in utero on GD 12 (24 μg/kg) and 6 h after initiating exposure to 1×10^{-9} M TCDD in medium (human and mouse cultures). The level of CYP1A1 induction was almost identical for mouse palates exposed either in vivo or in culture; however, expression in human palates was 1547 times lower after the same duration and exposure level in culture compared to the mouse. This difference in response of human palatal tissues may be a function of decreased affinity of the human receptor for binding of TCDD (Manchester et al., 1987; Ema et al., 1994). However, the level of TCDD required to produce the palatal cellular and morphological responses is also considerably higher in humans than in mice, suggesting that the level of expression of the receptor and its partner may also be involved.

CONCLUSIONS

In response to TCDD, human embryonic palates have fewer receptors, have different relative levels of AhR and ARNT, and show less induction of the biomarker enzyme CYP1A1. The levels of TCDD required to produce the morphological and cellular responses in the developing palate are unlikely to be achieved through exposure to existing environmental levels. There are effects of TCDD in animal models that occur at much lower exposure levels than those required to induce CP, and these may also be a concern for the developing human embryo and fetus. However, the conclusion from the preceding studies remains that a teratogenic response such as CP is unlikely in humans.

The research strategies outlined in the preceding section may require years of dedicated effort by many laboratories to evaluate even a single agent and the mechanisms through which it produces CP. There are advantages to using in vitro models for mechanistic research studies, and there can be applications for these culture models in the initial screening of candidate compounds under development for drug or commercial use. However, in vivo data are often essential to provide a basis for the design and selection of appropriate in vitro assays. Therefore, while culture data can be an important supplement, it is unlikely that these models will ever completely substitute for in vivo research. Recent advances in genomic research, human epidemiological studies, clinical research, and animal models represent an important component in the effort to reveal the etiology of CP.

The information in this document has been funded wholly (or in part) by the U.S. Environmental Protection Agency. It has been reviewed by the National Health and Environmental Effects Research Laboratory and approved for publication. Approval does not signify that the contents reflect the views of the agency, nor does mention of trade names or commercial products constitute endorsement or recommendation for use.

REFERENCES

Abbott, BD (1997). Developmental toxicity of dioxin: searching for the cellular and molecular basis of morphological responses. In: *Handbook of Experimental Pharmacology : Section III: Pathogenesis and Mechanisms of Drug Toxicity in Development,* edited by R Kavlock and G Daston. New York: Springer-Verlag, pp. 407–433.

Abbott, BD (1999). Palatal dysmorphogenesis: palate organ culture. In: *Methods in Molecular Biology: Developmental Biology Protocols,* Vol. II, edited by RS Tuan and CW Lo. Totowa, NJ: Humana Press, pp. 189–195.

Abbott, BD, Birnbaum, LS (1989). TCDD alters medial epithelial cell differentiation during palatogenesis. Toxicol Appl Pharmacol 99: 276–286.

Abbott, BD, Birnbaum, LS (1990). TCDD-induced altered expression of growth factors may have a role in producing cleft palate and enhancing the incidence of clefts after coadministration of retinoic acid and TCDD. Toxicol Appl Pharmacol 106: 418–432.

Abbott, BD, Birnbaum, LS (1991). TCDD exposure of human embryonic palatal shelves in organ culture alters the differentiation of medial epithelial cells. Teratology 43: 119–132.

Abbott, BD, Birnbaum, LS (1998). Dioxins and teratogenesis. In: *Molecular Biology of the Toxic Response,* edited by A Puga and K Wallace. Washington, DC: Taylor and Francis, pp. 439–447.

Abbott, BD, Birnbaum, LS, Diliberto, JJ (1996). Rapid distribution of 2,3,7,8-tetrachlorodibenzo-p-dioxin (TCDD) to embryonic tissues in C57BL/6N mice and correlation with palatal uptake in vitro. Toxicol Appl Pharmacol 141: 256–263.

Abbott, BD, Buckalew, AR (1992). Embryonic palatal responses to teratogens in serum-free organ culture. Teratology 45: 369–382.

Abbott, BD, Diliberto, JJ, Birnbaum, LS (1989). 2,3,7,8-Tetrachlorodibenzo-p-dioxin alters embryonic palatal medial epithelial cell differentiation in vitro. Toxicol Appl Pharmacol 100: 119–131.

Abbott, BD, Held, GA, Wood, CR, et al. (1999a). AhR, ARNT, and CYP1A1 mRNA quantitation in cultured human embryonic palates exposed to TCDD and comparison with mouse palate in vivo and in culture. Toxicol Sci 47: 62–75.

Abbott, BD, Lau, C, Buckalew, AR, et al. (1993). Effects of 5-fluorouracil on embryonic rat palate in vitro: fusion in the absence of proliferation. Teratology 47: 541–554.

Abbott, BD, Pratt, RM (1988). Influence of retinoids and EGF on growth of embryonic mouse palatal epithelia in culture. In Vitro Cell Dev Biol 24: 343–352.

Abbott, BD, Probst, MR, Perdew, GH, Buckalew, AR (1998). AH receptor, ARNT, glucocorticoid receptor, EGF receptor, EGF, TGF α, TGF β 1, TGF β 2, and TGF β 3 expression in human embryonic palate, and effects of 2,3,7,8-tetrachlorodibenzo-p-dioxin (TCDD). Teratology 58: 30–43.

Abbott, BD, Schmid, JE, Brown, JG, et al. (1999b). RT-PCR quantification of AHR, ARNT, GR, and CYP1A1 mRNA in craniofacial tissues of embryonic mice exposed to 2,3,7,8-tetrachlorodibenzo-p-dioxin and hydrocortisone. Toxicol Sci 47: 76–85.

Al-Obaidi, N, Kastner, U, Merker, HJ, Klug, S (1995). Development of a suspension organ culture of the fetal rat palate. Arch Toxicol 69: 472–479.

Birnbaum, LS (1994a). Evidence for the role of the Ah receptor in responses to dioxin. In: *Receptor-Mediated Biological Processes: Implications for Evaluating Carcinogens. Progress in Clinical and Biological Research,* edited by HL Spitzer, TL Slaga, WF Greenlee, and M McClain. New York: Wiley-Liss, pp. 139–154.

Birnbaum, LS (1994b). The mechanism of dioxin toxicity: relationship to risk assessment. Environ Health Perspect 102(Suppl 9): 157–167.

Birnbaum, LS (1995). Developmental effects of dioxins. Environ Health Perspect 103(Suppl 7): 89–94.

Birnbaum, LS, Abbott, BD (1996). Effect of dioxin on growth factor and receptor expression in developing palate. In: *Methods in Developmental Toxicology and Biology,* edited by S Klug and R Theil. Malden, MA: Blackwell, pp. 51–63.

Brown, NA, Fabro, S (1981). Quantitation of rat embryonic development in vitro: a morphological scoring system. Teratology 24: 65–78.

Brunet, CL, Sharpe, PM, Ferguson, MW (1995). Inhibition of TGF-β 3 (but not TGF-β 1 or TGF-β 2) activity prevents normal mouse embryonic palate fusion. Int J Dev Biol 39: 345–355.

Chai, Y, Sasano, Y, Bringas, P, Jr, et al. (1997). Characterization of the fate of midline epithelial cells during the fusion of mandibular prominences in vivo. Dev Dyn 208: 526–535.

Collins, TF (1987). Teratological research using in vitro systems. V. Nonmammalian model systems. Environ Health Perspect 72: 237–249.

Couture, LA, Abbott, BD, Birnbaum, LS (1990). A critical review of the developmental toxicity and teratogenicity of 2,3,7,8-tetrachlorodibenzo-p-dioxin: recent advances toward understanding the mechanism. Teratology 42: 619–627.

De Felice, M, Ovitt, C, Biffali, E, et al. (1998). A mouse model for hereditary thyroid dysgenesis and cleft palate. Nat Genet 19: 395–398.

Dixon, MJ, Ferguson, MW (1992). The effects of epidermal growth factor, transforming growth factors alpha and beta and platelet-derived growth factor on murine palatal shelves in organ culture. Arch Oral Biol 37: 395–410.

Ema, M, Ohe, N, Suzuki, M, et al. (1994). Dioxin binding activities of polymorphic forms of mouse and human arylhydrocarbon receptors. J Biol Chem 269: 27337–27343.

Ferguson, MW, Honig, LS, Slavkin, HC (1984). Differentiation of cultured palatal shelves from alligator, chick, and mouse embryos. Anat Rec 209: 231–249.

Flynn, TJ (1987). Teratological research using in vitro systems. I. Mammalian whole embryo culture. Environ Health Perspect 72: 203–210.

Gehris, AL, Pisano, MM, Nugent, P, Greene, RM (1994). Regulation of TGFβ3 gene expression in embryonic palatal tissue. In Vitro Cell Dev Biol Anim 30A: 671–679.

Greene, RM, Lloyd, MR (1985). Effect of epidermal growth factor on synthesis of prostaglandins and cyclic AMP by embryonic palate mesenchymal cells. Biochem Biophys Res Commun 130: 1037–1043.

Henry, KS, Kannan, K, Nagy, BW, et al. (1998). Concentrations and hazard assessment of organochlorine contaminants and mercury in smallmouth bass from a remote lake in the Upper Peninsula of Michigan. Arch Environ Contam Toxicol 34: 81–86.

Henry, TR, Spitsbergen, JM, Hornung, MW, et al. (1997). Early life stage toxicity of 2,3,7,8-tetrachlorodibenzo-p-dioxin in zebrafish (Danio rerio). Toxicol Appl Pharmacol 142: 56–68.

Holladay, SD, Luster, MI (1994). Developmental immunotoxicology. In: Developmental Toxicology, edited by CA Kimmel and J Buelke-Sam. New York: Raven Press, pp. 93–118.

Hornung, MW, Spitsbergen, JM, Peterson, RE (1999). 2,3,7,8-Tetrachlorodibenzo-p-dioxin alters cardiovascular and craniofacial development and function in sac fry of rainbow trout (Oncorhynchus mykiss). Toxicol Sci 47: 40–51.

Kaartinen, V, Cui, XM, Heisterkamp, N, et al. (1997). Transforming growth factor-beta3 regulates transdifferentiation of medial edge epithelium during palatal fusion and associated degradation of the basement membrane. Dev Dyn 209: 255–260.

Manchester, DK, Gordon, SK, Golas, CL, et al. (1987). Ah receptor in human placenta: stabilization by molybdate and characterization of binding of 2,3,7,8-tetrachlorodibenzo-p-dioxin, 3-methylcholanthrene, and benzo(a)pyrene. Cancer Res 47: 4861–4868.

Nebert, DW, Puga, A, Vasiliou, V (1993). Role of the Ah receptor and the dioxin-inducible (Ah) gene battery in toxicity, cancer, and signal transduction. Ann N Y Acad Sci 685: 624–640.

Nugent, P, Greene, RM (1995). Antisense oligonucleotides to CRABP I and II alter the expression of TGF-beta 3, RAR-beta, and tenascin in primary cultures of embryonic palate cells. In Vitro Cell Dev Biol Anim 31: 553–558.

Nugent, P, Greene, RM (1998). MSX-1 gene expression and regulation in embryonic palatal tissue. In Vitro Cell Dev Biol Anim 34: 831–835.

Nugent, P, Potchinsky, M, Lafferty, C, Greene, RM (1995). TGF-beta modulates the expression of retinoic acid-induced RAR-beta in primary cultures of embryonic palate cells. Exp Cell Res 220: 495–500.

Okey, AB, Riddick, DS, Harper, PA (1994). Molecular biology of the aromatic hydrocarbon (dioxin) receptor. Trends Pharmacol Sci 15: 226–232.

Peterson, RE, Theobald, HM, Kimmel, GL (1993). Developmental and reproductive toxicity of dioxins and related compounds: cross-species comparisons. Crit Rev Toxicol 23: 283–335.

Potchinsky, MB, Weston, WM, Lloyd, MR, Greene, RM (1997). TGF-beta signaling in murine embryonic palate cells involves phosphorylation of the CREB transcription factor. Exp Cell Res 231: 96–103.

Pratt, RM, Dencker, L, Diewert, VM (1984). 2,3,7,8-Tetrachlorodibenzo-p-dioxin–induced cleft palate in the mouse: evidence for alterations in palatal shelf fusion. Teratog Carcinog Mutagen 4: 427–436.

Pratt, RM, Goulding, EH, Abbott, BD (1987). Retinoic acid inhibits migration of cranial neural crest cells in the cultured mouse embryo. J Craniofac Genet Dev Biol 7: 205–217.

Pratt, RM, Willis, WD (1985). In vitro screening assay for teratogens using growth inhibition of human embryonic cells. Proc Natl Acad Sci USA 82: 5791–5794.

Proetzel, G, Pawlowski, SA, Wiles, MV, et al. (1995). Transforming growth factor-beta 3 is required for secondary palate fusion. Nat Genet 11: 409–414.

Romitti, PA, Lidral, AC, Munger, RG, et al. (1999). Candidate genes for nonsyndromic cleft lip and palate and maternal cigarette smoking and alcohol consumption: evaluation of genotype-environment interactions from a population-based case-control study of orofacial clefts. Teratology 59: 39–50.

Sadler, TW (1985). The role of mammalian embryo culture in developmental biology and teratology. In: Issues and Reviews in Teratology, edited by H Katter. Plenum Publishing Corporation, New York: pp. 273–294.

Sadler, TW, Horton, WE, Jr, Hunter, ES (1985). Mammalian embryos in culture: a new approach to investigating normal and abnormal developmental mechanisms. Prog Clin Biol Res 171: 227–240.

Schecter, A (1995). Dioxins and Health. Plenum Press, New York.

Schecter, A, Startin, J, Wright, C, et al. (1996). Concentrations of polychlorinated dibenzo-p-dioxins and dibenzofurans in human placental and fetal tissues from the U.S. and in placentas from Yu-Cheng exposed mothers. Chemosphere 32: 551–557.

Shah, RM, Crawford, BJ, Greene, RM, et al. (1985). In vitro development of the hamster and chick secondary palate. J Craniofac Genet Dev Biol 5: 299–314.

Sharpe, PM, Brunet, CL, Ferguson, MW (1992). Modulation of the epidermal growth factor receptor of mouse embryonic palatal mesenchyme cells in vitro by growth factors. Int J Dev Biol 36: 275–282.

Shiota, K, Kosazuma, T, Klug, S, Neubert, D (1990). Development of the fetal mouse palate in suspension organ culture. Acta Anat 137: 59–64.

Shuey, DL, Buckalew, AR, Wilke, TS, et al. (1994). Early events following maternal exposure to 5-fluorouracil lead to dysmorphology in cultured embryonic tissues. Teratology 50: 379–386.

Sun, D, Vanderburg, CR, Odierna, GS, Hay, ED (1998). TGFbeta3 promotes transformation of chicken palate medial edge epithelium to mesenchyme in vitro. Development 125: 95–105.

Taya, Y, O'Kane, S, Ferguson, MW (1999). Pathogenesis of cleft palate in TGF-beta3 knockout mice. Development 126: 3869–3879.

Tyler, MS, Pratt, RM (1980). Effect of epidermal growth factor on secondary palatal epithelium in vitro: tissue isolation and recombination studies. J Embryol Exp Morphol 58: 93–106.

Welsch, F, Stedman, DB, Carson, JL (1985). Effects of a teratogen on [3H]uridine nucleotide transfer between human embryonal cells and on gap junctions. Exp Cell Res 159: 91–102.

IV

Genetics of Cleft Lip and Palate

16

The Human Genome Project

JANEE GELINEAU-VAN WAES
RICHARD H. FINNELL

Technical advances in molecular genetics that were being developed in the 1970s led to the initiation of the Human Genome Project (HGP), a long-term international research effort to completely map and sequence the human genome. In 1988, U.S. Congress appropriated funds to the Department of Energy (DOE) and the National Institutes of Health (NIH) to begin the planning stages of this vast endeavor (Collins, 1999). The HGP objectives included construction of a detailed genetic and physical map of the human genome, determination of the complete nucleotide sequence of human DNA, and localization of the currently estimated 30,000 genes within the human genome. The completed HGP therefore comprises a resource of detailed information about the structure, organization, and function of human DNA. Similar analyses of the genomes of other model organisms used extensively in research laboratories are also being performed. This information will change the way medical services are provided in the future, including the treatment of individuals with oral-facial clefting disorders.

In addition to promoting the development of improved technologies for biomedical research and genomic analysis, project goals included training scientists to utilize tools and resources developed through the HGP to pursue biological studies that would ultimately improve human health. Specific additional benefits include an enhanced understanding of the genetic contributions to human disease and the development of rational strategies for minimizing or preventing disease phenotypes. Sequencing the human genome greatly improves our understanding of the genetic and molecular basis of disease mechanisms and suggests new therapeutic regimens for disease prevention or, at the very least, the targeting of specific treatment modalities to the individual patient on the basis of their genotype.

The potential long-term benefits for clinical science are tremendous, but the need to avoid potentially adverse consequences is also critical. Examination of the entire spectrum of implications of human genome research and development of policy options for public consideration are essential. An important component of the HGP is the goal of examining the ethical, legal, and social implications (ELSI) of these new gene-based technologies (Collins et al., 1998). Issues raised by the integration of genetic technologies and information into health care are being examined, as well as the ways in which this knowledge interacts with a variety of philosophical, theological, and ethical perspectives. The HGP's ELSI program is unique among technology programs in its mandate to consider and deal with these issues as societal and ethical considerations are crucial in determining the pace and acceptability of clinical developments.

HISTORY

The HGP is an international collaboration of research, involving the U.S. and several other countries, including Britain, France, Japan, and Germany. The HGP was established with the goal of mapping out the entire human genetic blueprint (genome) in order to give scientists a complete understanding of the genetic basis of evolution and the molecular events that take place in development, aging, and disease processes and to provide valuable knowledge for the development of new therapeutic strategies.

In late 1986, a committee on mapping and sequencing the human genome was commissioned by the National Academy of Sciences/National Research Council, and after considerable planning, initiation of the HGP was formalized in October 1990 (McKusick, 1997). In the United States, the NIH and the DOE have been the lead funding agencies, with the U.S. government responsible for developing and planning the project. The NIH-sponsored program was initially under the direction of the National Center for Human Genome Research, which became the National Human Genome Research Institute in January 1997. In Britain, the bulk of the DNA sequencing has been carried out at the Sanger Center in Cambridge, with funding from the Wellcome Trust and the Medical Research Council (Berger, 1998).

In addition to the basic sequencing of the genome and the plan to study human genetic variation and human susceptibility to disease, the project involves sequencing the genomes of other model organisms for comparative analysis. Some of these model organisms include the mouse *(Mus musculus)*, yeast *(Saccharomyces cerevisiae)*, the fruit fly *(Drosophila melanogaster)*, and the roundworm *(Caenorhabditis elegans)*. The genetic similarity between mice and humans makes identification of important regulatory genes in mice of particular interest and relevance. Scientists can use the mouse model to gather clues in order to subsequently go back to the human genome and identify sections of DNA that are likely to have a similar role in humans. The mouse model also provides a useful experimental tool. Knowledge of the mouse genome coupled with technological advances that allow for the creation of genetically engineered mice in which candidate genes of interest have been knocked out, lend considerable insight into gene functions and biological roles.

In October 1990, when the HGP officially began, the projected completion date was sometime in the year 2005. However, improvements in technology, success in achieving early mapping goals, and emerging research/funding opportunities prompted project leaders to promise the genetic blueprint ahead of schedule. New goals for the HGP were defined in October 1998, which included a commitment to complete a third of the human sequence and a "working draft" to cover 90% of the genome by 2001, with complete sequencing of the whole genome by 2003 (Collins, 1999).

In 1991, Craig Venter, a scientist at the NIH Neurological Institute, split off from the HGP to run The Institute for Genomic Research in Gaithersburg, Maryland. He decided that the best way to complete sequencing of the human genome was to utilize a "shotgun" sequencing approach. This basic strategy involved selecting cDNA clones at random and performing single automated sequencing reads from both ends of each insert (Schuler, 1997). These sequences were subsequently reassembled into the full genome using high-speed computers and novel software. In 1998, Venter formed a partnership with Applied Biosystems (now PE Biosystems, Foster City, CA), developer of the rapid, highly automated ABI Prism 3700 DNA sequencer. The joint venture was called Celera Genomics Corporation. Celera combined its sequencing data with data obtained from the international, publicly funded HGP, leading to a rapid acceleration of the project. In June 2000, scientists from Celera and the HGP announced jointly that they had finished sequencing the first working draft of the human genome. Well ahead of schedule, scientists announced that they had sequenced the human genome, deciphering essentially all of the 3.1 billion biochemical "letters" of human DNA.

GOALS/PERSPECTIVE

In 1990, the initial research plan for the HGP set out specific goals for the first 5 years of what was projected to be a 15-year research project. However, since progress was more rapid than initially anticipated, project goals were updated again in 1993 (Collins and Galas, 1993). In 1998, another NIH–DOE master plan was developed to cover completion of the original objectives of sequencing the human genome, as well as to expand the HGP to include the study of genetic variation and functional analysis (Collins et al., 1998).

In this new plan (1998–2003), the major emphasis of the HGP was outlined as DNA sequencing of the human genome. Additional goals addressed the development of both genetic and physical maps, improved DNA sequencing technology, the study of human sequence variation, gene identification, functional analysis, and comparative genomics through the use of model organisms. Bioinformatics and computational studies for the interpretation of data as well as training of genome scientists were also included. Study of the ethical, legal, and social implications of genomic research was defined as another project goal since acquisition of a high-quality human genome sequence would have an unprecedented impact on basic biology, biomedical research, biotechnology, and health care.

The 1998 5-year plan had eight major goals (Collins et al., 1998):

GOAL 1: Human DNA Sequence

a. Finish the complete human genome sequence by the end of 2003

b. Finish one-third of the human DNA sequence by the end of 2001

c. Achieve coverage of at least 90% of the genome in a working draft based on mapped clones by the end of 2001

d. Make the sequence totally and freely accessible

GOAL 2: Sequencing Technology

a. Continue to increase the throughput and reduce the cost of current sequencing technology

b. Support research on novel technologies that can lead to significant improvements in sequencing technology

c. Develop effective methods for the advanced development and introduction of new sequencing technologies into the sequencing process

GOAL 3: Human Genome Sequence Variation

a. Develop technologies for rapid, large-scale identification or scoring, or both, of single-nucleotide polymorphisms (SNPs) and other DNA sequence variants

b. Identify common variants in the coding regions of the majority of identified genes during this 5-year period

c. Create an SNP map of at least 10,000 markers

d. Develop the intellectual foundations for studies of sequence variation

e. Create public resources of DNA samples and cell lines

GOAL 4: Technology for Functional Genomics

a. Develop cDNA resources

b. Support research on methods for studying functions of non-protein-coding sequences

c. Develop technology for comprehensive analysis of gene expression

d. Improve methods for genomewide mutagenesis

e. Develop technology for global protein analysis

GOAL 5: Comparative Genomics

a. Complete the sequence of the *C. elegans* genome in 1998

b. Complete the sequence of the *Drosophila* genome by 2002

c. For the mouse genome:
Develop physical and genetic mapping resources
Develop additional cDNA resources
Complete the sequence of the mouse genome by 2005
Identify other model organisms that can make major contributions to the understanding of the human genome and support appropriate genomic studies

GOAL 6: Ethical, Legal, and Social Implications (ELSI)

a. Examine the issues surrounding the completion of the human DNA sequence and the study of human genetic variation

b. Examine issues raised by the integration of genetic technologies and information into health care and public health activities

c. Examine issues raised by the integration of knowledge about genomics and gene–environment interactions into nonclinical settings

d. Explore ways in which new genetic knowledge may interact with a variety of philosophical, theological, and ethical perspectives

e. Explore how socioeconomic factors and concepts of race and ethnicity influence the use, understanding, and interpretation of genetic information; the utilization of genetic services; and the development of policy

GOAL 7: Bioinformatics and Computational Biology

a. Improve content and utility of databases

b. Develop better tools for data generation, capture, and annotation

c. Develop and improve tools and databases for comprehensive functional studies

d. Develop and improve tools for representing and analyzing sequence similarity and variation

e. Create mechanisms to support effective approaches for producing robust, exportable software that can be widely shared

GOAL 8: Training

a. Nurture the training of scientists skilled in genomic research

b. Encourage the establishment of academic career paths for genomic scientists

c. Increase the number of scholars who are knowledgeable in both genomic and genetic sciences as well as ethics, law, or the social sciences

Accomplishing the goals outlined by the HGP should enhance our understanding of gene–environment interactions and aid in the development of highly accurate DNA-based medical diagnostics and therapeutics. Availability of the human genome sequence should also allow the study of natural genetic variation in humans and provide a basis for risk assessment among individuals with numerous medically important, genetically complex diseases. Furthermore, understanding the relationship between genetic variation and risk should provide valuable insight with respect to the prevention and treatment of illness.

MAPPING AND SEQUENCING

Genetic Map

Several essential stages preceded completion of the sequencing of the human genome. The first of these was the construction of an integrated genetic and physical map (Schuler et al., 1996). In principle, for any given segment of a chromosome, elucidation of the human genome has advanced by a series of maps. The *genetic map* consists of a series of sequence-based markers that can be used to pinpoint the location of an altered gene responsible for a disease phenotype or other trait. It provides information in which distances between map features represent their likelihood of co-inheritance (linkage) and can be used to identify and isolate highly penetrant gene mutations with Mendelian inheritance patterns. Genetic mapping involves recording the relationship between an extensive set of genetic markers, or segments of DNA, which vary in configuration between individuals (Schuler et al., 1996).

Markers on different chromosomes show no linkage as they sort randomly during meiosis, whereas markers on the same chromosome tend to be co-inherited. On the genetic map, the unit of distance is the centimorgan (cM), representing a 1% chance of recombination during a single meiosis or, in other words, a 99% probability that markers will stay together. On the average, 1 cM represents about 1 million bases (1 Mb). The initial goal of the HGP was to create a genetic map with markers spaced at intervals of 2 to 5 cM. For linkage studies, a screening set of 300 to 400 markers is generally used, followed by a more densely saturated map that is used to investigate the most promising areas (Collins, 1997).

If pairs of the various forms of markers are inherited together in families more than 50% of the time, these markers are considered to be genetically linked. By making multiple comparisons of this type with a large set of DNA-based genetic markers, it has been possible to put together a genetic linkage map of the human genome. The value of this map is that it allows examinations of linkage between sets of markers and putative disease loci that segregate in families. As the density of markers on the map improves, it will be possible to carry out large-scale, whole-genome association analyses that will supersede conventional linkage studies (Lanchbury, 1998).

The genetic map was then used to produce an integrated sequence-tagged site (STS) map, which offered extensive and detailed marker order across the human genome and provided a key tool for positional cloning.

Positional Cloning

Maps and other forms of genomic technology provide the tools for a gene-isolation technique known as *positional cloning*. The ability to locate and identify a gene coding for a disease advanced with the discovery of DNA markers such as restriction fragment length polymorphisms and the isolation and propagation of DNA fragments in bacterial or yeast cells. The traditional approach for the identification of disease genes involves positional cloning, in which researchers study a number of disease-affected families using a set of polymorphic DNA markers that span the entire genome (Hudson, 1998). When the transmission of certain markers is shown to correlate with the transmission of a disease, it is possible to locate or map the chromosomal interval that contains the responsible gene. The DNA from such an interval can then be isolated as a set of ordered and overlapping clones, referred to as a *physical map*, which serves as a template to identify the genes or transcripts localized in that specific region. These "candidate genes" are then examined for the presence of DNA sequence mutations in individuals with the disease.

Physical Map

The physical map gives the physical DNA base pair distances from one landmark to another and refers to an ordered set of DNA segments within the genome. Physical mapping provides cloned sets of contiguous DNA that represent regions of a chromosome. These overlapping DNA clone sets, or contigs, were used by the HGP to isolate genes located within a known region on a chromosome (Fink and Collins, 1997). Once genetic markers defined a region containing a sought-after gene, cloned pieces from the physical map provided a resource for the ultimate isolation and identification of the gene.

Physical mapping allows construction of overlapping sets of cloned DNA fragments spanning the genome, by providing a framework in which the DNA sequence can be arranged and the means to connect the linear DNA code of each chromosome. The HGP uses polymerase chain reaction-based markers, the STSs, as the cornerstone of its mapping strategy. Each STS represents the position of a unique DNA sequence in the human genome. The STSs are a universal tool for accessing the genome as they can be used to screen any type of genome resource, e.g., as yeast artificial chromosomes (YACs), bacterial artificial chromosomes (BACs), cosmids, or radiation hybrid panels. On physical maps, the distances between consecutive markers are defined not by probability of co-inheritance but by actual distances along the DNA, measured in bases. A goal of the HGP is to generate STSs that span the human genome at an average spacing of 100,000 bases and dissemination of this information by listing the sequence of the specific oligonucleotide primers on the Internet (Deloukas et al., 1998).

Sequencing

Detailed physical maps provided essential guidance for large-scale DNA sequencing, with the goal of identifying long, complete spans of DNA code. Under the original master plan, the NIH and the DOE were to sequence approximately 60% to 70% of the human genome, and the rest was to be sequenced by the Sanger Center in England and other sequencing centers around the world. The international sequencing community agreed to a policy of releasing data every 24 h into a free, publicly accessible database (GenBank, http://www.ncbi.nlm.nih.gov/GenBank), operated by the National Center for Biotech Information. The HGP began its sequencing efforts using the BAC-to-BAC method, also referred to as the map-based method (Lanchbury, 1998). This approach first creates a crude physical map of the whole genome before sequencing the DNA. Large blocks of genomic DNA (typically 150,000 bp) are inserted into BACs. The entire collection of BACs containing the human genome is called a BAC library. These pieces are fingerprinted to determine the location of each BAC along a chromosome. Each BAC is then broken into smaller pieces and sequenced.

In contrast, the privately funded company Celera Genomics took a different sequencing approach from that of the public consortium by adopting the "shotgun" technique, which utilized the basic strategy of selecting cDNA clones at random and performing single automated sequencing reads from both ends of each insert. The shotgun sequencing method was much faster since it bypassed the need for a physical map and went straight to the task of decoding. Computer algorithms were used to assemble the millions of sequenced fragments into a continuous stretch resembling each chromosome. Combining their own data with that publicly available on the NIH GenBank website, Celera reassembled millions of DNA base pairs with their supercomputer, fast outpacing the publicly funded HGP. In January 2000, Celera Genomics announced that it had sequenced 81% of the human genome, and when combined with publicly available data, it had accomplished enough sequencing to cover 90% of the human genome (Smaglik and Butler, 2000). This led to a rapid acceleration of the HGP, and on June 26, 2000, scientists from Celera and the HGP announced jointly that they had finished sequencing the first draft of the human genome.

With the completion of the working draft sequence of the human genome, the human genetic blueprint became available, consisting of thousands of linked pieces of DNA. The working draft met the HGP's goal for physical mapping, containing over 41,000 DNA markers (STSs) that properly align the pieces. With this density of markers, most genes in the human genome should lie within fewer than 100,000 bases of any given STS. The goal of the HGP is to produce the first complete, highly accurate reference sequence of the human genome by 2003, the year that marks the 50th anniversary of the discovery of the structure of DNA by James Watson and Francis Crick.

HUMAN GENOMIC VARIATION/GENETIC POLYMORPHISM

Genetic variation among individuals includes DNA mutations that give rise to disease or birth defects. The spectrum of diseases, or altered phenotype, being investigated using genetic technologies is shifting from "simple" genetic diseases, which can be caused by unique and highly penetrant mutations, toward "complex" genetic diseases, which are modulated by the action of many susceptibility alleles and environmental factors. Comprehensive genetic studies of common diseases require large-scale investigations of genomic variation among individuals, followed by large association studies comparing affected and unaffected individuals.

The HGP initiated new studies of genetic variation in the human population to provide a dense map of common DNA variants, including insertions and deletions of nucleotides, differences in the copy number of repeated sequences, and SNPs. The SNP variation, where one nucleotide is substituted for another, is the most common type in the genome, occurring at a rate of about 1/1000 bases of DNA (Hudson, 1998). While it often occurs without any physiological consequence, sometimes the variation, occurring in gene sequences or regulatory elements, does result in a biological effect. The SNPs can be used as markers in whole-genome linkage analysis of families with affected members as well as in association studies of individuals in a population. Association studies may directly test a variant with potential functional importance or may take advantage of the phenomenon of linkage disequilibrium, in which a marker and a gene are inherited together, to map gene variants associated with the disease of interest. Some SNPs may contribute directly to a trait or disease phenotype by altering function, particularly those within protein-coding sequences. As the importance of understanding genetic polymorphism and its relationship to disease became clear, so too did the need for large-scale analysis of millions of SNPs among individuals. Many SNPs have been identified by computer comparison of multiple sequences of the same gene using existing databases, and the recent development of DNA chip technology has further aided such studies in genetic variation.

GENE EXPRESSION/MICROARRAYS

DNA chips or arrays provide a promising approach to genome-scale studies of genetic variation, detection of heterogeneous gene mutations, and gene expression. Microarray technology can be applied to the detection of DNA variations as well as the expression of mRNA in individual cells and tissues, genomic comparisons across species, genetic recombination, and large-scale analysis of gene copy number and expression. This technology will also permit clinical geneticists to detect gene mutations. Baseline genome scans could provide helpful information about a person's risk profile and indicate prevention strategies (Lipshutz et al., 1995).

Gene expression profiles and genomic composition can be analyzed using high-density microarrays, generated by linking oligonucleotides or cDNA molecules to the surface of nylon filters, glass slides, or silicon chips. An RNA sample is isolated from the cell or tissue of interest, labeled with a fluorescent probe, and hybridized to the array. The intensity of hybridization, deduced from the fluorescence intensity at each position, enables determination of which genes have been up- or downregulated in a given experimental or clinical paradigm (Kozian and Kirschbaum, 1999; Graves, 1999).

The rapidly increasing power of bioinformatics and automation has resulted in substantial improvements in information gathering and interpretation, allowing better understanding of complex interactions and functional networks operating in living organisms (Zweiger, 1999). DNA chip technology enables large-scale comparisons to be made between related genes in one organism, genes and genomes of different organisms, genes in health and disease states in human beings and animal models, and analysis of gene expression profiles during development and aging. The expression levels of hundreds or thousands of genes from high-density microarrays will enable monitoring of the expression status of cells and tissues on a global basis and highlight induced and suppressed pathways by comparison with normal and diseased states. Expression profiling provides patterns of data and enables pattern recognition that will aid in the study of complex genotype–phenotype correlations and in elucidating the events between the primary mutation and the resulting disease state or alteration/dysfunction within the cell or organism (van Ommen et al., 1999).

COMPARATIVE GENOMICS

The genomic environment is specific to each organism. By comparing similar genes in different organisms, it is possible to determine how function and position have changed over the course of evolution. An understanding of evolutionary development through the use of comparative genomics provides necessary insight into the processes of genetics and inheritance.

Prior to 1996, the goals of DNA sequencing were largely targeted toward genomes of model organisms. Scientists sequenced the genomes of S. cerevisiae, a species of yeast, and numerous bacteria, including Escherichia coli. The first complete genomic sequence of a multicellular organism, the roundworm C. elegans, was finished in late 1998 and contains over 19,000 genes on six chromosomes (about 74% of named human genes have a definite C. elegans homologue) (Clark, 1999). Comparative mapping provides data on gene families, homologues, and gene environment. Evolutionarily conserved segments indicate regions of DNA where conservation of linkage has implications for gene control, and alteration in gene function can be correlated to positional changes within the genome.

The various genome projects are generating huge amounts of data, some in the form of finished sequences, either of single genes or of genomic regions, others in the form of expressed sequence tags (ESTs). Formation of an EST database and release of this information to the scientific community has accelerated the discovery and study of many new genes. The ESTs collected from GenBank are divided into clusters representing distinct genes and organized into a catalogue called *UniGene*. Map locations are determined by radiation hybrid mapping of one or more ESTs from a cluster. The increasing number of cDNA libraries and EST data represent a wealth of scientific information. Basically, genetics has been transformed from a data-poor to a data-rich discipline. Data are available in the public domain, and comparative databases and search engines have been constructed to take advantage of this information. Genomic similarities and differences have been exploited in studies of highly accurate sequences that have identified previously unrecognized exons, predicted gene enhancers, and found new genes; and the increasing use of cross-referencing has provided valuable comparative insights into gene structure and expression.

Many genes in humans have been identified through the exclusive use of computer programs and data-mining approaches, rather than through the more laborious wet lab approaches. The function of these human genes will become more apparent through comparisons with homologues in model organisms. Experimental data for analysis of gene function can be performed in model organisms using techniques such as mutation screens, reporter gene assays, and transgenic animals (Bouck et al., 2000). Comparative genomics enables the transfer of experimental results in model organisms to humans, which could provide potentially important consequences for health management.

Genetic studies of model organisms have elucidated numerous genes, their functions, and their association with human disease. One of the most widely used mammalian model systems is the mouse *(M. musculus)* (Meisler, 1996). Interspecies comparisons provide an excellent means to identify conserved regions of genomic DNA. Alignment of regions of shared homology between mice and humans has identified functionally important motifs, including exons, gene regulatory regions, and promoters. Considerable progress has been made in the efficiency of positional cloning of mutant mouse genes, induction of new mutants by teratogens or chemical mutagens, targeted mutation of cloned genes by homologous recombination, strategies for analysis of polygenic traits, and comparative mapping of human and mouse chromosomes (Pennisi, 1999).

CLEFT LIP WITH OR WITHOUT CLEFT PALATE

Cleft lip with or without cleft palate (CL/P) is a common congenital malformation. Nonsyndromic clefting of the lip and palate in humans has a highly complex etiology, with both multiple genetic loci and exposure to teratogens influencing individual susceptibility (Diehl and Erickson, 1997). The familial clustering of CL/P has been extensively characterized, and epidemiological studies have proposed monogenic models (putative major locus associated with reduced penetrance) (Hecht et al., 1991), multifactorial threshold models, and mixed major gene/multifactorial models to explain its inheritance (Farrall and Holder, 1992; Mitchell and Risch, 1992). Clefting can result from a single gene defect either as part of a syndrome (e.g., Van der Woude's syndrome, Treacher-Collins syndrome, velocardiofacial syndrome) or as an isolated phenotypic effect [e.g., X-linked cleft palate (CP); nonsyndromic, autosomal dominant orofacial clefting). Several studies have suggested that chromosome 6p is a candidate region for a locus involved in orofacial clefting (Davies et al., 1995), and linkage studies suggest another susceptibility locus on the long arm of chromosome 4 (Beiraghi et al., 1994). Although evidence for the involvement of a major gene in the etiology of CL/P has been reported, orofacial clefting is genetically complex, with no single gene being responsible for all forms. Molecular studies provide further insight into the genetic mechanism underlying CL/P, and these findings have important implications with regard to the feasibility of detecting linkage to loci conferring susceptibility to CL/P (Mitchell et al., 1995).

Genetic analysis and tissue-specific expression studies support a role for transforming growth factor-alpha *(TGF-α)* in craniofacial development. Numerous studies have confirmed an association at the *TGF-α* locus with nonsyndromic CL/P in humans (Farrall and Holder, 1992; Jara et al., 1995), extending the role for *TGF-α* in craniofacial morphogenesis and supporting an interrelated mechanism for this major gene in the etiology of nonsyndromic forms of CL/P (Shiang et al., 1993). In addition, a gene–environment interaction between maternal smoking, *TGF-α*, and clefting has been reported. Shaw et al. (1996) offered evidence that the risk for orofacial clefting in infants may be influenced by maternal smoke exposure alone as well as in combination (gene–environment interaction) with the presence of the uncommon *TGF-α* allele. This was supported in a study by Hwang et al. (1995), in which infants with isolated birth defects (CL/P and controls with nonclefting birth defects) were tested for an association among maternal exposures, genetic markers, and oral clefts. A modest increase in the less common C2 allele of the *TGF-α* locus was seen among CP only infants compared with the birth defect controls, and the association appeared to reflect an underlying interaction between maternal smoking and infant genotype. This apparent gene–environment interaction was also found among those reporting no family history of any birth defect.

Even though the first association studies of CL/P with candidate genes found an association with *TGF-α*, other candidate genes have also been identified. Association of CL/P with the retinoic acid receptor-alpha *(RAR-α)* locus has been reported (Mitchell et al., 1995), as well as associations with the *BCL-2* oncogene, *BCL-3* (Stein et al., 1995), *sonic hedgehog (Shh)*, epidermal growth factor receptor *(EGFR)* (Young et al., 2000), and several of the known homeobox genes (Chenevix-Trench et al., 1992). While some studies suggest that the familial aggregation of nonsyndromic CL/P is likely attributable to the effects of several susceptibility loci acting in a multiplicative fashion (Mitchell et al., 1995), others report no evidence of an interaction between the *TGF-α* and *RAR-α* polymorphisms, even though jointly they appear to account for almost half the attributable risk of clefting (Chenevix-Trench et al., 1992).

Another gene that has been identified as having a potential role in clefting is *TGF-β3*. Kaartinen et al. (1995), using *TGF-β3* null mutant mice, demonstrated an essential function for *TGF-β3* in normal morphogenesis of the palate, directly implicating a role for this gene in the epithelial–mesenchymal transformation necessary for palatal fusion (Proetzel et al., 1995). Mice lacking *TGF-β3* exhibit an incompletely penetrant failure of the palatal shelves to fuse, leading to CP. The defect appears to result from impaired adhesion of the apposing medial edge epithelia of the palatal shelves and subsequent elimination of the midline epithelial seam. Since these mutant mice exhibit no other craniofacial abnormalities, these results demonstrate that *TGF-β3* affects palatal shelf fusion by an intrinsic, primary mechanism rather than by effects secondary to craniofacial defects.

In addition to the identification of major genes involved in the etiology of nonsyndromic CL/P, information made available through the HGP and the use of animal models has facilitated the study of gene–environment interactions with respect to orofacial clefting. For example, an interaction between maternal periconceptual smoking and the *TGF-α* polymorphism leading to increased risk for CL/P has been shown (Shaw et al., 1996). In addition, it has been reported that maternal multivitamin supplementation may lead to a reduced risk for CL/P in infants having the *TGF-α* mutation (Shaw et al., 1998). Pharmaceutical compounds such as anticonvulsant drugs [phenytoin (Dilantin)] (Finnell and Dansky, 1991), hydrocortisone (Abbott, 1995), folate antagonists (methotrexate), and retinoids [isotretinoin (Accutane)], as well as alcohol, maternal hyperthermia, and organic solvents/agricultural chemicals have been shown to cause CL/P in exposed offspring (for review, see Wyszynski and Beaty, 1996). However, in spite of considerable effort on the part of the teratological community, the mechanism by which many of these compounds exert their teratogenic effect remains unknown. Recent technological advances, however, will allow critical changes in gene expression subsequent to teratogen exposure to be analyzed and promote the discovery of genetic polymorphisms that will enhance our ability to identify individuals at risk. The ability to identify individuals with inherent genetic susceptibility to environmentally induced malformations such as CL/P will have important medical implications in terms of diagnostic and preventive strategies.

CONCLUSION

Sequencing of the human genome has improved our understanding of the genetic and molecular mechanisms of disease and provided new opportunities for novel therapeutic regimens and disease-prevention research. Understanding genetic risk factors and their interaction with the environment may potentially provide the ability for diseases and developmental defects such as CL/P to be predicted and prevented, at both individual and population levels using environmental or behavioral interventions directed at genotypically susceptible individuals.

Genomics has accelerated our knowledge and understanding of mammalian biology through positional cloning of mutations in model organisms such as the mouse, and comparative genomics has further enabled the transfer of these experimental results to humans, providing important consequences for health management. In addition, the HGP has contributed to the understanding of developmental anomalies by providing informative and efficient genetic markers for the mapping of qualitative or complex traits, thereby allowing the subsequent mapping of variant genes that contribute to a given phenotype. Microarray technology permits baseline genome scans and analysis of individual expression patterns, which provides helpful information about a person's risk profile and indicates prevention strategies. Advanced technology for functional genomics provides a better understanding of the complex interactions between genetic and environmental factors and offers clinical benefits in the form of useful predictive or diagnostic tests for susceptibility genes.

The HGP has made it possible to map all of the individual nucleotides that make up the 23 human chromosomes. A catalogue of human gene sequences is a critical resource for both computational and experimental approaches to genomic analysis, and it provides a framework for organizing and understanding the information collected from these studies. The genetic research community now has access to numerous DNA markers, detailed chromosome maps, extensive online databases, and rapid DNA analysis technologies that can be used to identify genetic mutations. This information should lead to improved understanding of the causes of diseases and/or congenital malformations such as CL/P and to better approaches for the diagnosis, prevention, and treatment of human genetic disorders.

REFERENCES

Abbott, BD (1995). Review of the interaction between TCDD and glucocorticoids in embryonic palate. Toxicology *105:* 365–373.

Beiraghi, S, Foroud, T, Diouhy, S, et al. (1994). Possible localization of a major gene for cleft lip and palate to 4q. Clin Genet *46:* 255–256.

Berger, A (1998). Human genome project to complete ahead of schedule. BMJ *317:* 834.

Bouck, JB, Metzker, ML, Gibbs, RA (2000). Shotgun sample sequence comparisons between mouse and human genomes. Nat Genet *25:* 31–33.

Chenevix-Trench, G, Jones, K, Green, AC, et al. (1992). Cleft lip with or without cleft palate: associations with transforming growth factor alpha and retinoic acid receptor loci. Am J Hum Genet *51:* 1377–1385.

Clark, MS (1999). Comparative genomics: the key to understanding the Human Genome Project. Bioessays *21*: 121–130.

Collins, F (1997). Sequencing the human genome. Hosp Pract. Available from http://www.hosppract.com/genetics/9701/gen9701.html; INTERNET.

Collins, F (1999). Shattuck lecture. Medical and societal consequences of the human genome project. N Engl J Med *341*: 28–37.

Collins, F, Galas, D (1993). A new five-year plan for the U.S. Human Genome Project. Science *262*: 43–46.

Collins, F, Patrinos, A, Jordan, E, et al. (1998). New goals for the U.S. Human Genome Project: 1998–2003. Science *282*: 682–689.

Davies, AF, Stephens, RJ, Olavesen, MG, et al. (1995). Evidence of a locus for orofacial clefting on human chromosome 6p24 and STS content map of the region. Hum Mol Genet *4*: 121–128.

Deloukas, P, Schuler, GD, Gyapay, G, et al. (1998). A physical map of 30,000 human genes. Science *282*: 744–746.

Diehl, S, Erickson, R (1997). Genome scan for teratogen-induced clefting susceptibility loci in the mouse: evidence of both allelic and locus heterogeneity distinguishing cleft lip and cleft palate. Proc Natl Acad Sci USA *94*: 5231–5236.

Farrall, M, Holder, S (1992). Familial recurrence-pattern analysis of cleft lip with or without cleft palate. Am J Hum Genet *50*: 270–277.

Finnell, RH, Dansky, LV (1991). Parental epilepsy, anticonvulsant drugs, and reproductive outcome: epidemiologic and experimental findings spanning three decades. Reprod Toxicol *5*: 281–299.

Fink, L, Collins, F (1997). The Human Genome Project: view from the National Institutes of Health. J Am Med Womens Assoc *52*: 4–7.

Graves, DJ (1999). Powerful tools for genetic analysis come of age. Trends Biotechnol *17*: 127–134.

Hecht, JT, Yang, P, Michels, VV, Buetow, KH (1991). Complex segregation analysis of nonsyndromic cleft lip and palate. Am J Hum Genet *49(3)*: 674–681.

Hudson, T (1998). The Human Genome Project: tools for the identification of disease genes. Clin Invest Med *21*: 267–276.

Hwang, SJ, Beaty, TH, Panny, SR, et al. (1995). Association study of transforming growth factor alpha (TGFα) TaqI polymorphism and oral clefts: indication of gene–environment interaction in a population-based sample of infants with birth defects. Am J Epidemiol *141*: 629–636.

Jara, L, Blanco, R, Chiffelle, I, et al. (1995). Association between alleles of the transforming growth factor alpha locus and cleft lip and palate in the Chilean population. Am J Med Genet *57*: 548–551.

Kaartinen, V, Voncken, JW, Shuler, C, et al. (1995). Abnormal lung development and cleft palate in mice lacking TGF-β 3 indicates defects of epithelial–mesenchymal interaction. Nat Genet *11*: 415–421.

Kozian, DH, Kirschbaum, BJ (1999). Comparative gene-expression analysis. Trends Biotechnol *17*: 73–77.

Lanchbury, J (1998). The Human Genome Project. Br J Rheumatol *37*: 119–125.

Lipshutz, RJ, Morris, D, Chee, M, et al. (1995). Using oligonucleotide probe arrays to access genetic diversity. Biotechniques *19*: 442–447.

McKusick, VA (1997). Genomics: structural and functional studies of genomes. Genomics *45*: 244–249.

Meisler, M (1996). The role of the laboratory mouse in the human genome project. Am J Hum Genet *69*: 764–771.

Mitchell, LE, Healey, SC, Chenevix-Trench, G (1995). Evidence for an association between nonsyndromic cleft lip with or without cleft palate and a gene located on the long arm of chromosome 4. Am J Hum Genet *57*: 1130–1136.

Mitchell, LE, Risch, N (1992). Mode of inheritance of nonsyndromic cleft lip with or without cleft palate: a reanalysis. Am J Hum Genet *51*: 323–332.

Pennisi, E (1999). Mouse genome added to sequencing effort. Science *286*: 210.

Proetzel, G, Pawlowski, SA, Wiles, MV, et al. (1995). Transforming growth factor-beta 3 is required for secondary palate fusion. Nat Genet *11*: 409–414.

Schuler, G (1997). Pieces of the puzzle: expressed sequence tags and the catalog of human genes. J Mol Med *75*: 694–698.

Schuler, GD, Boguski, MS, Stewart, EA, et al. (1996). A gene map of the human genome. Science *274*: 540–546.

Shaw, GM, Wasserman, CR, Lammer, EJ, et al. (1996). Orofacial clefts, parental cigarette smoking, and transforming growth factor-alpha gene variants. Am J Hum Genet *58*: 551–561.

Shaw, GM, Wasserman, CR, Murray, JC, Lammer, EJ (1998). Infant TGF-alpha genotype, orofacial clefts, and maternal periconceptional multivitamin use. Cleft Palate Craniofac J *35*: 366–370.

Shiang, R, Lidral, AC, Ardinger, HH, et al. (1993). Association of transforming growth-factor alpha gene polymorphisms with nonsyndromic cleft palate only (CPO). Am J Hum Genet *53*: 836–843.

Smaglik, P, Butler, D (2000). Celera turns to public genome data to speed up endgame. Nature *403*: 119–120.

Stein, J, Mulliken, JB, Stal, S, et al. (1995). Nonsyndromic cleft lip with or without cleft palate: evidence of linkage to BCL3 in 17 multigenerational families. Am J Hum Genet *57*: 257–272.

van Ommen, J, Bakker, E, den Dunnen, J (1999). The Human Genome Project and the future of diagnostics, treatment, and prevention. Lancet *354*: 5–10.

Wyszynski, DF, Beaty, TH (1996). Review of the role of potential teratogens in the origin of human nonsyndromic oral clefts. Teratology *53*: 309–317.

Young, DL, Schneider, RA, Hu, D, Helms, JA (2000). Genetic and teratogenic approaches to craniofacial development. Crit Rev Oral Biol Med *11*: 304–317.

Zweiger, G (1999). Knowledge discovery in gene-expression-microarray data: mining the information output of the genome. Trends Biotechnol *17*: 429–436.

17

Twin studies in oral cleft research

LAURA E. MITCHELL

Twin studies of oral clefts (OCs) have in general been undertaken to address one of two questions: *(1)* Are OCs in twins related to or a consequence of the twinning process? and *(2)* What can twins tell us about the genetic contribution to OCs in the general population of, predominantly singleton (i.e., nontwin), affected individuals? Clearly, the answers to these two questions are not independent. If OCs in twins are a consequence of the twinning process, information from twins will not be useful in establishing the genetic contribution to OCs in the general population of affected individuals.

Prior to examining the literature, it is helpful to have an appreciation for some of the challenges presented by twin studies of OCs. Although OCs are relatively common malformations, the co-occurrence of twinning and OCs is rare. Population-based data from Denmark (Christensen and Fogh-Andersen, 1993a,b), which has a high ascertainment of OC cases (Christensen, 1999), suggests that only approximately 1/21,000 newborns will be a twin with an OC. Hence, it is extremely difficult to ascertain an unbiased sample of OC twins that is sufficiently large to address the questions of interest with any degree of precision. This problem is compounded by the fact that data from twins with cleft lip with or without cleft palate (CL/P) and those with cleft palate only (CP) must be evaluated separately since, with rare exceptions (e.g., Van der Woude's syndrome), the etiologies of these disorders differ (Fraser, 1970). In addition, twins with syndromic forms of CL/P and CP must be excluded from any analysis that focuses on the causes of nonsyndromic OCs, and *monozygotic twins* (i.e., identical twins derived from a single sperm and egg) and *dizygotic twins* (i.e., fraternal twins derived from the fertilization of two eggs) must be evaluated separately.

Accurate assessment of zygosity is an extremely important aspect of any twin study. Fortunately, recent advances in molecular genetics have made it possible to assign zygosity with a very high degree of accuracy in a relatively inexpensive and easy manner. DNA fingerprinting (Eufinger et al., 1993) or the evaluation of six to eight polymerase chain reaction (PCR) systems (Eufinger et al., 1995; Martin et al., 1997) can be used to obtain an accurate zygosity diagnosis. The latter approach is generally preferred since it can be performed using DNA from buccal swabs, blood spots (e.g., Guthrie card), or venous blood, whereas DNA fingerprinting requires 0.5 to 1.0 ml of ethylenediaminetetraacetic acid (EDTA) blood (Eufinger et al., 1995).

Unfortunately, the majority of published twin studies of CL/P and CP predate the use of DNA-based assignment of zygosity. In fact, many of these studies did not assess zygosity directly but, rather, used Weinberg's difference method to estimate the number of mono- and dizygotic twin pairs. This method estimates the number of monozygotic pairs by subtracting twice the number of opposite-sex pairs (which must be dizygotic) from the total number of pairs. The assumptions underlying this method are that the sexes of dizygotic twins are independent and that same-sex dizygotic pairs are representative of opposite-sex dizygotic pairs. The validity of the first of these assumptions has, however, been challenged (James, 1979; Allen, 1981; Boklage, 1985; James, 1992), and the validity of the second is questionable when dealing with conditions, such as CL/P, that exhibit distorted sex ratios. [Although some studies have detected a predominance of females among individuals with CP, there is evidence that this may be an artifact of ascertainment, which typically includes only cases requiring surgical intervention (Christensen

214

et al., 1992).] Hence, estimates of twin concordance for CL/P and CP based on Weinberg's difference method may be biased and must be interpreted with caution.

ORAL CLEFTS AND THE TWINNING PROCESS

Previous studies have suggested that twins are more likely than singletons to be affected with congenital malformations (Hay and Wehrung, 1970; Myrianthopoulos, 1976; Layde et al., 1980; Little and Nevin, 1989; Mastroiacovo et al., 1999), although such differences have not been identified in all studies (Windham and Bjerkedal, 1984; Ramos-Arroyo, 1991). When detected, the excess risk for congenital malformations in twins has generally been attributed to an increased risk only among monozygotic twins (Myrianthopoulos, 1976; Layde et al., 1980). It has been suggested that this may reflect either developmental disturbances associated with the monozygotic twinning process (Myrianthopoulos, 1978; Nance, 1981) or a common etiology for monozygotic twinning and specific malformations (Myrianthopoulos, 1978; Schinzel et al., 1979; Nance, 1981).

The conclusions that can be drawn from studies of the prevalence of congenital malformations in twins and singletons are limited by a number of factors. Several of these studies did not assess zygosity directly but, rather, compared the prevalence of malformations in same-sex twins and opposite-sex twins (Hay and Wehrung, 1970; Layde et al., 1980; Little and Nevin, 1989; Ramos-Arroyo, 1991). The rationale for this comparison is that all opposite-sex twins are dizygotic, whereas same-sex twins represent a mixture of monozygotic and dizygotic pairs. Hence, assuming that opposite-sex dizygotic twins are representative of same-sex dizygotic twins, any differences between same- and opposite-sex pairs must be attributed to the monozygotic twins. However, as previously stated, this assumption is questionable when dealing with conditions that exhibit distorted sex ratios. An additional limitation of these studies is that the risk to twins was assessed using information from both members of each twin pair. This will lead to an overestimate of the risk to twins relative to singletons since the members of a twin pair are not independent. Finally, most of these studies were based on relatively small samples and thus had limited statistical power to evaluate the relationship between twinning and specific malformations (Mastroiacovo et al., 1999).

A small number of studies have compared the prevalence of CL/P and CP in twin and singleton births and in same- and opposite-sex twin pairs. In general, these studies are limited by concerns regarding the completeness of case ascertainment and the potential for biased ascertainment of twin pairs (Christensen and Fogh-Andersen, 1993b). Based on these studies, there is some evidence that twins have a higher prevalence of CL/P, but not CP, relative to singletons (Table 17.1). However, in three of these studies (Layde et al., 1980; Little and Nevin, 1989; Ramos-Arroyo, 1991), the number of twins with CL/P was very small ($n < 10$), and the two largest studies (Hay and Wehrung, 1970; Mastroiacovo et al., 1999) provided conflicting results. Interpretation of the data from same- and opposite-sex twin pairs is also hampered by the small number of affected twins observed in the majority of studies. However, there appears to be no clear tendency for the prevalence of CL/P to be higher in same-sex than in opposite-sex twin pairs. Conclusions regarding differences in the prevalence of CP in same-sex and opposite-sex pairs are precluded by the small number of affected individuals in all but one study (Mastroiacovo et al., 1999).

Studies in Denmark have provided the most compelling evidence that the prevalence rates of CL/P and CP are not significantly different in twins and singletons (Christensen and Fogh-Andersen, 1993a,b). These studies had the advantage of near complete ascertainment since, in Denmark, individuals with CL/P or CP have been carefully registered for over five decades and treatment is both free and highly centralized (Christensen, 1999). In addition, zygosity was directly assessed (using 8–17 blood, serum, and enzyme types) in all twin pairs that included at least one affected individual, and the analyses were restricted to individuals who had nonsyndromic forms of CL/P and CP. Although a slight excess of twins with CL/P was detected in this population (33 expected vs. 47 observed), this difference was not statistically significant and there was no evidence that the risk of CL/P differed in monozygotic and dizygotic twins (Christensen and Fogh-Andersen, 1993a). Further, there was no significant difference in the observed and expected numbers of twins with CP (16 expected vs. 9 observed) and no evidence that the risk of this malformation differed by zygosity (Christensen and Fogh-Andersen, 1993b).

In summary, comparisons of the prevalence of CL/P and CP in singletons and twins, same-sex and opposite-sex twin pairs, and monozygotic and dizygotic pairs do not provide compelling evidence that these malformations are associated with twinning in general or with monozygotic twinning in particular. Additional evidence for or against such associations could be obtained by comparing other characteristics of CL/P and CP in twins and singletons. Specifically, demonstration of differences between affected singletons and twins with respect to well established characteristics of these

TABLE 17.1. *Prevalence per 10,000 of Cleft Lip with or without Cleft Palate (CL/P) and Cleft Palate (CP) in Singleton and Twin Births*

Condition	Reference	Singletons (No.)	All Twins (No.)	OR[A] (Twins vs. Singletons)	Opposite-Sex Twins (No.)	Same-Sex Twins (No.)	OR (Same vs. Opposite Sex)
CL/P	Mastroiacovo et al. (1999)	7.7 (9135)	10.2 (265)	1.31*	NA	NA	—
	Ramos-Arroyo (1991)	5.9 (196)	8.7 (5)	1.42	15.8 (2)	7.0 (3)	0.44[†]
	Little and Nevin (1989)	9.4 (146)	18.8 (6)	2.00	9.5 (1)	23.4 (5)	2.47
	Layde et al. (1980)[‡]	12.4 (173)	24.6 (6)	1.98	14.5 (1)	18.43 (3)	1.27
	Hay and Wehrung (1970)	7.7 (7714)	7.4 (147)	0.96	6.6 (43)	7.7 (104)	1.17
CP	Mastroiacovo et al. (1999)	3.8 (4480)	4.2 (110)	1.11	NA	NA	—
	Ramos-Arroyo (1991)	5.2 (173)	5.2 (3)	1.01	0.0 (0)	7.0 (3)	—
	Little and Nevin (1989)	4.0 (63)	0.0 (0)	—	0.0 (0)	0.0 (0)	—
	Layde et al. (1980)[‡]	6.7 (93)	8.2 (2)	1.23	0.0 (0)	6.1 (1)	—
	Hay and Wehrung (1970)	3.4 (3408)	3.4 (67)	0.99	3.5 (23)	3.3 (44)	0.93

[A]OR, odds ratio.
*Difference is significant at $p < 0.05$.
[†]This number was estimated from the reported prevalence per 10,000 in same- and opposite-sex twin pairs since the total number of such pairs was not provided.
[‡]The number of affected individuals was back-calculated from the total numbers and the reported prevalence.

conditions (e.g., sex ratio, pattern of familial recurrence, severity of defect) would provide some support for the hypothesis that these malformations are associated with the twinning process. Such differences have not been extensively investigated. However, the Danish data provide no evidence that the sex ratios among individuals with CL/P or CP differ in twins and singletons (Christensen and Fogh-Andersen, 1993a,b) or that either the distribution of CL/P types (i.e., unilateral vs. bilateral, cleft lip vs. cleft lip and palate) (Christensen and Fogh-Andersen, 1993a) or familial recurrence patterns for CL/P (Mitchell and Christensen, 1997) differ in twins and singletons.

In conclusion, additional, larger studies of the familial, clinical, and epidemiological characteristics of CL/P and CP in twins are required to definitively rule out the existence of an association between twinning and these conditions. Such studies should include accurate assessment of zygosity and samples of sufficient size to evaluate the characteristics of these conditions separately in monozygotic and dizygotic twins. Given that CL/P (and possibly CP) exhibits a distorted sex ratio, samples adequate for the analysis of zygosity and sex-specific subgroups would be particularly desirable. However, since the available data provide little evidence that the causes of CL/P or CP differ in twins and singletons, it appears likely that cautious use of twin data may provide important insights regarding the genetic contribution to these conditions in the general population of affected individuals.

WHAT TWINS TELL US ABOUT THE GENETIC CONTRIBUTION TO ORAL CLEFTS

In the classic twin design, concordance for a trait is measured in monozygotic twins (who are genetically identical) and dizygotic twins (who, on average, share only one-half of their genes) and the relative contribution of genetic and nongenetic factors to disease risk is estimated. A basic assumption of the classic twin approach is that the environment (both pre- and postnatal) of monozygotic and dizygotic twins is similar and, therefore, that any differences in their concordance rates must be attributable to differences in their degree of genetic similarity. Although this assumption has been challenged (Phillips, 1993), it appears to be valid in many circumstances (Duffy, 1993; Christensen et al., 1995). For additional information regarding the strengths and limitations of the classic twin approach, the reader is referred to the many reviews of this topic (Bundey, 1991; Bryan, 1992; LaBuda et al., 1992; Hall, 1996; Martin et al., 1997).

In many twin studies, only the subset of twin pairs that includes at least one affected member is sampled. Each independently ascertained twin is called a *proband*. Two methods are commonly employed to estimate twin concordance rates from such data. The *pairwise concordance rate*, which is the probability that both members of a twin pair are affected given that at least one is affected, and the *probandwise concordance rate*, which is the probability that a twin is affected given that the cotwin is a proband (Allen et al., 1967). The probandwise concordance rate is generally preferred over the pairwise rate because it provides estimates of risk for individuals rather than pairs. In addition, estimates of probandwise concordance are directly comparable to estimates of risk for other types of relatives and can be used to infer the relative importance of genetic factors for the trait of interest (McGue, 1992). In contrast to pairwise concordance rates, probandwise concordance rates can also be compared across studies with different ascertainment schemes (McGue, 1992).

Comparison of probandwise concordance rates in mono- and dizygotic twins can provide a number of clues regarding the genetic contribution to a trait. If a trait is determined by a single gene, the probandwise concordance rate for monozygotic cotwins should be no greater than four-fold higher than the corresponding rate for dizygotic cotwins. For example, concordance rates for a fully penetrant, autosomal dominant condition would be 100% and 50% in monozygotic and dizygotic twins, respectively, giving rise to a twofold difference in risk. The corresponding values for a fully penetrant, autosomal recessive condition would be 100% and 25%, corresponding to a fourfold difference. Hence, relative risks that exceed 4 are incompatible with simple, single-gene inheritance and indicate that more than one gene and/or environmental factor must impact on the disease risk.

Comparison of concordance rates in dizygotic twins with risks to full sibs also provides information regarding the influence of nongenetic factors. Specifically, an increase in risk to dizygotic cotwins relative to full sibs (who are genetically equivalent to cotwins) suggests that shared environmental factors must contribute to disease risk. Finally, monozygotic twin concordance rates less than 100% indicate that genetic alterations occurring after cleavage of the embryo and/or other noninherited factors (e.g., intrauterine environmental differences in the allocation of cells and in the placental vascular supply to each twin, stochastic events) influence disease risk.

Several studies have reported twin concordance rates for CL/P and CP (Metrakos et al., 1958; Hay and Wehrung, 1970; Shields et al., 1979; Christensen and

Fogh-Andersen, 1993a,b; Nordstrom et al., 1996; Natsume et al., 2000). However, estimates from the majority of these studies are largely inadequate for several reasons: concordance was assessed in same- and opposite-sex pairs and used to estimate the expected concordance rates in mono- and dizygotic twins (Hay and Wehrung, 1970), the number of available twin pairs was small (Table 17.2), and pairwise rather than probandwise concordance rates were reported (Metrakos et al., 1958; Hay and Wehrung, 1970; Shields et al., 1979; Nordstrom et al., 1996).

Probandwise concordance rates for CL/P suggest that the risk to monozygotic cotwins of affected individuals is less than 100% but six- to 19-fold higher than the risk to dizygotic cotwins (Table 17.2). In addition, the observed risk to dizygotic cotwins does not appear to be markedly different from the 3% to 5% risk generally quoted for the full sibs of individuals with CL/P (Mitchell and Risch, 1992). These observations suggest that CL/P is influenced by genetic factors but that it is unlikely to be determined by a single gene. Moreover, non-genetic factors (or postcleavage genetic alternations) are also implicated in the development of CL/P since the probandwise concordance rate for monozygotic twins is less than 100%.

Estimates derived from the most recent Danish study (Christensen and Fogh-Andersen, 1993a) suggest that as much as 73% of the variation in liability to CL/P (i.e., the heritability of CL/P) may be determined by genetic effects. This estimate is likely the most accurate assessment of the genetic contribution to CL/P since it is based on twins for whom zygosity was established using extensive typing of blood, serum, and enzymes, as well as an accurate estimate of the population prevalence of CL/P in Denmark during the relevant time period (Christensen et al., 1992).

Twin studies suggest that CP is also influenced by both genetic and nongenetic factors and unlikely to be inherited in a simple Mendelian fashion (Table 17.2). However, the relatively small number of dizygotic twin pairs in the individual studies makes it difficult to determine if the risk to dizygotic cotwins is similar to or greater than the risk to full sibs, which has been estimated to be approximately 2% to 3% (Fitzpatrick and Farrall, 1993; Christensen and Mitchell, 1996). Twin-based estimates of heritability for CP are also difficult to derive for this reason.

Additional, larger studies of twins with CL/P and CP will be required to obtain more precise estimates of twin concordance and heritability for these traits. Although heritability estimates provide useful information regarding the relative genetic contribution to a trait, such estimates can and have been obtained from other types of relative and it is generally recognized that the risk for both CL/P and CP is determined by genetic factors. Moreover, as the quest to identify the specific genes involved in these conditions has been initiated (Wyszynski et al., 1996a; Schutte and Murray, 1999), the availability of precise, twin-based estimates of heritability for CL/P and CP is unlikely to significantly influence the current direction of research regarding the etiology of these conditions. Hence, the ability to obtain heritability estimates does not by itself provide strong justification for additional twin studies of CL/P and CP. Twin studies of CL/P and CP can, however, provide information that would be useful for genetic counseling purposes [e.g., what is the risk that the unaffected member of a monozygotic twin pair discordant for CL/P will have an affected child? (Wyszynski et al., 1996b)]. In addition, information on probandwise twin concordance rates can be used to establish the mode of inheritance, which is helpful in determining the most appropriate methods for the identification of CL/P and CP susceptibility loci.

Several approaches (e.g., linkage, association studies) can be used to identify disease-causing or disease-predisposing genes (Lander and Schork, 1994). In general, linkage strategies are more appropriate for conditions determined by a small number of genes, each of which has a relatively major impact on risk. In contrast, association studies are better suited for conditions determined by a relatively large number of genes which have a modest impact on risk. Hence, it is helpful to have some understanding of the mode of inheritance of a trait (i.e., the number of genes involved and the magnitude of their effect) prior to undertaking studies aimed at disease-gene identification.

Analysis of the familial recurrence patterns exhibited by a trait can provide insight regarding the number of genes involved in determining a trait and the magnitude of their effect. Specifically, the pattern of decline in $\lambda_R - 1$, where λ_R is the ratio of risk to a relative of type R (R = M, 1, 2, 3 for monozygotic twin, parent/offspring, second-degree, and third-degree relatives, respectively) compared to the population prevalence is determined by the underlying genetic model, and analysis of the observed decline in $\lambda_R - 1$ from monozygotic cotwins to first-degree relatives, as well as from first- to second-, and second- to third-degree relatives, can be used to assess the mode of inheritance (Risch, 1990). (Additional detail regarding this approach is provided in Chapter 19.) The lack of good estimates of λ_R, for monozygotic twins has, however, limited the usefulness of this approach for establishing the mode of inheritance of CL/P and CP (Mitchell and Risch, 1992). Hence, an important goal of future twin studies of CL/P and CP should be the precise estimation of monozygotic probandwise concordance rates.

TABLE 17.2. *Monozygotic (MZ) and Dizygotic (DZ) Twin Concordance Rates for Cleft Lip with or without Cleft Palate (CL/P) and Cleft Palate (CP)*

Condition	Reference	Total pairs (concordant pairs)		Pairwise concordance rate		Probandwise concordance rate*	
		MZ	DZ	MZ	DZ	MZ	DZ
CL/P	Natsume et al. (2000)	26 (13)	NA[†]	0.50	NA	0.67	NA
	Nordstrom et al. (1996)	6 (1)	26 (0)	0.17	0.00	0.28	0.00
	Christensen and Fogh-Andersen (1993a)	14 (6)	19 (1)	0.43	0.05	0.60	0.05
	Fogh-Andersen (1942), Shields et al. (1979)	10 (4)	67 (1)	0.40	0.02	0.57	0.03
	Hay and Wehrung (1970)	51 (9)	84 (2)	0.18	0.02	0.30	0.05
	Total	107 (33)	196 (4)	0.31	0.02	0.47	0.04
CP	Natsume et al. (2000)	13 (5)	NA	0.31	NA	0.56	NA
	Nordstrom et al. (1996)	11 (6)	45 (5)	0.54	0.11	0.70	0.20
	Christensen and Fogh-Andersen (1993b)	2 (1)	8 (0)	0.50	0.00	0.67	0.00
	Fogh-Andersen (1942), Shields et al. (1979)	3 (1)	11 (0)	0.33	0.00	0.50	0.00
	Hay and Wehrung (1970)	15 (6)	42 (2)	0.40	0.05	0.57	0.09
	Total	44 (19)	106 (7)	0.43	0.07	0.60	0.12

*Probandwise concordance rates were estimated by assuming that all affected twins are probands.
[†]Natsume et al. (2000) evaluated only monozygotic twins.

Twin studies of CL/P and CP that incorporate the collection of DNA samples from both members of the twin pair and their parents may also help to determine the contribution of a specific genetic locus to disease risk. Information from monozygotic and dizygotic twins can be used to estimate the *coefficient of genetic contribution*, which measures the genetic contribution of a putative susceptibility locus to a multilocus disease (Rotter and Landaw, 1984). In addition, information from dizygotic twins can be used to estimate the relative increase in risk to sibs compared to the general population (λ_S) that is attributable to a putative susceptibility locus (Risch, 1987), and concordant dizygotic pairs can be used in affected sib pair or affected relative pair linkage analyses.

In conclusion, twin studies offer the opportunity to obtain additional insights regarding the genetic contribution to CL/P and CP. Such studies provide information that cannot be obtained by other methods and, hence, provide a useful complement to more traditional family-based and epidemiological investigations of these conditions.

SUMMARY

Twin studies have played an important role in attempts to unravel the genetic contribution to many diseases (Martin et al., 1997) but have not been extensively utilized to examine the genetic contribution to common congenital anomalies. The paucity of twin research on congenital anomalies is partly attributable to the commonly held belief that the causes of these conditions differ in twins and singletons. However, this belief is not well substantiated for either CL/P or CP.

The rarity of twins with specific malformations is also a limiting factor in twin studies of congenital anomalies. Ascertainment of twins with a specific malformation, from a single source, is unlikely to provide sufficient numbers to address the questions of interest. Hence, twin studies of CL/P and CP are likely to require multicenter, multinational collaborations. Such studies are subject to concerns regarding heterogeneity resulting from differences in case definition and ascertainment, as well as the potential for etiological heterogeneity across centers. Careful consideration of study design and the development of common protocols and diagnostic criteria will be essential factors in future twin studies of CL/P and CP. Although meta-analysis of observational data remains controversial, a well-designed prospective meta-analysis of OCs in twins may provide advantages over both retrospective meta-analyses of data from individual studies and stud-

ies coordinated through a single center (Margitic et al., 1995). One multicenter, international study of twins with CL/P is currently nearing completion (L.E. Mitchell, unpublished data). The results of this study should provide additional clues regarding the etiology of this condition and important insights regarding the design and implementation of future multicenter twin studies of OCs.

This work was supported in part by a grant (DE11388) from the National Institutes of Health.

REFERENCES

Allen, G (1981). Errors of Weinberg's difference method. Prog Clin Biol Res 69A: 71–74.

Allen, G, Harvarld, B, Sheilds, J (1967). Measures of twin concordance. Acta Genet 17: 475–481.

Boklage, CE (1985). Interaction between opposite-sex dizygotic fetuses and the assumptions of Weinberg's difference method in epidemiology. Am J Hum Genet 37: 591–605.

Bryan, EM (1992). The role in twins in epidemiologic research. Paediatr Perinat Epidemiol 6: 460–464.

Bundey, S (1991). Uses and limitations of twin studies. J Neurol 238: 360–364.

Christensen, K (1999). The 20th century Danish facial cleft population—epidemiological and genetic-epidemiological studies. Cleft Palate Craniofac J 36: 96–104.

Christensen, K, Fogh-Andersen, P (1993a). Cleft lip (+/− cleft palate) in Danish twins, 1970–1990. Am J Med Genet 47: 910–916.

Christensen, K, Fogh-Andersen, P (1993b). Isolated cleft palate in Danish multiple births. Cleft Palate Craniofac J 30: 469–474.

Christensen, K, Holm, NV, Olsen, J, et al. (1992). Selection bias in genetic-epidemiologic studies of cleft lip and palate. Am J Hum Genet 51: 654–659.

Christensen, K, Mitchell, LE (1996). Familial recurrence-pattern analysis of nonsyndromic isolated cleft palate—a Danish registry study. Am J Hum Genet 58: 182–190.

Christensen, K, Vaupel, JW, Holm, NV, Yashin, AI (1995). Mortality among twins after age 6: fetal origins hypothesis versus twin methods. BMJ 310: 432–436.

Duffy, DL (1993). Twin studies in the medical research. Lancet 341: 1418–1419.

Eufinger, H, Rand, S, Scholz, W, Machtens, E (1993). Clefts of the lip and palate in twins: use of DNA fingerprinting for zygosity determination. Cleft Palate Craniofac J 30: 564–568.

Eufinger, H, Schwartz, CE, Schutte, U (1995). Use of single- and multi-locus and polymerase chain reaction systems for zygosity determination—clinical applications in twins with clefts of the lip and palate. Acta Genet Med Gemellol (Roma) 44: 25–30.

Fitzpatrick, D, Farrall, M (1993). An estimation of the number of susceptibility loci for isolated cleft palate. J Craniofac Genet Dev 13: 230–235.

Fogh-Andersen, P (1942). *Inheritance of Harelip and Cleft Palate*. Copenhagen: Arnold Busck.

Fraser, FC (1970). The genetics of cleft lip and cleft palate. Am J Hum Genet 22: 336–352.

Hall, JG (1996). Twinning: mechanisms and genetic implications. Curr Opin Genet Dev 6: 343–347.

Hay, S, Wehrung, DA (1970). Congenital malformations in twins. Am J Hum Genet 22: 662–678.

James, WH (1979). Is Weinberg's differential rule valid? Acta Genet Med Gemellol (Roma) 28: 69–71.

James, WH (1992). The current status of Weinberg's differential rule. Acta Genet Med Gemellol (Roma) 41: 33–42.

LaBuda, MC, Gottesman, II, Pauls, DL (1992). Usefulness of twin studies for exploring the etiology of childhood and adolescent psychiatric disorders. Am J Med Genet 48: 47–59.

Lander, ES, Schork, NJ (1994). Genetic dissection of complex traits. Science 265: 2037–2048.

Layde, PM, Erickson, JD, Falek, A, McCarthey, BJ (1980). Congenital malformations in twins. Am J Hum Genet 32: 69–78.

Little, J, Nevin, N (1989). Congenital anomalies in twins in Northern Ireland. I. Anomalies in general and specific anomalies other than neural tube defects and defects of the cardiovascular sustem, 1974–1978. Acta Genet Med Gemellol (Roma) 38: 1–16.

Margitic, SE, Morgan, TM, Sager, MA, Furberg, CD (1995). Lessons learned from a prospective meta-analysis. J Am Geriatr Soc 43: 435–439.

Martin, N, Boomsma, D, Mackey, JF (1997). A twin-pronged attach on complex traits. Nat Genet 17: 387–392.

Mastroiacovo, P, Castilla, EE, Arpino, C, et al. (1999). Congenital malformations in twins: an international study. Am J Med Genet 83: 117–124.

McGue, M (1992). When assessing twin concordance, use the probandwise not the pairwise rate. Schizophr Bull 18: 171–176.

Metrakos, JD, Metrakos, K, Baxter, H (1958). Clefts of the lip and palate in twins. Plast Reconstr Surg 22: 109–122.

Mitchell, LE, Christensen, K (1997). Evaluation of family history data for Danish twins with non-syndromidic cleft lip with or without cleft palate. Am J Med Genet 72: 120–121.

Mitchell, LE, Risch, N (1992). Mode of inheritance of nonsyndromic cleft lip with or without cleft palate: a reanalysis. Am J Hum Genet 51: 323–332.

Myrianthopoulos, NC (1976). Congenital malformations in twins. Acta Genet Med Gemellol (Roma) 25: 331–335.

Myrianthopoulos, NC (1978). Congenital malformations: the contribution of twins studies. Birth Defects 14: 151–165.

Nance, WE (1981). Malformations unique to the twinning process. Prog Clin Biol Res 69A: 123–133.

Natsume, N, Sato, F, Hara, K, et al. (2000). Description of Japanese twins with cleft lip, cleft palate or both. Oral Surg Oral Med Oral Pathol Oral Radiol Endod 89: 6–8.

Nordstrom, REA, Laatikainen, T, Juvonen, TO, Ranta, RE (1996). Cleft-twin sets in Finland 1948–1987. Cleft Palate Craniofac J 33: 340–347.

Phillips, DIW (1993). Twin studies in medical research: can they tell us whether diseases are genetically determined? Lancet 341: 1008–1009.

Ramos-Arroyo, MA (1991). Birth defects in twins: study in a Spanish population. Acta Genet Med Gemellol (Roma) 40: 337–340.

Risch, N (1987). Assessing the role of HLA-linked and unlinked determinants of disease. Am J Hum Genet 40: 1–14.

Risch, N (1990). Linkage strategies for genetically complex traits. II. The power of affected relative pairs. Am J Hum Genet 46: 229–241.

Rotter, JI, Landaw, EM (1984). Measuring the genetic contribution of a single locus to a multilocus disease. Clin Genet 26: 529–542.

Schinzel, A, Smith, DW, Miller, JR (1979). Monozygotic twinning and structural defects. J Pediatr 95: 921–930.

Schutte, BC, Murray, JC (1999). The many faces and factors of orofacial clefts. Hum Mol Genet 8: 1853–1859.

Shields, ED, Bixler, D, Fogh-Andersen, P (1979). Facial clefts in Danish twins. Cleft Palate Craniofac J 16: 1–16.

Windham, GC, Bjerkedal, T (1984). Malformations in twins and their siblings, Norway, 1967–1979. Acta Genet Med Gemellol (Roma) 33: 87–95.

Wyszynski, DF, Beaty, TH, Maestri, NE (1996a). Genetics of nonsyndromic oral clefts revisited. Cleft Palate Craniofac J 33: 406–417.

Wyszynski, DF, Lewanda, AF, Beaty, TH (1996b). Phenotypic discordance in a family with monozygotic twins and non-syndromic cleft lip and palate. Am J Med Genet 66: 468–470.

18

Segregation analyses

MARY L. MARAZITA

Segregation analysis refers to statistical methods that are used to determine the mode of inheritance of a trait. Segregation in this context therefore is derived from Mendel's laws regarding the segregation of alleles in the formation of gametes (Mendel, 1866; translated by Bateson, 1902, 1909). According to the *Oxford English Dictionary* (Burchfield, 1986), the first usage of the word was by Weldon (1902) in his description of Mendel's laws. Therefore, segregation analysis originated from the assessment of Mendelian patterns of inheritance, i.e., testing whether family data were consistent with a single genetic locus. Today, the term is used more broadly, to encompass tests of many types of transmission of traits not limited to Mendelian patterns. *Complex* segregation analysis is sometimes used to describe statistical methods that incorporate two or more distinct, functionally independent parameters (Ellandt-Johnson, 1971).

The importance of inheritance in the etiology of cleft lip (CL) and cleft palate (CP) has been noted by scientists for more than 200 years. The first published description of a family with several affected members was in 1757 (Trew, 1757). Charles Darwin (1875) pointed out a publication of "the transmission during a century of hare-lip with a cleft-palate" by Sproule (1863) describing the author's family. Rischbieth (1910) summarized pre-1900 publications of familial cases of CL ("hare-lip") and CP (abridged facsimile of Rischbieth, 1910, and commentary putting Rischbieth's conclusions into historical perspective are provided by Melnick, 1997). Rischbieth (1910) epitomized the anti-Mendelian view of Pearson and the other members of the Galton Laboratory by concluding that inheritance of CL and CP was an expression of general physical and racial degeneracy which could be traced to poor protoplasm (Melnick, 1997). Bateson, however, was a leading proponent of Mendelism and included "hare-lip" as one of a group of "dominant hereditary diseases and malformations" (Bateson, 1909; Melnick, 1997).

The fundamental tenet of Mendelism, i.e., unit inheritance, has since been demonstrated to be correct and has led to today's burgeoning field of genetics. Rischbieth (1910), although fundamentally incorrect in his assessment of the meaning of familial cases of oral-facial clefts, did provide a pertinent charge to modern scientists studying the inheritance of CL and CP:

> The cause of these defects lies in the family tendency, but it is only when the family is considered as a whole, in all its branches and when normal as well as deformed individuals are included in the records, that we shall begin to understand the mode of working of the hereditary influence. This fact has long been known to students of insanity, but in the case of hare-lip and cleft palate inquiry has usually gone no further than to ask how many relatives (usually in the direct line) showed this defect.

This succinctly describes the key components of study designs of human disorders. When appropriate data are collected, statistical models can be applied to derive an unbiased conclusion regarding the inheritance pattern of a human trait.

Segregation analysis methods were developed to address the inherent biases of most studies of human family data. In studies of experimental animals, it is possible to design controlled matings that allow direct inference of the inheritance pattern of the trait of interest. The ideal human family study design would involve obtaining a large, random, population-based sample of families; taking a subset of the random families in which there are individuals with clefts; and then determining the genotypic mating type and offspring for each family. However, for a number of reasons, this ideal study design is not feasible for most human traits, including oral-facial clefts. The necessary fully informative matings are generally not available, and the genotypes of the family members are usually unknown. A further difficulty in studying inheritance patterns in humans is that the traits most often under study are relatively rare. Oral-facial clefts, for example, are common birth defects but still occur in only 1/500 to 1/1000 births. Therefore, it is generally not possible to take a random sample of a population and obtain the necessary numbers of families with cleft individuals. Families for study of human traits are most often ascertained through affected individuals, therefore requiring appropriate statistical correction to eliminate potential biases introduced by the mode of ascertainment.

CLASSICAL SEGREGATION RATIO ANALYSIS

To illustrate some important concepts in segregation analysis, I will focus on the first and simplest segregation analysis parameter, the segregation ratio. A *segregation ratio* is the proportion of affected children among the progeny of a particular mating type. Consider a two-allele autosomal genetic locus. There are six possible genotypic mating types, representing six phenotypically distinguishable mating types under codominance or three phenotypic mating types if dominance exists for the trait. Table 18.1 shows the possible matings and the expected proportions of affected children for each mating type. As can be seen, only some of the mating types are expected to produce affected children. Therefore, in the usual human study situation of ascertaining families through affected individuals, only some of the possible mating types will be represented in the resulting data set. This is one of the limitations that the statistical methods of segregation analysis are designed to address. The other major

limitation and source of potential bias that segregation analysis addresses is the mode of ascertainment.

There are two major classes of ascertainment, complete and incomplete ascertainment. The ascertainment probability is, conceptually, the proportion of probands among affected individuals. *Complete ascertainment* is the situation in which all possible offspring sets for a particular mating type will enter a study, i.e., independent of the phenotype of the offspring. An example of complete ascertainment is defining a sample of affected people and then estimating the segregation ratio in their children. *Incomplete ascertainment* refers to situations in which not all possible offspring sets are found. An example of incomplete ascertainment is defining a sample of affected people, their siblings, and parents and then estimating the segregation ratio in the children sets. This is incomplete because the only offspring sets entering the study will be those with at least one affected offspring. As can be seen in Table 18.1, many of the mating types that can produce affected offspring can also produce unaffected offspring. By chance, there will be an appreciable proportion of families with only unaffected offspring. Consider an autosomal recessive trait. If the affected allele is rare, the only genotypic mating type capable of producing affected children that is likely to be present in the data set will be AB × AB (Table 18.1). This mating type has an expected segregation ratio of 25%; therefore, the expected proportion of unaffected children is 75%. For three-child families, applying the multiplication rule of combining probabilities yields the probability of all three children being unaffected as $0.75^3 = 0.4219$. Therefore, ascertaining three-child families through affected children will miss 42.19% of the families that would be necessary for an unbiased estimate of the segregation ratio.

One of the first methods of correcting for ascertainment bias in segregation analysis was the Weinberg proband method, originally proposed by Weinberg

TABLE 18.1. *Expected Segregation Ratios for Mating Types at a Single Genetic Locus with Two Alleles, A and B, with A Representing the Affected Allele*

Phenotypic Mating Type	A dominant		A recessive	
	Genotypic Mating Type	Expected % Affected Offspring	Genotypic Mating Type	Expected % Affected Offspring
Affected × affected	AA × AA	100	AA × AA	100
	AA × AB	100		
	AB × AB	75		
Affected × unaffected	AA × BB	100	AA × AB	50
	AB × BB	50	AA × BB	0
Unaffected × unaffected	BB × BB	0	BB × BB	0
			AB × BB	0
			AB × AB	25

(1912, 1927) with standard error formulas derived by Fisher (1934). For Weinberg's method and for all subsequent methods of segregation analysis, it is crucial to define the term *proband* carefully. A *proband* (Weinberg, 1927; Morton, 1959; Wright, 1968) is an affected person who is necessary and sufficient to ascertain a family for study. Depending on the comprehensiveness of the sampling frame, there may be more than one proband per family. The first proband in a family is sometimes termed the *propositus* or *index case*. Additional nonproband affected individuals in a family are termed *secondary cases* (Morton, 1982). Careful delineation of probands and nonprobands in families is extremely important in correcting for ascertainment biases in the statistical genetic analysis of patterns of inheritance, although even then problems may arise (Greenberg, 1986; Vieland and Hodge, 1995). A dichotomy has developed in the use of the term *proband* by clinicians as opposed to researchers (Marazita, 1995). Clinicians tend to use *proband* and *index case* interchangeably (Thompson et al., 1991; Bennett et al., 1995a), implying that there would be only one proband indicated per family in clinical genetic records. This dichotomy would seriously bias analysis of such records (Marazita, 1995). Therefore, Bennett et al. (1995b) recommended that the research definition be followed in clinical genetic situations.

The essence of the Weinberg method is that the proband individuals provide the information that a particular mating type is segregating, i.e., capable of producing affected offspring. Therefore, Weinberg (1912, 1927) proposed calculating the segregation ratio in the nonproband children to obtain an unbiased estimate. Refinements were later introduced to incorporate a correction factor for large sibship sizes.

The next major advance in segregation analysis was by Morton (1959), in which the segregation ratio was assumed to follow the binomial probability distribution and likelihood methods were used to estimate the parameters and to test hypotheses. Morton also considered the ascertainment probability to be binomially distributed and estimable. Morton divided incomplete ascertainment into three categories: truncate, single, and multiple. Under single incomplete ascertainment, each family has only one proband (even if the family has multiple affected members) and the ascertainment probability is close to 0. Under truncate incomplete ascertainment, every affected individual in a family is a proband and the ascertainment probability is 1.0. Multiple incomplete ascertainment is intermediate between these two extremes, with some families having more than one proband but not all affected offspring being probands (ascertainment probability between 0 and 1.0). Table 18.2 summarizes the key points of incomplete ascertainment and the bias in the segregation ratio due to incomplete ascertainment. Table 18.3 summarizes the parameters that were estimated in classical segregation ratio analysis.

Segregation ratio analysis methods were limited to analysis of single-locus, Mendelian patterns in nuclear family data. Such analyses were amenable to analytic solution. The next wave of advances in segregation analysis included methods that were developed to address more complex models in larger family structures. The theoretical underpinnings of such methods were developed in the 1970s, before there were computers that were able to apply such methods fully. With improved computers, application of such models became a reality and laid the foundation for other important statistical methods in human genetics today, such as

TABLE 18.2. *General Incomplete Ascertainment Model of Morton (1959) for Selection through Affected Children*

	Type of incomplete ascertainment		
	Single	Multiple	Truncate
No. of probands/family	One proband per family	More than one proband in some families, but not every affected individual is a proband	Every affected individual is a proband
Value of π*	π close to 0	$0 < \pi \leq 1$	$\pi = 1$
Bias in segregation ratio	The segregation ratio is distorted because not every at-risk mating actually has an affected child		
Additional bias in segregation ratio	Extreme, families with r affected children appear r times more often than they should	Intermediate	No additional distortion
MLE† of segregation ratio (p)	Exact analytic MLE of p (true binomial distribution after omitting proband)	No analytic solution	No analytic solution (follows truncated binomial distribution)

*π, ascertainment probability: $0 < \pi \leq 1$.
†MLE, maximum likelihood estimate.

TABLE 18.3. *Parameters Estimated for Classical Single-Locus Segregation Analysis, Utilizing Segregation Ratios in Nuclear Families*

Method	Parameter	Description
Weinberg proband method (Weinberg, 1912, 1927)	p	Segregation ratio
	π	Ascertainment probability
Morton (1959)	p	Segregation ratio (binomial)
	X	Proportion of sporadic cases
	π	Ascertainment probability (binomial)

linkage analysis in extended kindreds (Ott, 1991). Related statistical methods for investigating the inheritance of oral-facial clefts are reviewed in other chapters (Chapters 17, 19, 21). In the discussion of complex segregation analysis methods, I will focus on those that have been applied to oral-facial cleft data, in particular, the major locus transmission model (Elston and Stewart, 1971; Elston, 1980), the mixed/unified model (Morton and MacLean, 1974; Lalouel and Morton, 1981; Lalouel et al., 1983), and regressive models (Bonney, 1984, 1986). Because the oral-facial cleft phenotypes analyzed to date have been qualitative in nature (i.e., "affected" vs. "unaffected"), I will focus on the qualitative application of these methods, though each method also has applications for quantitative traits.

Each of the approaches defines an underlying general model with assumptions as to the probability distributions and parameters of interest. The hypotheses to be tested are each nested within the underlying general model; i.e., each hypothesis corresponds to restrictions on the parameters of the underlying model. Likelihoods are calculated for each hypothesis; parameters are estimated by maximum likelihood (Edwards, 1992). The likelihood ratio criterion is used to compare the likelihood of each restricted hypothesis to that of the most general, unrestricted model. Twice the difference in ln-likelihoods between the unrestricted hypothesis and each of the restricted hypotheses is asymptotically distributed as a χ^2 with degrees of freedom corresponding to the difference in the numbers of pa-

rameters estimated between the restricted and unrestricted hypotheses. If there are multiple equally likely hypotheses, the Akaike information criterion (AIC; Akaike, 1974) is often applied. The AIC for any hypothesis equals -2(ln-likelihood) $+ 2$(number of parameters estimated). The model with the smallest AIC is the most parsimonious.

MAJOR LOCUS TRANSMISSION MODELS

Under the major locus transmission model of Elston and Stewart (1971), segregation at a major locus is parameterized by use of transmission probabilities for each of three possible types in the data (AA, AB, or BB). Two individuals have the same type if and only if the expected phenotypic distribution of their offspring by a mate of a given type is identical (Cannings et al., 1978). Genotypes are the special case of types (or "ousiotypes," following Cannings et al., 1978) that transmit to offspring in a Mendelian fashion. When there is no transmission from one generation to the next, the model allows for only a single type. Table 18.4 summarizes the parameters of the model.

Elston and Stewart (1971) also provided a major advance for genetic analysis of extended kindreds by developing an efficient computational algorithm for calculating the likelihoods of any general family structure (Lange, 1997). Their algorithm is the basis for the most widely used linkage analysis computer program, *LINKAGE* (Terwilliger and Ott, 1994).

TABLE 18.4. *Parameters for Major Locus Segregation Analysis of Qualitative Traits Utilizing Transmission Probabilities in General Pedigrees*

Method	Parameter	Description
Major locus segregation analysis (Elston and Stewart, 1971)	q	Gene frequency
	τ_1	Probability that an individual of type AA will transmit A
	τ_2	Probability that an individual of type AB will transmit A
	τ_3	Probability that an individual of type BB will transmit A
	f_1	Probability that an individual of type AA will be affected (penetrance)
	f_2	Probability that an individual of type AB will be affected (penetrance)
	f_3	Probability that an individual of type BB will be affected (penetrance)

TABLE 18.5. *Parameters Estimated for Complex Segregation Analysis of Qualitative Traits under the Mixed Model (i.e., Major Locus with Multifactorial and Sporadic Components) in General Pedigrees Broken Down into Their Component Nuclear Families*

Method	Parameter	Description
Mixed model, POINTER (Morton and MacLean, 1974)	d	Degree of dominance at the major locus
	t	Displacement between homozygotes, in standard deviation units
	q	Gene frequency
	b	Relative variance due to common sibling environment
	h^2	Polygenic heritability
	X	Proportion of sporadic cases
Unified mixed model (Lalouel et al., 1983), includes all of the above parameters plus the following transmission probabilities	τ_1	Probability that an individual of type AA will transmit A
	τ_2	Probability that an individual of type AB will transmit A
	τ_3	Probability that an individual of type BB will transmit A

MIXED/UNIFIED MODEL

Under the mixed/unified model, an individual's phenotype is assumed to be due to a major locus component and a multifactorial component (Morton and MacLean, 1974; Lalouel and Morton, 1981; Lalouel et al., 1983). This model has had particular appeal for segregation analyses of oral-facial clefting because of the desire to contrast multifactorial hypotheses with major locus hypotheses. The parameters of the model are summarized in Table 18.5. The original mixed model of Morton and MacLean (1974) was extended to incorporate the transmission probabilities of the Elston and Stewart (1971) major locus model to create the so-called unified model (Lalouel et al., 1983). Ascertainment corrections are done by breaking the extended kindreds into their component nuclear families and specifying the mode of ascertainment of each nuclear family. This method of ascertainment correction has the advantage of allowing multiple ascertainment schemes, each with its own ascertainment probability; however, some of the transmission information from extended kindreds is lost.

REGRESSIVE MODELS

Regression analysis methods were first applied to complex segregation analysis by Bonney (1984, 1986), who combined aspects of the transmission approach of Elston and Stewart (1971) with the flexibility of regression analysis. In regression models for complex segregation analysis as proposed by Bonney (1984), the dependence among family members is modeled as a Markovian process, where each individual's trait value (phenotype) is influenced by his or her own covariates, as well as the observed phenotypes of preceding family members. Class A, B, C, and D models were defined (Bonney, 1984, 1986), which differ in the assumptions regarding the dependence between siblings. In class A, B, and C models, the correlations between siblings differ depending on how close in age the siblings are. In the class D model, correlations between siblings are assumed not to differ by age relationships but, at the same time, are necessarily due to common parentage alone. The concept of types introduced by Elston and Stewart (1971) and summarized by Cannings et al. (1978) plus the structure of transmission probabilities was incorporated into the regressive models. Table 18.6 summarizes the primary parameters of the regression model. Ascertainment corrections were incorporated by conditioning on the subsets of proband individuals in each family.

FAMILY STUDIES OF ORAL-FACIAL CLEFTS

Oral-facial clefts are a major public health problem, affecting 1/500 to 1/1000 births worldwide (Murray, 1995). Therefore, many research groups have attempted to elucidate the etiology of oral-facial clefts, with limited success. Oral-facial clefts can occur as part of Mendelian syndromes, certain chromosomal anomalies include oral-facial clefts in the phenotype, and certain teratogens can increase the risk of having an offspring with a cleft. However, phenotypes of known etiology comprise only a small portion of all individuals with an oral-facial cleft; therefore, a major research focus has been on the genetics of nonsyndromic forms of clefting (the focus of this chapter).

There have been many essentially descriptive publications of oral-facial cleft families, summarized in Table 18.7. Each of the descriptive studies presented an hypothesis as to the inheritance of oral-facial clefts and described how their data fit the hypothesis, without attempting any statistical tests. In Rischbieth's (1910) summary of pre-1900 oral-facial cleft families, the hypothesis was that such families were the result of

TABLE 18.6. *Parameters Estimated for Complex Segregation Analysis of a Qualitative Trait under Regressive Models in General Pedigrees*

Method	Parameter	Description
Regressive model, complex segregation analysis (Bonney, 1986)	q	Gene frequency
	τ_1	Probability that an individual of type AA will transmit A
	τ_2	Probability that an individual of type AB will transmit A
	τ_3	Probability that an individual of type BB will transmit A
	β_1	Regression coefficient, type AA
	β_2	Regression coefficient, type AB
	β_3	Regression coefficient, type BB
	δ_{spouse}	Regressive effects for affected and unaffected spouse
	$\delta_{parents}$	Regressive effects (non-Mendelian) for affected and unaffected parents
	$\xi_1, \xi_2, \ldots \xi_v$	Regression coefficients for v covariates

general physical degeneracy. Bateson (1909), however, attributed the clefts in such families to dominantly inherited genes. Fogh-Andersen (1942) was the first to collect a systematic data set of cleft families and to evaluate the observed inheritance patterns. He concluded that the CL with or without CP (CL/P) families were consistent with segregation of alleles at a single genetic locus with variable penetrance and that CP families were consistent with autosomal dominant inheritance with greatly reduced penetrance.

In the 1960s and 1970s, there was a paradigm shift. A specific statistical model, termed the *multifactorial threshold model* (MFT), was described and invoked to explain the familial patterns of oral-facial clefts (Carter, 1976; Fraser, 1976). Under the MFT model, the occurrence of a cleft depends on a very large number of genes, each of equal, minor, and additive effect, plus environmental factors. An accumulation of these genes and environmental factors is tolerated by the developing fetus to a point, termed the *threshold*, beyond which there is the risk of malformation. This model has testable predictions and, in theory, could explain many of the features observed for oral-facial clefts in families. The early proponents of the MFT model published several large series of cleft families from a variety of populations, each concluding that the data were consistent with the MFT model (Table 18.7) (Woolf et al., 1963, 1964; Carter et al., 1982a,b; Hu et al., 1982). However, none of these early studies attempted any statistical tests of the MFT model.

The early descriptive studies were followed by studies that did test the predictions of the MFT model (Table 18.7) (Bear, 1976; Melnick et al., 1980; Marazita et al., 1984). In each of these studies, some or all of the predictions of the MFT model could be rejected. However, statistical tests of the predictions of a model do not constitute statistical tests of that model. Other investigators then formulated and parameterized

models to test the goodness-of-fit of the MFT model; a number of investigators applied such models to oral-facial cleft family data (Table 18.7) (Melnick et al., 1980; Mendell et al., 1980; Marazita et al., 1986b). The results of the goodness-of-fit studies were mostly inconclusive, with the MFT model being rejected for some portions of the parameter space in most studies.

In the late 1970s and early 1980s, investigators began to apply segregation analysis methods, such as mixed models, to test the MFT model and to evaluate the major locus alternative. Table 18.8 summarizes published segregation analyses of oral-facial clefting. Some of the first mixed-model studies of oral-facial clefts were inconclusive (Chung et al., 1974; Demenais et al., 1984) because the sample sizes were inadequate to distinguish between models. There were then a number of mixed or unified model studies of sufficient sample sizes (Table 18.8). In virtually every such study of CL/P, the MFT model could be rejected in favor of either a mixed model (major locus plus multifactorial background) (Marazita et al., 1984; Chung et al., 1986) or a major locus alone (Hecht et al., 1991; Marazita et al., 1992; Nemana et al., 1992). Most such studies were conducted in Caucasian populations, although there were a few in Asian populations (Table 18.8) (Marazita et al., 1992). Given these segregation analysis results, gene mapping studies of CL/P were then considered feasible and are a current focus of intensive research (see Chapters 20, 21, and 23).

There are many fewer segregation analyses of nonsyndromic CP than there are of CL/P. There are only three published studies, one in Hawaii (Chung et al., 1974) and two in Caucasian populations (Demenais et al., 1984; Clementi et al., 1997). Chung et al. (1974) and Demenais et al. (1984) could not distinguish between the MFT and major locus models; Clementi et al. (1997) concluded that a single recessive major locus with reduced penetrance was sufficient to explain

TABLE 18.7. *Summary of Published Family Studies of Cleft Lip with or without Cleft Palate (CL/P) and Cleft Palate Alone (CP) Using Methods Other Than Segregation Analysis*

Study Population	Analysis Method (Computer Program)*	Conclusion†	Reference
CL/P			
European Caucasian, compendium of pre-1900 reports: 74 multiplex pedigrees, summaries of 244 cases and other published reports, mixture of CL/P and CP cases	Descriptive	Hereditary, expression of general physical and racial degeneracy	Rischbieth (1910) (facsimile in Melnick, 1997)
Danish Caucasian, 703 surgical cases	Descriptive	Single gene with variable penetrance, either recessive or dominant based on genetic background	Fogh-Andersen (1942)
U.S. Caucasian (Utah), 533 surgical cases	Descriptive	Heterogeneity: dominant in some families, interaction of polygenes and nongenetic factors in other families, some phenocopies	Woolf et al. (1963)
U.S. Caucasian (Utah), 418 surgical cases	Descriptive	MFT	Woolf et al. (1964)
Japanese, number of cases not stated	Descriptive	MFT	Tanaka et al. (1969)
Danish and Canadian Caucasian, 805 surgical cases	Descriptive	MFT	Fraser (1970)
Hungarian Caucasian, 570 families	Descriptive	Polygenic, multifactorial	Czeizel and Tusnady (1972)
Hawaiian interracial crosses, 341 probands through registries and hospitals	Descriptive	No significant associations were found with demographic factors; hence, genetic control of CL/P was concluded	Ching and Chung (1974)
Japanese, 823 cases	Descriptive	MFT	Koguchi (1975)
British Caucasian, 324 surgical index cases	Predictions	MFT	Bear (1976)
U.S. Caucasian	Goodness-of-fit (PGOODFIT)	Assumed MFT	Spence et al. (1976)
Danish Caucasian, 1895 surgical cases with first-degree relatives	Predictions	Some predictions of the MFT were satisfied but others were not	Melnick et al. (1980)
	Goodness-of-fit (PGOODFIT)	Multiple-sex threshold model: neither MFT nor single-locus models fit well, proposed (but not tested) was a monogenic-dependent susceptibility locus	
U.S. Caucasian (North Carolina)	Goodness-of-fit (PGOODFIT)	MFT could be rejected at some points of the parameter space but not all	Mendell et al. (1980)
British Caucasian, 424 three-generation families, surgical probands	Descriptive	MFT	Carter et al. (1982b) (see also Marazita et al., 1986a)
Chinese, 163 surgical cases	Descriptive	MFT	Hu et al. (1982)
Danish Caucasian, 2027 nuclear families (all through surgical probands)	Goodness-of-fit (PGOODFIT)	MFT model was rejected (see also segregation analysis results in Table 18.8 below)	Marazita et al. (1984)
Danish Caucasian, 2686 surgical probands and their families; British Caucasian, 424 surgical probands and their three-generation families; Chinese, 163 surgical probands and their families	Predictions	All but one of the MFT predictions could be rejected	Marazita et al. (1986b)
	Goodness-of-fit (PGOODFIT)	MFT could be rejected in the Danish and Chinese data sets and at some points in the parameter space for the British data set (see also segregation analysis results in Table 18.8 below)	
British Caucasian, two multiplex families (affected members in three or four generations)	Descriptive	Apparently dominant transmission, but MFT could not be ruled out	Temple et al. (1989)
British Caucasian, 632 families	Recurrence risk	Oligogenic, four to seven loci	Farrall and Holder (1992)

(continued)

TABLE 18.7. *Summary of Published Family Studies of Cleft Lip with or without Cleft Palate (CL/P) and Cleft Palate Alone (CP) Using Methods Other Than Segregation Analysis (continued)*

Study Population	Analysis Method (Computer Program)*	Conclusion†	Reference
Combined Caucasian data from four studies (British, Danish, Canadian, U.S.)	Recurrence risk	Both MFT and single-locus models fit	Mitchell and Risch (1992)
India (Madras), 331 probands and their extended kindreds	Predictions	All but one of the MFT predictions could be rejected	Nemana et al. (1992)
	Goodness-of-fit (*PGOODFIT*)	MFT model could be rejected at the estimated ascertainment probability and heritability (see also segregation analysis results in Table 18.8 below)	
Danish Caucasian, 3073 probands	Recurrence risk	Single locus and additive multiplicative models could be excluded; model of multiple interacting loci could not be excluded	Mitchell and Christensen (1996)
CP			
European Caucasian, compendium of pre-1900 reports: 74 multiplex pedigrees, summaries of 244 cases and other published reports, mixture of CL/P and CP cases	Descriptive	Hereditary, expression of general physical and racial degeneracy	Rischbieth (1910) (facsimile in Melnick, 1997)
Danish Caucasian, 703 surgical cases	Descriptive	Single gene, dominant with greatly reduced penetrance	Fogh-Andersen (1942)
Hawaiian interracial crosses, 195 probands through registries and hospitals	Descriptive	No significant associations were found with demographic factors; hence, genetic control of CP was concluded	Ching and Chung (1974)
British Caucasian, 147 surgical index cases	Predictions	Heterogeneity, multiple genetic forms	Bear (1976)
U.S. Caucasian, one four-generation family	Descriptive	Single gene, X-linked recessive	Rushton (1979)
British Caucasian, 167 surgical probands	Descriptive	Heterogeneity, some families showing modified dominant inheritance	Carter et al. (1982a)
U.S. Caucasian, three multi-generation families	Descriptive	One family: single gene, autosomal dominant Two families: single gene, X-linked recessive One family: single gene, X-linked recessive but with some nonpenetrant males	Rollnick and Kaye (1986) Rollnick and Kaye (1986)
Combined Caucasian data from four studies (Scottish, Danish, U.S., French)	Recurrence risk	Oligenic model with six loci	Fitzpatrick and Farrall (1993)
Danish Caucasian, 1364 probands	Recurrence risk	Multiplicative interactions between CP-susceptibility loci, single gene, and MFT provide poor fit to the data	Christensen and Mitchell (1996)

*Descriptive, descriptive studies, no statistical tests; Predictions, statistical tests (usually χ^2) of the predictions of the multifactorial threshold (MF/T) model (note that such tests do not constitute a test of the model); Goodness-of-fit, goodness-of-fit tests of the MF/T model; Recurrence risk, analysis of the recurrence risk patterns in families. Reference for computer program: *PGOODFIT* (Gladstien et al., 1978).
†Conclusions drawn by the authors of each paper.

their data. There is also a significant subset of nonsyndromic CP families in which CP is X-linked, as evidenced by the descriptive studies of Rushton (1979) and Rollnick and Kaye (1986, 1987). The X-linked form of CP includes ankyloglossia and has been confirmed by linkage analysis (Moore et al., 1987, 1991; Bjornsson et al., 1989; Gorski et al., 1992, 1994) and physical mapping (Forbes et al., 1995, 1996).

In summary, segregation analyses of oral-facial clefts, both CL/P and CP, have consistently resulted in evi-

dence for genes of major effect. Although such studies imply a single major locus, hypotheses of multiple interacting loci or genetic heterogeneity cannot be ruled out and, indeed, have not been explicitly tested in any of the published segregation analyses to date (see Jarvik, 1998, for a summary review of this issue with respect to complex segregation analysis). Analyses of recurrence risk patterns (Table 18.7) (Farrall and Holder, 1992; Mitchell and Risch, 1992; Fitzpatrick and Farrall, 1993; Christensen and Mitchell, 1996;

TABLE 18.8. *Summary of Published Segregation Analyses of Cleft Lip with or without Cleft Palate (CL/P) and Cleft Palate Alone (CP)*

Study Population	Analysis Method (Computer Program)*	Conclusion†	Reference
CL/P			
Hawaiian, 240 probands from multiple ethnic backgrounds	Mixed	Could not distinguish between MFT with high heritability and major gene models, the high heritability being more consistent with a major gene	Chung et al. (1974)
French Caucasian, 458 surgical probands and their nuclear families	Unified mixed (*POINTER*)	Could not distinguish between MFT with high heritability and major gene models (dominant or additive)	Demenais et al. (1984)
Danish Caucasian, 2532 kindreds: 26 large multigenerational families with four or more affected members, 2027 nuclear families (all through surgical probands)	Classical (*SEGRAN*)	Consistent with autosomal recessive	Marazita et al. (1984)
	ML transmission (*GENPED*)	26 large families: eight fit autosomal recessive, three fit codominant, could not distinguish in 15	
	Unified mixed (*POINTER*)	MFT rejected, mixed model or major gene possible	
English Caucasian, 424 three-generation families	Unified mixed (*POINTER*)	MFT rejected, mixed model provided the best fit	Marazita et al. (1986a) (analysis of data in Carter et al., 1982b)
Danish Caucasian, 2686 surgical probands and their families; British Caucasian, 424 surgical probands and their three-generation families; Chinese, 163 surgical probands and their families	Classical (*SEGRAN*)	Segregation ratios were consistent with an autosomal recessive major gene in all three data sets, with significant admixture of sporadic cases in the Danish and British data sets	Marazita et al. (1986b)
	Mixed (*MIXMOD*)	Only performed in Danish and British data sets: a major gene alone fit well in the British data set, and the mixed model fit best in the Danish data set	
Chinese (Shanghai), 163 families through surgical probands	Mixed (*MIXMOD*)	MFT rejected, autosomal recessive provided best fit	Melnick et al. (1986)
Danish, 2998 families; Japanese, 627 families; all through surgical probands	Unified mixed (*POINTER*)	In the Danish families, the mixed model with a recessive major gene component fit best. In the Japanese families, MFT fit best	Chung et al. (1986)
Hawaiian: 189 Japanese probands and their families, 22 Chinese or Korean, 42 Caucasian, 122 Hawaiian, 59 Filipinos, 94 other	Mixed (*POINTER*)	Overall a mixed model provided the best fit, with no heterogeneity in the results based on high- or low-risk ethnic classifications or severity classifications	Chung et al. (1989)
U.S. Caucasian, 79 probands and families	Unified mixed (*POINTER*)	MFT, autosomal dominant and codominant fit equally well; the high heritability in the MFT model argues for a major locus	Hecht et al. (1991)
	Regressive (*SAGE*)	Autosomal dominant (or codominant) with reduced penetrance	
Chinese (Shanghai), 2255 nuclear families through surgical probands	Unified mixed (*POINTER*)	Autosomal recessive major locus	Marazita et al. (1992)
India (Madras), 331 probands and their extended kindreds	Unified mixed (*POINTER*)	Major gene with reduced penetrance	Nemana et al. (1992)
India (West Bengal), 90 extended kindreds	Unified mixed (*POINTER*)	Autosomal dominant or codominant	Ray et al. (1993)
Italian Caucasian, 549 probands from consecutive newborns plus their nuclear families	Unified mixed (*POINTER*)	MFT and major gene models fit equally well	Clementi et al. (1995)
	Two-locus (*COMDS*)	A single major gene could be rejected in favor of a two-locus model, one dominant major locus with a modifying locus	

(continued)

TABLE 18.8. *Summary of Published Segregation Analyses of Cleft Lip with or without Cleft Palate (CL/P) and Cleft Palate Alone (CP) (continued)*

Study Population	Analysis Method (Computer Program)*	Conclusion†	Reference
Chilean, Amerindian/Caucasian admixed, 67 multigenerational families with surgical probands	Unified mixed (PAP)	Autosomal dominant, reduced penetrance (25%)	Palomino et al. (1991, 1997)
Italian Caucasian, 46 extended kindreds with surgical probands	Unified mixed (POINTER) Two-locus (COMDS)	Mixed model with a dominant major locus component The highest likelihood was obtained for a dominant major locus with a recessive modifier locus	Scapoli et al. (1999)
CP			
Hawaiian, 113 probands from multiple ethnic backgrounds	Mixed (POINTER)	Could not distinguish between MFT and major gene models, MF/T had better fit	Chung et al. (1974)
French Caucasian, 156 surgical probands and their nuclear families	Unified mixed (POINTER)	Could not distinguish between MFT with high heritability and major gene models (recessive)	Demenais et al. (1984)
Italian Caucasian, 357 probands from consecutive newborns	Unified mixed (POINTER) Two-locus (COMDS)	Autosomal recessive major gene with reduced penetrance Single major locus (two-locus models did not improve the fit)	Clementi et al. (1997)

*Classical, classical segregation analysis (segregation ratio; Weinberg, 1912, or Morton, 1959); Mixed, mixed model (major locus and multifactorial components; Morton and MacLean, 1974); Unified mixed, unified mixed model (major locus and multifactorial components) incorporating transmission probabilities for the major locus (Lalouel et al., 1983); ML transmission, major locus transmission model (Elston and Stewart, 1971); Regressive, regressive major locus models incorporating the transmission probabilities of Elston and Stewart (1971), with residual variance and covariates (Bonney, 1984); Two-locus, extension of mixed model framework to evaluate oligenic or two-locus models. References for computer programs: SEGRAN (Morton et al., 1983); POINTER, COMDS (Morton and MacLean, 1974; Morton et al., 1983); GENPED (Elston and Stewart, 1971); SAGE (Case Western Reserve University, 1997); PAP (Hasstedt, 1994).
†Conclusion of the authors.

Mitchell and Christensen, 1996) (see also Chapter 17) have been consistent with oligenic models, with approximately four to seven interacting loci. Other potential limitations of complex segregation analysis include difficulty in determining the power of specific sample sizes and difficulty in appropriately adjusting for the method of ascertainment (Jarvik, 1998).

ROLE OF SEGREGATION ANALYSIS IN FUTURE STUDIES OF ORAL-FACIAL CLEFTS

Segregation analyses to date have primarily been concerned with testing the MFT hypothesis regarding the etiology of nonsyndromic oral-facial clefts. Although in some sense oral-facial clefts are due to multiple factors, the specific MFT statistical model that was invoked for several years (Carter, 1976; Fraser, 1976) was not well supported. As summarized in Table 18.8, in most studies, the MFT model either could be rejected or was equally as likely as major locus models.

In the current age of gene mapping, ultimate confirmation of the existence of major genetic loci for clefting may be at hand (see Chapters 20, 21, and 23 for progress to date). Until that time, there are still several

important roles for segregation analysis to play. Parametric linkage analysis methods require estimates of parameters such as gene frequency, which are obtained from segregation analyses. Most segregation analyses to date have been in Caucasian populations; thus, there is a need for studies in other ethnic/racial groups to determine if the family patterns are the same across groups. Furthermore, the lack of major gene mapping successes in oral-facial clefting highlights the fact that clefts are unlikely to be due to the proximate phenotypic expression of the genes involved. Segregation analyses can be used to refine the phenotype, with a focus on either subclinical expressions in unaffected relatives [e.g., anatomic differences in the obicularis oris muscle (Martin et al., 2000)] or associated phenotypic features that may be markers for developmental instability [e.g., handedness (Wentzlaff et al., 1997) or cephalometric features (Ward et al., 1994)]. Once genes have been identified, segregation analysis methods can also be used to help identify other factors that modify expression at those genes.

Despite over 200 years of interest in the familial aggregation of oral-facial clefts, we still do not have a definitive understanding of the genetic component of the familiality. Segregation analyses have provided significant insights, and the powerful statistical and molecular approaches available to geneticists today should continue to build on that foundation.

REFERENCES

Akaike, H (1974). A new look at the statistical model identification. IEEE Trans Automatic Control AC 19: 616–623.

Bateson, W (1902). Mendel's principles of heredity: a defence. Cambridge University Press, Cambridge, England.

Bateson, W (1909). Mendel's principles of hereditary. Cambridge University Press, Cambridge, England.

Bear, JC (1976). A genetic study of facial clefting in Northern England. Clinical Genetics 9: 277–284.

Bennett, RL, Steinhaus, KA, Uhrich, SB, O'Sullivan, CK, Resta, RG, Lochner-Doyle, D, Markel, DS, et al. (1995b). Reply to Marazita and Curtis. Am J Hum Genet 57: 983–984.

Bennett, RL, Steinhaus, KA, Uhrih, SB, O'Sullivan, CK, Resta, RG, Lochner-Doyle, D, Markel, DS et al. (1995a). Recommendations for standardized human pedigree nomenclature. Am J Hum Genet 56: 745–752.

Bjornsson, A, Arnason, A, Tippet, P (1989). X-linked cleft palate and ankyloglossia in an Icelandic family. Cleft Palate J 26 (1): 3–8.

Bonney, GE (1984). On the statistical determination of major gene mechanisms in continuous human traits: regressive models. Am J Hum Genet 18: 731–749.

Bonney, GE (1986). Regressive logistic models for familial disease and other binary traits. Biometrics 42: 348–353.

Burchfield, RW (1986). A supplement to the Oxford English dictionary: Volume IV, Se-Z. Clarendon Press, Oxford, England.

Cannings, C, Thompson, EA, Skolnick, MH (1978). Probability functions on complex pedigrees. Am Hum Genet 10: 26–61.

Carter, CO (1976). Genetics of common single malformations. Br Med Bull 32: 21–26.

Carter, CO, Evans, K, Coffey, R, Roberts, JA, Buck, A, Roberts, MF (1982a). A family study of isolated cleft palate. J of Medical Genetics 19: 329–331.

Carter, CO, Evans, K, Coffey, R, Roberts, JA, Buck, A, Roberts, MF (1982b). A three generation family study of cleft lip with or without cleft palate. J of Medical Genetics 19: 246–261.

Case Western Reserve University, Department of Epidemiology and Biostatistics (1997). SAGE (Statistical analysis for genetic epidemiology), Cleveland, OH.

Ching, GH, Chung, CS (1974). A genetic study of cleft lip and cleft palate in Hawaii. I. Interracial crosses. Am J Hum Genet 26: 162–176.

Christensen, K, Mitchell, LE (1996). Familial recurrence-pattern analysis of nonsyndromic isolated cleft palate-a Danish registry study. Am J Hum Genet 58: 182–190.

Chung, CS, Beechert, AM, Lew, RE (1989). Test of genetic heterogeneity of cleft lip with or without cleft palate as related to race and severity. Genetic Epidemiology 6: 625–631.

Chung, CS, Bixler, D, Watanabe, T, et al. (1986). Segregation analysis of cleft lip with or without cleft palate: a comparison of Danish and Japanese data. Am J Hum Genet 39: 603–611.

Chung, CS, Ching, GH, Morton, NE (1974). A genetic study of cleft lip and palate in Hawaii. II. Complex segregation analysis and genetic risks. Am J Hum Genet 26: 177–188.

Clementi, M, Tenconi, R, Collins, A, et al. (1995). Complex segregation analysis in a sample of consecutive newborns with cleft lip with or without cleft palate in Italy. Hum Hered 45: 157–164.

Clementi, M, Tenconi, R, Forabosco, P, et al. (1997). Inheritance of cleft palate in Italy. Evidence for a major autosomal recessive locus. Hum Genet 100: 204–209.

Czeizel, A, Tusnady, G (1972). A family study on cleft lip with or without cleft palate and posterior cleft palate in Hungary. Hum Hered 22: 405–416.

Darwin, C (1875). The variation of animals and plants under domestication, Vol. 1, second edition. New York: Appleton.

Demenais, F, Bonaiti-Pellie, C, Briard, ML, Feingold, J (1984). An epidemiological and genetic study of facial clefting in France. II. Segregation analysis. J Med Genet 21: 436–440.

Edwards, AWF (1992). Likelihood, Expanded Edition. Baltimore: Johns Hopkins University Press.

Ellandt-Johnson, RC (1971). Probability Models and Statistical Methods in Genetics. New York: John Wiley & Sons.

Elston, RC (1980). Segregation analysis. In: Current Developments in Anthropological Genetics, Vol. 1, edited by JH Mielke and MH Crawford. New York: Plenum Press, pp. 327–354.

Elston, RC, Stewart, J (1971). A general model for the genetic analysis of pedigree data. Hum Hered 21: 523–542.

Farrall, M, Holder, S (1992). Familial recurrence-pattern analysis of cleft lip with or without cleft palate. Am J Hum Genet 50: 270–277.

Fisher, RA (1934). The effect of methods of ascertainment upon the estimation of frequencies. Ann Eugen (Lond) 6: 13–25.

Fitzpatrick, D, Farrall, M (1993). An estimation of the number of susceptibility loci for isolated cleft palate. J Craniofac Dev Biol 13: 230–235.

Fogh-Andersen, P (1942). Inheritance of Harelip and Cleft Palate. Copenhagen: Arnold Busck.

Forbes, SA, Brennan, L, Richardson, M, et al. (1996). Refined mapping and YAC contig construction of the X-linked cleft palate and ankyloglossia locus (CPX) including the proximal X-Y homology breakpoint within Xq21.3. Genomics 31: 36–43.

Forbes, SA, Richardson, M, Brennan, L, et al. (1995). Refinement of the X-linked cleft palate and ankyloglossia (CPX) localisation by genetic mapping in an Icelandic kindred. Hum Genet 95: 342–346.

Fraser, FC (1970). Genetics of cleft lip and cleft palate. Am J Hum Genet 22: 336–352.

Fraser, FC (1976). The multifactorial threshold concept—uses and misuses. Teratology 14: 267–280.

Gladstien, K, Lange, K, Spence, MA (1978). A goodness-of-fit test for the polygenic threshold model: application to pyloric stenosis. Am J Med Genet 2: 7–13.

Gorski, SM, Adams, KJ, Birch, PH, et al. (1994). Linkage analysis of X-linked cleft palate and ankyloglossia in Manitoba Mennonite and British Columbia native kindreds. Hum Genet 94: 141–148.

Gorski, SM, Adams, KJ, Birch, PH, et al. (1992). The gene responsible for X-linked cleft palate (CPX) in a British Columbia native kindred is localized between PGKI and DXYSI. Am J Hum Genet 50: 1129–1136.

Greenberg, DA (1986). The effect of proband designation on segregation analysis. Am J Hum Genet 39: 329–339.

Hasstedt, SJ (1994). PAP, Pedigree Analysis Program. Salt Lake City: University of Utah Technical Report.

Hecht, JT, Yang, P, Michels, VV, Buetow, KH (1991). Complex segregation analysis of nonsyndromic cleft lip and palate. Am J Hum Genet 49: 674–681.

Hu, DN, Li, JH, Chen, HY, et al. (1982). Genetics of cleft lip and cleft palate in China. Am J Hum Genet 34: 999–1002.

Jarvik, GP (1998). Complex segregation analyses: uses and limitations. Am J Hum Genet 63: 942–946.

Koguchi, H (1975). Recurrence rate in offspring and siblings of patients with cleft lip and/or cleft palate. Jpn J Hum Genet 20: 207–221.

Lalouel, JM, Morton, NE (1981). Complex segregation analysis with pointers. Hum Hered 31: 312–321.

Lalouel, JM, Rao, DC, Morton, NE, Elston, RC (1983). A unified model for complex segregation analysis. Am J Hum Genet 35: 816–826.

Lange, K (1997). *Mathematical and Statistical Methods for Genetic Analysis.* New York: Springer-Verlag.

Marazita, M (1995). Defining proband. Am J Hum Genet 57: 981–982.

Marazita, ML, Goldstein, AM, Smalley, SL, Spence, MA (1986a). Cleft lip with or without cleft palate: reanalysis of a three-generation family study from England. Genet Epidemiol 3: 335–342.

Marazita, ML, Hu, DN, Spence, MA, et al. (1992). Cleft lip with or without cleft palate in Shanghai, China: evidence for autosomal major locus. Am J Hum Genet 51: 648–653.

Marazita, ML, Spence, MA, Melnick, M (1984). Genetic analysis of cleft lip with or without cleft palate in Danish kindreds. Am J Hum Genet 19: 9–18.

Marazita, ML, Spence, MA, Melnick, M (1986b). Major gene determination of liability to cleft lip with or without cleft palate: a multiracial view. J Craniofac Genet Dev Biol 2: 89–97.

Martin, RA, Hunter, V, Neufeld-Kaiser, W, et al. (2000). Ultrasonographic detection of orbicularis oris defects in first degree relatives of isolated cleft lip patients. Am J Med Genet 90: 155–161.

Melnick, M (1997). Cleft lip and palate etiology and its meaning in early 20th century England: Galton/Pearson vs. Bateson; polygenically poor protoplasm vs. Mendelism. J Craniofac Genet Dev Biol 17: 65–79.

Melnick, M, Bixler, D, Fogh-Andersen, P, Conneally, PM (1980). Cleft lip ± cleft palate: an overview of the literature and an analysis of Danish cases born between 1941 and 1968. Am J Med Genet 6: 83–97.

Melnick, M, Marazita, ML, Hu, DN (1986). Genetic analysis of cleft lip with or without cleft palate in Chinese kindreds. Am J Med Genet 21: 183–190.

Mendel, G (1866). Versuche uber pflanzenhybriden. Verhandenlungen des Naturforshenden Vereines Brunn 4: 3–17.

Mendell, NR, Spence, MA, Gladstien, K, et al. (1980). Multifactorial/threshold models and their application to cleft lip and cleft palate. In: *Etiology of Cleft Lip and Cleft Palate,* edited by M Melnick, D Bixler, and ED Shields. New York: Alan R. Liss, pp. 387–406.

Mitchell, LE, Christensen, K (1996). Analysis of the recurrence patterns for nonsyndromic cleft lip with or without cleft palate in the families of 3,073 Danish probands. Am J Med Genet 61: 371–376.

Mitchell, LE, Risch, N (1992). Mode of inheritance of nonsyndromic cleft lip with or without cleft palate: a reanalysis. Am J Hum Genet 51: 323–332.

Moore, GE, Ivens, A, Chambers, J, et al. (1987). Linkage of an X-chromosome cleft palate gene. Nature 326: 91–92.

Moore, GE, Williamson, R, Jensson, O, et al. (1991). Localization of a mutant gene for cleft palate and ankyloglossia in an X-linked Icelandic family. J Craniofac Genet Dev Biol 11: 372–376.

Morton, NE (1959). Genetic tests under incomplete ascertainment. Am J Hum Genet 11: 1–16.

Morton, NE (1982). *Outline of Genetic Epidemiology.* New York: Karger.

Morton, NE, MacLean, CJ (1974). Analysis of family resemblance. III. Complex segregation of quantitative traits. Am J Hum Genet 26: 489–503.

Morton, NE, Rao, DC, Lalouel, JM (1983). *Methods in Genetic Epidemiology.* Basel: Karger.

Murray, JC (1995). Face facts: genes, environment, and clefts. Am J Med Genet 57: 227–232.

Nemana, LJ, Marazita, ML, Melnick, M (1992). Genetic analysis of cleft lip with or without cleft palate in Madras, India. Am J Med Genet 42: 5–9.

Ott, J (1991). *Analysis of Human Genetic Linkage,* rev. ed. Baltimore: Johns Hopkins University Press.

Palomino, H, Cerda-Flores, R, Blanco, R, et al. (1997). Complex segregation analysis of facial clefting in Chile. J Craniofac Genet Dev Biol 17: 57–64.

Palomino, H, Li, SC, Palomino, HM, et al. (1991). Complex segregation analysis of facial clefting in Chile. Am J Med Genet Suppl 49: 154.

Ray, AK, Field, LL, Marazita, ML (1993). Nonsyndromic cleft lip with or without cleft palate in West Bengal, India: evidence for an autosomal major locus. Am J Hum Genet 52: 1006–1011.

Rischbieth, H (1910). Hare-lip and cleft palate. In: *Treasury of Human Inheritance. Part IV,* edited by K Pearson. London: Dulau, pp 79–123.

Rollnick, BR, Kaye, CI (1986). Mendelian inheritance of isolated nonsyndromic cleft palate. Am J Med Genet 24: 465–473.

Rollnick, BR, Kaye, CI (1987). A response: a further X-linked isolated nonsyndromic cleft palate family with a nonexpressing obligate affected male. Am J Med Genet 26: 241.

Rushton, AR (1979). Sex-linked inheritance of cleft palate. Hum Genet 48: 179–181.

Scapoli, C, Collins, A, Martinelli, M, et al. (1999). Combined segregation and linkage analysis of nonsyndromic orofacial cleft in two candidate regions. Am J Hum Genet 63: 17–25.

Spence, MA, Westlake, J, Lange, K, Gold, DP (1976). Estimation of polygenic recurrence risk for cleft lip and palate. Hum Hered 26: 327–336.

Sproule, J (1863). Hereditary nature of hare-lip. BMJ 1: 412.

Tanaka, K, Fujino, H, Fujita, Y, et al. (1969). Cleft lip and palate: some evidence for multifactorial trait and estimation of heritability based upon Japanese data. Jinrui Idengaku Zasshi 14: 1–9.

Temple, K, Calvert, M, Plint, D, et al. (1989). Dominantly inherited cleft lip and palate in two families. J Med Genet 26: 386–389.

Terwilliger, JD, Ott, J (1994). *Handbook of Human Genetic Linkage.* Baltimore: Johns Hopkins University Press.

Thompson, MW, McInnes, RR, Willard, HF (1991). *Thompson and Thompson: Genetics in Medicine,* 5th ed. Philadelphia: W.B. Saunders.

Trew, CJ (1757). Sistens plura exempla palati deficientis. Nova Acta Physico-Medica Academiae caesarae Leopoldion-Carolinae 1: 445–447.

Vieland, VJ, Hodge, SE (1995). Inherent intractability of the ascertainment problem for pedigree data: a general likelihood framework. Am J Hum Genet 56: 33–43.

Ward, RE, Bixler, D, Jamison, PL (1994). Cephalometric evidence for a dominantly inherited predisposition to cleft lip–cleft palate in a single large kindred. Am J Hum Genet 50: 57–63.

Weinberg, W (1912). Methode und fellerquellen der untersuhung auf Mendelsche Zahlen beim Menschen. Arch Rass Ges Biol 6: 165–174.

Weinberg, W (1927). Mathematische grundlagen der probandenmethode. Z Induktive Abstammungs Vererbungslehre 48: 179–228.

Weldon, WFR (1902). Mendel's laws of alternative inheritance in peas. Biometrika 1: 228–254.

Wentzlaff, KA, Cooper, ME, Yang, P, et al. (1997). Association between non-right-handedness and cleft lip with or without cleft palate in a Chinese population. J Craniofac Genet Dev Biol 17: 141–147.

Woolf, CM, Woolf, RM, Broadbent, TR (1963). A genetic study of cleft lip and palate in Utah. Am J Hum Genet 15: 209–215.

Woolf, CM, Woolf, RM, Broadbent, TR (1964). Cleft lip and heredity. Plast Reconstr Surg 34: 11–14.

Wright, S (1968). *Evolution and the genetics of populations. Genetic and biometric foundations,* Vol. 1. Chicago: University of Chicago Press.

19

Mode of inheritance of oral clefts

LAURA E. MITCHELL

Oral clefts (OCs), including cleft lip with or without cleft palate (CL/P) and isolated cleft palate (CP), comprise one of the most commonly occurring groups of human malformations. These malformations have a profound influence on the basic human condition, affecting appearance, nutrition, and communication, and require long-term, multidisciplinary treatment. Given the prevalence, severity, and economic consequences of OCs, it is not surprising that there has been extensive research into their etiology and inheritance.

It is generally recognized that CL/P and CP are, with rare exceptions (e.g., Van der Woude's syndrome), etiologically distinct conditions (Fogh-Andersen, 1942). Further, even within these two groups, there is causal heterogeneity; i.e., identical cleft malformations may occur as the result of different underlying factors. Over 300 recognized causes of OCs have been identified (Gorlin et al., 1990), including teratogenic exposures (e.g., antiepileptic medications), chromosomal abnormalities (e.g., deletion of chromosome 22q11), and single-gene disorders (e.g., Van der Woude's syndrome). However, such factors tend to be individually rare and are estimated to account for only 30% of CL/P and 50% of CP cases (Jones, 1988; Gorlin et al., 1990; Saal, 1998).

At present, a specific causative agent(s) cannot be identified for the majority (50%–70%) of OCs. In some cases, these OCs occur in association with additional malformations and are likely to be attributable to as yet unidentified teratogens, subtle chromosomal abnormalities (e.g., microdeletions), or unrecognized single-gene defects. However, in many cases, the OC occurs in isolation. This latter group constitutes the so-called nonsyndromic OCs and is the focus of the remainder of this chapter.

For both nonsyndromic CL/P and CP, the most consistently identified risk factor is the presence of a pos-

itive family history. The observed familial recurrence patterns provide strong evidence for a genetic contribution to both conditions since the risks to relatives of affected individuals are much higher than would be expected if familial aggregation was attributable to the effects of a shared environment (Khoury et al., 1988). However, the familial recurrence patterns for both CL/P and CP are also inconsistent with the segregation of a single fully penetrant Mendelian disease locus. Nonsyndromic CL/P and CP are, therefore, classified as genetically complex traits (Wyszynski et al., 1996), but their specific mode of inheritance has not been clearly defined.

MODE OF INHERITANCE

The ability to establish mode of inheritance for a given condition is important for at least two reasons. Knowledge of mode of inheritance allows for more accurate genetic counseling of affected individuals and their relatives. In particular, when mode of inheritance is known, recurrence risks can be based on an understanding of the underlying disease etiology rather than on empiric estimates. In addition, an understanding of mode of inheritance is important when designing studies aimed at the identification of disease-causing or predisposing loci.

One vs. Many

Efforts to determine the mode of inheritance of nonsyndromic CL/P and CP have been guided and limited by the methods that prevailed during a given period. Early investigators invoked modifications of simple Mendelian inheritance (Fogh-Andersen, 1942). However, such models were largely unsatisfactory to explain the observed familial recurrence patterns for these conditions, which are characterized by monozygotic twin concordance rates less than 100%, a nonlinear decline in risk to relatives with decreasing degree of genetic relationship to the proband, and recurrence risks that are dependent on the severity of the proband's defect as well as the number of affected family members (Carter, 1969).

During the 1960s, it was recognized that multifactorial threshold models, which were originally developed to explain the inheritance of continuously distributed traits, could also be applied to discrete traits such as CL/P and CP (Falconer, 1965). Under the multifactorial threshold model, liability to a discrete trait is assumed to be determined by the equal, additive, and relatively small effects of numerous genetic and environmental risk factors and to be normally distributed. Further, the observed dichotomy in phenotypic expression is determined by a threshold beyond which individuals are affected. Such models can account for monozygotic twin concordance rates of less than 100%, nonlinear declines in risk to relatives as a function of the degree of genetic relationship, and risks that are dependent on the severity of the proband's defect and/or the number of affected family members.

The multifactorial threshold model quickly gained acceptance as an appropriate model for the inheritance of many common congenital anomalies, including CL/P and CP. However, the assumptions underlying this model have been criticized as being unrealistic. In addition, it was not until the methods of complex segregation analysis were developed (see Chapter 18 for details) that the fit of multifactorial threshold and single-gene (i.e., Mendelian) models of inheritance to observed familial recurrence patterns could be directly compared.

Complex segregation analyses can explicitly evaluate single major locus vs. multifactorial threshold models of inheritance. Several such analyses of CL/P have been conducted (Demenais et al., 1984; Marazita et al., 1986, 1992; Chung et al., 1986, 1989; Hecht et al., 1991; Nemana et al., 1992; Ray et al., 1993; Clementi et al., 1995), but no clear picture had emerged from these studies (Mitchell, 1997). In those instances where it was possible to discriminate between alternate models of inheritance for CL/P, the best-fitting models varied widely and included multifactorial inheritance as well as both autosomal recessive and autosomal dominant single-gene models with and without an additional multifactorial component. Although fewer segregation analyses have been performed for CP (Chung et al., 1974; Demenais et al., 1984; Pietrzyk et al., 1985), conclusions regarding the best-fitting models of inheritance are also inconsistent. (A summary of the various modes of inheritance that have been proposed for CL/P and CP is provided in Chapter 18.)

The inconsistent results obtained from complex segregation analyses of CL/P and CP may be attributed to genetic heterogeneity; i.e., the genetic mechanisms underlying these conditions may differ across populations. However, given the similarity of CL/P and CP familial recurrence patterns across populations (particularly Caucasian populations), it is more likely that these differences reflect the relatively low power of segregation analyses to discriminate between single-locus and multifactorial models of inheritance (Smith, 1971; Ott, 1990).

Shifting Paradigms

The multifactorial threshold and single-gene models that are evaluated in the context of complex segregation analysis represent two extreme classes of inheritance. It is generally recognized that the mode of inheritance of many conditions, including CL/P and CP, is likely to lie between these two extremes. However, only in the very recent past has there been much interest in defining more precisely the mode of inheritance for such conditions. This interest follows from advances in molecular genetics that offer the possibility of identifying genes that contribute to the development of non-Mendelian or complex traits and the realization that an understanding of mode of inheritance is important when designing studies to identify such genes (Risch, 1990a,b; Lander and Schork, 1994).

Although mode of inheritance questions are difficult to answer definitively, familial recurrence studies can offer some clues (Risch, 1990b). For a dichotomous trait, such as CL/P or CP, familial recurrence is often expressed as the ratio of risk to relatives of an affected individual compared to the population prevalence, denoted λ_R. The subscript R denotes the type of relation (M, monozygotic twins; S, sib; 1, parent/offspring; 2, second-degree relative; 3, third-degree relative). For example, if the risk of CL/P in the offspring of affected individuals is 0.03 and the prevalence of CL/P in the population is 0.001, then λ_1 is 0.03/0.001 or 30.

The pattern of decline in $\lambda_R - 1$ with decreasing degree of unilineal relationship is determined by the underlying genetic model (Risch, 1990b). When a single gene contributes to disease risk, $\lambda_R - 1$ decreases by a factor of 2 with each degree of unilineal relationship, using the parent–offspring relationship for the first-degree relatives. If the parent–offspring risk is the same as the sib risk (i.e., the dominance variance is 0), this pattern will also hold for sibs and monozygotic twins. Under single-locus inheritance, the expected risk ratio to second-degree relatives is, therefore, obtained by solving the following equation for λ_2,

$$\lambda_2 - 1 = 0.5(\lambda_1 - 1)$$

$$\lambda_2 = 0.5\lambda_1 - 0.5 + 1 = 0.5\lambda_1 + 0.5 = 0.5(\lambda_1 + 1)$$

The expected risk ratio to third-degree relatives (λ_3) is obtained in a similar fashion. Hence, assuming a single-locus model of inheritance and $\lambda_1 = 30$, the risk ratios for second- and third-degree relatives of individuals with CL/P are expected to be 15.5 and 8.25, respectively.

If a trait is determined by multiple loci that act in an additive fashion or by multiple independent loci (i.e., loci that are each sufficient to cause disease), $\lambda_R - 1$ will also decline by a factor of 2 with each degree of unilineal relationship. Hence, the expected familial recurrence pattern is identical under single-locus, multiple additive loci, or multiple independent loci models of inheritance and familial recurrence studies cannot be used to discriminate between these models. If, however, the trait is determined by multiple loci acting in a multiplicative fashion, $\lambda_R - 1$ will decline by greater than a factor of 2 with each degree of relationship.

Under a multilocus, multiplicative model of inheritance, the rate of decrease of $\lambda_R - 1$ is determined by the number of underlying loci as well as the degree of interaction between loci; thus, it varies depending on the specifics of the underlying model. The predictions of various multiplicative models can, therefore, be compared to the observed familial recurrence pattern. In general, the power to discriminate between alternate multiplicative models of inheritance using this approach is low (Farrall and Holder, 1992). However, such comparisons are extremely helpful in defining the number of genes that contribute to a trait and the maximum plausible effect that any one gene may have on disease risk.

To estimate risk ratios under multiplicative models of inheritance, it is necessary to specify the number and magnitude of the effects at each locus in the model. For example, one multiplicative model of inheritance for CL/P might predict that the observed risk ratio, $\lambda_1 = 30$, is determined by two loci, one that increases the risk of CL/P in first-degree relatives by sixfold and a second that increases the risk by fivefold. Since these two loci are hypothesized to act multiplicatively, they are the only loci required to account for the overall increase in risk observed among first-degree relatives (i.e., $6 \times 5 = 30$). To calculate the risk to other types of relative, the increase in λ_R attributable to susceptibility locus i is determined in a manner analogous to that outlined above. For example, λ_{21} (the risk ratio for second-degree relatives attributable to the first locus) = $0.5(6 + 1) = 3.5$, $\lambda_{22} = 0.5(5 + 1) = 3.00$, and the overall risk to second-degree relatives (λ_2) is obtained

as the product of the effects of the individual loci, or $3.5(3.0) = 10.0$. Corresponding values for third-degree relatives are $\lambda_{31} = 2.25$, $\lambda_{32} = 2.00$, and $\lambda_3 = 4.5$. The expected decline in risk in λ_R is clearly more dramatic under this multiplicative model ($\lambda_1 = 30, \lambda_2 = 10, \lambda_3 = 4.5$) than under the single-locus model of inheritance ($\lambda_1 = 30, \lambda_2 = 15.5, \lambda_3 = 8.25$).

Familial Recurrence Pattern Analysis

Cleft Lip with or without Cleft Palate. Three analyses of the familial recurrence patterns observed for nonsyndromic CL/P, using the methods described above, have been published (Farrall and Holder, 1992; Mitchell and Risch, 1992; Mitchell and Christensen, 1996). Two of these studies were based on re-analyses of published data from multiple sources (Farrall and Holder, 1992; Mitchell and Risch, 1992), whereas the third was based on Danish data obtained by record linkage (Mitchell and Christensen, 1996). Despite differences in the types of bias that may have influenced the various data sets, the results from these studies are relatively consistent. In contrast to earlier segregation analyses, all three studies clearly excluded single-locus inheritance of CL/P. As the predictions of models with multiple additive loci and multiple independent loci are similar to those of the single major locus model, these models were also excluded in each of these studies.

Each of the familial recurrence studies of CL/P concluded that this condition is most likely determined by multiple genes acting in a multiplicative fashion. Further, these analyses suggest that there are likely to be two to eight CL/P susceptibility loci and that the maximum effect of any one of these loci would be to increase the risk to first-degree relatives of affected individuals by three- to sixfold. The analyses based on the Danish data (Mitchell and Christensen, 1996) are summarized in Table 19.1 and suggest that CL/P is likely to be determined by two to three loci, with no single locus accounting for more than a threefold increase in risk to first-degree relatives. This analysis is likely to provide the most accurate indication of the mode of inheritance of CL/P for several reasons: it is based on a single, well-defined population, estimates of risk were obtained by record linkage rather than self-reported family history, and an accurate estimate of the population prevalence of CL/P in Denmark was used to estimate values of λ_R.

Cleft Palate. Two analyses of the familial recurrence patterns observed for nonsyndromic CP have been published (Fitzpatrick and Farrall, 1993; Christensen and Mitchell, 1996). One was based largely on the re-analysis of published data from multiple sources (Fitz-

TABLE 19.1. *Familial Recurrence Pattern Analysis of Cleft Lip with or without Cleft Palate in Denmark*

	λ_1	λ_M	λ_2	λ_3
Observed values	24.7	461	4.2	7.6*
95% CI[Δ]		292–631	2.4–6.6	3.2–13.8
Predicted values				
Single-locus model		48	12.8	6.9
Multiplicative models†				
$\lambda_{11} = 2.0$		457	5.3	2.3
$\lambda_{11} = 3.0$		339	5.7	2.5
$\lambda_{11} = \lambda_{12} = 1.5$		482	5.2	2.3
$\lambda_{11} = \lambda_{12} = 2.0$		343	5.6	2.5
$\lambda_{11} = \lambda_{12} = \lambda_{13} = 1.25$		539	5.1	2.3
$\lambda_{11} = \lambda_{12} = \lambda_{13} = 1.5$		428	5.3	2.3

*Given the small number of affected second- (15/2738) and third- (8/809) degree relatives, the observed increase in risk to third-degree relatives, compared to second-degree relatives, is most likely attributable to random error. This pattern of risk is, however, incompatible with any genetic model of inheritance and limits the usefulness of third-degree relatives for familial recurrence pattern analysis.

[Δ]95% CI, 95% confidence interval.

†Under each multiplicative model of inheritance, the remainder of the increase in risk to first-degree relatives is attributable to a large number of loci, each with a very small effect on risk. See Risch (1990b) for details.

Source: Mitchell and Christensen (1996).

patrick and Farrall, 1993), whereas the other was based on Danish data obtained by record linkage (Christensen and Mitchell, 1996). Both studies provided strong evidence against single-locus inheritance of CP. Models of inheritance assuming multiple additive loci and multiple independent loci are, therefore, also unlikely for this condition.

The familial recurrence pattern exhibited by CP appears to be most consistent with an underlying multiplicative model of inheritance. The analyses based on the Danish data (Christensen and Mitchell, 1996) are summarized in Table 19.2 and suggest that CP is likely to be determined by several interacting loci. Under such a model, no single locus is likely to account for more

TABLE 19.2. *Familial Recurrence Pattern Analysis of Cleft Palate in Denmark*

	λ_1	λ_M	λ_2	λ_3
Observed values	47.2	1149	4.8	0.0
95% CI[Δ]		618–1681	1.0–11.9	
Predicted values				
Single-locus model		93	24.1	12.6
Multiplicative models*				
$\lambda_{11} = 2.0$		1671	7.3	2.8
$\lambda_{11} = 4.0$		975	8.6	3.2
$\lambda_{11} = 6.0$		681	9.8	3.8
$\lambda_{11} = \lambda_{12} = 2.0$		1253	7.7	2.9
$\lambda_{11} = \lambda_{12} = 3.0$		688	9.1	3.4
$\lambda_{11} = \lambda_{12} = \lambda_{13} = 1.5$		1566	7.3	2.8
$\lambda_{11} = \lambda_{12} = \lambda_{13} = 2.0$		940	8.2	3.0

[Δ]95% CI, 95% confidence interval.

*Under each multiplicative model of inheritance, the remainder of the increase in risk to first-degree relatives is attributable to a large number of loci, each with a very small effect on risk. See Risch (1990b) for details.

Source: Christensen and Mitchell (1996).

than a sixfold increase in risk to first-degree relatives of affected individuals.

CONCLUSIONS

The results of familial recurrence pattern analyses for CL/P and CP have important implications for the design of studies aimed at the identification of specific susceptibility loci. These analyses indicate that the strongest susceptibility loci for these conditions may be associated with values of λ_{1i} as large as 6 to 8 or as small as 2 to 3. Hence, the prospect of detecting such loci using traditional linkage approaches will be low, particularly if the latter estimates are correct. Moreover, even nonparametric linkage approaches (e.g. affected pedigree members, affected sib pairs) are likely to require sample sizes that will be difficult to achieve for these conditions (Risch, 1990c).

At present, association studies (see Chapter 20) targeted at specific candidate genes are likely to offer the most fruitful strategy for the identification of specific CL/P and CP susceptibility loci. Such studies should employ methods, such as the transmission disequilibrium test (Spielman et al., 1993), that eliminate concerns regarding false-positive findings attributable to population structure (Spielman et al., 1993; Ewens and Spielman, 1995) or focus on populations where such concerns are reduced. Association studies of CL/P and CP have begun to provide clues regarding the role of putative susceptibility loci (Wyszynski et al., 1996; Schutte and Murray, 1999). However, the full potential of this approach may not be realized until large-scale (i.e., genomewide) association studies for complex diseases become feasible.

Familial recurrence pattern analyses provide useful information regarding the genetic contribution to complex traits. However, such analyses do not consider all of the complexities that may be involved in the determination of a particular condition. For example, in the mouse, susceptibility to CL/P is influenced by both maternal genetic effects (Trasler and Trasler, 1984; Juriloff, 1986) and gene–environment interactions (Karolyi et al., 1987). Although such factors may also influence susceptibility to CL/P and CP in humans, their impact on familial recurrence patterns and on conclusions regarding mode of inheritance drawn from these patterns are difficult to predict. Hence, at present, mode of inheritance of CL/P and CP remains a vaguely defined concept that is unlikely to be fully elucidated until the specific causes of these conditions have been identified.

This work was supported in part by a grant (DE11388) from the National Institutes of Health.

REFERENCES

Carter, CO (1969). Genetics of common disorders. BMJ 25: 52–57.

Christensen, K, Mitchell, LE (1996). Familial recurrence-pattern analysis of nonsyndromic isolated cleft palate—a Danish registry study. Am J Hum Genet 58: 182–190.

Chung, CS, Beechert, AM, Lew, RE (1989). Test of genetic heterogeneity of cleft lip with or without cleft palate as related to race and severity. Genet Epidemiol 6: 625–631.

Chung, CS, Bixler, D, Watanabe, T, et al. (1986). Segregation analysis of cleft lip with or without cleft palate: a comparison of Danish and Japanese data. Am J Hum Genet 39: 603–611.

Chung, CS, Ching, GHS, Morton, NE (1974). A genetic study of cleft lip and palate in Hawaii. Complex segregation analysis and genetic risk. Am J Hum Genet 26: 177–188.

Clementi, M, Tenconi, R, Collins, ACE, Milan, M (1995). Complex segregation analysis in a sample of consecutive newborns with cleft lip with or without cleft palate in Italy. Hum Hered 45: 157–164.

Demenais, F, Bonaiti-Pellie, C, Briard, ML, Feingold, J (1984). An epidemiological and genetic study of facial clefting in France. II. Segregation analysis. J Med Genet 21: 436–440.

Ewens, WJ, Spielman, RS (1995). The transmission/disequilibrium test: history, subdivision, and admixture. Am J Hum Genet 57: 455–464.

Falconer, DS (1965). The inheritance of liability to certain diseases, estimated from the incidence among relatives. Ann Hum Genet 29: 51–76.

Farrall, M, Holder, SE (1992). Familial recurrence pattern analysis of cleft lip with or without cleft palate. Am J Hum Genet 50: 270–277.

Fitzpatrick, D, Farrall, M (1993). An estimation of the number of susceptibility loci for isolated cleft palate. J Craniofac Genet Dev Biol 13: 230–235.

Fogh-Andersen, P (1942). *Inheritance of Harelip and Cleft Palate.* Copenhagen: Arnold Busck.

Gorlin, RJ, Cohan MM, Lavin, LS (1990). *Syndromes of the Head and Neck.* New York: Oxford University Press.

Hecht, JT, Yang, PMVV, Buetow, KH (1991). Complex segregation analysis of nonsyndromic cleft lip and palate. Am J Hum Genet 49: 674–681.

Jones, MC (1988). Etiology of facial clefts: prospective evaluation of 428 patients. Cleft Palate Craniofac J 25: 16–20.

Juriloff, DM (1986). Major genes that cause cleft lip in mice: progress in the construction of a congenic strain and in linkage mapping. J Craniofac Genet Dev Biol 2(Suppl): 55–66.

Karolyi, IJ, Liu, S, Erickson, RP (1987). Susceptibility to phenytoin-induced cleft lip with or without cleft palate: many genes are involved. Genet Res Camb 49: 43–49.

Khoury, MJ, Beaty, TH, Liang, KY (1988). Can familial aggregation of disease be explained by familial aggregation of environmental factors. Am J Epidemiol 127: 674–683.

Lander, ES, Schork, NJ (1994). Genetic dissection of complex traits. Science 265: 2037–2048.

Marazita, ML, Goldstein, AM, Smalley, SL, et al. (1986). Cleft lip with or without cleft palate: reanalysis of a three-generation family study from England. Genet Epidemiol 3: 335–342.

Marazita, ML, Hu, D-N, Spence, MA, et al. (1992). Cleft lip with or without cleft palate in Shanghai, China: evidence for an autosomal major locus. Am J Hum Genet 51: 648–653.

Mitchell, LE (1997). Genetic epidemiology of birth defects: nonsyndromic cleft lip and neural tube defects. Epidemiol Rev 19: 61–68.

Mitchell, LE, Christensen, K (1996). Analysis of the recurrence patterns for nonsyndromic cleft lip with or without cleft palate in the families of 3,073 Danish probands. Am J Med Genet 61: 371–376.

Mitchell, LE, Risch, N (1992). Mode of inheritance of nonsyndromic cleft lip with or without cleft palate: a reanalysis. Am J Hum Genet 51: 323–332.

Nemana, LJ, Marazita, ML, Melnick, M (1992). Genetic analysis of cleft lip with or without cleft palate in Madras, India. Am J Med Genet 42: 5–9.

Ott, J (1990). Cutting a Gordian knot in linkage analysis of complex human traits. Am J Hum Genet 46: 219–221.

Pietrzyk, JJ, Rozanski, BS, Swisterska, E (1985). Genetic analysis of cleft lip and cleft palate in S. Poland: complex segregation analysis. Acta Anthropogenet 9: 140–152.

Ray, AK, Field, LL, Marazita, ML (1993). Nonsyndromic cleft lip with or without cleft palate in West Bengal, India: evidence for an autosomal major locus. Am J Hum Genet 52: 1006–1011.

Risch, N (1990a). Genetic linkage and complex diseases, with special reference to psychiatric disorders. Genet Epidemiol 7: 3–16.

Risch, N (1990b). Linkage strategies for genetically complex traits. I. Multilocus models. Am J Hum Genet 46: 222–228.

Risch, N (1990c). Linkage strategies for genetically complex traits. II. The power of affected relative pairs. Am J Hum Genet 46: 229–241.

Saal, HM (1998). Syndromes and malformations associated with cleft lip with or without clerft palate. Am J Hum Genet 63S: A118.

Schutte, BC, Murray, JC (1999). The many faces and factors of orofacial clefts. Hum Mol Genet 8: 1853–1859.

Smith, C (1971). Discriminating between different modes of inheritance in genetic disease. Clin Genet 2: 303–314.

Spielman, RS, McGinnis, RE, Ewens, WJ (1993). Transmission test for linkage disequilibrium: the insulin gene region and insulin-dependent diabetes mellitus (IDDM). Am J Hum Genet 52: 506–516.

Trasler, DG, Trasler, TA (1984). Left cleft lip predominance and genetic similarities of L line and CL/Fr strain mice. Teratology 30: 423–427.

Wyszynski, DF, Beaty, TH, Maestri, NE (1996). Genetics of nonsyndromic oral clefts revisited. Cleft Palate Craniofac J 33: 406–417.

20

Association studies

MARY L. MARAZITA
KATHERINE NEISWANGER

Association methods are used as an adjunct to linkage approaches for gene mapping, especially for complex traits. In association analysis, one compares the allele frequencies of a genetic marker or candidate gene between groups of affected individuals vs. controls. If allele frequencies differ significantly between the two groups, then a specific allele at the marker or candidate locus is said to be associated with the disease at the population level. Genetic linkage between a marker and a disease gene implies that alleles at the marker locus co-segregate with the disease allele within families. With linkage, different marker alleles may co-segregate with the disease allele in different families and the overall frequencies of the marker alleles, as calculated from population-based samples, need not vary between affected and control groups. For the purposes of this discussion, two loci are in linkage equilibrium when they are linked but not associated. *Linkage disequilibrium* occurs when two genes are both linked within families and associated in the population.

The procedures for mapping, cloning, and characterizing genes for rare, Mendelian diseases are now well established. Consequently, progress in mapping Mendelian traits has been dramatic over the past several years. In contrast, genes contributing to common, complex diseases such as oral-facial clefting have been much more difficult to isolate. Complex diseases are those for which no single dominant or recessive mode of inheritance adequately explains the observed patterns of transmission in families. In the absence of specific genetic models, the etiology of complex diseases is often conceptualized as being due to multiple factors, i.e., several genetic loci interacting with each other to produce an underlying susceptibility, which in turn interacts with additional environmental factors to produce an actual disease state. This concept does not exclude the possibility that Mendelian genes for a complex disorder segregate in atypical families or that one or a few of the underlying susceptibility genes exert relatively large effects. Indeed, for several complex disorders, including coronary artery disease (Ozturk and Killeen, 1999), breast cancer (Bennett et al., 1999), and Alzheimer's disease (St. George-Hyslop, 2000), linkage analysis has been used successfully to locate unusual genetic mutations that exert major effects in a subset of families.

However, for other complex traits, such as bipolar disorder (Berrettini, 2000), obesity (Chagnon et al., 1998), and oral-facial clefting (Murray, 1995; Carinci et al., 2000), linkage analysis has produced either negative results or a plethora of weak, positive results that are not easily replicated. Theoretical research suggests several reasons for the ambiguity of the linkage results in these cases. First, if a disease gene is neither necessary nor sufficient to cause a disease but rather is a "modifier" gene that elevates a non-zero baseline risk, conventional parametric linkage analysis may not detect it, even for close genetic linkage (Greenberg, 1993). Second, if the relative contribution of a gene to a disease phenotype is small, i.e., the disease susceptibility allele raises the risk by a factor of <2, linkage analysis using affected sib pairs will not be powerful enough to detect the gene, given realistic sample sizes (Risch and Merikangas, 1996). Thus, linkage analysis may not be a useful strategy to detect modifier genes or genes that exert small effects, precisely those genes which might operate in oral-facial clefting and many other complex disorders. In light of these issues, attention has shifted away from linkage analysis to association analysis as an alternative means of locating disease-susceptibility genes, especially since association studies can sometimes detect weaker effects than linkage analysis (Hodge, 1994).

Two types of association analysis are commonly employed in genetic studies: population-based and family-based (Hodge, 1993). The population-based approach utilizes a standard case-control design, in which marker allele frequencies are compared between cases (affected individuals) and controls (either unaffected individuals or individuals randomly chosen from the population). When a positive association is found, several interpretations are possible: *(1)* the associated allele itself is the disease-predisposing allele, *(2)* the associated allele is in linkage disequilibrium with the actual disease-predisposing locus, *(3)* the association is due to population stratification, or *(4)* the association is a sampling, or statistical, artifact.

The first two interpretations represent the alternative hypotheses of interest in a gene-mapping context. These two alternatives are not readily distinguishable using either population-based or family-based association strategies (Hodge, 1994). In case 1, the marker itself is the disease-susceptibility locus. This outcome is the rationale behind candidate-gene studies, in which the genes being tested have some a priori expectation of being directly involved in the disease process. A classic example is the human leukocyte antigen (HLA) system, in which various HLA haplotypes are associated with a number of diseases, including insulin-dependent diabetes mellitus, rheumatoid arthritis, and ankylosing spondylitis (Thomson, 1988).

Case 2 occurs if the actual disease-susceptibility mutation is at a second, unknown locus that is so close to the marker that it is still in linkage disequilibrium with it. This interpretation may be invoked if there is no obvious functional connection between the marker and the disease, e.g., if the associated allele is not located within the promoter or coding region of a gene. To fully appreciate the nature of associations due to linkage disequilibrium, it is necessary to consider carefully how linkage disequilibrium occurs. When a new mutation first appears in the genome, it occurs on one specific chromosome and is in complete linkage disequilibrium with any polymorphic markers in the adjacent DNA. For example, if a mutation, M, occurs near the $A1$ allele of genetic locus A (with allele frequencies of 0.6 and 0.4 for $A1$ and $A2$, respectively), $A1$ will be associated with 100% of the M mutations, while $A2$ is never associated with M mutations. This is a population-based association between M and $A1$, due to complete linkage disequilibrium between mutation M and locus A. With time, recombination will shuffle M and $A1$ so that eventually M will be on the same chromosome as $A1$ 60% of the time and on the same chromosome as $A2$ the other 40% of the time. Linkage still exists, but the population-based association due to linkage disequilibrium is gone; i.e., M and A have reached linkage equilibrium.

In the absence of selection, the degree of linkage disequilibrium depends on two factors: *(1)* the distance of the marker from the disease-susceptibility mutation and *(2)* the time elapsed since either the disease or the marker mutation occurred. A relatively recent disease-susceptibility mutation will be in linkage disequilibrium with its adjacent markers as a function of the genetic distance between disease mutation and marker. For example, disease mutations occurring up to 60,000 years ago demonstrate linkage disequilibrium with adjacent markers when the recombination rate between them is 1 in 1000 (Cavalli-Sforza and Bodmer, 1971). However, except for the most tightly linked markers, ancient disease-susceptibility mutations will show a pattern of linkage disequilibrium that does not depend solely on the distance to adjacent markers but also on the time at which the adjacent markers mutated. Recent marker mutations will be in varying degrees of linkage disequilibrium with the disease mutation, while older marker mutations will not, even when they are physically closer to it. Thus, lack of association still allows for the possibility that the marker is closely linked but in linkage equilibrium with the disease-susceptibility gene. A positive association suggests that the disease-susceptibility gene is close to the marker, probably within 1 cM and possibly within kilobases of it. However, the degree of linkage disequilibrium can vary throughout the genome or in different populations. In specific cases, such as genetically isolated populations, linkage disequilibrium can exist even if the distance between a marker and a disease locus is greater than 1 cM. However, a positive result from a population-based association test can also be artifactual, either because of population stratification (case 3 above) or sampling error (case 4). Stringent significance levels and larger sample sizes can help to reduce sampling error. Population stratification is more problematic. If the marker allele frequencies differ among ethnic groups and the case and control samples contain different proportions of these ethnic groups, an artifactual positive association due to allele frequency differences among ethnic groups may be misinterpreted as evidence for a disease-susceptibility gene. Thus, case and control groups should be matched as closely as possible for ethnicity, to avoid creating an association due to population stratification. The population-based association of alcoholism with the TaqI $A1$ allele from the dopamine D_2 receptor locus illustrates the difficulty in deciding among various possible interpretations (Neiswanger et al., 1995a,b).

To avoid the effects of unknown population stratification, alternative association analysis strategies that use family members as controls have been proposed. Such statistical methods are collectively known as family-based association studies (Hodge, 1993). Tests of this type include genotype- and haplotype-based haplotype relative risk methods (Falk and Rubinstein, 1987; Terwilliger and Ott, 1992), affected family-based controls (Thomson, 1995), the heterozygote transmission test (Swift et al., 1990), and the transmission disequilibrium test (TDT) (Spielman et al., 1993; Ewens and Spielman, 1995). Of these methods, the TDT has been widely applied in studies of complex traits, including a oral-facial clefting. The TDT determines whether a given marker allele is transmitted from a heterozygous parent to an affected child more often than the 50% expected frequency. The TDT cannot detect either linkage or association in the absence of linkage disequilibrium. Therefore, in general populations, the TDT will not detect linkage at distances much greater than 1 cM. However, neither will it generate an artifactual association due to population stratification.

Spielman and co-workers (Spielman et al., 1993; Ewens and Spielman, 1995) introduced the TDT in 1993, with modifications by several groups to extend the test to multiple alleles (Bickeboller and Clerget-Darpoux, 1995; Rice et al., 1995; Sham and Curtis, 1995; Cleves et al., 1997; Kaplan et al., 1997a,b; Sham, 1997). Cleves et al. (1997) and Kaplan et al. (1997a)

have proposed methods to obtain exact p values for TDTs for multiallelic markers. A sibship test has also been developed, in which unaffected siblings, rather than parents, are used as controls (Curtis, 1997; Boehnke and Langefeld, 1998; Horvath and Laird, 1998; Spielman and Ewens, 1998). Extensions of the TDT have been proposed that use nuclear family or pedigree data (Cleves et al., 1997; Martin et al., 1997, 2000), allow for incomplete data (Weinberg, 1999), incorporate covariates (Lunetta et al., 2000), and extend to quantitative traits (Allison, 1997; Rabinowitz, 1997; Fulker et al., 1999; Abecasis et al., 2000; Monks and Kaplan, 2000). As increasingly dense marker maps become available, many investigators advocate the TDT for genomewide screening. Camp (1997, 1999) reviewed the arguments, provided calculations of power under a range of assumptions for genome scans of complex traits, and demonstrated that TDT approaches have greater power than sib-pair identity-by-descent linkage methods. The TDT methods continue to develop rapidly; any such new approaches may become relevant to studies of oral-facial clefts in the future.

Gene-mapping studies of oral-facial clefts have utilized both linkage and association methods. Table 20.1 summarizes chromosomal regions that have shown positive results ($p < 0.05$, lod > 3.0) from at least one association or linkage study in humans, along with any additional evidence from animal models or chromosomal rearrangements [see also the reviews by Wyszyn-

TABLE 20.1. *Chromosomal Regions that Have Shown Positive Linkage or Association Results for Oral-Facial Clefting*

Region	Genetic Locus	CL/P or CP	Linkage Studies	Association studies		Other Evidence
				Case-Control	TDT or AFBAC	
2p13	TGFA	CL/P	−	+ +/−	+ +/−	EXP
		CP	−	+ +/−	−	
4p16	MSX1	CL/P	−	+/−	−	CH/KO/EXP
		CP	N/A	+/−	+/−	
4q31	anonymous	CL/P	+/−	+/−	−	
		CP	N/A	N/A	N/A	
6p23	anonymous	CL/P	+ +/−	N/A	N/A	CH/KO
		CP	N/A	N/A	N/A	
14q24	TGFB3	CL/P	−	−	−	KO/EXP
		CP	N/A	+/−	+/−	
17q21	RARA	CL/P	+/−	+ +/−	−	TG/EXP
		CP	N/A	N/A	−	
19q13	BCL3	CL/P	+/−	−	+ +/−	CH
		CP	N/A	−	−	

CL/P, cleft lip with or without cleft palate; CP, cleft palate; TDT, transmission disequilibrium test; AFBAC, family-based control; −, one or more negative studies; +, one positive study; ++, more than one positive study; CH, chromosome deletion (recurrent) or translocation; KO, knockout mouse; TG, transgenic mouse; EXP, expression studies; N/A, not available.

ski et al. (1996) and Carinci et al. (2000)]. Regions on chromosomes 2, 4, 6, 14, 17, and 19 have had positive findings. Chapter 21 provides more detail about linkage results in oral-facial clefting, Chapter 22 details animal model studies, and Chapter 23 summarizes gene–environment studies. This chapter provides a comprehensive review of the results from published allelic association studies.

Table 20.2 summarizes all published association studies with nonsyndromic cleft lip with or without cleft palate (CL/P) and cleft palate (CP), whether utilizing population-based or family-based controls. Presented in the table are all published studies of the regions with positive association results in at least one study. There are a few additional loci and chromosomal regions that have only negative results reported in the literature, although there are no comprehensive, genomewide association results. Also, there are many studies for some loci and few studies for others; this is not a reflection of the strength of the evidence for any particular association but merely a reflection of the interest in particular loci. In Table 20.2 we present the statistics reported in the original papers. Wyszynski et al. (1996), Mitchell (1996), and Carinci et al. (2000) instead present odds ratios calculated from the raw case-control data of the original references.

The first published association studies for oral-facial clefts evaluated association with alleles at loci within the major histocompatibility system (HLA) (Bonner et al., 1978; Van Dyke et al., 1980, 1983; Watanabe et al., 1984). They examined HLA because susceptibility to cortisone-induced CP in some mouse strains is associated primarily with genotypes at the H2 locus (Bonner and Slavkin, 1975; see also Chapter 22). Although several studies have been conducted in Caucasian and Asian populations, no overall positive associations between HLA and CL/P or CP have been found.

The first positive association with oral-facial clefts was a population-based association between CL/P and a TaqI restriction site polymorphism in the transforming growth factor-α locus *(TGFA)* (Ardinger et al., 1989). Interestingly, this locus was studied as a candidate because of its involvement in CP in the mouse. The *TGFA* association with CL/P has since been replicated in several studies, but several other studies have failed to confirm it (Table 20.2). An association of *TGFA* with CP has also been reported, although most studies of *TGFA* and CP have failed to find an association (Table 20.2).

There are many possible reasons for the conflicting *TGFA* association study results. Although the majority of the studies have been in Caucasian populations, the data sets are heterogeneous in several ways. There are differing proportions of cases with a family history of clefting: some studies included only familial cases, some studies included only sporadic cases, and many studies included both familial and sporadic cases in varying proportions. If there are different etiologic factors that are important in familial vs. sporadic clefting, then it is not surprising that association study results differ. Furthermore, there were different proportions of CL vs. CLP cases, different types of data (case-control vs. nuclear triads vs. nuclear families vs. extended kindreds), different types of analysis, and different *TGFA* markers employed. Sample size may also be a factor, although most of the published studies were sufficiently large for valid conclusions.

Any of these factors could account for the inconsistent results. However, there is no consistent correlation between any of the above factors and association; i.e., there are positive and negative associations with *TGFA* in each possible study design. In general, studies with fewer familial cases were less likely to exhibit a positive association with *TGFA*. There were also no positive results in Asians, although there were only two studies [Filipinos studied by Lidral et al. (1997) and Chinese studied by Marazita et al. (2001)], too few to draw any conclusion about *TGFA* and ethnicity. A meta-analysis of pre-1996 studies (Mitchell, 1996) concluded that there was positive evidence of association between CL/P and *TGFA* in Caucasians (odds ratio 1.43, 95% confidence interval 1.12–1.80). The meta-analysis found significant heterogeneity between Caucasian studies in the allele frequencies of cases but not controls. Thus, heterogeneity between studies is unlikely to be due to ethnicity differences; it is more likely to be due to the differing proportions of familial and/or severe cases of clefting (Mitchell, 1996).

There are additional etiologic clues from association studies of *TGFA* and clefting. A few studies were consistent, with *TGFA* modifying cleft severity, i.e., with significantly different *TGFA* allele patterns between CL and CLP cases. Also, some association studies reported an interaction between maternal smoking and *TGFA*, which increased the risk of clefts, although other studies failed to find such an interaction (see Chapter 23 for a summary of gene–environment interaction studies). Finally, as noted earlier, different *TGFA* markers have been assessed in different studies. Of possible etiologic significance, some studies tested multiple *TGFA* markers, with usually only one of the markers showing an association with clefting.

Machida et al. (1999) characterized the intron–exon boundaries in *TGFA*, as well as a substantial portion of additional untranslated sequence. They identified five regions of human–mouse homology outside of the coding sequence, with a particularly high degree of homology scattered throughout the 3′-untranslated region

TABLE 20.2. *Summary of Association Studies of Oral-Facial Clefting for Chromosomal Regions with at Least One Study Showing Positive Evidence of Association*

Association studies for cleft lip with or without cleft palate

Region	Polymorphic Locus	Analytic Method*	Results† OR (95% CI)	Results† p Value	Significant Association?	Population	Reference
2p13	TGFA, Taq1	Case-control	—	0.0047	Yes	U.S. Caucasian (80 cases, 102 controls), family history not reported	Ardinger et al. (1989)
	TGFA, BamH1	Case-control	—	0.0052	Yes	U.S. Caucasian (80 cases, 102 controls), family history not reported	
	TGFA, Taq1	Case-control	—	0.0003	Yes	Australian Caucasian (96 cases, 100 controls), 48 cases with a family history of clefting	Chenevix-Trench et al. (1991)
	TGFA, Taq1	Case-control	1.77 (1.00–3.26)	0.049	Yes	Australian Caucasian (117 cases, 113 controls), about 50% with a family history of clefting	Chenevix-Trench et al. (1992)‡
			2.23 (1.30–3.82)	0.005	Yes	Add 63 controls from Hayward et al. (1988)	
	TGFA, BamH1	Case-control	1.78 (0.89–3.50)	0.053	No	Australian Caucasian (115 cases, 112 controls), about 50% with a family history of clefting	
	TGFA, Taq1	Case-control, C2 allele	—	<0.001	Yes	British Caucasian (57 cases, 60 controls), 21 cases with a family history of clefting	Holder et al. (1992)‡
		Case-control, C2C2 genotype	—	<0.01	Yes		
	TGFA, BamH1	Case-control	—	0.85	No	British Caucasian (57 cases, 60 controls), 21 cases with a family history of clefting	
	TGFA, Taq1	Case-control	—	>0.05	No	Alsatian Caucasian (67 cases, 90 controls), sporadic cases only	Stoll et al. (1992)
	TGFA, BamH1	Case-control	—	>0.05	No	Alsatian Caucasian (67 cases, 90 controls) sporadic cases only	
	TGFA, TaqI	Case-control	—	>0.05	No	Alsatian Caucasian (98 cases, 99 controls), sporadic cases only	Stoll et al. (1993)‡ [includes data from Stoll et al. (1992)]
	TGFA, BamH1	Case-control	—	>0.05	No	Alsatian Caucasian (98 cases, 99 controls), sporadic cases only	
	TGFA, Taq1	Case-control	2.07 (1.06–4.04)	0.03	Yes	U.S. Caucasian (83 cases, 84 controls)	Sassani et al. (1993)‡·§

Gene, polymorphism	Study design	OR (95% CI)	p-value	Significant	Population	Reference
	Case-control	Pooled OR = 1.95	0.02	Yes	U.S. Caucasian (83 cases, 84 controls) plus Asian (6 cases, 6 controls) and African-American (11 cases, 8 controls, 14 with a family history of clefting	Feng et al. (1994) [the 36 simplex cases were derived from the subjects of Sassani et al. (1993)]
TGFA, Taq1	TDT	—	<0.005	Yes	U.S. and British Caucasian (13 multiplex families) U.S. Caucasian (36 simplex families)	Field et al. (1994) [overall results were nonsignificant but CL differed significantly from CLP]
TGFA, SSCP-K	Case-control (family member controls) AFBAC	—	0.407	No	West Bengal, Indian (34 affected individuals, 38 unaffected from 14 multiplex families)	
			0.581	No		
	CL vs. CLP AFBAC	—	0.00008	Yes	West Bengal, Indian (23 CL, 11 CLP)	Hwang et al. (1995)‡§
			0.002	Yes		
TGFA, Taq1	Case-control	1.20 (0.65–2.20)	0.51	No	U.S. Caucasian (114 cases, 284 noncleft, other birth defect controls)	
TGFA, Taq1	Case-control	—	0.97	No	Chilean admixed Caucasian/Amerindian (39 cases, 51 controls), 16 cases had a family history of clefting	Jara et al. (1995)§
TGFA, BamH1	Case-control	5.55 (1.14–36.83)	0.014	Yes	Chilean admixed Caucasian/Amerindian (39 cases, 51 controls), 16 cases had a family history of clefting	
TGFA, Taq1	Case-control	0.92 (0.54–1.50)	—	No	U.S. Caucasian (190 cases, 379 controls)	Shaw et al. (1996)‡§
	Case-control	1.6 (0.40–4.3)	—	No	U.S. Hispanic (85 cases, 175 controls)	
	Case-control	1.3 (0.04–23.9)	—	No	U.S. African-American (8 cases, 20 controls) All include some cases with a family history of clefts	
TGFA, Taq1	Case-control, Meta-analysis	1.43 (1.12–1.80)	—	Yes	Caucasian cases and controls	Mitchell (1996) [includes studies with Caucasians‡ and other groups§ plus controls from Hayward et al. (1988)]
	Case-control, Meta-analysis	1.42 (1.16–1.73)	—	Yes	All cases and controls	
TGFA, Taq1	Case-control, bilateral CLP cases	2.23 (0.51–9.75)	—	No	U.S. Caucasian (15 bilateral CLP cases, 86 controls)	Beaty et al. (1997)
TGFA, Taq1	Case-control, bilateral CL cases	2.09 (0.15–7.75)	—	No	U.S. Caucasian (22 bilateral CL cases, 86 controls)	

(continued)

TABLE 20.2. *Summary of Association Studies of Oral-Facial Clefting for Chromosomal Regions with at Least One Study Showing Positive Evidence of Association (continued)*

Region	Polymorphic Locus	Analytic Method*	Results† OR (95% CI)	Results† p Value	Significant Association?	Population	Reference
		Case-control, unilateral CL cases	0.81 (0.20–3.25)	—	No	U.S. Caucasian (38 unilateral CL cases, 86 controls) Mix of familial and non-familial cases	Lidral et al. (1997)§
	TGFA, Taq1	Case-control	—	0.84	No	Filipino (652 cases, 776 controls)	Maestri et al. (1997)
	TGFA (D2S443)	TDT, logistic regression, CL cases	OR from regression = 0.67	0.248	No	U.S., 87% Caucasian/13% other (28 CL case-parent triads)	
	TGFA (D2S443)	TDT, logistic regression, CLP cases	OR from regression = 5.50	0.013	Yes	U.S., 87% Caucasian/13% other (66 CLP case-parent triads)	
	TGFA (D2S443)	TDT	—	0.657	No	U.S. Caucasian (35 multiplex families)	Wyszynski et al. (1997a)
		TDT	—	0.457	No	Mexican (22 multiplex families)	
	TGFA, GGAA4D07	Case-control	—	0.84	No	U.S., 95% Caucasian (189 cases, 209 controls)	Lidral et al. (1998) [includes subjects of Ardinger et al. (1989)]
	TGFA, Taq1	Case-control	—	0.85	No	U.S., 95% Caucasian (182 cases, 251 controls)	Scapoli et al. (1998)
	TGFA, Taq1	TDT	—	0.847	No	Italian Caucasian (40 multiplex families	
		TDT, pooled with Feng et al. (1994)	—	0.297	No	40 Italian families plus 16 U.S. and British Caucasian families (Feng et al., 1994)	
	TGFA, Taq1	Case-control, nonsmoking mother (2 alleles)	1.20 (0.70–2.08)	—	No	Danish Caucasian (94 cases, 259 controls with nonsmoking mothers)	Christensen et al. (1999)
		Case-control, smoking mother (2 alleles)	1.03 (0.54–1.94)	—	No	Danish Caucasian (94 cases, 185 controls with smoking mothers)	
	TGFA, SSCP-K	Case-control	—	0.017	Yes	Japanese (43 cases, 73 controls)	Tanabe et al. (2000)
	TGFA, Taq1	Case-control	—	0.867	No		
	TGFA, SSCP	TDT, total	—	0.17	No	Chinese (Shanghai, 58 multiplex families	Marazita et al. (2001)
		TDT, CLP	—	0.34	No	Chinese (Shanghai, 41 multiplex families	
		TDT, CL	—	0.42	No	Chinese (Shanghai, 17 multiplex families	
4p16	MSX1	Case-control	—	0.26	No	Filipino (637 cases, 746 controls)	Lidral et al. (1997)
	MSX1, CA	Case-control	—	0.35	No	U.S., 95% Caucasian (198 cases, 275 controls/133 case-parent triads	Lidral et al. (1998) [includes subjects from Ardinger et al. (1989)]
		TDT	—	0.93	No		
		AFBAC	—	0.92	No		
	MSX1, X1.1	Case-control	—	0.80	No	U.S., 95% Caucasian (185 cases, 165 controls/133 case-parent triads	
		TDT	—	0.95	No		
		AFBAC	—	0.87	No		

Locus	Analysis	OR (95% CI)	p	Significant	Sample	Reference
MSX1, X1.3	Case-control	—	0.005	Yes	U.S., 95% Caucasian (197 cases, 159 controls/133 case-parent triads)	Marazita et al. (2001)
	TDT		0.41	No		
	AFBAC		0.46	No		
MSX1, X2.1	Case-control	—	0.44	No	U.S., 95% Caucasian (187 cases, 200 controls/133 case-parent triads)	
	TDT		0.68	No		
	AFBAC		0.55	No		
MSX1, X2.4	Case-control	—	0.68	No	U.S., 95% Caucasian (179 cases, 74 controls/133 case-parent triads)	
	TDT		0.41	No		
	AFBAC		0.60	No		
MSX1	TDT, total	—	0.26	No	Chinese (Shanghai, 22 multiplex families)	Marazita et al. (2001)
	TDT, CLP	—	0.75	No	Chinese (Shanghai, 15 multiplex families)	
	TDT, CL	—	0.25	No	Chinese (Shanghai, 7 multiplex families)	
4q31	Case-control, overall allele distribution	—	0.002	Yes	Australian Caucasian (95 cases, 254 controls, 59 patients had a family history of clefting)	Mitchell et al. (1995) [these cases and 94 of the controls are included in Chenevix-Trench et al. (1992)]
D4S192	Case-control, 2 high-risk alleles vs. all others	1.75 (1.24–2.47)	0.0013	Yes		
D4S192	Case-control, allele 87	1.98 (0.98–4.04)	0.0256	Yes	Chilean (78 total cases, 35 from simplex families, 43 from multiplex; 124 unaffected relatives; 85 controls)	Paredes et al. (1999)
D4S175	Case-control, allele 130	2.47 (0.99–6.31)	0.0088	Yes		
D4S175	TDT, total	—	0.98	No	Chinese (Shanghai, 28 multiplex families)	Marazita et al. (2001)
	TDT, CLP	—	0.99	No	Chinese (Shanghai, 22 multiplex families)	
	TDT, CL	—	1.00	No	Chinese (Shanghai, 6 multiplex families)	
D4S175	TDT, total	—	0.86	No	Chinese (Shanghai, 59 multiplex families)	
	TDT, CLP	—	0.92	No	Chinese (Shanghai, 42 multiplex families)	
	TDT, CL	—	0.34	No	Chinese (Shanghai, 17 multiplex families)	
14q24 TGFB3 (D14S61)	TDT, logistic regression, CL cases	OR from regression = 2.17	0.074	No	U.S., 87% Caucasian/13% other (27 CL case-parent triads)	Maestri et al. (1997)
	TDT, logistic regression, CLP cases	OR from regression = 1.62	0.057	No	U.S., 87% Caucasian/13% other (68 CLP case-parent triads)	
TGFB3	Case-control	—	0.92	No	Filipinos (282 cases, 440 controls)	Lidral et al. (1997)
TGFB3, CA	Case-control	—	0.27	No	U.S., 95% Caucasian (175 cases, 243 controls/133 case-parent triads)	Lidral et al. (1998) [includes subjects from Ardinger et al. (1989)]
	TDT		0.51	No		
	AFBAC		0.63	No		
TGFB3, 5' UTR.1	Case-control	—	0.45	No	U.S. 95% Caucasian (177 cases, 241 controls/133 case-parent triads)	
	TDT		0.11	No		
	AFBAC		0.11	No		

(continued)

TABLE 20.2. *Summary of Association Studies of Oral-Facial Clefting for Chromosomal Regions with at Least One Study Showing Positive Evidence of Association (continued)*

Region	Polymorphic Locus	Analytic Method*	Results† OR (95% CI)	Results† p Value	Significant Association?	Population	Reference
	TGFB3, X5.1	Case-control TDT AFBAC	—	0.63 0.05 0.08	No No No	U.S., 95% Caucasian (82 cases, 65 controls/133 case-parent triads)	
	TGFB3, CA	Case-control	—	0.52	No	Japanese (43 cases, 73 controls)	Tanabe et al. (2000)
17q21	RARA, Pst1	Case-control	2.11 (1.10–4.02)	—	Yes	Australian Caucasian (110 cases, 75 controls), about 50% with a family history of clefting	Chenevix-Trench et al. (1992)
	RARA (D17S579)	Case-control (family member controls)	—	0.44	No	West Bengal, Indian (35 affected individuals, 41 unaffected from 14 multiplex families)	Shaw et al. (1993) [overall results were nonsignificant, but CL differed significantly from CLP]
		CL vs. CLP	—	0.029	Yes	West Bengal, Indian (24 CL, 11 CLP)	
	RARA, Pst1	Case-control	1.34 (0.72–2.43)	—	No	British Caucasian (61 cases, 60 controls)	Vintiner et al. (1993)
	RARA Pst1	Case-control	1.60 (1.10–2.30)	—	Yes	Australian Caucasian (170 cases, 135 controls)	Mitchell et al. (1995)
	RARA (THRA1)	TDT, logistic regression CL cases	OR from regression = 2.00	0.088	No	U.S., 87% Caucasian/13% other (23 CL case-parent triads)	Maestri et al. (1997)
		TDT, logistic regression CLP cases	OR from regression = 1.32	0.208	No	U.S., 87% Caucasian/13% other (65 CLP case-parent triads)	
		TDT, logistic regression CL plus CLP cases	—	0.047	Yes	U.S., 87% Caucasian/13% other (88 CL/P case-parent triads)	
	D17S250	TDT, total	—	0.69	No	Chinese (Shanghai, 55 multiplex families)	Marazita et al. (2001)
		TDT, CLP	—	0.98	No	Chinese (Shanghai, 40 multiplex families)	
		TDT, CL	—	0.12	No	Chinese (Shanghai, 15 multiplex families)	
	D17S579	TDT, total	—	0.45	No	Chinese (Shanghai, 52 multiplex families)	
		TDT, CLP	—	0.72	No	Chinese (Shanghai, 38 multiplex families)	
		TDT, CL	—	0.83	No	Chinese (Shanghai, 14 multiplex families)	
19q13	BCL3	TDT, marginal homogeneity test, all affecteds TDT, 1 nuclear family/kindred	—	0.181 3 alleles 0.25	No [see Amos et al. (1996)]	U.S. multiplex, multigenerational families (38 Caucasian, 1 African-American)	Stein et al. (1995), Amos et al. (1996b)

Marker	Method	OR	p-value	Linkage/Association?	Sample	Reference
D19S178	TDT, marginal homogeneity test, all affecteds; TDT, 1 nuclear family/kindred	—	0.011	Yes [but was not re-tested by Amos et al. (1996)]	U.S. multiplex, multigenerational families (38 Caucasian, 1 African-American)	Stein et al. (1995), Amos et al. (1996b)
BCL3	TDT, marginal homogeneity test	—	3 alleles 0.006	Yes	U.S. sporadic cases (30 case-parent triads: 27 Caucasian, 1 Asian, 2 African-American)	Amos et al. (1996a)
	TDT	—	0.03			
D19S178	TDT, marginal homogeneity test	—	3 alleles, 0.03; 2 alleles, 0.004	Yes	U.S. sporadic cases (30 case-parent triads: 27 Caucasian, 1 Asian, 2 African-American)	Amos et al. (1996a)
	TDT	—	0.017			
BCL3	TDT	—	0.0005	Yes	U.S. Caucasian (58 proband-parent triads from 30 multiplex families)	Wyszynski et al. (1997b)
	TDT	—	0.0616	No	Mexican (32 proband-parent triads from 11 multiplex families)	
	TDT	—	<0.0001	Yes	Combined (90 trios from 41 U.S. and Mexican families)	
BCL3	TDT, logistic regression CL cases	OR from regression = 3.40	0.010	Yes	U.S., 87% Caucasian/13% other (20 CL case-parent triads)	Maestri et al. (1997)
	TDT, logistic regression CLP cases	OR from regression = 1.42	0.217	Yes	U.S., 87% Caucasian/13% other (40 CL case-parent triads)	
BCL3	Case-control	Results not presented in detail	—	No	U.S. 95% Caucasian (243 cases, controls not enumerated)	Lidral et al. (1998) [includes subjects from Ardinger et al. (1989)]
BCL3	TDT	—	0.768	No	Italian Caucasian (40 multiplex families)	Martinelli et al. (1998) [these are the same families reported in Scapoli et al. (1998)]
D19S574	TDT, alleles	—	0.065	No	Italian Caucasian (40 multiplex families)	Martinelli et al. (1998) [these are the same families reported in Scapoli et al. (1998)]
	TDT, genotypes	—	0.015	Yes		
ApoC2	TDT, total	—	0.49	No	Chinese (Shanghai, 48 multiplex families)	Marazita et al. (2001)
	TDT, CLP	—	0.29	No	Chinese (Shanghai, 36 multiplex families)	
	TDT, CL	—	0.45	No	Chinese (Shanghai, 12 multiplex families)	
D19S49	TDT, total	—	0.004	Yes	Chinese (Shanghai, 29 multiplex families)	
	TDT, CLP	—	0.09	No	Chinese (Shanghai, 20 multiplex families)	
	TDT, CL	—	0.25	No	Chinese (Shanghai, 9 multiplex families)	

(continued)

TABLE 20.2. *Summary of Association Studies of Oral-Facial Clefting for Chromosomal Regions with at Least One Study Showing Positive Evidence of Association (continued)*

Region	Polymorphic Locus	Analytic Method*	Results†		Significant Association?	Population	Reference
			OR (95% CI)	p Value			
Association studies of cleft palate alone							
2p13	TGFA, Taq1	Case-control	—	>0.05	No	Alsatian Caucasian (38 cases, 99 controls), sporadic cases only	Stoll et al. (1992)
	TGFA, BamH1	Case-control	—	>0.05	No	Alsatian Caucasian (38 cases, 99 controls), sporadic cases only	
	TGFA, Taq1	Case-control	—	>0.05	No	Alsatian Caucasian (57 cases, 99 controls), sporadic cases only	Stoll et al. (1993) [includes data from Stoll et al. (1992)]
	TGFA, BamH1	Case-control	—	>0.05	No	Alsatian Caucasian (57 cases, 99 controls), sporadic cases only	
	TGFA, Taq1	Case-control	2.64 (1.31–5.31)	—	Yes	U.S. Caucasian (43 cases, 170 controls)	Shiang et al. (1993)
	TGFA, Taq1	Case-control	2.17 (1.13–4.16)	0.015	Yes	U.S. Caucasian (69 cases, 284 noncleft, other birth defect controls)	Hwang et al. (1995)
	TGFA, Taq1	Case-control	1.6 (0.83–2.90)	—	No	U.S. Caucasian (77 cases, 379 controls)	Shaw et al. (1996)
		Case-control	0.65 (0.03–5.30)	—	No	U.S. Hispanic (24 cases, 175 controls)	
		Case-control	3.0 (0.08–79.3)	—	No	U.S. African-American (4 cases, 20 controls) All include some cases with family history of clefts	
	TGFA, Taq1	Case-control	—	0.37	No	Filipinos (97 cases, 776 controls)	Lidral et al. (1997)
	TGFA, Taq1	Case-control	1.40 (0.45–4.33)	—	No	U.S. Caucasians (46 cases, 86 controls), mix of familial and nonfamilial cases	Beaty et al. (1997)
	TGFA (D2S443)	TDT, logistic regression	OR from regression = 2.50	0.197	No	U.S., 87% Caucasian/13% other (47 CP case-parent triads)	Maestri et al. (1997)
	TGFA, GGAA4D07	Case-control	—	0.66	No	U.S., 95% Caucasian (57 cases, 209 controls)	Lidral et al. (1998) [includes subjects from Ardinger et al. (1989)]
	TGFA, Taq1	Case-control	—	0.62	No	U.S., 95% Caucasian (62 cases, 251 controls)	
	TGFA, Taq1	Case-control, with nonsmoking mothers	1.19 (0.55–2.57)	—	No	Danish Caucasian (40 cases, 259 controls with nonsmoking mothers)	Christensen et al. (1999)

Region	Gene/Marker	Method	OR (CI)	p	Significant	Population	Reference
4p16	MSX1	Case-control, with smoking mothers	0.72 (0.26–2.00)	—	No	Danish Caucasian (24 cases, 185 controls with smoking mothers)	Lidral et al. (1997)
	MSX1	Case-control	—	0.91	No	Filipino (92 cases, 746 controls)	Lidral et al. (1998) [includes subjects from Ardinger et al. (1989)]
	MSX1, CA	Case-control / TDT / AFBAC	—	0.027 / 0.11 / 0.04	Yes / No / Yes	U.S., 95% Caucasian (60 cases, 275 controls/61 case-parent triads)	
	MSX1, X1.1	Case-control / TDT / AFBAC	—	0.95 / 0.64 / 0.49	No / No / No	U.S., 95% Caucasian (51 cases, 165 controls/61 case-parent triads)	
	MSX1, X1.3	Case-control / TDT / AFBAC	—	0.0057 / 0.65 / 0.65	Yes / No / No	U.S., 95% Caucasian (61 cases, 159 controls/61 case-parent triads)	
	MSX1, X2.1	Case-control / TDT / AFBAC	—	0.53 / 0.36 / 0.35	No / No / No	U.S., 95% Caucasian (56 cases, 200 controls/61 case-parent triads)	
	MSX, X2.4	Case-control / TDT / AFBAC	—	0.37 / 0.68 / 0.51	No / No / No	U.S., 95% Caucasian (50 cases, 74 controls/61 case-parent triads)	
14q24	TGFB3	Case-control	—	0.86	No	Filipino (92 cases, 440 controls)	Lidral et al. (1997)
	D14S61	TDT, logistic regression	OR from regression = 2.09	0.024	Yes	U.S., 87% Caucasian/13% other (40 CP case-parent triads)	Maestri et al. (1997)
	TGFB3, CA	Case-control / TDT / AFBAC	—	0.85 / 0.80 / 0.97	No / No / No	U.S., 95% Caucasian (53 cases, 243 controls/61 case-parent triads)	Lidral et al. (1998) [includes subjects from Ardinger et al. (1989)]
	TGFB3, 5' UTR.1	Case-control / TDT / AFBAC	—	0.56 / 0.75 / 0.75	No / No / No	U.S., 95% Caucasian (53 cases, 241 controls/61 case-parent triads)	
	TGFB3, X5.1	Case-control / TDT / AFBAC	—	1.00 / 0.58 / 0.55	No / No / No	U.S., 95% Caucasian (35 cases, 65 controls/61 case-parent triads)	
17	RARA (THRA1)	TDT, logistic regression	OR from regression = 1.37	0.33	No	U.S., 87% Caucasian/13% other (41 CP case-parent triads)	Maestri et al. (1997)
19q13	BCL3	TDT, logistic regression	OR from regression = 1.70	0.250	No	U.S., 87% Caucasian/13% other (31 CP case-parent triads)	Maestri et al. (1997)
	BCL3	Case-control	Results not presented in detail	—	No	U.S, 95% Caucasian (77 cases, controls not enumerated)	Lidral et al. (1998) [includes subjects from Ardinger et al. (1989)]

*Case-control, standard population-based, cases with unrelated controls; AFBAC, family-based controls; TDT, transmission disequilibrium test; TGF, transforming growth factor; UTR, untranslated region; RAR, retinoic acid receptor.

†OR, odds ratio; CI, confidence interval. ORs are reported for population-based case-control methods; *p* values are reported for TDT and other family-based methods.

‡,§Studies included in Mitchell (1996) meta-analysis (‡indicates Caucasian data, §indicates other data).

(UTR). The 3′-UTR regions play a role in mRNA stability and are sites for RNA-binding proteins (Siomi and Dreyfuss, 1997). Machida et al. (1999) also found five rare variants (three in the 3′-UTR) among 250 nonsyndromic oral-facial cleft cases; none of these variants was found in any of 270 control samples. This may be an example of a rare mutation in control regions as at least one component of *TGFA* cleft susceptibility. Also of note is that *TGFA* knockout mice do not have a cleft (Luetteke et al., 1993). This result does not necessarily eliminate a role for *TGFA* in clefting because alterations in *TGFA* expression, rather than complete gene inactivation, could be involved.

In addition to *TGFA*, alleles at loci in several other chromosomal regions have shown positive association results with oral-facial clefting, although, like *TGFA*, none of these loci has given consistent results across all studies. Homeobox 7 (*MSX1*, chromosome 4p16) has one report of an association with CL/P and CP in Caucasians and two negative reports in Asians. Anonymous markers on 4q31 have one report of a positive association with CL/P in Caucasians and one negative report in Asians. Transforming growth factor-β3 (*TGFB3*, 14q24) has one positive association reported with CP (in Caucasians) and two negative reports (one Caucasian, one Asian). Retinoic acid receptor α (*RARA*, 17q21) has multiple reports of a positive association with CL/P (Caucasians) and negative reports (Caucasians and Asians), as well as one negative report with CP in Caucasians. Protooncogene *BCL3* (19q13) has multiple positive and negative reports with CL/P (Caucasians and Asians) and two negative reports with CP.

Association analysis in human genetics is coming of age, and the use of association analysis methods will have increasing utility in studies of oral-facial clefts. To clarify the inconsistent association study results, several study designs will be important, as will independent replication of any positive findings. To remove any possible biases due to unknown population stratification, family-based association studies, such as the TDT, should be pursued. Covariates such as gender, cleft severity, and pregnancy history should be included, e.g., using logistic regression methods (Schaid, 1996; Maestri et al., 1997). Additional studies should be done in ethnic groups other than Caucasians to clarify possible differences in association patterns. Future association studies of clefting should also focus on methods to incorporate gene–gene interactions, to assess the simultaneous effects of alleles at multiple loci on the risk of clefts. Statistical analysis of recurrence risk patterns is consistent with oligogenic models for oral-facial clefting, in which there are four to seven different etiologic genes (Farrall and Holder, 1992; Mitchell and Risch, 1992).

In addition, with the development of extremely dense marker maps, genomewide scans for cleft loci via linkage disequilibrium (at genetic distances much less than 1 cM) are becoming feasible. The major weakness of population-based analysis, that it has the potential to generate artifactual associations due to population stratification, has begun to be addressed by the use of genomic controls (Devlin and Roeder, 1999; Bacanu et al., 2000). Risch and Teng have compared the power of various population-based and family-based association methods, both when DNA samples are pooled (Risch and Teng, 1998) and for individual genotyping (Teng and Risch, 1999), and provide conditions under which different approaches will have the most power. Finally, methods that combine elements of both population- and family-based data are being proposed (Whittemore and Tu, 2000). With the development of new markers and new methods, progress in detecting cleft-susceptibility genes with small to moderate effects can be expected in the near future.

REFERENCES

Abecasis, GR, Cardon, LR, Cookson, WOC (2000). A general test of association for quantitative traits in nuclear families. Am J Hum Genet 66: 279–292.

Allison, DB (1997). Transmission-disequilibrium tests for quantitative traits. Am J Hum Genet 60: 676–690.

Amos, C, Gasser, D, Hecht, JT (1996a). Nonsyndromic cleft lip with or without cleft palate: new BCL3 information. Am J Hum Genet 59: 743–744.

Amos, C, Stein, J, Mulliken, JB, et al. (1996b). Nonsyndromic cleft lip with or without cleft palate: erratum. Am J Hum Genet 59: 744.

Ardinger, HH, Buetow, KH, Bell, GI, et al. (1989). Association of genetic variation of the transforming growth factor-alpha gene with cleft lip and palate. Am J Hum Genet 45: 348–353.

Bacanu, SA, Devlin, B, Roeder, K (2000). The power of genomic control. Am J Hum Genet 66: 1933–1944.

Beaty, TH, Maestri, NE, Hetmanski, JB, Wyszynski, DF (1997). Testing for interaction between maternal smoking and TGFA genotype among oral cleft cases born in Maryland 1992–1996. Cleft Palate Craniofac J 34: 447–454.

Bennett, IC, Gattas, M, Teh, BT (1999). The genetic basis of breast cancer and its clinical implications. Aust N Z J Surg 69: 95–105.

Berrettini, WH (2000). Genetics of psychiatric disease. Annu Rev Med 51: 465–479.

Bickeboller, H, Clerget-Darpoux, F (1995). Statistical properties of the allelic and genotypic transmission/disequilibrium test for multiallelic markers. Genet Epidemiol 12: 865–870.

Boehnke, M, Langefeld, CD (1998). Genetic association mapping based on discordant sib pairs: the discordant-alleles test. Am J Hum Genet 62: 950–961.

Bonner, JJ, Slavkin, HC (1975). Cleft palate susceptibility linked to histocompatibility-2 (H-2) in the mouse. Immunogenetics 2: 213–218.

Bonner, JJ, Terasaki, PI, Thompson, P, et al. (1978). HLA phenotype frequencies in individuals with cleft lip and/or cleft palate. Tissue Antigens 12: 228–232.

Camp, NJ (1997). Genomewide transmission/disequilibrium testing—consideration of the genotypic relative risks at disease loci. Am J Hum Genet 61: 1424–1430.

Camp, NJ (1999). Genomewide transmission/disequilibrium testing: a correction. Am J Hum Genet 64: 1485–1487.

Carinci, F, Pezzetti, F, Scapoli, L, et al. (2000). Genetics of nonsyndromic cleft lip and palate: a review of international studies and data regarding the Italian population. Cleft Palate Craniofac J 37: 33–40.

Cavalli-Sforza, LL, Bodmer, WF (1971). The Genetics of Human Populations. San Francisco: W.H. Freeman.

Chagnon, YC, Pérusse, L, Bouchard, C (1998). The human obesity gene map: the 1997 update. Obes Res 6: 76–92.

Chenevix-Trench, G, Jones, K, Green, AC, et al. (1992). Cleft lip with or without cleft palate: associations with transforming growth factor alpha and retinoic acid receptor loci. Am J Hum Genet 51: 1377–1385.

Chenevix-Trench, G, Jones, K, Green, AC, Martin, N (1991). Further evidence for an association between genetic variation in transforming growth factor alpha and cleft lip and palate. Am J Hum Genet 48: 1012–1013.

Christensen, K, Olsen, J, Norgaard-Pedersen, B, et al. (1999). Oral clefts, transforming growth factor alpha gene variants, and maternal smoking: a population-based case-control study in Denmark, 1991–1994. Am J Epidemiol 149: 248–255.

Cleves, MA, Olson, JM, Jacobs, KB (1997). Exact transmission-disequilibrium tests with multiallelic markers. Genet Epidemiol 14: 337–347.

Curtis, D (1997). Use of siblings as controls in case-control association studies. Ann Hum Genet 61: 319–333.

Devlin, B, Roeder, K (1999). Genomic control for association studies. Biometrics 55: 997–1004.

Ewens, WJ, Spielman, RS (1995). The transmission/disequilibrium test: history, subdivision, and admixture. Am J Hum Genet 57: 455–464.

Falk, CT, Rubinstein, P (1987). Haplotype relative risks: an easy reliable way to construct a proper control sample for risk calculations. Ann Hum Genet 51: 227–233.

Farrall, M, Holder, S (1992). Familial recurrence pattern analysis of cleft lip with or without cleft palate. Am J Hum Genet 42: 270–277.

Feng, H, Sassani, R, Bartlett, SP, et al. (1994). Evidence, from family studies, for linkage disequilibrium between TGFA and a gene for nonsyndromic cleft lip with or without cleft palate. Am J Hum Genet 55: 932–936.

Field, LL, Ray, AK, Marazita, ML (1994). Transforming growth factor alpha: a modifying locus for nonsyndromic cleft lip with or without cleft palate? Eur J Hum Genet 2: 159–165.

Fulker, DW, Cherny, SS, Sham, PC, Hewitt, JK (1999). Combined linkage and association analysis for quantitative traits. Am J Hum Genet 64: 259–267.

Greenberg, DA (1993). Linkage analysis of "necessary" disease loci versus "susceptibility" loci. Am J Hum Genet 52: 135–143.

Hayward, N, Nancarrow, D, Ellem, K, et al. (1988). A TaqI RFLP of the human TGFA gene is significantly associated with cutaneous malignant melanoma. Int J Cancer 42: 558–561.

Hodge, SE (1993). Linkage analysis versus association analysis: distinguishing between two models that explain disease–marker associations. Am J Hum Genet 53: 367–384.

Hodge, SE (1994). What association analysis can and cannot tell us about the genetics of complex disease. Am J Med Genet (Neuropsych Genet) 54: 318–323.

Holder, SE, Vintiner, GM, Farren, B, et al. (1992). Confirmation of an association between RFLPs at the transforming growth factor-alpha locus and nonsyndromic cleft lip and palate. Am J Med Genet 29: 390–392.

Horvath, S, Laird, NM (1998). A discordant-sibship test for disequilibrium and linkage: no need for parental data. Am J Hum Genet 63: 1886–1897.

Hwang, SJ, Beaty, TH, Panny, SR, et al. (1995). Association study of transforming growth factor alpha (TGFα) Taql polymorphism and oral clefts: indication of gene–environment interaction in a population-based sample of infants with birth defects. Am J Epidemiol 141: 629–636.

Jara, L, Blanco, R, Chiffelle, I, et al. (1995). Associations between alleles of the transforming growth factor alpha locus and cleft lip and palate in the Chilean population. Am J Med Genet 57: 548–551.

Kaplan, NL, Martin, ER, Weir, BS (1997a). Power studies for the transmission/disequilibrium tests with multiple alleles. Am J Hum Genet 60: 691–702.

Kaplan, NL, Martin, ER, Weir, BS (1997b). Reply to Sham. Am J Hum Genet 61: 778.

Lidral, AC, Murray, JC, Buetow, KH, et al. (1997). Studies of the candidate genes TGFB2, MSX1, TGFA, and TGFB3 in the etiology of cleft lip and palate in the Philippines. Cleft Palate Craniofac J 34: 1–6.

Lidral, AC, Romitti, P, Basart, AM, et al. (1998). Association of MSX1 and TGFB3 with nonsyndromic clefting in humans. Am J Hum Genet 63: 557–568.

Luetteke, NC, Qui, TH, Peiffer, RL, et al. (1993). TGFα deficiency results in hair follicle and eye abnormalities in targeted and waived-1 mice. Cell 73: 263–278.

Lunetta, KL, Faraone, SV, Biederman, J, Laird, NM (2000). Family-based tests of association and linkage that use unaffected sibs, covariates, and interactions. Am J Hum Genet 66: 605–614.

Machida, J, Yoshiura, Ki, Funkhauser, CD, et al. (1999). Transforming growth factor-alpha (TGFA): genomic structure, boundary sequences, and mutation analysis in nonsyndromic cleft lip/palate and cleft palate only. Genomics 61: 237–242.

Maestri, NE, Beaty, TH, Hetmanski, J, et al. (1997). Application of transmission disequilibrium tests to nonsyndromic oral clefts: including candidate genes and environmental exposures in the models. Am J Med Genet 73: 337–344.

Marazita, ML, Field, LL, Cooper, ME, et al. (2001). Non-syndromic cleft lip with or without cleft palate in China: assessment of candidate regions. Cleft Palate Craniofac J (in press).

Martin, ER, Kaplan, NL, Weir, BS (1997). Tests for linkage and association in nuclear families. Am J Hum Genet 61: 439–448.

Martin, ER, Monks, SA, Warren, LL, Kaplan, NL (2000). A test for linkage and association in general pedigrees: the pedigree disequilibrium test. Am J Hum Genet 67: 146–154.

Martinelli, M, Scapoli, L, Pezzetti, F, et al. (1998). Suggestive linkage between markers on chromosome 19q13.2 and nonsyndromic orofacial cleft malformation. Genomics 51: 177–181.

Mitchell, LE (1996). Transforming growth factor alpha locus and nonsyndromic cleft lip with or without cleft palate: a reappraisal. Genet Epidemiol 14: 231–240.

Mitchell, LE, Healey, SC, Chenevix-Trench, G (1995). Evidence for an association between nonsyndromic cleft lip with or without cleft palate and a gene located on the long arm of chromosome 4. Am J Hum Genet 57: 1130–1136.

Mitchell, LE, Risch, N (1992). Mode of inheritance of nonsyndromic cleft lip with or without cleft palate: a reanalysis. Am J Hum Genet 51: 323–332.

Monks, SA, Kaplan, NL (2000). Removing the sampling restrictions from family-based tests of association for a quantitative-trait locus. Am J Hum Genet 66: 576–592.

Murray, JC (1995). Face facts: genes, environment, and clefts. Am J Hum Genet 57: 227–232.

Neiswanger, K, Hill, SY, Kaplan, BB (1995a). Association and linkage studies of the TaqI *A1* allele at the dopamine D$_2$ receptor gene in samples of female and male alcoholics. Am J Med Genet (Neuropsych Genet) *60:* 267–271.

Neiswanger, K, Kaplan, BB, Hill, SY (1995b). What can the DRD2/alcoholism story teach us about association studies in psychiatric genetics? Am J Med Genet (Neuropsych Genet) *60:* 272–275.

Ozturk, IC, Killeen, AA (1999). An overview of genetic factors influencing plasma lipid levels and coronary artery disease risk. Arch Pathol Lab Med *123:* 1219–1222.

Paredes, M, Carreño, H, Solá, JA, et al. (1999). Association between nonsyndromic cleft lip/palate with microsatellite markers located in 4q [in Spanish]. Rev Med Chil *127:* 1431–1438.

Rabinowitz, D (1997). A transmission disequilibrium test for quantitative trait loci. Hum Hered *47:* 342–350.

Rice, JP, Newman, RJ, Hoshaw, SL, et al. (1995). TDT with covariates and genomic screens with MOD scores: their behavior on simulated data. Genet Epidemiol *12:* 659–664.

Risch, N, Merikangas, K (1996). The future of genetic studies of complex human diseases. Science *273:* 1516–1517.

Risch, N, Teng, J (1998). The relative power of family-based and case-control designs for linkage disequilibrium studies of complex human diseases I. DNA pooling. Genome Res *8:* 1273–1288.

Sassani, R, Bartlett, SP, Feng, H, et al. (1993). Association between alleles of the transforming growth factor-alpha locus and the occurrence of cleft lip. Am J Med Genet *45:* 565–569.

Scapoli, L, Pezzetti, F, Carinci, F, et al. (1998). Lack of linkage disequilibrium between transforming growth factor alpha taqI polymorphism and cleft lip with or without cleft palate in families from northeastern Italy. Am J Med Genet *75:* 203–206.

Schaid, DJ (1996). General score tests for association to genetic markers with disease using cases and their parents. Genet Epidemiol *13:* 423–449.

Sham, P (1997). Transmission/disequilibrium tests for multiallelic loci. Am J Hum Genet *61:* 774–778.

Sham, PC, Curtis, D (1995). An extended transmission/disequilibrium test (TDT) for multiallele marker loci. Ann Hum Genet *59:* 323–336.

Shaw, D, Ray, A, Marazita, M, Field, L (1993). Further evidence of a relationship between the retinoic acid receptor alpha locus and nonsyndromic cleft lip with or without cleft palate (CL ± P). Am J Hum Genet *53:* 1156–1157.

Shaw, GM, Wasserman, CR, Lammer, EJ, et al. (1996). Orofacial clefts, parental cigarette smoking, and transforming growth factor-alpha gene variants. Am J Hum Genet *58:* 551–561.

Shiang, R, Lidral, AC, Ardinger, HH, et al. (1993). Association of transforming growth factor alpha gene polymorphisms with nonsyndromic cleft palate only. Am J Hum Genet *53:* 836–843.

Siomi, H, Dreyfuss, G (1997). RNA-binding proteins as regulators of gene expression. Curr Opin Genet Dev *7:* 345–353.

Spielman, RS, Ewens, WJ (1998). A sibship test for linkage in the presence of association: the sib transmission/disequilibrium test. Am J Hum Genet *62:* 450–458.

Spielman, RS, McGinnis, RE, Ewens, WJ (1993). Transmission test for linkage disequilibrium: the insulin gene region and insulin-dependent diabetes mellitus (IDDM). Am J Hum Genet *52:* 506–516.

Stein, J, Mulliken, JB, Stal, S, et al. (1995). Nonsyndromic cleft lip with or without cleft palate: evidence of linkage to BCL3 in 17

multigenerational families. Am J Hum Genet *57:* 257–272; erratum: Amos, C, Stein, J, Mulliken, JB, et al. (1996b). Nonsyndromic cleft lip with or without cleft palate: erratum. Am J Hum Genet *59:* 744.

St George-Hyslop, PH (2000). Molecular genetics of Alzheimer's disease. Biol Psychiatry *47:* 183–199.

Stoll, C, Qian, JF, Feingold, J, et al. (1992). Genetic variation in transforming growth factor alpha: possible association of BamHI polymorphism with bilateral sporadic cleft lip and palate. Am J Hum Genet *50:* 870–871.

Stoll, C, Qian, JF, Feingold, J, et al. (1993). Genetic variation in transforming growth factor alpha: possible association of BamHI polymorphism with bilateral sporadic cleft lip and palate. Hum Genet *92:* 81–82.

Swift, M, Kupper, LL, Chase, CL (1990). Effective testing of gene–disease associations. Am J Hum Genet *47:* 266–274.

Tanabe, A, Taketani, S, Endo-Ichikawa, Y, et al. (2000). Analysis of the candidate genes responsible for non-syndromic cleft lip and palate in Japanese people. Clin Sci *99:* 105–111.

Teng, J, Risch, N (1999). The relative power of family-based and case-control designs for linkage disequilibrium studies of complex human diseases II. Individual genotyping. Genome Res *9:* 234–241.

Terwilliger, JD, Ott, J (1992). A haplotype-based "haplotype relative risk" approach to detecting allelic associations. Hum Hered *42:* 337–346.

Thomson, G (1988). HLA disease associations: models for insulin dependent diabetes mellitus and the study of complex human genetic disorders. Annu Rev Genet *22:* 31–50.

Thomson, G (1995). Mapping disease genes: family-based association studies. Am J Hum Genet *57:* 487–498.

Van Dyke, D, Goldman, A, Spielman, R, Zmijewski, C (1983). Segregation of HLA in families with oral clefts: evidence against linkage between isolated cleft palate and HLA. Am J Med Genet *15:* 85–88

Van Dyke, D, Goldman, A, Spielman, R, et al. (1980). Segregation of HLA in sibs with cleft lip or cleft palate: evidence against genetic linkage. Cleft Palate Craniofac J *17:* 189–193.

Vintiner, GM, Lo, KK, Holder, SE, et al. (1993). Exclusion of candidate genes from a role in cleft lip with or without cleft palate: linkage and association studies [see comments]. J Med Genet *30:* 773–778.

Watanabe, T, Ohishi, M, Tashiro, H (1984). Population and family studies of HLA in Japanese with cleft lip and cleft palate. Cleft Palate J *21:* 293–300.

Weinberg, CR (1999). Allowing for missing parents in genetic studies of case-parent triads. Am J Hum Genet *64:* 1186–1193.

Whittemore, AS, Tu, I-P (2000). Detection of disease genes by use of family data. I. Likelihood-based theory. Am J Hum Genet *66:* 1328–1340.

Wyszynski, DF, Beaty, TH, Maestri, NE (1996). Genetics of nonsyndromic oral clefts revisited. Cleft Palate Craniofac J *33:* 406–417.

Wyszynski, DF, Maestri, NE, Lewanda, A, et al. (1997a). No evidence of linkage for cleft lip with or without cleft palate to a marker near the transforming growth factor alpha locus in two populations. Hum Hered *47:* 101–109.

Wyszynski, DF, Maestri, NE, McIntosh, I, et al. (1997b). Evidence for an association between markers on chromosome 19q and nonsyndromic cleft lip with or without cleft palate in two groups of multiplex families. Hum Genet *99:* 22–26.

21

Locating genes for oral clefts in humans

DIEGO F. WYSZYNSKI

The identification of disease genes (genes whose aberrant alleles are responsible for defined clinical syndromes) has been a major focus of human genetics over the past 30 years as a natural consequence of significant improvements in DNA technology and genetic resources. To identify genes involved in inherited disease or predispositions, two general strategies are commonly applied: positional cloning and the candidate-gene approach. In the case of positional cloning, a physical map of the target region must be developed. All genes within the mapped region are considered candidates for the disease gene and are subject to screening for mutations in constitutional DNA from patients. In the candidate-gene approach, prior knowledge of specific genes is exploited by analyzing these genes for mutations (Groden and Albertsen, 1996). A subset of genes already shown to play an important role in the development of the head, with particular relevance to the development of the lip and palate, is listed in Table 21.1. Additional growth, signaling, and transcription factors that play a role in facial development include JAGGED1, sonic hedgehog, patched, cAMP response element (CRE)–binding protein, GLI3, fibroblast growth factor receptor 1 (FGFR1), calcium/calmodulin-dependent serine protein kinase (CASK), treacle, fibroblast grown factor receptor 2 (FGFR2), distalless homeo box (DLX)5/6, and paired box gene 3 (PAX3) (Schutte and Murray, 1999).

Many traits are not associated with cytogenetically detectable chromosomal abnormalities, and in these cases, linkage analysis on family material has to be performed to determine the chromosomal localization of the underlying mutant gene. Since chromosomal anomalies and linkage analysis are the mainstays of mapping technologies, they will be detailed and illustrated with relevant studies in the orofacial field.

CHROMOSOMAL ANOMALIES TO DETERMINE THE LOCATION OF DISEASE GENES

Chromosomal anomalies present in germline DNA, such as translocations, duplications, expansions, and deletions, are found either as de novo mutations or as transmissions in ova or sperm from parents to their offspring (Groden and Albertsen, 1996; Shaffer and Lupski, 2000). De novo, apparently balanced reciprocal translocation occurs in 1:2000 births, and close to 6% of these will be associated with major congenital malformations (Warburton, 1991). In a completely ascertained cohort of cases with oral clefting, apparently balanced chromosomal rearrangements were found in 1.05% (95% confidence interval 0.98%–1.12%) of patients (FitzPatrick et al., 1994).

As of November 2000, the Mendelian Cytogenetics Network database (http://mcndb.imbg.ku.dk/) contained information on 75 breakpoints in 25 individuals with cleft palate (CP). Among these cases, there were eight bands involved in more than one case (1p31, 4q21, 6p24, 7q36, 9p13, 16q24, 17q23, and 17p25). Table 21.2 presents published translocations and inversions associated with orofacial clefting. Systematic cloning of breakpoints associated with specific non-Mendelian developmental pathologies is now feasible and being undertaken by several investigators (Wirth et al., 1999).

TABLE 21.1. *Genes Regulating Development of the Head, in Particular of the Lip and Palate**

Gene	Type	Feature	Mouse	Human	References
TGFα	GF	L/P		LD	Ardinger et al. (1989), Mitchell (1997)
END1	SF	M	KO	Linkage	Kurihara et al. (1994)
RARα	SF	P/M	TG/EXP	LD, linkage	Chenevix-Trench et al. (1992)
TGFβ	GF	L/P	KO, EXP	LD	Lidral et al. (1998), Maestri et al. (1997)
SKI	GF	L/P/M	KO, EXP		Berk et al. (1997)
MSX1	HD	L/P	KO, EXP	LD, linkage	Lidral et al. (1998), van den Boogaard et al. (2000)
DLX1/2	HD	P/M	EXP		Qiu et al. (1997)
PITX2	HD	P/M	KO, EXP	Rieger	Semina et al. (1996)
PAX9	HD	P/M	KO, EXP		Peters et al. (1998)
AP2	TF	L/P/M	KO, EXP	Linkage	Nottoli et al. (1998)
TTF2	TF	P	KO	Thyroid dysgenesis	De Felice et al. (1998), Clifton-Bligh et al. (1998)
PVRL1	PVR	L/P		PC CL/P, ectodermal dysplasia	Suzuki et al. (2000), Sozen et al. (2001)

*GF, growth factor; HD, homeodomain; SF, signaling factor; TF, transcription factor; PVR, orthologue of the gene encoding the poliovirus receptor; lip; P, palate; M, maxilla and/or mandible; KO, knockout; TG, transgene; EXP, expression; LD, linkage disequilibrium; PC, positional cloning; CL/P, cleft lip with or without cleft palate.
Source: Schutte and Murray (1999).

TABLE 21.2. *Reported Translocations and Inversions Associated with Orofacial Clefting**

Reference	BP1	BP2	De novo?	Clinical Details
Cleft lip with/without cleft palate				
Yoshiura et al. (1998)	2q11.2	19q13.3†	Familial	
Davies et al. (1998)	6p23	7q36.1	?	Bilateral CLP
Donnai et al. (1992)	6p23‡	9q22.3	Familial	Oral clefts and features of ectodermal dysplasia
Hasegawa et al. (1991)	7p11.2	9q12	Familial	Familial case ectrodactyly, ectodermal dysplasia, and CL/P
Cowchock (1989)	2q23	10p13	?	Unilateral CLP
Cowchock (1989)	10p13	14q24	Familial	Father has bilateral CLP, son has VSD
Tinning et al. (1975)	1q23	6q27	?	MR and congenital glaucoma
Masuno et al. (1997)	Xq28	16q11.2	De novo	CL, pedunculated skin masses, short stature, MR
Akita et al. (1993)	7q22.1	7q36.3	De novo	Sparse hair, CLP, bilateral ectrodactyly of hands and feet
Viljoen and Smart (1993)	6q21	13q12	?	Severe MR, ectrodactyly of both feet, bilateral microphthalmia, bilateral CLP
Ikeuchi et al. (1991)	1q31.2	7p15	De novo	CLP, hypertelorism, microtia
Cleft palate only				
Wallace et al. (1994)	7q32.1	20q13.2	?	Cataracts, ptosis, CP, thickened alveolar ridges
Conte et al. (1992)	9p21.2	11p14.2	?	Dysmorphisms and CP
Brewer et al. (1999)	2q33‡	7p21	De novo	CP and mild MR
Brewer et al. (1999)	2q33‡	11p14	De novo	CP and mild MR
Pfeiffer et al. (1973)	Yq	15p	?	CP and MR
Davies et al. (1998)	6p24	9p23	?	CP and MR
Riccardi and Holmquist (1979)	13q12	13q22	?	

*BP, breakpoint; CLP, cleft lip and palate; CP, cleft palate; VSD, ventricular septal defect; MR, mental retardation.
†Breakpoint cloned and a gene identified.
‡Breakpoint currently being cloned by collaborating laboratories.
Source: D. David FitzPatrick (personal communication).

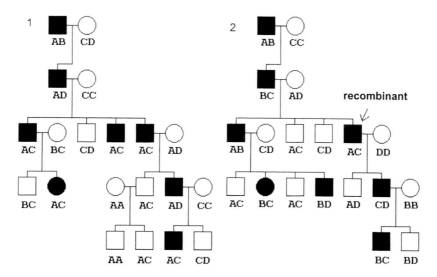

FIG. 21.1. In pedigree 1, the disease cosegregates with an *A* allele of the marker. In pedigree 2, the disease initially cosegregates with a *B* allele until there is a recombination, after which it cosegregates with a *C* allele.

LINKAGE ANALYSIS

Genetic linkage analysis refers to the ordering of genetic loci on a chromosome and to estimating genetic distances among them, where these distances are determined on the basis of a statistical phenomenon (i.e., the crossover frequency occurring between two points in a gamete) (Ott, 1999). Linkage analysis is a powerful methodology to help elucidate the underlying genetic mechanisms for inherited disorders (traits) and to find chromosomal locations for genes controlling susceptibility.

Genetic linkage is the phenomenon whereby alleles at loci close together on the same chromosome tend to be inherited together in a family, thus departing from

Mendel's law of independent assortment. The extent of linkage is a function of the distance between the two loci, which can be measured by the number of crossovers between them among the observed meioses (Xu et al., 1998).

In Figure 21.1, pedigree 1, the disease cosegregates with the *A* allele of the marker in all affected individuals. In pedigree 2, the disease cosegregates with the *B* allele of the marker. In this family, however, there is an affected individual who carries the genotype *AC*. This situation is referred to as *recombination*. A *non-recombinant* is an individual who inherited a haplotype (i.e., alleles at the marker locus and the disease locus) identical to that received by the parent from one grandparent. A *recombinant* is an individual who inherited

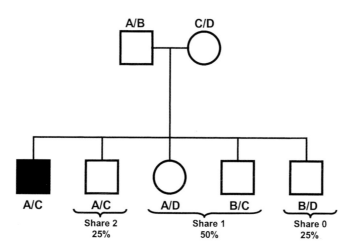

FIG. 21.2. DNA haplotypes shared by descent in siblings of affected individuals.

a haplotype not identical to that inherited from his or her grandparent. All individuals in pedigree 1 are non-recombinants, having received a paternal haplotype intact (i.e., *A* allele at the marker and disease allele at the trait locus). Individuals who inherited the *A* allele and are not affected are called *nonpenetrant*. In pedigree 2, there are two affected people who descend from the recombinant individual, both carriers of the *C* allele. This situation originated as a consequence of a genetic recombination during meiosis in the father of the recombinant individual.

The closer together two loci are, the less likely crossovers will be and the fewer recombinants will be observed. If loci are far apart or on different chromosomes, then recombination will occur by chance in 50% of meioses. The recombination fraction, also known as θ, ranges from 0 (complete linkage) to 0.5 (no linkage) and is a measure of genetic distance.

Linkage can be used to map disease genes by typing polymorphic DNA markers and seeing if their alleles cosegregate with disease among related subjects. Linkage can be studied in multiplex families, in which case the strength of evidence in favor of linkage can be measured as the log-odds or, as it is more frequently termed, the lod score. The *lod score* is the $\log_{10}$ of the ratio of the likelihood of the observed genotypes given linkage ($\theta < 0.5$) compared with the likelihood under nonlinkage (i.e., $\theta = 0.5$). Traditionally, a lod of 3.0 or more is taken as significant evidence for linkage, while a lod score of -2.0 or less is taken as evidence against linkage (Morton, 1955). These critical values correspond to 1000:1 odds for linkage and 100:1 odds against linkage, respectively, at some specified value of θ (Meyers, 1993). The actual rate of type I error (i.e., rejecting the true hypothesis that $\theta = 0.5$) using these values is very close to the conventional 5% level of significance, once the prior probability of two loci being linked is considered (Morton, 1955). Table 21.3 presents alterna-

tive approaches to judging significance when evaluating lod scores.

Xu et al. (1998) described four major advantages of lod score analysis over the genetic analysis methods described previously:

1. Statistically, it is a more powerful approach than any nonparametric method (see below).
2. It utilizes every family member's phenotypic and genotypic information.
3. It provides an estimate of the recombination fraction (genetic distance).
4. It provides a statistical test for linkage and for genetic heterogeneity.

It can be difficult to apply the lod score method to so-called complex diseases where there is non-Mendelian inheritance because the likelihood calculations require that an exact mode of inheritance and other parameters be specified and, of course, this may be unknown. When these parameters are correctly specified, linkage analysis remains a powerful approach for detecting genes. However, if the assumed genetic model is wrong, the true picture can be disguised, leading to either false-positive or false-negative evidence of linkage (Xu et al., 1998).

The MOD score analysis (also called maximized lod score), in which lod scores are maximized over several genetic parameters, not just θ, provides an alternative to lod score analysis when mode of inheritance is unknown. Simulation studies have shown that, in at least some cases, MOD score analyses have good power to detect linkage when the true mode of inheritance is complex (i.e., a single disease locus with reduced penetrance or two additive disease loci), but fairly simple genetic models are still assumed (Hodge and Elston, 1994; Greenberg et al., 1998).

A further limitation of the lod score method for the study of oral clefts is that it requires families with at

TABLE 21.3. *Proposed p Values for a Genomic Screen*

	Thomson (1994) Nominal *p* value (adjusted *p* value) [lod score]]	Lander and Kruglyak (1995) *p* value (lod score)		Haines (1998) *p* value (lod score)
Weak	3 data sets with *p* < 0.05 (0.0001) [2.9]	Suggestive	0.0007 (2.2)	Interesting	0.03 (1.0)
Moderate	2 data sets with *p* < 0.01 (0.0001) [3.0]	Significant	0.00002 (3.6)	Very interesting	0.0009 (2.0)
Strong	1 data set with *p* < 0.001 (0.001) [4.1]	Highly significant	0.0000003 (5.4)	Provisional linkage Confirmed linkage	0.00003 (3.0) 0.0000008 (4.0) (from at least 2 independent data sets)

Source: Haines (1998).

least two available affected individuals and DNA from both affected and unaffected family members. As most individuals with nonsyndromic cleft lip with or without cleft palate (CL/P) and CP do not have any family history of clefting, it is difficult to identify families that are suitable for lod score analyses. Hence, this approach is limited to investigators who have access to very large patient cohorts or who participate in multicenter collaborations (Mitchell et al., 2002).

SIB-PAIR METHODS OF ANALYSIS

An alternative approach to the lod score method is to examine allele sharing between pairs of affected relatives, and the simplest example of this is the sib-pair method. This approach was first described by Penrose (1935), who reasoned that if linkage existed, it would be reflected in the nonrandom association of two traits (i.e., a disease and a marker or two markers) in independent pairs of sibs.

In the absence of linkage between the unknown susceptibility locus and the marker locus, full sibs are expected to share two alleles at any marker 25% of the time, one allele 50% of the time, and zero alleles 25% of the time. Some terminology should be explained first. Two alleles are said to be *identical by state* (IBS) if they cannot be distinguished by means of a particular method of detection (Goldgar, 1998). *Identity by descent* (IBD), however, depends not only on whether the alleles appear the same but also on whether they were derived or inherited from a common ancestor (Goldgar, 1998). While IBD alleles must also be IBS, the converse is not necessarily true. Table 21.4 shows the expected proportion of alleles IBD for a number of other common relationships. Figure 21.2 illustrates the mating of two individuals with genotypes A/B and C/D. The proband carries the genotype A/C. He shares by descent both alleles with the first sibling, one allele with the following two sibs, and no alleles with his youngest sib, in perfect agreement with Mendelian expectation. If the marker is linked to the disease gene, however, alleles will be shared between affected sib pairs more often than expected. If the parents are genotyped, the inheritance of the marker alleles can be studied directly (IBD analysis). If the parents are unavailable, one can use population allele frequencies to test for increased allele sharing (IBS analysis). The strength of evidence in favor of linkage can be given by a χ^2 statistic or by a maximum likelihood score, the latter being on the same scale as a lod score. These allele-sharing statistics are commonly nonparametric approaches, primarily because no specific assumptions have been made about the mode of inheritance.

Nonparameteric Linkage Analysis

The nonparametric linkage (NPL) statistic is a measure of allele sharing among affected individuals within a pedigree. Introduced in 1996 by Kruglyak et al. (1996), this method is the only affected relative pair test that considers all affected relatives simultaneously, rather than as a combination of all possible pairs. This approach tests for excess allele sharing, however, as done in affected sib-pair analysis. This means that, e.g., if five affected individuals in a pedigree share the same allele IBD, this information should carry more weight than if each of the 15 possible pairs in the same pedigree shared some allele IBD but not necessarily the same allele.

While the major disadvantage of using the NPL method is that it is limited to relatively small and simple pedigrees, the NPL statistic can be used in several situations:

1. When pedigrees of moderate size are available
2. When many relatives other than siblings are available for a complex trait where the exact model of inheritance is unknown
3. When a large number of linked markers are being examined simultaneously (in this case, the NPL approach can be readily extended to multipoint analysis)

Relative to the lod score method, the main advantage of allele-sharing methods is that they provide valid tests of linkage without the need of specifying details of the mode of inheritance for the phenotype of inter-

TABLE 21.4. *Expected Percentage of Affected Pairs Showing 0, 1, or 2 Alleles Identical by Descent (IBD) at a Marker Locus if No Linkage Is Present*

Pair Type	Alleles IBD		
	0	1	2
Monozygotic twins	0	0	100
Siblings	25	50	25
Parent–child	0	100	0
Grandparent–grandchild	50	50	0
Half-siblings	50	50	0
Uncle–nephew, etc.	50	50	0
Cousins	75	25	0
Double first cousins	62	38	0

est. The main disadvantage of this method is that it can require a very large number (i.e., several hundred) of affected relative pairs (Mitchell et al., 2002).

The allele-sharing methods require DNA from pairs of affected relatives. To establish IBD, DNA is also required from additional relatives (e.g., for affected sib pairs, parental DNA samples are also required). As the recurrence rates for nonsyndromic CL/P and CP are relatively low, the accumulation of an adequate sample of affected relatives is likely to be restricted to investigators who have access to large patient cohorts or who participate in multicenter collaborations.

MULTIPOINT LINKAGE ANALYSIS

The term *multipoint mapping* refers to linkage analysis of more than two loci at a time. Considering multiple loci simultaneously gives substantial increases in information for both estimating the recombination fraction and establishing the order of linked loci (Meyers, 1993). Thus, linkage results are less sensitive to the uninformative or missing genotype at any single marker. Additionally, the multipoint mapping approach may be very useful to pinpoint the disease gene location when fine mapping. This technique may be used when applying the lod score method as well as the NPL statistic (Kruglyak and Lander, 1995), for both qualitative and quantitative traits, and in more general analyses of extended pedigrees (Kruglyak et al., 1996).

LINKAGE ANALYSIS OF NONSYNDROMIC ORAL CLEFTS

For the past 20 years, several research groups have evaluated multiplex families with CL/P using linkage analysis. The results, however, remain conflicting and nondefinitive. Table 21.5 presents some features of published linkage studies. No single locus has been shown conclusively to be etiologically related to nonsyndromic oral clefting in multiple studies.

It is widely accepted that nonsyndromic oral clefts are complex birth defects characterized by an uncertain mode of inheritance, incomplete penetrance, and heterogeneity both within and among populations (Maestri et al., 1997). Other non-mutually exclusive circumstances may produce conflicting linkage results as well:

- Clinical and etiological heterogeneity. Difference in clinical characteristics of oral cleft patients between studies could be a cause of discrepant linkage results if genetic markers are linked with different trait loci. A relatively large proportion of individuals with oral clefting have an underlying genetic or developmental syndrome (Jones, 1988; Gorlin, 1990; Saal, 1998; Stoll et al., 2000). Thus, it is necessary to distinguish between individuals with syndromic and nonsyndromic clefts when conducting studies of potential risk factors. Similarly, some oral clefts may be due to maternal exposures to teratogens. Identification of these cases is a challenge when conducting population-based research since both family history information and direct physical examination of affected individuals are needed and often unavailable (Mitchell et al., 2002).
- Ethnic variability. As shown by Wyszynski et al. (1997b) and Maestri et al. (1997), ethnic background may act as an effect modifier in the relationship between genetic polymorphisms and oral clefting.
- Insufficient statistical power. Attaining an adequate sample size to conduct definitive linkage analysis may be difficult in some populations. This situation is particularly critical if the genetic marker under study is not highly informative. An example is BCL3, on chromosome 19q13, which has a heterozygosity of only 0.47 (Wyszynski et al., 1997b). Also, large sample sizes are required if the contribution of the susceptibility locus to familial clustering of the trait is small, if oral clefts are determined by several susceptibility loci, and if the researcher is evaluating a modifier rather than a major gene. Results of analyses performed using an insufficient sample may produce ambiguous results (i.e., neither for nor against evidence of linkage).

In spite of these limitations and applying a biologically driven "complex disease approach," candidate genes are now used to test for interactions among genes and between genes and selected environmental factors (see Chapter 23). Sophisticated statistical methods to distinguish maternal genotypic effects from those of the fetus have been developed as well (Weinberg et al., 1998; Wilcox et al., 1998; Weinberg, 1999a,b; Wyszynski and Diehl, 2001). Finally, the growing number of robust statistical methods of linkage analysis incorporated in user-friendly computer software packages will allow researchers to overcome or at least minimize some of the limitations mentioned above.

TABLE 21.5. Results of Linkage Analyses on Candidate Genes for Nonsyndromic Cleft Lip and Cleft Palate

Chromosome Region	Locus Name	Results*	Population	References
1p36	Multipoint	MLS = 1.34	92 UK affected sib pairs	Prescott et al. (2000)
1q21	D1S104	$Z = 0.09$ at $\theta = 0.40$	3 European Caucasian families	Pierpont et al. (1995)
1q32	D1S245	$Z < -2$ for all markers (multipoint)	19 Swedish families	Wong et al. (2000)
	D1S471			
	D1S491			
	D1S3753			
	D1S205			
2p13	TGF-α	$Z = -2.1$ at $\theta = 0$	12 Families, ethnicity not specified	Hecht et al. (1993)
	TGF-α	$Z = 0.448$ at $\theta = 0$	8 Families, ethnicity not specified	Vintiner et al. (1993)
	TGF-α	$Z = 0.13$ at $\theta = 0.2$	14 West Bengal Indian families	Field et al. (1994)
	TGF-α	$Z = 0.22$ at $\theta = 0.3$	40 Caucasian Italian families	Scapoli et al. (1999)
	D2S443	$Z = 0.14$ at $\theta = 0.05$	32 U.S families	Wyszynski et al. (1997a)
	D2S443	$Z = -0.008$ at $\theta = 0.05$	22 Mexican families	Wyszynski et al. (1997a)
	D2S380	$Z = 1.15$ at $\theta = 0.3$	38 Italian Caucasian families	Pezzetti et al. (1998)
	D2S378	$Z = 0.001$	46 Italian Caucasian families	Scapoli et al. (1999)
	D2S123	$Z < -2$ for all markers (multipoint)	19 Swedish families	Wong et al. (2000)
	D2S378			
	D2S337			
	D2S380			
2q37	Multipoint	MLS = 0.66	92 UK affected sib pairs	Prescott et al. (2000)
	PAX3	$Z = -0.03$ at $\theta = 0.40$	3 European Caucasian families	Pierpont et al. (1995)
	Multipoint	MLS = 0.9	92 UK affected sib pairs	Prescott et al. (2000)
4q31	D4S175	$Z = 2.27$ at $\theta = 0$	1 U.S. Caucasian family	Beiraghi et al. (1994)
	D4S175	$Z = -0.64$ at $\theta = 0$	3 European Caucasian families	Pierpont et al. (1995)
6p23-24	F13A	$Z = 2.016$ at $\theta = 0.01$ for males	49 Danish Caucasian families	Eiberg et al. (1987)
	F13A	$Z = 0.224$ at $\theta = 0.001$	8 British Caucasian families	Vintiner et al. (1993)
	F13A	$Z = -0.29$ at $\theta = 0.3$	9 Families, different ethnic groups	Hecht et al. (1993)
	F13A	$Z \sim 1$ (multipoint)	19 Swedish families	Wong et al. (2000)
	D6S89	$Z = 4.48$ at $\theta = 0.001$	14 Families from northeastern Italy	Carinci et al. (1995)
	D6S89	$Z = -0.41$ at $\theta = 0.3$	12 Families, different ethnic groups	Hecht et al. (1993)
	D6S89	$Z < -2$ at $\theta < 0.3$	33 Families, different ethnic groups	Blanton et al. (1996)
	D6S259	$Z = 3.6$ at 1 cM, $\alpha = 0.6$	38 Italian Caucasian families	Scapoli et al. (1997)
	D6S259	$Z = 2.1$ at $\theta = 0.098$	46 Italian Caucasian families	Scapoli et al. (1999)
	D6S89+F13A	$Z = 2.03$ at $\theta = 0.001$ for males	14 Families from northeastern Italy	Carinci et al. (1995)
	D6S89+EDN1	$Z = 2.31$ at $\theta = 0.1$	14 Families from northeastern Italy	Carinci et al. (1995)
	EDN1	$Z < 1$ (multipoint)	19 Swedish families	Wong et al. (2000)

(continued)

TABLE 21.5. *Results of Linkage Analyses on Candidate Genes for Nonsyndromic Cleft Lip and Cleft Palate (continued)*

Chromosome Region	Locus Name	Population	Results*	References
	Multipoint	92 UK affected sib pairs	MLS = 1.34	Prescott et al. (2000)
6p23+2p13	D6S259–D2S378	30 Italian Caucasian families	$Z = 3.79$ at $\theta = 0.01$	Pezzetti et al. (1998)
6p23+19q13	D6S89–not stated	15 Families linked to 19q13.1	$Z = -0.835$ at $\theta = 0.3$	Blanton et al. (1996)
6p25	Multipoint	92 UK affected sib pairs	MLS = 1.50	Prescott et al. (2000)
11p12-q14	Multipoint	92 UK affected sib pairs	MLS = 2.09	Prescott et al. (2000)
16p13	Multipoint	92 UK affected sib pairs	MLS = 1.65	Prescott et al. (2000)
17q21	RAR-α	8 British Caucasian families	$Z = 0.048$ at $\theta = 0.05$	Vintiner et al. (1993)
	RAR-α	17 Families, different ethnic groups	$Z = 1.14$ at $\theta = 0$	Stein et al. (1995)
	D17S579	8 West Bengal Indian families	$Z = -2$ at $\theta < 0.1$	Shaw et al. (1993)
19q13	BCL3	17 Families, different ethnic groups	$Z = 7.00$ at $\theta = 0$ (multipoint)	Stein et al. (1995)
	BCL3	30 U.S. and 11 Mexican families	$Z = 0.89$ at $\theta = 0.2$	Wyszynski et al. (1997b)
	BCL3	38 Italian Caucasian families	$Z = 0.23$ at $\theta = 0.3$	Martinelli et al. (1998)
	BCL3	19 Swedish families	$Z < 1$ (multipoint)	Wong et al. (2000)
22q11.2	D22S156	3 European Caucasian families	$Z = -0.04$ at $\theta = 0.40$	Pierpont et al. (1995)
	D22S264	3 European Caucasian families	$Z = 0.43$ at $\theta = 0.20$	Pierpont et al. (1995)
Xcen	Multipoint	92 UK affected sib pairs	MLS = 2.89	Prescott et al. (2000)

*MLS, Maximum lod score from sib-pair analysis; Z, highest lod score from linkage analysis; θ, recombination fraction.

REFERENCES

Akita, S, Kuratomi, H, Abe, K, et al. (1993). EC syndrome in a girl with paracentric inversion (7)(q22.1;q36.3). Clin Dysmorphol 2: 62–67.

Ardinger, HH, Buetow, KH, Bell, GI, et al. (1989). Association of genetic variation of the transforming growth factor-alpha gene with cleft lip and palate. Am J Hum Genet 45: 348–353.

Beiraghi, S, Foroud, T, Diouhy, S, et al. (1994). Possible localization of a major gene for cleft lip and palate to 4q. Clin Genet 46: 255–256.

Berk, M, Desai, SY, Heyman, HC, Colmenares, C (1997). Mice lacking the ski proto-oncogene have defects in neurulation, craniofacial patterning, and skeletal muscle development. Genes Dev 11: 2029–2039.

Blanton, SH, Crowder, E, Malcolm, S, et al. (1996). Exclusion of linkage between cleft lip with or without cleft palate and markers on chromosomes 4 and 6. Am J Hum Genet 58: 239–241.

Brewer, CM, Leek, JP, Green, AJ, et al. (1999). A locus for isolated cleft palate, located on human chromosome 2q32. Am J Hum Genet 65: 387–396.

Carinci, F, Pezzetti, F, Scapoli, L, et al. (1995). Nonsyndromic cleft lip and palate: evidence of linkage to a microsatellite marker on 6p23. Am J Hum Genet 56: 337–339.

Chenevix-Trench, G, Jones, K, Green, AC, et al. (1992). Cleft lip with or without cleft palate: associations with transforming growth factor alpha and retinoic acid receptor loci. Am J Hum Genet 51: 1377–1385.

Clifton-Bligh, RJ, Wentworth, JM, Heinz, P, et al. Mutation of the gene encoding human TTF-2 associated with thyroid agenesis, cleft palate and choanal atresia. Nat Genet 19: 399–401.

Conte, RA, Sayegh, SE, Verma, RS (1992). An apparent balanced translocation [t(9;11)(p21.2;p14.2)] in a neonate with dysmorphic features. Ann Genet 35: 164–165.

Cowchock, S (1989). Apparently balanced chromosome translocations and midline defects. Am J Med Genet 33: 424.

Davies, AF, Imaizumi, K, Mirza, G, et al. (1998). Further evidence for the involvement of human chromosome 6p24 in the aetiology of orofacial clefting. J Med Genet 35: 857–861.

De Felice, M, Ovitt, C, Biffali, E, et al. (1998). A mouse model for hereditary thyroid dysgenesis and cleft palate. Nat Genet 19: 395–398.

Donnai, D, Heather, LJ, Sinclair, P, et al. (1992). Association of autosomal dominant cleft lip and palate and translocation 6p23;9q22.3. Clin Dysmorphol 1: 89–97.

Eiberg, H, Bixler, D, Nielsen, LS, et al. (1987). Suggestion of linkage of a major locus for nonsyndromic orofacial cleft with F13A and tentative assignment to chromosome 6. Clin Genet 32: 129–132.

FitzPatrick, DR, Raine, PA, Boorman, JG (1994). Facial clefts in the west of Scotland in the period 1980–1984: epidemiology and genetic diagnoses. J Med Genet 31: 126–129.

Goldgar, DE (1998). Sib pair analysis. In: Approaches to Gene Mapping in Complex Human Diseases, edited by JL Haines and MA Pericak-Vance. New York: Wiley-Liss, pp. 273–303.

Gorlin, RJ (1990). Syndromes of the Head and Neck. New York: Oxford University Press.

Greenberg, DA, Abrue, P, Hodge, SE (1998). The power to detect linkage in complex disease by means of simple LOD-score analyses. Am J Hum Genet 63: 870–879.

Groden, J, Albertsen, H (1996). Molecular approaches to the identification of disease genes. In: The Genetics of Asthma, edited by SB Liggett and DA Meyers. New York: Marcel Dekker, pp. 281–317.

Haines, JH (1998a). Affected relative pair analysis. In: Approaches to Gene Mapping in Complex Human Diseases, edited by JL Haines and MA Pericak-Vance. New York: Wiley-Liss, pp. 305–321.

Haines, JH (1998b). Genomic screening. In: Approaches to Gene Mapping in Complex Human Diseases, edited by JL Haines and MA Pericak-Vance. New York: Wiley-Liss, pp. 243–251.

Hasegawa, T, Hasegawa, Y, Asamura, S, et al. (1991). EEC syndrome (ectrodactyly, ectodermal dysplasia and cleft lip/palate) with a balanced reciprocal translocation between 7q11.21 and 9p12 (or 7p11.2 and 9q12) in three generations. Clin Genet 40: 202–206.

Hecht, JT, Wang, Y, Connor, B, et al. (1993). Nonsyndromic cleft lip and palate: no evidence of linkage to HLA or factor 13A. Am J Hum Genet 52: 1230–1233.

Hodge, SE, Elston, RC (1994). Lods, wrods and mods: the interpretation of lod scores calculated under different models. Genet Epidemiol 11: 329–342.

Ikeuchi, T, Motohashi, N, Yamamoto, K, Kuroda, T (1991). Refined determination of breakpoints of the translocation t(1;7) associated with signs of HMC syndrome. Jinrui Idengaku Zasshi 36: 155–158.

Jones, MC (1988). Etiology of facial clefts: prospective evaluation of 428 patients. Cleft Palate Craniofac J 25: 16–20.

Kruglyak, L, Daly, MJ, Reeve-Daly, M, Lander, ES (1996). Parametric and nonparametric linkage analysis: a unified multipoint approach. Am J Hum Genet 58: 1347–1363.

Kruglyak, L, Lander, ES (1995). Complete multipoint sib-pair analysis of qualitative and quantitative traits. Am J Hum Genet 57: 439–454.

Kurihara, Y, Kurihara, H, Suzuki, H, et al. (1994). Elevated blood pressure and craniofacial anomalies in mice deficient in endothelin-1. Nature 368: 703–710.

Lander, ES, Kruglyak, L (1995). Genetic dissection of complex traits: guidelines for interpreting and reporting linkage results. Nat Genet 11: 241.

Lidral, AC, Romitti, PA, Basart, AM, et al. (1998). Association of MSX1 and TGFB3 with nonsyndromic clefting in humans. Am J Hum Genet 63: 557–568.

Maestri, NE, Beaty, TH, Hetmanski, J, et al. (1997). Application of transmission disequilibrium tests to nonsyndromic oral clefts: including candidate genes and environmental exposures in the models. Am J Med Genet 73: 337–344.

Martinelli, M, Scapoli, L, Pezzetti, F, et al. (1998). Suggestive linkage between markers on chromosome 19q13.2 and nonsyndromic familial orofacial cleft malformation. Genomics 51: 177–181.

Masuno, M, Imaizumi, K, Fukushima, Y, et al. (1997). Median cleft of upper lip and pedunculated skin masses associated with de novo reciprocal translocation 46,X,t(X;16)(q28;q11.2). J Med Genet 34: 952–954.

Meyers, DA (1993). Genetic approaches to familial aggregation. III. Linkage analysis. In: Fundamentals of Genetic Epidemiology, edited by MJ Khoury, TH Beaty, and BH Cohen. New York: Oxford University Press, pp. 284–311.

Mitchell, LE (1997). Transforming growth factor alpha locus and nonsyndromic cleft lip with or without cleft palate: a reappraisal. Genet Epidemiol 14: 231–240.

Mitchell, LE, Beaty, TH, Lidral, AC, et al. (2002). Guidelines for the design and analysis of studies of nonsyndromic cleft lip and cleft palate in humans: summary report from a Workshop of the International Consortium for Oral Clefts Genetics. Cleft Palate Craniofac J 39: 93–100.

Morton, NE (1955). Sequential tests for the detection of linkage. Am J Hum Genet 7: 277–318.

Nottoli, T, Hagopian-Donaldson, S, Zhang, J, et al. (1998). AP-2-null cells disrupt morphogenesis of the eye, face, and limbs in chimeric mice. Proc Natl Acad Sci USA 95: 13714–13719.

Ott, J (1999). *Analysis of Human Genetic Linkage,* 3rd ed. Baltimore: Johns Hopkins University Press.

Penrose, LS (1935). The detection of autosomal linkage in data which consists of pairs of brothers and sisters of unspecified parentage. Ann Eugen 6: 133–138.

Peters, H, Neubuser, A, Kratochwil, K, Balling, R (1998). Pax9-deficient mice lack pharyngeal pouch derivatives and teeth and exhibit craniofacial and limb anomalies. Genes Dev 12: 2735–2747.

Pezzetti, F, Scapoli, L, Martinelli, M, et al. (1998). A locus in 2p13-p14 (OFC2), in addition to that mapped in 6p23, is involved in nonsyndromic familial orofacial cleft malformation. Genomics 50: 299–305.

Pfeiffer, RA, Bier, L, Majewski, F, Rager, K (1973). De novo translocation t(Yq−; 15p+) in a malformed boy. Humangenetik 19: 349–352.

Pierpont, JW, Storm, AL, Erickson, RP, et al. (1995). Lack of linkage of apparently dominant cleft lip (palate) to two candidate chromosomal regions. J Craniofac Genet Dev Biol 15: 66–71.

Prescott, NJ, Lees, MM, Winter, RM, Malcolm, S (2000). Identification of susceptibility loci for nonsyndromic cleft lip with or without cleft palate in a two stage genome scan of affected sib-pairs. Hum Genet 106: 345–350.

Qiu, M, Bulfone, A, Ghattas, I, et al. (1997). Role of the *Dlx* homeobox genes in proximodistal patterning of the branchial arches: mutations of *Dlx-1, Dlx-2,* and *Dlx-1* and *-2* alter morphogenesis of proximal skeletal and soft tissue structures derived from the first and second arches. Dev Biol 185: 165–184.

Riccardi, VM, Holmquist, GP (1979). De novo 13q paracentric inversion in a boy with cleft palate and mental retardation. Hum Genet 52: 211–215.

Saal, HM (1998). Syndromes and malformations associated with cleft lip with or without cleft palate. Am J Hum Genet 63S: A118.

Scapoli, C, Collins, A, Martinelli, M, et al. (1999). Combined segregation and linkage analysis of nonsyndromic orofacial cleft in two candidate regions. Ann Hum Genet 63: 17–25.

Scapoli, L, Pezzetti, F, Carinci, F, et al. (1997). Evidence of linkage to 6p23 and genetic heterogeneity in nonsyndromic cleft lip with or without cleft palate. Genomics 43: 216–220.

Schutte, BC, Murray, JC (1999). The many faces and factors of orofacial clefts. Hum Mol Genet 8: 1853–1859.

Semina, EV, Reiter, R, Leysens, NJ, et al. (1996). Cloning and characterization of a novel bicoid-related homeobox transcriptor factor gene, *RIEG*, involved in Rieger syndrome. Nat Genet 14: 392–399.

Shaffer, LG, Lupski, JR (2000). Molecular mechanisms for constitutional chromosomal rearrangements in humans. Annu Rev Genet 34: 297–329.

Shaw, D, Ray, A, Marazita, M, Field, L (1993). Further evidence of a relationship between the retinoic acid receptor alpha locus and nonsyndromic cleft lip with or without cleft palate (CL +/− P). Am J Hum Genet 53: 1156–1157.

Sozen, MA, Suzuki, K, Tolarova, MM, et al. (2001). Mutation of PVRL1 is associated with sporadic, non-syndromic cleft lip/palate in northern Venezuela. Nat Genet 29: 141–142.

Stein, J, Mulliken, JB, Stal, S, et al. (1995). Nonsyndromic cleft lip with or without cleft palate: evidence of linkage to BCL3 in 17 multigenerational families. Am J Hum Genet 57: 257–272.

Stoll, C, Alembik, Y, Dott, B, Roth, MP (2000). Associated malformations in cases with oral clefts. Cleft Palate Craniofac J 37: 41–47.

Suzuki, K, Hu, D, Bustos, T, et al. (2000). Mutations of PVRL1, encoding a cell–cell adhesion molecule/herpesvirus receptor, in cleft lip/palate-ectodermal dysplasia. Nat Genet 25: 427–430.

Thomson, G (1994). Identifying complex disease genes: progress and paradigms. Nat Genet 8: 189–194.

Tinning, S, Jacobsen, P, Mikkelsen, M (1975). A 1;6 translocation associated with congenital glaucoma and cleft lip and palate. Hum Hered 25: 453–460.

van den Boogaard, MJ, Dorland, M, Beemer, FA, van Amstel, HK (2000). *MSX1* mutation is associated with orofacial clefting and tooth agenesis in humans. Nat Genet 24: 342–343.

Viljoen, DL, Smart, R (1993). Split-foot anomaly, microphthalmia, cleft-lip and cleft-palate, and mental retardation associated with a chromosome 6;13 translocation. Clin Dysmorphol 2: 274–277.

Vintiner, GM, Lo, KK, Holder, SE, et al. (1993). Exclusion of candidate genes from a role in cleft lip with or without cleft palate: linkage and association studies. J Med Genet 30: 773–778.

Wallace, M, Zori, RT, Alley, T, et al. (1994). Smith-Lemli-Opitz syndrome in a female with a de novo, balanced translocation involving 7q32: probable disruption of an SLOS gene. Am J Med Genet 50: 368–374.

Warburton, D (1991). De novo balanced chromosome rearrangements and extra marker chromosomes identified at prenatal diagnosis: clinical significance and distribution of breakpoints. Am J Hum Genet 49: 995–1013.

Weinberg, CR (1999a). Allowing for missing parents in genetic studies of case-parent triads. Am J Hum Genet 64: 1186–1193.

Weinberg, CR (1999b). Methods for detection of parent-of-origin effects in genetic studies of case-parent triads. Am J Hum Genet 65: 229–235.

Weinberg, CR, Wilcox, AJ, Lie, RT (1998). A log-linear approach to case-parent-triad data: assessing effects of disease genes that act either directly or through maternal effects and that may be subject to parental imprinting. Am J Hum Genet 62: 969–978.

Wilcox, AJ, Weinberg, CR, Lie, RT (1998). Distinguishing the effects of maternal and offspring genes through studies of "case-parent triads." Am J Epidemiol 148: 893–901.

Wirth, J, Northwang, HG, van der Maarel, S, et al. (1999). Systematic characterization of disease associated balanced chromosomal rearrangements by FISH: cytogenetically and genetically anchored YACs identify microdeletions and candidate regions for mental retardation genes. J Med Genet 36: 271–278.

Wong, FK, Hagberg, C, Karsten, A, et al. (2000). Linkage analysis of candidate regions in Swedish nonsyndromic cleft lip with or without cleft palate families. Cleft Palate Craniofac J 37: 357–62.

Wyszynski, DF, Diehl, SR (2001). The mother-only method (MOM) to detect maternal gene–environment interactions. Paediatr Perinat Epidemiol 15: 317–318.

Wyszynski, DF, Maestri, N, Lewanda, AF, et al. (1997a). No evidence of linkage for cleft lip with or without cleft palate to a marker near the transforming growth factor alpha locus in two populations. Hum Hered 47: 101–109.

Wyszynski, DF, Maestri, N, McIntosh, I, et al. (1997b). Evidence for an association between markers on chromosome 19q and nonsyndromic cleft lip with or without cleft palate in two groups of multiplex families. Hum Genet 99: 22–26.

Xu, J, Meyers, DA, Pericak-Vance, MA (1998). Lod score analysis. In: *Approaches to Gene Mapping in Complex Human Diseases,* edited by JL Haines and MA Pericak-Vance. New York: Wiley-Liss, pp. 253–272.

Yoshiura, K, Machida, J, Daack-Hirsch, S, et al. (1998). Characterization of a novel gene disrupted by a balanced chromosomal translocation t(2;19)(q11.2;q13.3) in a family with cleft lip and palate. Genomics 1: 231–240.

22

Mapping studies in animal models

DIANA M. JURILOFF

Orofacial clefting has been observed sporadically in a variety of vertebrates, including monkeys (Stills and Bullock, 1981), gorillas (Siebert et al., 1998), cattle (Swartz et al., 1982), cats (Loevy and Feynes, 1968), dogs (Dreyer and Preston, 1974), and chickens (Juriloff and Roberts, 1975), but genetic studies have usually been limited. The most advanced animal models for genetic analysis and linkage mapping of orofacial defects are laboratory mice, where the extensive resources of specialized strains and crosses, spontaneous and targeted mutations, polymorphic markers, and well-developed linkage and physical maps can be used to identify genes and their effects on orofacial development. Conservation of genes and linkage relationships between mice and humans is well documented, and the chromosomal location of a gene in humans can often be predicted from its genetic map position in mice. Development of the orofacial complex is very similar between mouse and human embryos, and much of the understanding of developmental mechanisms in humans has been inferred from mice (Diewert and Wang, 1992).

Highly penetrant Mendelian defects of craniofacial development are relatively easily mapped in both mice and humans. The most common orofacial clefting in humans does not follow Mendelian transmission ratios, however, and is clearly genetically complex and not well understood (Mitchell and Risch, 1992; Schutte and Murray, 1999). Mapping and identification of mouse genes that participate in genetically complex ("multifactorial") causes of orofacial clefting will lead to knowledge of the gene-regulatory pathways important to nonsyndromic orofacial clefting and will identify candidate pathways, as well as candidate genes, for examination in studies of human genetic risk factors. The emphasis of this chapter is on the results of approaches to mapping the genetic components of the multifactorial nonsyndromic class of orofacial defects in mice.

DEVELOPMENTAL AND GENETIC INDEPENDENCE OF TYPES OF OROFACIAL CLEFTS IN MICE

Cleft lip with or without cleft palate (CL/P), isolated cleft palate (CP), and median cleft lip (MCL) are developmentally distinct malformations in mice. Cleft lip with or without cleft palate arises on embryonic days 10 to 11 of gestation, from the failure of a mesenchymal bridge to fuse the embryonic maxillary prominence with the lateral nasal prominence internally and with the lateral and medial prominences on the external surface of the prospective upper lip (Diewert and Wang, 1992; Millicovsky et al., 1982). The result is a unilateral or bilateral cleft between the maxilla and the premaxilla, extending into the nostril (see Figs. 1.3, 1.6, 1.7, and 1.12 in this volume). Cleft palate arises later, on days 14 to 16 of gestation in mice, from a failure of outgrowth of the palatal shelves from the medial aspect of the maxillary prominence or from a failure of the palatal shelves to elevate to a horizontal orientation to contact in the midline and fuse, resulting in a failure to form the roof of the mouth (see Fig. 2.1 in this volume). The cleft palate that usually accompanies cleft lip (CL) has been observed to originate in mechanical obstruction of palatal shelf elevation by the tongue, due to alterations in the shape of the oral cavity caused by the CL, and thus is secondary to the CL (Trasler and Fraser, 1963; Pourtois, 1967). Median cleft lip arises on gestational days 9 to 11 in mice, from

TABLE 22.1. *Genetic Causes of Cleft Lip with or without Cleft Palate in Mice*

Type of Liability	Loci	Location	Candidate Genes	Human Homologous Location*
Nonsyndromic multifactorial	*clf1*	Chr 11†	*Dlx3, Dlx7, Itgb3,* and others	17q21
	clf2	Chr 13‡	*Msx2, Madh5,* and others	Fragmented: 5q22, 5p, 9q22
Syndromic Mendelian	*Dc*	Chr 19	—	11q
	Tw	Chr 18	—	18q
	AP-2 chimera	Chr 13	Gene known: *Tcfap2a*	6p
	Xt^{bph}	Chr 13	Gene known: *Gli3*	7p13
	Lgl	Chr 12	—	7q
Liability to phenytoin-induced CL/P	*H2* complex	Chr 17	*H2*	6p21
	Nat1 region	Chr 8	*Nat1*	8p
	"A" liability loci 1–4§	Chr 3, 4, 7, 19	Many	4q, 9p, 11q/15q, 9q/11q
	"B" liability loci 5–8§	Chr 5, 8, 12, 12	Many	4p, 4q, 2p, 14q

*From the Mouse Genome Database (www.informatics.jax.org), 2001.
†Confirmed in two independent data sets.
‡Significant at $p < 0.05$ after correction for multiple tests of genome screen.
§Type I error reported as $p < 0.05$ was not corrected for the multiple tests of a genome screen; assuming that there are about 30 independent linkage tests in the mouse genome, the Bonferroni correction indicates that the type I error associated with each locus is $1.0 > p > 0.12$.

a midline defect of outgrowth of the mesenchyme between and merging with the medial prominences, leading to a midline cleft of the premaxilla.

Median CL and CL/P are different traits genetically as well as developmentally. Median CL occurs in syndromic mutants that do not have CL/P, such as patch (*Ph*) (Gruneberg and Truslove, 1960), doublefoot (*Dbf*) (Lyon et al., 1996), the *Rara* dominant-negative mutation (Damm et al., 1993), and the *MSX2* transgene (Winograd et al., 1997). Also, CL/P is usually genetically distinct from CP; they are caused by mutations at different loci, the exception being the twirler (*Tw*) syndromic mutant, where CL/P and CP can occur as alternative phenotypes (Lyon, 1958). Only five Mendelian mutations are known that cause CL/P, and all are syndromic (Table 22.1). Only a few Mendelian mutations cause nonsyndromic CP (Table 22.2), but numerous spontaneous and gene-knockout mutations cause syndromes that include CP; these will not be reviewed in detail. This pattern parallels the genetics of human orofacial clefting syndromes, and it is likely that the syndromic mouse mutants are homologs of human syndromes.

Nonsyndromic CL/P occurs spontaneously in some mouse strains, and nonsyndromic CP occurs spontaneously at unusually high frequencies in other strains (Table 22.3). This pattern indicates that they are genetically independent traits. The genetics and linkage mapping of CL/P and CP therefore will be discussed separately.

CLEFT LIP WITH OR WITHOUT CLEFT PALATE

Nonsyndromic

Occurrence Only in A-Strain Lineages. Spontaneous CL/P, i.e., not induced by teratogens, is very rare in most strains of mice. All stocks with frequent occurrence of spontaneous nonsyndromic CL/P trace to a single genetic origin, a closely related set of strains, referred to as the "A" strains. These strains share at least 30 generations of brother–sister inbreeding before their dispersion to different laboratories about 70 years ago and subsequent designation as substrains, and they are expected to be identical at nearly all of their loci.

All A strains examined produce CL/P at relatively high frequencies in their fetuses or newborns (Kalter, 1979; Juriloff, 1982). The frequency of CL/P varies among these strains. The A/J strain, with about 10% CL/P, was used in most genetic and developmental studies of CL/P until about 1980, when the A/WySnJ strain was discovered to have a higher risk of CL/P, 20% to 30% (Juriloff, 1982), and became the A strain of choice for CL/P studies. In the 1970s, outcrosses of the A/J strain, with subsequent selection for production of CL/P during inbreeding of descendants, led to two new stocks that also produced CL/P, the CL/Fr strain, with 20% to 25% CL/P in the offspring (Juriloff and Fraser, 1980), and the "L line," with about 10% CL/P (Trasler and Trasler, 1984).

An outcross of the A/J strain, to the normal C57BL/6J strain, was also the origin of a new set of re-

TABLE 22.2. *Genetic Causes of Liability to Nonsyndromic Cleft Palate (CP) in Mice*

Type of Liability	Loci	Location	Candidate Genes	Human Homologous Location*
Genetic CP	*Lhx8*	Chr 3	Gene known	—
	Gad1 (Gad67)	Chr 2	Gene known	2q
	Gabrb3	Chr 7	Gene known	15q
	Tgfb3	Chr 12	Gene known	14q24
Glucocorticoid-induced CP susceptibility	*Dcp1*	Chr 17	*H2-Eb*	6p21
	Dcp2	Chr 17	*H2*	6p21
	Acp	Chr 17	*H2*	6p21
	"*H3*" region	Chr 2	—	—
	Pgm1 region	Chr 5	—	4
	Nat1 region	Chr 8	*Nat1*	8p
	X-linked	Chr X	—	X
Phenytoin-induced CP susceptibility	*Dcp1*	Chr 17	*H2-Eb*	6p21
	Dcp2	Chr 17	*H2*	6p21
	Nat1 region	Chr 8	*Nat1*	8p
6-Aminonicotinamide-induced CP susceptibility	*Nat1* region	Chr 8	*Nat1*	8p
	"A" liability loci 1–3†	Chr 8, 11, 15	Many	4q, 5q/16p, 12q
	"B" liability loci 4–10†	Chr 4, 4, 5, 7, 9, 14, 17	Many	9p, 1p, 12q, 11q/15q, 11q/15q, 3p, 6q

*From the Mouse Genome Database (www.informatics.jax.org), 2001.

†Type I error reported as $p < 0.05$ was not corrected for the multiple tests of a genome screen; assuming that there are about 30 independent linkage tests in the mouse genome, the Bonferroni correction indicates that the type I error associated with each locus is $1.0 > p > 0.12$.

combinant inbred (RI) strains, descended from a series of closed lineages, each tracing back to a separate F2 breeding pair. These strains are called the AXB-1, AXB-2 . . . and the BXA-1, BXA-2 . . . strains; the AXB set has A/J cytoplasm and the BXA set has C57BL/6J cytoplasm. Each RI strain is expected to have a unique combination of pieces of its genome derived equally and randomly from the two parental strains, and half of the strains are expected to be homozygous for the A strain allele at any given locus (Sampson et al., 1998). Among these strains, only AXB-6/Pgn and BXA-8/Pgn have been reported to have spontaneous CL/P (Diehl and Erickson, 1997; Juriloff et al., 2001).

The cumulative understanding of the genetics and mapping of the liability to spontaneous CL/P of A-strain mice has been deduced in genetic contrasts with

TABLE 22.3. *Mouse Strains with High Frequencies of Spontaneous Nonsyndromic Orofacial Clefts*

Type of Cleft	Strain	Percent Affected*	References
Cleft lip with or without cleft palate	A/J	5–10	Kalter (1979), Juriloff and Fraser (1980)
	A/HeJ	5–10	Kalter (1979), Juriloff (1982)
	A/WySnJ	20–30	Juriloff (1982)
	CL/Fr	20–25	Juriloff and Fraser (1980)
	AXB-6/Pgn	5–10	Karolyi et al. (1987), Juriloff et al. (2001)
	BXA-8/Pgn	5	Juriloff et al. (2001)
	L line	10	Trasler and Trasler (1984)
Cleft palate	SW/Fr	5–10	Vekemans and Fraser (1979)
	CF1	3	Matsushima et al. (1992)
	J/Glw	"High"	Staats (1972)

*Both types of cleft are lethal at birth in mice. Frequencies are usually observed in fetuses.

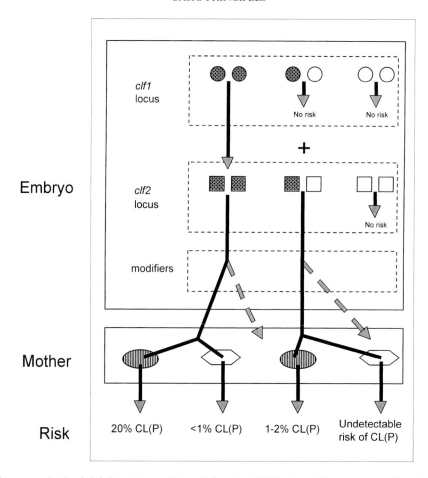

FIG. 22.1. Genetic architecture of risk of cleft lip with or without cleft palate (CL/P) derived from the A strains of mice. Two compartments influence risk: genes acting in the embryo and genes acting in the mother. *Filled circles and squares* denote alleles from the A strain; *open circles and squares* denote normal-strain alleles. Only a combination of *A* alleles across the *clf1* and *clf2* loci can cause risk of CL/P. The variety of specific risk levels created by subsequent modifiers is not shown; only the effect of A-strain modifiers is shown as the embryo risks are carried forward into the maternal effect compartment. Two types of maternal effect are shown: A/WySnJ mothers *(dark ovals)* and F1 mothers from A/WySnJ x C57BL/6J *(light polygons)*.

the normal C57BL/6J strain and the C57BL-related normal AEJ/GnRk strain. In the A strains, CL/P is a genetically complex trait but does not appear to have the polygenic additive basis often assumed of multi-factorial threshold traits. Historical assumptions about the number and nature of the CL/P genes acting directly in the embryos strongly influenced the approaches taken to linkage mapping, as discussed below. The genetic architecture of the trait has genetic components in two layers (Fig. 22.1): a layer of genes acting directly in the embryo to cause risk of CL/P and to influence expression of that risk and a layer of genes acting in the mother to indirectly modify the embryos' risk of CL/P.

Developmental Threshold. The developmental defect in A/J, CL/Fr, L Line, and A/WySnJ embryos is a minor quantitative change in the dynamic spatial rela-

tionships between the facial prominences (Trasler, 1968; Juriloff and Trasler, 1976). In particular, a delay in the forward growth of the maxillary prominence leads to its inadequate contact and fusion with the lateral and medial prominences (Diewert and Wang, 1992; Wang et al., 1995). By a critical time in the development of the face, the fusion (mesenchymal bridge) must reach a critical size or fail. Variation between embryos, stochastic or micro-environmental, distributes some embryos to the "failure" side of this threshold. Thus, among genetically identical embryos, some fail to successfully form one or both sides of the upper lip. The genes that cause risk of CL/P in the A strains therefore cause a quantitative change in the growth of embryonic facial prominences, which is not a severe abnormality in itself, although the potential consequence, CL/P, is severe. Embryos that successfully form the mesenchymal bridges go on to become normal adults. The genes causing risk of CL/P in the A strains are expected to be expressed in the cells that populate the maxillary prominence, and candidate loci identified in linkage studies can be evaluated by this criterion.

Maternal Effects. Every study of CL/P that has used reciprocal crosses has demonstrated that the genotype of the mother influences the frequency of CL/P in genetically liable embryos. The maternal effects do not cause CL/P; crosses of A-strain females to normal-strain males do not produce CL/P in the F1; the effect of the maternal genotype is to influence the risk of CL/P in embryos that have the CL/P-causing genes. Reciprocal crosses between A/HeJ and A/WySnJ, between A/J and CL/Fr, and between A/WySnJ and AXB-6/Pgn each indicated that the strain of the mother, not the genotype of the embryo, causes the differences in CL/P frequency between strains. The frequency of CL/P obtained in each cross was that of the maternal strain (Juriloff and Fraser, 1980; Juriloff, 1982; Juriloff et al., 2001). Maternal effects are not confined to strains that have CL/P liability; the standard normal C57BL/6J strain used in genetic studies of CL/P also differs from A/J, A/WySnJ, and CL/Fr by genetic maternal effects, detected in reciprocal backcrosses, where the frequency of CL/P is lower in progeny from F1 females than from F1 males (Davidson et al., 1969; Bornstein et al., 1970; Juriloff et al., 2001). The variety of strain combinations that demonstrate maternal effects indicates that multiple loci and/or at least three alleles are responsible for the maternal effects. None has been identified or mapped, and the mechanism is not known.

A Major Gene, *clf1*. Nonsyndromic spontaneous CL/P in mice was for many years thought to be a polygenic trait with low penetrance (Gruneberg, 1952; Davidson et al., 1969), leading to the assumption that linkage mapping of the genes involved would require impractically large sample sizes. However, in the 1980s, two separate studies showed that a major recessive gene in A/J, *clf1*, is necessary for risk of CL/P (Juriloff, 1980; Biddle and Fraser, 1986). In each study, after a cross between A/J and C57BL/6J and backcross of F1 to A/J, the resultant BC1 males were individually test-crossed with A/J and the frequency of CL/P in their progeny was observed. Two approximately equal groups of BC1 males were discerned, one producing CL/P in the progeny at about half the frequency of the other. This pattern is diagnostic of the presence of a major recessive variant necessary to risk of CL/P. If a set of closely spaced, highly polymorphic mapped linkage markers had been available at that time, it would have been possible to do a genome screen of marker genotypes in the sires or in BC1 segregants with CL/P to map *clf1*.

With evidence of a major gene, *clf1*, in hand, it was clearly feasible to construct a congenic strain pair, i.e., inbred strains differing only by the chromosomal segment containing *clf1*. This entailed transferring the CL/P liability trait from A/WySnJ by repeated backcrossing into the normal AEJ/GnRk strain background; segregants in each generation were testcrossed and the CL/P producers were used for further backcrossing. Simultaneously, assuming *clf1* to be a recessive essential mutation and using a variety of available markers in standard linkage crosses and other approaches, a significant part of the genome was excluded as the site of *clf1* (Juriloff, 1993). Later, when the ideal mapped polymorphic linkage markers, simple sequence length polymorphisms (SSLPs), became available, the A-strain alleles at passenger SSLP loci on the selected differential CL/P-causing chromosomal segment in the congenic strain were used to map *clf1* to mid-distal chromosome 11 near the marker, *D11Mit10* (Juriloff and Mah, 1995; Juriloff et al., 1996).

A Second Epistatic Gene, *clf2*. In addition to the evidence of a major recessive causative locus, *clf1*, historical genetic studies of CL/P indicated the presence of at least one other important contributing locus in A-strain mice because the frequencies of CL/P were consistently significantly lower in segregants after outcrosses than expected for segregation of a single locus (Davidson et al., 1969; Juriloff, 1980; Juriloff, 1995). Analysis of the CL/P frequencies recovered across all of the generations of testcrosses during construction of the congenic strain and comparison with expected patterns under various multigenic hypotheses excluded all additive genetic models and indicated that an allele from A strains at a second locus, *clf2*, was necessary to permit expression of CL/P caused by *clf1* homozygosity; heterozygotes at *clf2* permitted some CL/P at low frequencies, and homozygotes allowed high frequencies, similar to those of the A strains. With the map position of *clf1* in hand, a genome screen in a new independent genetic study was done to map *clf2*. It was based on a cross of A/WySnJ with C57BL/6J, followed by a backcross to A/WySnJ females to produce "BC1" embryos; 2.4% of the 1485 BC1 embryos had CL/P. The first 29 embryos with CL/P were used in a genome screen of informative mapped SSLP loci spaced 10 to 25 cM across the genome (Juriloff et al., 2001). For loci not linked to CL/P risk loci, half of the embryos were expected to be homozygous for the A allele; loci with an excess of A homozygotes with an uncorrected $p < 0.02$ were further typed in an additional seven CL/P BC1 embryos obtained later in the study. All 36 CL/P embryos were homozygous A at *D11Mit10* near *clf1*, confirming this locus. Of the 36, 32 were also homozygous A at *D13Mit13*, mapping *clf2* to mid-proximal chromosome 13 (Juriloff et al., 2001). Both were significant at $p < 0.001$ as individual tests and, when corrected for the multiple tests of a genome screen, at $p < 0.05$. No other regions were significant. The hypothesis (Juriloff, 1995) that the A strain-like high risk of CL/P requires both *clf1* and *clf2* simultaneously in homozygous A state and that homozygosity for the *clf1* causative gene in *clf2* heterozygotes leads to a detectable but lower risk of CL/P was supported by the data.

Epistatic Interaction between *clf1* and *clf2* and Finer Mapping of *clf2* in Testcrosses of the AXB/BXA RI Strain Set.

Gene mapping based on RI strains requires an observable phenotypic variation distributed among the strains, with several strains of each phenotype, to be correlated with the strain distribution pattern (SDP) of allelic alternatives at mapped marker loci throughout the genome. Although several strains have the *clf1* region from the A/J parent, CL/P occurs in only two of the several AXB/BXA RI strains examined, AXB-6/Pgn and BXA-8/Pgn; and their risk is similar to that of the A/J parental strain (Table 22.3). This SDP for CL/P has little statistical power for linkage mapping by a direct approach. The pattern, fairly high risk of CL/P in two RI strains and no detectable risk in all others examined, is not consistent with a polygenic additive genetic architecture, where a variety of levels of risk of CL/P would be expected to occur among the strains, but it is consistent with an epistatic genetic architecture, where A-strain alleles at a combination of particular loci must be reconstituted for the risk of CL/P to be present.

An indirect measure of the CL/P genotype of 10 of the RI strains was obtained by testcrossing them with A/WySnJ females. Testcross embryos are heterozygous for all CL/P risk loci not already present in the homozygous A allelic state in the RI strain itself and are within the most permissive maternal environment available. Consistent with the recessive epistatic model, only strains with the A allele at *D11Mit10* near *clf1* produced CL/P in testcrosses, and these strains produced CL/P at two distinct levels, one rate near 20% (two RI strains) and similar to that of the A/WySnJ strain, as expected for homozygotes for A alleles at both *clf1* and *clf2*, and one rate low, 0% to 2% (four RI strains), as expected for homozygotes for the A allele at *clf1* with heterozygosity at *clf2* (Fig. 22.1).

The A-strain derived chromosomal segments around *D11Mit10* in the RI strains that produced CL/P in testcrosses are relatively large (SDP database, www.informatics.jax.org/searches/riset_form.shtml) and cannot refine the map position of *clf1*. However, these strains

have a variety of recombination breakpoints in the broad region previously defined for *clf2*; and on the assumption that only the strains with the A allele at *clf2* produce high risk of CL/P in the testcross, they were used to refine the *clf2* candidate region as the subregion common to the two high risk–producing strains (Juriloff et al., 2001), between *D13Mit13* and *D13Mit231* (Fig. 22.2).

Modifiers. There are other modifier loci that influence risk levels for CL/P. The frequency of CL/P expected in the BC1 from A/WySnJ and C57BL/6J (in A/WySnJ mothers), if simultaneous homozygosity at two loci is required, is one-quarter of the A/WySnJ frequency, or about 6%, and the observed frequency of 2.4% was significantly lower (Juriloff et al., 2001). Furthermore, some RI strains whose genotypes at the *clf1* and *clf2* loci predicted 1% to 2% CL/P in testcrosses, produced none in samples of 130 to 225 embryos (Juriloff et al., 2001). The most promising candidate locations of modifier loci are near *D7Mit158* and *D18Mit4*, two genetic regions that had suggestive nonsignificant association with CL/P in the genome screen, with >75% probability of linkage after correction for multiple tests by a Bayesian approach (Silver, 1995; Juriloff et al., 2001). Both regions were homozygous for the A allele in the four BC1 CL/P embryos heterozygous at *clf2* and in the two RI strains with high risk of CL/P in testcrosses but not in strains with lower risk. The random probability of each genotype at each locus in each individual or strain is 0.5, and the random probability of the combination of the *AA* genotypes at the two loci across all six observations is <0.001. The human homologs of these two regions are on 19q and 18q.

Candidate Loci for *clf1*. The recombination and physical map for the region of *clf1* on chromosome 11 is summarized in Figure 22.2. The recombination map position of *clf1* is defined by an A-strain haplotype between *D11Mit360* and *D11Mit166* (Juriloff et al., 2001) held in common between congenic strain carriers of CL/P liability and BC1 embryos with CL/P from the genome screen. These markers flank an approximately 2 cM region, within which the genes *Crhr* and *Itgb3* have been located by recombination mapping in the same materials (Juriloff et al., 2001). Yeast artificial chromosome (YAC) contigs, marked by SSLP loci, indicate that the loci *Wnt15, Wnt3, Crhr,* and *Mtapt* are within the candidate region. The YAC contig is incomplete. One YAC that is well within the candidate region contains the loci *Itgb3, Dlx3,* and *Dlx7* (Juriloff et al., 2001). It is expected that a bacterial artificial chromosome (BAC) contig will extend through this region as part of the current Mouse Genome Project (Gra-

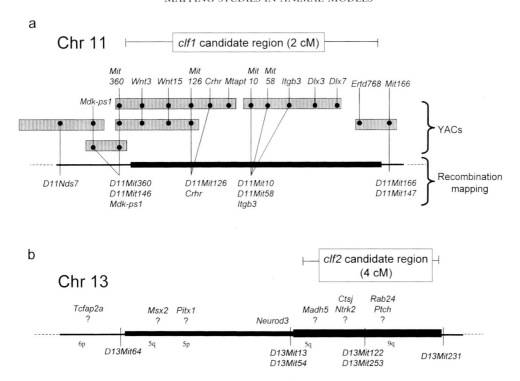

FIG. 22.2. Locations of *clf1* (a) and *clf2* (b) on the mouse linkage map. All known genes that map into the physical interval defined for *clf1* are shown. The order of genes mapped to yeast artificial chromosomes *(YACs)* but not by recombination mapping is arbitrary. For *clf2*, some potential candidate genes are shown; however, they have not been mapped against the interval defined for *clf2*, and their specific location is uncertain. For *clf2*, the *thickest bar* denotes the location defined by testcrosses of recombinant inbred strains; the *less thick bar* denotes the location from BC1 segregants (see text).

ham et al., 2001) and that more candidate genes for the *clf1* mutation may be identified. From the perspective that in knockout studies genes defined by a function in the maintenance of adult homeostasis have surprisingly demonstrated roles in embryogenesis, all of the loci in the candidate region can be considered to be candidate genes for *clf1*. Among these genes, embryonic expression of *Crhr* (corticotropin-releasing hormone receptor) and *Mtapt* (microtubule-associated protein tau) has not been described. *Wnt3* and *Wnt15* are members of a family of genes that encode secreted glycoproteins that act in signaling pathways to modulate cell behavior and fate in embryos (Moon et al., 1997). Expression domains have not been reported for *Wnt15*. In the embryonic period just before development of the facial prominences, *Wnt3* is expressed specifically in dorsal forebrain neuroepithelium, with a sharp rostral boundary between the prospective diencephalon and telencephalon, caudal to the part of the forebrain that will underlie the facial prominences, and not in the neural crest cells migrating to the facial prominences (Roelink and Nusse, 1991; Parr et al., 1993).

Dlx3 and *Dlx7* are members of the distal-less homeobox transcription factor gene family. *Dlx7* is said to be

expressed in the branchial arches and molar and incisor teeth (Nakamura et al., 1996), but details have not been published. As the maxillary prominence, the site of the primary defect in CL/P, is derived from the first branchial arch, *Dlx7* appears to be a good candidate for *clf1*. Another good candidate, *Dlx3*, is expressed in the distal tips of the first branchial arch; its knockout mutant dies during embryogenesis before lip formation due to placental defects (Kraus and Lufkin, 1999; Morasso et al., 1999); a frameshift mutation in humans causes trichodento-osseous (TDO) syndrome (Price et al., 1998).

Integrin $\beta3$ (*Itgb3*, also known as *Cd61*) is a member of a large family of genes coding for components of heterodimer transmembrane receptors for extracellular matrix proteins, and some are involved in cell migration during morphogenesis. The functional relationships among integrins are complex; each β protein can form functionally different heterodimers with different α proteins; each integrin locus produces multiple different proteins through alternative mRNA splicing sites. One of the heterodimers of $\beta3$ (αIIb, $\beta3$) is expressed on blood platelets, and human loss of function of the $\beta3$ gene causes Glanzmann's thrombasthenia, a bleeding disorder (Hynes, 1994). The embryonic expression domains of *Itgb3* have not been described in detail; one of the heterodimers, $\alpha_V\beta_3$, is expressed in the blastocyst and appears necessary for implantation (Illera et al., 2000). There is an interrelationship between $\alpha_V\beta_3$ and $\alpha_V\beta_1$ functions (Blystone et al., 1995), and it is a way that *Itgb3* could lead to CL/P: disruption of $\beta1$ function leads to deficient maxillary prominences (Baudoin et al., 1998), and $\alpha_V\beta_1$ with an expression domain in developing eyelids is associated with the defect open-eyelids-at-birth when deficient (Carroll et al., 1998). It is particularly interesting, therefore, that the CL-liable A strains and the CL/Fr strain occasionally have open-eyelids-at-birth (Kalter, 1979; Kadowaki et al., 1997), suggesting that they may have disruption of integrin signaling.

In summary, among the loci currently believed to be within the *clf1* region, the best candidates to be examined for mutations are *Dlx3*, *Dlx7*, and *Itgb3*. The human homologs of these loci are on 17q, which has been associated with CL/P in some studies (Chenevix-Trench et al., 1992; Huie et al., 1999).

Candidate Loci for clf2.

The identification of candidate loci for *clf2* is at an earlier stage than that for *clf1* (Fig. 22.2). Many of the gene loci around *clf2* have not been finely mapped or mapped against SSLPs, and their placement on the composite reference map MGD 2001 (Mouse Genome Database, www.informatics.jax.org), considered to be a work in progress, is expected to contain significant errors in the relative placement of loci. Consequently, loci shown on the current MGD map to be several centimorgans outside of the SSLP-defined *clf2* candidate interval are not necessarily excluded as candidate genes, and the number of potential candidates is large. An approach to identifying good candidate loci for *clf2* is based on the paralogy phenomenon. In mammals, a cluster of linked loci extending over several centimorgans and comprising several *Hox* genes, a pair of *Dlx* genes, and *Rar*, *Neurod*, *Evx*, *Crhr*, *Mdk*, *Itga*, *Wnt*, *Krt*, and *Scn* genes, is present in four copies, i.e., one on each of four mouse chromosomes (Chromosomes 2, 6, 11, 15), although not all loci are present in each of the four copies. It is thought that these conserved duplicated paralogous linkage groups originated in two sequential genome duplication events in the evolutionary path to mammals, with subsequent loss or sequence diversion of the duplicate loci. *clf1* maps into one of these paralogous linkage groups on chromosome 11 and interacts epistatically with *clf2* in the manner of duplicated loci. Although in mapping to chromosome 13, *clf2* is not located in one of the recognized paralogous gene clusters, the approach of paralogy need not be rejected. It appears that one of the clusters has broken up in the evolutionary lineage to

mice, and a piece of it, containing a *Neurod* locus, is on chromosome 13. *clf1* is linked to *Neurod2*, and *clf2* is linked to *Neurod3*. Thus, the possibility remains that *clf1* and *clf2* are functionally redundant paralogs. No pair of candidate paralogous loci have been recognized in the pair of candidate intervals, but more gene loci are expected to be identified in both.

Among the many loci currently known to map in the general region encompassing the *clf2* locus, some of the most interesting potential candidate loci are *Tcfap2a* (AP-2) and *Msx2*, although both appear to be outside of the segment most likely to contain *clf2* (Fig. 22.2). Locus AP-2 demonstrates a role in lip development by CL/P in mutants, as discussed below (Nottoli et al., 1998). *Msx2* is a transcription factor expressed in the maxillary prominence (MacKenzie et al., 1992; Wang et al., 1996). Knockout mutants have defects of skull ossification and other abnormalities but not CL/P (Satokata et al., 2000). As the *Msx2* knockout mutant has not been examined in the context of homozygosity for the requisite A-strain allele at *clf1*, it has not been examined in a context where it would be expected to cause CL/P. The homolog of a related gene, *Msx1*, has been associated with CL/P in humans (van den Boogaard et al., 2000). *Msx* gene products interact with candidates for *clf1*, *Dlx* products (Zhang et al., 1997), consistent with the epistatic relationship between *clf2* and *clf1*.

Other interesting possible candidate loci are within the *clf2* candidate region. These include *Madh5* (formerly *Smad5*), which codes for a protein involved in bone morphogenetic protein signaling and whose knockout mutant has forebrain and branchial arch deficiencies within a severe multifaceted embryonic lethal syndrome (Chang et al., 1999).

The *clf2* candidate interval is fragmented relative to human homologous linkage groups. *Tcfap2a* is on 6p, *Msx2* and *Madh5* are on 5q, and other loci in the region are reported to have homologs on 5p and 9q (MGD 2001).

Syndromic Mutants

Dancer. A semidominant mutation on proximal chromosome 19, *Dancer (Dc)* is characterized in heterozygotes by a circling behavior due to defects in the inner ear (Wenngren and Anniko, 1989). Homozygotes die at birth and often have CL/P due to deficiencies of the facial prominences (Trasler and Leong, 1982; Trasler et al., 1984). The human homologous region is on 11q.

Twirler. A semidominant mutation on proximal chromosome 18, *Twirler (Tw)* is characterized in heterozygotes by circling behavior due to defects of the inner ear and by obesity. Homozygotes die at birth and have CL/P (Lyon, 1958; Gong et al., 2000). The human homologous region is on 18q (Griffith et al., 1996).

AP-2 Null Chimeras. A widely expressed transcription factor, AP-2 (or AP-2α, *Tcfap2a*), has a strong expression domain in the facial prominences (Mitchell et al., 1991). Knockout homozygotes have multiple early, severe embryonic defects (Schorle et al., 1996; Zhang et al., 1996) that preclude observation of later defects such as CL/P. Embryos chimeric for AP-2 null cells have regions lacking in AP-2 activity; in many, CL/P was observed (Nottoli et al., 1998). As AP-2 has multiple transcripts (Meier et al., 1995), one can speculate that point mutations in a facial prominence-specific transcript could lead to nonsyndromic CL/P. The human homolog is on 6p.

Brachyphalangy (*Gli3^{Xt-Bph}*). A radiation-induced mutation, brachyphalangy, causes homozygotes to have abnormal digits and various other defects, including CL/P (Johnson, 1969). It is allelic to mutations at the *Gli3* locus, which is mapped to proximal chromosome 13 (Perou et al., 1997), clearly outside the candidate region for *clf2*. Only the *Bph* allele has been reported to cause CL/P, raising the possibility that the mutational event that caused this allele has also damaged *clf2* and is in linkage disequilibrium. The human homolog is on 7p.

Legless. A 600 kb deletion on distal chromosome 12 that probably spans multiple genes (Supp et al., 1999), the *legless (lgl)* mutation causes a recessive syndrome of skeletal, craniofacial, and visceral malformations, including absence of distal limb structures, and a variety of severe facial and brain defects, such as frontonasal encephalocele with severe midline clefts. As part of the phenotypic spectrum, some specimens have CL/P; illustrations of this mutant (McNeish et al., 1990) suggest that the premaxilla is abnormally small. The human homologous region is on 7q.

Genetic Liability to Teratogen-Induced Cleft Lip with or without Cleft Palate

Role of Genes that Influence Risk of Teratogen-Induced Cleft Lip with or without Cleft Palate. Heterozygotes for the CL/P liability gene *Dc* have greater risk of CL/P than genetically normal embryos when treated with 6-aminonicotinamide (Trasler et al., 1984). The CL/Fr strain, which has about 20% spontaneous CL/P, is easily induced to near 100% CL/P at dosages of 6-aminonicotinamide that cause less than

10% CL/P in the normal C57BL/6J strain (Juriloff, 1980). These differences are often explained on the basis of the multifactorial threshold model, where the effect of the teratogen adds to the initial genetic effect on risk (Fig. 22.3a). However, normal mouse strains that do not have risk of spontaneous CL/P also differ in the frequency of CL/P induced by treatment with a variety of teratogens (Biddle, 1988). Interpretation of the genetic basis of risk of teratogen-induced CL/P is complex; not only loci that affect craniofacial development but also loci influencing maternal, placental, and embryonic metabolism of the teratogen are expected to influence the risk of CL/P (Atlas et al., 1980; Lankas et al., 1998). Further complexity of interpretation derives from heterogeneity of defective developmental mechanisms; e.g., small lateral prominences (Sulik et al., 1979) vs. small maxillary prominences (Diewert and Wang, 1992; Wang et al., 1995) can result in CL/P. The developmental mechanism underlying the induced defect may differ from that underlying the spontaneous trait (Fig. 22.3b). A study of the genetic co-transmission of spontaneous CL/P risk and 6-aminonicotinamide–inducible CL/P indicated that the two traits are not controlled by the same genes (Juriloff, 1980).

Phenytoin-Induced Cleft Lip with or without Cleft Palate. The anticonvulsant phenytoin induces CL/P if administered to the pregnant mother in the 2 days prior to embryonic lip formation. The A strains are more liable to phenytoin-induced CL/P than the C57BL/10 and C57BL/6J strains (Goldman et al., 1983b; Karolyi et al., 1990). Differences in liability to phenytoin-induced CL/P in reciprocal congenic strains differing by the genomic region containing the major histocompatibility locus *H2* are present in the context of an A-strain background but not in a C57BL/10 background (Goldman et al., 1983b). Similarly, in other reciprocal congenic strains, a region that includes an *N*-acetyltransferase variant now called *Nat1* alters liability to phenytoin-induced CL/P in the context of the A/J strain background but not in the C57BL/6J background (Karolyi et al., 1990). There is another *N*-acetyltransferase locus, *Aanat*, linked to *clf1* about 20 cM distal (MGD 2001). The variant attributed to *Nat1* on chromosome 8 was transferred between backgrounds based on biochemical phenotype (Karolyi et al., 1990), raising the possibility that *Aanat* and *clf1* on chromosome 11 were also transferred in the congenic strains.

Another analysis to map loci influencing the risk of phenytoin-induced CL/P was done in the AXB and BXA RI strains (Diehl and Erickson, 1997). The parental strain C57BL/6J (B) had about 1% phenytoin-induced CL/P at the dosage used, whereas the A/J strain had about 43% CL/P. Nine RI strains with CL/P responses

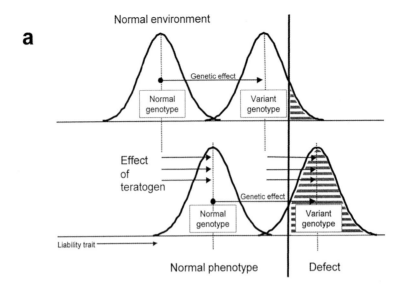

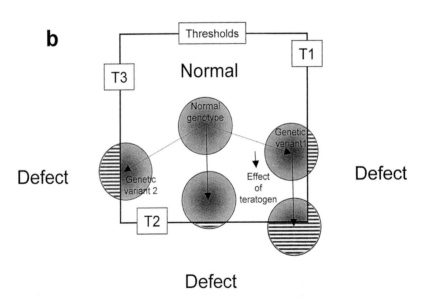

FIG. 22.3. Conceptual models for the interpretation of genetic liability to teratogen-induced orofacial clefts. *(a)* Threshold model assumes additivity of genotypes and teratogens for risk of clefting. Gaussian curves represent relative frequencies of individuals, within a given genotype, having each value of a quantitative liability trait, shown on the x axis. The liability trait impinges on a critical threshold value, denoted by a *bold vertical line,* beyond which malformation occurs. Both the effect of genetic variants that increase liability and the effect of teratogens move the distributions toward the same threshold, and the effects of genes and teratogens act by the same developmental mechanism. *(b)* Threshold model assumes that there is mechanistic heterogeneity of various types of genetic and teratogen-induced orofacial cleft. Each *circle* represents a distribution of individuals within a given genotype. Normal development occupies a range of values for several liability traits, and the borders of "normal" space represent three different mechanistic thresholds (*T1, T2, T3*; e.g., small lateral prominences vs. late growth of maxillary prominences). In this model, genetic liability may be created by mechanisms at least partly different from the mechanism of effect of the teratogen.

ranging from 0% to 34 % were used. A novel analytical method contrasted the set of risk values for strains with the *A* allele at a marker locus with the risk values for the strains with the *B* allele at the locus. The threshold value for type I error for linkage (false-positives) was estimated from the values obtained from all possible random distributions of marker alleles at that locus. By this strategy, a genome screen for linkage to closely spaced marker loci was done. Eight chromosomal regions were significant by the criterion of $p < 0.05$ for each test; among these regions, the *B* allele from the low-risk strain, C57BL/6J, was associated with high risk of CL/P in the RI strains at four of these eight loci (Table 22.1). None of the eight regions coincided with the spontaneous CL/P loci *clf1* and *clf2* or with the *Dc*, *Tcfap2a*, or *Gli3* gene loci; however, one with an *A*-susceptibility allele coincided with the vicinity of the *Tw* locus on chromosome 19, one with a *B*-susceptibility allele coincided with the region of the *lgl* mutation, and one with a *B*-susceptibility allele coincided with the *Nat1* region for which *B* in the previous congenic study conferred resistance.

The four regions (Table 22.1) with *B* alleles (from the low-risk strain) that contribute to high risk are difficult to interpret. If both parental strains have alleles conferring relative risk at various loci, it is expected that the frequencies of induced CL/P for some RI strains will fall beyond the parental strain range because of new allelic combinations across loci; but this expectation is not met. Each of the eight regions has a high likelihood of being a false "hit." Genome screens for linkage involve many statistical analyses of one data set, and there is a high risk of false-positives at the standard $p < 0.05$ threshold for type I error. For example, if 100 independent markers are used, at $p < 0.05$, five false-positive linkages are expected; therefore, in this study using 342 markers at $p < 0.05$, many of the eight loci "mapped" may well be false-positives. Various approaches to identify the *P* value for each marker locus that corresponds to a functional value of $p < 0.05$ per locus in genome screens have been described (Silver, 1995; Belknap et al., 1996); these values tend to be around $p < 0.001$ or less, a criterion not met by any of the linkages indicated. On the basis of balancing the risk of false-positives against overlooking loci of moderate effect, Diehl and Erickson (1997) endorse a two-step mapping strategy to confirm these suggested linkages in new intercross or backcross data. In the meantime, it is premature to attempt to further interpret the genetic architecture implied by participation of several low-risk strain alleles in causing high risk, as well as the very large number of potential candidate loci within 15 cM of each of the eight marker loci.

CLEFT PALATE

A wide variety of perturbations of the developing craniofacial complex can, singly or in combinations, lead to CP (Fraser, 1976, 1980; Diewert, 1986). Some of these factors, e.g., small size of the palatal shelves, delayed timing of elevation of the shelves, and lack of fusion of apposed shelves, are intrinsic to the palate. Other factors, such as excessive head width, abnormal head posture, lack of tongue movement, lack of jaw movement, and deficient size of the lower jaw, are ex-

trinsic to the palate but also contribute to risk of CP. This multifactorial and heterogeneous set of developmental factors predicts that the genetic factors involved also will be heterogeneous.

Nonsyndromic

Some genetically normal inbred strains of mice have a fairly high risk of spontaneous nonsyndromic CP at birth (Table 22.3): the SW/Fr strain was reported to have 6% CP (Vekemans and Fraser, 1979); several stocks of CF1 mice in Japan have 3% CP (Matsushima et al., 1992); and the J/Glw strain was said to have a "high" risk of CP (Staats, 1972), estimated to be up to 25% (S. Gluecksohn-Waelsch, personal communication, 1978). Generally, sporadic CP is not rare in genetically normal stocks of laboratory mice, and it is occasionally documented (Gasser et al., 1981; Proetzel et al., 1995). The genetic cause of a relatively high risk of spontaneous CP in mouse strains has not been studied, and there appear to be no mapping studies of sporadic, probably multifactorial, nonsyndromic CP in mice.

A few mutations that cause nonsyndromic CP in mice are known (Table 22.2). These are promising models for definition of the gene-regulatory pathways involved in human nonsyndromic multifactorial CP. Loss of function of a transcription factor on chromosome 3, *Lhx8*, leads to CP in about half of homozygotes, through failure of the elevated palatal shelves to make contact (Zhao et al., 1999); the moderate penetrance suggests that genetic and environmental modifiers could influence risk, as would be expected in its human counterpart. Similarly, loss of function of the γ-aminobutyric acid (GABA)-synthesizing enzyme *Gad1* (also *Gad67*) on chromosome 2 leads to failure of fusion of elevated shelves in most homozygotes (Condie et al., 1997); loss of the β3 subunit for a GABA receptor (*Gabrb3*) on chromosome 7 also causes CP (Culiat et al., 1995). Lack of transforming growth factor-β3 (*Tgfb3*) on chromosome 12 also leads to CP, through failure of fusion of the apposed palatal shelves (Proetzel et al., 1995; Kaartinen et al., 1995; Taya et al., 1999). The human homologous regions are listed in Table 22.2.

Syndromic Mutants

More than 50 mapped mutations in mice cause syndromes of malformations that include CP. Many probably correspond to human syndromes caused by mutations at homologous loci. Searches of the TBASE (tbase.jax.org) and DHMHD (www.hgmp.mrc.ac.uk/DHMHD/dysmorph.html) electronic databases for "cleft palate" lead to lists of many of these mutants, and their human linkage homologies can be found in the MGD 2001 database; they will not be reviewed in detail here. In many of these syndromic mutants, the CP appears to be secondary to other defects. For example, defects in cartilage growth that cause short limbs and short snouts probably lead to mechanical obstruction of palatal closure by the tongue because of inadequate space in the oral cavity for the tongue, as in *cmd* (Rittenhouse et al., 1978), *cho* (Seegmiller and Fraser, 1977), and *Col2a1* (Maddox et al., 1998) mutants. A similar obstructive mechanism may be present in mutants with a small mandible, such as the δEF1 transcription factor knockout (Takagi et al., 1998), the activin receptor II knockout (Matzuk et al., 1995a), and the *Hoxa2* knockout with abnormal tongue movement (Barrow and Capecchi, 1999). In several other mutants, the cause of CP seems to be an independent pleiotropic effect of loss of function of genes with key roles in other developmental pathways. Among these are activin-βA (*Inhba*) (Matzuk et al., 1995b), follistatin (*Fst*) (Matzuk et al., 1995c), *Tgfb2* (Sanford et al., 1997), *Egfr* (Miettinen et al., 1995, 1999), the regulator of *Hox* gene expression *Edr1* (formerly *rae28*) (Takihara et al., 1997), and the transcription factors *Titf2* (De Felice et al., 1998), *Msx1* (Satokata and Maas, 1994), and *Pax9* (Peters et al., 1998). In some syndromic mutants, the effect on palatal shelves appears to be direct; severe deficiency of the palatal shelves is the cause of CP in the *Dlx2* transcription factor knockout (Qiu et al., 1997) and the *Far* mutant (Juriloff and Harris, 1983). A genetic complexity of CP risk may be introduced by the participation of imprinted loci from the genomic region on chromosome 7 homologous to Beckwith-Wiedemann syndrome loci (Eggenschwiler et al., 1997; Wise and Pravatcheva, 1997; Caspary et al., 1999).

Genetic Liability to Teratogen-Induced Cleft Palate

Complexities of Interpretation of the Genetics of Liability to Teratogen-Induced Cleft Palate. Palatal closure is one of the last major morphogenetic events during development. The critical period for inducing CP by teratogens is usually after most other morphogenetic events are completed, and the CP is therefore usually nonsyndromic. Genetic liability to spontaneous CP expressed as late palatal closure can cause elevated liability to teratogen-induced CP, as demonstrated by the SW/Fr strain response to cortisone (Vekemans and Fraser, 1979). A/J, a strain with spontaneous CL/P, is more susceptible than C57BL/6J to isolated CP induced

by various teratogens such as glucocorticoids, 6-aminonicotinamide, and phenytoin. A common preconception has been that liability to teratogen-induced CP is caused by a weakness in craniofacial development in A/J arising from the same loci as spontaneous CL/P. The available evidence indicates that the apparent convergence of these traits in A/J may be a misinterpretation. There are several avenues of evidence. A/J has neither an unusually high risk of spontaneous isolated CP, with less than 0.5% (Hackman and Brown, 1972; Brown et al., 1974; Gasser et al., 1981) (Table 22.3), nor a uniquely high risk of either cortisone- or 6-aminonicotinamide–induced CP. Another strain, SWV/Bc, has a genetic liability to cortisone-induced CP as high as that of A/J and a high liability to 6-aminonicotinamide–induced CP but never has CL/P (Biddle, 1978; Juriloff, 1987). The mechanisms leading to CP in A/J differ between cortisone and 6-aminonicotinamide, as demonstrated by their different critical periods and by their different dose-response slopes (Biddle, 1978), indicating that these two types of CP are different traits. In backcrosses descended from a cross of A/J and C57BL/6J, liability to CL/P and liability to either type of induced CP segregate independently (my analysis of combined data from Biddle and Fraser, 1979, 1986). Among the 12 RI strains derived from A/J and C57BL/6J that were tested for liability to 6-aminonicotinamide–induced CP, the only one that produced spontaneous CL/P, AXB-6, ranked ninth for CP, also indicating the genetic independence of spontaneous CL/P and 6-aminonicotinamide–induced CP (Diehl and Erickson, 1997).

Few genetic analyses have attempted to detect the number of differential loci responsible for a strain difference in liability to teratogen-induced CP. The A/J–C57BL/6J difference in liability to cortisone-induced CP may be due to two loci acting additively (Biddle and Fraser, 1977), and that for 6-aminonicotinamide–induced CP may be due to three loci interacting epistatically (Biddle, 1977). Another strain difference in susceptibility to cortisone-induced CP, between DBA/2J and C57BL/6J, where DBA/2J is the more susceptible strain, may be largely due to one gene (Vekemans et al., 1981).

Mapping studies (Table 22.2) for loci controlling liability to teratogen-induced CP are expected to detect a heterogeneity of types of locus, some involved in a variety of craniofacial mechanisms that lead to CP and some in teratogen binding or metabolism (Lankas et al., 1998; Atlas et al., 1980).

Glucocorticoid-Induced Cleft Palate. Several genomic regions, identified in different strain comparisons, influence liability to glucocorticoid-induced CP. The regions include at least three loci within the major histocompatibility gene (*H2*) complex, *Dcp1*, *Dcp2*, and *Acp* (Gasser et al., 1988, 1991; Tyan and Tyan, 1993), which were detected in congenic strains on the C57Bl/10 background. On this background, in other congenic strains, another immune response gene region, *H3*, also influences susceptibility (Gasser et al., 1981). The *H2*-region loci do not appear to affect palatal development directly (Vekemans and Fraser, 1982), they seem to cause differences in palate binding of glucocorticoids (Katsumata et al., 1981), and biochemical studies indicate that the mechanism of teratogenesis is through the anti-inflammatory activity of glucocorticoids and consequent differences in inhibition of arachidonic acid release (Gupta et al., 1984). In contrast to the congenic strains, the DBA/2J-C57BL/6J strain difference in susceptibility to glucocorticoid-induced CP is not detectably influenced by the genes in the *H2* complex, and a major susceptibility locus difference was mapped in the BXD RI strains to chromosome 5 near the *Pgm1* marker locus (Vekemans et al., 1981). Another strain difference in susceptibility to glucocorticoid-induced CP, between A/J and C57BL/6J, where A/J is the relatively susceptible strain, was shown by reciprocal congenic strains to be strongly influenced by functional variants of N-acetyltransferase, attributed to *Nat1* on chromosome 8 or closely linked loci (Karolyi et al., 1990). An effect of genes on the X chromosome also was demonstrated for the susceptibility differences between A/J, C57BL/6J, and C3H/HeJ, using comparisons of risk in specific categories of reciprocal backcrosses that differ only in X chromosome genes (Francis, 1973).

Phenytoin-Induced Cleft Palate.

In many strains of mice, CP is induced when the anticonvulsant phenytoin is given to the mother during the 3 days before palatal closure in the fetus. Although phenytoin is not chemically similar to glucocorticoids, at least some of the same genes appear to influence strain susceptibilities to CP induced by both teratogens. On the C57BL/10 background, at least two loci in the *H2* complex and a gene at or near the *H3* locus strongly influence susceptibility to phenytoin-induced CP (Goldman et al., 1983a,b). The biochemical mechanism of the *H2* genetic effect on susceptibility to phenytoin-induced CP has been observed to be the same as for glucocorticoids, involving an *H2* effect on the degree of inhibition of arachidonic acid release (Gupta et al., 1984). Other loci are also implicated: the A/J background confers a higher degree of inhibition of arachidonic acid by phenytoin than the C57BL/10 background (Gupta et al., 1984). One of

these loci may be the *Nat1* region, also involved in glucocorticoid susceptibility, as shown by a significant increase in phenytoin-induced CP when the A/J N-acetyltransferase trait was substituted into a congenic C57BL/6J background (Karolyi et al., 1990).

6-Aminonicotinamide-Induced Cleft Palate.

Liability to 6-aminonicotinamide–induced CP is much higher in A/J than C57BL/6J mice and is in part attributable to the variant in the *Nat1* region. Substitution of the C57BL/6J variant into A/J in a congenic strain significantly reduced the frequency of CP induced; however, this effect was limited to the context of the A/J background, and the reverse substitution into the C57BL/6J background had no detectable effect (Karolyi et al., 1990). This epistatic phenomenon is consistent with the independent genetic analysis that estimated that a combination of three recessive epistatic loci in A/J cause its high response to 6-aminonicotinamide (Biddle, 1977) as the epistasis would enable the dominant allele from C57BL/6J at any one of the three loci to suppress the effects of the other two loci, whereas the homozygous recessive state at one of the three loci would have no effect, as demonstrated by the reverse congenic on C57BL/6J.

In another approach (Diehl and Erickson, 1997) to mapping loci responsible for the A/J–C57BL/6J strain difference (54% CP vs. 9% CP at the 6-aminonicotinamide dosage used), the CP response and genome screen of markers from a set of nine AXB/BXA RI strains were analyzed by a novel method, as described above for the parallel study done on phenytoin-induced CL/P. Ten genomic regions were identified at $p < 0.05$; however, as discussed above, the lack of correction for the multiple tests of a genome screen increases the actual risk of false linkages greatly, and it is likely that as many as half of the "hits" could be false-positives. Among the 10 potential linkages found, in three the higher-susceptibility allele was from the A/J strain (Table 22.2); in the rest, it was the *B* (low-risk strain) allele. Although the RI strains do exceed the parental range in CP response, predicting some *B*-susceptibility alleles, it is difficult to reconcile the very low risk of the C57BL/6J strain with its contributing most of the high-risk alleles to the cross, and this argues that many are false linkages. In keeping with the recommended two-step mapping strategy for genome surveys in RI strains (Belknap et al., 1996; Diehl and Erickson, 1997), which relaxes the criterion for significance on the first pass on condition that the suggested linkages be tested in independent segregating crosses, it is premature to extrapolate to genetic architecture or to candidate loci from these data.

POTENTIAL FUTURE ROLES FOR QUANTITATIVE TRAIT LOCUS APPROACHES

Measurable characteristics that normally vary among individuals on a continuous scale are termed *quantitative traits*. The normal variation in agriculturally important traits such as milk production, egg production, fruit yield, and growth rate appears to be due to the additive effects of numerous polymorphic gene loci. A theoretical base and statistical methods were developed to study and manipulate these traits (Falconer, 1981). An individual locus that contributes to the variation in a quantitative trait is termed a *quantitative trait locus* (QTL). Quantitative genetic methodology has been developed to use highly polymorphic mapped molecular markers in a genome screen of genetic segregants to identify chromosomal regions that contain QTLs (Lander and Botstein, 1989; Tanksley, 1993). In principle, the core of these methods is concerned with statistical detection of the impacts on variation in the quantitative trait by the QTL variants present in marked chromosomal regions. Several statistical approaches to QTL mapping have been developed and the available software packages reviewed (Manly and Olson, 1999). Generally, BC1 and F2 generations are more efficient for detection of QTLs than are RI strains; BC1 segregants are more efficient than F2s for mapping major QTLs, but F2s give a more accurate picture of genetic architecture (Darvasi, 1998).

Approaches to QTL mapping have been applied to diseases with complex inheritance that are expressed as observable extremes of quantitative physiological variables, such as hypertension (Jacob et al., 1991) or frequency of seizures induced by specific environments (Frankel et al., 1994). Application of the statistical methods for QTL mapping both to normal variation and to disease states tends to obscure some fundamental genetic questions. Whether there is a systematic difference in the genetic architecture and type of genetic variants or loci that contribute to the two situations is not known. It has become conventional to refer to the loci involved in genetically complex traits as QTLs, although their role may not be quantitative.

A longstanding quantitative genetic hypothesis (Fraser, 1976; Falconer, 1981) explains the complexity of heredity of some "all-or-none" (qualitative) birth defects such as CL/P and CP. It proposes that an underlying polygenic quantitative trait in a developmental process is translated into the observed binary trait by a critical threshold value, such as timing or size (Fig. 22.3a). This threshold hypothesis has been supported by observations of embryos. The polygenic aspect of the hypothesis has not been supported by mouse models; the genetic complexity originates in nonadditive in-

teractions among a few loci rather than segregation of a large number of QTL's.

The QTL mapping programs that are based on statistical assumptions for quantitative variables are generally not directly applicable to the low-penetrance binary data for orofacial clefting in segregants. A function of the *MAPMAKER/QTL* program, termed a *penetrance scan,* can be used with binary data to map QTLs of large effect, as demonstrated by *Cadfar* in cadmium-induced forelimb malformations (Hovland et al., 2000). However, if a small number of loci of relatively large effect are involved, they can be mapped by direct analysis of marker segregation ratios in a genome screen of affected segregants, as demonstrated by *clf1* and *clf2* (Juriloff et al., 2001).

The goal of mapping QTLs is to identify the genes. Mapping is the first step. Because there is not a direct relationship between the genotype at a particular QTL and the phenotype, it is not possible, among segregants, to distinguish the rare recombinants that refine the definition of the QTL map position. Therefore, QTL map positions begin as large chromosomal segments (e.g., 10 cM) containing dozens of genes. A prerequisite to gene identification is more precise mapping of the QTL (e.g., a 1–2 cM segment). Precise mapping requires additional mapping strategies (reviewed in Darvasi, 1998). Some approaches that are applicable to binary threshold traits are as follows. In the recombinant progeny testing method, segregants are screened for the flanking markers surrounding the QTL interval, recombinants within the QTL interval are testcrossed, and the phenotypes of their progeny indicate which part of the interval contains the QTL. For example, if high risk of CL/P were associated with the *A* allele at the QTL, the recombinants retaining the *A* haplotype through the part of the interval containing the QTL would transmit a higher risk of CL/P to their testcross progeny than the recombinants that had been changed by recombination to *B* in this region. In the interval-specific congenic strain approach, the flanking markers are used to assist in transferring the QTL interval from one parental strain to the other, by repeated backcrossing. Then, individuals with recombinant haplotypes between the flanking markers are used as founders of homozygous strains, each containing a different section of the transferred interval, identified by a series of closely spaced markers. Comparison of the phenotypes of these strains is used to identify the fraction of the original interval that contains the QTL. Other, more complex approaches may also be taken (Darvasi, 1998).

With a precisely defined map position in hand, the gene at the QTL can be identified by examination of the sequence of candidate genes already known in the region.

SUMMARY

Mouse models offer some insight into the gene-regulatory pathways involved in nonsyndromic noninduced CL/P and CP. For CL/P, these are *clf1* and *clf2*, which are naturally occurring variants that need to be identified at the molecular genetic level by examination of candidate genes or by positional cloning and sequencing. For CP, the genes are knockout mutations of known genes: *Lhx8*, *Gad1*, *Gabrb3*, and *Tgfb3*. Their reduced penetrance offers an access point to identification of genetic modifiers.

As there likely is a role of environment in risk of orofacial clefting (Schutte and Murray, 1999), the loci important to susceptibility to environmentally induced CL/P and CP offer a clue to other mechanisms of susceptibility. The loci identified for susceptibility to CL/P or CP induced by the anticonvulsant phenytoin, particularly those in the major histocompatibility complex and the *N*-acetyltransferase candidates, are attractive, clinically relevant entry points.

One of the very strong themes emerging from studies of genetics and mapping of genes for nonsyndromic orofacial clefting in mice is genetic complexity due to epistatic interaction between loci. Whether a particular allelic substitution at a locus important to the risk of orofacial clefting will have a detectable effect depends on the genetic context of the substitution. Although this is sometimes called the "strain background," genetic analyses have demonstrated that large strain differences that appear genetically complex can be due to a small number of loci with epistatic interactions, as for the A/J–C57BL/6J difference for spontaneous CL/P or 6-aminonicotinamide–induced CP. The contextual background effect therefore may be due to the effect of a specific allele at a specific locus, rather than the amorphous situation implied by *background*. It will be interesting to explore the mechanistic nature of these interactions using targeted alterations of known genes.

Mouse models provide a powerful tool that can be of immense value in unraveling the genetic complexity of human CL/P and CP. It remains to be seen whether the particular mutant gene loci identified in mice have human mutant counterparts responsible for a significant fraction of human orofacial clefts. More important is the identification in mice of gene-regulatory pathways important to orofacial clefting as these are expected to be highly conserved and will identify a series of candidate genes that may contribute to risk of human orofacial clefting. Future candidate genes can be targeted for mutagenesis in mice and the specific molecular, cellular, and developmental effects of the candidate gene isolated in congenic strains. The molecular developmental mechanisms and genetic mechanisms of interaction that lead to complexity of transmission patterns of orofacial clefts will likely be identified first in mice.

REFERENCES

Atlas, SA, Zweier, JL, Nebert, DW (1980). Genetic differences in phenytoin pharmacokinetics. In vivo clearance and in vitro metabolism among inbred strains of mice. Dev Pharm Ther *1:* 281–304.

Barrow, JR, Capecchi, MR (1999). Compensatory defects associated with mutations in *Hoxa1* restore normal palatogenesis to *Hoxa2* mutants. Development *126:* 5011–5026.

Baudoin, C, Goumans, MJ, Mummery, C, Sonnenberg, A (1998). Knockout and knockin of the beta1 exon D define distinct roles for integrin splice variants in heart function and embryonic development. Genes Dev *12:* 1202–1216.

Belknap, JK, Mitchell, SR, O'Toole, LA, et al. (1996). Type I and type II error rates for quantitative trait loci (QTL) mapping studies using recombinant inbred mouse strains. Behav Genet *26:* 149–160.

Biddle, FG (1977). 6-Aminonicotinamide–induced cleft palate in the mouse: the nature of the difference between the A/J and C57BL/6J strains in frequency of response and its genetic basis. Teratology *16:* 301–312.

Biddle, FG (1978). Use of dose-response relationships to discriminate between the mechanisms of cleft-palate induction by different teratogens: an argument for discussion. Teratology *18:* 247–252.

Biddle, FG (1988). Genetic differences in the frequency of acetazolamide-induced ectrodactyly in the mouse exhibit directional dominance of relative embryonic resistance. Teratology *37:* 375–388.

Biddle, FG, Fraser, FC (1977). Cortisone-induced cleft palate in the mouse. A search for the genetic control of the embryonic response trait. Genetics *85:* 289–302.

Biddle, FG, Fraser, FC (1979). Genetic independence of the embryonic reactivity difference to cortisone- and 6-aminonicotinamide–induced cleft palate in the mouse. Teratology *19:* 207–211.

Biddle, FG, Fraser, FC (1986). Major gene determination of liability to spontaneous cleft lip in the mouse. J Craniofac Genet Dev Biol (Suppl) *2:* 67–88.

Blystone, SD, Lindberg, FP, LaFlamme, SE, Brown, EJ (1995). Integrin beta3 cytoplasmic tail is necessary and sufficient for regulation of alpha5beta1 phagocytosis by alphavbeta3 and integrin-associated protein. J Cell Biol *130:* 745–754.

Bornstein, S, Trasler, DG, Fraser, FC (1970). Effect of the uterine environment on the frequency of spontaneous cleft lip in CL/Fr mice. Teratology *3:* 295–298.

Brown, KS, Johnston, MC, Murphy, PF (1974). Isolated cleft palate in A/J mice after transitory exposure to drinking water deprivation and low humidity in pregnancy. Teratology *9:* 151–158.

Carroll, JM, Luetteke, NC, Lee, DC, Watt, FM (1998). Role of integrins in mouse eyelid development: studies in normal embryos and embryos in which there is a failure of eyelid fusion. Mech Dev *78:* 37–45.

Caspary, T, Cleary, MA, Perlman, EJ, et al. (1999). Oppositely imprinted genes *p57(Kip2)* and *igf2* interact in a mouse model for Beckwith-Wiedemann syndrome. Genes Dev *13:* 3115–3124.

Chang, H, Huylebroeck, D, Verschueren, K, et al. (1999). Smad5 knockout mice die at mid-gestation due to multiple embryonic and extraembryonic defects. Development *126:* 1631–1642.

Chenevix-Trench, G, Jones, K, Green, AC, et al. (1992). Cleft lip with or without cleft palate: associations with transforming growth factor alpha and retinoic acid receptor loci. Am J Hum Genet 51: 1377–1385.

Condie, BG, Bain, G, Gottlieb, DI, Capecchi, MR (1997). Cleft palate in mice with a targeted mutation in the gamma-aminobutyric acid-producing enzyme glutamic acid decarboxylase 67. Proc Natl Acad Sci USA 94: 11451–11455.

Culiat, CT, Stubbs, LJ, Woychik, RP, et al. (1995). Deficiency of the beta3 subunit of the type A gamma-aminobutyric acid receptor causes cleft palate in mice. Nat Genet 11: 344–346.

Damm, K, Heyman, RA, Umesono, K, Evans, RM (1993). Functional inhibition of retinoic acid response by dominant negative retinoic acid receptor mutants. Proc Natl Acad Sci USA 90: 2989–2993.

Darvasi, A (1998). Experimental strategies for the genetic dissection of complex traits in animal models. Nat Genet 18: 19–24.

Davidson, JG, Fraser, FC, Schlager, G (1969). A maternal effect on the frequency of spontaneous cleft lip in the A-J mouse. Teratology 2: 371–376.

De Felice, M, Ovitt, C, Biffali, E, et al. (1998). A mouse model for hereditary thyroid dysgenesis and cleft palate. Nat Genet 19: 395–398.

Diehl, SR, Erickson, RP (1997). Genome scan for teratogen-induced clefting susceptibility loci in the mouse: evidence of both allelic and locus heterogeneity distinguishing cleft lip and cleft palate. Proc Natl Acad Sci USA 94: 5231–5236.

Diewert, VM (1986). Craniofacial growth during human secondary palate formation and potential relevance of experimental cleft palate observations. J Craniofac Genet Dev Biol (Suppl)2: 267–276.

Diewert, VM, Wang, KY (1992). Recent advances in primary palate and midface morphogenesis research. Crit Rev Oral Biol Med 4: 111–130.

Dreyer, CJ, Preston, CB (1974). Classification of cleft lip and palate in animals. Cleft Palate J 11: 327–332.

Eggenschwiler, J, Ludwig, T, Fisher, P, et al. (1997). Mouse mutant embryos overexpressing IGF-II exhibit phenotypic features of the Beckwith-Wiedemann and Simpson-Golabi-Behmel syndromes. Genes Dev 11: 3128–3142.

Falconer, DS (1981). Introduction to Quantitative Genetics, 2nd ed. New York: Longman, pp. 270–280.

Francis, BM (1973). Influence of sex-linked genes on embryonic sensitivity to cortisone in three strains of mice. Teratology 7: 119–126.

Frankel, WN, Taylor, BA, Noebels, JL, Lutz, CM (1994). Genetic epilepsy model derived from common inbred mouse strains. Genetics 138: 481–489.

Fraser, FC (1976). The multifactorial/threshold concept—uses and misuses. Teratology 14: 267–280.

Fraser, FC (1980). The William Allan Memorial Award address. Evolution of a palatable multifactorial threshold model. Am J Hum Genet 32: 796–813.

Gasser, DL, Goldner-Sauve, A, Katsumata, M, Goldman, AS (1991). Restriction fragment length polymorphisms, glucocorticoid receptors, and phenytoin-induced cleft palate in congenic strains of mice with steroid susceptibility differences. J Craniofac Genet Dev Biol 11: 366–371.

Gasser, DL, Mele, L, Lees, DD, Goldman, AS (1981). Genes in mice that affect susceptibility to cortisone-induced cleft palate are closely linked to Ir genes on chromosomes 2 and 17. Proc Natl Acad Sci USA 78: 3147–3150.

Gasser, DL, Yadvish, KN, Trammell, MA, Goldman, AS (1988). Recombinants in the H-2S/H-2D interval of mouse chromosome 17 define the map position of a gene for cleft palate susceptibility. Teratology 38: 571–577.

Goldman, AS, Baker, MK, Gasser, DL (1983a). Susceptibility to phenytoin-induced cleft palate in mice is influenced by genes linked to H-2 and H-3. Immunogenetics 18: 17–22.

Goldman, AS, Fishman, CL, Baker, MK (1983b). Phenytoin teratogenicity in the primary and secondary mouse embryonic palate is influenced by the H-2 histocompatibility locus. Proc Soc Exp Biol Med 173: 82–86.

Gong, SG, White, NJ, Sakasegawa, AY (2000). The Twirler mouse, a model for the study of cleft lip and palate. Arch Oral Biol 45: 87–94.

Graham, B, Battey, J, Jordan, E (2001). Report of second follow-up workshop on priority setting for mouse genomics. Mamm Genome 12: 1–2.

Griffith, AJ, Radice, GL, Burgess, DL, et al. (1996). Location of the 9257 and ataxia mutations on mouse chromosome 18. Mamm Genome 7: 417–419.

Gruneberg, H. (1952). Harelip and cleft palate. In: The Genetics of the Mouse, 2nd ed., edited by H Gruneberg. The Hague: Martinus Nijhoff, pp. 363–370.

Gruneberg, H, Truslove, GM (1960). Two closely linked genes in the mouse. Genet Res 1: 69–90.

Gupta, C, Katsumata, M, Goldman, AS (1984). H-2 influences phenytoin binding and inhibition of prostaglandin synthesis. Immunogenetics 20: 667–676.

Hackman, RM, Brown, KS (1972). Corticosterone-induced isolated cleft palate in A/J mice. Teratology 6: 313–316.

Hovland, DN, Cantor, RM, Lee, GS, et al. (2000) Identification of a murine locus conveying susceptibility to cadmium-induced forelimb malformations. Genomics 63: 193–201.

Huie, ML, Kasper, JS, Arn, PH, et al. (1999). Increased occurrence of cleft lip in glycogen storage disease type II (GSDII): exclusion of a contiguous gene syndrome in two patients by presence of intragenic mutations including a novel nonsense mutation Gln58Stop. Am J Med Genet 85: 5–8.

Hynes, RO (1994). Genetic analyses of cell–matrix interactions in development. Curr Opin Genet Dev 4: 569–574.

Illera, MJ, Cullinan, E, Gui, Y, et al. (2000). Blockade of the alpha(v)beta(3) integrin adversely affects implantation in the mouse. Biol Reprod 62: 1285–1290.

Jacob, HJ, Lindpaintner, K, Lincoln, SE, et al. (1991). Genetic mapping of a gene causing hypertension in the stroke-prone spontaneously hypertensive rat. Cell 67: 213–224.

Johnson, DR (1969). Brachyphalangy, an allele of extra-toes in the mouse. Genet Res 13: 275–280.

Juriloff, DM (1980). Genetics of clefting in the mouse. Prog Clin Biol Res 46: 39–71.

Juriloff, DM (1982). Differences in frequency of cleft lip among the A strains of mice. Teratology 25: 361–368.

Juriloff, DM (1987). Maternal treatment with cortisone accelerates eyelid closure and other developmental fusion processes in fetal mice. Development 100: 611–618.

Juriloff, DM (1993). Current status of genetic linkage studies of a major gene that causes CL/P in mice: exclusion map. J Craniofac Genet Dev Biol 13: 223–229.

Juriloff, DM (1995). Genetic analysis of the construction of the AEJ.A congenic strain indicates that nonsyndromic CL/P in the mouse is caused by two loci with epistatic interaction. J Craniofac Genet Dev Biol 15: 1–12.

Juriloff, DM, Fraser, FC (1980). Genetic maternal effects on cleft lip frequency in A/J and CL/Fr mice. Teratology 21: 167–175.

Juriloff, DM, Harris, MJ (1983). Abnormal facial development in the mouse mutant first arch. J Craniofac Genet Dev Biol 3: 317–337.

Juriloff, DM, Harris, MJ, Brown, CJ (2001). Unravelling the complex genetics of cleft lip in the mouse model. Mamm Genome 12: 426–435.

Juriloff, DM, Harris, MJ, Mah, DG (1996). The *clf1* gene maps to a 2- to 3-cM region of distal mouse chromosome 11. Mamm Genome 7: 789.

Juriloff, DM, Mah, DG (1995). The major locus for multifactorial nonsyndromic cleft lip maps to mouse chromosome 11. Mamm Genome 6: 63–69.

Juriloff, DM, Roberts, CW (1975). Genetics of cleft palate in chickens and the relationship between the occurrence of the trait and maternal riboflavin deficiency. Poult Sci 54: 334–346.

Juriloff, DM, Trasler, DG (1976). Test of the hypothesis that embryonic face shape is a causal factor in genetic predisposition to cleft lip in mice. Teratology 14: 35–41.

Kaartinen, V, Voncken, JW, Shuler, C, et al. (1995). Abnormal lung development and cleft palate in mice lacking TGF-beta3 indicates defects of epithelial–mesenchymal interaction. Nat Genet 11: 415–421.

Kadowaki, S, Sakamoto, M, Kamiishi, H, Tanimura, T (1997). Embryologic features of term fetuses and newborns in CL/Fr mice with special reference to cyanosis. Cleft Palate Craniofac J 34: 211–217.

Kalter, H (1979). The history of the A family of inbred mice and the biology of its congenital malformations. Teratology 20: 213–232.

Karolyi, IJ, Liu, S, Erickson, RP (1987). Susceptibility to phenytoin-induced cleft lip with or without cleft palate: many genes are involved. Genet Res 49: 43–49.

Karolyi, J, Erickson, RP, Lui, S, Killewald, L (1990). Major effects on teratogen-induced facial clefting in mice determined by a single genetic region. Genetics 126: 201–205.

Katsumata, M, Baker, MK, Goldman, AS, Gasser, DL (1981). Influence of H-2-linked genes on glucocorticoid receptors in the fetal mouse palate. Immunogenetics 13: 319–325.

Kraus, P, Lufkin, T (1999). Mammalian *Dlx* homeobox gene control of craniofacial and inner ear morphogenesis. J Cell Biochem Suppl 32–33: 133–140.

Lander, ES, Botstein, D (1989). Mapping Mendelian factors underlying quantitative traits using RFLP linkage maps. Genetics 121: 185–199.

Lankas, GR, Wise, LD, Cartwright, ME, et al. (1998). Placental P-glycoprotein deficiency enhances susceptibility to chemically induced birth defects in mice. Reprod Toxicol 12: 457–463.

Loevy, H, Feynes, V (1968). Spontaneous cleft palate in a family of Siamese cats. Cleft Palate J 5: 57–60.

Lyon, MF (1958). Twirler: a mutant affecting the inner ear of the house mouse. J Embryol Exp Morphol 6: 105–116.

Lyon, MF, Quinney, R, Glenister, PH, et al. (1996). Doublefoot: a new mouse mutant affecting development of limbs and head. Genet Res 68: 221–231.

MacKenzie, A, Ferguson, MWJ, Sharpe, PT (1992). Expression patterns of the homeobox gene *Hox-8* in the mouse embryo suggest a role in specifying tooth initiation and shape. Development 115: 403–420.

Maddox, BK, Garofalo, S, Horton, WA, et al. (1998). Craniofacial and otic capsule abnormalities in a transgenic mouse strain with a Col2a1 mutation. J Craniofac Genet Dev Biol 18: 195–201.

Manly, KF, Olson, JM (1999). Overview of QTL mapping software and introduction to Map Manager QT. Mamm Genome 10: 327–334.

Matsushima, Y, Ohne, M, Irino, T, Maki, M (1992). Spontaneous cleft palate in CF:1/Ohu mice. Jikken Dobutsu 41: 83–85.

Matzuk, MM, Kumar, TR, Bradley, A (1995a). Different phenotypes for mice deficient in either activins or activin receptor type II. Nature 374: 356–360.

Matzuk, MM, Kumar, TR, Vassalli, A, et al. (1995b). Functional analysis of activins during mammalian development. Nature 374: 354–356.

Matzuk, MM, Lu, N, Vogel, H, et al. (1995c). Multiple defects and perinatal death in mice deficient in follistatin. Nature 374: 360–363.

McNeish, JD, Thayer, J, Walling, K, et al. (1990). Phenotypic characterization of the transgenic mouse insertional mutation, legless. J Exp Zool 253: 151–162.

Meier, P, Koedood, M, Philipp, J, et al. (1995). Alternative mRNAs encode multiple isoforms of transcription factor AP-2 during murine embryogenesis. Dev Biol 169: 1–14.

Miettinen, PJ, Berger, JE, Meneses, J, et al. (1995). Epithelial immaturity and multiorgan failure in mice lacking epidermal growth factor receptor. Nature 376: 337–341.

Miettinen, PJ, Chin, JR, Shum, L, et al. (1999). Epidermal growth factor receptor function is necessary for normal craniofacial development and palate closure. Nat Genet 22: 69–73.

Millicovsky, G, Ambrose, LJ, Johnston, MC (1982). Developmental alterations associated with spontaneous cleft lip and palate in CL/Fr mice. Am J Anat 164: 29–44.

Mitchell, LE, Risch, N (1992). Mode of inheritance of nonsyndromic cleft lip with or without cleft palate: a reanalysis. Am J Hum Genet 51: 323–332.

Mitchell, PJ, Timmons, PM, Hebert, JM, et al. (1991). Transcription factor AP-2 is expressed in neural crest cell lineages during mouse embryogenesis. Genes Dev 5: 105–119.

Moon, RT, Brown, JD, Torres, M (1997). WNTs modulate cell fate and behavior during vertebrate development. Trends Genet 13: 157–162.

Morasso, MI, Grinberg, A, Robinson, G, et al. (1999). Placental failure in mice lacking the homeobox gene *Dlx3*. Proc Natl Acad Sci USA 96: 162–167.

Nakamura, S, Stock, DW, Wydner, KL, et al. (1996). Genomic analysis of a new mammalian distal-less gene: *Dlx7*. Genomics 38: 314–324.

Nottoli, T, Hagopian-Donaldson, S, Zhang, J, et al. (1998). AP-2-null cells disrupt morphogenesis of the eye, face, and limbs in chimeric mice. Proc Natl Acad Sci USA 95: 13714–13719.

Parr, BA, Shea, MJ, Vassileva, G, McMahon, AP (1993). Mouse *Wnt* genes exhibit discrete domains of expression in the early embryonic CNS and limb buds. Development 119: 247–261.

Perou, CM, Perchellet, A, Jago, T, et al. (1997). Comparative mapping in the beige-satin region of mouse chromosome 13. Genomics 39: 136–146.

Peters, H, Neubuser, A, Kratochwil, K, Balling, R (1998). Pax9-deficient mice lack pharyngeal pouch derivatives and teeth and exhibit craniofacial and limb abnormalities. Genes Dev 12: 2735–2747.

Pourtois, M (1967). Influence of cleft lip upon palatal closure in A/Jax mice. Cleft Palate J 4: 120–123.

Price, JA, Bowden, DW, Wright, JT, et al. (1998). Identification of a mutation in *DLX3* associated with tricho-dento-osseous (TDO) syndrome. Hum Mol Genet 7: 563–569.

Proetzel, G, Pawlowski, SA, Wiles, MV, et al. (1995). Transforming growth factor-beta3 is required for secondary palate fusion. Nat Genet 11: 409–414.

Qiu, M, Bulfone, A, Ghattas, I, et al. (1997). Role of the *Dlx* homeobox genes in proximodistal patterning of the branchial arches: mutations of *Dlx-1, Dlx-2*, and *Dlx-1* and *-2* alter morphogenesis of proximal skeletal and soft tissue structures derived from the first and second arches. Dev Biol 185: 165–184.

Rittenhouse, E, Dunn, LC, Cookingham, J, et al. (1978). Cartilage matrix deficiency (cmd): a new autosomal recessive lethal mutation in the mouse. J Embryol Exp Morphol 43: 71–84.

Roelink, H, Nusse, R (1991). Expression of two members of the Wnt family during mouse development—restricted temporal and spatial patterns in the developing neural tube. Genes Dev 5: 381–388.

Sampson, SB, Higgins, DC, Elliot, RW, et al. (1998). An edited linkage map for the AXB and BXA recombinant inbred mouse strains. Mamm Genome 9: 688–694.

Sanford, LP, Ormsby, I, Gittenberger-de Groot, AC, et al. (1997). TGFbeta2 knockout mice have multiple developmental defects that are non-overlapping with other TGFbeta knockout phenotypes. Development 124: 2659–2670.

Satokata, I, Ma, L, Ohshima, H, et al. (2000). Msx2 deficiency in mice causes pleiotropic defects in bone growth and ectodermal organ formation. Nat Genet 24: 391–395.

Satokata, I, Maas, R (1994). Msx1 deficient mice exhibit cleft palate and abnormalities of craniofacial and tooth development. Nat Genet 6: 348–356.

Schorle, H, Meier, P, Buchert, M, et al. (1996). Transcription factor AP-2 essential for cranial closure and craniofacial development. Nature 381: 235–238.

Schutte, BC, Murray, JC (1999). The many faces and factors of orofacial clefts. Hum Mol Genet 8: 1853–1859.

Seegmiller, RE, Fraser, FC (1977). Mandibular growth retardation as a cause of cleft palate in mice homozygous for the chondrodysplasia gene. J Embryol Exp Morphol 38: 227–238.

Siebert, JR, Williams, B, Collins, D, et al. (1998). Spontaneous cleft palate in a newborn gorilla (Gorilla gorilla gorilla). Cleft Palate Craniofac J 35: 436–441.

Silver, LM (1995). Classical linkage analysis and mapping panels. In: Mouse Genetics, edited by LM Silver. New York: Oxford University Press, pp. 195–263.

Staats, J (1972). Standardized nomenclature for inbred strains of mice: fifth listing. Cancer Res 32: 1609–1646.

Stills, HF, Jr, Bullock, BC (1981). Congenital defects of squirrel monkeys (Saimiri sciureus). Vet Pathol 18: 29–36.

Sulik, KK, Johnston, MC, Ambrose, LJ, Dorgan, D (1979). Phenytoin (dilantin)–induced cleft lip and palate in A/J mice: a scanning and transmission electron microscopic study. Anat Rec 195: 243–255.

Supp, DM, Brueckner, M, Kuehn, MR, et al. (1999). Targetted deletion of the ATP binding domain of left–right dynein confirms its role in specifying development of left–right asymmetries. Development 126: 5495–5504.

Swartz, HA, Vogt, DW, Kinter, LD (1982). Chromosome evaluation of Angus calves with unilateral congenital cleft lip and jaw (cheilognathoschisis). Am J Vet Res 43: 729–731.

Takagi, T, Moribe, H, Kondoh, H, Higashi, Y (1998). DeltaEF1, a zinc finger and homeodomain transcription factor, is required for skeleton patterning in multiple lineages. Development 125: 21–31.

Takihara, Y, Tomotsune, D, Shirai, M, et al. (1997). Targeted disruption of the mouse homologue of the Drosophila polyhomeotic gene leads to altered anteroposterior patterning and neural crest defects. Development 124: 3673–3682.

Tanksley, SD (1993). Mapping polygenes. Annu Rev Genet 27: 205–233.

Taya, Y, O'Kane, S, Ferguson, MW (1999). Pathogenesis of cleft palate in TGF-beta3 knockout mice. Development 126: 3869–3879.

Trasler, DG (1968). Pathogenesis of cleft lip and its relation to embryonic face shape in A-J and C57BL mice. Teratology 1: 33–49.

Trasler, DG, Fraser, FC (1963). Role of the tongue in producing cleft palate in mice with spontaneous cleft lip. Dev Biol 6: 45–60.

Trasler, DG, Kemp, D, Trasler, TA (1984). Increased susceptibility to 6-aminonicotinamide–induced cleft lip of heterozygote Dancer mice. Teratology 29: 101–104.

Trasler, DG, Leong, S (1982). Mitotic index in mouse embryos with 6-aminonicotinamide-induced and inherited cleft lip. Teratology 25: 259–265.

Trasler, DG, Trasler, TA (1984). Left cleft lip predominance and genetic similarities of L line and CL/Fr strain mice. Teratology 30: 423–427.

Tyan, ML, Tyan, DB (1993). Vitamin A–enhanced cleft palate susceptibility gene maps between C4 and B144 within the H-2 complex. Proc Soc Exp Biol Med 202: 482–486.

van den Boogaard, MH, Dorland, M, Beemer, FA, van Amstel, HKP (2000). MSX1 mutation is associated with orofacial clefting and tooth agenesis in humans. Nat Genet 24: 342–343.

Vekemans, M, Fraser, FC (1979). Stage of palate closure as one indication of "liability" to cleft palate. Am J Med Genet 4: 95–102.

Vekemans, M, Fraser, FC (1982). Susceptibility to cleft palate and the major histocompatibility complex (H-2) in the mouse. Teratology 25: 267–270.

Vekemans, M, Taylor, BA, Fraser, FC (1981). The susceptibility to cortisone-induced cleft palate of recombinant inbred strains of mice: lack of association with the H-2 haplotype. Genet Res 38: 327–331.

Wang, KY, Juriloff, DM, Diewert, VM (1995). Deficient and delayed primary palatal fusion and mesenchymal bridge formation in cleft lip-liable strains of mice. J Craniofac Genet Dev Biol 15: 99–116.

Wang, W, Chen, X, Xu, H, Lufkin, T (1996). Msx3: a novel murine homologue of the Drosophila msh homeobox gene restricted to the dorsal embryonic central nervous system. Mech Dev 58: 203–215.

Wenngren, BI, Anniko, M (1989). Vestibular hair cell pathology in the dancer mouse mutant. Acta Otolaryngol (Stockh) 107: 182–190.

Winograd, J, Reilly, MP, Roe, R, et al. (1997). Perinatal lethality and multiple craniofacial malformations in MSX2 transgenic mice. Hum Mol Genet 6: 369–379.

Wise, TL, Pravatcheva, DD (1997). Perinatal lethality in H19 enhancers-Igf2 transgenic mice. Mol Reprod Dev 48: 194–207.

Zhang, H, Hu, G, Wang, H, et al. (1997). Heterodimerization of Msx and Dlx homeoproteins results in functional antagonism. Mol Cell Biol 17: 2920–2932.

Zhang, J, Hagopian-Donaldson, S, Serbedzija, G, et al. (1996). Neural tube, skeletal and body wall defects in mice lacking transcription factor AP-2. Nature 381: 238–241.

Zhao, Y, Guo, YJ, Tomac, AC, et al. (1999). Isolated cleft palate in mice with a targeted mutation of the LIM homeobox gene lhx8. Proc Natl Acad Sci USA 96: 15002–15006.

23

Gene–environment interaction and risk to oral clefts

JOANNA S. ZEIGER

TERRI H. BEATY

Oral clefts include cleft lip (CL), cleft palate (CP), and cleft lip and palate (CLP); and collectively these constitute a heterogeneous group of nonfatal birth defects known to be multifactorial in origin, in that both genes and environmental factors contribute to their etiology (Mitchell et al., 2001). It is possible to reduce heterogeneity in a sample of oral cleft cases by eliminating infants with recognized malformation syndromes (genetic or teratogenic) that can include oral clefts and infants with multiple anomalies that may not fall into any recognized malformation syndrome. Even so, isolated, nonsyndromic oral clefts represent a complex and heterogeneous group of birth defects where there is strong evidence of an etiologic role for both genetic and environmental factors. It is imperative, therefore, to design studies of oral clefts so that the effects of both genes and environmental factors, as well as their possible interaction, are considered. A variety of study designs are available, each with its own advantages and limitations. Here, we review how these different study designs can be used to test for gene–environment interaction and then describe published studies of oral clefts which incorporate gene–environment interactions to one degree or another.

In epidemiologic studies, interaction occurs when the joint effect of two risk factors is greater *(synergism)* or less than a simple combination of their individual effects (Rothman, 1986). In the context of gene–environment interaction, the isolated effects of a genotype (or of an allele) and of some observed environmental exposure fail to predict the effect seen when both are present. While interactions are commonly described as syner-

gistic effects, it is important to realize that a number of patterns of risk in the presence of the gene alone, environment alone, and both are possible, including negative or protective effects (Khoury et al., 1993). Ottman (1996) described five "biologically plausible" models of relationships between genotype, environmental exposure, and disease risk. These models include situations where *(1)* the genotype increases expression of the risk factor, which can act on its own; *(2)* the high-risk genotype exacerbates the effect of the risk factor, but the genotype has no effect in unexposed individuals; *(3)* the exposure exacerbates the effect of a high-risk genotype, but there is no effect in exposed individuals without this genotype; *(4)* both exposure and the high-risk genotype are needed to alter risk; and *(5)* both the exposure and the genotype affect disease risk separately, but the risk is higher (or lower) when they occur simultaneously.

The marginal effects of the gene or the environment may or may not be apparent when interaction exists. A number of epidemiologic study designs can be used to test for gene–environment interaction, as discussed below, and several of these have been used to demonstrate gene–environment interaction in studies of oral clefts.

METHODS FOR IDENTIFYING GENE–ENVIRONMENT INTERACTION

It is possible to model gene–environment interaction in formal genetic analysis by considering genotype-specific effects of covariates on the risk of having an oral cleft (where the covariate represents some observable environmental factor), but this has significant limitations. In particular, information about the covariate will be needed for all family members (affected and unaffected), not just on the proband who brings the family into the study. When the covariate is something simple like gender (which does influence risk for oral clefts), this may be possible; but in utero environmental exposures, such as maternal smoking, will be difficult to collect on older relatives. Thus, analysis of extended pedigrees is rarely used to detect gene–environment interaction. Rather, retrospective epidemiologic designs are commonly extended to incorporate genetic information and used to test for gene–environment interactions (Weinberg and Umbach, 2000).

The most common epidemiologic design used to detect gene–environment interaction is the case-control design. Cases with the birth defect of interest are compared to controls with no known birth defects or with a birth defect other than the one under study. Cases and controls are genotyped for the markers of interest, and environmental exposure information is collected, typically by direct interview of parents.

This retrospective design allows broad inferences under two conditions: *(1)* when it is population-based, i.e., when the sampled cases are representative of all infants with oral clefts and the controls are representative of all infants without oral clefts, and *(2)* these two samples are sufficiently comparable to conclude that differences in either gene frequencies or environmental exposures could reflect causality. It is important to remember, however, that when a genetic marker is used in any case-control study, a statistically significant association could represent direct causality (i.e., the genetic marker could be part of the causal pathway) or indirect causality (i.e., the marker could be in linkage disequilibrium with a causal allele at some unobserved susceptibility locus).

A critical weakness of the case-control design for testing for association between genetic markers and case or control status (and thus the possibility of gene–environment interaction) is the distinct possibility of confounding due to population stratification. Confounding arises when the sample of cases and controls consists of genetically distinct subgroups that vary in both disease frequency and marker allele frequency. Such heterogeneity among unrecognized subgroups can, under the right circumstances, create a completely spurious statistical association, a phenomenon known as *Simpson's paradox*. The resulting bias in estimates of any odds ratio (OR) due to confounding can be substantial (Witte et al., 1999), although Wacholder et al. (2000) argued that observed differences in marker al-

TABLE 23.1. *Contrasts Needed to Test for Gene–Environment Interaction in a Case-Control Study*

Genotype and Exposure	Cases	Controls	Notation
G^+E^+	a_1	b_1	OR_{ge}
G^+E^-	a_2	b_2	OR_g
G^-E^+	a_3	b_3	OR_e
G^-E^-	c	d	Reference

G^+E^+, presence of high-risk genotype and environmental exposure; G^+E^-, presence of high-risk genotype and no exposure; G^-E^+, presence of low-risk genotype and environmental exposure; G^-E^-, reference group, low-risk genotype and no exposure.

lele frequencies across most European populations are too modest to justify such concern.

When testing for gene–environment interaction in the case-control design, the standard 2×2 table comparing exposure to case or control status expands to consider all combinations of genetic and environmental factors (Yang and Khoury, 1997), as shown in Table 23.1.

From this table, three distinct ORs can be constructed: *(1)* the effect of the genotype (G) in the absence of the environmental exposure (E) [G^+E^- vs. G^-E^-, $OR_g = (a_2{}^*d)/(b_2{}^*c)$], *(2)* the effect of exposure in the absence of the genotype [G^-E^+ vs. G^-E^-, $OR_e = (a_3{}^*d)/(b_3{}^*c)$], and *(3)* their interaction [G^+E^+ vs. G^-E^-, $OR_{ge} = (a_1{}^*d)/(b_1{}^*c)$]. If gene–environment interaction is present, OR_{ge} will not be a simple function of OR_e and OR_g, under either an additive or a multiplicative model. Under an additive model, the null hypothesis of no interaction would imply $(OR_g + OR_e) - OR_{ge} = 1$ (i.e., $OR_{ge} = OR_g + OR_e$); while under a multiplicative model, the null hypothesis would be $OR_{ge}/(OR_e * OR_g) = 1$ (i.e., $OR_{ge} = OR_g{}^*OR_e$).

An alternative method to look at the joint effects of genotype and environment in the context of a case-control design is multiple logistic regression (Umbach and Weinberg, 1997). An interaction term is added to the standard predictive model that tests for the marginal effects of genotype (x_1) and environment (x_2). This interaction term is generated by multiplying the outcomes of the two variables of interest, x_1 and x_2 [e.g., transforming growth factor-α (*TGFA*) genotype and smoking] to create a new variable $(x_1 x_2)$:

$$\text{logit}[\theta] = \ln[P(Y)/(1 - P(Y)] =$$
$$\alpha + \beta_1 x_1 + \beta_2 x_2 + \beta_3 (x_1 x_2)$$

A model testing for interaction between *TGFA* genotype and maternal smoking would look like the following:

$$\text{logit}[\theta] = \ln[P(Y)/(1 - P(Y))] = \alpha + \beta_1(TGFA) + \beta_2(\text{smoking}) + \beta_3(TGFA * \text{smoking})$$

This logistic model tests not only for the independent effects of smoking and *TGFA* genotype but also for the effect of smoking in the presence of the high-risk genotype (Pagano and Gauvreau, 1993).

The three ORs presented in Table 23.1 along with the prevalence of the genotype, the prevalence of exposure to the environmental factors, and the number of controls recruited per case combine to determine statistical power. A number of reports have presented methods to estimate statistical power and the minimum sample sizes needed to achieve predetermined levels of power in case-control designs (Hwang et al., 1994; Khoury et al., 1995; Foppa and Speigelman, 1997; Garcia-Closas and Lubin, 1999). The assumptions made in each study differ, however, so subsequent calculations of minimum sample size often vary.

One key assumption of all of these tests for gene–environment interaction is the independence of the genotype and exposure. While this assumption is by no means guaranteed, it seems reasonable for many situations involving birth defects. A more subtle possibility is that the prevalence of a genotype and exposure to an environmental factor could vary across unrecognized subgroups sufficiently to create a correlation between genotype and exposure in the total sample (Weinberg and Umbach, 2000).

A variation on the case-control design is the case-only design, which can be used to test for gene–environment interaction (Khoury and Flanders, 1996; Yang et al., 1997). Paradoxically, this approach can be more statistically efficient than the traditional case-control design but faces its own strict limitations. Piegorsch et al. (1994) showed that case-only designs can actually provide greater statistical efficiency in testing for interaction within the framework of a log-linear model and should thus be more powerful at detecting gene–environment interaction. The gain in efficiency occurs primarily because case-only designs do not consider the variance contributed by controls. However, it is impossible to test for isolated effects of either genotype or environmental factors in case-only designs. Furthermore, the case-only approach relies strictly on the assumption of independence in the distribution of genotypes and environmental exposure and on a multiplicative model.

Family-based case-control studies offer an alternative to either case-only or traditional case-control designs since they avoid the pitfall of confounding by matching a control to the genetic background of the case (Andrieu and Goldstein, 1998). When, e.g., the control is an unaffected sib or cousin, the potential for confounding is minimized; but use of related controls rep-resents "overmatching" and, thus, will reduce statistical power to detect isolated genetic and environmental effects. Witte et al. (1999) noted that sib controls are more closely matched for genetic factors than are cousin controls and, thus, minimize the possibility of confounding but provide less statistical power to detect genetic effects due to overmatching. Furthermore, full sibs will be closely matched for shared maternal environmental factors. In addition to this loss of power, the practical issue of availability of a sib or a cousin must be considered. Given today's relatively small family sizes, not all oral cleft cases will have a sib or first cousin available. For example, Beaty et al. (1997) found that almost 40% of all case infants were firstborn and had no sib.

A more intriguing family-based study design, which traces its roots back to work by Falk and Rubinstein (1987), has generated much interest (Schaid, 1998). This approach has been variously termed the "case-parent trio" design, the "case-parental control" design, or the "triad" design. The case-parent trio is comprised of the case and two parents and involves comparing the genes observed in the case with those present in the parental mating type, thus eliminating the requirement of a separate individual as a control. Spielman et al. (1993) proposed an allelic version of this design called the transmission disequilibrium test (TDT). As demonstrated in Figure 23.1, the father with alleles 1 and 2 transmitted allele 1 and did not transmit allele 2 to the child. The mother, whose genotype was 2,2 transmitted one allele 2 to the child but not the other allele 2. The subsequent genotype of the child was 1,2 (where the three alternative genotypes were 1,2; 2,2; and 2,2).

The case-parent trio design (in either an allelic or a genotypic form) allows tests for deviation from expected transmission of marker alleles (or genotypes) to the affected child and represents a composite null hy-

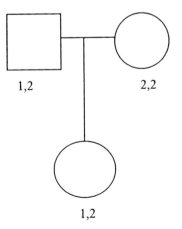

FIG. 23.1. Pedigree illustrating transmitted vs. nontransmitted alleles.

TABLE 23.2. *Allelic Transmission Disequilibrium Test (TDT)*

	Allele not transmitted	
Allele Transmitted	M_1	M_2
M_1	a	b
M_2	c	d

H_0: P(transmitting M_1) = 0.5, McNemar's $\chi^2 = (b - c)^2/(b + c)$.

pothesis that there is neither linkage nor association (i.e., no disequilibrium due to linkage) between the observed marker locus and an unobserved trait locus. The original TDT, e.g., constructs a 2×2 table comparing alleles transmitted and not transmitted to the affected child and uses McNemar's χ^2 statistic to test for deviation from the expected 50% transmission of any one marker allele from a heterozygous parent (as shown in Table 23.2).

The null hypothesis implies both no disequilibrium due to linkage (i.e., the target allele M_1 is not associated with the high-risk allele at the trait locus in the population) and that the marker is not linked to the trait locus; thus, transmission of the marker allele to the affected child has a 50% probability from a heterozygous parent, i.e., $b = c$ under the null hypothesis. While this is a valid test of linkage (Speilman and Ewens, 1996) in the presence of disequilibrium, it could well miss a linked susceptibility locus if two-locus Hardy-Weinberg equilibrium existed (so there would be no association between alleles at the marker and trait loci).

Maestri et al. (1997) expanded the allelic TDT to test for gene–environment interaction and oral clefts using conditional logistic regression models to include covariates. An interaction term was created by obtaining the product of the indicator variable for the target al-lele and an observed environmental risk factor variable. Covariates were then added to the original logistic model individually, and the likelihood ratio test was used to calculate the impact of the exposure on the odds of transmission to the case.

Umbach and Weinberg (2000) have criticized this allelic approach as too narrow. An alternative approach is to compare the observed genotype of the case to the three possible genotypes from the parental mating type (Schaid, 1998). Again, logistic regression models can be used to predict the log-odds of being the affected infant as a function of marker genotypes and then expand these models to include gene–environment or even gene–gene interaction.

As Lake et al. (2000) noted, the original case-parent trio design was developed for the composite null hypothesis of no linkage or no linkage disequilibrium; however, a related approach is to test for linkage disequilibrium (association) given prior evidence of linkage. In this situation, the alternative hypothesis is the same, i.e., that both linkage and linkage disequilibrium exist. Generalized test statistics for both of these null hypotheses have been developed for nuclear family designs and for case-parent trios (Laird et al., 2000). A summary of study designs to test for gene–environment interaction is presented in Table 23.3.

STUDIES EXAMINING GENE–ENVIRONMENT INTERACTION AND ORAL CLEFTS

It is very important to investigate possible gene–environment interaction because, if present, it opens up the option of effective intervention programs to prevent birth defects through modification of the environmental risk factor alone. There are several examples of potential gene–environment interaction in studies of oral clefts; however, the observed associations are modest

TABLE 23.3. *Study Designs to Test for Gene–Environment Interaction*

Study Design	Advantages	Disadvantages
Case-control (unrelated)	Broad inferences about causality possible for population-based samples	Confounding due to population stratification could lead to spurious results
Case-control (related)	Minimizes potential for confounding due to population stratification	Constitutes overmatching on genetic factors and possibly on environmental factors; not all cases will have available sib/cousin
Case only	Greater statistical power than case-control possible, cheaper without controls	Cannot test for isolated genotypic or environmental effects
Case-parent trios	Avoids confounding due to population heterogeneity	Cannot test for environmental factors only

TABLE 23.4. *Studies of Oral Clefts that Tested for Gene–Environment Interactions*

Reference	Candidate Gene	Environmental Factor	Subjects	Results	Interaction Odds Ratio (95% Confidence Interval)
Hwang et al. (1995), Maryland	TGFA	Smoking	114 CL/P 69 CP 284 birth defect controls	Gene–smoking interaction for CP	CP: 5.5 (2.1–14.6)
Shaw et al. (1996), California	TGFA	Smoking	348 CL/P 141 CP cases 734 normal controls	Gene–smoking interaction for heavy smokers	CL/P: 6.1 (1.1–36.6) CP: 9.0 (1.4–61.9)
Maestri et al. (1997), Maryland	TGFA TGFB3, RARA, BCL3	Smoking	160 case-parent trios	Gene–smoking interaction for TGFA and TGFB3 for all clefts	Nonsmokers: TGFA 1.46 TGFB3 1.54 Smokers: TGFA 9.00 ($p = 0.06$)* TGFB3 5.33 ($p = 0.04$)
Shaw et al. (1998), California	TGFA	Multivitamin use	348 CL/P 141 CP cases 734 normal controls	Gene–nutrient interaction for both C and CL/P	CL/P: 3.0 (1.4–6.6) CP: 2.6 (0.97–7.7)
Shaw et al. (1998), California	MTHFR, C677T	Multivitamin use	310 CL/P 383 controls	No evidence of gene–nutrient interaction	Nonusers: 1.4 (0.54–3.6) Uses 0.74 (0.39–1.4)
Romitti et al. (1999), Iowa	TGFA, MSX1, TGFB3	Smoking and alcohol	154 CL/P 60 CP 373 controls	CP: gene–smoking interaction (MSX1 and CL/P: gene–alcohol interaction (MSX1)	CP: MSX1 2.7 (1.1–6.3) TGFB3 18.8 (1.3–469.5) CL/P: 19.3 (2.9–274.7)
Christensen et al. (1999), Denmark	TGFA	Smoking	233 CL/P 83 CP 604 controls	No increased risk for CP or CL/P; no evidence for gene–smoking interaction	Not available

CL/P, cleft lip with or without cleft palate; CP, cleft palate.
*p-values based on likelihood ratio test.

and somewhat inconsistent across studies (Table 23.4). The single most widely studied genetic marker is the *TGFA* gene, although several other candidate genes have been examined. Environmental exposures examined to date include modifiable risk factors such as smoking and alcohol consumption and dietary factors such as vitamin supplementation.

Hwang et al. (1995) first studied the association between the *Taq*1 site marker in the *TGFA* gene and isolated oral clefts. Both cases and controls were ascertained from the Birth Defects Registry Information System, a passive birth defect registry maintained by the Maryland Department of Health and Mental Hygiene. Hwang et al. (1995) used these data in a retrospective case-control study design to examine whether there was an association between the rarer *C2* allele at the *Taq*1 site in the *TGFA* gene and oral clefts. Cases with isolated oral clefts were compared to controls with

an isolated, noncleft defect. They showed *(1)* a slight but nonsignificant increase in the number of CP only infants carrying the rare *C2* allele compared to the birth defects control group and *(2)* a significantly increased risk of CP among infants carrying the *C2* allele if the mother smoked [OR = 5.5, 95% confidence interval (CI) = 2.1–14.6], thus suggesting gene–environment interaction between the infant's genotype at this *TGFA* locus and maternal smoking.

Shaw et al. (1996) confirmed these findings in a population-based case-control study from California, in which control infants had no birth defect. Mothers who smoked more than 20 cigarettes/day showed an increased risk for having a child with CP or CL with or without CP (CL/P); this risk increased when the infant carried the rare *C2* allele.

Christensen et al. (1999) performed a large population-based case-control study in Denmark. This study had the advantages of a high participation rate, a homogeneous population, and exposure information on smoking collected soon after the birth of the child. Controls were non-malformed infants born at the same hospital as the case infant. Twenty-five percent of all CL/P cases ($n = 233$), CP cases ($n = 83$), and controls ($n = 316$) carried the rare Taq1 allele. There was a slight increased risk of having a CL/P infant among mothers who smoked during pregnancy (OR = 1.40, 95% CI 0.99–2.00); however, these authors found no evidence of interaction between *TGFA* genotype of the infant and maternal smoking. Romitti et al. (1999) also failed to find any evidence of gene–environment interaction between this rare *C2* allele at the Taq1 site and maternal smoking during pregnancy in a study of 366 cases (161 with CL/P and 64 with CP) and 393 controls from Iowa. Thus, the evidence for gene–environment interaction between *TGFA* and maternal smoking remains ambiguous.

Shaw et al. (1998) found evidence for an interaction between this same *TGFA* marker and nutrient intake. Cleft cases ($n = 731$) and non-malformed controls ($n = 734$) were obtained from a population-based case-control study performed in California. Cases included 348 with CL/P, 141 with CP, 99 with CL/P and other anomalies, 74 with CP and other anomalies, and 69 with some known syndrome. Women who reported taking multivitamins containing folic acid during the periconceptual period were at reduced risk for delivering a child with an oral cleft; i.e., there was a marginal protective effect of vitamin use. There were no increased risks for oral clefts when considering the rare Taq1 allele alone, however. Gene–environment interaction was suggested since there was an increased risk for having a child with an oral cleft if the mother did not use multivitamins during the periconceptual period and the infant carried the rare *C2* allele at *TGFA*. This risk was highest for CL/P (OR = 3.0, 95% CI 1.4–6.6).

In the above-mentioned Iowa study, Romitti et al. (1999) examined three candidate genes *(TGFA, MSX1, TGFB3)* and two environmental factors (smoking, alcohol) to determine their combined effects on oral clefts. Cases ($n = 60$ CP, $n = 154$ CL/P) were identified through the Iowa Birth Defects Registry from 1987 through 1994, and controls ($n = 373$) were selected from all Iowa births during this same time period. No marginal allelic effects for markers at any of these candidate genes were observed. Small increases in risk were seen among CP infants if the mother smoked more than 10 cigarettes/day (OR = 2.3, 95% CI 1.1–4.6), but these risks were even higher if the infant carried allelic variants at the *MSX1* or *TGFB3* gene. Increases in risk for CL/P were also observed if the mother consumed alcohol (OR = 2.8, 95% CI 1.2–6.6), and this risk was magnified if the infant carried an allelic variant at the *MSX1* site. As mentioned above, there was no evidence of gene–smoking interaction for either type of cleft phenotype at the *TGFA* locus in this Iowa study.

Shaw et al. (1998) tested for an association between the C677T mutation in the methyltetrahydrofolate reductase (*MTHFR*) gene, maternal multivitamin use, and risk of CL/P. Cases ($n = 310$) and controls ($n = 383$) were obtained from a cohort of California births from 1987 through 1989. There was no increased risk for CL/P among infants carrying the mutant *T* allele. In addition, there was no evidence for an interaction between infant's genotype at the *MTHFR* locus and maternal multivitamin use affecting risk of CL/P.

In a review of different methodologies to test for gene–environment interaction, Yang and Khoury (1997) utilized the data from Hwang et al. (1995) to illustrate the case-only design. Using the standard case-control method, Hwang et al. (1995) found an OR of interaction for CP, maternal smoking, and *TGFA* genotype of 5.5 (95% CI 2.1–14.6). This is quite comparable to the OR of 5.1 (95% CI 1.5–18.5) computed by Yang and Khoury (1997) using only cases. However, when reanalyzing the data from Shaw et al. (1996), which also examined the effects of maternal smoking and *TGFA* on oral clefts, we found less agreement between these two designs. For CP, Shaw et al. (1996) found an OR of interaction of 9.0 (95% CI 1.4–61.9), which was quite different from the case-only OR of 2.92 (95% CI 0.64–13.34). Likewise, for CL/P, Shaw et al. (1996) found an OR of interaction of 6.1 (95% CI 1.1–36.6), which deviated considerably from the case-only OR of 2.01 (95% CI 0.60–6.55). Schmidt and Schaid (1999) suggested that case-only analysis to test for gene–environment interaction may lead to underestimated ORs in some circumstances.

Although Lidral et al. (1998) incorporated TDT analysis into their Iowa study, Maestri et al. (1997) performed one of the few studies using case-parent trios to test explicitly for gene–environment interaction. Using 160 case-parent trios from Maryland, they utilized conditional logistic regression models to extend the traditional allelic TDT to include an interaction term for gene–environment interaction. Markers at *TGFA* (D2S443), *TGFB3* (D14S61), *BCL3*, and *RARA* were genotyped; and information about maternal smoking was included as an environmental exposure. There was some evidence of increased transmission of allele 4 among smoking mothers for the *TGFA* marker D2S443. In addition, the *TGFB3* marker D14S61 showed increased transmission of allele 6 only among smoking mothers. Both of these results raise the possibility that gene–environment interaction at several loci may contribute to risk of oral clefts.

DISCUSSION

Despite their sometimes ambiguous results, it is evident from the preceding examples that genetic factors and environmental factors do play a role in the etiology of oral clefts, both independently and jointly. When studying complex diseases, such as birth defects, it is important to explore the effects of both genetic and environmental factors and whether they interact, not only to better understand the etiology of oral clefts but also to identify when modifiable environmental factors may increase risk. Such situations present a real opportunity for intervention. Several different methods and study designs exist to examine gene–environment interaction, ranging from family-based studies to traditional epidemiologic studies incorporating data on genetic markers. The choice of study design depends both on the availability of subjects and on the hypothesis being tested, but the etiology of oral clefts will not be fully understood without serious consideration of both genes and environmental factors, as well as their interaction.

REFERENCES

Andrieu, N, Goldstein, AM (1998). Epidemiologic and genetic approaches in the study of gene–environment interaction: an overview of available methods. Epidemiol Rev 20: 137–147.

Beaty, TH, Maestri, NE, Hetmanski, JB, et al. (1997). Testing for gene–environment interaction among oral cleft cases born in Maryland in 1992–1996. Cleft Palate Craniofac J 34: 447–454.

Christensen, K, Olson, J, Norgaard-Pedersen, B, et al. (1999). Oral clefts, transforming growth factor alpha gene variants, and maternal smoking: a population-based case-control study in Denmark, 1991–1994. Am J Epidemiol 149: 248–255.

Falk, CT, Rubinstein, P (1987). Haplotype relative risks: an easy reliable way to construct a proper control sample for risk calculations. Am J Hum Genet 51: 227–233.

Foppa, I, Speigelman, D (1997). Power and sample size calculations for case-control studies of gene-environment interactions with a polytomous exposure variable. Am J Epidemiol 146: 596–604.

Garcia-Closas, M, Lubin, JH (1999). Power and sample size calculations in case-control studies of gene-environment interactions: comments on different approaches. Am J Epidemiol 149: 689–692.

Hwang, SJ, Beaty, TH, Liang, KY, et al. (1994). Minimum sample size estimation to detect gene–environment interaction in case-control designs. Am J Epidemiol 140: 1029–1037.

Hwang, SJ, Beaty, TH, Panny, SR, et al. (1995). Association study of transforming growth factor alpha (TGF-α) Taq1 polymorphism and oral clefts: indication of gene–environment interaction in a population-based sample of infants with birth defects. Am J Epidemiol 141: 629–636.

Khoury, MJ, Beaty, TH, Cohen, BH (1993). Fundamentals of Genetic Epidemiology. New York: Oxford University Press.

Khoury, MJ, Beaty, TH, Hwang, SJ (1995). Detection of gene-environment interaction in case-control studies of birth defects: how big a sample size? Teratology 51: 336–343.

Khoury, MJ, Flanders, WD (1996). Non-traditional epidemiologic approaches in the analysis of gene-environment interaction: case-control studies with no controls. Am J Epidemiol 144: 207–213.

Laird, NM, Horvath, S, Xu, X (2000). Implementing a unified approach to family based tests of association. Genet Epidemiol Suppl 19: S36–S42.

Lake, SL, Blacker, D, Laird, NM (2000). Family based tests of association in the presence of linkage. Am J Hum Genet 67: 1515–1525.

Lidral, AC, Romitti, PA, Basart, AM, et al. (1998). Association of MSX1 and TGFB3 with nonsyndromic clefting in humans. Am J Hum Genet 63: 557–568.

Maestri, NE, Beaty, TH, Hetmanski, J, et al. (1997). Application of transmission disequilibrium tests to nonsyndromic oral clefts: Including candidate genes and environmental exposures in the models. Am J Med Genet 73: 337–344.

Mitchell, LE, Beaty, TH, Lidral, AC, et al. (2001). Guidelines for the design and analysis of studies on non-syndromic cleft lip and cleft palate in humans. Summary report from a workshop of the International Consortium for Oral Clefts Genetics. Cleft Palate Craniofac J (in press).

Ottman, R (1996). Gene–environment interaction: definitions and study designs. Prev Med 25: 764–770.

Pagano, M, Gauvreau, K (1993). Principles of Biostatistics. Belmont, CA: Duxbury Press.

Piegorsch, WW, Weinberg, CR, Taylor, JA (1994). Non-hierarchial logistic models and case-only designs for assessing susceptibility in population-based case-control studies. Stat Med 13: 153–162.

Romitti, PA, Lidral, AC, Munger, RG, et al. (1999). Candidate genes for nonsyndromic cleft lip and palate and maternal cigarette smoking and alcohol consumption: evaluation of genotype–environment interactions from a population-based case-control study of orofacial clefts. Teratology 59: 39–50.

Rothman, KJ (1986). Modern Epidemiology. Boston: Little, Brown.

Schaid, DJ (1998). Transmission disequilibrium, family controls, and great expectations. Am J Hum Genet 63: 935–941.

Schmidt, S, Schaid, DJ (1999). Potential misinterpretation of the case-only study to assess gene-environment interaction. Am J Epidemiol 150: 878–885.

Shaw, GM, Wasserman, CR, Lammer, EJ, et al. (1996). Orofacial clefts, parental cigarette smoking, and transforming growth factor-alpha gene variants. Am J Hum Genet 58: 551–561.

Shaw, GM, Wasserman, CR, Murray, JC, Lammer, EJ (1998). Infant TGF-alpha genotype, orofacial clefts, and maternal periconceptional multivitamin use. Cleft Palate Craniofac J 35: 366–370.

Speilman, RS, Ewens, WJ (1996). The TDT and other family-based tests for linkage disequilibrium and association. Am J Hum Genet 59: 983–989.

Spielman, RS, McGinnis, RE, Ewens, WJ (1993). Transmission test for linkage equilibrium: the insulin gene region and insulin-dependent diabetes mellitus. Am J Hum Genet 52: 506–516.

Umbach, DM, Weinberg, CR (1997). Designing and analysing case-control studies to exploit independence of genotype and exposure. Stat Med 16: 1731–1743.

Umbach, DM, Weinberg, CR (2000). The use of case-parent triads to study joint effects of genotype and exposure. Am J Hum Genet 66: 251–261.

Wacholder, S, Rothman, N, Caporaso, N (2000). Population stratification in epidemiologic studies of common genetic variants and cancer. J Natl Cancer Inst 19: 1151–1158.

Witte, JS, Gauderman, WJ, Thomas, DG (1999). Asymptotic bias and efficiency in case-control studies of candidate genes and gene-environment interactions: basic family designs. Am J Epidemiol 149: 693–705.

Yang, Q, Khoury, MJ (1997). Evolving methods in genetic epidemiology. III. Gene–environment interaction in epidemiologic research. Epidemiol Rev 19: 33–43.

Yang, Q, Khoury, MJ, Flanders, WD (1997). Sample size requirements in case-only designs to detect gene-environment interaction. Am J Epidemiol 146: 713–720.

II

TREATMENT

24

Developing a cleft palate or craniofacial team

RONALD P. STRAUSS

Cleft palate and other craniofacial conditions are widely cared for in the context of a multi-specialty healthcare team (Strauss, 1999). Various types of healthcare team organization exist, and effective team-based healthcare delivery has the ability to address the fragmentation and dehumanization that can result when a spectrum of specialists and disciplines are needed to provide assessment and technical care. The organization and delivery of cleft palate and craniofacial health services vary according to national and health system characteristics. Economic development and sociopolitical structures define the resources and health delivery system within which craniofacial care is rendered. In developed nations, organized healthcare teams largely deliver craniofacial care, although individual specialists outside of the team context render some care. In some nations, regional or national centers of clinical care have been organized to aggregate clinical service delivery and facilitate regionalization. In recent years, efforts such as the "Eurocleft" study have resulted in more regionalized care delivery. In many nations, such as the United States, a competitive market system exists that allows as many teams to develop as the market for services will bear. Reimbursement mechanisms, cultural factors, and health system characteristics define the craniofacial health delivery system.

HEALTHCARE TEAMS

Research has examined the roles (Horwitz, 1970; Furnham et al., 1981; Logan and McKendry, 1982; Nason, 1983; Temkin-Greener, 1983; Ovretveit, 1996; Jones, 1992) and ideology (Nagi, 1975; Brill, 1976; Dingwall, 1980; Kane, 1980; Payne, 1982; Feinstein, 1983; Margolis and Fiorelli, 1984) of the interdisciplinary healthcare team as well as the settings for interdisciplinary team practice (Briggs, 1980; Campbell and Whitenack, 1983; DeSantis, 1983). The cleft palate or craniofacial team has been studied as an organization (Koepp-Baker, 1979; Day, 1981; MacGregor, 1982; Strauss and Broder, 1985, 1990; Nackashi and Dixon-Wood, 1989; Ellis, 1993) with specific focus on issues related to team communication (Lillywhite, 1957) and function (Mason and Riski, 1982; Noar, 1992). In particular, the mental health and support functions of the interdisciplinary healthcare team have been examined (Lonsdale et al., 1980; Webb and Hobdell, 1980; Cluff and Cluff, 1983; DeSpirito and Grebler, 1983; Mc-Keganey and Bloor, 1987; Strauss and Ellis, 1996; Strauss, 1997).

Cleft palate and craniofacial care has been described as optimally delivered by organized teams (Strauss and Ellis, 1996). The benefits of healthcare teams include the ability to coordinate complex services, meet the psychological and social needs of families, and provide multifaceted evaluations (Koepp-Baker, 1979; Morris et al., 1978; Nackashi and Dixon-Wood, 1989; Pannbacker et al., 1992; Strauss, 1997). Typically, cleft or craniofacial teams include medical, surgical, speech, psychosocial, and dental professionals; but large sample profiles of these organizations did not appear in the literature until recently (Strauss and The ACPA Team Standards Committee, 1998).

The literature on healthcare teams suggests that there is little agreement on what comprises a healthcare team, how it is organized, and what its goals and objectives should be. However, the need for integrating various specialized disciplinary perspectives in the care of persons with complex health issues results in increasing numbers of clinical settings in which teamwork is employed. Attention has been paid to team decision-making, the authority structure of teams (Nagi, 1975), and team cost effectiveness in terms of personnel and other resources (Strauss and Broder, 1985). Research on the attitudes and perspectives of team professionals (Noar, 1992) suggests that most teams function by agreement or consensus, even though each profession may view the needs of patients differently. Healthcare teams form when a sizable number of professionals and other health workers become involved in complex patient care that demands the insights and skills of various specialists. Teams, such as cleft palate or craniofacial teams, are a response to increasingly specialized knowledge and to the advancing technology of medicine. Teams are organized when a variety of specialists are required for the treatment of patients, as occurs in facial birth defects. Some have hypothesized that the availability of intensive care units and life support for newborns with craniofacial conditions has improved their survival and resulted in greater and more specialized treatment demands on the cleft or craniofacial team (Strauss and Ellis, 1996). If such is the case, the future model of team care delivery will need to fit increasingly complex clinical needs. Teams may find themselves incorporating professionals with expertise in swallowing disorders, pediatric anesthesiology, pulmonary function, neuropsychology, dental implantology, and intensive care medicine. This elaboration of team function will depend on the healthcare system providing resources and a payment mechanism. Market forces, including managed care, may limit the ability to expand the services of the team as they seek to control the costs of team care.

The specialization and complexity of health professional practice have been seen as causing fragmentation of care, with dehumanizing results (Feinstein, 1983). To humanize care, teams often include several psychosocial specialists, such as social workers, psychologists, therapists, and nurses. Commenting on the complex nature of craniofacial problems and the need for specialists to work together, Nackashi and Dixon-Wood (1989) point out that the cleft lip and palate rehabilitative process includes medical, social, psychological, and vocational factors and that a holistic approach to the patient or client is needed.

When medical or human problems cluster in a family (Nagi, 1975), they need to be treated in a way that integrates both medical and social interventions (Phillips and Whitaker, 1979; Dingwall, 1980). Mc-Keganey and Bloor (1987) argue that teamwork emerged particularly in those specialties where social problems are most evident. Teamwork in healthcare delivery has sometimes evolved as a result of the recognition by healthcare professionals of the social and behavioral aspects of medical conditions (Ovretveit, 1996; Cluff and Cluff, 1983; Day, 1981, 1984; MacGregor, 1982, Brantley and Clifford, 1979).

Cleft palate and craniofacial teams have been developed around the appreciation that all professionals, as well as patients and their families, can make meaningful contributions to treatment and management. MacGregor (1982) notes that all team healthcare workers must demonstrate an awareness of the behavioral and social structural aspects of the sickness experience; this function cannot be the exclusive concern of behavioral professionals. It is important to involve family members, especially parents, in craniofacial team decision-making and treatment planning (Hill, 1956; MacDonald, 1979; Temkin-Greener, 1983; Jones, 1992). Craniofacial teams have formed to efficiently meet the clinical and psychosocial needs of a complex patient population. The health outcomes of craniofacial team management have not as yet been established in the research literature, though clinicians and administrators report many advantages of team-based care over fragmented, community-based, multispecialty care.

MODELS OF TEAM ORGANIZATION

There has been disagreement about whether or not a health team is a distinct social unit (Temkin-Greener, 1983; Margolis and Fiorelli, 1984; Strauss and Ellis, 1996). Most health teams are established and operate for particular and specialized purposes (Campbell and Whitenack, 1983; Nason, 1983; Ellis, 1993, Logan and McKendry, 1982). Specific organizational or institutional arrangements may also force some professionals to work together as a "team" (Furnham et al., 1981). Distinctions are drawn by some between intradisciplinary, multidisciplinary, and interdisciplinary teams (Briggs, 1980; DeSpirito and Grebler, 1983; Horwitz, 1970; Kane, 1980; Ovretveit, 1996). The exact disciplinary composition of the team specialties may determine the categorization of a team. Furthermore, team categorization has to do with cohesiveness, level of cooperation between members, quality of relationships, and maintenance of professional authority and autonomy.

An *intradisciplinary team* is composed of more or less similar specialists within a very narrow field of specialization. It has been described as a team in which each discipline makes an initial independent assessment, information is later shared, and team members are not permitted to cross over traditional role boundaries between disciplines (Nackashi and Dixon-Wood, 1989). An intradisciplinary team operates with a narrow focus and has members whose orientation is to one discipline but who speak to different aspects of that discipline (Brill, 1976).

Multidisciplinary teams may be specifically set up to allow a number of professionals to cooperate in a particular area while maintaining autonomy from each other (Payne, 1982; Bardach et al., 1984; Ovretveit, 1996; Jones, 1992; Strauss and Ellis, 1996). Nackashi and Dixon-Wood (1989) indicate that on multidisciplinary teams the members work independently because they involve established, defined roles for the professional and permit only limited communication among professionals. Multidisciplinary teams may be seen as work units where a number of varied professionals are involved in a treatment situation (Temkin-Greener, 1983). They form a loose collection of specialists treating various aspects of a patient's clustered problems without constructing mutually agreed on plans. Payne (1982) calls these "work groups," as distinguished from a "collaborative team."

In comparing interdisciplinary and multidisciplinary teams, Day (1981) suggests that a multidisciplinary approach may involve isolated evaluations by a series of disciplines and does not imply the merger of thinking or the formation of a shared treatment plan. An *interdisciplinary team* is one in which a number of professionals from related, but not necessarily similar, disciplines are involved in conducting a joint evaluation and developing a treatment plan in which expertise is pooled and decision-making is collective (Day, 1981; Strauss and Broder, 1985). Nackashi and Dixon-Wood (1989) indicate that interdisciplinary teams meet often to plan, with each professional member forming an independent opinion, followed by the sharing of findings, the construction of recommendations, and the writing of a report summarizing all recommendations. The team leader facilitates and coordinates the treatment plan and then communicates this to the patient and family.

TEAM LEADERSHIP

The scientific literature deals with team organization by describing hierarchical and egalitarian teams (Nagi, 1975). Horwitz (1970) distinguishes between a "leader-centered coordinated" team and a "fraternally oriented integrated" team, or a "hierarchical" and a "participative" team. It appears that teams might be divided into those with a structured hierarchy of authority and power and those which share authority, allocating power to the group. Hierarchical teams may be considered efficient because individual disciplines can maintain autonomy and conflicts are limited, while egalitarian teams allow for joint participation and decision-making (Strauss and Broder, 1985; Ellis, 1986). There are important implications of team structure on team communication and cooperation. Multidisciplinary teams are often assumed to be hierarchical and interdisciplinary teams to be egalitarian in nature. Temkin-Greener (1983) questioned the existence of egalitarian interdisciplinary teams, claiming that the structure of teams reflects traditional status arrangements in which physicians dominate. Bardach et al. (1984) also regarded certain medical specialists as "cornerstones" of the team, while others were portrayed as contributing less central, but necessary, "support and treatment."

The role of the physician/surgeon is often critical to the function of healthcare teams. Some may expect that physicians will dominate on healthcare teams (Nagi, 1975). For instance, on a surgical operating team, a hierarchy of professionals may be engaged but final authority and decision-making may be given to the surgeon (Dingwall, 1980). Medicine's traditional authority and status among the professions usually account for the strength of physician influence. The effects of medical training, the doctor–patient relationship, and the bureaucratic structure and technological nature of hospitals and medical schools reinforce status and power relationships on teams (Strauss and Ellis, 1996). A subservient and auxiliary role for other nonphysician professionals may occur on some healthcare teams (Mason and Riski, 1982; De Santis, 1983). The interdisciplinary team may present a direct challenge to physician dominance as it emphasizes "role blurring" (Kane, 1980). This does not mean that differences between team specialists are eliminated with respect to roles. Legal accountability mandates specific disciplinary roles and a clear division of labor (Logan and McKendry, 1982). Ambiguous professional or team member roles may lead to team conflict. The need for shared understanding and acceptance of role definitions is important to healthcare team function (Strauss, 1994). A lack of such understanding can cause suspicion about other specialists and their methods (Lillywhite, 1957). An ethical concern has arisen about where responsibility resides when a group or team renders care. It is important that a team leader be seen as ultimately responsible for the outcomes and complications or care and that this person be identified clearly to the family.

On contemporary cleft palate and craniofacial teams, there have been interprofessional tensions related to common domains of expertise. Such overlapping expertise may occur between mental health and psychosocial professionals, such as psychologists, social workers, and nurses. Most commonly, interprofessional boundary disputes have occurred between surgical specialties in the United States. The oral-maxillofacial surgeon, the plastic/reconstructive surgeon, and the otolaryngologist may be trained and capable in performing cleft palate and craniofacial surgery. In centers where all three disciplines coexist, there may sometimes be rivalry for access to patients and tensions may erupt along professional boundaries. Such tensions have the potential for being detrimental to the team process and to the quality and continuity of patient care. Successful resolutions of interprofessional rivalries may require mediation by disinterested parties and will depend on the various professionals holding high-quality patient care as a prime value.

Some observers hold that treatment decisions are often made unilaterally by team leaders, often physicians, who hold a dominant place on the hierarchy of the team (Bardach et al., 1984; Mason and Riski, 1982). Others have found that joint decision-making takes place when teams have more egalitarian and collegial structures (Strauss and Broder, 1985). In the case of joint decision-making, there is sharing of status and knowledge with colleagues and a willingness to learn about other disciplines (Ellis, 1986). To achieve true interdisciplinary function, it is necessary that communicative openness and a shared vocabulary exist (Lillywhite, 1957; Margolis and Fiorelli, 1984; Koepp-Baker, 1979).

Where the formulation of a joint plan of action is the desired team goal, as in interdisciplinary teams, insistence on the dominance of one specialty can become counterproductive. Leadership on healthcare teams can vary according to the nature of the team, the patient's problem(s), the institutional set-up, personal leadership style, and individual personalities. Horwitz (1970) viewed team leadership primarily as "facilitating the achievement of common goals." Margolis and Fiorelli (1984) also viewed the leader as an "impartial facilitator," who ensures efficiency in the team's operation. Logan and McKendry (1982) referred to a coordinator, rather than a leader, whose role should be clearly distinguished from the professional roles on the team, to avoid being dominating. Leadership can also be granted to the person who serves as the administrator of the team.

In some craniofacial team settings, team leadership is rotated between disciplines and their various members (Strauss and Broder, 1985; Horwitz, 1970). This style may reduce interprofessional barriers and assist in diminishing professional status hierarchies. The rotation of the position of team leader assures that several disciplines experience being at the helm of the team. They will certainly become more aware of the challenge of leadership and will appreciate how hard it is to develop an interprofessional plan at the team conference.

Team leadership often implies the ability to resolve team conflict. Conflicts resulting from the structural constraints of a team organization can be dealt with by a team leader who can arbitrate differing positions (Lonsdale et al., 1980); however, conflicts that reflect larger interprofessional rivalries, or "turf battles," may be more difficult to resolve on a team-specific basis. On teams where plastic surgeons, otolaryngologists, and oral-maxillofacial surgeons try to negotiate their specific boundaries and responsibilities, conflicts may occur over the division of labor in patient care. The team leader must recognize such conflicts, but their resolution may actually depend on the role definitions of the specific professionals involved and the "turf" definitions supported by professional organizations.

The team interaction approach to conflict resolution allows the leader to facilitate team members in the settling of their differences, thus reducing role clashes, conflicting professional judgments, and class, cultural, and gender differences (Strauss and Broder, 1985; Strauss, 1985; Nason, 1983). Tensions within the team and in team deliberations may be natural, inevitable, and productive. The expression of tension may, if carefully managed, enhance the probability of emerging with superior patient care plans (Margolis and Fiorelli, 1984). Nonprofessional actors in team deliberations are the patient, the family, and the funder of care. Their perspectives will often be woven into the team deliberations, and in some settings patients or parents may sit in on team discussions. In other team settings, an interpretive meeting is held between a designated team member and the parent or patient, to transmit the treatment plans and team findings. Both strategies allow for parents or patients to voice their concerns and to determine if the team has responded to their questions. Teams that meet with patients only in a group or that do not find time to interpret findings and recommendations may fail to meet consumer expectations.

The healthcare funder has increasingly been perceived as a party to the team's decisions about care. In the United States, managed care organizations and other funders have increasingly mandated treatment options and even have determined which team professionals will be engaged in a patient's evaluation and treatment (Herelinger, 1997).

The cost and quality of cleft palate and craniofacial care are receiving increasing attention in the health policy arena (Strauss, 1994). Little has been written about the emergence of managed care into the care of persons with cleft and craniofacial conditions in the United States. The managed care organization has sometimes been seen as providing effective levels of gatekeeping to assure that overutilization of care does not occur (Kutner, 1998). The managed care organization generally will guide entrance to team services for their clients and will restrain clinical activism. The managed care organization has much at stake in preventing unnecessary procedures, radiographs, or laboratory tests. In the name of controlling costs, the managed care organization has sought to limit the number of professionals that evaluate a person with a health condition (Kutner, 1998; Nelson, 1997). Furthermore, they may mandate that only their own providers can evaluate clients of their managed care organization. In the case of "closed-panel" managed care organizations or health maintenance organizations, there is often a reluctance to allow a client to seek services or evaluation "out of system." The primary care provider assigned to, or selected by, the client is portrayed as serving in an advocacy role, wherein the provider seeks needed services for the client. Critics of the managed care organization point out that there are often incentives for the primary care provider to reduce the number of specialty referrals made, especially "out of system." In some managed care organizations, there are direct economic disincentives for specialty referral, even for evaluation purposes (Povar and Moreno, 1995; Simon and Emmons, 1997). Clients of some managed care organizations report that they have a difficult time accessing their primary care physician due to the long wait for nonemergency appointments or consultations. Some cleft palate and craniofacial teams work with managed care organizations that wish to "unbundle" the team evaluation. In other words, they seek to use several team professionals and several of their own in-house professionals. Some teams have resisted this move by arguing that they function effectively when they can work as an experienced and complete unit or team. Another challenge associated with the current health system relates to the ability of patients to access comprehensive coverage for craniofacial conditions (Strauss, 1994). Some states have passed legislation to mandate coverage, but the results have been uneven across the United States. One issue that has arisen is when health coverage is provided by an employer who self-insures workers (Nelson, 1997). In that situation, the insurer is often not covered under state-specific insurance legislation and cannot be affected by state legislation. National legislation has sought to permit Americans portability of health insurance and to protect them from denial of coverage when changing jobs (Kutner, 1998). Some managed care organizations have been selective in who they enroll. When this occurs, it has been called "skimming the cream," in that the lowest-risk patient population is covered while more complex populations are left uncovered. To deal with this, many states have begun to cover Medicaid services (care for primarily low-income persons) under managed care. Thus, poor adults and children may also receive care under the guidelines of a managed care organization. The advent of managed care may have fundamentally changed the relationship between the patient and the provider by inserting the managed care organization between them (Povar and Moreno, 1988; Reinhardt, 1993; Emmanuel and Dubler, 1995).

Issues of the quality of care (Inglehardt, 1996) have also emerged as the healthcare system in the United States changes. The National Committee for Quality Assurance has taken on the role of evaluating and accrediting managed care organizations and health plans using specified outcome measures and parameters of care (Inglehardt, 1996). Such standards of care and clinical pathways or guidelines have been developed to rationalize care patterns. The emphasis on evidence-based practice suggests that technological advances will need to demonstrate their effectiveness and that outcomes research will guide future clinical practices.

EVALUATING THE CHARACTERISTICS OF TEAMS

The American Cleft Palate-Craniofacial Association (ACPA) (1993) has revised its mechanism for listing teams in the ACPA *Membership-Team Directory* (2001). This began when it became apparent that public funding agencies and many health insurance or managed care providers would set criteria for cleft palate and craniofacial team care. Believing that a professional association should provide leadership in such matters, the ACPA initiated efforts to define basic and minimal standards for team listing that include categorization of teams. The resulting ACPA Team Self-Assessment Instrument employs specific criteria to list teams. Team categorization is achieved through a self-rating process with no examiners or site visitors. Standards for listings permit the specification of two principal types of team, the cleft palate team and the craniofacial team. A given center may be listed in either or both of these categories. Strauss and The ACPA Team Standards Committee (1998) reported that all known ($n = 296$)

TABLE 24.1. *American Cleft Palate-Craniofacial Association (ACPA) Standards for Listing the Cleft Palate Team (CPT)**

Basic Criteria

1. The CPT meets face-to-face for regularly scheduled meetings for treatment planning and case review, at least six times per year, with at least four specialties represented.
2. The CPT evaluated at least fifty new or recall patients with cleft lip/palate in the past year.
3. The CPT keeps a central and shared file on each patient.
4. The CPT has at least an actively involved Surgeon, Orthodontist and Speech-Language Pathologist, who attend team meetings. As a minimum, patients evaluated by the CPT are seen by these specialties plus at least one additional team specialty that attends the CPT meetings.
5. The CPT assures that each child has health evaluation by a primary care Physician (Pediatrician, Family Physician or General Internist) in the community or on the team. The CPT uses the findings from the health evaluation to guide its treatment planning and team meeting deliberations.
6. Evaluations at the CPT include a screening hearing test and tympanogram. All patients with clefts of the palate, or hearing concerns, or abnormal tympanograms or hearing tests, are referred to an Otolaryngologist (E.N.T.) for examination, consultation or treatment.
7. At least one Surgeon on the CPT operated on ten or more patients for primary repairs of a cleft lip and/or cleft palate in the past year.
8. For patients requiring facial skeletal surgery, the CPT has or refers to a surgeon whose education, training and experience has adequately prepared him/her to provide facial skeletal surgery (bone graft, orthognathic surgery) and who has performed ten or more major maxillary or mandibular osteotomies in the past year (not necessarily on patients with cleft lip and/or cleft palate.

Additional CPT Criteria

1. The CPT has a Speech-Language Pathologist(s) who attends team meetings and whose education, training and experience have adequately prepared him/her for the diagnosis and treatment of patients with cleft lip/palate.
2. At least one Speech-Language Pathologist on the CPT provided speech therapy and/or a complete speech and language evaluation to a minimum of 10 patients (team or other patients) with cleft lip/palate in the past year.
3. The CPT Speech-Language Pathologist performs a structured speech assessment during team evaluations.
4. The CPT uses clinical speech instrumentation (such as endoscopy, pressure flow, videofluoroscopy, etc.) to assess velopharyngeal function, when indicated.
5. CPT has an Orthodontist who attends team meetings and whose education, training and experience have adequately prepared him/her for the diagnosis and treatment of patients with cleft lip/palate.
6. At least one Orthodontist on the CPT provided orthodontic treatment for a minimum of 10 patients with cleft lip/palate in the past year.
7. The CPT refers patients requiring orthognathic treatment to an Orthodontist(s) whose education, training and experience have adequately prepared him/her for the provision of orthodontic care as a part of orthognathic treatment.
8. Orthognathic surgical treatments are adequately documented with intraoral dental casts, facial and intraoral photographs, and appropriate radiographs.
9. Orthognathic surgical planning and outcomes are routinely discussed at the CPT meetings for patients requiring such care.
10. The CPT has, or refers to, a Pediatric Dentist/General Dentist/Prosthodontist(s) whose education, training and experience have adequately prepared him/her for the dental diagnosis and treatment of patients with cleft lip/palate.
11. CPT has a Surgeon(s) who attends team meetings and whose education, training and experience have adequately prepared him/her for the diagnosis and treatment of patients with cleft lip/palate.
12. The CPT has a Psychologist, Clinical Social Worker, or other Mental Health Professional(s) who evaluates all patients on a regular basis.
13. The CPT routinely tests or screens patients for learning disabilities and developmental, psychological, and language skills.
14. The CPT collects school reports and other information relative to learning in school-age patients, when indicated.
15. The CPT has a nurse or other trained professional who regularly provides supportive counseling and instruction (feeding, developmental) to parents of newborns.
16. The CPT sponsors or makes referrals to a parent support group or parent network in the community (if available), as desired by families.
17. The CPT regularly provides supportive counseling and instruction to parents and patients pre- and post-operatively.
18. The CPT provides for formal genetic counseling or a clinical genetic evaluation for parents and patients.
19. The CPT evaluation includes a hearing test by an Audiologist(s) beginning before one year of age.
20. The CPT has an Otolaryngologist(s) whose education, training and experience have adequately prepared him/her for the diagnosis and treatment of patients with cleft lip/palate. The Otolaryngologist provides examination, consultation and treatment to patients evaluated by your team.
21. The CPT evaluation includes ear examinations by an otolaryngologist(s) on a routine basis beginning before one year of age.
22. After a CPT evaluation, the patient and family have an opportunity to ask questions and discuss the treatment plan with a team representative.
23. The CPT routinely (for each evaluation) writes reports or summary letters, containing a treatment plan, which are sent to the family in a timely manner.
24. CPT reports are routinely sent in a timely manner to the patient's care providers in the community (schools, health department,local professionals) with the family's permission.
25. The CPT record includes a diagnosis(es).
26. The CPT team record includes a complete medical history.
27. The CPT record includes a treatment plan or goals which are reviewed periodically on a formal basis.
28. The CPT record includes a social and psychological history.
29. The CPT record includes dental and orthodontic findings and history.
30. The CPT makes intraoral dental casts on patients, when indicated.

(continued)

TABLE 24.1. *American Cleft Palate-Craniofacial Association (ACPA) Standards for Listing the Cleft Palate Team (CPT)* (continued)*

31. The CPT takes facial photographs on patients in treatment or evaluation.
32. The CPT obtains appropriate radiographs, including lateral cephalometric radiographs on patients, when indicated.
33. The CPT has an office and coordinator or secretary.
34. The CPT supports, encourages, or offers continuing education in cleft lip/palate care for its members.
35. The CPT provides case management (follow-up, referral, and coordination of care) and benefits advocacy/assistance (help families obtain financial or programmatic support), as needed.

*The CPT provides coordinated and interdisciplinary evaluation and treatment to patients with cleft lip and/or cleft palate. The CPT meets the 8 basic criteria defined by the ACPA Committee on Team Standards, plus 30 of the 35 additional criteria.
Source: American Cleft Palate-Craniofacial Association. Parameters for evaluation and treatment of patients with Cleft Lip/Palate or other Craniofacial Anomalies. Pittsburgh: American Cleft Palate-Craniofacial Association, 1993.

North American cleft and craniofacial teams were contacted for team listing purposes using a self-assessment method developed by an interdisciplinary committee of national stature. Team clinical leaders classified their centers and provided data on team care. The response rate was 83.4% ($n = 247$), and the distribution of listed teams was 105 (42.5%) cleft palate teams, 102 (41.3%) craniofacial teams (includes craniofacial teams that are both cleft palate and craniofacial teams), and 12 (4.9%) geographically listed teams. There were 28 (11.3%) other teams that included interim cleft palate teams (new teams of less than 5 years' duration), low-density teams (teams in states with low population density), or evaluation and treatment review cleft palate teams (teams that provide no direct clinical treatment but only evaluation and quality assurance). They noted that 85% of all teams systematically collected and stored clinical data on their team's patient population in the past year. Furthermore, 50% of all North American teams had a quality assurance program in place to measure treatment outcomes. Other findings included the annual number of face-to-face team meetings; new and follow-up patient censuses; and surgical rates for initial repair of cleft lip/palate, orthognathic/osteotomy procedures, and intracranial/craniofacial procedures. The authors concluded that two out of five North American teams classify themselves as having the capacity to provide both cleft palate and craniofacial care. An additional two out of five teams limit their primary role to cleft palate care.

In evaluating a team, one might consider the questions included on the ACPA Team Self-Assessment Instrument (Strauss and The ACPA Team Standards Committee, 1998). As shown in Tables 24.1 and 24.2, there are different criteria for cleft palate teams and craniofacial teams. In developing a team, a potential team leader might use these criteria to guide planning.

As the U.S. health system changes, it is predictable that increasing attention will be paid to the rationale and value of cleft and craniofacial teams. Health planners are likely to ask the following:

1. How can cleft/craniofacial teams be most productive?
2. Are limitations on the numbers of cleft/craniofacial teams in a region effective at controlling cost and improving the quality of care?
3. Is team care more cost-effective than fragmented care? Does it result in improved outcomes for patients?
4. What constitutes a minimal team? an excellent team?

The cleft palate and craniofacial team can be understood as a way to organize complex, multi-specialty care in a humanistic and cost-effective manner. It is not difficult to endorse the vision of teams of professionals working together to reduce fragmentation and to make specialized care more personal. It is clear that getting a group to work together, e.g., to perform several different surgical procedures with one hospitalization and one anesthesia in one operating room, makes intuitive sense. A team approach reduces costs, minimizes school and work time loss, and promotes a more comprehensive view of care. The team approach implies quality peer review on a continuous basis. Constructing the most effective team possible is a challenge, but the rewards lie in the shared group interaction, the esprit-de-corps, and the families and patients who express satisfaction with the experience and outcomes of care.

Team standards criteria were developed by the ACPA Team Standards Committee: Samuel Berkowitz, DDS, MS (Orthodontics, Miami, FL); Philip J. Boyne, DMD, MS (Oral and Maxillofacial Surgery, Loma Linda, CA); Arthur Brown, MD (Plastic Surgery, Camden, NJ); John Canady, MD (Plastic Surgery, Iowa City, IA); Marilyn Cohen, BA (Team Coordinator, Speech Pathology, Camden, NJ); Linda Hallman, DDS, PhD (Orthodontist, Washington, DC); Robert Hardesty, MD (Plastic Surgery, Loma Linda, CA); Marilyn Jones, MD (Pediatrics and Genetics, San Diego, CA); Kathleen Kapp-Simon, MA, PhD (Psychology, Chicago, IL); Pat Landis, MA (Speech Pathology and Administration, Baltimore, MD); James Lehman, MD (Plastic Surgery, Akron, OH); Lynda Power, RN (Nursing, Toronto, Canada); Craig Senders, MD (Otolaryngology, Sacramento, CA); He-

TABLE 24.2. *American Cleft Palate-Craniofacial Association (ACPA) Standards for Listing Craniofacial Team (CFT)**

1. The Operating Surgeon(s), Orthodontist(s), Mental Health Professional(s) and Speech-Language Pathologist(s) on the CFT meet face-to-face at a scheduled team meeting or conference to evaluate patients with craniofacial anomalies or syndromes at least six times per year. The meeting may or may not coincide with CPT meetings.
2. The CFT evaluated at least 20 patients with craniofacial anomalies or syndromes in the past year.
3. The CFT assures that each child has health evaluation by a primary care Physician (Pediatrician, Family Physician or General Internist) in the community or on the team. The CPT uses the findings from the health evaluation to guide its treatment planning and team meeting deliberations. A community or team-based primary care Physician evaluates all patients prior to craniofacial surgery.
4. Craniofacial surgical treatments are adequately documented with facial and intraoral photographs, and appropriate radiographs.
5. Craniofacial treatment plans and treatment outcomes (results) for patients with craniofacial anomalies or syndromes are discussed at CFT meetings.
6. The CFT has a Surgeon(s) who attends team meetings and whose education, training and experience have adequately prepared him/her for the diagnosis and treatment of patients requiring craniofacial surgery.
7. At least one Surgeon on the CFT provided craniofacial surgical treatment (surgical procedures in which the intracranial approach to the midfacial segment -includes the orbit and/or supraorbital rim-is used) for a minimum of 10 patients with craniofacial anomalies or syndromes in the past year.
8. The CFT has an Orthodontist(s) who attends team meetings and whose education, training and experience have adequately prepared him/her for the orthodontic diagnosis and treatment of patients with craniofacial anomalies or syndromes.
9. At least one Orthodontist on the CFT provided orthodontic evaluation or treatment for a minimum of 10 patients with craniofacial anomalies or syndromes in the past year.
10. The CFT has a Speech-Language Pathologist(s) who attends team meetings and whose education, training and experience have adequately prepared him/her for speech and language diagnosis and treatment of patients with craniofacial anomalies or syndromes.
11. At least one Speech-Language Pathologist on the CFT provided speech therapy and/or a complete speech and language evaluation to a minimum of 10 patients (team or other patients) with craniofacial anomalies or syndromes (or cleft lip/palate) in the past year. The CFT Speech-Language Pathologist performs a structured speech assessment during team evaluations.
12. The CFT uses clinical speech instrumentation (such as endoscopy, pressure flow, videofluoroscopy, etc.) to assess velopharyngeal function, when indicated.
13. The CFT has a Mental Health Professional(s) (Psychologist, Social Worker, Developmental Pediatrician, Psychiatrist) who attends team meetings and whose education, training and experience have adequately prepared him/her for the psychological and psychosocial diagnosis and treatment of patients with craniofacial anomalies or syndromes.
14. The CFT has a Mental Health Professional(s) who evaluates all patients on a regular basis.
15. The CFT routinely tests or screens patients for learning disabilities and developmental, psychological, and language skills.
16. The CFT collects school reports and other information relative to learning in school-age patients, when indicated.
17. The CFT has a nurse or other trained professional who regularly provides supportive counseling and instruction (feeding, developmental) to parents of newborns.
18. The CFT sponsors or makes referrals to a parent support group or parent network in the community, as desired by families.
19. The CFT regularly provides supportive counseling and instruction to parents and patients pre- and post-operatively.
20. The CFT has a Neurosurgeon(s) whose education, training and experience have adequately prepared him/her for the neurosurgical diagnosis and treatment of patients with craniofacial anomalies or syndromes and who provides examination, treatment and consultation for CFT patients with craniofacial anomalies or syndromes.
21. The CFT has an Ophthalmologist(s) whose education, training and experience have adequately prepared him/her for the ophthalmological diagnosis and treatment of patients with craniofacial anomalies or syndromes and who provides examination, treatment and consultation for CFT patients with craniofacial anomalies or syndromes.
22. The CFT has an Otolaryngologist(s) whose education, training and experience have adequately prepared him/her for the otolaryngologic diagnosis and treatment of patients with craniofacial anomalies or syndromes and who provides examination, treatment and consultation for CFT patients with craniofacial anomalies or syndromes.
23. The CFT evaluation routinely includes hearing evaluation by an audiologist and\or otologic evaluations by an otolaryngologist.
24. The CFT has a Radiologist(s) whose education, training and experience have adequately prepared him/her for the radiological evaluation of patients with craniofacial anomalies or syndromes and who provides examination and consultation for CFT patients with craniofacial anomalies or syndromes.
25. The CFT facility has C.T. capability and access to M.R.I.
26. The CFT obtains lateral cephalometric radiographs (or the equivalent) on patients, when indicated.
27. The CFT has a Pediatric Dentist/General Dentist/Prosthodontist(s) whose education, training and experience have adequately prepared him/her for the dental diagnosis and treatment of patients with craniofacial anomalies or syndromes and who provides examination, treatment and consultation for CFT patients with craniofacial anomalies or syndromes.
28. The CFT makes intraoral dental casts on patients, when indicated.
29. The CFT has an Audiologist(s) whose education, training and experience have adequately prepared him/her for the audiologic diagnosis and treatment of patients with craniofacial anomalies or syndromes and who provides examination, treatment and consultation for CFT patients with craniofacial anomalies or syndromes.
30. The CFT has a Geneticist(s) whose education, training and experience have adequately prepared him/her for the genetic diagnosis and treatment of patients with craniofacial anomalies or syndromes and who provides examination, treatment and consultation for CFT patients with craniofacial anomalies or syndromes.
31. The CFT provides for formal genetic counseling or a clinical genetic evaluation for parents and patients.
32. The CFT facility has a Pediatric Intensive Care Unit (P.I.C.U.) in the facility where they perform craniofacial surgery.
33. After a CFT evaluation, the patient and family have an opportunity to ask questions and discuss the treatment plan with a team representative.
34. The CFT (for each evaluation) writes reports or summary letters, containing a treatment plan, which are sent to the family in a timely manner.

(continued)

TABLE 24.2. *American Cleft Palate-Craniofacial Association (ACPA) Standards for Listing Craniofacial Team (CFT)* (continued)*

35. CFT reports are sent in a timely manner to the patient's care providers in the community (schools, health department, local professionals) with the family's permission.
36. The CFT keeps a central and shared file on each patient.
37. The CFT record includes a diagnosis(es).
38. The CFT record includes a complete medical history.
39. The CFT record includes a treatment plan or goals which are reviewed periodically.
40. The CFT record includes a social and psychological history.
41. The CFT record includes dental and orthodontic findings and history.
42. The CFT takes facial photographs on patients in treatment or evaluation.
43. The CFT has an office and coordinator or secretary.
44. The CFT supports, encourages, or offers continuing education in craniofacial care for its members.
45. The CFT provides case management (follow-up, referral, and coordination of care) and benefits advocacy/assistance (help families obtain financial or programmatic support), as needed.

*The CFT provides coordinated and interdisciplinary evaluation and treatment for patients with a range of craniofacial anomalies or syndromes.

For the purposes of the categorization, craniofacial anomalies or syndromes are defined as congenital conditions other than cleft lip/palate, unless cleft lip/palate is a feature of another condition, anomaly or syndrome. The specific definition of craniofacial surgery being used states that "craniofacial surgery consists of the diagnosis, treatment planning, and surgical procedures in which the intracranial approach to the midfacial segment (includes the orbit and/or supraorbital rim) is used."

The CFT meets all of the following criteria defined by the ACPA Committee on Team Standards.

Source: American Cleft Palate-Craniofacial Association. Parameters for evaluation and treatment of patients with cleft lip/palate or other craniofacial anomalies. Pittsburgh: American Cleft Palate-Craniofacial Association, 1993.

len Sharp, MS (Speech Pathology/Ethics, Iowa City, IA); Barry Steinberg, DDS, MD, PhD (Oral and Maxillofacial Surgery, Ann Arbor, MI); Ronald P. Strauss, DMD, PhD (Dentistry and Sociology, Chapel Hill, NC, Chair); Timothy Turvey, DDS (Oral and Maxillofacial Surgery, Chapel Hill, NC); Duane VanDemark, PhD (Speech Pathology, Iowa City, IA). The ACPA Team Standards Committee conducted this work with the assistance of the ACPA National Office. The Allegheny Marketing Group (Pittsburgh, PA) performed data entry and data management.

REFERENCES

American Cleft Palate-Craniofacial Association (1993). *Parameters for Evaluation and Treatment of Patients with Cleft Lip/Palate or other Craniofacial Anomalies.* Pittsburgh: American Cleft Palate-Craniofacial Association.

American Cleft Palate-Craniofacial Association (2001). *2001–2002 Membership-Team Directory.* Chapel Hill: American Cleft Palate-Craniofacial Association.

Bardach, J, Morris, H, Olin, W, et al. (1984). Late results of multidisciplinary management of unilateral cleft lip and palate. Ann Plast Surg *12:* 235.

Brantley, HT, Clifford, E (1979). Cognitive self-concept and body image measures of normal, cleft palate, and obese adolescents. Cleft Palate J *16:* 177.

Briggs, TL (1980). Research an intra-professional social work teams in the United States of America. In: *Teamwork in the Personal Social Services and Health Care,* edited by S Lonsdale, A Webb, and TL Briggs. London: Croom Helm.

Brill, NI (1976). *Teamwork: Working Together in the Human Services.* Philadelphia: JB Lippincott.

Campbell, LS, Whitenack, DC (1983). An interdisciplinary approach for consultation on multiproblem patients. N C Med J *44:* 81–87.

Cluff, CB, Cluff, LF (1983). Informal support for disabled persons: a role for religious and community organizations. J Chron Dis *36:* 815–820.

Day, DW (1981). Perspectives on care: the interdisciplinary team approach. Otolaryngol Clin North Am *14:* 769–775.

Day, DW (1984). Genetics of congenital lip defects. Clin Plast Surg *11:* 693.

De Santis, G (1983). From teams to hierarchy: a short-lived innovation in a hospital for the elderly. Soc Sci Med *17:* 1613–1618.

DeSpirito, AP, Grebler, J (1983). Interdisciplinary approach to developmental pediatrics in a hospital-based child evaluation center. J Med Soc N J *80:* 906–908.

Dingwall, R (1980). Problems of teamwork in primary care. In: *Teamwork in the personal social services and health care,* edited by S Lonsdale, A Webb, and TL Briggs. London: Croom Helm, pp. 111–137.

Ellis, JHP (1986). Psychosocial Aspects in Health Care Teamwork: The Dynamics of Interaction in an Interdisciplinary Cleft Lip and Palate Team. Chapel Hill: Univ. of North Carolina. Dissertation.

Ellis, JHP (1993). Health Care Decision-Making Involvement of Patients and Medical Ideology. Chapel Hill: Univ. of North Carolina. Dissertation.

Emmanuel, EJ, Dubler, NN (1995). Preserving the physician–patient relationship in the era of managed care. JAMA *273:* 323–329.

Feinstein, AR (1983). On the coordination of care. J Chron Dis *36:* 813–814.

Furnham, A, Pendleton, D, Manicom, C (1981). The perception of different occupations within the medical profession. Soc Sci Med *15:* 289–300.

Herzlinger, R (1997). *Market Driven Health Care.* Reading MA: Addison-Wesley.

Hill, MJ (1956). An investigation of the attitudes and information possessed by parents of children with clefts of the lip and palate. Cleft Palate Bull *6:* 3.

Horwitz, JJ (1970). *Team Practice and the Specialist. An Introduction to Interdisciplinary Teamwork.* Springfield, IL: Charles Thomas.

Inglehart, JK (1996). The National Committee for Quality Assurance. N Engl J Med *335:* 995–999.

Jones, R (1992). Teamwork in primary health care: how much do we know about it? J Interprofessional Care *6:* 25–29.

Kane, RA (1980). Multi-disciplinary teamwork in the United States: trends, issues and implications for the social worker. In: *Teamwork in the Personal Social Services and Health Care,* edited by

S Lonsdale, A Webb, and TL Briggs. London: Croom Helm, pp. 138–151.

Koepp-Baker, H (1979). The craniofacial team. In: *Communicative Disorders Related to Cleft Lip and Palate,* 2nd ed. edited by KR Bzoch. Boston: Little, Brown, pp. 52–61.

Kutner, R (1998). The commercialization of Prepaid Group Health Care. N Engl J Med *338:* 1558–1563.

Lillywhite, H (1957). Communication problems in the cleft palate rehabilitation team. Cleft Palate Bull *7:* 8–10.

Logan, RL, McKendry, M (1982). The multi-disciplinary team: a different approach to patient management. N Z Med J *95:* 883–884.

Lonsdale, S, Webb, A, Briggs, TL (eds) (1980). *Teamwork in the Personal Social Services and Health Care.* London: Croom Helm.

MacDonald, SK (1979). Parental needs and professional responses: a parental perspective. Cleft Palate J *16:* 188.

MacGregor, FC (1982). Foreword. Social psychological considerations in plastic surgery. Past, present and future. Clin Plastic Surg *9:* 283–288.

Margolis, H, Fiorelli, JS (1984). An applied approach to facilitating interdisciplinary teamwork. J Rehabil *50:* 13–17.

Mason, RM, Riski, JE (1982). The team approach to orofacial management. Ann Plast Surg *8:* 71–78.

McKeganey, NP, Bloor, MJ (1987). Teamwork, information control and therapeutic effectiveness: a tale of two therapeutic communities. Sociol Health Illness *9:* 154–158.

Morris, HL, Jakobi, P, Harrington, D (1978). Objectives and criteria for the management of cleft lip and palate and the delivery of management services. Cleft Palate J *15:* 1.

Nackashi, JA, Dixon-Wood, VL (1989). The craniofacial team: medical supervision and coordination. In: *Communicative Disorders Related to Cleft Lip and Palate,* 3rd ed., edied by KR Bzoch. College Hill, pp. 63–74.

Nagi, SS (1975). Teamwork in health care in the United States: a sociological perspective. Milbank Mem Fund Q Health Soc *53:* 75–91.

Nason, F (1983). Diagnosing the hospital team. Soc Work Health Care *9:* 25–45.

Nelson, H (1997). *Nonprofit and For-Profit HMOs: Converging Practices but Different Goals?* New York: Milbank Memorial Fund.

Noar, JH (1992). A questionnaire survey of attitudes and concerns of three professional groups involved in the cleft palate team. Cleft Palate Craniofac J *29:* 92–95.

Ovretveit, J (1996). Five ways to describe a multidisciplinary team. J. Interprofessional Care *10:* 163–171.

Pannbacker, M, Lass, NJ, Scheurle, JF, et al. (1992). Survey of services and practices of cleft palate-craniofacial teams. Cleft Palate Craniofac J *29:* 164.

Payne, M (1982). *Working in Teams.* London: MacMillan.

Phillips, J, Whitaker, LA (1979). The social effects of cranofacial deformity and its correction. Cleft Palate J *16:* 7.

Povar, G, Moreno, J (1988). Hippocrates and the health maintenance organization: a discussion of ethical issues. Ann Intern Med *109:* 419–424.

Reinhardt, UE (1993). Reforming the health care system: the universal dilemma. Am J Law Med *19:* 21–36.

Simon, C, Emmons, DW (1997). Physician earnings at risk. Health Affairs *16:* 120–126.

Strauss, RP (1985). Culture, rehabilitation and facial birth defects: international case studies. Cleft Palate J *22:* 56–62.

Strauss, RP (1994). Health policy and craniofacial care: issues in resource allocation. Cleft Palate Craniofac J *31:* 78–80.

Strauss, RP (1997). Social and psychological perspectives on cleft lip and palate. In: *Communicative Disorders Related to Cleft Lip and Palate,* 4th ed., edited by KR Bzoch. Austin, TX: Pro Ed, pp. 95–113.

Strauss, RP (1999). The organization and delivery of craniofacial health services: the state of the art. Cleft Palate Craniofac J *36:*

Strauss, RP, Broder, H (1985). Interdisciplinary team care of cleft lip and palate: social and psychological aspects. Clin Plast Surg *12:* 543–551.

Strauss, RP, Broder, H (1990). Social and psychological aspects of cleft lip and palate. In: *Multidisciplinary Management of Cleft Lip and Palate,* edited by J Bardach and H Morris. Philadelphia: WB Saunders, pp. 831–837.

Strauss, RP, Ellis, JHP (1996). Comprehensive team management. In: *Facial Clefts and Craniosynostosis: Principles and Management,* edited by TA Turvey, KWL Vig, and RJ Fonseca. Philadelphia: WB Saunders, pp. 130–142.

Strauss, RP, The ACPA Team Standards Committee (1998). Cleft palate and craniofacial centers in the United States and Canada: a national survey of team organization and standards of care. Cleft Palate Craniofac J *35:* 473–480.

Temkin-Greener, H (1983). Interprofessional perspectives on teamwork in health care: a case-study. Milbank Mem Fund Q Health Soc *61:* 641–658.

Webb, AL, Hobdell, M (1980). Coordination and teamwork in the health and personal social services. In: *Teamwork in the Personal Social Services and Health Care,* edited by S Lonsdale, A Webb, and TL Briggs. London: Croom Helm, pp. 97–110.

25

Health care for children with cleft lip and palate: comprehensive services and infant feeding

JOHN A. NACKASHI

E. ROSELLEN DEDLOW

VIRGINIA DIXON-WOOD

Children with cleft lip with or without palate (CL/P) have a wide array of needs. The most obvious consequence of CL/P is the facial difference. The impact of the cleft condition on the child and family can vary considerably. The child's long-term outcome is influenced by many factors, which include the underlying condition, strengths of the child and family, access to services, and completion of a comprehensive treatment plan. Children with CL/P have all of the needs and strengths of typical children, but many have special needs related to the cleft condition. Children with clefts can be referred to as children with special health care needs, i.e., "those who have or are at elevated risk for chronic physical, developmental, behavioral, or emotional conditions and who also require health and related services of a type or amount not usually required by children" (Maternal and Child Health Bureau, 1995). This definition helps to identify children who may need increased services. Through this identification process and to provide care, government agencies and health policymakers are given the foundation to build systems of care, health benefit packages, and services. For the clinician, recognizing that a child has special needs directs and emphasizes the importance of comprehensive and coordinated services.

The presence of CL/P is a marker indicating that there may be associated concerns, which may be more significant and of greater consequence to the child than the cleft itself. Clefts may be associated with syndromes, early feeding problems, airway compromise, growth and developmental abnormalities, speech disorders, recurrent ear infections, and psychosocial concerns. An understanding of the underlying condition helps in predicting the complexity of the child's needs and possible outcomes. A child may have essentially no major concerns or may be unusually complicated. Early identification of a syndrome is extremely important and represents the first step in determining the child's needs and the complexity of care. Due to the increased risk for medical, developmental, psychological, surgical, and dental problems, a team of CL/P specialists can best serve the child and family. A team can also support the child's community providers in the provision of local healthcare services. Pediatric primary care providers, specialists, and cleft palate teams need to recognize that children with CL/P have the same needs as typical children in addition to their special needs. This conceptual framework provides the foundation for care.

KEY TIMES FOR CARE: A GENERAL PERSPECTIVE

There are key times for the child and family that are associated with significant medical, development, psychosocial, surgical, and dental needs. The care for children with CL/P is very age-dependent. This is important to know because the final outcome is dependent on the correct timing of evaluations and procedures. As a child becomes older, the next step in care is built upon the prior completed step. During the life of the child, there are periods of time, which extend from weeks to years, in which a specific type of need (i.e., feeding, surgical, speech, or dental services) best describes the goals of treatment. There are also periods of time in which the only intervention is monitoring. Recognition of these key times is very useful in communicating with families to help them develop a frame of reference about their child's care and the treatment plan. These key times are linked to the specific goals and interventions.

There is a great commonality of needs among children and across cleft conditions and associated health concerns, but there also may be great variation of needs depending on the specific child and family. The following is a simplified way to view care for children with CL/P, providing a big-picture perspective that should be helpful to families. There is some variation in the timing of surgery by various centers and teams.

First Month

The first month is the time for evaluations to make the diagnosis, counsel families, and provide instruction to safely feed the infant. Weekly weight checks are recommended to monitor weight gain and ensure that the infant reaches birth weight by at least 3 weeks of age. A critical role for healthcare professionals is communication, information sharing, and referral to services.

Birth to 2 Years

For many children, the majority of surgery is completed by 18 months. In many centers, the lip is repaired by 3 months and the palate by 1 year. For all children, this is a time for screening growth and development with a special emphasis on language and speech, growth, middle ear disease, and hearing.

Age 2 to 7 Years

Screening of development with a special emphasis on speech and cognitive and psychosocial functioning is a pivotal need between the ages of 2 and 7. Initiation of dental care sets the stage for most of the treatment needs for the adolescent and teenage years. For many children, the occurrence of otitis media begins to wane. Some children continue to have middle ear disease and hearing loss. There are a significant number of children who require interventions for speech, development, and cognitive and psychosocial needs. Some children require surgical procedures to correct speech. Some families choose to have minor surgical lip and nose revisions.

Age 7 to Teenage Years

For children who have completed the needed and appropriately timed procedures, the primary needs are now dental. Dental care provides the final and necessary step to have the best long-term outcome. From the age of 7 to the teen years a period of extensive dental bracing is required. Bone grafting is routinely done to allow teeth to be moved into the cleft. Many families will choose this time period to have minor, "touch-up" surgery on the nose and lip. Due to a significant dental malocclusion, some children will have orthognathic surgery when they are finished growing, usually after 16 years of age. For most children, the treatment is now complete.

THE BIRTH EXPERIENCE AND FIRST CLINICAL ENCOUNTER

The birth of an infant with CL/P is usually unexpected. Prenatal diagnosis is becoming more common with transvaginal sonography. Accurate detection of a cleft lip is possible at 13 to 16 weeks' gestation. Cleft palate is difficult to detect in utero due to its posterior and midcephalic location (Habel et al., 1996). Prenatal diagnosis of CL/P represents only a very small number of children. As a result, families and healthcare providers are not prepared. In addition, healthcare providers commonly do not know the significance of the CL/P, what to tell the family, and how to provide care for the infant. Families are looking for a healthy baby and certainly not one that looks different and is difficult to feed. They are expecting healthcare providers who are confident and reassuring rather than confused and uncertain.

Many parents will describe their reaction to the birth of their baby with a cleft, especially when it involves a cleft lip, as one of "shock." A consistent finding in studies involving the birth and diagnosis of CL/P is the families reporting shock, guilt, anxiety, and depression (Strauss, 1997). Families commonly state that there appears to be a great deal of confusion associated with the birth of their baby. Factors contributing to the difficulties encountered during the birth include cultural beliefs, the birthing experience, the level of experience of healthcare providers with CL/P infants, and the quality of communication with the family. Typically, the medical and nursing staff has little opportunity to develop competency in the early management of infants with CL/P, even though it is one of the most frequent congenital defects. The incidence of infants with CL/P is approximately 1/700 births in North America. Numerous community hospitals may have fewer than 1 or 2/1000 births in a year. Based on the incidence of cleft lip and palate, there may be only one or two such infants born in a year. In some community hospitals, a baby with CL/P may be delivered only every few years. Due to the limited number of births, physicians do not develop a high level of experience in providing care for the infant with CL/P. Typically, there is turnover of nursing and other hospital staff, which adds to the problem of developing competency in the care of newborns with clefts.

For many years, literature on children with disabilities has shown that families have expressed major concerns about how physicians communicate and deliver needed information. A study on parental recall about how they were told of their child's diagnosis of CL/P (Strauss, 1997) revealed that there were significant differences between what parents experienced and what they wanted in their communication with physicians. Parents related the need for more time to talk, more of an opportunity to show their feelings, and more of an effort on the part of the physician to make them feel better. Parents wanted more information, referral to another parent of a child with CL/P, and more opportunity to discuss the possibility of mental retardation (Strauss et al., 1995).

The first clinical encounter with healthcare providers has profound significance for the child and family. Since the birth of an infant with CL/P is typically unexpected, the role of the pediatrician or other healthcare providers is complicated by the special needs of the infant and the emotional and psychosocial impact on the family.

Pediatric providers have a critical role that involves evaluating the medical and feeding needs of the infant. The first responsibility is to evaluate the infant's medical stability and need for immediate treatment, referral to specialists, and/or transferral to a neonatal intensive care unit (NICU). Once it is determined that the infant is medically stable (which represents the majority of infants), the next step is to search for the presence of major and minor malformations or findings suggesting an associated syndrome. This involves a detailed review of the infant's medical history and the family's history of CL/P, syndromes, congenital defects, or conditions that have affected children. The prenatal history is important to elicit information about prenatal care, illnesses, chronic conditions, use of medications, use of alcohol, use of tobacco, or substance abuse during pregnancy. A newborn is examined with an emphasis on detecting subtle variations and obvious anomalies while focusing on the craniofacial, cardiac, skeletal, and genitourinary systems. Meticulous observation and documentation is the key to quickly determining the correct diagnosis. At the same time, the pediatrician should not feel pressured to make a definitive diagnosis. Geneticists and cleft palate team experts are best at making a final diagnosis. The detailed birth history and physical examination will enable the geneticist to determine if the cleft is a sporadic occurrence, associated with a syndrome, genetically transmitted through single-gene or multifactorial inheritance, chromosomal in nature, or caused by teratogens (Domet, 1986). References are available which will be of assistance in determining whether physical exam findings suggest a syndrome (Pashayan, 1983; Smith, 1997) and which link major and minor anomalies with syndromes (Pashayan, 1983; Smith, 1997). For the infant who has findings suggesting the presence of a syndrome, genetic consultation should be obtained as soon as possible.

If the history reveals no concerns and the physical exam is normal, the pediatric provider can tell the family that the baby most likely has an isolated CL/P. The family can be told that the infant can be referred to a cleft palate team and that comprehensive services directed by the team can maximize the outcome for the child. Even though a child appears to have only an isolated CL/P, many infants will benefit from a genetics evaluation, which can be scheduled at a convenient time for the family. This is an important time for families to gain information about CL/P in general and about their infant's specific needs. They may also have questions about future childbearing, which can be addressed by the genetics counselor. Pamphlets, web sites, and contact with families who have a child with CL/P are a great help to the family. These resources are an effective way to provide information and support to the family. A critical responsibility at the first clinical encounter is assessing the infant's feeding skills.

PROVISION OF PEDIATRIC HEALTH SERVICES: COMMUNITY AND CLEFT PALATE TEAM

All children with oral clefts should have primary care through a community medical home that provides continuity of care which is accessible, compassionate, and culturally competent. The American Academy of Pediatrics and the National Center of Medical Home Initiatives for Children with Special Health Care Needs promote this concept for children with special healthcare needs. The primary care well-child evaluation consists of a history, review of medications, allergies, immunizations, development and psychosocial status, family and social history, complete physical exam, anticipatory guidance, laboratory tests, immunizations, clinical impression, plan, and follow-up.

Coordinated, comprehensive services are best provided by a partnership between the primary care provider, the cleft palate team, and the family. This partnership is critical for the optimum outcome. Pediatric healthcare providers may be pediatricians, family practitioners, pediatric nurse practitioners, and physician assistants. The functions of the community and team pediatric healthcare providers overlap, but the roles are different. The community pediatrician uses this comprehensive approach to provide primary care. The cleft palate team pediatrician uses this comprehensive approach to gain a familiarity with the child and to support the team's evaluation and the development of an appropriate and safe treatment plan. The team benefits from the pediatrician's ability to give advise about special health concerns, the need for diagnostic evaluations and treatments for known or previously undetected problems, general developmental and psychosocial functioning, and the determination that surgery and procedures can be safely conducted. The team pediatrician has a unique role of overseeing the total needs of the child during the team evaluation and treatment process.

ROLES AND RESPONSIBILITIES OF THE PRIMARY CARE PROVIDER

Provide Early Identification and Diagnosis of Cleft Lip with or without Palate and Associated Conditions and Refer to Appropriate Specialists

The primary care provider can support the family following the prenatal diagnosis by collaborating with geneticists and specialists. Key responsibilities include aiding the communication and parental education process so that the family understands the significance of the suspected condition for the life of the child and family, required treatments, complexity of care, probable outcome with appropriate care, and the family's options. The primary care provider's role is to facilitate communication with experts in the field and to listen to the family's concerns and questions. The primary care provider may have a unique role as gatekeeper, to support the family's search for expert care. The most important initial responsibility at birth is determining that the infant is medically stable or has complex health conditions requiring special support or transfer to an NICU experienced with children with CL/P. The next step is to provide a medical diagnosis. Early commu-

nication with a cleft palate team can be important in determining the need for special testing (i.e., renal ultrasounds, cardiac consultation, immediate genetic evaluations, and cranial computed tomographic scans). Infants with isolated CL/P may need only a genetic evaluation, which can be scheduled at a time convenient for the family. Other infants may need early or immediate extensive evaluation.

Evaluate Infant's Ability to Feed and Refer to a Professional with Expertise in Feeding of Infants with Cleft Lip with or without Palate

The vast majority of infants with CL/P will need assistance to be successfully fed orally. The primary care provider, through the initial medical examination, needs to determine that the infant can protect the airway and coordinate feeding and breathing. Consultation with a professional, knowledgeable about feeding infants with CL/P, is important to instruct the family, nurses, and hospital staff how to feed the infant (see Feeding Infants with Cleft Lip with or without Palate, below, for specific information).

Provide Screening and Monitoring with Each Well-Child Visit for Early Detection of Problems for which Children with Cleft Lip with or without Palate Are at Increased Risk

Weight Gain in the First Month of Life. In general, feeding an infant with CL/P is initially difficult and stressful for the family, but with appropriate instruction and monitoring, the infant will do fine. Parents can be told to expect that their infant will not only take longer to feed but be a noisy feeder compared to the typical newborn. A weekly weight check for the first month of life ensures that the infant is gaining weight adequately. Birth weight should be regained by 2 to 3 weeks of life. Documented weekly weight gain is of importance to the infant's physiological health and the psychological well-being of the family, indicating that the infant is growing normally. Usually, after the first 4 to 5 weeks of age, the baby develops the ability to effectively orally feed. Infants with isolated CL/P should be able to orally feed and not require tube feedings. Infants who are unable to successfully feed without tube-feeding support should be evaluated for associated anomalies, perinatal illnesses, or injuries. Children who drop off their own growth curve need to be evaluated for failure to thrive.

Stature. Investigators have reported on the relationship between CL/P and children's stature. Short stature is defined as height less than two standard deviations below the mean or height below the third percentile for same sex and age peers. An expected outcome for children with CL/P is attainment of normal stature consistent with the family. A review of the literature shows great variability of findings about the stature and growth patterns of children with CL/P.

Increased incidence of short stature has been reported (Ranalli and Mazaheri, 1975; Roitman and Laron, 1978; Rudman et al., 1978; Duncan et al., 1983; Cunningham and Jerome, 1992; Felix-Schollaart et al., 1992). Investigators have found variations in the growth patterns, e.g., poor early growth with attainment of normal growth by 2 years of age (Roitman and Laron, 1978; Rudman et al., 1978; Duncan et al., 1983, Felix-Schollaart et al., 1992; Nystrom et al., 1992). Increased incidence of severe short stature due to associated growth hormone deficiency has been reported (Roitman and Laron, 1978; Rudman et al., 1978). Normal growth has also been reported (Nackashi et al., 1988). The variation in findings may be due to sample size, accuracy of measurements, ascertainment bias, cultural differences (country of origin), and definition of short stature.

Explanations for growth pattern variations and excessive short stature include feeding difficulties during the neonatal period and infancy (Drillen et al., 1966; Jensen et al., 1983) and decreased feeding after palatal surgery (Drillen et al., 1966; Ranalli and Mazahari, 1975; Hunter, 1981; Jensen et al., 1983, 1988; Seth and McWilliams, 1988). Felix-Schollaart et al. (1992) reported that feeding difficulties, airway infections, and surgery affect growth but did not account for differences among the CL/P groups and controls reported in the literature. Danish infants with some combination of CL/P were found to have birth weights and lengths close to those considered average for Danish newborns, but infants with severe palatal clefts demonstrated increased incidence of delayed growth.

Due to the variation in findings, many suggesting that children with CL/P have short stature, it is wise to view these children as at risk for being somewhat short but not meeting the criteria for short stature. The primary care provider, through continuity of care, is afforded the best opportunity to monitor growth by serial measurements and standardized growth charts.

After the newborn period, weight and length, in particular length, need to be closely monitored. Families need to be informed that children with syndromes commonly are small for age. Children with true short stature (height less than two standard deviations below the mean or below the third percentile) should be referred for an endocrinological evaluation. Children who are smaller than their peers or family members but are between the 5th and 95th percentiles for stature, have adequate nutrition, and have no other health risks need to be routinely monitored. The family and child should be counseled that the child is normal and healthy.

Development, Behavior, and Psychosocial Functioning. Children with CL/P experience many psychosocial stressors starting in early childhood. Multiple investigators have examined a diverse set of psychological factors, including emotional and behavioral adjustments (Padwa et al., 1991); peer relationships (Krueckeberg et al., 1993), learning disabilities, and neuropsychological development (Kapp-Simon et al., 1993; Richman and Eliason, 1993; Kapp-Simon, 1994); self-perception and body image (Broder and Strauss, 1989; Leonard et al., 1991; Kapp-Simon et al., 1992; Pope and Ward, 1997); and social interaction patterns (Kapp-Simon and McGuire, 1997). An extensive review of the literature on CL/P and other craniofacial anomalies involving parental acceptance, social competence, self-concept, emotional adjustment, and cognitive functioning indicates that 30% to 40% of children in most studies experience difficulties with internalizing and/or externalizing problems, learning disorders, and social competence (Endriga and Kapp-Simon, 1999).

Screening of development and behavior by the primary care provider involves standard developmental approaches. Appropriate approaches include parental report of skills and concerns, use of milestones and developmental screening tools (e.g., the Denver II), and clinical observation to detect developmental delay and affirm particular strengths of the infant and young child. Screening by a cleft palate team is also of great help to the primary care provider. The team has the advantage of seeing many children with CL/P, resulting in a rich experience and expertise. When concerns arise, referral to a developmental pediatrician, psychologist, speech–language pathologist, and other specialists is critical to reduce morbidity and improve outcome.

Developmental screening of school-aged children focuses on learning problems, school-related issues, and psychosocial functioning. The primary care provider can screen the child and family for psychosocial stressors and well-being by asking about family and peer relationships, social and educational concerns, and strengths. Recommendations to the family to intervene with peer-related concerns by visiting with schoolteachers and counselors can be helpful. Parents can talk to their child's classmates about CL/P with the hope that an understanding of the condition will extinguish negative behaviors and teasing. The primary care provider should counsel the family prospectively through anticipatory guidance. Persistent, disturbing, and pervasive psychological problems may require referral to a psychologist or licensed mental health professional.

Speech–Language Skills. Cleft palate puts the child at high risk for a speech disorder known as velopharyngeal insufficiency (VPI), the cause of classic "cleft palate speech." Even after surgery, the velum (soft palate) and pharyngeal walls may be unable to create a velopharyngeal port that regulates the correct amount of airflow through the nose. Excess airflow through the nose results in hypernasality. If not treated, the hypernasality contributes to the development of compensatory speech patterns, which can be severe and lifelong. Most speech pathologists are not trained in the care of VPI, and this makes the involvement of an experienced cleft palate team even more important. The role of the primary care provider is to conduct routine speech–language screening and to refer to professionals for therapy when indicated. Indications for referral include speech–language delay, articulation problems, hypernasality, and unintelligible speech.

Otitis Media and Hearing Loss. Children with CL/P are at increased risk for otitis media and hearing loss. Most children with CL/P experience some degree of middle ear inflammation, otitis media, or recurrent middle ear pathology during their early childhood years. Eustachian tube dysfunction is the physiological cause for this increased incidence of middle ear pathology and hearing loss. It is generally thought that eustachian tube dysfunction is caused by disruption of the entire muscular sling of the soft palate due to the formation of the posteriorly located cleft. This results in abnormal muscle attachments of the tensor veli palatini to the eustachian tubes. The tensor veli palatini muscles cannot contract effectively, resulting in inadequate opening of the eustachian tubes, which leads to middle ear disease. One of the goals of early palatal repair is to create a palate that is functional for speech and improves eustachian tube function. Investigators have reported that eustachian tube function improves after cleft palate repair (Doyle et al., 1986; Sweitzer et al., 1968). Children with a cleft palate can recover normal eustachian tube function after repair of the palate, but the recovery may take many years (Smith et al., 1994). For children who do not regain normal eustachian tube function, recurring otitis media or chronic otitis media with effusion continues to be a problem. Paradise et al. (1969) found that the most prevalent form of otitis media in children with cleft palate is chronic otitis media with effusion (COME). Persistent

middle ear effusion increases the risk of conductive hearing loss, especially during the first year of life, increasing the chance of delayed speech and language development (Habel et al., 1996).

This is even more problematic since it is generally painless and therefore can go undetected except by an otological evaluation. In addition, the child with cleft palate may have COME, which increases the chances for serious middle ear pathology, including tympanic membrane atelectasis, perforation, and cholesteatoma (Bluestone and Kline, 1990).

Otological and audiological monitoring to detect middle ear pathology and hearing loss need to begin in infancy and continue through the teenage years. Children should receive biannual otological and audiological testing consisting of at least an ear exam, tympanometry, and audiogram during the first year of life and preferably up through 3 years of age. This same battery of screening tests should continue annually until care is completed. Many children have stabilization of their middle ear status by 7 years of age and primarily require monitoring. Depending on the complexity of the child's otological and audiological status, testing may need to be more frequent and extensive.

Contemporary approaches for the treatment of acute otitis media include minimizing the use of antibiotics in asymptomatic cases. Antibiotics are used for febrile episodes and when hearing loss is detected. If otitis media persists or continues to recur regardless of antibiotic treatment, the child needs more extensive follow-up. Recurrent otitis media, COME, and hearing loss are commonly treated by placement of tympanostomy tubes. Tympanostomy tubes can be effective at clearing middle ear effusion and correcting hearing impairment, but they can also cause sequelae, including scarring and tympanic membrane perforation. Adenoidectomy is contraindicated because it can exacerbate VPI. The outcome for middle ear function and hearing is maximized by long-term monitoring and testing as part of the comprehensive care provided by a cleft palate team.

Dental. The primary care provider can emphasize the importance of developing good dental hygiene habits toward the long-term outcome of cleft care. Weaning from the bottle early in the second year of life can enhance dental care. Other important strategies involve introduction of early cleaning and brushing of teeth. Since dental malocclusion is common, long-term use of a pacifier and thumb sucking should be discouraged. The family needs to know that the child's care from around 6 years of age to the completion of treatment in the mid-teens is primarily dental. Completion of properly timed dental care and procedures results in the best outcome. Families need to understand that dental care is a necessary component of the total treatment plan and that a combination of surgery and dental care will result in the best outcome for the child.

Special Conditions

There are over 300 syndromes associated with CL/P. All children with CL/P can benefit from a genetics evaluation and referral to a cleft palate team. Two of the more common associated conditions have implications for the primary care provider.

Velocardiofacial syndrome (VCFS) is the most frequent clefting condition (Shprintzen et al., 1981). There are numerous features, which are not always present, including cleft palate, cardiac anomalies, typical facial features, slender hands and digits, ophthalmological abnormalities, psychiatric illness, VPI, and medial displacement of the internal carotid arteries. The condition is caused by deletions of the human chromosome 22q11 region. These deletions are also common in DiGeorge syndrome, suggesting an etiological connection. DiGeorge syndrome is considered a sequence found in VCFS and involves thymic aplasia, immune deficiency, hypocalcemia, and congenital heart defects. Children who have these clinical features and 22q11 deletions have VCFS. The implications of VCFS are broad, spanning physical, cognitive, psychosocial, speech, and developmental domains. These children are at high risk for poor outcomes, including school failure, behavioral concerns, and psychiatric illness. This is an example of a condition that can be missed at birth and has long-term consequences.

Robin sequence (RS) is a well-known condition that includes micrognathia, cleft palate, and glossoptosis, causing airway obstruction. Many infants with RS have some degree of airway compromise and are at risk for airway-related feeding problems. A large number of infants are managed with positioning, careful feeding, and close monitoring. When calm, infants are generally engaged in quiet breathing and appear well. Upper respiratory infections, vigorous crying, and feeding can cause obstruction or partial obstruction of the airway, which leads to airway compromise.

At birth, infants with severe airway compromise need NICU management, which may include tracheal intubation, supplemental oxygen, mechanical ventilation, orogastric tube feedings, and 24 h monitoring. Surgical management of the airway may involve tracheostomy, tongue–lip adhesion, or mandibular distraction. Some infants may require months of hospitalization before they are stable enough to be discharged home. The vast majority of infants will stabilize and have normal breathing and feeding abilities although, some will require a protracted period of time to outgrow their need

for airway and nutrition support. Some children with RS may also have Stickler syndrome, which involves orofacial findings consistent with RS along with myopia and musculoskeletal abnormalities. After many years, arthritis may become a significant problem and progressive myopia may lead to retinal detachment and blindness. Some children are at risk for mitral valve prolapse. Children with RS, and especially those thought to have Stickler syndrome, should have a chest x-ray, electrocardiogram, genetic evaluation, eye examination, and a sleep study. Robin sequence is an example of a condition often apparent at birth, due to the airway compromise and feeding difficulties, but that can have an excellent outcome with appropriate supportive care. Stickler syndrome is an example of a condition that cannot be fully evaluated at birth because the features evolve over time. Children with this condition are at risk for worsening vision and need regular vision screening in the primary care office.

Feeding Infants with Cleft Lip with or without Palate

The goal of feeding the newborn is to provide adequate calories to support life, growth, and development. Mother–infant bonding is an important, but physiologically secondary, part of the feeding process. It has been suggested by Rybski et al. (1984) that feeding the newborn is contingent on the coordinated interaction of a complex set of behaviors, including the participation of a caregiver. It is a common clinical observation that parents of a newborn with CL/P often experience considerable anxiety due to the problems they encounter when attempting to feed their baby and that these feelings can interfere with the normal interaction between parent and child.

BIOLOGY OF SUCKING

Normal Sucking

Sucking, one of the earliest organized behaviors, and rhythmical bursts of jaw opening and closing associated with movements of the tongue have been identified even in fetal life (de Vries et al., 1988). Fetuses have been observed in activities of nonnutritive sucking of thumbs and toes as early as 28 weeks while in utero (Shaker, 1990; Medoff-Cooper and Ray, 1995).

For the neonate of 32 to 34 weeks, the mechanisms of creating a partial vacuum intraorally, controlling an effective stripping motion of the nipple by the tongue, and coordinating an efficient swallow have matured into a well-integrated system (Goldson, 1987; Shaker, 1990). The infant encompasses the nipple with the lips, creating an airtight seal around the nipple or areola. With an effective anterior seal, the mandible is pulled down along with the central dorsum part of the tongue, resulting in more space intraorally and subsequently a decreased or negative intraoral air pressure (suction). The infant then presses the nipple against the alveolus and hard palate and, with a rolling or stripping movement of the tongue tip across the nipple from front to back, extracts milk from the nipple. The milk bolus is forced by this rolling action of the tongue into the pharynx, where it enters into the esophagus, and through the process of peristalsis (and gravity), is carried to the stomach (Bu'Lock et al., 1990).

Suction or the Partial Vacuum Created Intraorally as Part of the Sucking Process

Various techniques have been utilized to define the sucking and swallowing process, including cineradiography (Ardran et al., 1958a,b), ultrasound (Smith et al., 1985; Weber et al., 1986; Bu'Lock et al., 1990; Nowak et al., 1995), videofiberoscopy (Eishima, 1991; Iwayama and Eishima, 1997), and assessment of pressure changes intraorally, with or without measurement of fluid flow, using pressure transducers (Goldson, 1987; Jain et al., 1987; Medoff-Cooper et al., 1989, 1993; Fadavi et al., 1997; Waterland et al., 1998). Of the three primary components in feeding [lip seal, tongue stripping, and intraoral negative pressure (suction)], it is suction with its several dimensions that can be relatively easily and objectively measured.

Research has been directed at quantifying various components of sucking, such as the intensity of each suck, the duration of each suck, and the duration of rest periods between sucks. These measures have been obtained using a pressure transducer to determine changes in air pressure within the bottle while the infant is feeding (Linder, 1991; McGowan et al., 1991; Medoff-Cooper, 1991; Palmer, 1993; Medoff-Cooper and Ray, 1995). As growth occurs, the infant can generate greater negative intraoral pressure and stripping pressure (Linder, 1991; Medoff-Cooper et al., 1993). By the end of the first year, there is generally a change in diet and a weaning off the bottle, with sucking activities and reflexes becoming repressed (Iwayama and Eishima, 1997).

Biology of Sucking during Breast-Feeding

Functionally, breast-feeding differs from bottle-feeding in the wide-open position of the jaw, the position of the nipple in the mouth, the muscles used, and the response or elasticity of the nipple in the mouth in response to the sucking (Turgeon-O'Brien et al., 1996). Most of the research on sucking has been done on infants fed from bottles equipped with transducers. Great care is taken to remove confounding variables by offering the same nipple, the same fluid, in the same position, etc., to all infants in a study. Research on breast-fed infants is more complex as it is harder to measure negative intraoral pressure and the infant–mother interaction and physiological responses of the mother to sucking cannot be quantified. Research and clinical observation indicate that the sucking pattern of infants changes over the course of the feed, as do the availability and composition of the breast milk (Chetwynd et al., 1998). The amount of milk extracted is not determined solely by the baby and the sucking pressure patterns but is affected by the let-down reflex and other maternal variables (Prieto et al., 1996). Infants who are breast-fed use negative intraoral pressure to position and stabilize the breast in the mouth. A combination of negative intraoral pressure, the stripping action of the tongue against the breast supported by the palate, and the pumping movements of the jaw and gums empties the milk ducts (Clarren et al., 1987; BuLock et al., 1990).

Biology of Sucking in a Neonate with a Cleft

There has been extensive research in the sucking patterns of preterm and term infants, and descriptions of the developmental stages of the sucking pattern to the age of 14 months (DeMonterice et al., 1992; Medoff-Cooper and Ray, 1995; Turgeon-O'Brien et al., 1996; Fadavi et al., 1997; Hafström et al., 1997; Iwayama and Eishima, 1997; Finan and Barlow, 1998; Waterland et al., 1998). There has been very little research on the sucking patterns of infants with cleft lip or cleft palate preoperatively or postoperatively (Choi et al., 1991). One report examined palatal motor movement pre- and postoperatively (Igawa et al., 1998). The sucking characteristics of these groups must be described prior to comparison to noncleft children. Dixon-Wood et al. (1999) measured the intraoral pressure of infants with CL/P during feeding. Special nipples were developed (Medoff-Cooper et al., 1993), which contained two tubes connected to a transducer. Intraoral pressure was measured during bottle-feeding. None of the children with cleft palate were able to generate any negative intraoral pressure. An interesting finding was that these children learned very early to position the nipple in the mouth so as to mechanically strip it with the tongue against the alveolus, cheek, or palate.

This supports what we know about anatomy, the development of negative intraoral pressure during sucking, and the effect of cleft palate on the ability to develop negative intraoral pressure. Therefore, we can assume that a child with a cleft palate preoperatively cannot create effective negative intraoral pressure due to the open communication between mouth and nose.

Additionally, infants with cleft palate lack the support against which the tongue can effectively strip the nipple or breast. Depending on the position of the premaxilla and its stability, the infant may be further hampered by an inability to use movements of the jaw and gums to assist with feeding. Clarren et al. (1987) separated subjects into groups by diagnosis and made feeding recommendations for each cleft type. This technique has been adapted Table 25.1.

DETERMINING AN INFANT'S ABILITY TO BE ORALLY FED

After the birth of an infant with CL/P, the physician and newborn nursery staff need to make a rapid determination of the infant's ability to be safely and successfully fed by breast or bottle. The clinician can use Table 25.1 to guide the feeding evaluation by asking four physiological questions: *(1)* Can the infant protect the airway and coordinate swallowing with breathing? *(2)* Is the ability to swallow intact? *(3)* Can the infant generate negative intraoral pressure? *(4)* Is the sucking mechanism normal? Table 25.1 lists a series of cleft conditions and compares them across these four physiological elements.

A review of Table 25.1 reveals the following basic concepts:

- Most infants with CL/P can be safely and successfully orally fed using breast or bottle, usually bottle.
- The presence of a syndrome, multiple anomalies, perinatal illness, or neurological complications puts the infant at risk for not being able to be safely orally fed.
- Infants with RS may be unable to generate negative intraoral pressure or even suck/swallow normally due to anatomy (a posteriorly placed tongue due to micrognathia).
- Infants with isolated cleft lip are the easiest to feed.
- The presence of an isolated cleft palate suggests that an infant can safely orally feed but will need assistance due to an inability to generate negative intraoral pressure.
- Some infants with symptomatic submucous cleft palate may have difficulty generating negative intraoral pressure.

FEEDING PRACTICES IN A CLINICAL SETTING

What to Feed Infants with Cleft Lip with or without Palate

Breast Milk is Best. The American Academy of Pediatrics (1997) guidelines state "human milk is uniquely superior" nutritionally for both sick and well infants, and every mother should be encouraged to breast-feed. Research has shown breast milk to have multiple health benefits, including a decreased incidence of diarrhea and otitis media (Scariati et al., 1997), inhibition of colonization by respiratory bacterial pathogens (Hokama et al., 1999), and increased protection against viral illness (Englund et al., 1998), among many others. Breast milk provides protection against otitis media even in otitis-prone infants with CL/P (Paradise et al., 1994). Several researchers have even found breast-feeding to be responsible for improved cognitive development (Anderson et al., 1999; Uauy and Peirano, 1999). In addition to health benefits for the infant, health benefits for the mother and socioeconomic benefits for families, employers, and the nation are expounded (American Academy of Pediatrics, 1997; Ball and Wright, 1999). The primary care provider's role is to provide parents with complete and current information about the benefits of breast-feeding so that a fully informed decision can be made. Mothers of infants with CL/P should be encouraged to provide breast milk as the preferred source of nutrition if they are able to do so.

Encouraging breast-feeding has been a controversial subject in this population (Chibbaro, 1998). Societal parenting pressures and breast-feeding expectations compounded by the difficulties in feeding an infant with CL/P, anxieties about the infant's underlying condition, concerns about upcoming surgeries, and the already stressful postpartum period leave many parents feeling overwhelmed, anxious, and guilty. Professional concerns about already fragile parent–infant attachment in infants with a facial difference and about further increasing stress in this difficult postpartum period have led some to suggest that breast-feeding should not be recommended. The increasing findings of health benefits from breast milk cannot be ignored. Some parents have reported feeling good about expressing breast milk because they know this is something they can do for their child's health. Individual preference is paramount; however, the American Academy of Pediatrics (1997) states "before advising against breastfeeding or recommending premature weaning, the practitioner should weigh thoughtfully the benefits of breastfeeding against the risks of not receiving human milk."

Formula Is Satisfactory. Although not providing all of the health benefits attributed to breast milk, formula feeding is an acceptable alternative. Historically, formula supplementation and assisted feeding techniques have been the mainstay of feeding an infant with CL/P. Extended periods of time to directly breast-feed, then express additional breast milk, give expressed milk by assisted feeding, followed by the additional time-consuming chores of cleaning the breast pump, the bot-

TABLE 25.1. *Feeding Characteristics and Suggested Feeding Techniques by Orofacial Diagnosis**

Diagnosis	Expected Ability to Protect Airway and Coordinate Swallow with Breathing	Expected Presence of Intact Swallow	Ability to Generate Negative Intraoral Pressure	Ability to Make Normal Mechanical Movements of Sucking	Feeding Techniques
Orofacial clefts with syndromic conditions or multiple anomalies	+/−	+/−	+/−	+/−	Require careful evaluation of physiological and neurological conditions which might affect feeding in addition to impact of type of cleft
Orofacial clefts with prematurity, perinatal infection, or injury with possible neurological sequelae	+/−	+/−	+/−	+/−	
Robin sequence	+/−	+/−	−	−	Direct breast-feeding unlikely, nipple position critical, needs assisted feeding
Isolated cleft lip	+	+	+	+	Direct breast-feeding best, soft artificial nipple with a large base works well, does not need assisted feeding
Isolated cleft lip and palate	+	+	−	+	Direct breast-feeding unlikely, needs assisted feeding
Isolated cleft of hard and soft palate only	+	+	−	+	Direct breast-feeding unlikely, needs assisted feeding
Isolated cleft of soft palate only	+	+	−	+	Direct breast-feeding unlikely but depends on size of cleft, artificial nipple shape may assist with palate function, probably needs assisted feeding
Submucous cleft palate (symptomatic)	+	+	+/−	+	Direct breast-feeding best, nipple shape may assist with palate function by support, may need assisted feeding

*Based on Herbst (1983), Clarren et al. (1987), Bu'Lock et al. (1990), and Kaufman (1991).

tles, and the baby's bottom, all while keeping the mother well fed, rested, and hydrated are minimized. In households where other children also require care, the demands of breast-feeding an infant with a cleft may contribute to family stress or neglect of other family members. Benefits of formula include the ability to accurately measure the volume and caloric intake and to provide changes in concentration or additives to increase the caloric density. Under a pediatric nutritionist's guidance, formula has the unique ability to be reconstituted from concentrate or powder to create a more concentrated formulation. Pediatric nutritionists can also prescribe a variety of substances to add to formulas and expressed breast milk to increase caloric density. Simple sugars, Polycose®, corn oil, and medium chain triglycerides (MCT oil®) oil are just a few.

At first glance, a calorically dense formula is inviting since the infant needs less volume to meet caloric needs. A careful balance is necessary, however. If too dense, the fluid is hard to digest. This can increase transit time, causing constipation and other gastrointestinal symptoms. Maintaining enough free water for adequate hydration and protection of the kidneys is another important factor.

Whatever feeding method is chosen by the family, the primary care provider's responsibility is to support the decision and put the family in contact with the appropriate community support professionals. The American Cleft Palate-Craniofacial Association maintains a registry of cleft and craniofacial teams that provide care for people with clefts. The Cleft Palate Foundation (1992) has written educational materials for parents, healthcare providers, and hospitals.

Recommended Feeding Strategies

Initial feeding instruction is often provided to parents of a newborn with CL/P at a time when they are experiencing shock, anxiety, and grief. Newborn nursery staff, who may have little experience with feeding an infant with CL/P, often provide this initial instruction. All too often, parents are discharged to take their baby home without having received any training in feeding or time to practice these techniques. However, when feeding instruction is provided by cleft palate teams, it is generally based on trial-and-error strategies that may have worked for some families, rather than on proven physiological principles of sucking/feeding (Richard, 1994). Most instruction is limited to positioning the infant during feeding so as to minimize choking and gagging. Parents also are often advised to assist fluid flow from the bottle by enlarging or cross-cutting the hole in the nipple or by using a plastic bottle that can be squeezed to force a more rapid flow (Elster et al., 1994).

Such instruction is offered, knowing that parents run the risk of "flooding" their baby in a flow of milk. This may result in undesired compensatory oral motor strategies in an attempt to cope with the excess flow and prevent choking and gagging and/or to gain momentary control to enable swallowing and breathing. Finan and Barlow (1998) and Fadavi et al. (1997) demonstrated the disruptive impact of such environmental stimuli on sucking motor patterns.

Rather than espousing only one feeding technique, it is important to communicate to parents that there is no "right" way to feed an infant with cleft. Each infant and parent dyad will develop their own relationship and strategy during feeding, which works best for them. Infants (especially those with a cleft) are very adaptable and can tolerate being fed in a variety of ways by different care providers, parents, and other family members. However, some general guidelines or strategies are commonly used.

Direct Breast-Feeding. Infants with cleft lip or cleft lip with incomplete cleft of the alveolus may have some difficulty with the orolabial seal around the breast or bottle. These infants may respond best to breast-feeding since the breast tissue is more malleable and can fill the opening, allowing for a tight seal. If there is no associated cleft palate, the infant should be able to strip the nipple against the roof of the mouth normally and seal the soft palate against the posterior pharyngeal wall to create negative intraoral pressure (suction). These infants should be able to feed and grow normally, and their intake is not affected by their cleft (Clarren et al., 1987; Coulter-Danner, 1992; Elster et al., 1994).

Infants who have clefts of the palate can provide some stripping action, depending on the size and placement of the cleft, but cannot create negative intraoral pressure. The breast must be held in the infant's mouth and the infant held up to the breast. Supporting the baby on pillows will decrease the strain on the mother. Experimenting with the infant body and head position, to get the best compression of the breast within the mouth, will assist with the mechanical emptying of the milk ducts. These infants can still be directly breast-fed by mothers with a strong let-down reflex who have a stream of milk from the breast. Massaging the breast to assist the letdown reflex or manually expressing milk from the breast into the infant's mouth are additional strategies (Cleft Palate Foundation, 1992). This may be easier in mothers who have previously breast-fed other infants. Using these strategies may allow a parent and infant to have some direct breast-feeding time but rarely provides adequate calories. Accurate measurement of actual intake (not just minutes of feeding on each breast) is essential since feeding efficiency is reduced. One way to estimate this is by obtaining prefeeding and postfeeding weights. The higher-calorie "hind milk" is not expressed by these methods, and the infant may miss out on the nutrient-dense portion of the feeding while expending higher calories over a longer period of time than with direct breast-feeding alone. This puts the infant at increased risk of dehydration, hyperbilirubinemia, failure to thrive, and weight loss (Clarren et al., 1987; Coulter-Danner, 1992; McCartney, 1996; Wide Smiles, 1997).

Subsets of the population at greatest risk for breast-feeding failure include infants with symptomatic but undiagnosed submucous cleft palate. Most children with submucous cleft palate are asymptomatic, and this is often not diagnosed until later. In this age group, symptomatic submucous cleft palate puts these infants at risk because the palatal musculature is not able to effectively and consistently seal against the posterior pharyngeal wall, impairing the ability to produce negative intraoral pressure and increasing feeding inefficiency. When the baby is put to breast or to bottle, appropriate rooting and sucking movements occur. If a gloved finger is placed in the mouth, appropriate placement of the tongue with normal peristaltic muscular movements and compression against the roof of the mouth are felt. This may mislead a healthcare provider or parent into believing that effective sucking is occurring. If a symptomatic submucous cleft palate is not diagnosed by physical exam at birth, it may not be diagnosed until feeding difficulty progresses to failure to thrive or poor weight gain.

Expressed Breast-Feeding. A combination of direct breast-feeding and expressed breast milk by assisted feeding or expressed breast milk by assisted feeding alone is the preferable way to feed most infants with CL/P. A mother's desire to provide breast milk to an infant is a commitment of time, energy, and fortitude. She will need the full support of the hospital staff, family, primary care provider, and cleft palate team to accomplish it. She needs better than average nutrition, adequate sleep, forced hydration, and a great breast pump. She will, in essence, be taking the time for two feedings for each infant feeding. She will need assistance from a spouse or family member to feed the infant with assisted feeding techniques while she expresses breast milk to be fed later. She will benefit from a lactation consultant familiar with feeding infants with cleft and from a friend who will support her decision to breast-feed or to begin formula supplementation if breast-feeding becomes too difficult for her.

For each feeding, a careful diary must be maintained with the number of minutes at breast, the volume of milk given by assisted feeding, and the length of time needed. In this way, if an infant shows poor weight gain at a follow-up visit, the energy expenditure at the breast and the total time of feeding with assistance can be evaluated and recommendations made to decrease energy expenditure or increase intake. It is important to stress to mothers that every infant is different and, in some ways, every feeding is different. Infants will vary in their ability to feed efficiently depending on many variables, including the extent of the cleft, their level of arousal at the time of feeding, development of respiratory infections, or just a change in schedule. By doing their best at each feeding and monitoring weight gain every week or so, mothers will be doing all they can to ensure that their baby has the best nutrition for growth and development (Wide Smiles, 1996).

Assisted Feeding. Assisted feeding can reduce calorie expenditure. Assisted feeding techniques use pulse-squeezed bottles, droppers, cups, and other devices to get the milk into the infant's mouth without sucking and with decreased energy expenditure. It should take approximately 15 to 30 min for infants to complete a feeding (Sidoti and Shprintzen, 1995). If an infant takes longer than 30 min, valuable calories needed for growth are being used and the infant may tire, fail to gain weight, or even lose weight (Balluff, 1986). Because infants with CL/P are inefficient feeders due to the structural problems of the cleft, assisted feeding is recommended to compensate for the decreased or absent negative intraoral pressure. The choice of feeding equipment must be based on what works well for the infant, is readily available in the community, and is affordable for the parent. Some examples are described below.

The Mead Johnson (Evansville, IN) Cleft Lip/Palate Nurser is a compressible bottle with a cross-cut straight nipple. It can be fitted with an orthodontic nipple. The orthodontic nipple is wider and has a larger surface to be compressed, but care must be taken to turn the nipple upside down so the stream of fluid is directed toward the tongue or the posterior pharnyx, not up into the cleft. This bottle works best with nipples that have the porthole on the tip. If a vertical slice is made on the tip, the formula will flow through the enlarged hole when the infant compresses the nipple between the gums, even without negative intraoral pressure. Alternatives are a horizontal slice for a lower flow rate or a cross-cut for a faster flow rate. The bottle can also be pulse-squeezed by the caregiver along with the infant's mouthing pattern to simulate sucking. The Mead Johnson CL/P Nurser is a disposable bottle and cannot be sterilized. It can be reused in the home by washing it in warm water with soap and sterilizing the nipples or washing it in the top rack of the dishwasher. Standard baby bottle nipples by most manufacturers fit.

These bottles are the least expensive and require replacement after 15 uses. To increase the life of the Mead Johnson CL/P Nurser, do not heat milk or formula on the stove or in the microwave. Use a regular bottle to heat the milk or formula in a cup of warm or hot water, then transfer it to the Mead Johnson CL/P Nurser (Dixon-Wood, 1997; Mead Johnson Nutritionals, personal communication, 2000).

The Haberman Feeder (Medela, McHenry, IL) is a rigid bottle with an elongated, compressible nipple. It has an adjustable flow rate depending on the direction the nipple is inserted into the mouth. Making this adjustment does not require any alteration of the nipple hole. The feeder has a one-way valve between the nipple and the bottle to prevent formula from being pushed back into the bottle by compression and to decrease the amount of air ingested through the nipple. Some infants are able to adequately compress the enlarged nipple and do not need pulse-assisted feeds; however, the nipple can be pulse-squeezed for infants who need additional assistance. Due to the one-way valve, this nipple does not do well for infants who require thickened feedings for gastroesophageal reflux. The Haberman Feeder and nipple can be sterilized. As with the Mead Johnson CL/P Nurser, do not heat milk or formula in a Haberman Feeder in the microwave. The Haberman nipple is recommended for room-temperature liquids only. Complaints about this feeder center around the price (currently about $16 each if purchased directly from the manufacturer), the unusual appearance, and the lack of a travel cap (Medela, Inc., 1994; Wide Smiles, 1996).

The Cleft Palate Nipple System (Children's Medical Ventures, Norwell, MA) is a compressible bottle with a larger-than-usual tri-cut nipple that is stiffer on one side and very pliable on the other. It is positioned in the infant's mouth with the stiff side toward the cleft. The tongue then strips along the very pliable side, compressing against the stiffer side and maximizing each attempt at sucking. The bottle can also be pulse-squeezed by the caregiver along with the infant's mouthing pattern to simulate sucking. It also has a one-way valve between the nipple and the bottle to prevent milk from flowing back into the bottle by compression. Flow rate can be adjusted by tightening or loosening the cap, which opens or closes dual air holes. If the infant does not require pulse-squeezed assistance, this nipple will fit on any baby bottle. The Pigeon Feeder can be boiled or gas-sterilized. As with the Haberman Feeder, the one-way valve precludes the use of thickened feedings for infants with gastroesophogeal reflux (Children's Medical Ventures, 1999).

A review of the literature reveals a variety of other feeding innovations and anecdotal stories of infants fed successfully with eyedroppers, Dixie cups, shot glasses, and syringes with all manner of bulbs, catheters, and other attachments. An interesting adaptation of the Playtex Nurser with its wide-based nipple and collapsible formula bag was made by cutting away part of the hard plastic sleeve so the liner could be compressed by the parent. There is not room to review all of the possibilities here. Suffice it to say that if it gets a sufficient quantity of breast milk or formula in the baby with little calorie expenditure or risk of choking, it has probably been tried. If the infant fails to grow with conventional feeding strategies and after medical, psychosocial, and nutritional evaluations the growth failure is still felt to be a mechanical problem due to the cleft, then unconventional feeding techniques can be tried.

Additional Helpful Feeding Strategies

Feed in More Upright Position. Positioning the infant with CL/P in a more upright position (>65 degrees) is recommended for several reasons. One is that the more upright position allows gravity to assist with moving the formula bolus to the back of the mouth and down the esophagus. This gravity assistance helps to reduce infant energy expenditure and fatigue during feeding. It also reduces the amount of nasal regurgitation. Nasal regurgitation is common since the infant's tongue reflexively pushes up into the cleft when attempting to strip the nipple. Although nasal regurgitation is a sign of swallowing dyscoordination in children without clefts, it is not an indication of swallowing problems in an infant with a cleft palate (Clarren et al., 1987; Cleft Palate Foundation, 1992).

Frequent Burping. The soft palate cannot form an airtight seal during swallowing, and air freely flows through the nose during feeding and swallowing. In addition, coordination between the parent pulsing the formula (with an assisted feeding device) and the infant swallowing and breathing may not be fully developed for several weeks. For these reasons, infants with CL/P swallow more air during feeding. They require more frequent burping than infants without a cleft and may have more "wet burps," nasal regurgitation, vomiting, or colic-like symptoms. Thankfully, as the infant grows and muscle tone, swallow–breath coordination, and parental skill at feeding and reading subtle cues from the infant improve, these symptoms usually resolve. Colic-like symptoms from air swallowing are common in this population and do not necessarily mean that true colic is developing. Antiflatulence drops (e.g., simethicone) are one possible medical intervention to consider.

At the same time, if feeding and burping are going well and the typical symptoms of colic continue, then counseling the parents on the development of colic in babies with or without CL/P may be indicated. A trial of some of the other common interventions for treatment of colic may work. In addition, the possibility of other etiologies (other than the cleft) should be explored. It cannot be too strongly stressed that infants with CL/P have the same incidence rates of associated problems like colic, reflux, and pyloric stenosis as the general population.

Plain Water for Mouth and Nose Rinse. Mucus may line the nasal area and cleft prior to a feeding. Formula (and later foods) may get trapped in the cleft after a feeding. A few sips or spoonfuls of water before and after feedings will rinse trapped mucus and food/formula particles away (Muir and Burton, 2000).

Obturators ("Feeding Appliances"). Presurgical palatal appliances were at one time advocated because it was hoped that they would help the infant with CL/P feed more efficiently (Balluff and Udin, 1986; Jones, 1988). In as much as these appliances provide a solid surface against which the infant can compress the nipple, they do improve the ability to feed. Currently, these presurgical appliances are used to direct palatal segments into position for surgical repair or to prevent dental arch collapse from the pressure of the cheeks. These appliances do not allow the infant to create negative intraoral pressure, however, and the infant still needs assisted feeding (Choi et al., 1991). A palatal appliance may improve, but will not solve, feeding problems in an infant with CL/P. The benefit of a solid surface on which to compress the nipple must be weighed against the large percentage of intraoral space the appliance occupies. Infants with retrognathia, whose tongues are posteriorly positioned, are poor candidates for palatal appliances because of the risk for airway occlusion. In addition, palatal appliances must be monitored closely and refitted with growth, thus becoming expensive and time-consuming (Cleft Palate Foundation, 1992; Berkowitz, 1996).

REFERENCES

American Academy of Pediatrics (1997). Breastfeeding and the use of human milk. Pediatrics *100*: 1035–1039.

Anderson, JW, Johnstone, BM, Remley, DT (1999). Breast-feeding and cognitive development: a meta-analysis. Am J Clin Nutr *70*: 525–535.

Ardran, GM, Kemp, FH, Lind, J (1958a). A cineradiographic study of bottle-feeding. Br J Radiol *31*: 11–22.

Ardran, GM, Kemp, FH, Lind, J (1958b). A cineradiographic study of breast feeding. Br J Radiol *31*: 156–162.

Ball, TM, Wright, AL (1999). Health care costs of formula feeding in the first year of life. Pediatrics *103*: 870–876.

Balluff, MA (1986). Nutritional needs of an infant or child with a cleft lip or palate. Ear Nose Throat J *65*: 44/311–49/315.

Balluff, MA, Udin, RD (1986). Using a feeding appliance to aid the infant with cleft palate. Ear Nose Throat J *65*: 50/316–55/320.

Berkowitz, S (ed) (1996). *Cleft Lip and Palate: Perspectives in Management.* San Diego: Singular Publishing Group.

Bluestone, CD, Klein, JO (1990). Intratemporal complications and sequelae of otitis media. In: *Pediatric Otolaryngology,* Vol. 1, edited by CD Bluestone, SE Stool, and MA Kenna. Philadelphia: WB Saunders, pp. 583–635.

Broder, H, Strauss, R (1989). Self concept of early primary school age children with visible or invisible defects. Cleft Palate J *26*: 111–118.

Bu'Lock, F, Woolridge, MW, Baum, JD (1990). Development of coordination of sucking, swallowing and breathing: ultrasound study of term and pre-term infants. Dev Med Child Neurol *32*: 669–678.

Chetwynd, AG, Diggle, PJ, Drewett, RF, Young, B (1998). A mixture model for sucking patterns of breast-fed infants. Stat Med *17*: 395–405.

Chibbaro, P (moderator) (1998). The great debate: be it resolved that early palate closure allows effective breastfeeding. Presented at the 55th annual meeting of the American Cleft Palate-Craniofacial Association, Baltimore, Maryland, April 24, 1998.

Children's Medical Ventures, Inc (1999). *Technical Information Bulletin. Pigeon Corporation Nursing Bottles and Nipples.* Norwell, MA: Children's Medical Ventures.

Choi, BH, Kleinheinz, J, Joos, U, Komposch, G (1991). Sucking efficiency of early orthopaedic plate and teats in infants with cleft lip and palate. Int J Oral Maxillofac Surg *20*: 167–169.

Clarren, SK, Anderson, B, Wolf, LS (1987). Feeding infants born with cleft lip, cleft palate, or cleft lip and palate. Cleft Palate J *24*: 244–249.

Cleft Palate Foundation (1992). *Feeding an Infant with Cleft.* Chapel Hill: Cleft Palate Foundation.

Coulter-Danner, S (1992). Breast feeding the infant with a cleft defect. NAACOG Clin Issues Perinat Womens Health *3*: 634–639.

Cunningham, ML, Jerome, JT (1997). Linear growth characteristics of children with cleft lip and palate. J Pediatr *131*: 707–711.

DeMonterice, D, Meier, PP, Engstrom, JL, et al. (1992). Concurrent validity of a new instrument for measuring nutritive sucking in preterm infants. Nurs Res *41*: 342–346.

de Vries, JIP, Visser, GHA, Prechtl, HFR (1988). The emergence of fetal behavior. III. Individual differences and consistencies. Early Hum Dev *16*: 85–103.

Dixon-Wood, VL (1997). Counseling and early management of feeding and language skill development for infants and toddlers with cleft palate. In: *Communicative Disorders Related to Cleft Lip and Palate,* 4th ed., edited by KR Bzoch. Austin, TX: Pro-Ed, pp. 465–474.

Dixon-Wood, VL, Williams, WN, Clapper, DC, Gibbs C (1999). Nutritive sucking characteristics of infants with cleft lip and palate. Presented at the 56th annual meeting of the American Cleft Palate-Craniofacial Association, Scottsdale, Arizona, April 1999.

Domet, MJ (1986). The general pediatrician and the craniofacial defects team. Ear Nose and Throat J *65*: 25–33.

Doyle, WJ, Reilly, JS, Jardini, L, Roonak, S (1986). Effect of palatoplasty on the function of the eustachian tube in children with cleft palate. Cleft Palate J *23*: 63–68.

Drillen, CM, Ingram, TTS, Wilkinson, EM (1966). *The Causes and Natural History of Cleft Lip and Palate.* Edinburgh: Livingstone.

Duncan, PA, Shapiro, LR, Soley, RL, Turet, SE (1983). Linear growth patterns in patients with cleft lip or palate or both. Am J Disabled Child *137*: 159–163.

Eishima, K (1991). The analysis of sucking behavior in newborn infants. Early Hum Dev *27*: 163–173.

Elster, BA, Richard, ME, Maksud, DP (1994). Feeding infants with cleft lip and/or palate. Plast Surg Nurs 14: 101–112.

Endriga, MC, Kapp-Simon, K (1999). Psychological issues in craniofacial care: state of the art. Cleft Palate Craniofac J 36: 3–11.

Englund, J, Glezan, WP, Piedra, PA (1998). Maternal immunization against viral disease. Vaccine 16: 1456–1463.

Fadavi, S, Punwani, I, Jain, L, Vidyasagar, D (1997). Mechanics and energetics of nutritive sucking: a functional comparison of commercially available nipples. J Pediatr 130: 740–5.

Finan, DS, Barlow, SM (1998). Intrinsic dynamics and mechanosensory modulation of non-nutritive sucking in human infants. Early Hum Dev 52: 181–97.

Felix-Schollaart, B, Hoeksma, JB, Prahl-Andersen, B (1992). Growth comparison between children with cleft lip and/or palate and controls. Cleft Palate Craniofac J 29: 186–191.

Goldson, E (1987). Non-nutritive sucking in the sick infant. J Perinatol 7: 30–34.

Green, J (1991). Cleft and nursing: the basic facts. Wide Smiles Cleft Links. Available from http://www.widesmiles.org; INTERNET.

Habel A, Sell, D, Mars, M (1996). Management of the lip and palate. Arch Disabled Child 74: 360–366

Hafström, M, Lundquist, C, Lindecrantz, K, et al. (1997). Recording non-nutritive sucking in the neonate. Description of an automatized system for analysis. Acta Paediatr 86: 82–90.

Herbst, JJ (1983). Development of suck and swallow. J Pediatr Gastroenterol Nutr 3(Suppl 1): S131–S135.

Hokama, T, Yara, A, Hirayama, K, Takamine, F (1999). Isolation of respiratory bacterial pathogens from the throats of healthy infants fed by different methods. J Trop Pediatr 45: 173–176.

Hunter, WS (1981). The Michigan cleft twin study. J Craniofac Genet Dev Biol 1: 235–242.

Igawa, HH, Nishizawa, N, Sugihara, T, Inuyama, Y (1998). A fiberscopic analysis of velopharyngeal movement before and after primary palatoplasty in cleft infants. Plast Reconstr Surg 102: 668–674.

Iwayama, K, Eishima, M (1997). Neonatal sucking behavior and its development until 14 months. Early Hum Dev 47: 1–9.

Jain, L, Sivieri, E, Abbasi, S, Bhutani, V (1987). Energetics and mechanics of nutritive sucking in the preterm and term neonate. Pediatrics 111: 984–989.

Jensen, BL, Dahl, E, Kreiborg, S (1983). Longitudinal study of body height, radius length and skeletal maturity in Danish boys with cleft lip and palate. Scand J Dent Res 91: 473–481.

Jensen, BL, Kreilborg, DE , Fogh-Andersen P (1988). Cleft lip and palate in Denmark 1976–1981: epidemiology, variability, and early somatic development. Cleft Palate J 25: 258–269.

Jones, WB (1988). Weight gain and feeding in the neonate with a cleft: a three-center study. Cleft Palate J 25: 379–384.

Kapp-Simon, K, McGuire, DE (1997). Observed social interaction patterns in adolescents with and without craniofacial conditions. Cleft Palate Craniofac J 34: 380–384.

Kapp-Simon, KA (1994). Mental development in infants with nonsyndromic craniosynostosis with and without cranial release and reconstruction. Plast Reconstr Surg 94: 408–410.

Kapp-Simon, KA, Figueroa, A, Jocher, CA, Schafer, M (1993). Longitudinal assessment of mental development in infants with nonsyndromic craniosynostosis with and without cranial release and reconstruction. Plast Reconstr Surg 92: 831–839.

Kapp-Simon, KA, Simon, DJ, Kristovich, S (1992). Self-perception, social skills, adjustment and inhibition in young adolescents with craniofacial anomalies. Cleft Palate Craniofac J 29: 352–356.

Kaufman, FL (1991). Managing the cleft lip and palate patient. Pediatr Clin North Am 38: 1127–1147.

Krueckeberg, SM, Kapp-Simon, KA, Ribordy, SC (1993). Social skills

of preschoolers with and without craniofacial anomalies. Cleft Palate Craniofac J 30: 475–481.

Leonard, BJ, Brust, JD, Abrahams, G, Sielaff, B (1991). Self-concept of children and adolescents with cleft lip and/or palate. Cleft Palate Craniofac J 28: 347–353.

Linder, A (1991). Measurement of intraoral negative air pressure during dummy sucking in human newborn. Eur J Orthod 13: 317–321.

Maternal and Child Health Bureau (1995). Definition of Children with Special Health Care Needs. Rockville, MD: Division of Services for Children with Special Health Care Needs.

McCartney, J (1996). Supplementing the breastfed infant with a cleft. Wide Smiles Cleft Links. Available from http://www.widesmiles.org; INTERNET.

McGowan, JS, Roger, RR, Fowler, SM, Levy, SE, Stallings, VA (1991). Developmental patterns of normal nutrative sucking in infants. Dev Med Child Neurol 33: 891–897.

Medela, Inc (1994). The Haberman Feeder: Instructions for Use. McHenry, IL: Medela.

Medoff-Cooper, B (1991). Changes in nutritive sucking patterns with increasing gestational age. Nurs Res 40: 245–247.

Medoff-Cooper, B, Ray, W (1995). Neonatal sucking behaviors. J Nurs Schol 27: 195–200.

Medoff-Cooper, B, Verklan, T, Carlson, S (1993). The development of nutritive sucking patterns and physiological correlates in very-low-birth-weight infants. Nurs Res 42: 100–105.

Medoff-Cooper, B, Wenninger, S, Zukowsky, K (1989). Neonatal sucking as a clinical assessment tool: preliminary findings. Nurs Res 42: 162–165.

Muir, TL, Burton, L (2000). Successful feeding interventions for infants with cleft lip and palate and craniofacial anomalies. Presented at the 57th annual meeting of the American Cleft Palate-Craniofacial Association, Atlanta, Georgia, April 13, 2000.

Nackashi, JA, Rosenbloom, AL, Marks, R, et al. (1988). Stature of Russian children with isolated cleft lip and palate. Cleft Palate J 35: 500–502.

Nowak, AJ, Smith, WL, Erenberg, A (1995). Imaging evaluation of breast-feeding and bottle-feeding systems. J Pediatr 126: S130–S134.

Nystrom, M, Ranta, R, Kataja, M (1992). Sizes of dental arches and general body growth up to six years of age in children with isolated cleft palate. Scand J Dent Res 100: 123–129.

Padwa, BL, Evans, CA, Pillemier, FC (1991). Psychosocial adjustment in children with hemifacial microsomia and other craniofacial deformaties. Cleft Palate Craniofac J 28: 354–359.

Palmer, MM (1993). Identification and management of the transitional suck pattern in premature infants. J Perinat Neonat Nurs 7: 66–75.

Paradise, JL, Bluestone, CD, Felder, H (1969). The universality of otitis media in 50 infants with cleft palate. Pediatrics 44: 35–42.

Paradise, JL, Elster, BA, Tan, L (1994). Evidence in infants with cleft palate that breast milk protects against otits media. Pediatrics 94: 853–860.

Pashayan, HM (1983). What else to look for in a child born with a cleft of the lip and/or palate. Cleft Palate J 20: 54–82.

Pope, AW, Ward, JW (1997). Self-perceived facial appearance and psychosocial adjustment in preadolescents with craniofacial anomalies. Cleft Palate Craniofac J 34: 396–401.

Prieto, CR, Cardenas, H, Salvatierra, AM, et al. (1996). Sucking pressure in relationship to milk transfer during breastfeeding in humans. J Reprod Fertil 108: 69–74.

Ranalli, DN, Mazaheri, M (1975). Height–weight growth of cleft children, birth to six years. Cleft Palate J 11: 400–404.

Richard, M (1994). Weight comparisons of infants with complete cleft lip and palate. Pediatr Nurs 20: 191–196.

Richman, LC, Eliason, MJ (1995). Disorders of communications, developmental language disorders and cleft palate. In: *Handbook of Child Clinical Psychology*, edited by CE Walker and MC Roberts. New York: Wiley, pp. 697–722.

Roitman, A, Laron, Z (1978). Hypothalamo-pituitary hormone insufficiency associated with cleft lip and palate. Arch Disabled Child 53: 952–955.

Rudman, D, Davis, T, Prest, JH, et al. (1978). Prevalence of growth hormone deficiency in children with cleft lip or palate. Pediatrics 93: 378–382.

Rybski, DA, Almli, CR, Gisel, EG, et al. (1984). Sucking behaviors of normal 3-day old female neonates during a 24-hr period. J Dev Psychobiol 17: 79–86.

Scariati, PD, Grummer-Strawn, LM, Fein, SB (1997). A longitudinal analysis of infant morbidity and the extent of breast-feeding in the United States. Pediatrics 99: E5.

Seth, AK, McWilliams, BJ (1988). Weight gain in children with cleft palate from birth to two years. Cleft Palate J 25: 146–150.

Shaker, C (1990). Nipple feeding premature infants: a different perspective. Neonat Network 8: 9–17.

Shprintzen, RJ, Goldberg, RB, Young, D, et al. (1981). The velo-cardio-facial syndrome: a clinical and genetic analysis. Pediatrics 67: 167–172.

Sidoti, EJ, Shprintzen, RJ (1995). Pediatric care and feeding of the newborn with a cleft. In: *Cleft Palate Speech Management: A Multidisciplinary Approach*, edited by RJ Shprintzen and J Bardack. Mosby: St. Louis.

Smith, LT, DiRugiero, DC, Lones, KR (1994). Recovery of eustachian function and hearing outcome inpatients with cleft palate. Otolaryngol Head Neck Surg 111: 423–429.

Smith, WL, Erenburg, A, Nowak, A, Franken, EA (1985). Physiology of sucking in the normal term infant using real-time ultrasound. Radiology 156: 379–381.

Strauss, RP (1997). Social and psychological perspectives on cleft lip and palate. In: *Communicative Disorders Related to Cleft Lip and Palate*, 4th ed., edited by KR Bzoch. Austin, TX: Pro-Ed, pp. 95–113.

Strauss, RP, Sharp, MC, Lorch, SC, Kachalia, B (1995). Physicians and communication of "bad news"—parent experiences of being informed of their child's cleft lip/palate. Pediatrics 96: 82–89.

Sweitzer, RS, Melrose, J, Morris, HL (1968). The air–bone gap as a criterion for identification of hearing loss. Cleft Palate J 141–152.

Turgeon-O'Brien, H, Lachapelle, D, Gagnon, PF, et al. (1996). Nutritive and non-nutritive sucking habits: a review. J Dent Child 63: 321–7.

Uauy, R, Peirano, P (1999). Breast is best: human milk is the optimal food for brain development. Am J Clin Nutr 70: 433–434.

Waterland, RA, Berkowitz, RI, Stunkard, AJ, Stallings, VA (1998). Calibrated-orifice nipples for measurement of infant nutritive sucking. J Pediatr 132: 523–526.

Weber, F, Woolridge, MW, Baum, JD (1986). An ultrasonographic study of the organization of sucking and swallowing by newborn infants. Dev Med Child Neurol 28: 19–24.

Wide Smiles (1996). Breast feeding the cleft-affected newborn: making it safe. Wide Smiles Cleft Links. Available from http://www.widesmiles.org; INTERNET.

26

Staging of cleft lip and palate reconstruction: infancy through adolescence

JEFFREY C. POSNICK

RAMON L. RUIZ

The satisfactory rehabilitation of a child born with cleft lip and palate (CLP) presents unique challenges. Close cooperation is required among the specialists who integrate their talents for the child's overall well-being. A coordinated approach is required to achieve ideal speech, occlusion, facial aesthetics, and individual self-esteem (Adams, 1981; Berry et al., 1997; Broder and Strauss, 1989; Harper, 1995; Richman and Eliason, 1982; Richman et al., 1985). The effective cleft palate (CP) team is patient-, family-, and community-oriented rather than physician-, specialty-, and hospital-centered (Benacerraf and Mulliken, 1993; Slutsky, 1969).

Koop (1987), then the Surgeon General of the United States, issued a report, *Children with Special Health Care Needs*, that called for a family-centered, community-based, coordinated healthcare delivery system for children with special needs (Christensen and Fogl-Andersen, 1993; Jensen et al., 1983; Jones, 1988; Laatikainen et al., 1996).

The American Cleft Palate-Craniofacial Association (ACPA) (1993) responded by developing parameters of care designed to facilitate the rehabilitation of patients with CLP. The parameters developed by the ACPA support the concept of interdisciplinary care for the CLP patient, encouraging the use of treatment protocols that emphasize the thoughtful timing of interventions (surgery, speech and language therapy, dental and psychosocial treatment) to coincide with the child's physical, cognitive, dental, and psychosocial development (Bowers et al., 1987; Gould, 1990). The parameters of

care emphasize the need for the team of cleft specialists to organize for maximum long-term patient benefit, taking into account the child's growth intervals and levels of need in the individual's life.

Whenever surgery is contemplated for the reconstruction of CLP deformities, the benefit-to-risk (and -cost) ratio should be considered (Leonard et al., 1991; Strauss, 1994). Windows of opportunity may exist for maximum advantage (improved benefit-to-risk ratio) at different stages in the patient's growth and development. The goal of the CLP surgeon, orthodontist, speech therapist, and team is to work with the family, carry out periodic reassessments, and make suggestions about the timing and sequencing of care to ensure long-term benefits and to minimize complications and costs (Cohen et al., 1995).

The child born with either a complete unilateral or bilateral CLP (UCLP or BCLP, respectively) or cleft of the palate only (ICP) will face a series of hurdles related to speech, occlusion, facial appearance, and self-development. Reviewing the basic decision-making process of treatment options prospectively provides a reconstructive outline for the family and team members.

ROBIN SEQUENCE

The French stomatologist Pierre Robin is best known for his description of an anomaly consisting of micrognathia with glossoptosis, CP, and respiratory obstruction (Jeresaty et al., 1969; Perlman and Robin,

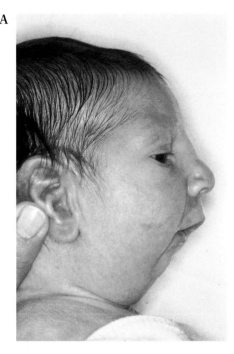
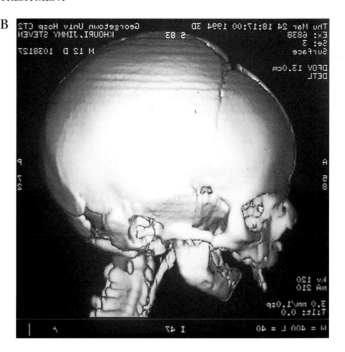

FIG. 26.1. A child born with Robin sequence consisting of micrognathia with glossoptosis, clefting of the secondary palate, and a degree of respiratory distress. *A:* Profile view indicating micrognathia. *B:* Profile view of three-dimensional craniofacial computed tomographic reconstruction indicating micrognathia but with all of the components of the jaw present. For this child, the small mandible is the result of deforming forces during fetal development rather than of a malformation. Catch-up growth of the mandible is anticipated during childhood. (From Posnick, 2000a, with permission.)

1992; Randall et al., 1965; Robin, 1923, 1934) (Fig. 26.1), but the condition had been described earlier by St. Hilaire in 1822 (Dennison, 1965), Fairbairn (1846), and Shukowsky (1911). Birth prevalence estimates of Robin sequence have ranged from 1/200 to 1/30,000 (Bush and Williams, 1983; Carroll et al., 1971; Cohen, 1976). Definitions of this sequence of events also vary, making it difficult to obtain a more precise estimate of the birth prevalence and the ratio of syndromes said to be associated with the Robin sequence (Cohen, 1997). Cohen (1997) indicated that the clinical data are most consistent with etiologic and pathogenetic heterogeneity (Stoll et al., 1992). The most common genetic syndrome associated with Robin sequence is Stickler's syndrome (Turner, 1974). Prompt ophthalmologic assessment of the newborn with Stickler's syndrome is required to detect a myopia because blindness, resulting from retinal detachment, is associated with this syndrome (Turner, 1974; Schreiner et al., 1973; Smith and Stowe, 1961).

In animal models, intrauterine mandibular constraint with secondary failure of the tongue to descend and resultant CP has been described (Cocke, 1966; Edwards and Newall, 1985). Some instances of Robin sequence have been associated with oligohydramnios. It is thought that reduced amniotic fluid results in compression of the fetal chin against the sternum, restrict-

ing mandibular growth and impacting the elevated tongue between the palatal shelves (Poswillo, 1968; Rintala et al., 1984). This deformational cause of Robin sequence has been supported by several authors (Beers and Pruzansky, 1955). Pruzansky (1969) and Pruzansky and Richmond (1954) have shown that mandibular catch-up growth is likely to result in a normal profile by 4 to 6 years of age, when the cause of micrognathia is deformation rather than malformation. Hanson and Smith (1975) found specific syndromes in 25% of their Robin sequence patients, multiple anomalies but no specific syndrome in 35%, and isolated Robin sequence in the remaining 40%. A diversity of specific syndromes and associated malformations have been reported (Bezirdjian and Szucs, 1989; Bruce and Winship, 1993; Carey et al., 1982; Chitayat et al., 1991; Dykes et al., 1985; Glander and Cisneros, 1992; Robinow et al., 1986; Schimke et al., 1993; Schrander-Stumpel et al., 1991; Shprintzen, 1992).

Caouette-Laberge and co-workers (1994) reviewed all children admitted to Montreal Children's Hospital between 1964 and 1991 with the diagnosis of Robin sequence. Each child was placed into one of three groups according to the severity of symptoms: group I comprised children with adequate respiration in the prone position and bottle-feeding (*n* = 56, 44.8%), group II had adequate respiration in the prone position but feeding difficulties requiring gavage feeding ($n =$ 40, 32%), group III consisted of children with respiratory distress requiring endotracheal intubation and gavage feeding ($n = 29$, 23.2%). Interestingly, 17 children (13.6%) died during the first year of life. The mortality rate increased with the severity of symptoms (breathing and swallowing), associated anomalies, and the prematurity of the newborn. Among the 108 survivors in the study, 25 presented with psychomotor impairment (23.1%).

The results of Caouette-Laberge and colleagues (1994) contrasts somewhat with those of Lehman and associates (1995). The latter reviewed a consecutive series of Robin sequence newborns presenting over an 18-year period (1972–1990) to their tertiary care pediatric center located in the midwestern United States. Thirty-six patients were included in this study. Only two infants required a tracheostomy, and 34 patients underwent CP repair. At follow-up several years later, only 17.4% of the repaired CP patients required a secondary pharyngoplasty and 11.8% had palatal fistula. No deaths were reported. The discrepancy in these two studies likely reflects differences in referral patterns to each hospital center. Other authors have reported various airway difficulties and have recommended a variety of treatment protocols (Abramson et al., 1997; Argamaso, 1992; Frohberg and Lange, 1993; James and Ma, 1997; LeBlanc and Golding-Kushner, 1992; Moos, 1997; Moyson, 1961; Sher, 1992).

CLEFT LIP REPAIR

A cleft that occurs through at least the lip and alveolus (primary palate) produces distortions in all tissue layers, including skin, muscle, cartilage, mucous membranes, teeth, and bone. With repair of the UCL, e.g., the surgeon is expected to create a structure directly adjacent to its normal mirror image located in the most conspicuous area of the human body (Figs. 26.2, 26.3). There are many reasons for the observed differences in the aesthetic results of the repaired CL. Surgeons vary in their ability to achieve a symmetrical and proportionate lip repair. Furthermore, there is a wide variety of presenting cleft malformations and potentials for healing. Although clefts usually follow a pattern, some are narrow while others are wide. There are differences in the severity of distortion of the cupid's bow in UCL and in the amount of philtrum to work with in BCL (Latham, 1993; Mulliken et al., 1993) (Figs. 26.4, 26.5). It is an advantage for the surgeon to have experience in CLP care and a broad range of techniques from which to choose.

Timing

Cleft lip repair is generally carried out when the child is 2 to 3 months of age (Thompson, 1912). The general rule is to proceed when the child is approximately 10 weeks of age, weighs 10 lb, and has achieved a serum hemoglobin of 10 mg/ml. These guidelines have stood the test of time and, in general, place the child at reduced anesthetic risk, ensure successful wound healing, and allow enough time to determine if other malformations are present and to establish comfortable feeding and airway routines for the child and parents (Marsh, 1996).

Some surgeons and cleft teams have advocated other protocols, including "immediate" repair of the cleft, just after birth and prior to discharge from the newborn nursery (Van Boven et al., 1993). Their rationale for doing so is twofold: first, to take advantage of the benefits of "fetal-like" wound healing and, second, to avoid any psychosocial trauma to the parents of having to live with their baby with an unrepaired CL (Marsh, 1996). Unfortunately, the desired long-term facial aesthetic advantages of "neonatal" lip repair with reduced scarring have not been realized (Longaker et al., 1992; Sullivan et al., 1996). Furthermore, studies have failed to show improved bonding between the child and mother when immediate lip repair is performed (Field and Vega-Lahr, 1984). It is therefore difficult to justify the increased anesthetic and surgical risks of neonatal surgery (Eaton et al., 1994).

Techniques

Placing tape or an elastic band across the segmented lip or cheeks to encourage soft tissue lip alignment and alveolar segment remodeling has been performed in preparation for lip repair for centuries. One of the earliest proponents of this procedure was Gaspare Tagliacocci, who in the 16th century described the use of a linen splint with "agglutination" material, under which the approximated prepared (CL) edges could heal with less tension (Gnudi and Webster, 1950). Poole and Farnworth (1994) described their experience with "lip taping" to approximate the segments prior to repair. It is their belief that the soft tissue approximation and bony alignment achieved by lip taping can be as effective as lip adhesion for those who believe that alignment of the lip and alveolar segments prior to repair provides long-term advantages to lip and nose aesthetics.

Controversy continues as to whether it is advantageous to use passive or more aggressive presurgical orthopedic regimens and, if so, to what extent (Ross and MacNamera, 1994; Shaw and Semb, 1990). The purpose of these techniques is to improve the alignment of

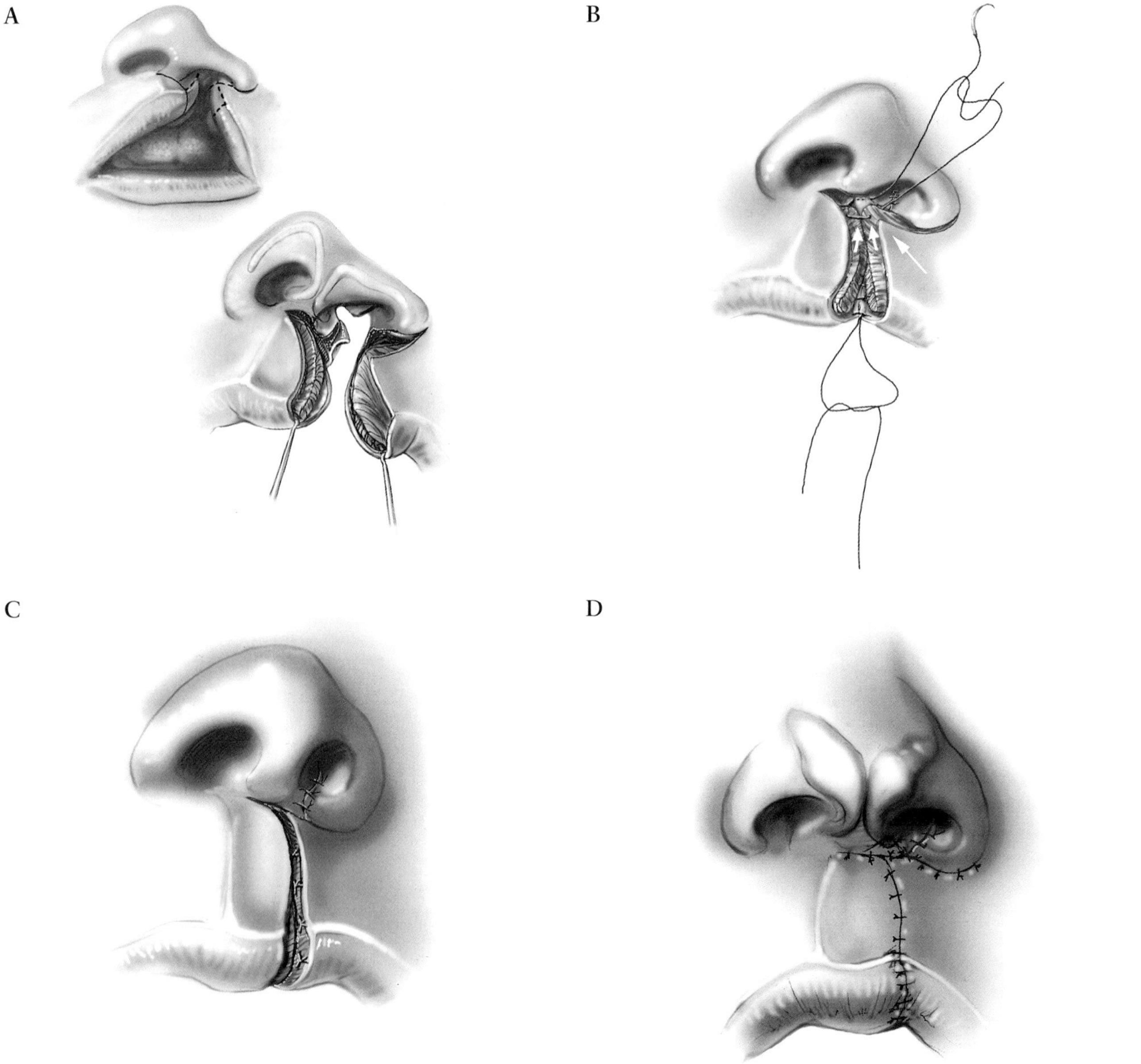

A

B

C

D

FIG. 26.2. Illustration of the basic components of the Millard rotation and advanced flap technique used by the authors for unilateral cleft lip repair. *A:* The rotation flap (greater lip segment) and the advancement flap (lesser lip segment) are outlined. Flaps are incised, redundant tissue is excised, and initial flap dissection is completed. The three tissue layers (skin, orbicularis oris muscle, and underlying mucosa) are separated. *B:* The orbicularis oris muscle, having been released from its abnormal bony attachments, is sutured across the midline and to the base of the columella. The underlying oral mucosa is sutured with reestablishment of a normal intraoral vestibule. *C:* Once the orbicularis oris muscle has been sutured, the cutaneous flaps approximate without tension for wound closure. The floor of the nose flaps are sutured to establish the nasal sill. *D:* Precise approximation of anatomic landmarks with fine sutures is undertaken to align the philtral columns, vermilion–cutaneous junction, and vermilion–mucosa/junction. (From Posnick, 2000a, with permission.)

the maxillary segments and overlying soft tissues prior to lip repair. Ross and MacNamara (1994) reviewed the long-term CL and nasal soft tissue aesthetics in two groups of teenagers who were born with BCLP. The first group underwent presurgical orthopedic procedures (lip taping) prior to lip repair, and the second

group did not. When facial photographs were judged by double-blinded impartial observers, no statistical difference in lip or nasal aesthetics between the two groups was found.

A lip adhesion is a partial CL repair that converts a wide, complete cleft into an incomplete one (Millard,

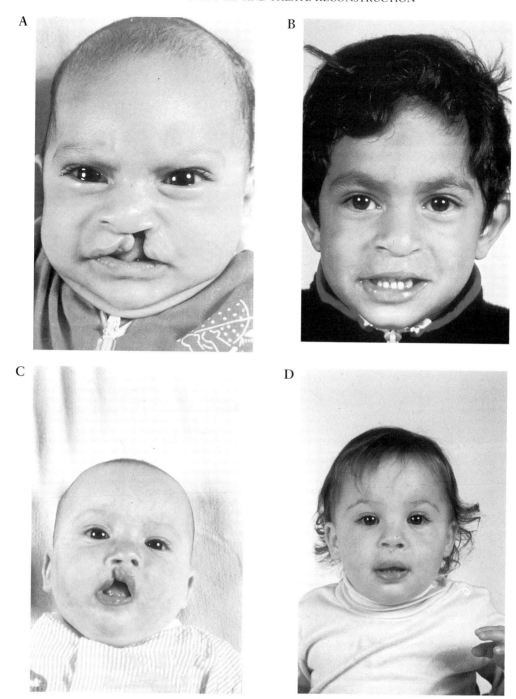

FIG. 26.3. A spectrum of children born with varied degrees of unilateral cleft lip/alveolus and palate (UCLP) before and after initial repairs. *A:* Child with complete UCLP before surgery. *B:* Child 2 years later. *C:* Child with incomplete UCL before surgery. *D:* Child 6 months later. (From Posnick, 2000a, with permission.)

1976a; Randall, 1965). Advocates of lip adhesion suggest that it be used as a first stage only for those patients with very wide clefts where a primary repair might not be possible. A lip adhesion is said to recreate the natural compression forces and can be expected to narrow a wide cleft and to encourage the alignment of the alveolar arches. Those who advocate a lip ad-

hesion usually carry it out when the child is 3 to 4 months of age (Randall, 1965). They then allow 3 to 6 months for the scar tissue of the lip to soften before undertaking definitive lip repair. Lip adhesion has the disadvantage of adding a second operation with additional anesthetic and hospital recovery. Potential complications associated with lip adhesion include wound

A   B

C   D

E   F

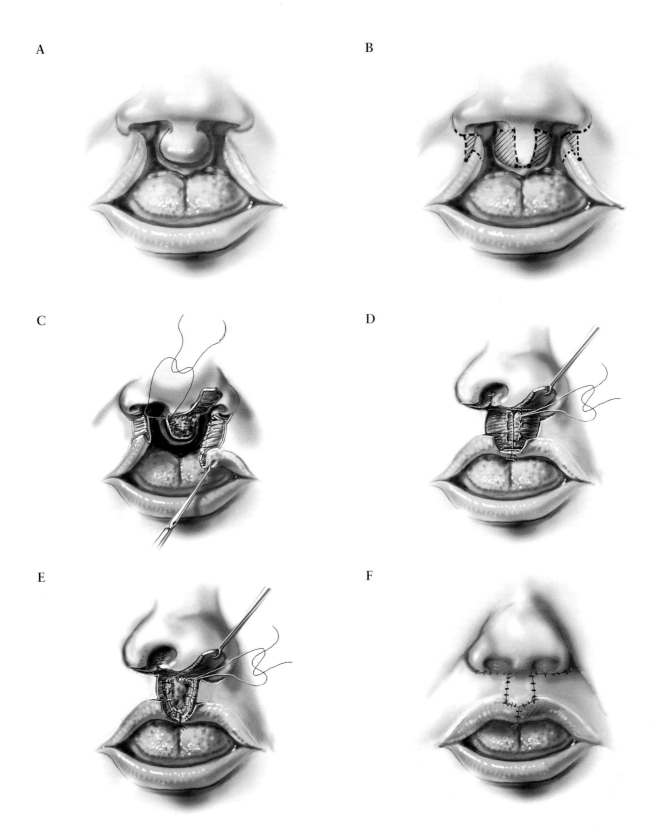

FIG. 26.4. Illustration of the basic components of the Millard technique used by the authors for bilateral cleft lip repair. *A:* Typical complete bilateral cleft lip deformity. *B:* Incisions for bilateral cleft lip repair are indicated (*dotted lines*), with tissue to be excised (*diagonal lines*). *C:* The philtral (skin) flap has been elevated, with circulation maintained on its columellar base. Lateral lip flaps have been elevated with addition dissection of lateral vermilion mucosal flaps to be used for reconstruction of the central red lip region. The orbicularis oris muscle has been dissected free of its abnormal bony attachments. *D:* The anterior portion of the nasal floor has been reconstructed by suturing of the medial and lateral nasal floor flaps. The intraoral mucosa and oral vestibule have been carefully sutured with excision of redundant red lip from the philtral flap. *E:* The orbicularis oris muscle is approximated across the midline and sutured to the columellar base. *F:* The vermilion–cutaneous junction is sutured on each side, and the vermilion–mucosal junction is aligned in the midline by approximating the lateral red lip flaps. Lateral cutaneous flaps are advanced and sutured to the columellar base on each side. Philtral columns and nasal sills are sutured. (From Posnick, 2000a, with permission.)

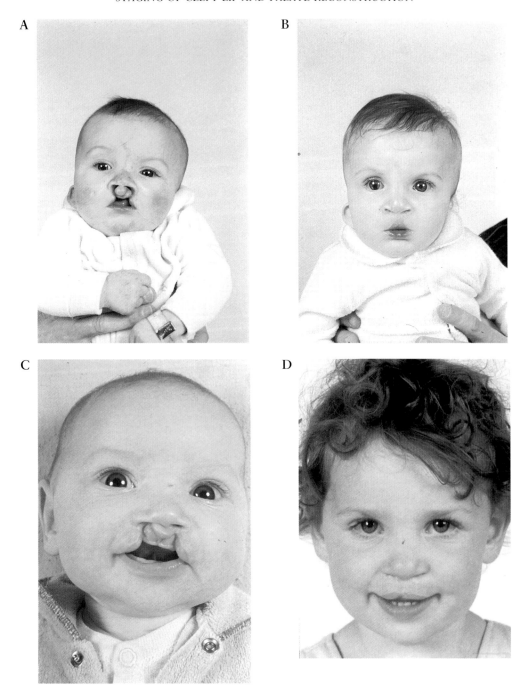

FIG. 26.5. A spectrum of children born with bilateral cleft lip/alveolus and palate (BCLP) before and after initial repairs. *A:* Child born with multiple malformations, including complete BCLP, before surgery. *B:* Child 8 months later. *C:* Child born with BCLP before surgery. *D:* Child 2 years later. (From Posnick, 2000a, with permission.)

dehiscence and excess scar formation, which may leave the tissue less supple for the definitive lip repair.

Every CL surgeon has a favorite technique for repairing the unilateral and bilateral cleft types (Abbe, 1898; Brauer, 1985; Davies, 1966; LeMesurier, 1955; McComb, 1985; Millard, 1960, 1964, 1976b; Mohler, 1987; Skoog, 1969). Refinements in lip repair were pre-

sented by LeMesurier (1955), whose approach gave advantages over the previously advocated straight line closure. This was followed by the Tennison (1952) triangular flap technique, the Skoog (1969) high triangular insertion of the lateral lip segment method, and the modifications introduced by Randall (1990) and Brauer (1985). Finally, in the early 1950s, Millard, realized that the popular triangular flap technique often aligned the peak of the cupid's bow in its normal position but violated the natural lines of the philtrum dimple (Millard, 1957). Rather than merely rotating the lower third of the central lip, he conceptualized the high release and subsequent rotation of the whole medial lip segment, thereby returning it to its normal position. The lateral lip segment was then prepared and advanced to meet the leading edge of the rotated medial lip segment. Through the years, Millard and others have added various refinements to his initial technique (Millard, 1960, 1964, 1976a,b). Today, the Millard rotation and advancement flap technique remains the gold standard by which other lip repairs are judged.

Millard's method of UCL repair (the rotation and advancement flap technique) is the most frequently employed method of CL repair in the United States and throughout the world (Fig. 26.2). The rotation and advancement flap repair can be applied to a wide variety of UCL deformities, with flexibility and consistency of results. Other options for CL repair remain the straight-line closure (Rose, 1976), the Tennison-Randall triangular flap technique (Randall, 1990), and the LeMesurier (1955) approach. Whichever basic technique is used, the goal is to achieve a symmetrical and proportionate upper lip in repose with dynamic mimetic function.

In unilateral clefts, the alar cartilage is splayed out (laterally) and rotated caudally (downward). The lower border of the lateral crus produces an oblique ridge in the nasal vestibule and the nostril rim droops. The alar dome is pulled laterally and downward, causing irregularity of the nasal tip and shortening of the columella on the cleft side.

At the time of primary CL repair, if the nostril on the cleft side is repositioned without lifting the alar cartilage, a curve is further accentuated in the nostril that may result in the typical flare of the CL nose. Lifting the slumped alar cartilage is thought to be a useful step in limiting this problem. McComb considers the essential features of primary CL nasal repair to be wide undermining of the nasal skin envelope (separating the lower lateral cartilage from the overlying skin) on the side of the cleft, avoidance of incisions in the nasal lining (to limit nostril cicatrization), and placement of sutures to bolster the lower lateral cartilage on the cleft side into its preferred position (McComb, 1985, 1990, 1994; McComb and Coghlan, 1996). The details of surgical technique should be expected to differ from surgeon to surgeon (Takato et al., 1995a; Trier, 1995).

Key elements unique to BCL repair include repairing both cleft sides at one operative sitting, achieving a successful orbicularis oris muscle repair, bringing in adequate vermilion and mucosa from the lateral lip seg-

ments to reconstruct the central red lip, reconstructing a relatively small philtrum as it tends to stretch and expand with growth, and restoring a sufficient inner lip vestibule (Figs. 26.4, 26.5). Millard's concepts of preserving tissue led him to suggest the "banking of forked flaps" in each nasal sill, to be used later to lengthen the columella in the BCLP patient. It has been the experience of many that, in the short run, the banked forked flaps may obstruct the infant's nasal breathing. In the long run, the flaps contract and are unlikely to provide useful tissue for later nasal reconstruction.

Mulliken (1995) has advanced our understanding of the BCLP patient's nasal deformities and has added several key refinements to BCL repair. He believes that "the bilateral cleft lip nasal deformity is both intrinsic (a primary malformation deficiency) and deformational (extrinsic, secondary to the surgeon's well-intended closure of the lip)." He states that the "malformed alar cartilages are rotated caudally and subluxed from their normal position overlying the upper lateral cartilage. The lower lateral cartilages and alar soft tissues are hypoplastic and widely separated." Unlike the majority, he believes that early repositioning of the alar cartilage under direct vision through an open technique at the time of primary lip repair is essential to correct BCL nasal deformity. He does not believe that the columella is intrinsically deficient and recommends against lengthening procedures. While the final word is not in, we prefer the McComb approach to nasal reconstruction at the time of lip repair and recommend against columellar (skin) lengthening procedures.

CLEFT PALATE REPAIR

While the optimal age of the patient and method of closure of the CP remain unresolved, available information suggests a limited range of acceptable options for timing and technique. A surgical objective of the primary repair is to reconstruct the hard and soft palate with closure of all existing oronasal communication from the incisal foramen back through the uvula. Another goal is the creation of a dynamic soft palate, capable of interfacing with the lateral and posterior pharyngeal walls to achieve sufficient velopharyngeal (VP) closure and, thus, "normal" speech (Broomhead, 1957; Maher, 1977; Ross and Johnstone, 1972).

Timing

Ideally, a decision about the appropriate age for palatal repair should be based on the child's stage of phonemic development or articulation age (language or speech age), as opposed to chronologic age (Copeland, 1990; Dalston, 1992; Denk and Magee, 1996; Evans and Renfrew, 1974; Haapanen and Rantala, 1992; Kemp-Fincham et al., 1990; Randall et al., 1983; Riski and DeLong, 1984). A child with either an unrepaired palate or an inadequately closed palate who approaches a level of phonemic development (articulation age) that requires VP competence will be left vulnerable to the development of compensatory articulations. These maladaptive speech patterns interfere with intelligibility and may be difficult to eliminate once developed (Blijdorp and Muller, 1984; Chapman and Hardin, 1992; Grobbelaar et al., 1995; Harding and Campbell, 1989; Herman, 1995; Riski, 1996; Rohrich et al., 1996).

Most studies indicate that the nonsyndromic normally developing infant who is without hearing impairment or cognitive delay will develop significantly fewer compensatory articulations and maladaptive speech patterns if the palate is repaired before 2 years of age. Furthermore, Dorf and Curtin (1982) reported startlingly different speech results in a group of 21 children whose clefts were closed before 12 months of age compared with a group of 59 children who underwent palatal repair after 12 months of age. In their study, speech was assessed only for the presence or absence of compensatory articulations. Only 10% of children in the early-repair group developed these patterns compared with 86% in the late-repair group. In a later follow-up study of an expanded series of patients, Dorf and Curtin (1990) reported an even greater discrepancy in speech performance between the early- and late-repair groups. The independent studies of Peterson-Falzone (1990, 1995) and Dalston (1992) failed to confirm the Dorf and Curtin findings of 12 months being a watershed age for CP repair. While these authors did find an overall prevalence of compensatory articulations in their CP study group similar to that found by Dorf and Curtin, there were no statistical significances when the CP was closed at or before 12 months vs. between 12 and 24 months of age. The two studies did confirm that repair of the palate after 24 months resulted in a much higher prevalence of compensatory articulations than repair at less than 24 months of age. Unfortunately, none of the CP "timing" studies to date have controlled for the variable *language or speech age*. Riski (1996) and Riski and DeLong (1984) believe that children who develop speech early may be more prone to incorporate maladaptive misarticulations since they attempt pressure consonants even before palatal repair. For most children, CP repair to close down the oronasal opening and establish a competent VP sphincter by 9 to 12 months of age minimizes the development of irreversible pathologic compensatory speech patterns as

well as the surgical risks and potential for growth restriction of the upper jaw (Dorf and Curtin, 1990; Devlin, 1990).

Techniques

Options for repositioning the displaced cleft maxillary segments prior to CP repair include no preoperative orthopedic procedures (no active segment repositioning), a conservative preoperative orthopedic treatment (lip taping and a passive palatal plate), or use of the Latham presurgical orthopedic appliance (Bitter, 1992; Georgiade and Latham, 1975; Millard and Latham, 1990; Nguyen and Sullivan, 1993; Pruzansky, 1955, 1964; Ross and MacNamera, 1994). Despite several decades of experience with the Latham appliance and other less aggressive preoperative orthopedic options, no convincing studies have demonstrated long-term comparative benefits in lip or nose aesthetics, arch alignment, or occlusion (Millard, 1980). The potential for morbidity when aggressive preoperative orthopedic options are selected must also be considered.

Berkowitz (1996) compared conservative presurgical orthopedic treatment in complete BCLP patients to use of the Millard-Latham (M-L) method. In the conservatively treated group, external elastic traction was sometimes used to apply gentle pressure to the premaxilla prior to surgical lip closure. The M-L method involves mechanical traction of the protruded premaxilla using the pinned Latham palatal appliances followed by a Millard gingivoperiosteoplasty. In both study groups, the palatal cleft (hard and soft) was closed between 18 and 30 months of age using a modified Langenbeck procedure.

As part of the Berkowitz (1996) study, the children who underwent each regimen were followed similarly into the early teenage years. The conservative presurgical orthopedic group underwent secondary alveolar bone grafting between the ages of 6 and 9 years. Ninety percent of the children in the M-L group demonstrated bony bridging across the alveolar cleft with partial or complete closure of the lateral incisor gap. By 10 to 12 years of age, only two of the 29 patients in the conservatively treated group (6%) demonstrated an anterior crossbite suggestive of maxillary retrusion. *All* of the patients that underwent the M-L method demonstrated maxillary retrusion by 9 years of age, indicative of maxillary hypoplasia. The results of Berkowitz (1996) confirm that a *major disadvantage* of using the latham palatal appliance followed by the Millard gingivoperiosteoplasty technique for palatal repair is maxillary growth restriction, with a need for orthognathic surgery in the teenage years anticipated in the majority of patients.

CP centers have advocated earlier protocols for the timing of initial repair (Copeland, 1990; Denk and Magee, 1996). When contemplating early repair of the palate (before 6 months of age), three additional factors are important to consider (Bardach and Salyer, 1991a; Hedrick et al., 1996). First, there is a known potential for maxillary or midfacial growth restriction resulting from surgery carried out in the immature maxilla (Copeland, 1990; Pruzansky, 1964; Bishara, 1973; Canady et al., 1997; Derijcke et al., 1994; Heidbuchel et al., 1994; Kramer et al., 1996; McCance et al., 1993; Motohashi et al., 1994; Roberg and Koblin, 1973; Semb, 1991; Shaw et al., 1992; Trotman and Ross, 1993). Second, the need for blood transfusion at the time of palatal repair and the potential for airway complications are inherently greater when the procedure is carried out at a very young age. Third, for the general CP population, there are no known long-term functional advantages (speech, airway, dental) to carrying out palatal repair before 9 to 12 months of age.

There are three basic surgical options for palatal repair: the modified Langenbeck procedure (von Langenbeck, 1861), the two-flap Bardach technique (Bardach and Salyer, 1991a; Bardach and Nosal, 1987; Bardach et al., 1990), and the Furlow Z-plasty (Furlow, 1986, 1992, 1997; Horswell et al., 1993; Upton, 1993). There are no confirmed inherent advantages of one method over the other, and each has theoretical benefits and technical limitations which the surgeon must understand and master. Other methods of CP repair have been advocated over the years (Kilner, 1937, 1958; Millard et al., 1970; Perko, 1979; Schweckendiek, 1978; Skoog, 1965; Veau, 1931; Wardill, 1928, 1937; Wood et al., 1997). Whichever technique the surgeon prefers, the objectives of primary repair remain the same: achievement of an intact palate (from the anterior incisive foramen through the uvula) without oronasal communication and creation of a dynamic soft palate that is able to achieve VP closure during normal phonation (Abyholm, 1979; Amaratunga, 1988; Emory et al., 1997; Posnick and Getz, 1987). Whenever possible, complete soft tissue closure over the hard palate should be achieved in the operating room without leaving raw lateral bone surfaces open to heal with granulation tissue formation. Healing of the hard palate by secondary intention likely results in increased palatal scarring, maxillary growth restrictions, and the need for orthognathic surgery in the teenage years.

Another often discussed issue related to CP repair is whether to complete a one- or two-stage palatoplasty. The aim of the one-stage palatoplasty (whether using the Langenbeck method, the Bardach two-flap technique, or the Furlow Z-plasty) is straightforward: complete closure of the palatal cleft in one operation, creating adequate conditions for normal speech. There remain some cleft surgeons who continue to advocate a two-stage palatoplasty, in which the velum (soft palate) is repaired first, leaving the hard palate unrepaired for a period ranging from several months to several years. Advocates of the two-stage palatoplasty, a concept presented by Schweckendiek in the late 1930s, believe that this approach achieves two goals simultaneously: creation of a functional soft palate and unrestricted maxillary growth. Advocates of the one-stage palatoplasty believe their approach to be more efficient as it obviates the need for a second palatal procedure and prevents the need to constantly wear a palatal plate, which must be frequently modified to ensure satisfactory speech. Many prominent CP speech pathologists (Morris, Shprintzen, Witzel, and others) report more favorable speech outcomes following the one-stage palatoplasty than following the two-stage approach (Witzel et al., 1984). Interestingly, studies have not documented advantages in maxillary growth with the two-stage technique. The one-stage palatoplasty remains the most frequently performed technique for CP repair throughout the world (Bardach and Salyer, 1991a; von Langenbeck, 1861; Bardach et al., 1990; Furlow, 1986, 1992, 1997; Horswell et al., 1993; Upton, 1993).

The basic principles of the Bardach two-flap palatoplasty technique include (1) complete closure of the entire palatal cleft as a one-stage procedure; (2) two-layer closure (nasal and oral layers) of the hard palate and three-layer closure (nasal mucosa, soft palatal muscles, and oral mucosa) of the soft palate; (3) release of the muscles of the soft palate from the posterior edge of the hard palate and from the periosteum on the nasal side, allowing creation of a more physiologic soft palate muscle sling; and (4) in wide clefts, when an area of bare bone must be left exposed on the hard palate, covering of the open areas with Avitene (microfibrillar collagen) Hemostat to limit healing time and scar formation (Bardach and Salyer, 1991a; Bardach and Nosal, 1987; Bardach et al., 1990) (Fig. 26.6).

The *Furlow Z-plasty* is also a one-stage palatoplasty (Furlow, 1986, 1992, 1997; Horswell et al., 1993). The Furlow technique provides for closure of the hard palate in one procedure without push-back or lateral relaxing incisions and repair of the soft palate with mirror-image Z-plasties to retroposition and overlap the soft palatal muscles, forming a muscle sling (Fig. 26.7). Furlow believes that if there is some lengthening of the soft palate it is by the Z-plasties, which do not take tissue from the hard palate. If the Z-plasties in fact lengthen the palate, they do so at the expense of palatal tissue, which would otherwise be used for approximation at the junction of the hard and soft palate. This may be the reason for the reported in-

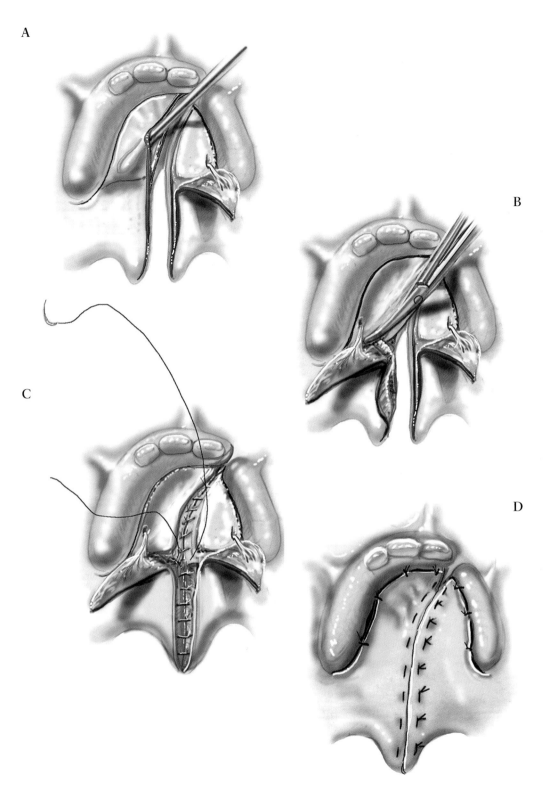

FIG. 26.6. Illustration of the basic technique of the Bardach two-flap palatal repair. *A:* Oral and nasal mucosae are incised and separated from the uvula forward to the incisal foramen on each side of the cleft. A second incision is completed on each palatal shelf to allow for flap elevation. The second set of incisions is from the anterior extent of the previous incision, continuing posteriorly at the junction of the palatal mucosa and alveolar mucosa. Relaxing incisions are made behind each maxillary tuberosity. Each full-thickness mucoperiosteal flap is elevated, with care taken to preserve the greater palatine vascular pedicle within each flap. *B:* With each full-thickness flap elevated and the greater palatine vessels preserved, the soft palatal musculature is taken off its abnormal attachments to the posterior palatine bones. *C:* Nasal mucosa is sutured for a water-tight closure from the incisal foramen to the junction of the hard and soft palate. The nasal side of the soft palate is then closed from the uvula forward to the junction of the hard and soft palate. The soft palatal musculature is also sutured across the midline. *D:* Oral mucosa is closed from the uvula forward to the incisal foramen. Finally, each mucoperiosteal flap is sutured back to its original location, limiting exposed bone whenever feasible. (From Posnick, 2000a, with permission.)

329

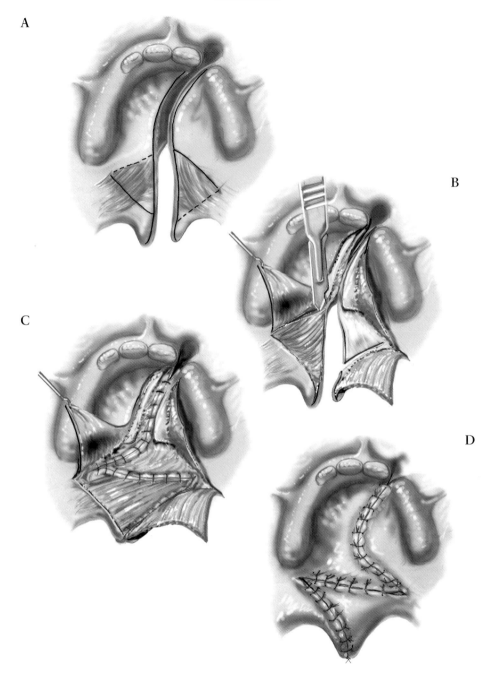

FIG. 26.7. Illustration of the basic technique of the Furlow double-opposing Z-plasty palatal repair. *A:* Location of planned incisions. *B:* Flaps are elevated. *C:* Nasal side closure is achieved using opposing Z-plasty flaps in the soft palate and nasal flap closure over the hard palate. *D:* Oral side closure of hard and soft palate is completed. (From Posnick, 2000a, with permission.)

creased incidence of oronasal fistulae when using the Furlow technique.

The *Langenbeck palatoplasty* calls for elevation of two bipedicled mucoperiosteal flaps, one off of each palatal shelf (von Langenbeck, 1861) (Fig. 26.8). The theoretical advantage is the maintenance of an anterior

pedicle for improved flap circulation. Unfortunately, with maintenance of the anterior pedicle, direct visualization for nasal side closure is limited. In addition, flap elevation and relaxation for advancement to the midline to close the cleft at the junction of the hard and soft palate may be difficult.

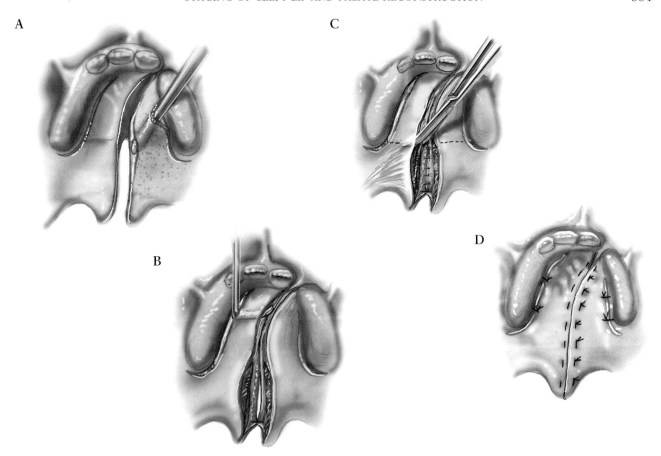

FIG. 26.8. Illustration of the basic technique of Langenbeck's cleft palate repair. *A, B:* Incisions and initial elevation of bipedicled, full-thickness mucoperiosteal palatal flaps. *C:* After separation of nasal and oral mucosae, nasal side closure is achieved from the incisal foramen back to the uvula. Release of the soft palatal musculature off of its abnormal attachment to the palatine bones is completed, and the soft palatal musculature is approximated in the midline with sutures. *D:* Oral side closure is completed with interrupted sutures from the incisal foramen back through the uvula. Laterally, the palatal flaps are sutured back to their origin. This prevents exposed bone, which would then have to heal by secondary intention. (From Posnick, 2000a, with permission.)

SECONDARY CLEFT PALATE PROCEDURES FOR MANAGEMENT OF VELOPHARYNGEAL DYSFUNCTION

Velopharyngeal dysfunction (VPD) is one of the most complex secondary problems related to CP treatment. It affects the ability of the patient to communicate coherently with others and may be considered more debilitating than many other secondary lip, nose, and dental deformities that primarily affect physical appearance.

When carrying out initial CP repair, the surgeon will try to restore the palatal anatomy for optimal VP closure and eventual normal speech production (Cutting et al., 1995; Morris, 1973). Unfortunately, present knowledge does not allow prediction of the eventual speech outcome in individual patients after initial palatal repair (Ainoda et al., 1985; Hartzel et al., 1994;

Morris et al., 1989; Peterson-Falzone, 1995; Riski, 1995). It must be remembered that all aspects of VP valve function are not based solely on the palate. The CP itself is only one factor contributing to VP function, and even this single aspect cannot be managed optimally in every patient because of the varying degrees of severity of cleft and hypoplasia as well as differences in surgical techniques used, surgeon expertise, and individual factors related to the local wound-healing process (McCance et al., 1993; Ren and Wang, 1993).

Timing

Additional surgical intervention is recommended after initial palatal repair when VP dysfunction is consistent and determined to be related to an anatomic problem (Henningsson and Isberg, 1986; Isberg and Henningsson, 1987; Lohmander-Agerskov et al., 1996). In patients 2.5 to 4 years of age, it is difficult for the surgeon, but occasionally possible for the speech and language pathologist, to draw definitive conclusions about VP function or dysfunction. Riski (1997a,b) believes that many children who suffer marked VP dysfunction after CP repair can be critically assessed at 3 years of age. According to Shprintzen and Bardach (1995a) and Shprintzen and Golding-Kushner (1989), this judgment generally cannot be made until the child is 4 to 5 years of age. They specify several reasons for delaying surgery until this age, including the child's language and articulation development, the ability to accurately assess VP function, and patient compliance. All agree that preoperative diagnostic accuracy is critical to achieving a good clinical outcome. Secondary palatal surgery should not be planned until reliable and consistent assessment of the patient's speech is possible (Riski, 1997b; D'Antonio et al., 1989; Golding-Kushner et al., 1990; Siegel-Sardewitz and Shprintzen, 1986; Warren, 1975, 1994; Warren et al., 1994). Pharyngeal flap surgery is reportedly successful approximately 80% of the time when applied randomly to repaired CP patients with subjective hypernasality who have not undergone advanced preoperative diagnostic tests (i.e., nasopharyngoscopy or multiview videofluoroscopy) (Argamaso et al., 1994; Shprintzen et al., 1979). However, a success rate of 97% was reported when the same surgeons applied their operations based on the preoperative diagnostic information provided by nasendoscopy, multiview videofluoroscopy, and discussion with the evaluating speech therapist (Argamaso et al., 1994; Shprintzen et al., 1979). The major advantage of nasendoscopy is the ability to dynamically observe the internal anatomy of the nose, pharynx, and larynx in detail. Decisions regarding the advisability of surgery, the choice of operation, and treatment alternatives are influenced by observations of the VP valve and surrounding structures and are best made after discussion with the speech pathologist (Argamaso et al., 1994; Croft et al., 1981; Peat et al., 1994; Riski et al., 1984; Shprintzen, 1990; Shprintzen and Bardach, 1995b).

Techniques

Various pharyngoplasty techniques have been designed to improve VP function following initial CP repair (Bardach and Salyer, 1991b; Barone et al., 1994; Blocksma, 1963; Bluestone et al., 1968; Brauer et al., 1990; Chen et al., 1994; Denny et al., 1993; Graivier et al., 1992; Hogan, 1973; Jackson, 1990; Morris et al., 1995; Orticochea, 1968, 1984; Witt et al., 1995, 1997; Wolford et al., 1989). The basic goal of any pharyngoplasty is to allow complete VP sphincter closure with specific speech sounds, eliminating hypernasality. At present, there are only limited clinical data to support any one surgical technique as the optimal choice for a particular form of VP dysfunction (Riski, 1979; Riski et al., 1984, 1989, 1992a,b; Witt et al., 1997; Witzel et al., 1989). The basic techniques of pharyngoplasty include the inferiorly based pharyngeal flap, the superiorly based pharyngeal flap, the sphincter pharyngoplasty, and augmentation of the posterior pharyngeal wall.

The custom-designed, superiorly based pharyngeal flap remains the standard for the surgical resolution of VP dysfunction after initial palatal repair (Argamaso et al., 1994; Shprintzen et al., 1979) (Fig. 26.9). With the superiorly based flap technique, a long flap can be designed to ensure a tension-free insertion and fixation of the flap into a bed created in the soft palate. The width of the flap is varied to accommodate individual VP needs (Argamaso et al., 1994). Proper elevation of the pharyngeal flap to place its base at a level higher than the posterior edge of the soft palate is preferred, to avoid a downward pull on the soft palate. This problem is avoided with a superiorly based flap but occurs frequently when an inferiorly based flap is used. Randall and others in the 1970s (Randall et al., 1978) documented greater morbidity without improved speech outcomes when using the inferiorly based flap compared with the superiorly based flap. For this reason, the inferiorly based flap is rarely used. Using a tailored approach to the elevation and insertion of the superiorly based flap designed to accommodate individual patient needs, Argamaso and colleagues (1994) described effective resolution of VPI in 97% of their patients. Bardach and Salyer (1991b) reported the use of a superiorly based pharyngeal flap tailored according to preoperative objective findings and demonstrated a 95% success rate.

The so-called dynamic sphincter pharyngoplasty is another option (Jackson, 1990; Jackson and Silverton, 1977). Its aim is to substitute the two lateral ports that would be created by a superiorly based pharyngeal flap with one central port with improved VP valve function. This is achieved by elevating and inserting mucomuscular flaps into the lateral walls, to create a functional sphincter. The dynamic sphincteroplasty technique has no proven advantage over the superiorly based flap in the elimination of VP dysfunction but may be the preferred method to prevent the postoperative airway obstruction and mucus trapping sometimes seen with the latter (Croft et al., 1981; Brouilette et al., 1984; Caouette-Laberge et al., 1992; Gray, 1990; Guilleminault and Stoohs, 1990; Shprintzen et al., 1987; Sirois et al., 1994; Witt et al., 1996; Ysunza et al., 1993).

Augmentation of the posterior pharyngeal wall represents another option in the treatment of VPI recog-

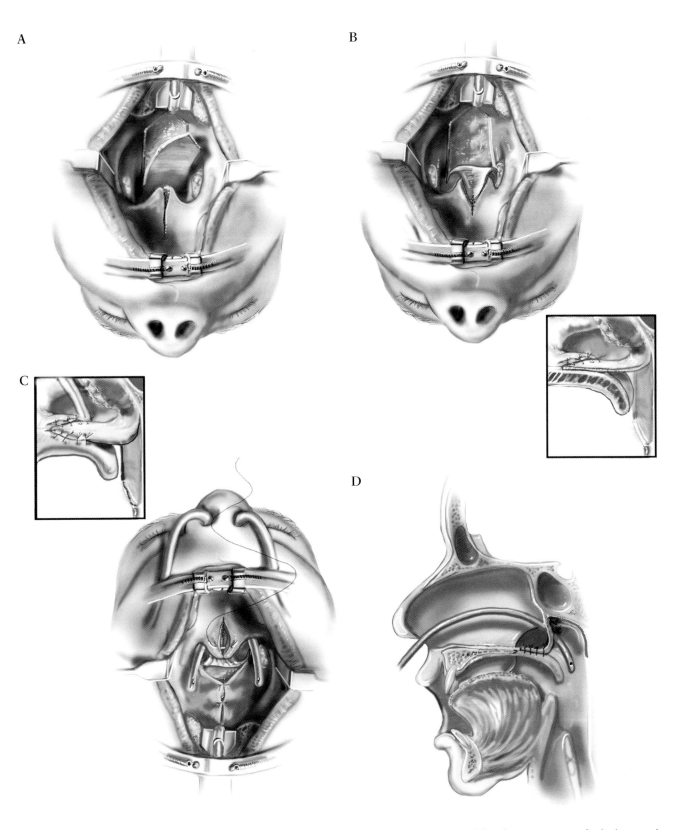

FIG. 26.9. Illustration of the basic technique of elevation and inset of a superiorly based pharyngeal flap for management of velopharyngeal insufficiency. *A:* Intraoperative view of soft palate and posterior pharyngeal wall with Dingman mouth gag in place. The soft palate is incised in the sagittal midline from the uvula forward to the junction of the hard and soft palate. The superiorly based pharyngeal flap is elevated off the prevertebral fascia. *B:* The superiorly based pharyngeal flap is inset to the soft palate and sutured to the nasal side of the soft palate with interrupted sutures. This is also demonstrated in the cross-sectional view (*inset*). *C:* The pharyngeal wall donor site is partially closed with 2-0 Vicryl interrupted sutures. Nasopharyngeal airways are placed through each lateral pharyngeal port for sizing and for post-operative airway support as needed. With the flap inset and the nasal side closed, the soft palatal musculature is further dissected and approximated as indicated. The oral side of the soft palate is then closed with interrupted sutures. A cross-sectional view (*inset*) demonstrates the separate oral and nasal side closure of the soft palate. *D:* Cross-sectional sagittal view of the face indicates the location of the nasopharyngeal airway in relationship to the soft palate and inset pharyngeal flap. (From Posnick, 2000a, with permission.)

333

nized in the child after first-stage palatal repair. (Blocksma, 1963; Bluestone et al., 1968; Brauer et al., 1990; Witt et al., 1997). When successful, this procedure moves the posterior pharyngeal wall forward so that the mobile but poorly functioning palate can more easily make contact with the posterior wall to prevent nasal air escape with certain speech sounds. Unfortunately, the ideal material to use for augmentation of the posterior pharyngeal wall has not been found. Homologous or autologous cartilage, Silastic implants, Teflon injections, and Dacron-wrapped silicone gel implants have been tried but without reliable long-term success. Outcome studies demonstrating the long-term efficacy of these augmentation techniques have not been forthcoming.

Witt and co-workers (1996) reported on the use of autogenous posterior pharyngeal wall augmentation using a "rolled superiorly based pharyngeal myomucosal flap." This procedure was originally described by Wardill (1928). Witt and colleagues (1996) used this technique on a series of 14 consecutive patients who had VP dysfunction not responsive to speech therapy and a less than 20% coronal gap on VP nasendoscopy. All patients were evaluated preoperatively and 3 months postoperatively with recorded (audiovisual tape) perceptual, nasendoscopic, and fluoroscopic standardized speech and airway tests. Preoperatively, the majority of these patients had nasal turbulence and all had variable degrees of hypernasality ranging from intermittent to pervasive. Unfortunately, there were no statistically significant tendencies for patients' speech to be rated as closer to normal after the augmentation procedure than before it. The authors concluded that autogenous posterior pharyngeal wall augmentation by the techniques selected does not result in speech improvement.

In another attempt to resolve the problem of VPI, Marsh and Wray (1980) reported the results of 34 children, aged 3 to 13 years, who were randomized to manage their VPI with either a speech bulb ($n = 12$) or superiorly based pharyngeal flap ($n = 22$). The speech bulb was effective in 11 of 12 and the pharyngeal flap in 20 of 22 cases. All patients randomized to surgery complied, while 29% of the prosthesis patients did not. In addition, 33% of patients randomized to the speech prosthesis later had a pharyngeal flap placed. For a variety of reasons (e.g., cost, time, expertise, compliance, and family preference for surgery), use of a speech bulb to solve the problem of VPI is almost always a secondary choice (Ross et al., 1996).

Our clinical impression is in agreement with the objective findings of Shprintzen et al. (1979), Argamaso et al. (1994), and Salyer and others. For the majority of patients, a superiorly based pharyngeal flap tailored in both height and width according to the preoperative findings gives the most reliable results with an acceptable degree of morbidity.

MANAGEMENT OF ALVEOLAR AND PALATAL (CLEFT) SKELETAL DEFECTS AND RESIDUAL ORONASAL FISTULA

When the congenital cleft runs through the alveolar ridge, as it does in 75% of CLP patients, a residual perialveolar oronasal fistula and bony defect through the alveolar ridge, floor of the nose, and hard palate will remain despite satisfactory lip and palatal repair (Millard, 1980). In addition, by early childhood there will be a variable degree of collapse of the two maxillary segments in the UCLP patient and of the lateral and premaxillary segments in the BCLP patient, resulting in lateral crossbites and the potential for a negative overjet at the incisors (Preuzansky, 1964; Derijcke et al., 1994; Jolleys, 1954; Jolleys and Robertson, 1972; Lebert, 1962; McCance et al., 1993; Nelson et al., 1988; Nylen et al., 1974; Rehrmann, 1971; Robertson and Jolleys, 1968).

Timing

The most efficient way to achieve the objectives of eruption of the (permanent) canine tooth through the grafted cleft with normal alveolar ridge development, improved skeletal support for the base of the nose, effective closure of all residual labial and palatal oronasal fistulae, and unity of the cleft maxillary segments is through properly sequenced and timed interceptive orthodontic treatment and secondary alveolar and palatal skeletal and soft tissue surgery (Pruzansky, 1964; Abyholm et al., 1981; Assuncao, 1993; Bergland et al., 1986; Bertz, 1981; Boyne, 1970, 1974, 1985; Boyne and Sands, 1972, 1976; Correa Normando et al., 1992; El Deeb et al., 1982; Hall and Posnick, 1984; Henderson and Jackson, 1975; Koberg, 1973; Nique et al., 1987; Posnick, 1991; Rosenstein et al., 1982, 1991a,b; Rudman, 1997; Sindet-Pedersen and Enemark, 1990; Troxell et al., 1982; Turvey et al., 1984; Waite and Kersten, 1980). There are two advantages to waiting until the eruption of the permanent maxillary first molars before proceeding. First, reliable and efficient orthodontic anchorage is achieved for rapid arch expansion just prior to the surgical procedure. Second, waiting allows maximal transverse (posterior) growth of the maxilla prior to bone grafting. The preferred age at treatment is therefore dependent on dental age rather than chronologic age (Abyholm et al., 1981; Hall and

Posnick, 1984). It is important to remember that in the CLP patient the maxillary dental eruption pattern is often delayed.

Techniques

The interceptive phase of orthodontic treatment will achieve expansion of the posterior arch width in both BCLP and UCLP patients and will reposition the premaxilla in BCLP patients. Once these orthodontic objectives are completed, surgery is carried out to place the patient's own cancellous iliac (hip) bone within the skeletal defects in the hard palate, alveolar ridge, and nasal floor with closure of all residual labial and palatal oronasal fistulae (Canady et al., 1993; Catone et al., 1992; Fonseca, 1997; Posnick, 2000a,b) (Figs. 26.10–26.12). While some CLP teams believe that placement of the bone graft within the skeletal defect prior to eruption of the permanent central or lateral incisors at the cleft site is an advantage, all agree that a successful graft is best placed prior to eruption of the permanent canine tooth through the cleft (Abyholm et al., 1981; Hall and Posnick, 1984).

There is no long-term advantage to achieving orthodontic expansion of the cleft segments until just prior to grafting. Arch expansion is generally achieved with

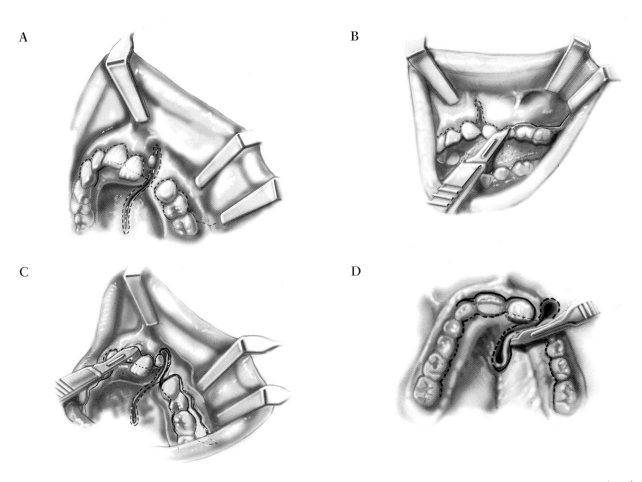

(continued)

FIG. 26.10. Illustrations of techniques for bone grafting and management of residual oronasal fistula in the patient with unilateral cleft lip and palate. *A:* Location of planned left and right labial and bilateral palatal incisions prior to flap elevation. *B:* Close-up view of left labial mucogingival incision in progress. *C:* Left labial mucogingival incision completed and right labial incision in progress. *D:* Attention is turned to the palate for elevation of the palatal flaps and separation of the oral and nasal mucosae at the site of the fistula. *E:* Subperiosteal elevation of palatal flaps. *F:* With palatal flaps elevated, the nasal mucosa is separated from the floor of the nose on each side for later closure. *G:* Left and right labial flaps have been elevated. The nasal mucosa is further separated from its bony surface along the distal aspect of the central incision for later suturing. *H:* Suturing of nasal flaps for water-tight closure. A hemostat is placed through the left nostril to demonstrate the sutured nasal floor. *I:* Once the nasal flaps are sutured, lilac cancellous bone graft is packed into palatal, alveolar, and floor-of-the-nose skeletal defects. *J:* The left labial flap is scored at the periosteum to allow advancement for wound closure over the cleft site. *K:* Left and right labial flaps and palatal flaps are closed for water-tight seal. By advancing the left labial mucogingival flap, keratinized tissue has been placed over the alveolar ridge where the permanent canine tooth will eventually erupt. (From Posnick, 2000b, with permission.)

E

G

F

H

I

J

K

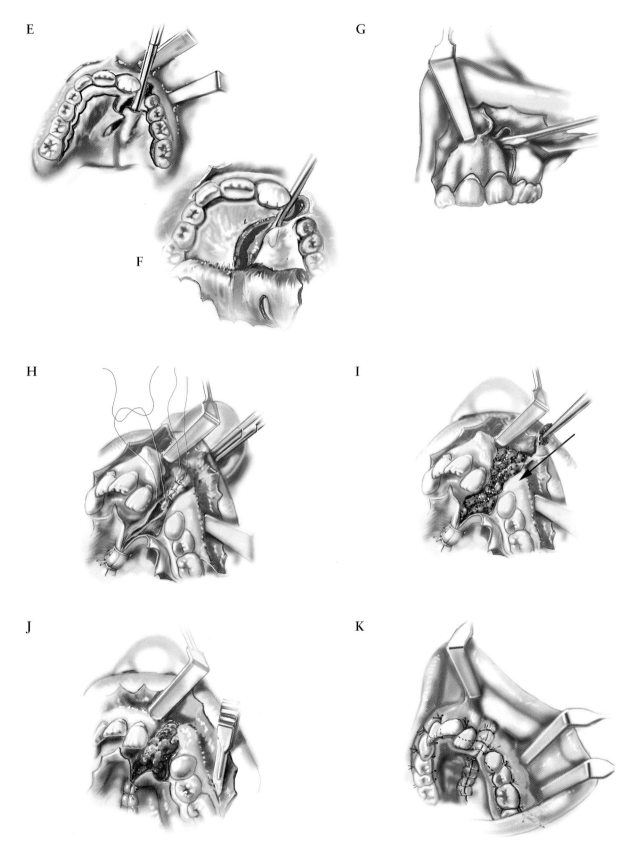

FIG. 26.10. *Continued*

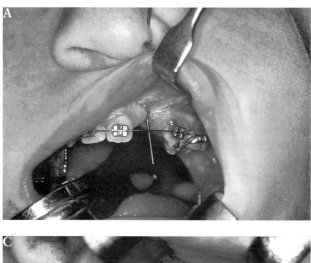
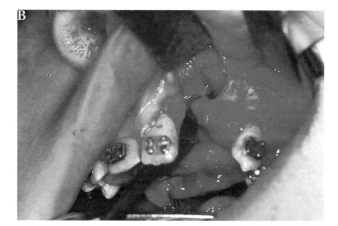
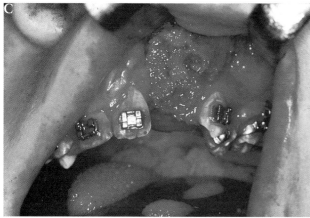
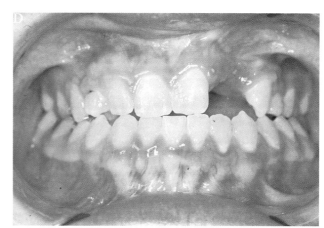

FIG. 26.11. A child in the mixed dentition born with unilateral cleft lip and palate who underwent lip and palatal repair in infancy and early childhood. He presented in the mixed (transitional) dentition with an alveolar/palatal defect and residual labial and palatal oronasal fistulae. He underwent interceptive orthodontic treatment to expand the maxillary arch width, followed by autogenous lilac bone grafting and fistula closure. *A:* Intraoperative close-up view with nasolacrimal probe placed through the floor of the nose into the oral cavity, demonstrating oronasal fistula. *B:* Close-up view of skeletal defect after flap elevation. *C:* Same view with cancellous (lilac) bone graft packed into defect. *D:* Occlusal view after bone grafting and completion of interceptive orthodontic treatment. (From Posnick, 2000b, with permission.)

a Quadhelix or Hyrax appliance over a 3- to 6-month period. Approximately 6 to 8 weeks following bone grafting, the orthodontist may proceed with additional segment repositioning and tooth movement in and around the grafted area. Only rarely will the rudimentary lateral incisor tooth at the cleft site have long-term value (Abyholm et al., 1981; Hall and Posnick, 1984). Even if the (lateral incisor) crown is sufficient to hold a restoration, its root length and volume are generally insufficient to warrant its preservation. The decision of whether to retain or extract the lateral incisor tooth must be made early in the mixed dentition, with extraction carried out prior to or at the time of bone grafting.

An important aspect of the surgical procedure is management of the intraoral soft tissue as part of the oronasal fistula closure. A labial mucogingival flap is elevated and advanced anteriorly, bringing keratinized mucosa to the cleft site, where the permanent canine tooth will erupt (Adell, 1974). It is important to elevate and advance the flap to achieve closure of the fistula without destruction of the vestibular architecture, as would occur if a buccal (cheek) flap were used. The erupted canine tooth is then surrounded by gingiva and develops a normal periodontal sulcus.

ORTHOGNATHIC DEFORMITIES IN CLEFT LIP AND PALATE

Unfortunately, one long-term negative effect of CP repair is a 25% incidence of maxillary growth restriction that produces secondary deformities of the jaws and occlusion, which will also have a negative impact on speech and self-esteem to the extent that further skeletal surgery will be required (Harper, 1995; Correa Normando et al., 1992; Bardach et al., 1994; Kapp-Simon,

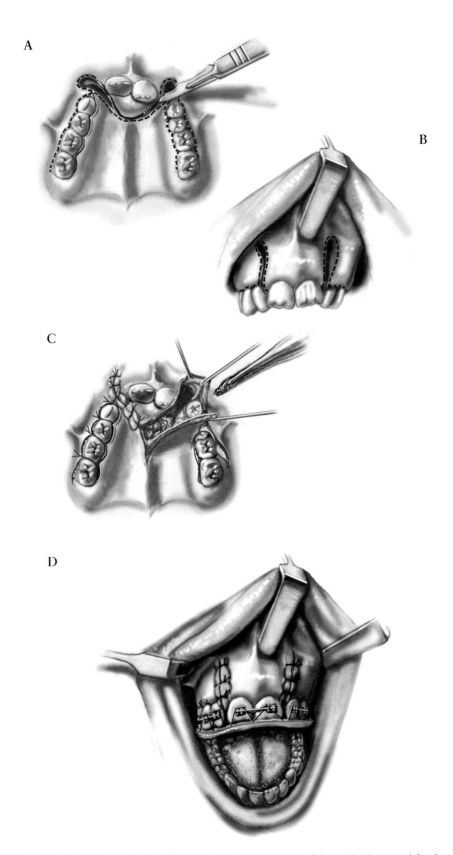

FIG. 26.12. Illustration of the technique modifications for bone graft and management of the residual oronasal fistula in the patient with bilateral cleft lip and palate. *A:* Palatal view indicating location and extent of planned incisions for secondary bone grafting and fistula closure. *B:* Frontal view indicating location and extent of planned labial incisions. Note the importance of maintaining the integrity of the labial mucosa to the premaxillary bone. Without doing so, the circulation requirements to the premaxilla would be compromised. *C:* After nasal side closure and bone graft placement, the oral wounds are closed. View of palate indicating final placement of bone graft prior to closure. *D:* Frontal view of patient at end of bone grafting procedure. A prefabricated acrylic splint is used to secure the three maxillary segments to one another to allow for bone graft healing. (From Posnick, 2000b, with permission.)

1995). The maxillary hypoplasia is the result of surgical intervention and is not attributable to the congenital clefting. Jaw reconstruction is needed for these patients, which must be coordinated with the final phase of orthodontic treatment. Jaw surgery, if required, is preferably carried out at the time of skeletal maturity of the patient (age 14–16 in girls and 16–18 in boys).

Unfortunately, there remains a subgroup of adolescents who present with a jaw deformity requiring orthognathic surgery as well as residual CLP, alveolar and palatal defects, oronasal fistulae, and dental gaps of the maxilla. For these patients, modification of the standard Le Fort I osteotomy allows for independent repositioning of the cleft maxillary segments according to the type of presenting cleft (UCLP or BCLP), the specific residual deformities, and individual variation (Hall and Posnick, 1984; Posnick, 1991, 2000c,d; Proffitt, 1991). These unique anatomic abnormalities should be seen as technical challenges rather than obstacles to the satisfactory rehabilitation of the patient. For either the isolated CP patient or the UCLP or BCLP patients who achieved a successful bone graft in the mixed dentition, a more standard Le Fort I type osteotomy provides the desired skeletal reconstruction of the maxilla and dental rehabilitation.

Cleft-Orthognathic Surgery: Unilateral Cleft Lip and Palate

Residual deformities in the adolescent born with unilateral cleft lip and palate. The prevalence of residual clefting deformities in adolescents born with UCLP who present with a jaw discrepancy varies widely, depending on the center's philosophy in regard to the staging of reconstruction and its available surgical expertise. In addition, despite a center's preferred method of management in infancy, childhood, and early adolescence, a subgroup of UCLP patients presenting with multiple clefting problems includes the following:

1. *Maxillary hypoplasia.* The maxilla is often vertically short, resulting in an edentulous look, and the occlusal plane is often canted (up on the cleft side). Arch width deficiency resulting in crossbite may be present in the transverse plane. The maxillary dental midline may be shifted off the facial midline, usually toward the cleft side. The hypoplastic maxilla is retruded in the horizontal plane, resulting in a concave midfacial profile, Angle class III malocclusion, and negative overjet. Greater and lesser maxillary segments vary in degree of dysplasia, making it difficult to achieve a satisfactory appearance by repositioning the maxilla in one unit rather than with segmental osteotomies.

2. *Residual oronasal fistula.* Despite the general preference for oronasal fistula closure and bone grafting in the mixed dentition, the UCLP candidate for orthognathic surgery will often have residual labial and palatal fistulae. Previous attempts at closure may have failed. Furthermore, buccal mucosa may have been placed over the cleft site, resulting in a lack of attached gingiva in the tooth-bearing surface region and loss of vestibular depth.

3. *Residual bony defects.* In the UCLP patient who has not been successfully bone-grafted in the mixed dentition, there remain significant bony defects, not just at the alveolus but throughout the palate and floor of the nose along the cleft site. This results in an inferiorly and posteriorly displaced floor of the nose and nasal sill.

4. *Cleft-dental gap.* The lateral incisor is frequently congenitally absent at the cleft site. A hypoplastic tooth may be present but with inadequate root development or bony impaction in the cleft. Orthodontic closure of this gap with movement of the canine tooth into the bone-grafted lateral incisor location is the preferred approach in the mixed dentition. Unfortunately, this is not always accomplished and often there is mesial angulation of the canine tooth into a nongrafted cleft site. The result is often a dental gap at the cleft site between the central incisor and canine teeth.

5. *Chin dysplasia.* The UCLP patient will frequently be a mouth-breather with the resulting open-mouth posture. Addition of a pharyngeal flap in childhood may increase this tendency. The result is a vertically long and retrognathic chin.

6. *Mandibular dysplasia.* True mandibular prognathism is uncommon in the UCLP patient. The need for mandibular osteotomies should be limited to facial asymmetries, occlusal plane canting, and the occasional true anteroposterior discrepancy (Laspos et al., 1997).

Technique. We have described modifications of the Le Fort I osteotomy for the UCLP deformity, placing the soft tissue incisions to permit direct exposure for dissection, osteotomies, disimpaction, fistula closure, bone graft, and application of plate-and-screw fixation but without risk of circulation injury to the dento-osseous-musculo-mucosal flaps (Posnick, 2000c; Posnick and Tompson, 1992). The increased visibility provided by these incisions makes it possible to incorporate routine surgical closure of the cleft-dental gap through differential maxillary segmental repositioning (Figs. 26.13, 26.14). This method of approximating the gap in the maxillary segments also closes the cleft dead space and brings together the labial and palatal flaps

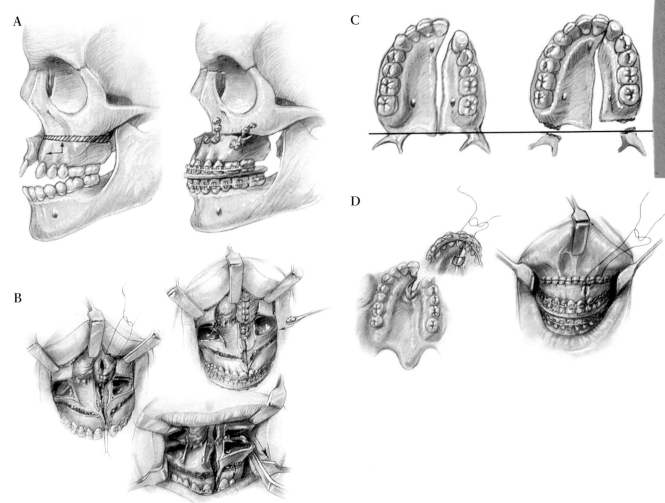

FIG. 26.13. Illustrations of modified Le Fort I osteotomy, performed in two segments, in a patient with unilateral cleft lip and palate. *A:* Lateral view of maxillofacial skeleton before and just after osteotomies and fixation of modified Le Fort I osteotomy. *B:* Illustration of downfractured Le Fort I osteotomy in two segments after submucous resection of septum, reduction of inferior turbinate through the nasal mucosa opening, and watertight nasal side closure. *C:* Palatal view of bony segments before and after repositioning. *D:* Oral-side wound closure on both labial and palatal aspects after differential segmental repositioning. (From Posnick, 1991b, with permission.)

to permit closure of recalcitrant oronasal fistulae without tension.

Cleft-Orthognathic Surgery: Bilateral Cleft Lip and Palate Deformity

Residual deformities in the adolescent born with bilateral cleft lip and palate. The BCLP adolescent presenting with a jaw discrepancy may have several or all of the following residual clefting problems (Posnick, 2000d). These deformities, when present, must be addressed to achieve improved facial aesthetics, function, and dental rehabilitation.

1. *Maxillary hypoplasia.* The premaxilla may be either vertically long, resulting in a gummy smile, or vertically short, with an edentulous look. There may be a negative overjet, indicating horizontal deficiency. The arch width of the lateral segments is generally deficient in the transverse plane, with bilateral posterior crossbites and a degree of horizontal deficiency, with an Angle class III malocclusion.

2. *Residual oronasal fistula.* Despite a preference for fistula closure and bone grafting in the mixed dentition, the BCLP candidate for orthognathic surgery will often have residual labial and palatal fistulae with loss of fluid through the nose while drinking and air leakage while speaking. Previous attempts at fistula closure may have failed because of inadequate available soft tissue for wound closure.

3. *Cleft-dental gaps.* Lateral incisors are most frequently absent at the cleft site. Rudimentary teeth

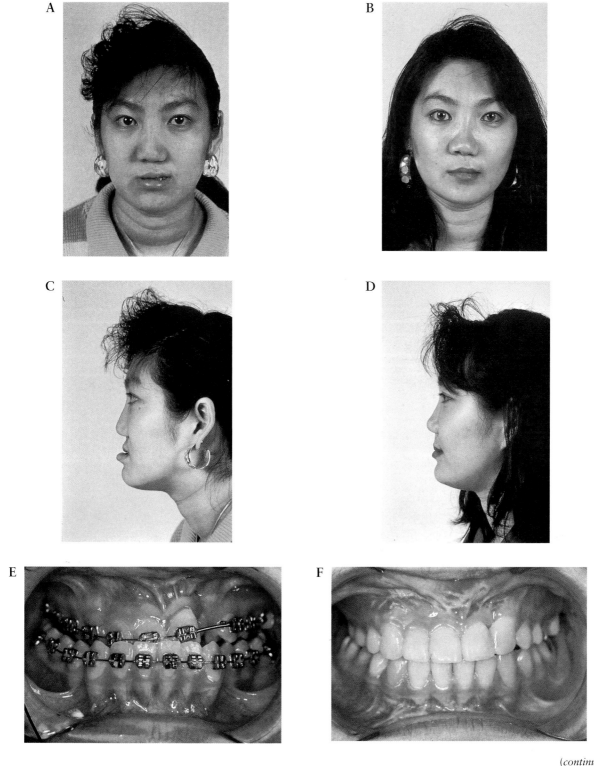

(continued)

FIG. 26.14. A 16-year-old girl born with unilateral cleft lip and palate underwent a combined orthodontic and orthognathic surgical approach including a modified Le Fort I osteotomy in two segments (differential repositioning of the segments, correction of occlusal canting, and closure of oronasal fistula, alveolar defect, and cleft-dental gap), bilateral sagittal split osteotomies of the mandible (correction of asymmetry), and osteoplastic genioplasty (vertical reduction and horizontal advancement). Stabilization was accomplished with iliac graft and miniplate and screw fixation. *A:* Frontal view in repose before surgery. *B:* Frontal view in repose after reconstruction. *C:* Profile view before surgery. *D:* Profile view after reconstruction. *E:* Occlusal view before surgery. *F:* Occlusal view after reconstruction. *G:* Oblique occlusal view before surgery. *H:* Oblique occlusal view after reconstruction. *I:* Lateral view of articulated dental casts before surgery. *J:* Lateral view of articulated dental casts after model surgery. *K:* Lateral cephalometric radiograph before surgery. *L:* Lateral cephalometric radiograph after reconstruction. (From Posnick and Tompson, 1995, with permission.)

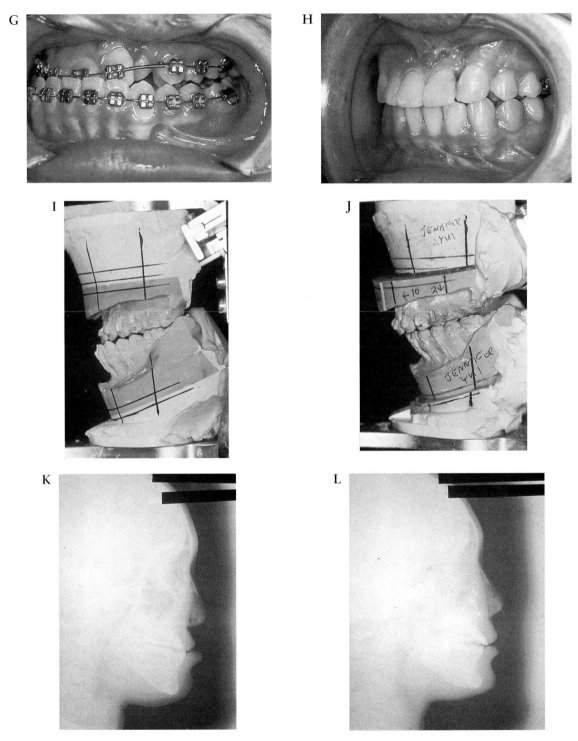

FIG. 26.14. *Continued*

may also be impacted within the cleft and, if so, are of no functional value. If hypoplastic lateral incisors do erupt in the lateral segments, they rarely have adequate root support for long-term functioning. The result is often a dental gap at the cleft site between the central incisor and canine teeth on each side.

4. *Residual bony defects.* Significant residual bony defects through the alveolus, floor of the nose, and palate are frequent, resulting in a mobile premaxilla secured only to the nasal septum.
5. *Chin dysplasia.* The BCLP patient will frequently be a mouth-breather with the resulting open-mouth

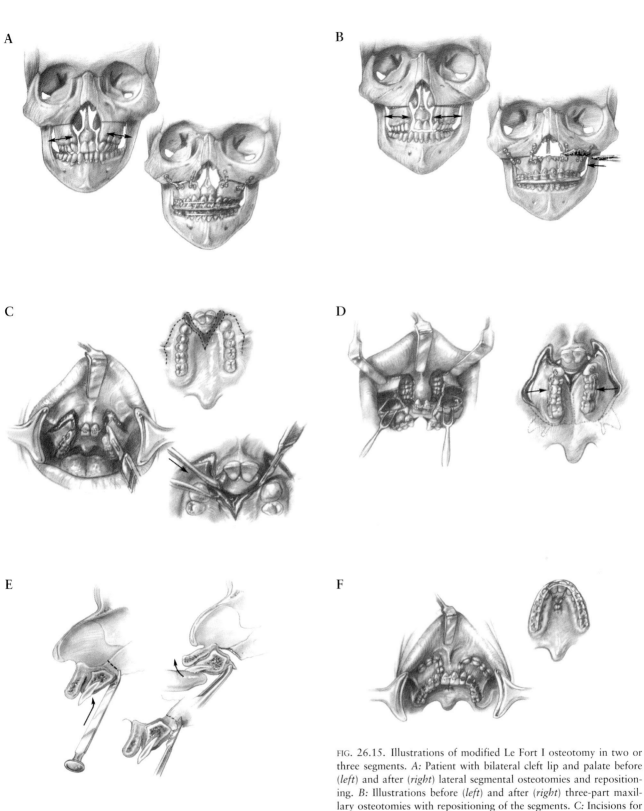

FIG. 26.15. Illustrations of modified Le Fort I osteotomy in two or three segments. *A:* Patient with bilateral cleft lip and palate before (*left*) and after (*right*) lateral segmental osteotomies and repositioning. *B:* Illustrations before (*left*) and after (*right*) three-part maxillary osteotomies with repositioning of the segments. *C:* Incisions for modified Le Fort I in three segments. *D:* Downfractured lateral segments demonstrating exposure of nasal-side closure of oronasal fistula and additional view of oral mucosal incisions. *E:* Premaxillary osteotomy from palatal side using either a chisel, a rongeur, or a reciprocating saw. *F:* Oral wounds sutured at end of procedure. *G:* Palatal view of bone segments before (*left*) and after (*right*) repositioning for closure of cleft-dental gaps. (From Posnick, 1991b, with permission.)

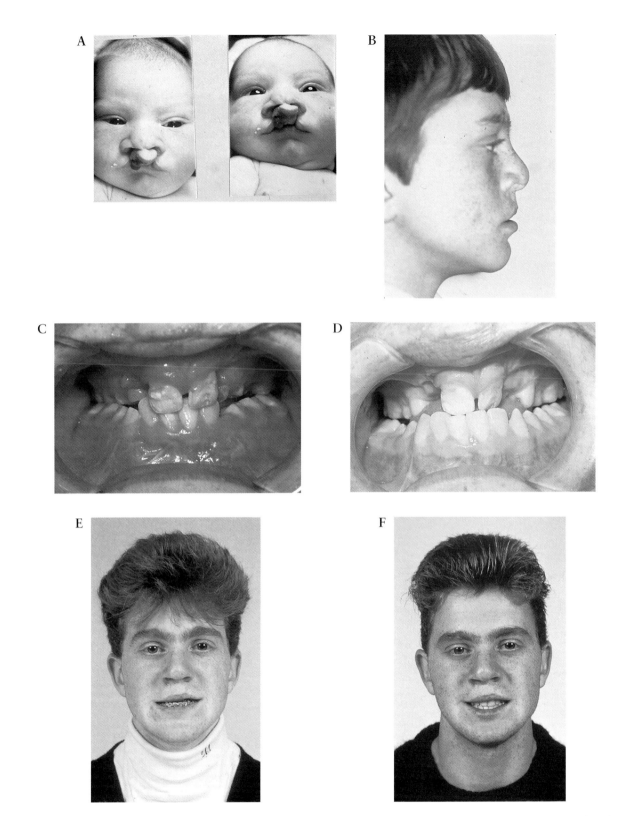

(continued)

FIG. 26.16. An 18-year-old boy born with bilateral cleft lip and palate underwent a combined orthodontic and orthognathic surgical approach including a modified Le Fort I osteotomy in three segments (differential repositioning of segments; closure of oronasal fistula, alveolar defects, and cleft-dental gaps; and stabilization of premaxilla), bilateral sagittal split osteotomies of the mandible (correction of asymmetry), and an osteoplastic genioplasty (vertical reduction and horizontal advancement). Stabilization was accomplished with iliac bone graft and miniplate and screw fixation. *A:* Frontal view prior to cleft lip and palate repair. *B:* Profile view in the mixed dentition developmental stage. *C:* Occlusal view early in the mixed dentition stage. *D:* Occlusal view later in the mixed dentition stage. *E:* Frontal view with smile before surgery. *F:* Frontal view with smile after reconstruction. *G:* Profile view before surgery. *H:* Profile view after reconstruction. *I:* Occlusal view before surgery. *J:* Occlusal view after reconstruction. *K, L:* Lateral views of articulated dental casts after model surgery. *M:* Lateral cephalometric radiographs before surgery. *N:* Lateral cephalometric radiograph after reconstruction. (From Posnick and Tompson, 1993, with permission.)

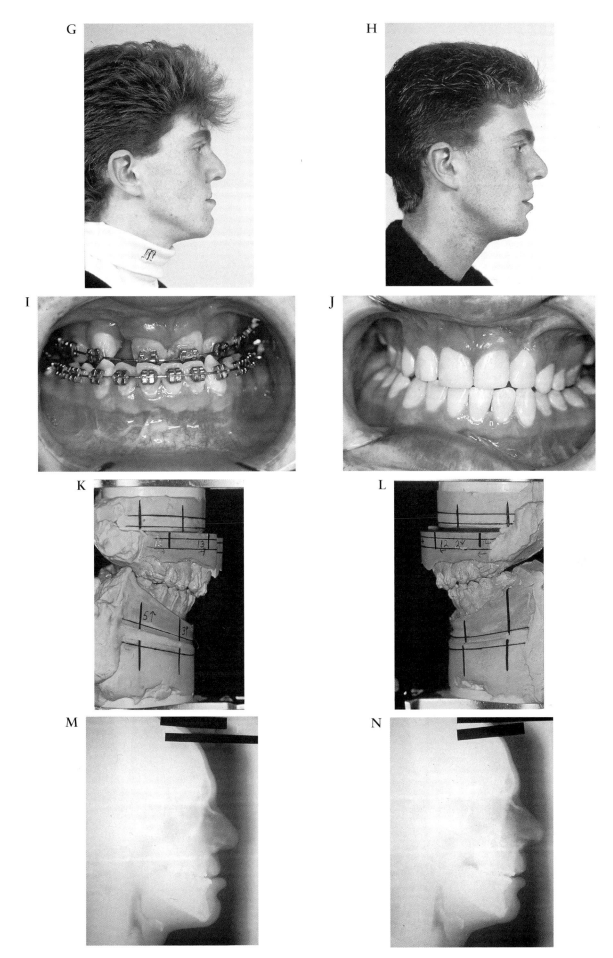

FIG. 26.16. *Continued*

posture. The result is a vertically long and retrognathic chin.

6. *Mandibular dysplasia.* True manidular prognathism in the BCLP patient is uncommon. The need for mandibular osteotomy should be limited to facial asymmetries, occlusal plane canting, and actual anteroposterior discrepancy.

Technique. Precise incision placement is critical in the modified Le Fort I osteotomy for midfacial advancement in the BCLP patient (Posnick, 2000d; Posnick and Tompson, 1993) (Figs. 26.15, 26.16). Buccal incisions are made in the depth of the vestibules and extend from the zygomatic buttress forward to the location of the residual labial oronasal fistula on each side. The premaxillary segment labial incisions are placed adjacent to the distal line angle of the central incisor on each side to separate the oral and nasal mucosae. Care is required to prevent any disruption of, or incision into, the mucosa on the labial vestibule of the premaxilla. It is imperative that the labial vestibule mucosa in the premaxilla remain connected to its underlying periosteum and the bone since blood flows through this pedicle into the premaxillary bone and teeth. The nasal and oral mucosae are also sharply incised and separated on the palatal aspect of the premaxilla and on each lateral segment.

A subperiosteal soft tissue dissection provides direct exposure of the anterolateral maxilla on each (lateral segment) side. Routine Le Fort I osteotomies are then performed through the lateral, anterior, and medial maxillary walls with a reciprocating saw. The pterygomaxillary sutures are separated with a mallet and osteotome. The lateral segments are downfractured with finger pressure, then disimpacted with Tessier hooks to release scar tissue for three-dimensional repositioning. The vomer may be attached to the lateral segments. If it is, an osteotomy is also required before the downfracture. The lateral maxillary segments are advanced and ligated into the prefabricated acrylic occlusal splint, along with the premaxillary segment. Through this procedure, the cleft-dental gap on each side and the dead space associated with the bony clefts are closed. All three segments are placed into a prefabricated acrylic splint, and the desired horizontal advancement is achieved. The ideal vertical dimension, determined preoperatively, is achieved at the maxillary osteotomy sites to improve the lip-to-tooth relationship and the appearance of the smile.

Cleft-Orthognathic Surgery: Isolated Cleft Palate Deformity

Residual deformities in the adolescent born with an isolated cleft palate. The isolated CP adolescent presenting with a jaw discrepancy may have one or more of the following residual maxillofacial deformities (Posnick, 2000e).

1. *Maxillary dysplasia.* When maxillary dysplasia occurs, it generally follows one of two patterns. The first and most frequently seen is horizontal maxillary retrusion, generally with a degree of vertical hypoplasia. The second is vertical maxillary excess with a degree of horizontal retrusion. The latter tends to occur in mouth-breathers, especially if a pharyngeal flap was placed in childhood.

2. *Residual oronasal (palatal) fistula.* There may be a residual midline palatal fistula located in the region between the incisal foramen and the soft palate.

3. *Residual bony defects.* The alveolus is not cleft, but generally there are bony defects of the hard palate.

4. *Chin dysplasia.* The isolated CP patient will frequently be a mouth-breather with the resulting open-mouth posture. The end result is a vertically long and retrognathic chin. If Robin sequence is present, retrogenia is also expected.

5. *Mandibular dysplasia.* True mandibular prognathism is rare. Mandibular retrognathism may be part of a Robin sequence but is rarely seen in the adolescent. The need for mandibular osteotomies in addition to maxillary osteotomy is limited, but each patient's unique jaw deformities must be evaluated independently.

REVISION OF THE CLEFT LIP SCAR AND CORRECTION OF THE NASAL DEFORMITY

Cleft Nasal Reconstruction

A congenital cleft, either unilateral or bilateral, extending through the lip, nasal base, and alveolar ridge results in a significant nasal malformation affecting both function and appearance (McComb, 1990, 1994; Horswell and Pospisil, 1995; Sandham and Murray, 1993). Despite effective initial CL repair with or without primary nasal maneuvers, a significant functional and displeasing nasal malformation or deformation frequently persists, which, for psychological reasons, will benefit from further reconstruction.

Some surgeons take an aggressive posture to correction of both the nasal dysfunction and less-than-ideal facial aesthetics, carrying out additional surgery once the problem is recognized, regardless of the child's age. Others take a long-range approach and selected a preferred window of opportunity to achieve maximal long-term nasal function and facial aesthetics, with the creation of minimal scar tissue and a limited need for additional procedures.

The final (secondary) nasal reconstruction will likely be carried out through an open (columella-splitting) technique to achieve maximal exposure of the nasal dorsum, tip, and septum. Through this approach, nasal osteotomies, dorsal reduction, lower lateral cartilage repositioning or sculpting, and harvesting of septal cartilage for augmentation of the nasal tip to improve nasal symmetry and projection can be performed under direct vision (Gubiscla, 1990; Takato et al., 1995b). If the need for orthognathic surgery seems likely, then it is best to postpone the final rhinoplasty until after the jaw reconstruction. The cleft surgeon must remember that cartilage grafting is an essential component of the final rhinoplasty and that septal cartilage provides the best source and will be available in sufficient quantity only one time. The use of ear or rib cartilage is another option.

Standard thinking holds that the columella in the BCL patient is short and requires secondary lengthening. The teaching is that there are two ways to accomplish this goal: using banked forked flaps (Millard, 1967; van der Meulin, 1992) and lengthening the columella with medial rotation of the bilateral nasal floor and alar flaps (Cronin, 1958). Unfortunately, these techniques result in an unnatural, sharp columellar–labial angle, excessive columellar length, a broad nasal tip, further deformity to the nostrils, and a wide and scarred columella. Trier (1995), agreeing with Mulliken (1995), abandoned the secondary columellar lengthening procedures as unsightly and cosmetically counterproductive. We prefer to reshape and augment the lower lateral cartilage of the nose with a septal cartilage strut graft secured to the caudal portion of the septum under direct vision via the open technique. By doing this, a stretching of the overlying soft tissue envelope rather than a direct lengthening of the skin of the columella is possible.

Cleft Lip Scar Revision

The majority of children who undergo initial CL repair in infancy will require at least one lip scar revision in childhood or adolescence (Harper, 1995; Cohen et al., 1995). The extent of revision required is dependent on the success of the primary CL repair and the degree to which subsequent growth has affected the initial results (Chen et al., 1995; Randall, 1995). Cleft lip revision will often require a complete takedown with excision of scar tissue (skin, vermilion, and mucosa), removal of redundant and residual hypoplastic tissue, and reapproximation of the obicularis oris muscle. It may also require reapproximation of key anatomic landmarks, including the vermilion–cutaneous junction and the vermilion–mucosal junction. Additional objectives include leveling of the lip lengths (philtral columns) and establishment of a normal upper lip oral vestibule. Ideally, only one major lip scar revision will be required, and it is best accomplished when the child is between 5 and 15 years of age, with psychosocial needs taken into account. The exact age at revision is dependent on the family's and patients' preference, the extent of the deformity, and the potential for surgical improvements.

CONCLUSIONS

The successful rehabilitation of a child born with CLP requires close cooperation among the specialists that make up the CLP team. Each specialist has a level of involvement at different stages of the patient's growth and development. A coordinated approach is essential to help the child achieve ideal speech, occlusion, facial appearance, and self-esteem. Unnecessary, unproductive, and unproven interventions, whether speech therapy, orthodontic or prosthetic treatment, or surgical procedures, should be avoided as they exhaust the patient, family, and healthcare system, produce unfulfilled expectations, and often introduce secondary deformities which may limit the eventual success of rehabilitation. Maximizing the patient's ability to pursue and achieve personal success in his or her life without special regard to the original CLP malformation is the ultimate objective.

REFERENCES

Abbe, R (1898). A new plastic operation for the relief of deformity due to double hare lip. Med Rec 53: 477.

Abramson, DL, Marrinan, EM, Muiilken, JB (1997). Robin sequence: obstructive sleep apnea following pharyngeal flap. Cleft Palate Craniofac J 34: 256.

Abyholm, F, Bergland, O, Semb, G (1981). Secondary bone grafting of alveolar clefts. Scand J Plast Reconstr Surg 15: 127.

Abyholm, FE (1979). Palatal fistulae following cleft palate surgery. Scand J Plast Reconstr Surg 13: 295.

Adams, GR (1981). The effects of physical attractiveness on the socialization process. In: Lucker GW, Psychological Aspects of Facial Form. Craniofacial Growth Series 11, edited by GW Lucker, KA Ribbens, and JA McNamara. Ann Arbor: University of Michigan Press, pp. 25–47.

Adell, R (1974). Regeneration of the periodontium. Scand J Plast Reconstr Surg Hand Surg Suppl 11: 1–177.

Ainoda, N, Yamashita, Y, Tsukada, S (1985). Articulation at age 4 in children with early repair of cleft palate. Ann Plast Surg 15: 415.

Amaratunga, NA (1988). Occurrence of oronasal fistulas in operated cleft palate patients. J Oral Maxillofac Surg 46: 834.

American Cleft Palate-Craniofacial Association (1993). Parameters for the evaluation and treatment of patients with cleft lip/palate or other craniofacial anomalies. Cleft Palate Craniofac J 30(Suppl 1): 4.

Argamaso, RV (1992). Glossopexy for upper airway obstruction in Robin sequence. Cleft Palate Craniofac J 29: 232.

Argamaso, RV, Levandowski, G, Golding-Kushner, KJ, et al. (1994).

Treatment of asymmetric velopharyngeal insufficiency with skewed pharyngeal flap. Cleft Palate Craniofac J *31*: 287.

Assuncao, AGA (1993). The design of tongue flaps for the closure of palatal fistulas. Plast Reconstr Surg *91*: 806.

Bardach, J, et al. (1990). The Iowa–Hamburg project. In: *Multidisciplinary Management of Cleft Lip and Palate*, edited by J Bardach and HL Morris. Philadelphia: WB Saunders, pp. 98–112.

Bardach, J, Kelly, KM, Salyer, KE (1994). Relationship between the sequence of lip and palate repair and maxillary growth: an experimental study in beagles. Plast Reconstr Surg *93*: 269.

Bardach, J, Nosal, P (1987). Geometry of the two-flap palatoplasty. In: *Surgical Techniques in Cleft Lip and Palate*, edited by J Bardach and K Salyer. St. Louis: Mosby Year Book, pp. 192–197.

Bardach, J, Salyer, K (1991a). *Surgical Techniques in Cleft Lip and Palate*, 2nd ed. St. Louis: Mosby Year Book.

Bardach, J, Salyer, K (1991b). Pharyngoplasty. In: *Surgical Techniques in Cleft Lip and Palate*, 2nd ed., edited by J Bardach and K Salyer. St. Louis: Mosby Year Book.

Barone, CM, Shprintzen, RJ, Strauch, B, et al. (1994). Pharyngeal flap revisions: flap elevation from a scarred posterior pharynx. Plast Reconstr Surg *93*: 279.

Beers, MD, Pruzansky, S (1955). The growth of the head of an infant with mandibular micrognathia: glossoptosis and cleft palate following the Beverly Douglas operation. Plast Reconstr Surg *16*: 189.

Benacerraf, BR, Mulliken, JB (1993). Fetal cleft lip and palate: sonographic diagnosis and postnatal outcome. Plast Reconstr Surg *92*: 1045.

Bergland, O, Semb, G, Abyholm, FE, et al. (1986). Elimination of the residual alveolar cleft by bone graft and subsequent orthodontic treatment. Cleft Palate J *23*: 175.

Berkowitz, S (1996). The comparison of treatment results in complete cleft lip/palate using conservative approach vs Millard-Latham PSOT procedure. Semin Orthod *2*: 169.

Berry, LA, Witt, PD, Marsh, JL, et al. (1997). Personality attributions based on speech samples of children with repaired cleft palates. Cleft Palate Craniofac J *34*: 385–9.

Bertz, JE (1981). Bone grafting of alveolar clefts. J Oral Surg *39*: 874.

Bezirdjian, DR, Szucs, R (1989). Sickle-shaped scapulae in a patient with the Pierre Robin syndrome. Br J Radiol *62*: 171.

Bishara, SE (1973). Cephalometric evaluation of facial growth in operated and unoperated individuals with isolated clefts of the palate. Cleft Palate J *10*: 239.

Bitter, K (1992). Latham's appliance for presurgical repositioning of the protruded premaxilla in bilateral cleft lip and palate. J Craniomaxillofac Surg *20*: 99.

Blijdorp, P, Muller, H (1984). The influence of the age at which the palate is closed on speech in the adult cleft patient. J Maxillofac Surg *12*: 239.

Blocksma, R (1963). Correction of velopharyngeal insufficiency by Silastic pharyngeal implants. Plast Reconstr Surg *31*: 268.

Bluestone, CD, Musgrave, RH, McWilliams, BJ (1968). Teflon injection pharyngoplasty: status 1968. Laryngoscope *78*: 558.

Bowers, EJ, Mayro, RF, Whitaker, LA, et al. (1987). General body growth in children with clefts of the lip, palate and craniofacial structure. Scand J Plast Reconstr Surg *21*: 7.

Boyne, PJ (1970). Autogenous cancellous bone and marrow transplants. Clin Orthop *73*: 199.

Boyne, PJ (1974). Use of marrow–cancellous bone grafts in maxillary alveolar and palatal clefts. J Dent Res *53*: 821.

Boyne, PJ (1985). Correction of dentofacial deformities associated with residual alveolar and palatal clefts. In: *Surgical Correction of Dentofacial Deformities*, Vol. 3, edited by WH Bell. Philadelphia: WB Saunders, pp. 560–591.

Boyne, PJ, Sands, NR (1972). Secondary bone grafting of residual alveolar and palatal clefts. J Oral Surg *30*: 87.

Boyne, PJ, Sands, NR (1976). Combined orthodontic–surgical management of residual palatoalveolar cleft defects. Am J Orthod *70*: 21.

Brauer, RO (1985). Repair of unilateral cleft lip: triangular flap repairs. Clin Plast Surg *12*: 595.

Brauer, RO, Fox, DR, Humphreys, D. (1990). Augmentation of the posterior pharyngeal wall. In: *Multidisciplinary Management of Cleft Lip and Palate,* edited by J Bardach and HL Morris. Philadelphia: WB Saunders.

Broder, H, Strauss, RP (1989). Self-concept of early primary school age children with visible or invisible defects. Cleft Palate J *26*: 114.

Broen, PA, Doyle, SS, Bacon, CK (1993). The velopharyngeally inadequate child: phonologic change with intervention. Cleft Palate Craniofac J *30*: 500.

Broomhead, I (1957). The nerve supply of the soft palate. Br J Plast Surg *10*: 81.

Brouilette, R, Hanson, D, David, R, et al. (1984). A diagnostic approach to suspected obstructive sleep apnea in children. J Pediatr *105*: 10.

Bruce, A, Winship, I (1993). Radial ray defect and Robin sequence: a new syndrome? Clin Dysmorphol 2:241.

Bush, PG, Williams, AJ (1983). Incidence of the Robin anomalad (Pierre Robin syndrome). Br J Plast Surg *36*: 434.

Canaday, JW, Thompson, SA, Colburn, A (1997). Craniofacial growth after iatrogenic cleft palate repair in a fetal ovine model. Cleft Palate Craniofac J *34*: 69.

Canady, JW, Zeitler, DP, Thompson, SA, et al. (1993). Suitability of the iliac crest as a site for harvest of autogenous bone grafts. Cleft Palate Craniofac J *30*: 579.

Caouette-Laberge, L, Bayet, B, Larocque, Y (1994). The Pierre Robin sequence: review of 125 cases and evolution of treatment modalities. Plast Reconstr Surg *93*: 934.

Caouette-Laberge, L, Egerszegi, EP, de Remont, A-M, et al. (1992). Long-term follow-up after division of a pharyngeal flap for severe nasal obstruction. Cleft Palate Craniofac J *29*: 27.

Carey, JC, Fineman, RM, Ziter, FA (1982). The Robin sequence as a consequence of malformation, dysplasia, and neuromuscular syndromes. J Pediatr *101*: 858.

Carroll, DB, Peterson, RA, Worton, EW, Birnbaum, LM (1971). Hereditary factors in the Pierre Robin syndrome. Br J Plast Surg *24*: 43.

Catone, GA, Reimer, BL, McNeir, D, et al. (1992). Tibial autogenous cancellous bone as an alternative donor site in maxillofacial surgery. J Oral Maxillofacial Surg *50*: 1258.

Chapman, KL, Hardin, MA (1992). Phonetic and phonologic skills of 2-year-olds with cleft palate. Cleft Palate Craniofac J *29*: 435.

Chen, KT, Noordhoff, MS, Chen, Y-R, et al. (1995). Augmentation of the free border of the lip in cleft lip patients using temporoparietal fascia. Plast Reconstr Surg *95*: 781.

Chen, PK-T, Wu, JTH, Chen, Y-R, et al. (1994). Correction of secondary velopharyngeal insufficiency in cleft palate patients with the Furlow palatoplasty. Plast Reconstr Surg *94*: 933.

Chitayat, D, Meunier, CM, Hodgkinson, KA, et al. (1991). Robin sequence with facial and digital anomalies in two half-brothers by the same mother. Am J Med Genet *40*: 1167.

Christensen, K, Fogh-Andersen, P (1993). Isolated cleft palate in Danish multiple births, 1970–1990. Cleft Palate Craniofac J *30*: 469.

Cocke, WJ (1966). Experimental production of micrognathia and glossoptosis associated with cleft palate (Pierre Robin syndrome). Plast Reconstr Surg *38*: 395.

Cohen, MM, Jr (1976). The Robin anomalad—its nonspecificity and associated syndromes. J Oral Surg *34*: 587.

Cohen, MM, Jr (1997). Need for velopharyngeal management following palatoplasty: an outcome analysis of syndromic and nonsyndromic patients with Pierre Robin. Plast Reconstr Surg 99: 1530.

Cohen, SR, Corrigan, M, Wilmot, J, et al. (1995). Cumulative operative procedures in patients aged 14 years and older with unilateral or bilateral cleft lip and palate. Plast Reconstr Surg 96: 267.

Copeland, M (1990). The effect of very early palatal repair on speech. Br J Plast Surg 43: 676.

Correa Normando, AD, da Silva Filho, OG, Capelozza Filho, L (1992). Influence of surgery on maxillary growth in cleft lip and/or palate patients. J Craniomaxillofac Surg 20: 111.

Croft, CB, Shprintzen, RJ, Ruben, RJ (1981). Hypernasal speech following adenotonsillectomy. Otolaryngol Head Neck Surg 89: 179.

Cronin, TD (1958). Lengthening columella by use of skin from nasal floor and alae. Plast Reconstr Surg 21: 417.

Cutting, CB, Rosenbaum, J, Rovati, L (1995). The technique of muscle repair in the cleft soft palate. Operative Tech Plast Reconstr Surg 2: 215.

Dalston, RM (1992). Timing of cleft palate repair: a speech pathologist's viewpoint. In: Problems of Plastic Surgery in Cleft Palate Surgery, edited by JA Lehman. Philadelphia: JB Lippincott, pp. 30–38.

D'Antonio, L, Marsh, JL, Province, M, et al. (1989). Reliability of flexible fiberoptic nasopharyngoscopy for evaluation of velopharyngeal function in a clinical population. Cleft Palate J 26: 217.

Davies, D (1966). The one-stage repair of unilateral cleft lip and palate: a preliminary report. Plast Reconstr Surg 38: 129.

Denk, MJ, Magee, WP, Jr (1996). Cleft palate closure in the neonate: preliminary report. Cleft Palate Craniofac J 33: 57.

Dennison, WM (1965). The Pierre Robin syndrome. Pediatrics 36: 336.

Denny, AD, Marks, SM, Oliff-Carneol, S (1993). Correction of velopharyngeal insufficiency by pharyngeal augmentation using autologous cartilage: a preliminary report. Cleft Palate Craniofac J 30: 46.

Derijcke, A, Kuijpers-Jagtman, AM, Lekkas, C, et al. (1994). Dental arch dimensions in unoperated adult cleft palate patients: an analysis of 37 cases. J Craniofac Genet Dev Biol 14: 69.

Devlin, HB (1990). Audit and the quality of clinical care. Ann R Coll Surg Engl 72(Suppl 1): 3.

Dorf, DS, Curtin, JW (1982). Early cleft palate repair and speech outcome. Plast Reconstr Surg 70: 74.

Dorf, DS, Curtin, JW (1990). Early cleft palate repair and speech outcome: a ten year experience. In: Multidisciplinary Management of Cleft Lip and Palate, edited by J Bardach and HL Morris. Philadelphia: WB Saunders, pp. 341–348.

Dykes, EH, Raine, PA, Arthur, DS (1985). Pierre Robin syndrome and pulmonary hypertension. Pediatr Surg 20: 49.

Eaton, AC, Marsh, JL, Pilgram, TK (1994). Does reduced hospital stay affect morbidity and mortality rates following cleft lip and palate repair in infancy? Plast Reconstr Surg 94: 911.

Edwards, JRG, Newall, DR (1985). The Pierre Robin syndrome reassessed in the light of recent research. Br J Plast Surg 38: 339.

El Deeb, M, Messer, LB, Lehnert, MW, et al. (1982). Canine eruption into grafted bone in maxillary alveolar cleft defects. Cleft Palate J 19: 9.

Emory, RE, Jr, Clay, RP, Bite, U, et al. (1997). Fistula formation and repair after palatal closure: an institutional perspective. Plast Reconstr Surg 99: 1535.

Evans, D, Renfrew, C (1974). The timing of primary cleft palate repair. Scand J Plast Surg 8: 153.

Fairbairn, P (1846). Suffocation in an infant from retraction of the base of the tongue, connected with defect of the frenum. Monthly J Med Sci 6: 280.

Field, TM, Vega-Lahr, N (1984). Early interactions between infants with craniofacial anomalies and their mothers. Infant Behav Dev 7:527.

Fonseca, RJ (1997). Prospective evaluation of morbidity associated with iliac crest harvest for alveolar cleft grafting. J Oral Maxillofac Surg 55: 223.

Frohberg, U, Lange, R-T (1993). Surgical treatment of Robin sequence and sleep apnea syndrome: case report and review of the literature. J Oral Maxillofac Surg 51: 1274.

Furlow, LT (1986). Cleft palate repair by double opposing Z-plasty. Plast Reconstr Surg 78: 724.

Furlow, LT (1992). The double opposing Z-plasty for palate closure. Part I. In: Recent Advances in Plastic Surgery, edited by I Jackson and B Sommerlad. Edinburgh: Churchill Livingstone, pp. 29–42.

Furlow, LT (1997). Bilateral buccal flaps with double opposing Z-plasty for wider palatal clefts. Plast Reconstr Surg 100: 1144.

Georgiade, NG, Latham, RA (1975). Maxillary arch alignment in the bilateral cleft lip and palate infant, using the pinned coaxial screw appliance. Plast Reconstr Surg 52: 52.

Glander, K II, Cisneros, GJ (1992). Comparison of the craniofacial characteristics of two syndromes associated with the Pierre Robin sequence. Cleft Palate Craniofac J 3: 210.

Gnudi, MT, Webster, JP (1950). The Life and Times of Gaspare Tagliococci: Surgeon of Bologna. New York: Herbert Reichner, 1950.

Golding-Kushner, KJ, Argamaso RV, Cotton, RT, et al. (1990). Standardization for the reporting of nasopharyngoscopy and multiview videofluoroscopy: a report from an international working group. Cleft Palate J 27: 337.

Gould, HJ (1990). Hearing loss and cleft palate: the perspective of time. Cleft Palate J 27:36.

Graivier, MH, Cohen, SR, Kawamoto, HK, et al. (1992). A new operation for velopharyngeal insufficiency: the palatoglossus myomucosal pharyngoplasty. Plast Reconstr Surg 90: 707.

Gray, S (1990). Airway obstruction and apnea in cleft palate patients. In: Multidisciplinary Management of Cleft Lip and Palate, edited by J Bardach and HL Morris. Philadelphia: WB Saunders.

Grobbelaar, AO, Hudson, DA, Fernandes, DB, et al. (1995). Speech results after repair of the cleft soft palate. Plast Reconstr Surg 95: 1150.

Gubiscla, W (1990). How to obtain symmetries in a unilaterally cleft nose. Eur J Plast Surg 13: 241.

Guilleminault, C, Stoohs, R (1990). Chronic snoring and obstructive sleep apnea syndrome in children. Lung 168(Suppl): 912.

Haapanen, ML, Rantala, SL (1992). Correlation between the age at repair and speech outcome in patients with isolated cleft palate. Scand J Plast Reconstr Surg Hand Surg 26: 71.

Hall, HD, Posnick, JC (1984). Early results of secondary bone grafts in 106 alveolar clefts. J Oral Maxillofac Surg 41: 289.

Hanson, J, Smith, DW (1975). U-shaped palatal defect in the Robin anomaly: developmental and clinical relevance. J Pediatr 87: 30.

Harding, A, Campbell, RC (1989). A comparison of the speech results after early and delayed hard palate closure: a preliminary report. Br J Plast Surg 42: 187.

Harper, DC (1995). Children's attitudes to physical differences among youth from Western and non-Western cultures. Cleft Palate Craniofac J 32: 114.

Hartel, J, Gundlach, KKH, Ruickoldt, K (1994). Incidence of velopharyngoplasty following various techniques of palatoplasty. J Craniomaxillofac Surg 22: 272.

Hedrick, MH, Rice, HE, Vander Wall, KJ, et al. (1996). Delayed in utero repair of surgically created fetal cleft lip and palate. Plast Reconstr Surg 97: 900.

Heidbuchel, KLWM, Kuijpers-Jagtman, AM, Freihofer, HPM (1994). Facial growth in patients with bilateral cleft lip and palate. A cephalometric study. Cleft Palate Craniofac J *31*: 210.

Henderson, D, Jackson, IT (1975). Combined cleft lip revision, anterior fistula closure and maxillary osteotomy: a one-stage procedure. Br J Oral Surg *13*: 33.

Henningsson, G, Isberg, A (1986). Velopharyngeal movements in patients alternating between oral and glottal articulation: a clinical and cineradiographical study. Cleft Palate J *23*: 1.

Herman, LT (1995). An evaluation of verlopharyngeal ring ligation in cleft palate repair. J Oral Maxillofac Surg *53*: 655.

Hogan, VM (1973). A clarification of the surgical goals in cleft palate speech and the introduction of the lateral port control (LPC) pharyngeal flap. Cleft Palate J *10*: 331.

Horswell, BB, Castiglione, CL, Poole, AE, et al. (1993). The double-reversing Z-plasty in primary palatoplasty: operative experience and early results. J Oral Maxillofac Surg *51*: 145.

Horswell, BB, Pospisil, OA (1995). Nasal symmetry after primary cleft lip repair: comparison between Delaire cheilorhinoplasty and modified rotation-advancement. J Oral Maxillofac Surg *53*: 1025.

Isberg, A, Henningsson, G (1987). Influence of palatal fistula on velopharyngeal movements: a cineradiographic study. Plast Reconstr Surg *79*: 525.

Jackson, IT (1990). Pharyngoplasty: Jackson technique. In: *Multidisciplinary Management of Cleft Lip and Palate,* edited by J Bardach and HL Morris. Philadelphia: WB Saunders.

Jackson, IT, Silverton, JS (1977). The sphincter pharyngoplasty as a secondary procedure in cleft palates. Plast Reconstr Surg *59*: 518.

James, D, Ma, L (1997). Mandibular reconstruction in children with obstructive sleep apnea due to micrognathia. Plast Reconstr Surg *100*: 1131.

Jensen, BL, Dahl, E, Kreiborg, S (1983). Longitudinal study of body height, radius length and skeletal maturity in Danish boys with cleft lip and palate. Scand J Dent Res *91*: 473.

Jeresaty, RM, Huszar, RJ, Basu, S (1969). Pierre Robin syndrome. Am J Dis Child *117*: 710.

Jolleys, A (1954). A review of the results of operations on cleft palates with reference to maxillary growth and speech function. Br J Plast Surg *7*: 229.

Jolleys, A, Roberston, NR (1972). A study of the effects of early bone grafting in complete clefts of the lip and palate: five year study. Plast Reconstr Surg *25*: 229.

Jones, WB (1988). Weight gain and feeding in the neonate with cleft: a three-center study. Cleft Palate J *25*: 379.

Kapp-Simon, KA (1995). Psychological interventions for the adolescent with cleft lip and palate. Cleft Palate Craniofac J *32*: 104.

Kemp-Fincham, SI, Kuehn, DP, Trost-Cardamone, JE (1990). Speech development and the timing of primary palatoplasty. In: Bardach J, Morris HL (eds): *Multidisciplinary Management of Cleft Lip and Palate,* edited by J Bardach and HL Morris. Philadelphia: WB Saunders.

Kilner, TP (1937). Cleft lip and palate repair techniques. St Thomas Hosp Rep *2*: 127.

Kilner, TP (1958). The management of the patient with cleft lip and/or palate. Am J Surg *93*: 204.

Koberg, WR (1973). Present view on bone grafting in cleft palate. J Maxillofac Surg *1*: 185.

Koop, CE (1987). *Surgeon General's Report: Children with Special Health Care Needs,* 184-020/65654. Washington, DC: Government Printing Office.

Kramer, GJC, Hoeksma, JB, Prahl-Andersen, B (1996). Prediction of early palatal growth and development in children with cleft lip and palates. Cleft Palate Craniofac J *33*: 112.

Laatikainen, T, Ranta, R, Nordstrom, R (1996). Craniofacial mor-

phology in twins with cleft lip and palate. Cleft Palate Craniofac J *33*: 96.

Laspos, CP, Kyrkanides, S, Moss, ME, et al. (1997). Mandibular and maxillary asymmetry in individuals with unilateral cleft lip and palate. Cleft Palate Craniofac J *34*: 232.

Latham, FA (1993). The anatomy of cupid's bow in normal and cleft lip. Plast Reconstr Surg *92*: 404.

Lebert, L (1962). Growth change of the palate. J Dent Res *41*: 1391.

LeBlanc, SM, Golding-Kushner, KJ (1992). Effect of glossopexy on speech sound production in Robin sequence. Cleft Palate Craniofac J *29*: 239.

Lehman, JA, Fishman, JRA, Neiman, GS (1995). Treatment of cleft palate associated with Robin sequence: appraisal of risk factors. Cleft Palate Craniofac J *32*: 25.

LeMesurier, AB (1955). Quadrilateral Mirault flap operation. Plast Reconstr Surg *16*: 425.

Leonard, BJ, Brust, JD, Abrahams, G, et al. (1991). Self-concept of children and adolescents with cleft lip and/or palate. Cleft Palate Craniofac J *28*: 347.

Lohmander-Agerskov, A, Dotevall, H, Lith, A, et al. (1996). Speech and velopharyngeal function in children with an open residual cleft in the hard palate, and the influence of temporary covering. Cleft Palate Craniofac J *33*: 324.

Longaker, MT, Stern, M, Lorenz, HP, et al. (1992). A model for fetal cleft lip repair in lambs. Plast Reconstr Surg *90*: 750.

Maher, W (1977). Distribution of palatal and other arteries in cleft and non-cleft human palates. Cleft Palate J *14*: 1.

Marsh, JL (1996). Craniofacial surgery: the experiment on the experiment of nature. Cleft Palate Craniofac J *33*: 1.

Marsh, JL, Wray, RC (1980). Speech prosthesis versus pharyngeal flap: a randomized evaluation of the management of velopharyngeal incompetence. Plast Reconstr Surg *65*: 592.

McCance, A, Roberts-Harry, D, Sherriff, M, et al. (1993). Sri Lankan cleft lip and palate study model analysis: clefts of the secondary palate. Cleft Palate Craniofac J *30*: 227.

McComb, H (1985). Primary correction of unilateral cleft lip nasal deformity: a 10-year review. Plast Reconstr Surg *75*: 791.

McComb, H (1990). The nasal deformity in clefts. In: Kernahan DA, Rosenstein SW (eds): *Cleft Lip and Palate: A System of Management,* edited by DA Kernahan and SW Rosenstein. Baltimore: Williams and Wilkins, pp. 68–73.

McComb, H (1994). Primary repair of the bilateral cleft lip nose: a 4-year review. Plast Reconstr Surg *94*: 37.

McComb, HK, Coghlan, BA (1996). Primary repair of the unilateral cleft lip nose: completion of a longitudinal study. Cleft Palate Craniofac J *33*: 23.

Millard, DR, Jr (1957). A primary camouflage in the unilateral harelip. In: *Transactions of the International Congress of Plastic Surgeons.* Baltimore: Williams and Wilkins, p. 160.

Millard, DR, Jr (1960). Complete unilateral clefts of the lip. Plast Reconstr Surg *25*: 595.

Millard, DR, Jr (1964). Refinements in rotation-advancement cleft lip technique. Plast Reconstr Surg *33*: 26.

Millard, DR (1967). Bilateral cleft lip and a primary forked flap: a preliminary report. Plast Reconstr Surg *30*: 50.

Millard, DR, Jr (1976a). A preliminary adhesion. In: *Cleft Craft. The Unilateral Deformity,* Vol. 1, edited by DR Millard. Boston: Little, Brown. pp 17–51.

Millard, DR, Jr (1976b). How to rotate and advance in a complete cleft. In: *Cleft Craft. The Unilateral Deformity,* Vol. 1, edited by DR Millard. Boston: Little, Brown, pp. 449–486.

Millard, DR, Jr (1980). *Cleft Craft: The Evolution of Its Surgery. Alveolar and Palatal Deformities,* Vol. 3. Boston: Little, Brown.

Millard, DR, Jr, Batstone, J, Heycock, M, et al. (1970). Ten years with the palatal island flap. Plast Reconstr Surg *46*: 540.

Millard, DR, Jr, Latham, RA (1990). Improved surgical and dental treatment of clefts. Plast Reconstr Surg 86: 856.

Mohler, LR (1987). Unilateral cleft lip repair. Plast Reconstr Surg 80: 511.

Moos, KF (1997). Mandibular reconstruction in children with obstructive sleep apnea due to micrognathia. Plast Reconstr Surg 100: 1138.

Morris, H, Bardach, J, VanDermark, D, et al. (1989). Results of two-flap palatoplasty with regard to speech production. Eur J Plast Surg 12: 19.

Morris, HL (1973). Velopharyngeal competence and primary cleft palate surgery, 1960–1971: a critical review. Cleft Palate J 10: 62.

Morris, HL, Bardach, J, Jones, D, et al. (1995). Clinical results of pharyngeal flap surgery: the Iowa experience. Plast Reconstr Surg 95: 652.

Motohashi, N, Kuroda, T, Filho, LC, et al. (1994). P-A cephalometric analysis of nonoperated adult cleft lip and palate. Cleft Palate Craniofac J 31: 193.

Moyson, F (1961). A plea against tracheotomy in the Pierre Robin's syndrome. Br J Plast Surg 14: 187.

Mulliken, JB (1995). Bilateral complete cleft lip and nasal deformity: an anthropometric analysis of staged to synchronous repair. Plast Reconstr Surg 96: 9.

Mulliken, JB, Pensler, JM, Kozakewich, HPW (1993). The anatomy of cupid's bow in normal and cleft lip. Plast Reconstr Surg 92: 395.

Nelson, CL, Chemello, PD, Jones, JE, et al. (1988). The effect of primary alveolar cleft bone grafting on facial growth. J Oral Maxillofac Surg 46: 33.

Nguyen, PN, Sullivan, PK (1993). Issues and controversies in the management of cleft palate. Clin Plast Surg 20: 671.

Nique, T, Fonseca, RJ, Upton, LG, et al. (1987). Particulate allogeneic bone grafts into maxillary alveolar clefts in humans: a preliminary report. J Oral Maxillofac Surg 45: 386.

Nylen, B, Korlof, B, Arnander, C, et al. (1974). Primary, early bone grafting in complete clefts of the lip and palate. Scand J Plast Reconstr Surg 8: 79.

Orticochea, M (1968). Construction of a dynamic muscle sphincter in cleft palate. Plast Reconstr Surg 41: 323.

Orticochea, M (1984). A rationale for modifying the site of insertion of the Orticochea pharyngoplasty. Plast Reconstr Surg 73: 892.

Peat, BG, Albery, EH, Jones, K, et al. (1994). Tailoring velopharyngeal surgery. The influence of etiology and type of operation. Plast Reconstr Surg 93: 948.

Perko, MA (1979). Two-stage closure of cleft palate. J Maxillofac Surg 7: 76.

Perlman, C, Robin, P (1992). A personal diary. Cleft Palate Craniofac J 29: 201.

Peterson-Falzone, SJ (1990). A cross-sectional analysis of speech results following palatal closure. In: Multidisciplinary Management of Cleft Lip and Palate, edited by J Bardach and HL Morris. Philadelphia: WB Saunders, pp. 750–757.

Peterson-Falzone, SJ (1995). Speech outcomes in adolescents with cleft lip and palate. Cleft Palate Craniofac J 32: 125.

Pigott, RW (1974). The results of nasopharyngoscopic assessment of pharyngoplasty. Scand J Plast Reconstr Surg 8: 148.

Poole, R, Farnworth, TK (1994). Preoperative lip taping in the cleft lip. Ann Plast Surg 32: 243.

Posnick, JC (1991a). Orthognathic surgery in cleft patients treated by early bone grafting. Plast Reconstr Surg 87: 840.

Posnick, JC (1991b). Orthognathic surgery in the cleft patient. In: Instructional Courses. Plastic Surgery Education Foundation, Vol. 4, edited by RC Russel. St. Louis: Mosby-Year Book, pp. 129–157.

Posnick, JC (2000a). The staging of cleft lip and palate reconstruction: infancy through adolescence. In: Craniofacial and Maxillofacial Surgery in Children and Young Adults, edited by JC Posnick. Philadelphia: WB Saunders.

Posnick, JC (2000b). Cleft lip and palate: bone grafting and management of the residual oronasal fistula. In: Craniofacial and Maxillofacial Surgery in Children and Young Adults, edited by JC Posnick. Philadelphia: WB Saunders.

Posnick, JC (2000c). Cleft-orthognathic surgery: the unilateral cleft lip and palate deformity. In: Craniofacial and Maxillofacial Surgery in Children and Young Adults, edited by JC Posnick. Philadelphia: WB Saunders.

Posnick, JC (2000d). Cleft-orthognathic surgery: the bilateral cleft lip and palate deformity. In: Craniofacial and Maxillofacial Surgery in Children and Young Adults, edited by JC Posnick. Philadelphia: WB Saunders. pp. 908–950.

Posnick, JC (2000e). Cleft-orthognathic surgery: the isolated cleft palate deformity. In: Craniofacial and Maxillofacial Surgery in Children and Young Adults, edited by JC Posnick. Philadelphia: WB Saunders. pp. 951–980.

Posnick, JC, Getz, SB, Jr (1987). Surgical closure of end-stage palatal fistulas using anteriorly-based dorsal tongue flaps. J Oral Maxillofac Surg 45: 907.

Posnick, JC, Tompson, B (1992). Modification of the maxillary Le Fort I osteotomy in cleft-orthognathic surgery: the unilateral cleft lip and palate deformity. J Oral Maxillofac Surg 50: 666.

Posnick, JC, Tompson, B (1993). Modification of the maxillary Le Fort I osteotomy in cleft-orthognathic surgery: the bilateral cleft lip and palate deformity. J Oral Maxillofac Surg 51: 2.

Poswillo, D (1968). The aetiology and surgery of cleft palate with micrognathia. Ann R Coll Surg Engl 43: 61.

Proffitt, WR (1991). Orthodontic treatment of clefts: yesterday, today and tomorrow. In: Proceedings of the 48th Annual Meeting, American Cleft Palate-Craniofacial Association, Hilton Head, South Carolina, March 1991, p. 32.

Pruzansky, S (1955). Factors determining arch form in cleft of the lip and palate. Am J Orthod 41: 827.

Pruzansky, S (1964). Pre-surgical orthopaedics and bone grafting for infants with cleft lip and palate: a dissent. Cleft Palate J 1: 154.

Pruzansky, S (1969). Not all dwarfed mandibles are alike. Birth Defects 5: 120.

Pruzansky, S, Richmond, JB (1954). Growth of the mandible in infants with micrognathia. Am J Dis Child 88: 29.

Randall, P (1965). A lip adhesion operation in cleft lip surgery. Plast Reconstr Surg 35: 371.

Randall, P, Whitaker, LA, Noone RB, Jones, WD. The case for the inferiorly based pharyngeal flap. Cleft Palate Craniofac J. 1978; 15(3):262–5.

Randall, P (1990). Long-term results with the triangular flap technique for unilateral cleft lip repair. In: Multidisciplinary Management of Cleft Lip and Palate, edited by J Bardach and H Morris. Philadelphia: WB Saunders, p. 173.

Randall, P (1995). Augmentation of the free border of the lip in cleft patients using temporoparietal fascia. Plast Reconstr Surg 95: 789.

Randall, P (1965). Pierre Robin and the syndrome that bears his name. Cleft Palate J 2: 237.

Randall, P, Larossa, DD, Fakhraee, SM, et al. (1983). Cleft palate closure at 3 to 7 months of age: a preliminary report. Plast Reconstr Surg 71: 624.

Rehrmann, AH (1971). The effects of early bone grafting on the growth of the upper jaw in cleft lip and palate children: a computer evaluation. Minerva Chir 26: 874.

Ren, Y-F, Wang, G-H (1993). A modified palatopharyngeous flap operation and its application in the correction of velopharyngeal incompetence. Plast Reconstr Surg 91: 612.

Richman, LC, Eliason, M (1982). Psychological characteristics of children with cleft lip and palate: intellectual achievement, behavioral and personality variables. Cleft Palate J 19: 249.

Richman, LC, Holmes, CS, Eliason, MJ (1985). Adolescents with cleft lip and palate: self-perceptions of appearance and behavior related to personality adjustment. Cleft Palate J 22: 93.

Rintala, A, Ranta, R, Stegars, T (1984). On the pathogenesis of cleft palate in the Pierre Robin syndrome. Scand J Plast Reconstr Surg 18: 237.

Riski, JE (1979). Articulation skills and oral–nasal resonance in children with pharyngeal flaps. Cleft Palate J 16: 421.

Riski, JE (1995). Speech assessment of adolescents. Cleft Palate J 32: 109.

Riski, JE (1996). Speech outcome following palatoplasty in primary school children: do lay peer observers agree with speech pathologists? Plast Reconstr Surg 98: 966.

Riski, JE (1997a). Principles of speech pathology in the cleft lip and palate child. In: Georgiade Plastic, Maxillofacial and Reconstructive Surgery, 3rd ed., edited by GS Georgiade, R Riefkohl and LS Levin. Philadelphia: JB Lippincott.

Riski, JE (1997b). Secondary surgical procedures to correct postoperative velopharyngeal incompetencies found after primary palatoplasties. In: Communicative Disorders Related to Cleft Lip and Palate, 4th ed., edited by KR Bzoch. Austin, TX: Pro-Ed, p. 121.

Riski, JE, DeLong, E (1984). Articulation development in children with cleft lip/palate. Cleft Palate J 21: 57.

Riski, JE, Hoke, JA, Dolan, EA (1989). The role of pressure flow and endoscopic assessment in successful palatal obturator revision. Cleft Palate J 26: 56.

Riski, JE, Ruff, GL, Georgiade, GS, et al. (1992a). Evaluation of failed sphincter pharyngoplasties. Ann Plast Surg 28: 545.

Riski, JE, Ruff, GL, Georgiade, GS, et al. (1992b). Evaluation of the sphincter pharyngoplasty. Cleft Palate Craniofac J 29: 254.

Riski, JE, Serafin, D, Rictkohl, R, et al. (1984). A rationale for modifying the site of insertion of the Orticochea pharyngoplasty. Plast Reconstr Surg 73: 882.

Roberg, W, Koblin, I (1973). Speech development and maxillary growth in relation to technique and timing of palatoplasty. J Maxillofac Surg 1: 44.

Robertson, NR, Jolleys, A (1968). Effects of early bone grafting in complete clefts of the lip and palate. Plast Reconstr Surg 42: 414.

Robin, P (1923). La chute de la base de la langue consideree comme une nouvelle cause de gene dans la respiration naso-pharyngienne. Bull Acad Med (Paris) 89: 37.

Robin, P (1934). Glossoptosis due to atresia and hypotrophy of the mandible. Am J Dis Child 48:541.

Robinow, M, Johnson, GF, Apesos, J (1986). Robin sequence and oligodactyly in mother and son. Am J Med Genet 25: 293.

Rohrich, RJ, Rowsell, AR, Johns, DF, et al. (1996). Timing of hard palatal closure: a critical long-term analysis. Plast Reconstr Surg 98: 236.

Rose, W (1976). Harelip and Cleft Palate. London: HK Lewis.

Rosenstein, S, Dado, DV, Kernahan, D, et al. (1991a). The case for early bone grafting in cleft lip and palate: a second report. Plast Reconstr Surg 87: 644.

Rosenstein, SW, Kernahan, D, Dado, D, et al. (1991b). Orthognathic surgery in cleft patients treated by early bone grafting. Plast Reconstr Surg 87: 835.

Rosenstein, SW, Monroe, CW, Kernahan, DA, et al. (1982). The case for early bone grafting in cleft lip and cleft palate patients. Plast Reconstr Surg 70: 297.

Ross, RB, Johnston, MC (1972). Cleft Lip and Palate. Baltimore: William and Wilkins.

Ross, RB, MacNamera, MC (1994). Effect of presurgical infant orthopedics on facial esthetics in complete bilateral cleft lip and palate. Cleft Palate Craniofac J 31: 68.

Ross, DA, Witzel, MA, Armstrong, DC, et al. (1996). Is pharyngoplasty a risk in velocardiofacial syndrome? An assessment of medially displaced carotid arteries. Plast Reconstr Surg 98: 1182.

Rudman, RA (1997). Prospective evaluation of morbidity associated with iliac crest harvest for alveolar cleft grafting. J Oral Maxillofac Surg 55: 219.

Sandham, A, Murray, JAM (1993). Nasal septal deformity in unilateral cleft lip and palate. Cleft Palate Craniofac J 30: 222.

Schimke, RN, Collins, DL, Hiebert, JM (1993). Congenital nonprogressive myopathy with Mobius and Robin sequence: the Carey-Fineman-Ziter syndrome. A confirmatory report. Am J Med Genet 46: 721.

Schrander-Stumpel, C, Fryns, JP, Beemer, FA, et al. (1991). Association of distal arthrogryposis, mental retardation, whistling face, and Pierre Robin sequence: evidence for nosologic heterogeneity. Am J Med Genet 38: 557.

Schreiner, RL, McAlister, WH, Marshall, RE, Shearer, WT (1973). Stickler syndrome in a pedigree of the Pierre Robin syndrome. Am J Dis Child 126: 86.

Schweckendiek, W (1978). Primary veloplasty: long-term results without maxillary deformity. A twenty-five year report. Cleft Palate J 15: 268.

Semb, G (1991). A study of facial growth in patients with bilateral cleft lip and palate treated by the Oslo CLP team. Cleft Palate Craniofac J 28: 22.

Shaw, WC, Asher-McDade, C, Brattshrtom, V, et al. (1992). The RPS: a six-centre international study of treatment outcome in patients with clefts of the lip and palate: Part 5. General discussion and conclusions. Cleft Palate Craniofac J 29: 413.

Shaw, WC, Semb, G (1990). Current approaches to the orthodontic management of cleft lip and palate. J R Soc Med 83: 30.

Sher, AE (1992). Mechanisms of airway obstruction in Robin sequence: implications for treatment. Cleft Palate Craniofac J 3: 224.

Shprintzen, RJ (1992). The implications of the diagnosis of Robin sequence. Cleft Palate Craniofac J 3: 205.

Shprintzen, RJ (1990). Conceptual framework for pharyngeal flap surgery. In: Multidisciplinary Management of Cleft Lip and Palate, edited by J Bardach and HL Morris. Philadelphia: WB Saunders.

Shprintzen, RJ, Bardach, J (1995a). Communicative impairment associated with clefting. In: Cleft Palate Speech Management: A Multidisciplinary Approach. St. Louis: Mosby Year Book, p. 137.

Shprintzen, RJ, Bardach, J (1995b). The use of information obtained from speech and instrumental evaluations in treatment planning for velopharyngeal insufficiency. In: Cleft Palate Speech Management: A Multidisciplinary Approach. St. Louis: Mosby Year Book, p 257.

Shprintzen, RJ, Golding-Kushner, K (1989). Evaluation of velopharyngeal insufficiency. Otolaryngol Clin North Am 22: 519.

Shprintzen, RJ, Lewin, ML, Croft, CB, et al. (1979). A comprehensive study of pharyngeal flap surgery: tailor-made flaps. Cleft Palate J 16: 46.

Shprintzen, RJ, Sher, AE, Croft, CB (1987). Hypernasal speech caused by hypertrophic tonsils. J Pediatr Otorhinolaryngol 14: 45.

Shukowsky, WP (1911). Zur Atiologie des Stridor inspiratorius congenitus. Z Kinderheilkd 73: 459.

Siegel-Sardewitz, VL, Shprintzen, RJ (1986). Changes in velopharyngeal valving with age. Int J Pediatr Otorhinolaryngol *11*: 171.

Sindet-Pedersen, S, Enemark, H (1990). Reconstruction of alveolar clefts with mandibular or iliac crest bone graft: a comparative study. J Oral Maxillofac Surg *48*: 554.

Sirois, M, Caouette-Laberge, L, Spier, S, et al. (1994). Sleep apnea following a pharyngeal flap: a feared complication. Plast Reconstr Surg *93*: 943.

Skoog, T (1965). The use of periosteal flaps in the repair of the primary palate. Cleft Palate J *2*: 332.

Skoog, T (1969). Repair of unilateral cleft lip deformity. Maxilla, nose and lip. Scand J Plast Reconstr Surg *3*: 109.

Slutsky, H (1969). Maternal reaction and adjustment to birth and care of cleft palate child. Cleft Palate J *6*: 425.

Smith, JL, Stowe, FR (1961). The Pierre Robin syndrome (glossoptosis, micrognathia, cleft palate): a review of 39 cases with emphasis on associated ocular lesions. Pediatrics *27*: 128.

Stoll, C, Kieny, JR, Dott, B, et al. (1992). Ventricular extrasystoles with syncopal episodes, perodactyly, and Robin sequence in three generations: a new inherited MCA syndrome? Am J Med Genet *42*: 480.

Strauss, RP (1994). Health policy and craniofacial care: issues in resource allocation. Cleft Palate Craniofac J *31*: 78.

Sullivan, WG, Hedrick, MH, Rice, HE, et al. (1996). Delayed in utero repair of surgically created fetal cleft lip and palate. Plast Reconstr Surg *97*: 906.

Takato, T, Yonehara, Y, Mori, Y, et al. (1995a). Early correction of the nose in unilateral cleft lip patients using an open method: a 10-year review. J Oral Maxillofac Surg *53*: 28.

Takato, T, Yonehara, Y, Mori, Y, et al. (1995b). Columella lengthening using a cartilage graft in the bilateral cleft lip-associated nose: choice of cartilage according to age. J Oral Maxillofac Surg *53*: 149.

Tennison, C (1952). The repair of the unilateral cleft lip by the stencil method. Plast Reconstr Surg *9*: 115.

Thompson, JE (1912). An artistic and mathematically accurate method of repairing the defect in cases of harelip. Surg Gynecol Obstet *14*: 498.

Trier, WC (1995). Bilateral complete cleft lip and nasal deformity: an anthropometric analysis of staged to synchronous repair. Plast Reconstr Surg *96*: 24.

Trotman, C-A, Ross, RB (1993). Craniofacial growth in bilateral cleft lip and palate: ages six years to adulthood. Cleft Palate Craniofac J *30*: 261.

Troxell, JB, Fonseca, RJ, Osbon, DB (1982). A retrospective study of alveolar cleft grafting. J Oral Maxillofac Surg *40*: 721.

Turner, G (1974). The Stickler syndrome in a family with the Pierre Robin syndrome and severe myopia. Aust Paediatr J *10*: 103.

Turvey, TA, Vig, K, Moriarty, J, et al. (1984). Delayed bone grafting in the cleft maxilla and palate: a retrospective multidisciplinary analysis. Am J Orthod 86:244.

Upton, LG (1993). The double-reversing Z-plasty in primary palatoplasty: operative experience and early results. J Oral Maxillofac Surg *51*: 149.

Van Boven, MJ, Pendeville, PE, Veyckemans, F, et al. (1993). Neonatal cleft lip repair: the anesthesiologist's point of view. Cleft Palate Craniofac J *30*: 574.

van der Meulin, JC (1992). Columellar elongation in bilateral cleft lip repair: early results. Plast Reconstr Surg *59*: 6.

Veau, V (1931). *Division Palatine*. Paris: Masson, pp. 6–8, 51–53.

von Langenbeck, B (1861). Operation der angeborenen totalen Spaltung des harten Gaumens nach einer neuen Methode. Dtsch Klin *8*: 231.

Waite, DE, Kersten, RB (1980). Residual alveolar and palatal clefts. In: *Surgical Correction of Dentofacial Deformities*, edited by WH Bell, WR Proffit, and RP White Jr. Philadelphia: WB Saunders, p. 1335.

Wardill, W (1937). The technique of operation for cleft palate. Br J Surg *25*: 117.

Wardill, WFM (1928). Cleft palate: results of operation for cleft palate. Br J Plast Surg *16*: 127.

Warren, DW (1975). The determination of velopharyngeal incompetency by aerodynamic and acoustical techniques. Clin Plast Surg *2*: 299–304.

Warren, DW (1994). Should velopharyngoplasty and tonsillectomy in the cleft palate child be performed simultaneously? J Oral Maxillofac Surg *52*: 930.

Warren, DW, Dalston, RM, Mayo, R (1994). Hypernasality and velopharyngeal impairment. Cleft Palate Craniofac J *31*: 257.

Witt, PD, Marsh, JL, Marty-Grames, L, et al. (1995). Management of the hypodynamic velopharynx. Cleft Palate Craniofac J *32*: 179.

Witt, PD, Marsh, JL, Muntz, HR, et al. (1996). Acute obstructive sleep apnea as a complication of sphincter pharyngoplasty. Cleft Palate Craniofac J *33*: 183.

Witt, PD, O'Daniel, TG, Marsh, JL, et al. (1997). Surgical management of velopharyngeal dysfunction: outcome analysis of autogenous posterior pharyngeal wall augmentation. Plast Reconstr Surg *99*: 1287.

Witzel, MA, Salyer, KE, Ross, RB (1984). Delayed hard palate closure: the philosophy revisited. Cleft Palate J *21*: 263.

Witzel, MA, Tobe, J, Salyer, KE (1989). The use of videonasopharyngoscopy for biofeedback therapy in adults after pharyngeal flap surgery. Cleft Palate J *26*: 129.

Wolford, LM, Oelschlaeger, M, Deal, R (1989). Proplast as a pharyngeal wall implant to correct velopharyngeal insufficiency. Cleft Palate J *26*: 119.

Wood, RJ, Grayson, BH, Cutting, CB (1997). Gingivoperiosteoplasty and midfacial growth. Cleft Palate Craniofac J *34*: 17.

Ysunza, A, Garcia-Velasco, M, Garcia-Garcia, M, et al. (1993). Obstructive sleep apnea secondary to surgery for velopharyngeal insufficiency. Cleft Palate Craniofac J *30*: 387.

27

Evaluation and management of speech, language, and articulation disorders

JOHN E. RISKI

Cleft palate (CP) is the most common cause of velopharyngeal incompetence (VPI). Hypernasality, nasal air emission, and other forms of aberrant speech mark the failed primary management of the patient with CP. Despite the best attempts, primary palatal management is successful in only 70% to 80% of individuals with CP (Morris, 1973; Riski, 1979). Significant efforts have been devoted to better understand, evaluate, and manage the problem, as well as to achieve the goal of velopharyngeal competence. However, many challenges and issues remain concerning evaluation of the velopharyngeal mechanism, physical management, and speech therapy. The purpose of this chapter is to discuss these challenges and issues by reviewing our current understanding of this area.

ISSUES AND CHALLENGES OF CRANIOFACIAL DISORDERS

Specialists who routinely deal with oral clefts face several challenges that impact labeling and identification of some disorders. We must meet these challenges with education, to improve the quality of care and outcomes.

Although oral clefts are among the most common birth defects, they remain a low-incidence disorder in pediatric practice. The prevalence is approximately 1/750 to 1/1000 newborns in the Caucasian population and even higher in other populations. It is estimated that there are 4000 new cleft lip with or without palate (CL/P) cases in the United States annually. Despite the relative prevalence of oral clefts, these patients still represent a small part of the pediatric case-

load outside of craniofacial centers. Hypernasality, nasal air emission, and compensatory articulation are also low-incidence speech disorders and may result from structural, neurological, or functional (learned) etiologies. The rate of hypernasality after initial CP closure is only 20% to 30% (Riski, 1979; Riski and De-Long, 1984). Low-incidence disorders such as oral clefts and hypernasality offer few educational or clinical opportunities for developing clinical expertise. We are challenged to educate other healthcare workers about appropriate identification, diagnosis, and management.

A challenge to evaluation is that the etiologies of hypernasality and nasal airflow disorders are often occult or hidden. In reviews, of patients receiving surgical correction for hypernasality, approximately 30% did not have CP (Riski et al., 1992; Riski, 1995). The etiology in these children is an anatomically deep nasopharynx, which can be diagnosed accurately only by lateral cephalometric (radiographic) assessment. Normal dimensions and growth of the velopharynx were described after cephalometric analysis by Subtelny (1957) and highlighted by Zemlin (1997). The disproportionately deep pharynx, an occult anatomical defect, was described by Calnan (1971).

An issue in speech pathology that may have its origin in the low incidence and occult nature of the disorder is that noncleft hypernasality is erroneously labeled as a voice disorder. Labeling hypernasality as a voice disorder implies that it is a disorder of the larynx and results in delayed identification, labeling, referral, and management. Because the physical defect is not recognized, ineffective speech therapies are often undertaken (Ruscello, 1997). This further delays identification and referral to specialists at craniofacial teams. A CP is identified at birth, and surgical closure is before 1 year of age (Riski, 1995). In stark contrast, the average age at referral to our center for children with noncleft hypernasality resulting from velocardiofacial syndrome (VCFS) is 9.2 years of age.

Delayed management of VPI leads to increased failure of surgical intervention and refractory speech deficits. The rate of complete success when VPI is managed before 6 years of age is 90.9%. Success rates fall to 73.9% between 6 and 12 years, 70.0% between 12 and 18 years, and 47.0% after 18 years (Riski et al., 1992).

Oral clefts and hypernasality are evaluated by specialists in craniofacial clinics. However, Public Laws 94-142 and 99-457 have mandated that speech therapy be provided through specialists in schools and developmental centers. Professionals in these settings often have limited experience with cleft-related problems because these problems usually form a very small part of their caseload. This separation of evaluation and therapy can lead to poor communication between the evaluator and the therapist. The result can be therapy plans that do not directly address the needs of the patient. There is an unmistakable need for partnerships between the evaluation centers and the settings in which the therapy is conducted.

NASOPHARYNGEAL ANATOMY AND PHYSIOLOGY

Many surgical procedures have been devised to take advantage of the presumed function of the velopharyngeal portal. In addition, some surgical strategies and techniques have been criticized as inconsistent with the neuroanatomy and physiology of the velopharyngeal mechanism. Further, understanding of the motor control of the velopharyngeal mechanism is paramount to establishing effective speech therapy regimens. There are many excellent descriptions of normal velopharyngeal anatomy and physiology (Zemlin, 1997). The purpose of this section is to comment on the specific aspects of anatomy, physiology, and motor control which are pertinent to the evaluation and management of the velopharyngeal mechanism.

The levator veli palatini is the primary elevator of the velum for speech. The levator palatini has been implicated as the sole muscle responsible for velopharyngeal closure in speech (Bell-Berti, 1976; Fritzell, 1979). Innervation of the velum is generally conceded through the pharyngeal plexus by way of the pharyngeal branch of cranial nerve X, the vagus. However, Sedlackova (1967) proposed a two-stage theory of innervation. whereby velopharyngeal function for swallowing is innervated through the vagus but speech function is innervated through cranial nerve VII, the facial nerve. This proposal has been supported by Ibuki et al. (1978), who traced facial nerve fibers of rhesus monkeys through the greater petrosal nerve to the levator palatini.

The superior constrictor narrows the pharynx during swallowing (Bell-Berti, 1976; Fritzell, 1979.) Some have proposed that the superior constrictor is also responsible for mesial movement of the lateral pharyngeal walls for speech (Shprintzen et al., 1975; Iglesias et al., 1980). In contrast, Maue-Dickson and Dickson (1980) argued that the levator veli palatini leads to lateral pharyngeal wall motion. Niimi et al. (1982) suggested that we do not know what muscle(s) contributes to the mesial movement of the lateral pharyngeal walls.

Since the fibers of the superior constrictor are divided in a pharyngeal flap pharyngoplasty, postoperative movement of the lateral pharyngeal walls has been questioned. Some have observed reduced postoperative lateral wall motion (Zwitman, 1982a,b) and some have not (Shprintzen et al., 1980).

The musculus uvulae is a paired muscle that occupies the midline of the nasal surface of the velum. Its role during speech appears to be to provide midline mass and to assist in obturating the nasopharynx. Absence of the musculus uvulae leads to a midline defect on the nasal surface of the velum (Huang et al., 1997). The tensor veli palatini is generally regarded as the primary muscle of eustachian tube dilation (Bell-Berti, 1976).

The bilateral palatopharyngeus muscles form the posterior faucial pillars; their function is to narrow the posterior oral cavity during swallowing. The muscles do not consistently function with the levator for velopharyngeal closure. The palatopharyngeus muscles are used in the sphincter pharyngoplasty. Superiorly based flaps are created and then raised from a vertical to a horizontal position and inserted into a transverse incision made into the posterior pharyngeal wall. This provides a static buttress for the elevating velum to contact. There has been speculation that active sphinctering also develops. Ysunza et al. (1999) used pre- and postoperative electromyograms of this muscle to determine that any movement of the palatopharyngeus flaps remains passive postoperatively. The bilateral palatoglossus muscles form the anterior faucial pillars. They contribute to posterior tongue elevation for the lingual–velar sounds. They are antagonistic to the levator and can lower the velum. In one isolated instance, these muscles were substituted for the palatopharyngeus in a sphincter pharyngoplasty (Graiver et al., 1992).

Kuehn and Moon (1995) have conducted a series of studies to evaluate the role and limits of velopharyngeal function. They reported that subjects with CP use a relatively high activation level for the levator muscle during speech, in relation to their total activation range, compared to subjects without CP (Kuehn and Moon, 1995); i.e., speakers with CP have less reserve palatal strength. They also found that the electromyographic response of the levator increases with increased oral pressure for blowing (Kuehn and Moon, 1994). This is consistent with frequent clinical observations that there is greater velopharyngeal function when speech sounds are aspirated with more force, i.e., increased oral pressure. Lastly, Kuehn and Moon (2000) investigated the ability of the velum to close against nasal air pressure. They found that it was possible to induce such fatigue in most subjects and that greater rates of fatigue generally occurred at the higher levels of external loading, i.e., 25 and 35 cm H_2O.

Patterns of velopharyngeal function have been identified. Shprintzen et al. (1974) examined velopharyngeal function by videofluoroscopy for speech and nonspeech tasks. They observed that patterns of closure were different for pneumatic (speech) and nonpneumatic (nonspeech) tasks. Tasks involving airflow (blowing, whistling, and speech) showed focal closure of the velopharyngeal port. In contrast, nonpneumatic tasks demonstrated more complete closure of the entire pharynx. Skolnick and colleagues (Skolnick, 1970; Skolnick and McCall, 1972) first described and labeled the velopharyngeal closure patterns for speech as coronal, circular, and sagittal. A *coronal* pattern included active velar elevation with some simultaneous mesial movement of the lateral pharyngeal walls; closure was in the coronal plane. A *circular* pattern was demonstrated by relatively greater lateral wall motion than velar movement. Finally, lateral wall movement and contact with little velar elevation characterized a *sagittal* pattern.

Some theories of motor control have developed from research of compensatory speech in speakers with CP. These theories are an application of the theory of motor equivalence. *Motor equivalence* was initially described as "variability of specific muscular responses, with circumstance, in such a way as to produce a single result" (Tolman, 1932; Hebb, 1949). Motor equivalence was applied to speech production by MacNeilage (1970) to refer to the adjustment of speech motor commands to assure that individual articulators reach semi-invariant target positions. A further adaptation of motor equivalence is the pressure regulation/control theory forwarded by Warren and Hinton (1983) and Warren (1986). This theory is based on compensations to VPI in the CP population and ob-

servations of normal vocal tract function. They proposed that the vocal tract is regulated during speech to maintain pressure. Vocal tract pressure is controlled by adjusting respiratory airflow and vocal tract (e.g., laryngeal) valving.

Vocal tract adjustments during breathing or speech should require continual adjustments of laryngeal valving and respiratory support. These adjustments appear to require instantaneous knowledge of vocal tract status from receptors within the vocal tract. Morr et al. (1988) speculated that certain respiratory receptors found in the trachea, larynx, and nasopharynx may also operate in the regulation of vocal tract pressures during speech. While these receptors have not been identified, investigations in humans and laboratory animals (reported in the experimental pulmonary physiology literature) offer some possible explanations regarding the location and nature of the receptors. Possible sites include the nasopharynx (McBride and Whitelaw, 1981), bronchi (Gonzalez-Baron et al., 1989), C-fiber afferents in the extrathoracic trachea and larynx (Sant'Ambrogio et al., 1983; Szereda-Przestaszewska, 1989), pulmonary stretch receptors (Harding, 1984), receptors responding to rate of lung volume change and/or upper airway pressure (Giering and Daubenspeck, 1990), and receptors of expiratory resistive loads and changes in respiratory pattern (Insalaco et al., 1991).

In response to Warren's pressure regulation/control theory, Netsell (1990) suggested an acoustic regulation hypothesis, which suggested that the goal of speech is to produce meaningful acoustics. A speaker with VPI valves at the larynx to generate acoustic distinctions that cannot be produced downstream from the VPI. In a test of the acoustic and pressure regulation theories, Moon and Folkins (1991) disrupted auditory feedback with noise. This yielded only small increases in oral pressure, leading the investigators to conclude that auditory regulation alone does not explain pressure maintenance. Additional study of speech compensations for various deficits may provide greater insight into speech motor control.

SPEECH SOUND SYSTEM

Articulation

Understanding the normal speech system is necessary to assess the outcome of treatment and to understand compensatory articulation. American English includes approximately 46 sounds or phonemes. The sounds are learned, beginning in the first year of life and continuing through 6 to 7 years of age. The neurologically simple sounds (vowels) are learned first and the more complex sounds (affricates, i.e., *ch* and *dg*) are learned last. Normal speech learning requires adequate hearing and a competent velopharyngeal mechanism. Both may be compromised because of a CP. The severity of articulation disorders increases with the severity of clefting (Riski, 1979; Riski and DeLong, 1984; Laitinen et al., 1998).

All vowels are voiced and described by the position of the tongue in the oral cavity. The vertical position is described as high, middle, or low. The horizontal position is described as front, mid, or back. For example, *ee* requires a high-front tongue position and *ah* requires a low-back position. A high tongue carriage offers more resistance to sound energy as it exits the oral cavity. In the presence of even a small VPI, high vowels are more susceptible to hypernasal resonance than low vowels.

Two parameters are used to describe consonants. The *place of articulation* describes the location of articulators in the oral cavity. For example *p* is bilabial, *t* is a lingual-alveolar, and *k* is a lingual-velar. The *manner of articulation* describes the way in which the sound is produced. Stop-plosive sounds such as *p*, *t*, and *k* are made by a brief interruption or stop of the airstream and then a release. Fricative sounds such as *s*, *f*, and *th* are made by constricting the airstream. The affricate sounds *ch* and *dg* are considered combinations of stops and fricatives. There are three nasal sounds, *m*, *n*, and *ng*. Lastly, several sounds are labeled as glides or semivowels, including the sounds *w*, *y*, *l*, and *r*.

All vowels and the nasal and glide consonants are voiced. The stops, fricatives, and affricates exist in voiced and voiceless pairs. For example, the sound *s* is voiceless and made only with a constriction of the airstream between the tongue and alveolar ridge. The addition of voicing to the *s* creates the *z*. All stops, fricatives, and affricates require intraoral air pressure. Intraoral air pressure requires appropriate coordination of velopharyngeal competence with adequate respiratory pressure and oral articulatory function.

Nasal Coupling

The terminology used to describe the characteristics of nasal coupling has been described (Riski and Millard, 1979). Resonance qualities are associated with the voiced elements of speech, while nasal air emission is associated with the unvoiced elements of speech.

Oral–nasal resonance is the balance of oral and nasal acoustic (voiced) energies. It is achieved by the appropriate coupling or isolation of the nasal cavity from the remainder of the vocal tract during speech by movements of the velopharyngeal valve. Three English sounds require the nasal cavity to be coupled with the vocal tract: *m*, *n*, and *ng*. All other sounds require the

velopharyngeal valve to isolate the nasal cavity from the vocal tract. *Hypernasality* is the quality perceived by the listener caused by inappropriate nasal coupling with the vocal tract during speech. It is most easily perceived on vowel sounds. In contrast, *hyponasality* is perceived as inadequate coupling or obstruction of the nasal tract during production of those sounds normally associated with nasal energy. The obstruction may be posterior (e.g., hypertrophied adenoids) or anterior (e.g., hypertrophied turbinates). Further, a speaker may also demonstrate a mixed *hyper-hyponasality* when velopharyngeal closure is incomplete but the nasal cavity is occluded anteriorly.

Nasal air emission is most easily perceived on the unvoiced consonants. Nasal air emission may be inaudible in patients with patent nasal cavities. In these patients, the air passes through the nasal cavity without creating any audible turbulence. Oral pressure is required for the frication associated with the fricative consonants (e.g., *s* and *f*) or the stop and release of pressure associated with the plosive consonants (e.g., *p* and *t*). Oral pressure is often inversely related to nasal air emission, which represents loss of pressure out of the nose. Posterior nasal frication in association with attempts at oral airflow generally represents touch velopharyngeal contact. Velopharyngeal closing force is not maintained, and the air leak through the port creates the posterior nasal frication. Air flows simultaneously through the oral and nasal cavities.

Compensatory Articulation

Children born with CL/P often learn articulation compensatory to the loss of oral pressure or dental arch collapse. The classic compensatory misarticulations described are glottal stops and pharyngeal fricatives. Trost (1981) added the following:

- *Pharyngeal stop*, point of stop is tongue base to posterior pharyngeal wall, used as substitute for *k* or *g*.
- *Midpalatal stop*, point of stop is midpalate, between position of *t* and *k*, used as substitute for *t*, *d*, *k*, or *g*.
- *Posterior nasal fricative*, point of frication is velopharyngeal valve, tongue stops airstream and nasal airflow is the only airflow, used as a substitute for *s*, *z*, and other fricative and affricate sounds.

We might also consider the *anterior nasal fricative*, which is similar to the posterior nasal fricative except that the point of frication is the anterior nostrils. Nasal grimacing may accompany this substitution.

The posterior nasal fricative is often observed in speakers without CP and with normal velopharyngeal function. Other hallmarks of speech include normal oral–nasal resonance, normal aspiration of stop-plosive consonants, and ability to learn a normal oral *s*. For such cases, the terms *sound-specific VPI* and *functional VPI* have been coined (Riski, 1984). However, the posterior nasal fricative does not reflect anatomical or neurological dysfunction of the velopharyngeal mechanism but, rather, a unique sound substitution. The clinician's differential diagnosis of the nasal airflow associated with the posterior nasal fricative and a true VPI is critical to developing an appropriate treatment plan, the former requiring speech therapy and the latter possible surgical or prosthetic intervention.

The etiology of the posterior nasal fricative is somewhat elusive. One theory is that it develops to compensate for conductive hearing loss (Riski, 1984). The vibration produced at the velopharynx could be easily transmitted by bone conduction up the cervical vertebrae to the skull and the cochlea. The sound *s* may be more susceptible since it is one of the earliest learned sibilants and requires a lesser degree of hearing loss to impact perception.

ASSESSMENT OF VELOPHARYNGEAL FUNCTION

Assessing velopharyngeal function may be approached as a multilevel problem. The first level should include the perceptual evaluation of oral pressure, oral–nasal resonance, nasal air escape, and articulatory precision. The trained ear is still the gold standard of the evaluation. Resonance should be neither hypernasal nor hyponasal (Riski et al., 1989). The second level is the screening of velopharyngeal closure. This step can use inexpensive tools and is underutilized by clinicians. Patients who fail these two steps should undergo the third step of objective assessment with computerized instruments for acoustic (Fletcher, 1978) and nonacoustic (Warren and DuBois, 1964; Warren and Devereux, 1966) assessment of velopharyngeal function. Finally, imaging should account for the three-dimensional nature of the velopharyngeal port. This can be achieved by some combination of flexible fiberoptic nasendoscopy (Pigott, 1974; Gilbert and Pigott, 1982; Zwitman, 1982a,b), radiography, or fluoroscopy (Skolnick, 1970, 1975; Williams, 1979; Williams and Eisenbach, 1981) during speech. Articulatory precision should be evaluated separately with special attention to any compensatory misarticulations and the age appropriateness of articulation.

Each technique has its advantages and disadvantages. No one instrument can provide all of the necessary information. An ad hoc committee of the American Cleft Palate-Craniofacial Association suggested minimal standards for the evaluation of velopharyngeal func-

tion, including a perceptual evaluation of resonance and assessment using at least one instrument during connected speech (i.e., fluoroscopy or pressure-flow) (Dalston et al., 1988). A consensus conference of 71 individuals experienced in the diagnosis and treatment of individuals with craniofacial anomalies developed the *Parameters for Evaluation and Treatment of Patients with Cleft Lip/Palate or Other Craniofacial Anomalies* (American Cleft Palate-Craniofacial Association, 1993).

The American Speech–Language Hearing Association (1997) has also produced a resource for evaluation of the velopharyngeal mechanism, listing procedures to assess oral, nasal, and velopharyngeal functions for speech production. It advocates perceptual and instrumental assessment.

Longitudinal study of velopharyngeal port function has demonstrated instability in children as the phonological system develops and craniofacial growth and adenoid involution occur (Van Demark and Morris, 1983; Van Demark et al., 1988). Some children develop VPI as the adenoids involute (Mason and Warren, 1980; Riski and Mason, 1994). In contrast, some children eventually resolve hypernasality, which is identified immediately following palatoplasty (Fox et al., 1988). These studies demonstrate the need for longitudinal assessment of velopharyngeal function and the need to exercise caution before performing a pharyngoplasty.

Velopharyngeal function impacts speech proficiency. However, speech proficiency is not an adequate measure of velopharyngeal function (Riski, 1979). These two areas should be evaluated separately. It is possible to have severely defective speech and a competent velopharyngeal mechanism. However, normal speech usually cannot be produced without a competent velopharyngeal mechanism.

Nasopharyngeal Patency

Aerodynamic assessment has demonstrated the requirements of adequate nasal airway patency (Warren, 1984). Nasal deformities decrease nasal patency in the CP population (Warren et al., 1969), and pharyngeal flap surgery further decreases nasal airway patency in children but not in adults (Warren et al., 1974). Both children and adults with CL/P demonstrate increased nasal resistance (15%–30%) compared to the noncleft population (Hairfield et al., 1988). Furthermore, the minimal cross-sectional area of the nose can be estimated from differential oral–nasal pressure and nasal flow measures and has been reported for individuals with and without CP (Warren et al., 1992). Surgeons have become so successful in addressing and managing hypernasality that hyponasality may now be a more frequent velopharyngeal dysfunction (Riski, 1995).

Evaluation Protocol

There are many procedures and instruments for evaluating speech and velopharyngeal function. Evaluation can take the form of a perceptual exam, clinical screening of velopharyngeal closure, computer instrumental evaluation, imaging, or diagnostic therapy. Each instrument offers advantages and disadvantages that the clinician should consider. A problem-oriented protocol can lead the clinician in the process.

Perceptual Evaluation

The perceptual evaluation is the most common form of evaluating speech. The result of this evaluation is still the standard from which speech surgeries are recommended. The scale studied by Subtelny et al. (1972) is especially useful since it allows functional analysis of speech qualities associated with oral clefts. Hypernasality is often used as a standard of success. However, there are advantages to rating the aspiration or oral pressure of the pressure consonants. Van Demark (1979) demonstrated that correct production of the oral pressure bilabial consonants p and b is predictive of future velopharyngeal competence.

The advantage of perceptual evaluation is that it provides an accepted standard for speech qualities. Ratings of oral–nasal resonance, nasal air escape, oral pressure, and articulation are the standards by which surgical outcomes are evaluated. The disadvantage is that these qualities are not easily quantified and validity is difficult to establish without extensive listener training (Keunig et al., 1999). However, nasal air escape is not always audible, so some VPIs might escape detection without instrumental evaluation. The quality of voice or articulation may influence the rating of resonance. The presence of articulation disorders may negatively influence ratings of resonance, while the presence of hoarseness may preclude an accurate assessment of resonance.

Screening Velopharyngeal Closure

Numerous devices are available to screen velopharyngeal closure. Generally, anything that is sensitive to airflow can be used. Examples of these devices include the See-Scape© (Pro-Ed, Austin, TX), nasal listening tubes (Blakeley, 1972; Riski and Millard, 1979), nasal mirrors, and paper paddles. Nasal airflow is monitored during the pronunciation of words such as *puppy*, *puppy*, which should be devoid of nasal airflow. The presence of any airflow indicates some degree of velopharyngeal opening and that further objective testing is warranted.

The advantages of these devices are that they are inexpensive, portable, noninvasive, and very accurate for determining the presence or absence of nasal airflow. In addition, they require little training and clinicians with little experience can become adept users. The disadvantage is that they lack quantification.

Objective Assessment of Velopharyngeal Function

The two most common computer instruments for evaluating velopharyngeal function are pressure-flow and nasometry. Pressure-flow evaluates nonvocalic elements, and nasometry documents vocalic elements. The two measures are taken consecutively, and correlations are reported in the 0.70 range. Powerful personal computers and improved multichannel software now allow simultaneous recording of vocalic and nonvocalic elements.

Pressure Flow

Pressure-flow instrumentation measures the oral–nasal pressure differential and the volume–velocity of nasal airflow. It provides quantifiable data about velopharyngeal port function for speech. The hydrokinetic equation has been modified by Warren and Dubois (1964) for estimating velopharyngeal port orifice area. This modification of the hydrokinetic equation has withstood vigorous study (Smith and Weinberg, 1980, 1982). Pressure-flow study is an objective and reliable method for repeated, noninvasive measures of velopharyngeal port function. The palatal efficiency rating computed instantaneously-Speech Aeromechanical Research System (Perci-SARS; MicroTronics, Carrboro, NC) allows six channels of input, including two pressure channels, two flow channels, a high-speed voice channel, and a low-speed DC channel. Software is included for velopharyngeal function, nasopharyngeal airway patency, laryngeal airway resistance, and several other voice-analysis measures (Riski et al., 1995).

Advantages of pressure-flow assessment are that it quantifies oral pressure and nasal air escape. It also provides an objective estimate of the size of the velopharyngeal opening. Disadvantages are that it is relatively expensive and does not quantify the shape of the velopharyngeal opening. In addition, the speech sample is restricted to unvoiced, stop-plosive consonants (i.e., p), and measures of velopharyngeal area do not always correlate with perception of hypernasality.

Acoustic Measures

The Nasometer (Kay Elemetrics, Lincoln Park, NJ) has become a popular and useful instrument for evaluating the acoustic elements (i.e., hypernasality) of velopharyngeal function. The Nasometer provides an objective measure of nasality, termed *nasalance,* which is the ratio of nasal acoustic energy divided by nasal plus oral acoustic energy. Hardin et al. (1992) reported 91% agreement of nasalance with listener ratings of hypernasality. In addition, nasalance values greater than 26 were correlated with hypernasality, values between 26 and 39 were correlated with mild hypernasality, and values greater than 40 were correlated with moderate to severe hypernasality. Dalston et al. (1991a) reported sensitivity of 0.89 and specificity of 0.99 for listeners' ratings of mild hypernasality. Dalston and Warren (1986) observed that nasalance and velopharyngeal area estimates change in concert. Normative nasalance values were reported by Adams et al. (1989). A completely oral passage ("zoo passage") yielded an average nasalance of 15.53 [standard deviation (SD) = 4.86]. A mixed oral and nasal passage ("rainbow passage") yielded an average nasalance of 35.69 (SD = 5.20). Nasal-laden sentences yielded an average nasalance of 61.06 (SD = 6.94).

The correlation of nasalance with hyponasality has also been reported. Dalston et al. (1991b) reported sensitivity of 0.48 and specificity of 0.79. The measure may have been influenced by nasal air escape in some patients since the measures improved to 1.0 and 0.95, respectively, when patients with nasal air escape were eliminated. Hardin et al. (1992) reported that listeners' perception of hyponasality was related to nasalance scores of less than 50.

An advantage of nasometry is that it reliably quantifies oral–nasal resonance. The instrument also provides feedback in real time and, thus, is useful as a therapy tool as well as a diagnostic tool. A disadvantage is that the speech sample must be restricted to voiced sound elements. Another disadvantage is that the instrument does not discriminate between hypernasality and nasal air escape. In a study that simultaneously recorded nasalance and nasal airflow, Riski (1996) found that 33/92 (35.9%) airflow peaks had recordable nasalance. These findings supported the observation of Karnell (1995) that the combination of turbulent nasal airflow during pressure consonant productions with nasal acoustic energy during vowel productions resulted in elevated nasalance values.

Imaging

Lateral still cephalometric radiographs and videofluoroscopy have been used for some time to assess velopharyngeal function. Sphincteric function during speech has been demonstrated using multiview videofluoroscopy by Skolnick and colleagues (Skolnick, 1970, 1975; Skolnick and McCall, 1972), who described and labeled the velopharyngeal closure patterns:

coronal, circular, and sagittal (see above, NASOPHARYNGEAL ANATOMY AND PHYSIOLOGY). These patterns are significant because pharyngoplasties have been designed and their success reviewed with reference to the type and amount of movement. Videofluoroscopy allows assessment of velar function in its dynamic state for connected speech. Still radiographs often misrepresent velar function because of the limited speech sample that can be employed (Williams and Eisenbach, 1981). In addition, shadows and the two-dimensional nature of the still radiograph can distort the true nature of velopharyngeal function.

Advantages of the lateral radiograph are that the image it produces provides good resolution of the velopharyngeal port and allows assessment of the ratio of nasopharyngeal depth to velar length. These measures can be compared to normative age-matched data (Subtelny, 1957). The average normal ratio of nasopharyngeal depth, measured along the palatal plane, compared to the length of the velum, measured from the posterior nasal spine to the tip of the uvula, ranges from 0.6 to 0.7. This ratio is maintained through growth and development.

Despite being two-dimensional and static, the depth:length ratio appears to have some value in predicting VPI. Wu et al. (1996) reported differences in cephalometric measures between groups of patients differentiated by velopharyngeal competence. Specifically, noncleft patients with velopharyngeal competence demonstrated a significantly smaller depth:length ratio (0.66) compared to CP patients with VPI (1.02).

Velopharyngeal closure is achieved using adenoids in all preadolescent speakers (Gereau and Shprintzen, 1988). Lateral radiographs can assess the contribution of the adenoids to, and changes in, the depth:length ratio to velopharyngeal closure. In one reported series, 11/121 (9.1%) speakers with CP developed VPI with involution of the adenoids (Riski et al., 1996). The depth:length ratio was 0.76 when nasal air escape was first detected at an average age of 5.7 years. The ratio increased to 0.91 with adenoidal involution at an average age of 8.6 years. A matched control group with normal velopharyngeal function demonstrated a depth:length ratio of 0.75.

The relationship of attempted velopharyngeal closure to the cervical spine can be determined and is important for targeting the height of insertion of the sphincter pharyngoplasty (Riski et al., 1984b). Lateral radiographs were used to determine the height of attempted velopharyngeal contact relative to the cervical spine. The information was used by the surgeon to guide the insertion of the sphincter flaps to the height of the attempted closure. The success of resolving VPI increased from 61% to 93%. Disadvantages of lateral radiographs are that the image is static and two-dimensional and requires irradiation.

Advantages of videofluoroscopy are the same as those for lateral radiographs but also include the ability to evaluate the movements of the velopharyngeal mechanism and the mechanism in multiple views. Disadvantages include exposure to irradiation and the inability of young children to cooperate.

Fiberoptic Nasendoscopy

The flexible fiberoptic nasal endoscope is a popular tool for evaluating velopharyngeal function because there is no irradiation and it allows direct observation of the portal during connected speech. There are rigid endoscopes and flexible endoscopes. Rigid scopes provide better optics, but flexible scopes are more comfortable to the patient. Each allows recording of the image using 35 mm or videotape format.

The advantages of fiberoptic nasendoscopy include direct visualization of velopharyngeal movement and evaluation of the nasal surface of the velum for the prominence of the musculus uvulae or defects. It also allows observation of the size and shape of velopharyngeal opening and evaluation of the larynx and pharynx, which are innervated through the vagus nerve. Disadvantages include its invasive nature and the possibility that young children will not be able to comply. The vertical component may be difficult to evaluate. Another disadvantage is that, although most speech pathologists working in the field of oral clefts believe that nasendoscopy is important in the assessment of velopharyngeal function, surveys have revealed that they are not well trained in the use of a nasopharyngoscope. In a survey, 40% had no academic preparation and 20% had no clinical experience in nasopharyngoscopy (Pannbacker et al., 1993).

In summary, no single instrument can provide all of the necessary information about velopharyngeal function. A combination of instruments, each selected after assessing the advantages and disadvantages, is advocated (Van Demark et al., 1975; Hirschberg and Van Demark, 1997).

Articulation Assessment

There have been numerous studies of articulation development in the CLP population (Van Demark et al., 1979; Riski and DeLong, 1984). Articulation is a very important part of speech assessment. Analysis of an articulation test provides data for the speech clinician to develop a therapy program that is realistic and structured. Articulation tests also help clinicians evaluate the child's progress (Van Demark, 1997).

There is a positive relationship between the extent of clefting and articulation deficiency. Children with any one type of cleft demonstrate heterogeneous development of articulation skills (Riski and DeLong, 1984). The type of cleft may affect early sound development. Lohmander-Agerskov et al. (1994) found that noncleft and CP only children first learned anteriorly placed sounds, e.g., bilabial, dental, and alveolar sounds. In contrast, children with cleft lip and palate first learned posteriorly placed sounds.

Under normal valving conditions, a fairly constant pressure is maintained along the vocal tract during speech articulation. The unique misarticulations associated with VPI (e.g., glottal stops and pharyngeal fricative sound substitutions) may be attempts to maintain a constant resistance in the presence of a loss of pressure through the velopharyngeal port. It has been suggested that the vocal tract functions with the use of pressure-sensing regulators (Warren, 1986). Some of the receptors needed for feedback may be in the oral mucosa (Furusawa et al., 1994).

In contrast to the errors that compensate for VPI, errors such as *tat/cat*, *wabbit/rabbit*, and *teef/teeth* are examples of normal developmental errors. Children are expected to outgrow these errors; however, excessive errors (given the age of the child) should be treated with speech therapy.

When compensatory errors are concomitant with VPI, the course of management is two-pronged: first, the VPI must be treated; second, the speech problem must be treated. In some cases, speech therapy can begin before the VPI is managed. In such cases, the nostrils can be occluded manually to direct the airstream orally. The child usually cannot employ newly learned sounds without holding the nose. Therapy before surgery can assist learning after surgery (Riski et al., 1984a). Speech therapy has a limited role in treating VPI. Increasing oral air pressure increases muscular activity of the levators and may increase velopharyngeal movements (Kuehn et al., 1993), and continuous positive nasal airway pressure may be used to increase velopharyngeal closure (Kuehn, 1991). With these few exceptions, a review of velopharyngeal exercises demonstrates their ineffectiveness (Ruscello, 1982, 1989).

SPECIAL CONCERNS AND TREATMENT STRATEGIES

Palatoplasty

Children who have their palate closed early (before 1 year) often develop normal speech earlier and more easily than children who have the palate closed later (after 1 year) (Dorf and Curtin, 1982). This may be especially true for early learning of oral stop-plosive sounds (O'Gara et al., 1994). The best timing of palatoplasty has not been defined, possibly because studies have controlled only for chronological age and not for language age at the time of palatoplasty (O'Gara and Logemann, 1988). The coordination of palatal closure with the development of babbling is intuitive. It is at this point in speech and language development that a child must learn to coordinate velopharyngeal function with respiratory pressure, laryngeal abduction and adduction, and oral articulation to produce consonants. In short, the child's first *dada* is much more complicated than it appears.

Palatoplasty successfully creates a competent velopharyngeal mechanism in 80% of children. This 80% success rate may or may not be influenced by the initial type of cleft (Riski, 1979; Riski and DeLong, 1984; Karnell and Van Demark, 1986). One report demonstrated that the dimensions of the unoperated nasopharynx vary within each type of cleft and suggested that the type and extent of palatoplasty should be tailored to the preoperative dimensions of the nasopharynx (Komatsu et al., 1982). Furlow (1986) first described the double opposing Z-plasty for primary repair of CP with good results.

Long-term follow-up of palatal surgery has been reported by Becker et al. (2000). They reported on 66 adults who had isolated CP closed by either the von Langenbeck or Wardill repair. Speech problems were primarily residual hypernasality, which was moderate or severe in seven (16%) of the patients in the von Langenbeck group and in seven (32%) in the Wardill group. Patients in the Wardill group had fewer fistulas closed and fewer velopharyngoplasties. There were no significant differences between the two methods regarding speech in adulthood.

Oronasal Fistula

Loss of air through an oronasal fistula can be detected and quantified with the assessment tools described previously. It is wise to repeat these measures once with the fistula open and a second time with the fistula temporarily occluded with dental wax (Bless et al., 1980) or chewing gum. With the fistula successfully occluded, velopharyngeal port function can also be adequately tested. Accurate assessment of airflow through the fistula is often confounded by obstructing turbinates or a deviated nasal septum. If the fistula is not patent for speech, surgical intervention may not be warranted. A patent fistula allows the loss of air for speech sounds produced anterior to its site. These are usually the *p*, *b*, *f*, *v*, and *th* sounds, although others may be affected, depending on the location of the fistula and the place-

ment of the tongue. Fistulas should be managed when testing indicates air loss sufficient to undermine speech or when there is a nasal hygiene problem from nasal regurgitation. Research suggests that only larger fistulas are capable of such air loss (Shelton and Blank, 1984). Further Tachimura et al. (1997) reported that the magnitude of the effect is greater for subjects with adequate velopharyngeal function than for subjects who demonstrate VPI. Fistulas may be covered with a dental appliance or closed surgically. Surgical intervention might be delayed until after any planned maxillary arch expansion because this might reopen any fistula closed under tension.

Submucous Cleft Palate

Children with submucous CP are unique in the CP population. The frequency is reported to be between 1:10,000 and 1:20,000. Velopharyngeal incompetence is more common in the coronal closure pattern (Velasco et al., 1988). The speech of individuals with submucous CP should be monitored and management initiated only when VPI is diagnosed. A large percentage (44%) remain unsymptomatic through adulthood (McWilliams, 1991).

Reading Disabilities

Investigation of reading abilities has revealed that children with CL/P display a prevalence for reading disabilities similar to the general population (9%). In contrast, children with CP only demonstrate a much higher rate of reading disabilities (33%) (Richman et al., 1988). Ceponiene et al. (1999) explored auditory short-term memory in children with oral clefts. A measure of detection of change in auditory input was used. They reported a deficiency in auditory short-term memory trace maintenance in cleft children and contend that this dysfunction may contribute to their language and learning disabilities.

SURGICAL MANAGEMENT OF VELOPHARYNGEAL INCOMPETENCE

Posterior Pharyngeal Flap Pharyngoplasty

The concept of a surgical procedure to manage VPI was first introduced by Passavant (1862), who surgically tethered the uvula to the posterior pharyngeal wall in an attempt to restore a competent valving mechanism for speech. This was modified to the superiorly based flap by Bardenheur (1892) and Sanvenero-Rosselli (1934).

Postoperative studies of pharyngeal flap surgery using electromyographic analysis and endoscopic and videofluoroscopic imaging have suggested several methods by which the nasopharynx is obturated. The primary method of velopharyngeal closure is by active mesial movement of the lateral pharyngeal walls against the static, obturating flap (Shprintzen et al., 1980). Secondarily, circumferential scar contracture narrows the pharynx. Finally, contracture of the flap itself elevates the velum into the pharynx, diminishing the anterior–posterior dimension. Crockett et al. (1988) suggested that three variables should be controlled for successful pharyngeal flap surgery: flap width, height or level of flap, and lateral port size. Strategies have been developed to cope with these variables. The size of the lateral ports has been controlled (Hogan and Schwartz, 1977), and the width of the pharyngeal flaps have been tailored to the amount of wall motion (Shprintzen et al., 1979). Some have suggested that little strategy, if any, is needed for small VPI. Randall et al. (1978) observed that if the VPI is small, any method should have a good result.

Posterior Pharyngeal Wall Augmentation and Muscle Transposition

Augmentation of the posterior pharyngeal wall was first reported by Wardill (1928, 1933). He created a permanent ridge of fibrous tissue on the posterior pharyngeal wall by making transverse incisions through the superior constrictor at the level of Passavant's ridge. The tissue was sutured vertically, creating a ridge for the elevated velum to contact. Hynes (1951, 1953) and Orticochea (1968, 1970, 1983) advocated pharyngoplasties by muscle transposition that were similar in design but differed in their intended function. Each procedure has undergone modification and refinement (Jackson and Silverton, 1977; Huskie and Jackson, 1977; Pigott, 1993; Riski et al., 1984b, 1992; Roberts and Brown, 1983; Stratoudakis and Bambace, 1984; Moss et al., 1987; Mirrett et al., 1993).

Orticochea (1968) recommended elevating the height of insertion for the sphincter pharyngoplasty from the low insertion. Several others have recommended elevating the height of insertion as high as possible (Jackson and Silverton, 1977; Roberts and Brown, 1983). Riski et al. (1992) offered a rationale for tailoring the height of flap insertion. The height of attempted velopharyngeal contact was identified relative to the anterior tubercle of the first cervical vertebra, the atlas. The atlas was identified by palpation at the time of surgery, and the flaps were surgically inset at that predetermined height. Success improved from 61% to 93% when the height of the flaps was elevated to the level of attempted velopharyngeal contact.

Debate has continued over whether closure of the sphincter orifice is active or passive. Ysunza et al.

(1999) reported the results of electromyographic analysis before and after sphincter pharyngoplasty in 25 patients. None of the patients demonstrated electromyographic activity in the palatopharyngeus muscle. In contrast, all patients showed normal electromyographic activity at the superior constrictor and the levator veli palatini muscles. Videonasopharyngoscopy demonstrated that lateral pharyngeal wall movements, which ranged from 25% to 40%, were related to strong electromyographic activity at the superior constrictor muscle. They concluded that the flaps of the sphincter pharyngoplasty do not seem to create an active diaphragm for velopharyngeal closure. Moreover, the observed sphinctering appeared to be passive, caused by contraction of the superior constrictor pharyngeus.

Sie et al. (1998) reported the results of sphincter pharyngoplasty on children with VCFS. Three (12.5%) required a revision because of residual hypernasality, and three (12.5%) were hyponasal. After revision, they reported an overall success rate of 18/24 (75.0%).

Treatment strategies are compared infrequently. Pensler and Reich (1991) compared the outcome of 75 patients undergoing pharyngeal flaps with only 10 patients undergoing sphincter pharyngoplasties. Surgeries were done over a 31-year span, from 1958 to 1989. The authors reported a failure rate of 30% for each type of surgery. They concluded that either procedure could be used with equal effectiveness. de Serres et al. (1999) evaluated speech outcomes and complications of sphincter pharyngoplasties and pharyngeal flaps. Patients who underwent sphincter pharyngoplasties had a higher rate of resolution of VPI than those who had pharyngeal flaps, although this was not statistically significant. Postoperative hyponasality and obstructive sleep symptoms were present in both groups. However, only patients who underwent pharyngeal flaps and had postoperative obstructive sleep symptoms had obstructive sleep apnea.

Combined Pharyngoplasty and Primary Palatoplasty

Because the initial palatoplasty may not be completely successful, a number of investigators have incorporated a primary pharyngoplasty. The procedure remains controversial. Most report more patients with normal resonance than with palatoplasty alone (Bingham et al., 1972; Dalston and Stutteville, 1975; Dorf and Curtin, 1982) but not all (Morris, 1973). One study demonstrated that 54% of children receiving a combined procedure did not require the pharyngoplasty (Riski et al., 1987). Mazaheri and colleagues (1994) could not identify any differences in velar length or nasopharyngeal depth between one group of children with clefts who required pharyngeal flaps and a second group of children with clefts who did not. Although it is clear that some children born with CP will require a pharyngoplasty, we cannot accurately identify those children at the time of palatoplasty.

Furlow Z-Plasty

Chen et al. (1994) reported their results with the Furlow Z-plasty as a secondary procedure. They documented velopharyngeal closure in 16/18 patients. Furlow (1994), in a review of the series, observed that retroposition of the levator muscle sling appeared to be the chief benefit of the procedure and that any lengthening of the velum may be an incidental benefit. Gunther et al. (1998) evaluated the results of Furlow's double reversing z-plasty (Furlow, 1986) compared to intravelar veloplasty. Intravelar veloplasty patients demonstrated a 34% higher incidence of hoarseness, nasal escape, and hypernasality at 3 years of age compared to Furlow patients. These same patients likewise required significantly more secondary pharyngoplastic procedures.

Complications of Pharyngoplasty

Complications with pharyngoplasties are not uncommon. Some complications are immediate and some develop in the long term. Obstruction may be severe enough to warrant takedown of the flap (Caouette-Laberge et al., 1992). Ren et al. (1992) suggested that loss of tongue–lip balance might be one factor causing midfacial retrusion. Sturim (1974) reported hemorrhaging from pharyngeal flap surgery in two patients who previously had a Teflon injection for VPI. Zaworski (1981) reported anorexia nervosa in a 15-year-old female after pharyngeal flap surgery. Hoffman (1985) reported surgical revision followed by dilation and stenting with a dental prosthesis to prevent repeat contracture of a pharyngeal flap that stenosed. Drew et al. (1985) reported that 12/25 pharyngeal flap patients demonstrated elevated serum antidiuretic hormone levels, low serum osmolity, and hyponatremia in the postoperative period.

Obstructive Sleep Apnea

Kravath et al. (1980) reported on three patients who developed obstructive sleep apnea (OSA) immediately following pharyngeal flap surgery. Thurston et al. (1980) reported significant nasal obstruction in 8/85 patients following pharyngeal flap. Obstruction was often occult and identified only after careful questioning. Seven of the eight patients required surgical revision to relieve airway obstruction.

Orr et al. (1987) observed OSA in 9/10 patients at 2 to 3 days post-surgery. Apnea resolved in 7/9 patients by 3 months. Shprintzen (1988) identified OSA by polysomnography in 30/300 patients following pharyngeal flap surgery; OSA lasted longer than 6 months in three and resolved in the remaining patients. Narrow and wide flaps had the same incidence of OSA. They postulated that the causes of OSA were obstruction of the portals by large tonsils, contraction of the nasopharynx around the flap, postoperative nasopharyngeal edema, or a sudden change in breathing pattern. Sirois et al. (1994) reported on 14/40 (35%) patients with abnormal polysomnograms after pharyngeal flap surgery. Six had OSA, six had central sleep apnea, and two had both types. Long-term follow-up demonstrated residual central apneas. Witsell et al. (1994) showed decreased nasal patency in 5/7 patients after a pharyngeal flap.

Shprintzen et al. (1992) modified pharyngeal flaps (shorter) for less contracture below the flap, in an attempt to lessen airway obstruction. They also suggested using nasopharyngeal tubes for nasal respiration until the patient is awake and can breathe orally. The authors reported that the protocol reduced all complications: OSA was eliminated in all patients, snoring was reduced from 82% to 10.5%, and hospital stay was reduced from 7 to 3 days.

SPEECH THERAPY

Before Palatal Closure

Parents are counseled regarding what to expect from their child's early speech attempts. Resonance will be hypernasal, and the child will be able to say correctly words with a nasal sound, such as *mama*, but will not correctly say words with pressure sounds, such as *dada*. Parents are instructed in play activities which focus on verbal interaction between parent and child and appropriate modeling of speech and language.

After Palatal Closure

Speech and language stimulation should continue with age-appropriate games, vocabulary, and syntax. Parents are now asked to monitor the sounds that the child makes. If there are no confounding developmental problems, we expect the child to begin making crisp, pressure consonants such as *p, b, t, d, k,* and *g.* Often, parents are asked to occlude the child's nose manually while playing "sound games," such as repeating the syllable *ba, ba, ba, ba.* Occluding the nose prevents any nasal airflow and directs the airstream to the oral cavity. Parents are also asked to observe any signs of velopharyngeal dysfunction or oral–nasal fistulas. These include nasal reflux while eating or drinking, nasal airflow or facial grimacing, or the continued use of nasal sounds and the lack of pressure consonants while talking.

Speech therapy for the child with CP is unique because the child may present with unique misarticulations not found in the noncleft population (Trost, 1981). Unique speech therapy strategies and facilitating postures are used to correct misarticulations in the CL/P child. Moreover, exercises are generally unsuccessful at increasing velopharyngeal movements except in some very specific situations (Ruscello, 1982, 1989). Maximizing oral pressure for pressure consonants will maximize velopharyngeal elevation and may gain velopharyngeal closure for small VPIs. Kuehn (1991) developed a unique therapy technique using continuous positive airway pressure to the nasal surface of the soft palate. Velar elevation for speech under the resistance of continuous positive airway pressure may improve velopharyngeal closure.

The importance of parental involvement in the therapeutic process has been demonstrated. Broen et al. (1993) and Pamplona et al. (1996) evaluated the effectiveness of speech therapy provided by parents and directed by a speech–language pathologist. Broen et al. (1993) reported that the mother was able to change the child's speech so that more of the child's productions were at the correct place of articulation. After structural management, nasal and glottalized productions disappeared from the child's speech but glottal stops did not (Pamplona et al., 1996). Patients accompanied by their mothers showed significantly higher linguistic advance compared to patients receiving therapy without their mothers. The results of this study support the statement that linguistic development in the CP child is strongly related to adult–child modes of interaction.

Pamplona et al. (1999) studied whether a phonological intervention may reduce the total time of speech therapy necessary for correcting compensatory articulation in CP children compared to an articulatory intervention. They demonstrated that the total time of speech intervention was significantly reduced ($p <$ 0.001) when a phonological intervention was utilized.

Once a VPI is diagnosed as adversely affecting speech or speech development, it should be managed. Articulation skills improve immediately following management of VPI (Riski, 1979). Patients with VPI make little or no progress in speech therapy until the VPI is managed (Van Demark, 1974; Riski and DeLong, 1984; Van Demark and Hardin, 1985). When a VPI is suspected or documented, speech therapy should be considered diagnostic and short-term. Referral to a CP-craniofacial team is appropriate after no more than several weeks of ineffective speech therapy.

SPECIAL POPULATIONS

Functional or Sound-Specific Velopharyngeal Incompetence

The practicing clinician should also recognize that there are a small number of cleft (and noncleft) children with normal soft palate function who use some form of nasal air emission as a sound substitute (Peterson, 1975; Riski, 1984). This is termed a *functional VPI* or a *sound-specific VPI*. The characteristics include normal resonance, sound-specific use of some form of nasal air escape (usually a posterior nasal fricative), normal velopharyngeal function for correctly produced sounds, and the ability to correctly produce the errored sound without nasal air escape. These patients present a special diagnostic challenge, and the differential diagnosis of an organic VPI from a functional VPI is the key to appropriate management.

Velocardiofacial Syndrome

Shprintzen et al. (1978) first described VCFs. Over 100 characteristics have been reported. The most common features include facial dysmorphology, conotruncal heart defects, palatal abnormalities or hypernasality, learning disabilities, and behavioral abnormalities. Phenotypically, VCFS overlaps with DiGeorge syndrome, and both are associated with hemizygous deletion of 22q11.2. Yamagishi et al. (1999) reported that VCFs might be related to the gene *Ufd1*.

The incidence of VCFS is reported to be 1/4000. It is thought to be the most common form of syndromic clefting. Riski et al. (1999) demonstrated that 20% of children with VCFS at two different centers had CP. There is also a high incidence of noncleft hypernasality found in VCFS, which may vary from center to center because of referral patterns. One center, with a high rate of referral from the public schools, found hypernasality in 19/25 (76%) VCFS children without clefts. The second center, with a high rate of referral from a heart center, found hypernasality in only 5/22 (23%) VCFS children without clefts (Riski et al., 1999).

Other investigations have found a high incidence of Chiari malformation, cervical spine anomalies, and neurological deficits in a series of patients with VCFS (Hultman et al., 2000). Four of 16 (25%) children demonstrated Chiari malformation type I, 2/16 (12.5%) had occipitalization of the atlas, 1/16 (8.25%) had spina bifida occulta and subluxation on extension, and

1/16 (8.25%) had narrowing of the foramen magnum with basilar invagination of the odontoid. One patient required suboccipital craniectomy with laminectomy and decompression. Orofacial neurological deficits were identified in 14/41 (34%). Ten demonstrated velar paralysis, which was unilateral in six and bilateral in four.

SUMMARY

The child with an oral cleft or related disorder represents a special challenge. Correct identification and labeling of occult disorders such as noncleft hypernasality requires careful imaging of the velopharynx. Successful evaluation and management of the structural and behavioral problems requires special knowledge, special tools, and most importantly close communication among professionals. While craniofacial teams pride themselves on their skills and expertise, there is an obligation to partner with the community specialist in caring for these children. The past decade has seen a marked advancement in computer and imaging instrumentation. These instruments can provide the clinician with objective measures of velopharyngeal dynamics, including the size, shape, and position of a velopharyngeal opening. Each of these instruments has specific advantages and disadvantages that should be appreciated. It appears that surgical outcome is often improved by applying information obtained from preoperative imaging to patient selection and surgical procedure. Finally, our understanding of speech motor control for the velum is improving. This is leading to a better understanding of appropriate speech therapy and to the development of new management paradigms.

Despite some advances, success rates are not much better than described in reviews from more than two decades ago (Yules and Chase, 1971). This is especially disheartening given the advances in computer instrumentation and imaging during the same time. Surgeons, and possibly teams, are slow to learn from the mistakes of others and appear more content to follow their own learning curve. There appears to be greater improvement in individual results over time than there is in the collective management of hypernasality. Further, a pharyngoplasty is not without risk to the patient. The benefits of pharyngoplasty should be weighed against possible complications.

A number of clinical research challenges remain, including early identification of children who require a pharyngoplasty, development of criteria for selecting a pharyngeal flap or a sphincter pharyngoplasty in individual situations, and management of VPI without creating hyponasality and obstruction. Hyponasality has been considered more socially acceptable than hypernasality, and many consider hyponasality an improvement over hypernasality (Crockett et al., 1988).

A pharyngoplasty should have a physiological basis, and evaluation of velopharyngeal physiology has been the responsibility of the speech pathologist. The clinician is challenged to incorporate available instrumentation into the evaluation process. The clinician may be guided by experience and by documents of the American Speech–Language, Hearing Association and the American Cleft Palate-Craniofacial Association. The American Speech–Language, Hearing Association (1997) offers specific recommendations for the evaluation of nasal resonance and nasal airflow. The American Cleft Palate-Craniofacial Association (1993) offers several recommendations for evaluation and treatment, including "secondary palatal and pharyngeal surgery for velopharyngeal inadequacy should be performed only after evaluation of the velopharyngeal mechanism and review by the team." This includes "in-depth analysis of articulatory performance, aerodynamic measures, videofluoroscopy, nasopharyngoscopy, and nasometric studies, all of which should be conducted with the participation of the team speech–language pathologist."

REFERENCES

Adams, L, Fletcher, S, McCutcheon, M (1989). Cleft palate speech assessment through oral-nasal acoustic measures. In: *Communicative Disorders Related to Cleft Lip and Palate*, 3rd ed., edited by K Bzoch. Boston: College Hill Press, pp. 246–257.

American Cleft Palate-Craniofacial Association (1993). *Parameters for Evaluation and Treatment of Patients with Cleft Lip/Palate or Other Craniofacial Anomalies*. Pittsburgh: American Cleft Palate-Craniofacial Association.

American Speech–Language, Hearing Association (1997). Preferred practice patterns for the profession of speech–language pathology. *Resonance and Nasal Airflow Assessment*. Rockville, MD: Author.

Bardenheur, D (1892). Vorschlage zu plastischen operationen bei chirurgischen eingriffen in der mundhohle. Arch Klin Chir 43: 32.

Becker, M, Svensson, H, Sarnas, K, Jacobsson, S (2000). Von Langenbeck or Wardill procedures for primary palatal repair in patients with isolated cleft palate: speech results. Scand J Plast Reconstr Surg Hand Surg 34: 27–32.

Bell-Berti, F (1976). An EMG study of VP function in speech. J Speech Hear Res 19: 225–240.

Bingham, HG, Suthunyara, P, Richards, S (1972). Should the pharyngeal flap be used primarily with palatoplasty? Cleft Palate J 9: 319.

Blakeley, RW (1972). *The Practice of Speech Pathology: A Clinical Diary*. Springfield, IL: Charles C. Thomas.

Bless, DM, Ewanowski, SJ, Dibbell, DG (1980). A technique for temporary obturation of fistulae: a clinical note. Cleft Palate J 17: 297.

Broen, PA, Doyle, SS, Bacon, CK (1993). The velopharyngeally inadequate child: phonologic change with intervention. Cleft Palate Craniofac J 30: 500–507.

Calnan, JS (1971). Permanent nasal escape after adenoidectmy. Br J Plast Surg 24: 197–204.

Caouette-Laberge, L, Egerszegi, EP, de Remont, AM, Ottenseyer, I (1992). Long-term follow-up after division of a pharyngeal flap for severe nasal obstruction. Cleft Palate Craniofac J 29: 27–31.

Ceponiene, R, Hukki, J, Cheour, M, et al. (1999). Cortical auditory dysfunction in children with oral clefts: relation with cleft type. Clin Neurophysiol 110: 1921–1926.

Chen, PK-T, Wu, JTH, Chen, YR, Noordhoff, S (1994). Correction of velopharyngeal insufficiency in cleft palate patients with the Furlow palatoplasty. Plast Reconstr Surg 94: 933–941.

Crockett, DM, Bumstead, RM, Van Demark, DR (1988). Experience with surgical management of velopharyngeal incompetence. Otolaryngol Head Neck Surg 99: 1–9.

Dalston, RM, Marsh, JL, Vig, KW, et al. (1988). Minimal standards for reporting the results of surgery on patients with cleft lip, cleft palate, or both: a proposal. Cleft Palate J 25: 3.

Dalston, RM, Stutteville, OM (1975). A clinical investigation of the efficacy of primary nasopalatal pharyngoplasty. Cleft Palate J 12: 177.

Dalston, RM, Warren, DW (1986). Comparison of Tonar II, pressure flow, and listener judgements of hypernasality in the assessment of velopharyngeal function. Cleft Palate J 23: 108.

Dalston, RM, Warren, DW, Dalston, ET (1991a). Use of nasometry as a diagnostic tool for identifying patients with velopharyngeal impairment. Cleft Palate J 28: 184.

Dalston, RM, Warren, DW, Dalston, ET (1991b). A preliminary investigation concerning the use of nasometry in identifying patients with hyponasality and/or nasal airway impairment. J Speech Hear Res 34: 11.

de Serres, LM, Deleyiannis, FW, Eblen, LE, et al. (1999). Results with sphincter pharyngoplasty and pharyngeal flap. Int J Pediatr Otorhinolaryngol 48: 17–25.

Dorf, DS, Curtin, JW (1982). Early cleft palate repair and speech outcome. Plast Reconstr Surg 70: 74.

Drew, GS, Tripathi, S, Lehman, JA, Jr (1985). The syndrome of inappropriate secretion of antidiuretic hormone in the pharyngeal flap operation. Cleft Palate J 22: 88–92.

Fletcher, SC (1978). Diagnosing Speech Disorders from Cleft Palate. New York: Grune and Stratton.

Fox, DR, Lynch, JI, Cronin, TD (1988). Change in nasal resonance over time: a clinical study. Cleft Palate J 25: 245.

Fritzell, B (1979). Electromyography in the study of velopharyngeal function: a review. Folia Phoniatr 31: 93–102.

Furlow, LT (1986). Cleft palate repair by double opposing Z-plasty. Plast Reconstr Surg 78: 724–738.

Furlow, LT (1994). Correction of velopharyngeal insufficiency in cleft palate patients with the Furlow palatoplasty. Plast Reconstr Surg 94: 942–943.

Furusawa, K, Yamaoka, M, Ichikawa, N (1994). Responsiveness of single afferents in the infraorbital nerve to oral air pressure generated by consonants. Cleft Palate J 31: 161.

Gereau, SA, Shprintzen, RJ (1988). The role of adenoids in the development of normal speech following palate repair. Laryngoscope 98: 299–303.

Giering, RW, Daubenspeck, JA (1990). Time course of laryngeal aperture response to expiratory resistance loading in humans. Respir Physiol 81: 371–379.

Gilbert, STJ, Pigott, RW (1982). The feasibility of nasal pharyngoscopy using the 70° Storz-Hopkins nasopharyngoscope. Br J Plast Surg 35: 14.

Gonzalez-Baron, S, Dawid-Milner, MS, Lara, JP, Calvijo, E (1989). Changes in laryngeal resistance and bronchial tonus. Rev Esp Fisiol 45: 191–196.

Graiver, MH, Cohen, SR, Kawamoto, HK, Fromwiller, S (1992). A new operation for velopharyngeal insufficiency: the palatoglossus myomucosal flap. Plast Reconst Surg 90: 707–710.

Gunther, E, Wisser, JR, Cohen, MA, Brown, AS (1998). Palatoplasty: Furlow's double reversing Z-plasty versus intravelar veloplasty. Cleft Palate Craniofac J 35: 546–549.

Hairfield, WM, Warren, DW, Seaton, DL (1988). Prevalence of mouthbreathing in cleft lip and palate. Cleft Palate J 25: 135.

Hardin, MA, Van Demark, DR, Morris, HL, Payne, MM (1992). Correspondence between nasalance scores and listener judgements of hypernasality and hyponasality. Cleft Palate J 29: 346.

Harding, R (1984). Function of the larynx in the fetus and newborn. Annu Rev Physiol 46: 645–659.

Hebb, DO (1949). The Organization of Behavior: A Neuropsychological Theory. New York: John Wiley and Sons.

Hirschberg, J, Van Demark, DR (1997). A proposal for standardization of speech and hearing evaluations to assess velopharyngeal function. Folia Phoniatr Logop 49: 158–167.

Hoffman, S (1985). Correction of lateral port stenosis following a pharyngeal flap operation. Cleft Palate J 22: 51–55.

Hogan, VM, Schwartz, MF (1977). Velopharyngeal incompetence. In: Converse, JM Reconstructive Plastic Surgery, 4th ed., edited by JM Converse. Philadelphia: WB Saunders, pp. 2268–2283.

Huang, MH, Lee, ST, Rajendran, K (1997). Structure of the musculus uvulae: functional and surgical implications of an anatomic study. Cleft Palate Craniofac J 34: 466–474.

Hultman, CS, Riski, JE, Cohen, SR, et al. (2000). Chiari malformation, cervical spine anomalies, and neurologic deficits in velocardiofacial syndrome. Plast Reconstr Surg 106: 16–24.

Huskie, CF, Jackson, IT (1977). The sphincter pharyngoplasty—a new approach to the speech problem of velopharyngeal incompetence. Br J Disord Commun 12: 31–35.

Hynes, W (1951). Pharyngoplasty by muscle transposition. Br J Plast Surg 3: 128–135.

Hynes, W (1953). The results of pharyngoplasty by muscle transplantation in "failed cleft palate" cases, with special reference to the influence of the pharynx on voice production. Ann R Coll Surg Engl 13: 17–35.

Ibuki, K, Matsuya, T, Nishio, J, et al. (1978). The course of the facial nerve for the levator veli palatini muscle. Cleft Palate J 15: 209.

Iglesias, A, Kuehn, DP, Morris, HL (1980). Simultaneous assessment of pharyngeal wall and velar displacement for selected speech sounds. J Speech Hear Res 23: 429.

Insalaco, G, Kuna, ST, Costanza, BM, et al. (1991). Thyroarytenoid muscle activity during loaded and nonloaded breathing in adult humans. J Appl Physiol 70: 2410–2416.

Jackson, IT, Silverton, JS (1977). The sphincter pharyngoplasty as a secondary procedure in cleft palates. Plast Reconstr Surg 59: 518–524.

Karnell, MP (1995). Nasometric discrimination of hypernasality and turbulent nasal airflow. Cleft Palate Craniofac J 32: 145–148.

Karnell, MP, Van Demark, DR (1986). Longitudinal speech performance in patients with cleft palate: comparisons based on secondary management. Cleft Palate J 23: 278.

Keuning, KH, Wieneke, GH, Dejonckere, PH (1999). The intrajudge reliability of the perceptual rating of cleft palate speech before and after pharyngeal flap surgery: the effect of judges and speech samples. Cleft Palate Craniofac J 36: 328–333.

Komatsu, Y, Genba, R, Kohama, G (1982). Morphological studies of the velopharyngeal orifice in cleft palate. Cleft Palate J 19: 275.

Kravath, RE, Pollak, CP, Borowiecki, B, Weitzman, ED (1980). Obstructive sleep apnea and death associated with surgical correction of velopharyngeal incompetence. J Pediatr 96: 645–648.

Kuehn, DP (1991). New therapy for treating hypernasal speech using continuous positive airway pressure (CPAP). Plast Reconstr Surg 88: 959–966.

Kuehn, DP, Moon, JB (1994). Levator veli palatini muscle activity in relation to intraoral air pressure variation. J Speech Hear Res 37: 1260–1270.

Kuehn, DP, Moon, JB (1995). Levator veli palatini muscle activity in relation to intraoral air pressure variation in cleft palate subjects. Cleft Palate Craniofac J 32: 376–381.

Kuehn, DP, Moon, JB (2000). Induced fatigue effects on velopharyngeal closure force. J Speech Lang Hear Res 43: 486–500.

Kuehn, DP, Moon, JB, Folkins, JW (1993). Levator veli palatini muscle activity in relation to intranasal air pressure variation. Cleft Palate J 30: 361.

Laitnen, J, Haapanen, ML, Paaso, M, et al. (1998). Occurrence of dental consonant misarticulations in different cleft types. Folia Phoniatr Logop 50: 92–100.

Lohmander-Agerskov, A, Söderpalm, E, Friede, H, et al. (1994). Pre-speech in children with cleft lip and palate or cleft palate only: phonetic analysis related to morphologic and functional factors. Cleft Palate J 31: 271.

MacNeilage, PF (1970). Motor control of serial ordering of speech. Psychol Rev 77: 182–196.

Mason, RM, Warren, DW (1980). Adenoid involution and developing hypernasality in cleft palate. J Speech Hear Dis 45: 469.

Maue-Dickson, W, Dickson, DR (1980). Anatomy and physiology related to cleft palate: current research and clinical implications. Plast Reconstr Surg 65: 83.

Mazaheri, M, Athanasiou, AE, Long, RE (1994). Comparison of velopharyngeal growth between cleft lip and/or palate patients requiring or not requiring pharyngeal flap surgery. Cleft Palate J 31: 452–460.

McBride, B, Whitelaw, WA (1981). A physiologic stimulus to upper airway receptors in humans. J Appl Physiol 51: 1179.

McWilliams, BJ (1991). Submucous clefts of the palate: how likely are they to be symptomatic? Cleft Palate J 28: 247–248.

Mirrett, P, Georgiade, GS, Riski, JE (1993). Tailoring the Sphincter Pharyngoplasty Presented at the April 22 annual meeting of the American Cleft Palate-Craniofacial Association, Pittsburgh, Pennsylvania,

Moon, J, Folkins, JW (1991). The effects of auditory feedback on intraoral air pressure during speech. J Acoust Soc Am 90: 2992–2999.

Morr, KE, Warren, DW, Dalston, RM, et al. (1988). Intraoral pressure measures after experimental loss of velar resistance. Folia Phoniatr 40: 284–289.

Morris, HL (1973). Velopharyngeal competence and primary cleft palate surgery, 1960–1971: a critical review. Cleft Plate J 10: 62.

Moss, AL, Pigott, RW, Albery, EH (1987). Hynes pharyngoplasty revisited. Plast Reconstr Surg 79: 346–355.

Netsell, R (1990). Commentary on maintaining speech pressures in the presence of velopharyngeal impairment regulation. Cleft Palate J 27: 58–60.

Niimi, S, Bell-Berti, F, Harris, KS (1982). Dynamic aspects of velopharyngeal closure. Folia Phoniatr 34: 246.

O'Gara, MM, Logemann, JA (1988). Phonetic analyses of the speech development of babies with cleft palate. Cleft Palate J 25: 122.

O'Gara, MM, Logemann, JA, Rademaker, AW (1994). Phonetic features by babies with unilateral cleft lip and palate. Cleft Palate Craniofac J 6: 446–451.

Orr, WC, Levine, NS, Buchanan, RT (1987). Effect of cleft palate repair and pharyngeal flap surgery on upper airway obstruction during sleep. Plast Reconstr Surg 80: 226–232.

Orticochea, M (1968). Construction of a dynamic muscle sphincter in cleft palates. Plast Reconstr Surg 41: 323–327.

Orticochea, M (1970). Results of the dynamic muscle sphincter operation in cleft palates. Br J Plast Surg 23: 108–114.

Orticochea, M (1983). A review of 236 cleft palate patients treated with dynamic muscle sphincter. Plast Reconstr Surg 71: 180–188.

Pamplona, MC, Ysunza, A, Espinosa, J (1999). A comparative trial of two modalities of speech intervention for compensatory articulation in cleft palate children, phonologic approach versus articulatory approach. Int J Pediatr Otorhinolaryngol 49: 21–26.

Pamplona, MC, Ysunza, A, Uriostegui, C (1996). Linguistic interaction: the active role of parents in speech therapy for cleft palate patients. Int J Pediatr Otorhinolaryngol 37: 17–27.

Pannbacker, MD, Lass, NJ, Hansen, GG, et al. (1993). Survey of speech–language pathologists' training, experience, and opinions on nasopharyngoscopy. Cleft Palate Craniofac J 30: 40–45.

Passavant, G (1862). Ueber die operation der angeborenen spalten des harten gaumens und der damit complicirten hasenscharten. Arch Ohr Nas Kehlkopfheilk 3: 193.

Pensler, JM, Reich, DS (1991). A comparison of speech results after the pharyngeal flap and the dynamic sphincteroplasty procedures. Ann Plast Surg 26: 441–443.

Peterson, SJ (1975). Nasal emission as a component of the misarticulation of sibilants and affricates. J Speech Hear Disord 40: 106.

Pigott, RW (1974). The results of nasopharyngoscopic assessment of pharyngoplasty. Scand J Plast Surg 8: 148.

Pigott, RW (1993). The results of pharyngoplasty by muscle transplantation by Wilfred Hynes. Br J Plast Surg 46: 440–442.

Randall, P, Whitaker, LA, Noone, RB, Jones, WD (1978). The case for the inferiorly-based posterior pharyngeal flap. Cleft Palate J 15: 262–265.

Ren, YF, Isberg, A, Henningsson, G, Larson, O (1992). Tongue posture in cleft palate patients with a pharyngeal flap. Scand J Plast Reconstr Surg Hand Surg 26: 307–312.

Richman, LC, Eliason, MJ, Lindgren, SD (1988). Reading disability in children with clefts. Cleft Palate J 25: 21.

Riski, JE (1979). Articulation skills and oral–nasal resonance in children with pharyngeal flaps. Cleft Palate J 16: 421–428.

Riski, JE (1984). Functional velopharyngeal incompetence: diagnoses and management. In: Treating Articulation Disorders: For Clinicians by Clinicians, edited by H Winitz. Baltimore: University Park Press, pp. 224–234.

Riski, JE (1995). Assessment of speech in adolescents with cleft palate. Cleft Palate J 32: 109–113.

Riski, JE (1996). The relationship of nasal air turbulence and nasalance in speakers with VPI. Presented at the annual meeting of the American Cleft Palate-Craniofacial Association, San Diego, California, April 26.

Riski, JE, DeLong, E (1984). Articulation development in children with cleft lip/palate. Cleft Palate J 21: 57–64.

Riski, JE, Millard, RT (1979). The process of speech evaluation and treatment. In: Cleft palate and cleft lip: A team approach to clinical management and rehabilitation of the patient, edited by HK Cooper, RL Harding, WM Krogman, et al. Philadelphia: WB Saunders, pp. 431–484.

Riski, JE, Cohen, SR, Burstein, F, et al. (1999). Pressure flow and nasometric evaluation of velopharyngeal function in velo-cardio-facial syndrome at two centers. Presented at the annual meeting of the American Cleft Palate-Craniofacial Association, Scottsdale, Arizona, April 16.

Riski, JE, Georgiade, NG, Serafin, D, et al. (1987). The Orticochea pharyngoplasty and primary palatoplasty: an evaluation. Ann Plast Surg 18: 303–309.

Riski, JE, Hoke, JA, Dolan, EA (1989). The role of pressure-flow and endoscopic assessment in successful palatal obturator revision. Cleft Palate J 26: 1.

Riski, JE, Kunze, LH, Mann, J, Nailling, KR (1984a). Speech patterns and disturbances associated with clefts and craniofacial anomalies. In: *Pediatric Plastic Surgery*, edited by D Serafin and NG Georgiade. St. Louis: Mosby, p. 246–258.

Riski, JE, Mason, RM (1994). Adenoid involution as a cause of velopharyngeal incompetence in children with cleft palate. Presented at the annual meeting of the American Cleft Palate-Craniofacial Association, Toronto, Canada.

Riski, JE, Ruff, GL, Georgiade, GS, et al. (1992). Evaluation of the sphincter pharyngoplasty. Cleft Palate Craniofac J 29: 254–261.

Riski, JE, Serafin, D, Riefkohl, R, et al. (1984b). A rationale for modifying the site of insertion of the Orticochea pharyngoplasty. Plast Reconstr Surg 73: 882–894.

Riski, JE, Stewart, M, Mason, R, Simms, C (1996). Analysis of the craniofacial skeleton in cleft palate children with and without adenoids. Program of the annual meeting of the American Cleft Palate-Craniofacial Association, San Diego, California.

Riski, JE, Warren, DW, Lutz, RL, Zajac, D (1995). Application of Perci-SARS for speech evaluation. Study session at the annual meeting of the American Cleft Palate-Craniofacial Association, Tampa, Florida.

Roberts, TMF, Brown, BSJ (1983). Evaluation of a modified sphincter pharyngoplasty in the treatment of speech problems due to palatal insufficiency. Ann Plast Surg 10: 209–213.

Ruscello, DM (1982). A selected review of palatal training procedures. Cleft Palate J 19: 181.

Ruscello, DM (1989). Modifying velopharyngeal closure through training procedures. In: *Communicative Disorders Related to Cleft Lip and Palate*, 3rd ed., edited by K Bzoch. Austin, TX: Pro-Ed, pp. 338–349.

Ruscello, DM (1997). Considerations for behavioral management for velopharyngeal closure for speech. In: *Communicative Disorders Related to Cleft Lip and Palate*, 4th ed., edited by KR Bzoch. Austin, TX: Pro-Ed, pp. 509–528.

Sant'Ambrogio, G, Matthew, OP, Fisher, JT, Sant'Ambrogio, FB (1983). Laryngeal receptors responding to transmural pressure, airflow and local muscle activity. Respir Physiol 54: 317.

Sanvenero-Rosselli, G (1934). Divisione palatina e sua cura chirurgica. Rome: Casa Editrice Luigi Pozzi.

Sedlackova, E (1967). The syndrome of the congenitally shortened velum. The dual innervation of the soft palate. Folia Phoniatr 19: 441–450.

Shelton, RL, Blank, JL (1984). Oronasal fistulas, intraoral air pressure, and nasal air flow during speech. Cleft Palate J 21: 91.

Shprintzen, RJ (1988). Pharyngeal flap surgery and the pediatric upper airway. Int Anesthesiol Clin 26: 79–88.

Shprintzen, RJ, Lencione, RM, McCall, GN, Skolnick, ML (1974). A three dimensional cinefluoroscopic analysis of velopharyngeal closure during speech and nonspeech activities in normals. Cleft Palate J 11: 412–428.

Shprintzen, RJ, Lewin, ML, Croft, CB, et al. (1979). A comprehensive study of pharyngeal flap surgery: tailor-made flaps. Cleft Palate J 16: 46–55.

Shprintzen, RJ, McCall, GN, Skolnick, ML (1980). The effect of pharyngeal flap surgery on the movements of the lateral pharyngeal walls. Plast Reconstr Surg 66: 570–573.

Shprintzen, RJ, McCall, GN, Skolnick, ML, Lencione, RM (1975). Selective movement of the lateral aspects of the pharyngeal walls during velopharyngeal closure for speech, blowing, and whistling in normals. Cleft Palate J 12: 51.

Shprintzen, R, Goldberg, R, Lewin, M, et al. (1978). A new syndrome involving cleft palate, cardiac anomalies, typical facies, and learning disabilities. Cleft Palate J 5: 56–62.

Shprintzen, RJ, Singer, L, Sidoti, EJ, Argamaso, RV (1992). Pharyngeal flap surgery: postoperative complications. Int Anesthesiol Clin 30: 115–124.

Sie, KC, Tampakopoulou, DA, de Serres, LM, et al. (1998). Sphincter pharyngoplasty: speech outcome and complications. Laryngoscope 108: 1211–1217.

Sirois, M, Caouette-Laberge, L, Spier, S, et al. (1994). Sleep apnea following pharyngeal flap: a feared complication. Plast Reconstr Surg 93: 943–947.

Skolnick, ML (1970). Videofluoroscopic examination of the velopharyngeal portal during phonation in lateral and base projections—a new technique for studying the mechanics of closure. Cleft Palate J 7: 803–816.

Skolnick, ML (1975). Velopharyngeal function in cleft palate. Clin Plast Surg 2: 285.

Skolnick, ML, McCall, GN (1972). Velopharyngeal competence and incompetence following pharyngeal flap surgery: videofluoroscopic study in multiple projections. Cleft Palate J 9: 1–12.

Smith, BE, Weinberg, B (1980). Prediction of velopharyngeal orifice size: a re-examination of model experimentation. Cleft Palate J 17: 277.

Smith, BE, Weinberg, B (1982). Prediction of modeled velopharyngeal orifice areas during steady flow conditions and during aerodynamic stimulation of voiceless stop consonants. Cleft Palate J 19: 172.

Stratoudakis, AC, Bambace, C (1984). Sphincter pharyngoplasty for correction velopharyngeal incompetence. Ann Plast Surg 12: 243–248.

Sturim, HS (1974). Bleeding complications with pharyngeal flap construction in humans following Teflon pharyngoplasty. Cleft Palate J 11: 292–294.

Subtelny, JD (1957). A cephalometric study of the growth of the soft palate. J Plast Reconstr Surg 19: 49–62.

Subtelny, JD, Van Hattum, RJ, Myers, BB (1972). Ratings and measures of cleft palate speech. Cleft Palate J 9: 18–27.

Szereda-Przestaszewska, M (1989). Effects of serotonin on laryngeal resistance and respiratory timing in lung denervated rabbits. Mater Med Pol 21: 297–300.

Tachimura, T, Hara, H, Koh, H, Wada, T (1997). Effect of temporary closure of oronasal fistulae on levator veli palatini muscle activity. Cleft Palate Craniofac J 34: 505–511.

Thurston, JB, Larson, DL, Shanks, JC, et al. (1980). Nasal obstruction as a complication of pharyngeal flap surgery. Cleft Palate J 17: 148–154.

Tolman, EC (1932). *Purposive Behavior in Animals and Men*. New York: Century.

Trost, JE (1981). Articulatory additions to the classical description of the speech of persons with cleft palate. Cleft Palate J 18: 193.

Van Demark, DR (1974). A comparison of articulation abilities and velopharyngeal competence between Danish and Iowa children with cleft palate. Cleft Plate J 11: 463.

Van Demark, DR (1979). Predictability of velopharyngeal competency. Cleft Palate J 16: 429.

Van Demark, DR (1997). Diagnostic value of articulation tests with individuals having clefts. Folia Phoniatr Logop 49: 147–157.

Van Demark, DR, Hardin, MA (1985). Longitudinal evaluation of articulation and velopharyngeal competence of patients with pharyngeal flaps. Cleft Palate J 22: 163–172.

Van Demark, DR, Hardin, MA, Morris, HL (1988). Assessment of velopharyngeal competence: a long-term process. Cleft Palate J 25: 362.

Van Demark, RV, Kuehn, DP, Tharp, RF (1975). Prediction of velopharyngeal competency. Cleft Palate J 12: 5–11.

Van Demark, DR, Morris, HL (1983). Stability of velopharyngeal competency. Cleft Palate J 20: 18.

Van Demark, DR, Morris, HL, VandeHaar, C (1979). Patterns of articulation abilities in speakers with cleft palate. Cleft Palate J *16:* 230.

Velasco, MG, Ysunza, A, Hernandez, X, et al. (1988). Diagnosis and treatment of submucous cleft palate: a review of 108 cases. Cleft Palate J *25:* 171.

Wardill, WEM (1928). Results of operation for cleft palate. Br J Surg *16:* 127.

Wardill, WEM (1933). Cleft palate. Br J Surg *21:* 347.

Warren, DW (1984). A quantitative technique for assessing nasal airway impairment. Am J Orthod *86:* 306.

Warren, DW (1986). Compensatory speech behaviors in individuals with cleft palate: a regulation/control phenomenon? Cleft Palate J *23:* 251–260.

Warren, DW, Devereux, JL (1966). An analog study of cleft palate speech. Cleft Palate J *3:* 103.

Warren, DW, Drake, AF, Davis, JU (1992). Nasal airway in breathing and speech. Cleft Palate Craniofac J *29:* 511–519.

Warren, DW, Duany, LF, Fischer, ND (1969). Nasal pathway resistance in normal and cleft lip and cleft palate subjects. Cleft Palate J *6:* 134.

Warren, DW, DuBois, AB (1964). A pressure flow technique for measuring velopharyngeal orifice area during continuous speech. Cleft Palate J *1:* 52.

Warren, DW, Hinton, VA (1983). Compensatory speech behaviors in cleft palate: a regulation/control phenomenon? ASHA *25:* 107.

Warren, DW, Trier, WC, Bevin, AG (1974). Effect of restorative procedures on the nasopharyngeal airway in cleft palate. Cleft Palate J *11:* 367.

Williams, WN (1979). Radiological measures of abnormal speech physiology. In: *Communicative Disorders Related to Cleft Lip and Palate,* edited by KR Bzoch. Boston: Little, Brown, pp. 249–262.

Williams, WN, Eisenbach, OR (1981). Assessing VP function: the lateral still technique vs. cinefluorography. Cleft Palate J *18:* 45.

Witsell, DL, Drake, AF, Warren, DW (1994). Preliminary data on the effect of pharyngeal flaps on the upper airway in children with velopharyngeal inadequacy. Laryngoscope *104:* 12–15.

Wu, JT, Huang, G, Huang, CS, Noordhoff, MS (1996). Nasopharyngoscopic evaluation of cephalometric analysis of velopharynx in normal and cleft palate patients. Ann Plast Surg *36:* 117–123.

Yamagishi, H, Garg, V, Matsuoka, R, et al. (1999). A molecular pathway revealing a genetic basis for human cardiac and craniofacial defects. Science *283:* 1158–1161.

Ysunza, A, Pamplona, MC, Molina, F, et al. (1999). Velopharyngeal motion after sphincter pharyngoplasty: a videonasopharyngoscopic and electromyographic study. Plast Reconstr Surg *104:* 905–910.

Yules, RB, Chase, RA (1971). Secondary techniques for correction of palatopharyngeal incompetence. In: *Cleft Lip and Palate,* edited by K Bzoch, Grabb, Rosenstein. Boston: Little, Brown.

Zaworski, RE (1981). Anorexia nervosa following a pharyngeal flap operation. Cleft Palate J *18:* 223–224.

Zemlin, WR (1997). *Speech and Hearing Science: Anatomy and Physiology,* 4th ed. New York: Prentice-Hall.

Zwitman, DH (1982a). Velopharyngeal physiology after pharyngeal flap surgery as assessed by oral endoscopy. Cleft Palate J *19:* 36–39.

Zwitman, DH (1982b). Oral endoscopic comparison of velopharyngeal closure before and after pharyngeal flap. Cleft Palate J *19:* 40–46.

28

Pediatric dental care

FRANK FARRINGTON

Optimum dental health is essential for the total health of the child. The basic dental care needs of children with oral clefts are the same as those for anyone of the same age, with the addition of the special needs resulting from the cleft. Early evaluation and preventive care are extremely important as the primary and developing permanent dentitions provide the basic framework for future dental, orthodontic, and prosthetic treatment. However, parents are often so overwhelmed by other aspects of their children's care that dental needs are given a rather low priority. Emphasizing the fact that their child with an oral cleft needs the same basic dental care as any child the same age brings an element of normalcy to parents' thinking regarding their children's needs. The dental needs of the child can be divided into four stages, based on oral development, preventive needs, and treatment:

1. The infant and toddler need early assessment, and parents need to be oriented toward the prevention of oral disease.
2. The needs of the child during the primary dentition center around the establishment of regular dental care, assessment of the developing dentition, development of a preventive program, and treatment needs related to the cleft.
3. Mixed dentition presents a time of transition as the child becomes more involved in dental care, including the temporary replacement of missing teeth as well as regular dental care.
4. The needs of the adolescent during the development of the young permanent dentition center around the dental needs associated with supporting orthodontic and prosthetic care.

During each of these stages, the management of the child is a prime concern. Management of the child's be-

havior and attitude toward dental care is as important as the actual dental treatment in the child's overall care. Past dental and medical experience, the age of the child, the extent of care needed, and the child's attitudes and fears must be of major concern in developing a good dental patient. The American Cleft Palate-Craniofacial Association (1993) provides guidelines for the optimum care of individuals with craniofacial anomalies, regardless of the specific type of disorder. The underlying principle of these guidelines is that patients with craniofacial anomalies are best managed by an interdisciplinary team of specialists.

THE INFANT AND TODDLER

The infant should be seen for initial oral evaluation shortly after birth and, preferably, as part of an interdisciplinary team evaluation. Evaluation of factors that may influence surgical management, such as arch form, displacement of the arch segments, and presence of natal or neonatal teeth, needs to be done. Evaluation of airway and feeding problems also needs to be done early. In some programs, the use of an oral appliance is an option as a noninvasive method of management. Dental evaluation and preventive care should begin with this initial team evaluation of the infant. The importance the profession puts on this early evaluation is seen in the American Academy of Pediatric Dentistry (1999) recommendation that all children be seen for a first general dental visit 6 months after the eruption of the first tooth or at 1 year of age, whichever comes first.

The early oral healthcare visit provides the foundation for a lifetime of preventive and corrective dental care and helps to assure optimal oral health during childhood and into adulthood. Oral examination, anticipatory guidance including preventive education, and appropriate therapeutic care are essential during the entire period of oral development, to provide the necessary specialty care needed because of the oral cleft. Following are several recommendations related to infant oral health:

1. Ideally, infant oral healthcare begins with prenatal oral health counseling for parents. An initial oral evaluation should occur within 6 months of the eruption of the first primary tooth and no later than 12 months of age.
2. At the infant oral evaluation visit, the dentist should do the following:
   a. Record a thorough medical and dental history, covering the prenatal, perinatal, and postnatal periods
   b. Complete a thorough oral examination
   c. Assess the patient's risk of developing oral and dental disease and determine an appropriate interval for periodic re-evaluation based on that assessment
   d. Discuss and provide anticipatory guidance regarding dental and oral development, fluoride status, nonnutritive oral habits, injury prevention, oral hygiene, and effects of diet on the dentition
3. Dentists who perform such services for infants should be prepared to provide therapy when indicated or should refer the patient to an appropriately trained individual for necessary treatment (American Academy of Pediatric Dentistry, 1999).

The general development of the dentition is the same in children with and without clefts. Abnormal findings are usually isolated to the areas in and adjacent to the cleft itself. Eruption of the dentition occurs at the usual time and in the usual sequence.

Infant Oral–Facial Orthopedics

The break in the continuity of the alveolar arch may lead to a collapse of the arch segments and the development of anterior and posterior crossbites. Closure of the lip can lead to pressure on the alveolar segments, resulting in remolding of the bony segments and/or collapse of the posterior portions of the arch, creating a unilateral or bilateral crossbite. Depending on the treatment philosophy of the interdisciplinary team and the actual deformity of the alveolar arch, early appliance therapy may be indicated. Use of tape or a combination of tape and orthodontic elastics to close the gap between the anterior and posterior segments of a unilateral cleft allows for less stretching of lip tissue at the

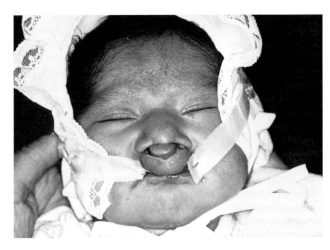

FIG. 28.1. Retraction of the premaxillary segment in a bilateral cleft with tape and elastics.

time of lip repair. In bilateral clefts, the retraction and centering of the premaxillary segment also makes lip closure easier (Fig. 28.1). To prevent collapse of the arch from the tension of the tape or elastics, a palatal prosthesis, essentially a denture base without teeth, can be used. The appliance is usually tolerated well by infants during the period prior to lip repair. If the appliance is used after the lip repair to stabilize the segments or cover the hard palate defect, the eruption of teeth makes retention of the appliance difficult. Intraoral appliances to stabilize and realign cleft segments have been used for over 50 years. McNeil (1950) used a chewing or feeding plate to realign segments. A model of the cleft arch was progressively modified to reposition the segments. As the infant chewed or nursed, the appliance acted similarly to an orthodontic positioner to move the segments. Removable appliances using expansion screws to slowly expand and reposition the dental arch have been used since the 1960s. To gain more control of the movement of segments, Latham (1980) designed an acrylic palatal appliance containing an elaborate combination of screws and hinges, which was anchored to the maxillary palatal shelves with metal pins. A number of variations of pinned palatal appliances have been developed over the years. A modification developed by Mylin used sliding plastic palatal shelves to keep the hard palate defect sealed during expansion (Farrington, 1998) (Fig. 28.2).

Treatment of these crossbites is usually not needed until the child is older. In a few cases, treatment may be advised if there are functional problems associated with the crossbite. The lack of proper anterior development of the maxilla can lead to a pseudo-class III malocclusion. By 2.5 to 3 years of age, the primary dentition should be complete, as it would be in the normal child without a cleft.

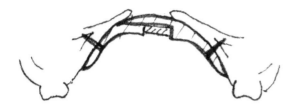

FIG. 28.2. Pinned palatal appliance showing sliding shelves to seal palatal cleft during expansion.

For the child with a cleft, this early evaluation is even more important than for the average child. Erupted natal or neonatal teeth that may be malformed in the area of the cleft need to be identified early. The lateral incisor is located directly in the plane of the suture of the maxillary and premaxillary segments. The primary lateral incisor may be absent or malformed. In some cases, a supernumerary lateral incisor may develop. The tooth may erupt early and can appear anywhere along the cleft line (Figs. 28.3, 28.4).

The teeth on either side of the cleft are at increased risk for caries. Their location makes them hard to keep clean and susceptible to plaque accumulation.

Feeding problems related to the cleft and the surgery over the first year increase the risk for early childhood caries. Concerns that the child is well nourished and comfortable, especially after surgery, may keep the child on the bottle past 10 to 12 months, when it is recommended that the child go to a cup. Parents need to be informed of the problems related to prolonged and ad lib. use of the bottle, especially at naptime and at night.

Streptococcus mutans and lactobacilli are important pathogens in the development of dental caries. Usually,

S. mutans are not detected before eruption of the primary teeth, and there is a gradual increase in the frequency of *S. mutans* with age as the number of teeth increases. Seeding of the organism seems to come from the mother, with the time of greatest infectability being around 18 months of age. If the mother has a high *Streptococcus* count, the child is likely to have a high count as well (Kohler et al., 1979).

Children colonized with *S. mutans* before the age of 2 years run a higher risk of developing dental caries than children colonized with the organism at a later age. Almost 50% of children with oral clefts had been colonized with *S. mutans* and 16% with lactobacilli at the age of 18 months compared to children without clefts, who showed 13% *S. mutans* colonization. Kohler et al. (1983) found that 24% of 15-month-old children with mothers who had high levels of *S. mutans* were colonized with *S. mutans*.

Children with clefts who took a bottle to bed have shown an increased risk for developing early childhood or nursing bottle caries. In a study by Lin and Tsai (1999), 39% of children reported a bottle-feeding habit. The overall prevalence of baby bottle nursing caries was 15.4%. The decayed–extracted–filled primary teeth (def) scores of bottle-fed children were significantly higher than those of children who were not bottle-fed. Parents and caregivers of bottle-fed babies showed a lack of motivation to perform regular preventive dental home care. Parents of non-bottle-fed children demonstrated significantly better dental care than parents of bottle-fed children regarding brushing frequency and brushing before bed.

Dental treatment of the infant and toddler centers on evaluation, prevention, education of parents, and man-

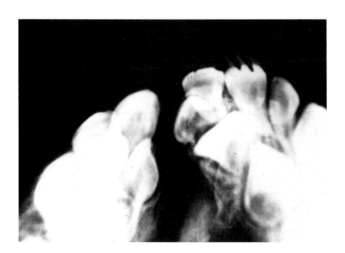

FIG. 28.3. Radiography of unilateral cleft showing a wide defect in the area of the lateral incisor, which is shown with no supporting bone on the entire mesial surface.

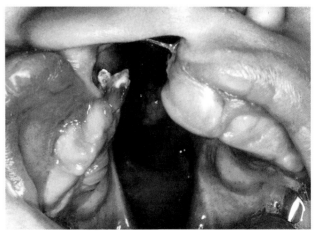

FIG. 28.4. Unilateral cleft lip and palate showing a malformed tooth erupting ectopically along the cleft margin.

agement of dental problems resulting from the cleft. Prevention of dental disease is a major goal. The fluoride content of the child's water supply needs to be evaluated early. If the water supply has less than the optimum of 0.7 to 1.2 ppm, supplementation needs to be considered at 6 months of age. The level of supplementation is based on the fluoride level of the water and the child's age. A number of families use bottled water for drinking and cooking. If the child's major water intake is from nonfluoridated bottled water, complete or partial supplementation needs to be considered. The bottled water label usually will not indicate if the water is fluoridated. As soon as the first teeth erupt, parents should be instructed to clean them with a cloth when bathing the child.

Anticipatory Guidance

Anticipatory guidance, as used in pediatric health care, is the process of providing practical, developmentally appropriate health information about children to their parents in anticipation of significant physical, emotional, and psychological milestones. This information guides parents by alerting them to impending change, teaching them their role in maximizing their children's developmental potential, and identifying their children's special needs.

Areas of concern in anticipatory guidance in pediatric dentistry are oral development, fluoride adequacy, oral hygiene and diet, habits, nutrition, and injury prevention. Early evaluation and education of the parents as to the dental needs of their child is extremely important if comprehensive dental care is to be provided (Nowak and Casamassimo, 1995).

Special Needs

A small number of infants with cleft palate also present with glossoptosis, resulting in difficulty in managing the airway. Usually, this is a transitory problem that resolves itself in a short time as the child grows. Oral appliances to assist in the maintenance of an airway can be used in some cases, thus alleviating the need for other techniques, such as long-term intubation or tracheotomy. Appliances similar to denture bases without teeth have been developed. Impressions can be taken with either alginate or compound. Alginate gives a clearer impression of the cleft defect but runs the risk of material being left in the defect. Compound does not give as detailed an impression but is easier to remove when set. For short-term use, it is usually not necessary to use the undercuts of the defect for retention. With the use of denture adhesive as needed, the appliance does not have to extend into the cleft. The pur-

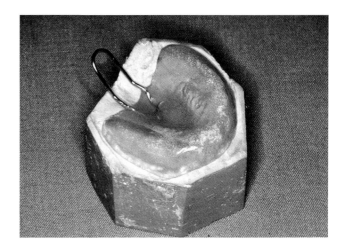

FIG. 28.5. Basic palatal appliance with posterior wire loop to hold tongue down.

pose in managing the airway is to use the appliance to hold endotracheal tubes or a wire loop extending posteriorly to hold the tongue forward off the posterior pharyngeal wall. The tube not only holds the tongue forward but also establishes a mechanical airway (Farrington, 1998). Once the basic appliance is complete, a loop of orthodontic wire can be attached with acrylic (Fig. 28.5). The exact length of the wire and amount of curvature will vary in each case. As a starting point, the wire loop should extend posterior to the appliance to a length that is about the same as the anterior–posterior length of the appliance. An endotracheal tube can be attached to the appliance by forming self-cure acrylic around a well-lubricated tube (Fig. 28.6). The tube should be of the same size as one that would be used to intubate that child. The natural curve will help to direct the tube down behind the tongue (Fig. 28.7).

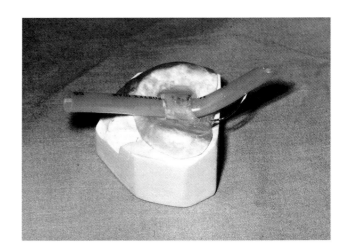

FIG. 28.6. Basic palatal appliance with endotracheal tube added to aid in maintaining airway.

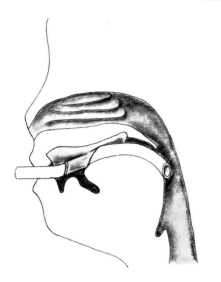

FIG. 28.7. Position of appliance showing the endotracheal tube extending over the tongue to maintain the airway.

Starting with the tube extending about the same length posterior to the appliance as with the wire loop, it can be extended or retracted as needed. The tube should extend back as far as the child will allow. At this point, it should be retracted a few millimeters. In some cases, use of a tube and a wire loop may be considered. The wire loop extends behind the tube and is used to increase the curvature of the tube and to keep it from irritating the posterior pharyngeal wall. The effectiveness of the appliance can be measured using a pulse oxymeter to measure saturation levels with and without the appliance.

PRIMARY DENTITION

As mentioned before, prevention and caries control are the same for the child with a cleft as for other children at the same age and state of development. Hence, more frequent recalls, at 3- to 4-month intervals, may be necessary to monitor oral health. Topical fluoride needs to be professionally applied regularly. In areas without optimal water fluoridation, prescription fluoride supplements should be considered. Use of pit and fissure sealants should be considered in selected cases. Oral hygiene instructions and dietary advice must be checked and reinforced.

Restorative care should be provided before carious lesions become extensive. Loss of a single tooth can complicate the overall treatment. Use of stainless steel crowns on carious primary teeth should be considered, especially if the tooth is to be banded as part of appliance therapy (King and Wei, 1988).

Establishment of a fairly normal occlusion is the overall dental goal. The pure mechanics of treatment must be tempered by the behavioral development and ability of the child to accept treatment and cooperate (Farrington, 1998).

Close supervision is needed because of the added risk the child has for dental disease, especially in the area of the cleft. Parents initially, and the child at the appropriate age, should be instructed in proper oral hygiene techniques. Ectopic eruption of teeth in the area of the cleft and redundant gingival and alveolar tissue make good plaque control difficult (Figs. 28.8, 28.9). Children with cleft lip and/or palate have more decayed and filled teeth in the primary dentition than do children without clefts. Almost 50% of children with an oral cleft had *S. mutans* colonization by 18 months of age. This compares with studies of children without clefts, who had colonization rates of between 13% and 36%. Such early colonization indicates a high risk for dental caries in the primary dentition for children with cleft lip and/or palate (Bokhout et al., 1996).

Eruption of the primary dentition and occlusal development need to be followed closely. A high incidence of natal/neonatal teeth was found in unilateral (2.02%) and bilateral (10.6%) cleft groups. The findings in both groups were higher than the incidence reported in a noncleft group (0.05%) (Machado de Almeida and Gomide, 1996).

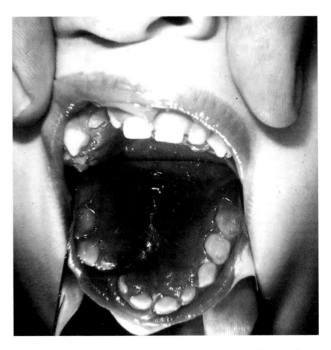

FIG. 28.8. Eruption of the lateral incisor into the site of the cleft, resulting in a crossbite; poor plaque control increases the risk of cervical caries.

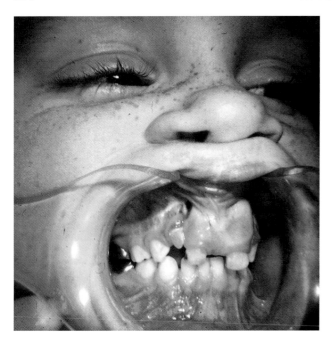

FIG. 28.9. The alveolar defect has resulted in the lateral incisor failing to properly erupt into occlusion.

Dental treatment at this age centers on prevention, caries control, and support for the other disciplines involved. This includes removal of malformed teeth and replacement of teeth that may be needed to help with speech therapy. Occasionally, a child will be seen with an unrepaired hard palate or a hard palate fistula that cannot be closed.

A major concern should be patient management. The small child does not always distinguish between the examination and treatment of the various team members. To the young child, there is no difference between dental treatment and other care that involves the face and oral cavity. This is of special concern when the child needs restorative or oral surgical care. If the child needs extensive restorative care, consideration should be given to combining the dental care with some other surgical care, such as ear, nose, and throat surgery. In treating any young child where behavior is an issue, consideration should be given to restoration with stainless steel crowns on primary molars rather than alloys or composites. The goal in the restoration of any primary tooth should be that, with proper oral hygiene, a tooth should have to be restored only once.

MIXED DENTITION

With the eruption of the first permanent molars, caries of the occlusal surfaces and morphological defects that require restoration or sealing may be expected (McDonald et al., 2000). Gray et al. (1991) found that the best predictor of dental caries in the first permanent molars of 7-year-olds was caries in three or more primary molars by 5 years of age.

Eruption of the permanent dentition during the elementary school years must be carefully observed. In boys with unilateral cleft lip and palate, eruption of the permanent maxillary lateral incisors and the permanent maxillary second molar is retarded on the cleft side. In boys with bilateral cleft lip and palate, the highest retardation of eruption was found in the permanent maxillary lateral incisor and the permanent maxillary first molar (Peterka et al., 1996). Ectopic eruption of both primary and permanent incisors is common. Lateral incisors may erupt in the cleft defect without periodontal support. These teeth are usually very unstable, are lost prematurely, or have to be extracted (Fig. 28.10).

Dental treatment centers on caries control, temporary replacement of missing teeth, general dental care, and support for the other services involved in the child's care. Preventive care centers on the expanded use of fluorides and occlusal sealants. Plaque control in the areas of the cleft can be difficult, and following surgery or grafts, the child and parents may be reluctant to adequately clean the areas. Prevention at this age is marked by acceptance of increasing responsibility by children for their own oral health. Parental involvement is still needed; however, the parents' role moves from one of performing the child's oral hygiene to that of active supervision. By the start of middle school, most children can provide their own basic oral hygiene. Parents do need to actively inspect the results of their children's oral hygiene practices. As the child gets older, home-applied fluoride gels and rinses need to be considered, especially in children with poor plaque control

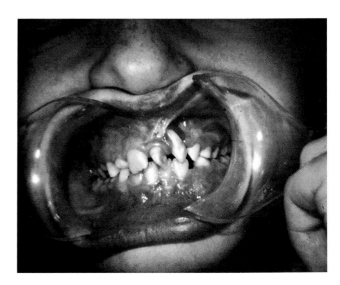

FIG. 28.10. The alveolar defect has resulted in the lateral incisor erupting into the arch without periodontal support. Note the rotation of the central incisor and the scar tissue from the lip repair.

and a history of caries. The child must be able to follow instructions and properly expectorate before home-applied gels and rinses should be introduced. Fluoride rinses have been shown to be very effective when orthodontic and prosthetic appliances are used and plaque control is difficult (McDonald et al., 2000).

Alveolar grafts are usually carried out as the permanent maxillary canines begin their initial eruption. The graft provides a bed of bone into which the canine on the cleft side can erupt. Prior to grafting, expansion of the maxillary arch to correct crossbites and to align the alveolar segments is usually completed. Appliances to stabilize the arch, such as a transpalatal arch, may be placed for retention. It is critically important that oral hygiene and home care be excellent to reduce caries risk factors. Use of sealants on teeth being banded, especially molars, and frequent checking for loose bands are essential in caries prevention.

As the child grows older, appearance and replacement of missing teeth become more important to the child and parents. Removable and fixed appliances each have drawbacks. Removable appliance use for long-term tooth replacement has problems of compliance and proper care by the preteen child. Loss of appliances, when removed for eating and sports at school, is common. The frequently changing dentition at this age affects the fit and comfort of removable appliances. Fixed appliances, such as the lingual arch to hold replacement teeth, work well at this age (Figs. 28.11, 28.12). Compliance issues are removed, but oral hygiene and increased caries risk become concerns. Banding permanent molars increases caries risk and makes oral hygiene more difficult; however, if the risk is recognized and a sound preventive program established, these appliances are very effective. When possible, consideration should be given to banding second primary molars instead of permanent molars. Although the

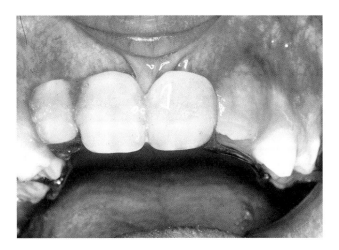

FIG. 28.12. Maxillary lingual arch in place. Note the partial-eruption appearance of the lateral incisor to match the contralateral side.

caries and hygiene problems still exist, the long-term risk is reduced.

YOUNG PERMANENT DENTITION

The dental needs of the adolescent with a cleft are similar to the needs of children of the same age without a cleft except for the additional facial and oral problems caused by the cleft. Care mainly centers on the repair of malformed teeth and the replacement of missing teeth. Many children in this age group undergo orthodontic treatment. Incorporation of prosthetic teeth is an easy way to temporarily replace teeth and give the child an appearance similar to that of his or her peers (Figs. 28.13–28.15).

Dental caries continue to be the major dental infectious disease problem for adolescents. A rise in the caries attack rate continues with the eruption of the

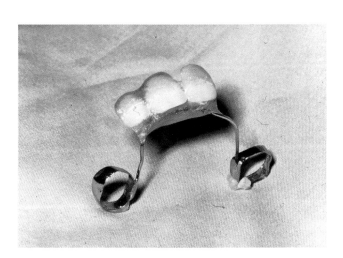

FIG. 28.11. Maxillary lingual arch with prosthetic teeth attached.

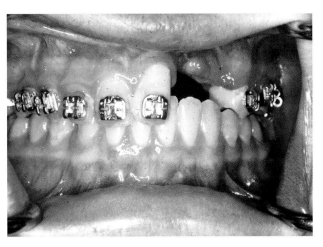

FIG. 28.13. During orthodontic treatment, a large space has been created due to missing teeth in the area of the cleft.

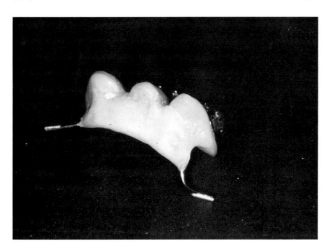

FIG. 28.14. Prosthetic teeth to be incorporated into an orthodontic appliance. The acrylic ridge overlap and lingual wires prevent the teeth from rotating on the arch wire.

second permanent molars and premolars. Adolescents are still prone to tooth decay. Immature permanent teeth, an increase in susceptible tooth surfaces, and factors such as diet, independence in seeking or avoiding care, poor oral hygiene practices, and failure to comply with preventive recommendations contribute to dental and periodontal disease.

The adolescent can still benefit from fluoride throughout the teenage years. Although the systemic benefit of fluoride for developing enamel is not considered necessary after the age of 16, the topical benefits of remineralization and antimicrobial activity still can be obtained through water fluoridation, professionally applied or prescribed fluoride, and fluoridated toothpaste.

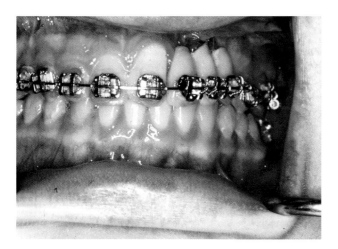

FIG. 28.15. Prosthetic teeth wired into place in the orthodontic appliance.

The American Academy of Pediatric Dentistry (1999) recommends that the adolescent benefit from a preventive dental program consisting of the following:

1. Fluorides
   a. Systemic fluoride intake via optimal fluoridation of drinking water or professionally prescribed supplements to age 16 years or eruption of the second permanent molars is needed.
   b. A fluoride dentifrice is recommended, to provide continuous topical fluoride benefit.
   c. Regular professionally applied fluoride treatments through adolescence should be based on the individual patient's caries pattern and fluoride status of the community water.
   d. Topical supplementation by home-applied fluoride is indicated by an individual's dental caries pattern or caries risk.
2. Oral Hygiene and Diet Management
   a. Adolescents should be educated and motivated to maintain personal oral hygiene through daily plaque removal, including flossing. Professional cleaning and calculus removal is recommended, with a frequency determined by the dentist.
   b. Dietary analysis and management should consider dental disease patterns, overall nutrient and energy needs, psychological aspects of adolescent nutrition, dietary carbohydrate intake, and wellness.
3. Sealants
   Pit and fissure sealants can be of significant benefit. The occlusal surfaces of second permanent molars are highly prone to caries. Sealants are an effective decay-preventing measure that should be used on an individual basis.

PERIODONTAL DISEASE

Adolescence seems to be a critical period in periodontal health. Data suggest that irreversible periodontal damage begins in late adolescence and early adulthood. Pubertal changes characteristically affect the periodontium with an increase in inflammation, which in most cases is managed by oral hygiene and professional care. Periodontal disease in patients with cleft palate is similar in extent to the general population. Patients with cleft lip, palate, and alveolus had a predisposition to deep periodontal destruction of teeth adjacent to the cleft (Schultes et al., 1999).

Crowded or malpositioned teeth, hypertrophic gingiva, orthodontic appliances, and prosthetic replacements can impede proper plaque removal and thus perpetuate periodontal disease. It is important to incorporate periodontal treatment into the comprehensive treatment as early as possible.

MISSING TEETH

A significant concern in the dental care of the adolescent with a craniofacial cleft is missing teeth. As part of the team evaluation, the permanent replacement of missing teeth must be considered. As the permanent dentition is complete, decisions as to how to replace missing teeth must be made. Temporary replacement of anterior teeth, usually maxillary lateral incisors, may continue to be needed during orthodontic care or during the period of alveolar and periodontal grafting, to establish the continuity of the dental arch. Pontics may be incorporated into orthodontic appliances, and teeth may be replaced with removable or fixed appliances, such as acid etch bridges. Use of dental implants is becoming a standard of care for single tooth replacement. Although implants have been placed in the early teen years, this treatment is usually delayed until late adolescence, when growth and development, surgical treatment, and orthodontic care are complete.

Caring for the adolescent patient with a cleft is a rewarding endeavor. Science is unable to provide a decisive answer to many of the questions that guide treatment, so it becomes obligatory to let the patient have an expanded role in determining the course of treatment. This may require spending time listening to a patient who may not want to tell us anything at the time we want to hear it. With more time and more patience, a course can usually be plotted which will get both the practitioner and the patient to a desired destination (Canady, 1995).

Periodontal therapy should be an integral part of the total restoration of the function and esthetics of the cleft palate patient. Periodontal treatment should begin early and continue as supportive therapy.

The amount of periodontal destruction is more pronounced in the cleft lip and palate patient than in noncleft patients. Bacterial plaque accumulation is enhanced due to irregularly positioned teeth or displaced teeth, difficulty in closing the lips, mouth breathing, and inadequate personal oral hygiene care. It is important to appreciate the etiology of periodontal disturbances in cleft lip and palate patients so that periodontal disease can be diagnosed early and treatment initiated and maintained before, during, and after surgical, orthodontic, and prosthetic treatments (Santi et al., 1995).

In prosthetic treatment of cleft lip and palate patients, it is imperative to prevent regression and collapse of the alveolar segments and teeth after surgical and orthodontic correction, but it is also important that the treatment provide equal functional loading capabilities for the upper and lower jaws. Accordingly, some of the teeth in the upper jaw must be splinted across the cleft, to increase the functional loading capability and to prevent regression. Use of multiple-unit fixed prostheses, however, may create a number of problems, including extensive loss of sound tooth structure and increased difficulty with oral hygiene. It is desirable to include as few teeth as possible in the fixed prosthesis (Suzuki et al., 1995). Single tooth implants can be considered when esthetically and functionally restoring the dental arch. Cosmetically, the single tooth replacement is more acceptable than a multiunit bridge. Tooth structure is spared on healthy adjacent teeth, and the problem presented by large pulp chambers on abutment teeth in teenage patients is circumvented. A possible disadvantage is the necessity of adequate graft height and width to support the implant. In the case of placement of implants in grafted sites, it seems likely that the success of osseointegration would approach that of implants in nongrafted areas. Early failure of the implant should be evident in the first year after implantation (Verdi et al., 1991).

Once the permanent dentition has erupted and facial growth is complete, treatment of the adolescent is directed at prosthetic care to permanently replace missing teeth. The reason teeth are missing is not as important at this stage as the design and construction of the prosthesis.

FAMILY SUPPORT

There are a number of excellent resources available to the family that provide information on the management of the child's oral health needs. The American Academy of Pediatric Dentistry web site provides information to parents, children, and professionals regarding proper oral health care for children of all ages. The American Dental Association also has an extensive array of information for the lay public and professionals on all aspects of oral healthcare, new products, and research. The American Dental Association can be contacted by phone, mail, or through its web site. The information available from these organizations addresses children with special needs but is basically directed at the needs of the average child. There are two organizations providing programs and support specifically related to individuals with cleft defects and other facial differences: *(1)* AboutFace in Canada (http://www.interlog.com/~abtface/aface.html) and AboutFace U.S.A. (http://www.interlog.com/~abtface/AUSA.html) and *(2)* the American Cleft Palate-Craniofacial Association (http://www.cleftline.org). The goal of the foundation is to provide information to parents of newborns with clefts and other craniofacial birth defects and to healthcare professionals. Both organizations provide a wealth of information through published material, web sites, and chapters throughout the United States and Canada. A major service these organizations offer parents and families is the opportunity to interact with parents of other children with similar problems. Chances for new parents to talk or correspond with others who "have been there" can help. The opportunity to see children who have been through the various levels of surgery and the results that may seem impossible to achieve when the newborn is first seen can help parents and other family members adjust to the initial trauma of this unexpected problem.

Regardless of the interaction an individual has in the oral healthcare of a child with a craniofacial defect, the goal of all those involved is to provide the general and specialty care needed for the child to pass through the various stages of oral development as easily and normally as possible.

REFERENCES

Ameican Academy of Pediatric Dentistry (2001). American Academy of Pediatric Dentistry Reference Manual 2000–01. Pediatr Dent 22. Guidelines for Dental Health of the Adolescent, pp. 52–54.

American Cleft Palate-Craniofacial Association (1993). *Parameters for Evaluation and Treatment of Patients with Cleft Lip/Palate or Other Craniofacial Anomalies.* Pittsburgh: American Cleft Palate-Craniofacial Association.

Bokhout, B, van Loveren, C, Xavier, F, et al. (1996). Prevalence of *Streptococcus mutans* and lactobacilli in 18-month-old children with cleft lip and/or palate. Cleft Palate Craniofac J 33: 5, pp. 424–428.

Canady, J (1995). Emotional effects of plastic surgery on the adolescent with a cleft. Cleft Palate Craniofac J 32: 2, pp. 120–124.

Farrington, FH (1998). Management of the child with cleft lip and palate. In: *Clinical Dentistry,* Vol. 2, edited by J Clark. St. Louis: Mosby, Chapter 14, pp. 1–18.

Gray, MM, Marchment, MD, Anderson, RJ (1991). The relationship between caries experience in the deciduous molars at 5 years and in first molars of the same child at 7 years. Community Dent Health 8: 3–7.

King, NM, Wei, SH (1988). The management of children with cleft lip and palate. In: *Pediatric Dentistry—Total Patient Care,* edited by SH Wei. Philadelphia: Lea and Febiger, pp. 374–387.

Kohler, B, Bratthall, D, Krasse, B (1979). Intrafamilial levels of *Strep. mutans* and some aspects of the bacterial transmission. Scand J Dent Res 86: 35–42.

Kohler, B, Bratthall, D, Krasse, B (1983). Preventive measures in mothers influence the establishment of the bacterium *Streptococcus mutans* in their infants. Arch Oral Biol 28: 225–231.

Latham, RA (1980). Orthopedic advancement of the cleft maxillary segment: a preliminary report. Cleft Palate J 17: 227–233.

Lin, YJ, Tsai, C (1999). Caries prevalence and bottle-feeding practices in 2-year-old children with cleft lips, cleft palate, or both in Taiwan. Cleft Palate Craniofac J 36: 622–626.

Machado de Almeida, C, Gomide, MR (1996). Prevalence of natal/ neonatal teeth in cleft lip and palate infants. Cleft Palate Craniofac J 33: 4. pp. 397–399.

McDonald, RE, Avery, DR, Stookey, GK (2000). Dental caries in the child and adolescent. In: *Dentistry for the child and adolescent,* edited by RE McDonald and DR Avery. St. Louis: Mosby, pp. 209–246.

McNeil, CK (1950). Orthopedic procedures in the treatment of congenital cleft palate. Dent Rec 70: 126–132.

Nowak, AJ, Casamasssimo, PS (1995). Using anticipatory guidance to provide early dental intervention. J Am Dent Assoc 126: 1156–1163.

Peterka, M, Peterlpva, R, Likovsky, Z (1996). Timing of exchange of the maxillary deciduous and permanent teeth in boys with three types of orofacial clefts. Cleft Palate Craniofac J 33: 4, pp. 318–323.

Santi, E, Weinberg, MA, Abitol, TE (1995). Periodontal and prosthetic treatment of a cleft lip and palate patient: a case report. Cleft Palate Craniofac J 32: 4, pp. 346–349.

Schultes, G, Gaggl, A, Karcher, H (1999). Comparison of periodontal disease in patients with clefts of palate and patients with unilateral clefts of lip, palate, and alveolus. Cleft Palate Craniofac J 36: 4, pp. 322–327.

Suzuki, R, Taniguchi, H, Ohyama, T (1995). Prosthodontic abutment in four patients with unilateral cleft lip and palate. Cleft Palate Craniofac J 32: 5, pp. 346–349.

Verdi, FJ, Lanzi, GL, Cohen, SR, Powell, R (1991). Use of the Branemark implant in the cleft palate patient. Cleft Palate Craniofac J 28: 3, pp. 301–304.

29

Role of the orthodontist in the management of patients with cleft lip and/or palate

ANDREW C. LIDRAL

KATHERINE W. L. VIG

The role of the orthodontist on a cleft palate team was defined when the cleft palate team approach was recognized as the most appropriate method to manage the care of patients with facial clefts. In the past, individuals with clefts and craniofacial anomalies underwent a succession of evaluations and hospitalizations by their independent caregivers. This individualized delivery of care was considered in the best interest of the patients in spite of additional hospital admissions and general anesthetics. However, this led to the fragmentation of care and higher costs and risks. A team approach for providing care has been developed and is the contemporary standard endorsed by the American Cleft Palate Association, which was established in 1943. In 1972, craniofacial teams became established as an extension to the cleft palate team, and the organization was renamed the American Cleft Palate–Craniofacial Association. This was a natural development to the cleft palate team as clinical geneticists and dysmorphologists became increasingly aware that facial clefts were part of a phenotypic spectrum of craniofacial anomalies (Shprintzen et al., 1985).

The team approach to comprehensive care requires the orthodontist to work in a collaborative way to determine the timing and sequencing of treatment interventions. This patient-centered care by an interactive and evidence-based team of caregivers provides the basis for a rational approach to diagnosis and treatment planning and delivery. Because there are multiple methods and alternative treatment interventions available, the team approach to management requires that pa-

tients and their parents be aware of the choices with a risk/cost/benefit appraisal so that they can make an informed decision, understanding the consequences of the different options available, especially in light of emerging technologies and treatment modalities for which long-term outcomes are not available. The "Parameters for evaluation and treatment of patients with cleft lip/palate or other craniofacial anomalies," which was the product of a consensus conference on recommendations for the care of patients with craniofacial anomalies, serves as a guideline for the clinical management of these anomalies in a patient-oriented manner (American Cleft Palate-Craniofacial Association, 1993).

The purpose of this chapter is to discuss the orthodontic management of the patient with cleft lip and/or palate in the context of a team approach. Orthodontic intervention should be confined to discrete stages in skeletodental development of the craniofacial complex and should not be considered a continuum of treatment from birth to adulthood.

THE TEAM APPROACH

The timing and sequencing of orthodontic care may conveniently be divided into four distinct developmental periods. These are defined by age and dental development and should be considered time frames for the accomplishment of specific objectives. This avoids the all too common tendency to allow an early phase of treatment intervention to extend through childhood

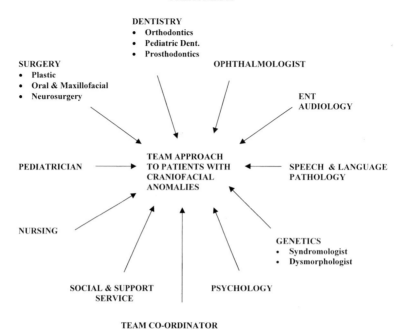

FIG. 29.1. Members of a cleft palate-craniofacial team.

into adolescence and beyond. The timing and sequencing of orthodontic treatment are not carried out in isolation from other members of the team but as a result of collaborative decisions made in a coordinated manner (Fig. 29.1). Several texts provide specific details of treatment intervention, but the overall care of affected infants should rely on team decisions rather than a series of conflicting events sequenced by individual specialists on a team (Surgeon General's Report, 1987). The orthodontist serving on a cleft palate team should consider additional priorities other than malocclusion. The timing and sequencing of treatment should be sensitive to other interventions by specialists on the team, to provide the affected individual with a patient-centered interdisciplinary approach that follows critical pathways (Vig and Turvey, 1985; Turvey et al., 1995). These have been well defined in a document on critical elements of care for children with special health problems, which was developed by the Washington State Department of Health (1997). These guidelines were developed through a consensus process including primary and tertiary care providers, family members, and representatives from a health plan.

With the understanding that children born with cleft lip and/or palate should be treated by an interdisciplinary team approach, the following four time periods in the child's development will be used as a framework for discussing and recommending defined objectives in the care of this special group of patients.

THE NEONATE

Presurgical orthopedics or neonatal maxillary orthopedics typically is initiated during the first week following birth unless there are complications due to other congenital anomalies or medical problems (Burston, 1958; McNeil, 1964; Pruzansky, 1964; Jolleys and Robertson, 1972; Hotz et al., 1978; Rosenstein et al., 1982). This treatment is usually carried out by the orthodontist, the pediatric dentist, or the prosthodontist. The goals of presurgical orthopedics are to align both the soft and hard tissues of the cleft segments to approximate the normal neonatal anatomy. This would presumably facilitate closure of the cleft lip and result in fewer postoperative complications such as dehiscence and scarring. In addition, for surgeons advocating primary bone grafting or periosteoplasty, infant orthopedics is a necessity to allow for closure of the alveolar segments. Claims have also been made that restoring the anatomy to normal leads to normalization of future growth. The popularity of infant orthopedics and primary bone grafting was at its height in the 1960s (Long et al., 2000), but reports that primary bone grafting adversely affected the potential growth of the midface and that no long-term benefit was achieved led to a decrease in the use of infant orthopedics by most teams as a routine intervention before surgical lip repair (Pruzansky, 1964; Jolleys and Robertson, 1972; Hotz et al., 1978; Millard et al., 1999). Furthermore, studies comparing various treatment regimens suggested that neonatal maxillary orthopedics produced little effect on developing malocclusions if assessed when the child was 10 years old, especially if treatment had included primary bone grafting to stabilize and prevent maxillary collapse in the infant (Molsted et al., 1993).

However, as an adjunctive procedure to primary definitive lip repair, the procedure was recognized by plastic surgeons as having benefits and its popularity has recently returned but with objectives different from eliminating orthodontic treatment later in development. Specifically, nasal molding has been advocated as a mechanism to restore normal nasal symmetry and anatomy, while eliminating the need for future nasal revisions. Numerous articles regarding neonatal orthopedics have been published, and the enthusiasm of many clinicians in this field attests to the variety and complexity of the appliances created (Molsted et al., 1993; Winters and Hurwitz, 1995; Grayson et al., 1999). The one feature that all of these appliances have in common is that they adjust the position of the cleft segments into a more ideal relationship prior to definitive surgical repair of the lip (Fig. 29.2). Some are fixed using pins inserted into the maxilla (Millard et al., 1999). This requires at least two general anesthesia procedures, and there is the risk of damaging a developing tooth bud by the inserted pin. This remains a controversial topic, although there are several institutions that continue neonatal maxillary orthopedics and primary bone grafting with substantial benefits reported (Rosenstein et al., 1982; Millard et al., 1999). However, the emerging evidence is only of short-term benefit for presurgical orthopedic appliances, and this needs to be weighed against the increased burden of care due to the multiple number of clinic visits necessary to adjust the appliance during the first year of life (Ross and MacNamera, 1994; Santiago et al., 1998; Severens et al., 1998; Grayson et al., 1999). Long-term outcomes assessing the growth of the midface and both nasal and lip esthetics will be necessary to determine the benefits of presurgical orthopedics and nasal molding.

Although neonatal maxillary orthopedics continues to be practiced in a number of centers in both the United States and Europe, it is not generally considered an essential or desirable routine intervention for treatment of the infant with a cleft. Nonetheless, the molding of segments achieved by these appliances does make definitive lip repair easier for the plastic surgeon, especially in patients with a severely protruding premaxilla due to a bilateral cleft lip (Vig and Turvey, 1985).

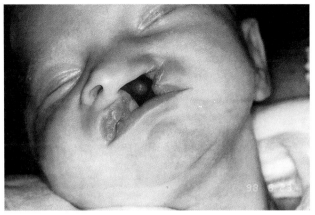

A

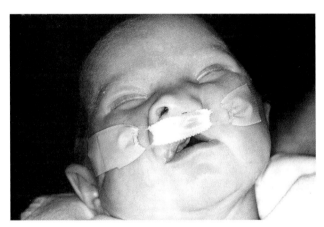

B

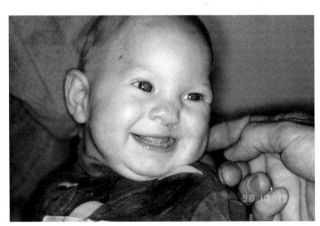

C

FIG. 29.2. *A:* Neonate with complete unilateral cleft lip and palate. *B:* Neonatal with presurgical orthopedics via lip taping to approximate the segments before cleft lip repair. *C:* Postsurgical view of definitive lip repair.

Surgical lip adhesion in infancy is another technique employed to align the segments, yielding results similar to those obtained with infant orthopedic appliances. When the segments have been aligned following lip adhesion, definitive lip repair, including ensuring muscle continuity, is performed. This early surgical repair of the lip by an adhesion technique has much to commend it as the parents are not required to remove or adjust appliances, the cosmetic appearance is improved with a relatively minor initial surgical procedure, and postoperative care by the parents is minimal. The most serious problem with this approach is the potential of wound dehiscence and the need for an additional surgery (Hotz et al., 1978). Currently, lip adhesion is not universally accepted as a method of realigning the segments before definitive repair of the lip.

Although definitive repair of the lip is usually achieved by the time the infant is 3 to 6 months old, repair of the palate is typically delayed until 12 months to 2 years of age. This is also a controversial issue, and many methods are available for repairing either just the soft palate or both the hard and soft palate simultaneously. The rationale for the timing of palatal repair is related to the speech and language development of the child, which is usually in conflict with the effect of early surgical repair and the constraints of scar tissue on the growth and development of the maxillary complex

(Long et al., 2000). Early repair of the palate may have a profound effect on the developing maxilla and dentition. The most common malocclusion of patients who have had repair of a cleft lip or palate is a dental crossbite of anterior and/or posterior teeth, due to maxillary hypoplasia as a result of surgical scaring. The severity of the malocclusion may be associated with certain methods of surgical repair of the palate.

PRIMARY DENTITION

At 2 to 3 years of age, the establishment of the primary dentition permits classification of the type of developing malocclusion. This may be part of the diagnostic regime in which the contribution of the skeletal and dental components is specified relative to the etiology of the malocclusion.

The facial soft tissues may mask the underlying skeletal deficiency of the midface in young children (Fig. 29.3). With growth of the intermaxillary space in three dimensions, redistribution of the facial soft tissue changes as the chubby face of infancy takes on the more mature and defined proportions of the child. These facial characteristics reflect the underlying skeletal discrepancy more accurately than in the younger child. The dentition often reflects the skeletal discrepancy, es-

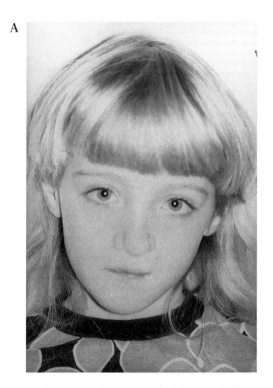

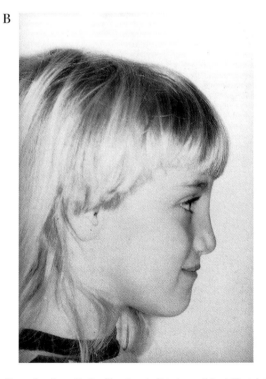

FIG. 29.3. *A:* Frontal view of a 6-year-old girl with repaired bilateral cleft lip and palate. *B:* Profile view indicating mild midfacial deficiency in the paranasal and infraorbital regions.

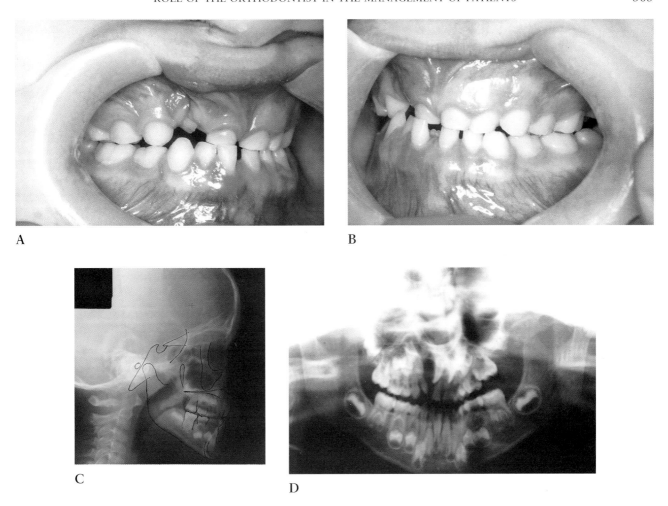

A

B

C

D

FIG. 29.4. *A*: Intraoral view in occlusion of the same child shown in Figure 29.3. Note the normal occulsion on the nonaffected side and the anterior crossbite on the affected side. *B*: Panorex radiograph indicating congenitally absent maxillary lateral incisor associated with the cleft site. *C*: Lateral skull radiograph in early mixed dentition with superimposed tracing.

pecially if the dentoalveolar component has not compensated for the skeletal relationship and the axial inclination of the teeth reflects the skeletal discrepancy. Typically, dental compensation for maxillary skeletal deficiency results in retroclination of mandibular incisors with proclination of the maxillary incisors to eliminate the anteroposterior discrepancy (Fig. 29.4).

The more upright primary incisors may result in an anterior crossbite and/or posterior crossbite, which may be unilateral or bilateral and with or without a functional shift of the mandible. This shift occurs when the child closes the teeth together. To eliminate mandibular shifts, orthodontic treatment may be indicated to remove the interfering contact by tooth movement. This may involve the maxillary incisors if an anterior crossbite exists or expansion of the posterior segments to eliminate a posterior crossbite (Fig. 29.5). The dental crossbite relationship is a continuing problem once the dentition is established and may be a reflection of the

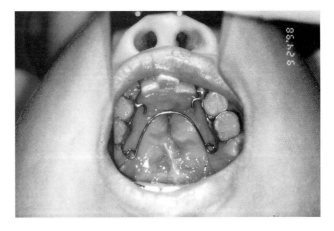

FIG. 29.5. Palatal expander with bands cemented on the maxillary second premolars and canines with palatal hooks to attach the protraction face mask.

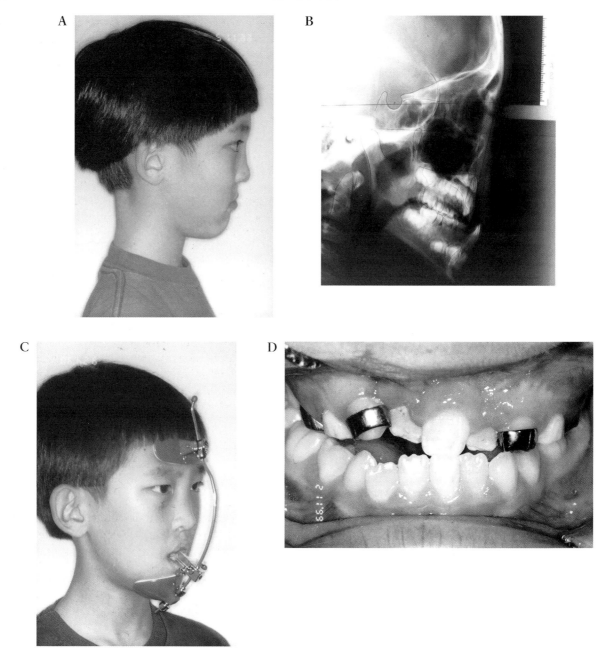

FIG. 29.6. *A:* Eight-year-old boy with repaired unilateral complete cleft lip and palate with sagittal and transverse maxillary deficiency. *B:* Lateral skull radiograph of the same boy. Note the 7 mm reverse overjet. *C:* Protraction face mask with elastics attached to palatal hooks (see Fig. 29.5). *D:* Lateral and anterior crossbites improving with palatal expansion and maxillary and dental protraction.

underlying skeletal discrepancy for which growth modification and redirection may be indicated with a facial mask (Fig. 29.6) Many factors need to be considered in determining whether to initiate orthodontic treatment during this stage, including the ability of the child to cooperate, severity of the malocclusion, timing of any secondary bone grafts, psychosocial issues, speech considerations, and the need for future orthodontic treatment in either the early mixed or permanent den-

tition. Given that typically there will be a need for orthodontic treatment in the early mixed and permanent dentitions and there is no evidence for a benefit of treating during the primary dentition, orthodontic treatment may be best deferred until it can be combined with other treatment goals to shorten the overall length of time a patient is in orthodontic treatment.

Severe sagittal skeletal discrepancies in the primary dentition, most commonly caused by maxillary hy-

A

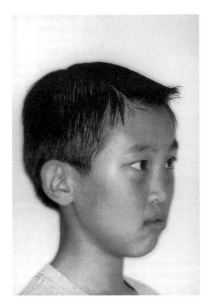

B

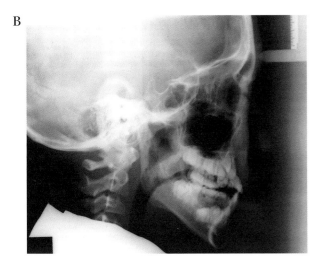

C

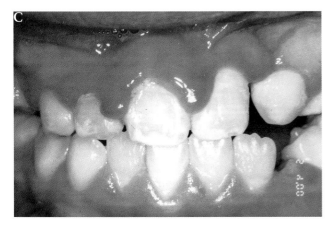

FIG. 29.7. *A:* Facial profile after 9 months of protraction face mask therapy and palatal expansion (same patient shown in Fig. 29.6). *B:* Lateral skull radiograph demonstrating anterior crossbite correction. *C:* Intraoral view with correction of anterior and posterior crossbites.

poplasia, are a more complex problem. Modification or redirection of growth has been advocated, and use of functional or orthopedic appliances and the forward protraction face mask, as promoted by Delaire, has had some success (Rygh and Tindlund, 1995). More commonly, the "apparent correction" is achieved by a transient change in the position of the teeth only so that, with subsequent growth, the skeletal discrepancy is once again reflected in the re-establishment of the malocclusion. Early treatment procedures, in common with neonatal maxillary orthopedics, require a long-term follow-up period to evaluate the outcome of treatment when the child reaches adolescence (Figs. 29.6, 29.7). Excessive changes attributable to therapeutic growth modification are now considered the exception rather than a predictable outcome of this early intervention (Tindlund, 1989, 1994; Ishikawa et al., 2000). Careful consideration must be given to the severity of the skeletal discrepancy, to determine the likelihood of successful growth modification and subsequent long-term results vs. conventional orthognathic surgery at a later stage. It may be more conservative to provide a combined orthodontic/orthognathic surgical treatment plan than to promote long-term growth-modification strategies that may not ultimately be successful.

MIXED DENTITION

The mixed dentition stage starts at approximately 6 years of age with the eruption of the first permanent molars and incisors. Further growth of the craniofacial complex often accentuates a previously mild skeletal discrepancy. As the permanent incisor teeth erupt adjacent to the cleft site, they will typically be rotated, misplaced, or malformed (hypoplastic). In addition, there may be supernumerary, absent, or peg-shaped incisors. This is considered a result of early disruption of the dental lamina at the cleft site, which subsequently affects the developing tooth germs (Figs. 29.8, 29.9a). As deficiency of tissue is an inevitable consequence of clefting, not only may there be missing teeth but also the supporting alveolar bone at the cleft site is variable. In the past, rehabilitation of the maxillary dentition was dependent on the expertise of the prosthodontist to replace the missing teeth and alveolus in the cleft defect with a fixed or removable partial denture, or in the most severe cases, an overdenture. This challenge to restore the cleft site was resolved with the advent of secondary alveolar bone grafting in the 1970s (Boyne, 1974; Boyne and Sands, 1976; Abyholm et al., 1981). This provided the orthodontist with one of the most important milestones in managing the cleft site, allowing for the orthodontic movement of teeth across the

A

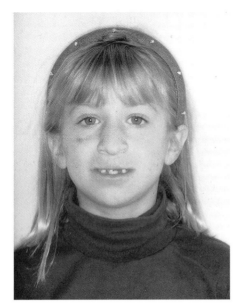

B

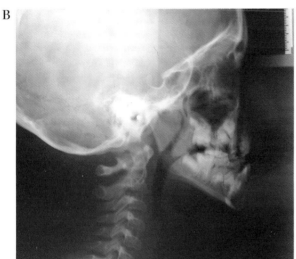

C

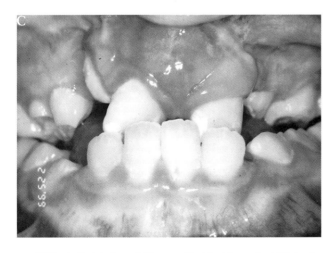

FIG. 29.8. *A:* Facial view of 10-year-old girl with repaired bilateral cleft lip and palate. *B:* Lateral skull radiograph of mixed dentition with anterior crossbite. *C:* Intraoral photograph with bilateral posterior and anterior crossbites.

intact alveolus or the placement of implants for the prosthetic replacement of missing teeth in the cleft site (Fig. 29.9). Elimination of the residual cleft provided a major advance in the contemporary management of the cleft maxilla and is an example of the outcome of a coordinated and problem-oriented approach to developing new strategies of treatment (Turvey et al., 1984; Vig et al., 1995; Vig, 1999).

Alveolar Bone Grafting

The success of alveolar bone grafting requires collaborative treatment planning between the orthodontist, surgeon, and other team members (Troxell et al., 1982; Bergland et al., 1986; Semb, 1991). Secondary alveolar bone grafting offers the following five main benefits:

1. Bone support for unerupted teeth and those teeth adjacent to the cleft. If a bone graft is placed before eruption of teeth adjacent to the cleft, it will improve their periodontal support. If a bone graft is placed after eruption of the canine, the bone will not improve the crestal height of support and will quickly resorb to its original level.
2. Closure of oral–nasal fistulas. By utilizing a three-layered closure technique, with the graft sandwiched between the two soft tissue planes, a high success rate of fistula closure has been observed.
3. Support and elevation of the alar base on the cleft side. This benefit helps to achieve nasal and lip symmetry and provides a stable platform on which the nasal structures are supported. If this procedure is performed alone or combined with alar cartilage revision, satisfactory esthetic changes occur.
4. Construction of a continuous arch form and alveolar ridge. This benefits the orthodontist by moving teeth into the cleft site and the surgeon and prosthodontist by enabling a more esthetic and hygienic prosthesis or implants to be placed when teeth are missing.
5. Stabilization and some repositioning of the premaxilla in the bilateral cleft patient.

Controversies concerning alveolar bone grafting require a rational and evidence-based approach for resolution. These relate to the timing of the alveolar bone graft, the sequencing of orthodontic treatment to correct a transverse discrepancy with palatal expansion, and the sites and types of bone for the graft (Zins and Whittaker, 1979; Vig, 1990, 1999).

Timing of Bone Graft. The timing of the bone graft surgery is more dependent on dental development than on chronological age. Ideally, the permanent cuspid

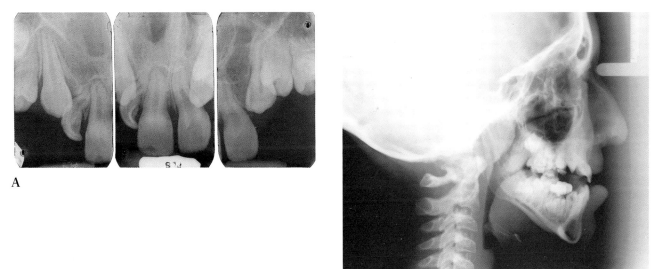

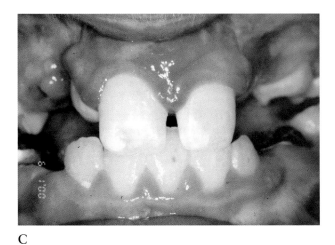

FIG. 29.9. *A:* Intraoral radiograph demonstrating successful bone grafting (same patient shown in Fig. 29.8). Note missing permanent lateral incisor on the left with the canine erupting through the graft adjacent to the central incisor and a malformed right lateral incisor, which will be extracted to allow the permanent canine to erupt adjacent to the right central incisor. *B:* Central incisors moved labially to correct the anterior crossbite. Note the mild maxillary deficiency, which has been camouflaged by proclining the maxillary incisors. *C:* Intraoral view following correction of the anterior crossbite. *D:* Facial appearance following labial movement of the maxillary incisors to correct the crossbite.

root should be approximately one-half to two-thirds formed at the time the graft is placed (Fig. 29.9a). This generally occurs between the ages of 8 and 11 years (Vig, 1992). Rarely is the graft placed prior to this time, although occasionally it may be placed at an earlier age to improve the prognosis of a lateral incisor. Once teeth have erupted into the cleft site, their periodontal support will not improve with a bone graft. Instead, the height of the crest of alveolar bone resorbs to its orig-

inal level. It is for this reason that it is essential to perform the graft prior to the eruption of the permanent cuspid, or if the lateral incisor will erupt into the cleft, the graft should be placed earlier. Although results from primary bone grafting have indicated a significant adverse effect on maxillary development, performing a secondary bone graft at an age when maxillary growth is almost complete has resulted in no effect on subsequent facial development (Semb et al., 1988).

Sequencing of Treatment. Secondary bone grafting has been divided into the categories of early (2–5 years of age), intermediate (6–15 years of age), and late (16 years to adult). Since the results of an Oslo study, in which 378 consecutive patients who had undergone alveolar bone grafting, were published (Bergland et al., 1986), contemporary opinion supports the intermediate period as the most appropriate time for grafting. This has the greatest benefit and least risk for interfering with midfacial and skeletodental growth and development. This sequencing of procedures, including presurgical orthodontics, requires interdisciplinary communication and cooperation, but the benefit is improved and more predictable patient care.

Surgical Technique. The surgical procedure utilizes tissue lining the cleft defect to construct a nasal floor and close the nasal side of the oral–nasal fistula. The cleft lining is elevated in a subperiosteal plane, which leaves bare the osseous margins of the cleft. Cancellous bone taken from the ilium, cranium, or mandibular symphysis is then packed into the cleft defect. Cortical bone is avoided because the cancellous bone revascularizes quickly and is less likely to become infected (Zins and Whittaker, 1979). Once the cleft defect is packed with bone and the margins are overpacked, soft tissue coverage of the graft is required. The donor site is chosen by the surgeon. Traditionally, the iliac crest, ribs, and tibia have been utilized because of their abundant supply of cancellous bone. The morbidity of harvesting bone from these sites results in most patients being hospitalized postsurgically because of complications associated more with the donor site than the oronasal recipient site. The cranium has become an alternative site from which to harvest cancellous bone because of the lack of associated pain and the reduced hospitalization time involved. However, the operating risks are higher and the abundance of cancellous bone reduced. The mandibular symphysis is another donor site that is associated with relatively little pain and allows for early hospital discharge. This site should be utilized only when the permanent mandibular cuspids have been carefully located so as to minimize the chances of injuring these developing teeth.

Orthodontic Considerations Associated with Secondary Bone Grafting

Transverse Dimension. Orthodontic expansion of the posterior segments (Fig. 29.5) preoperatively may improve the occlusion but also may widen an existing fistula. The larger fistula in most cases is favorable because it provides better access at surgery, and closure of the palatal and vestibular fistulas occurs following the cancellous bone graft. Retention of the corrected crossbite with orthodontic appliances postsurgically may be indicated as the bone graft is unlikely to maintain the expansion initially.

Incisor Alignment. Alignment of the incisors adjacent to the cleft will be limited by the available bone into which the roots of the teeth can be moved. Appliances may be placed presurgically but not activated. This permits the initiation of orthodontic tooth movements within 3 to 6 weeks following placement of the bone graft. The early movement of the roots into the grafted bone appears clinically to consolidate the alveolar bone and improve the crestal height.

Canine Eruption. The maxillary canine erupts through the grafted bone following surgery (Fig. 29.9a). With orthodontic movement, enough space is created in the arch to allow the cuspids to erupt successfully. Supernumerary teeth are removed at the time that the bone graft is placed, to create an unobstructed path of eruption for the cuspid. Often, the canine will erupt rapidly once the bone is available, and if the lateral incisors are malformed or absent, especially in patients with bilateral clefts, the canine is encouraged to erupt adjacent to the central incisors. This is an advantage in closing space as it avoids the need for prosthetic replacement of the absent lateral incisors. However, canine substitution needs to be considered in light of the occlusion and the need for orthognathic surgery.

PERMANENT DENTITION

Following eruption of the canines and premolars, the permanent dentition is established. During this time, the adolescent growth spurt and onset of puberty occur. The skeletal discrepancy becomes accentuated, and both facial appearance and occlusal relationships deteriorate (Fig. 29.10). This occurs at a time when the individual is most self-conscious of his or her appearance. Facial scars already detract from the cosmetic appearance, and derogatory comments by peers may have a profound psychological effect. At this time, involution of the adenoidal lymphoid tissue occurs, often with a consequent impairment of speech and hyper-nasality. With a decline in both cosmetic appearance and speech communication, many patients have a special need for early intervention by surgeons, orthodontics, and speech therapists.

Growth Considerations

Unilateral complete clefts of the lip and palate typically become more maxillary-deficient and mandibu-

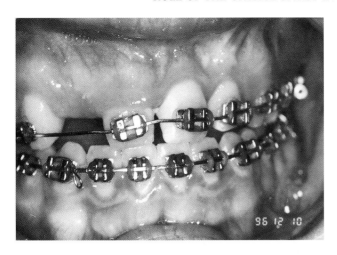

FIG. 29.10. Intraoral view of the same patient illustrated at 6 years of age in Figure 29.3. Note anterior crossbite re-establishing as patient undergoes her pubertal growth spurt.

A

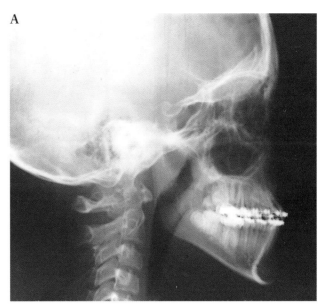

B

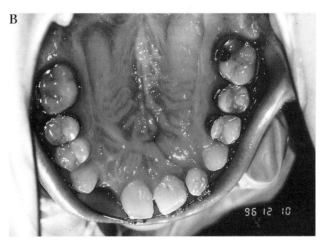

C

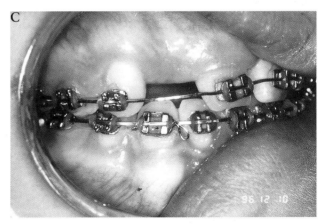

FIG. 29.11. *A:* Comprehensive orthodontic treatment with camouflage for stabilized skeletal discrepancy (same patient shown in Figs. 29.3 and 29.10). Note the proclined maxillary incisors and retroclined mandibular incisors. *B:* Occlusal view showing missing right lateral incisor and left lateral incisor, which is smaller than normal. *C:* Intraoral lateral view showing class I canine relationship and stable overjet and overbite.

lar-prognathic in appearance. Typically, this is a result of sagittal maxillary deficiency (Kuijpers-Jagtman and Long, 2000; Will, 2000). However, vertical maxillary deficiency may also accentuate the class III tendency, resulting in overclosure of the mandible to achieve occlusion of the teeth. It is important to evaluate clinically the extent of overclosure and to measure the interocclusal clearance at the premolar region with the patient in a resting posture. Alternatively, a class III skeletal relationship can be camouflaged by increasing the vertical dimension to rotate the mandible down and back. Careful consideration must be made to ensure that any camouflage treatment is an acceptable option, depending on the patient's desires, esthetics, occlusion, and biological limits. The class III dental relationship also accentuates the transverse discrepancy. To evaluate the occlusion, study models of the teeth will be necessary so that the relationship of the maxillary to mandibular dentition can be accurately assessed in all three dimensions, taking into account the final sagittal occlusion. Facial growth is the result of the interaction of genetic and environmental factors. Continued growth in early adulthood may enhance or detract from treatment results obtained during childhood and adolescence. These dynamic properties of the face make the management of facial growth both challenging and rewarding (Rygh and Tindlund, 1995; Kuijpers-Jagtman and Long, 2000; Will, 2000). A patient whose orthodontic treatment in the permanent dentition allowed camouflage of the mild skeletal discrepancy and prosthetic replacement of the maxillary right lateral incisor is shown in Figures 29.11–29.13.

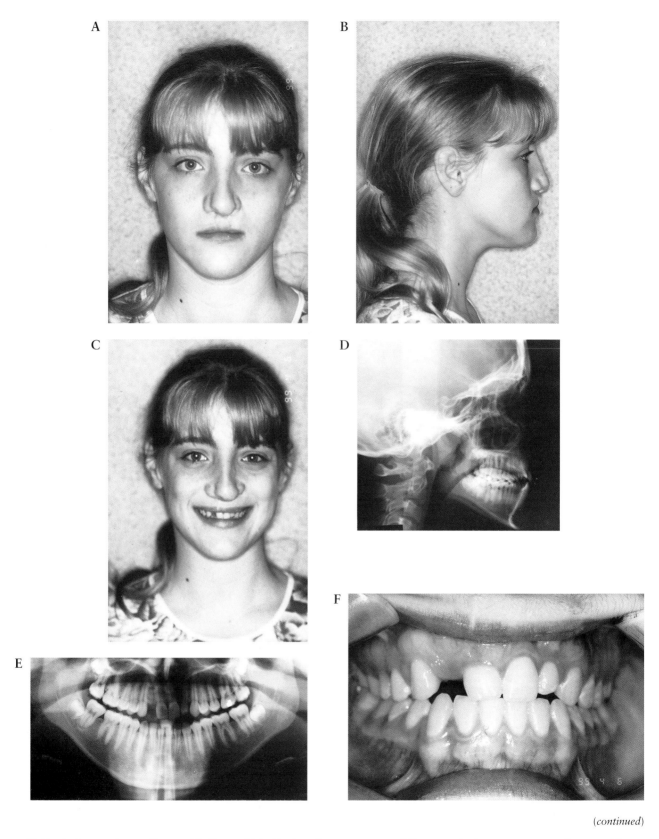

(*continued*)

FIG. 29.12. *A:* Same patient as illustrated in Figures 29.3, 29.10, and 29.11 at age 13 following orthodontic treatment and nose and lip revisions. *B:* Profile view showing mild midfacial deficiency and paranasal flattening. *C:* Facial view of patient smiling. Note the symmetry of the upper lip in function. The patient is very satisfied with the facial and dental outcomes. *D:* Lateral skull radiograph demonstrating class I camouflaged occlusion. *E:* Panorex radiograph with cleft site successfully bone-grafted and adequate space for implant placement to prosthetically replace the congenitally missing lateral incisor due to the cleft alveolus. *F:* Class I incisal relationship with some overbite reduction. *G:* Maxillary occlusal view demonstrating closure of palatal oronasal fistula and adequate bony ridge depth for an implant replacement of the missing lateral incisor. *H:* Mandibular occlusal view illustrating a well-aligned and symmetrical arch form.

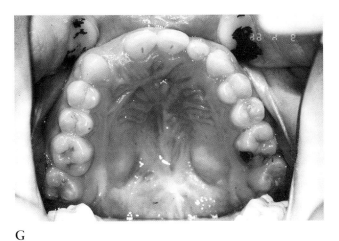

G

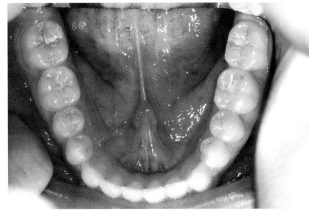

H

FIG. 29.12. *Continued*

Skeletal–Facial Considerations

Examination of facial balance and proportions is essential in determining a treatment plan that combines surgery and orthodontics. This clinical evaluation should be carried out with the patient standing so that the overall stature can be taken into consideration. Full-face and profile assessments will provide a database incorporating all three dimensions, and this information should be documented with the patient in a resting position, smiling, animated, and in occlusion. Cephalometric analysis and surgical prediction tracings will provide further information for deciding whether a patient should be treated by orthodontics alone or in combination with a surgical orthognathic procedure. If the skeletal discrepancy is mild and esthetic concerns are minimal, dental compensation by orthodontic treatment alone may be recommended (Figs. 29.9, 29.11–

A

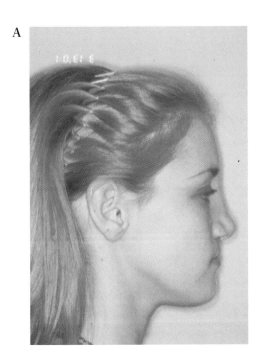

B

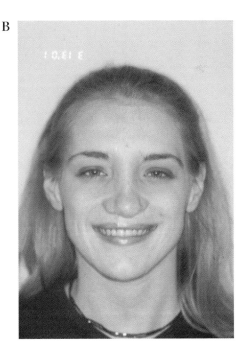

(continued)

FIG. 29.13. *A:* Profile of the same patient at age 16 showing stability of the skeletal relationship. *B:* Smiling view after prosthodontic treatment via an implant for tooth number 7 and esthetic recountouring of tooth number 10. *C:* Intraoral view of prosthodontic treatment in combination with gingivoplasty to restore the tissue contours and position for an improved tooth display and better gingival symmetry. *D:* Radiograph showing complete osteointegration of implant prosthesis in the former site of the cleft alveolus.

C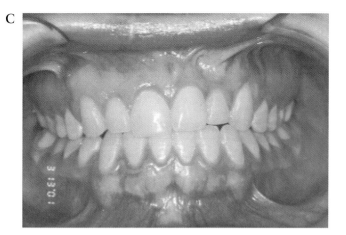

D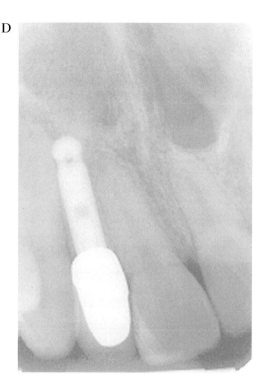

FIG. 29.13. *Continued*

29.13). Alterations in the axial inclination of the teeth may adequately camouflage the skeletal relationship. However, caution should be taken as the individual may outgrow the dental correction so that ultimately skeletal surgery may be necessary to obtain a normal occlusion.

If surgery is necessary, the presurgical phase of orthodontic treatment will require decompensation of the dentition so that the maxillary and mandibular teeth are placed in their correct relationship to the underlying skeletal bases. If orthodontic therapy has achieved the ideal relationship of the dentition to their skeletal bases, surgical correction of the skeletal discrepancy will result in normal class I occlusion and a normal skeletal relationship. In the past, using conventional orthognathic surgical techniques for patients with severe maxillary hypoplasia, it was not uncommon to advance the maxilla as much as possible, with the limit being the scar tissue from the lip and palatal repairs. The remaining skeletal discrepancy would then be corrected with a mandibular setback. Essentially, this was a surgical compromise due to the inability to predictably correct the underlying maxillary hypoplasia. With the advent of distraction osteogenesis, it may be possible to correct severe maxillary hypoplasia solely by advancing the maxilla (Cohen et al., 1997; Polley and Figueroa, 1998). This would be accomplished by tissue expansion of the scar tissue at the same time distrac-

tion osteogenesis is performed. However, this is an emerging treatment modality that currently has no long-term follow-up results. Questions related to how much to overcorrect the occlusion if utilized on a growing child and the effects of surgery on any remaining growth remain. Also, distraction osteogenesis may not negate the need for a conventional osteotomy to detail the occlusion due to the inability to precisely control the maxilla during distraction. Again, the treatment benefits need to be weighed vs. the burden of care and considered in light of the scientific evidence of positive outcomes (Dalston et al., 1988; Shaw et al., 1995).

Treatment Coordination

The timing and sequencing of orthodontic treatment require close communication with the team. Deciding to delay surgical orthodontic treatment until growth is stabilized may be sound judgment but not always in the patient's best interest, especially when psychosocial development is affected. In some instances, skeletal surgery may be indicated before growth is completed, knowing that a further procedure may be necessary should the patient outgrow the correction. As a general rule, skeletal surgery, orthodontic intervention, and final prosthetic rehabilitation should be completed before soft tissue revision or rhinoplasty is instituted. The outcome of soft tissue surgical procedures when combined with surgical orthognathic movement of the maxilla and mandible is unpredictable.

Orthodontic Intervention

A coordinated approach to the presurgical phase of orthodontic treatment will be indicated before the surgical procedure. Approximately 12 to 18 months of orthodontics will usually be necessary to align the teeth, correct any midline discrepancy, coordinate arches, and localize space for prosthetic replacement of the teeth. The provision of space for surgical cuts between both the crown and the roots of adjacent teeth is also an important part of the presurgical preparations. Placement of full-sized arch wires with lugs provides a means of intermaxillary fixation at the time of surgery as rigid internal fixation is performed. The goal of the postsurgical phase of orthodontics is to detail the occlusion in coordination with any future prosthodontic treatment, and this should be completed within 4 to 6 months.

SUMMARY

The orthodontist's role on the cleft palate team requires close collaboration with the other team members. The rationale of timing and sequencing orthodontic treatment has been discussed in four periods of development: *(1)* neonatal or infant maxillary orthopedics, *(2)* orthodontic considerations in the primary dentition, *(3)* mixed dentition orthodontics to include presurgical recommendations before an alveolar bone graft and its rationale for use, and *(4)* final treatment in the permanent dentition using orthodontics alone or orthognathic surgery combining an orthodontic and surgical approach to the correction of dental and skeletal components of malocclusion as well as facilitating any necessary prosthodontic treatment.

Speech considerations and the communicative skills of the patient with a cleft are important aspects in planning orthognathic surgery for this group of patients. Also, subsequent nose and lip revisions for cosmetic improvement must not be underestimated in the enhancement of the final result following correction of the skeletal and dental discrepancies. Provided the timing and sequencing of appropriate treatment modalities are planned in a closely coordinated, problem-oriented approach by the team members, patients with clefts should have optimal functional and esthetic results. Outcome measures for reporting the results of surgical interventions require that valid and reliable measures be identified and implemented (Dalston et al., 1988; Shaw et al., 1995). The ultimate outcome of team-based care is to have a fully rehabilitated patient who is satisfied with the treatment outcomes in terms of speech, hearing, occlusion, facial, and dental esthetics such that he or she needs only conventional dental and medical preventive therapies typical of any adult and possesses optimal self-esteem to develop to his or her full potential.

We are indebted to Dr. Jack Lude for permission to publish Figure 29.2 and to the patients and their families for agreeing to participate in this publication. In addition, we extend gratitude to the orthodontic residents and to the members of the cleft palate team at Children's Hospital of Columbus, Ohio, including Drs. Robert Ruberg, Peter Larsen, Brent Buchele, Rafael Villolobos, Ron Berggren, James Ferraro, Gregory Wiet, Michael Martyn, Darryl Willett, Lisa Knobloch, Christine Halket, and Annemarie Sommer as well as Ms. Leslie Justice, CPNP; Ms. Christina Ferguson, MS, CCC-SLP; Ms. Nancy Neal, RN, BSN, CPN, and Ms. Katy Nash Krahn, MS, CGC for their cooperative management of the patients illustrated in this chapter.

REFERENCES

Abyholm, FE, Bergland, O, Semb, G (1981). Secondary bone grafting of alveolar clefts. Scand J Plast Reconstr Surg 15: 127–140.

American Cleft Palate-Craniofacial Association (1993). Parameters for the evaluation and treatment of patients with cleft lip/palate or other craniofacial anomalies. Cleft Palate Craniofac J 30(Suppl 1): 4.

Bergland, O, Semb, G, Abyholm, FE (1986). Elimination of the residual alveolar cleft by secondary bone grafting and subsequent orthodontic treatment. Cleft Palate J 23: 175–205.

Boyne, PJ (1974). Use of marrow-cancellous bone grafts in maxillary alveolar and palatal clefts. J Dent Res 53: 821.

Boyne, PJ, Sands, NR (1976). Combined orthodontic–surgical management of residual palato-alveolar cleft defect. Am J Orthod 70: 20.

Burston, WR (1958). The early treatment of cleft palate conditions. Dent Pract 9: 41–52.

Cohen, SR, Burstein, FD, Stewart, MB, Rathbun, MA (1997). Maxillary-midface distraction in children with cleft lip and palate: a preliminary report. Plast Reconstr Surg 9: 1421–1428.

Dalston, RM, Marsh, JL, Vig, KWL, et al. (1988). Minimal standards for reporting the results of surgery on patients with cleft lip, palate or both. A proposal. Cleft Palate J 25: 3–7.

Grayson, BH, Santiago, PE, Brecht, LE, Cutting, CB (1999). Presurgical nasoalveolar molding in infants with cleft lip and palate. Cleft Palate Craniofac J 36: 486–98.

Hotz, MM, Gnoinski, WM, Nussbaumer, H, Kistler, E (1978). Early maxillary orthopedics in cleft lip and palate cases: guidelines for surgery. Cleft Palate J 15: 405–411.

Ishikawa, H, Kitazawa, S, Iwasaki, H, Nakamura, S (2000). Effects of maxillary protraction combined with chin-cap therapy in unilateral cleft lip and palate patients. Cleft Palate Craniofac J 37: 92–97.

Jolleys, A, Robertson, NRE (1972). A study of the effects of early bone grafting in complete clefts of the lip and palate—five year study. Br J Plast Surg 25: 229–237.

Kuijpers-Jagtman, AM, Long, RE, Jr (2000). The influence of surgery and orthopedic treatment on maxillofacial growth and maxillary arch development in patients treated for orofacial clefts. Cleft Palate Craniofac J 37: 527.

Long, RE, Jr, Semb, G, Shaw, WC (2000). Orthodontic treatment of the patient with complete clefts of lip, alveolus, and palate: lessons of the last 60 years. Cleft Palate Craniofac J 37: 533.

McNeil, CK (1964). Orthopedic principles in the treatment of lip and palate clefts. In: *International Symposium on Early Treatment of Cleft Lip and Palate,* edited by RP Hotz. Berne: Hans Huber.

Millard, DR, Latham, R, Huifen, X, et al. (1999). Cleft lip and palate treated by presurgical orthopedics, gingivoperiosteoplasty, and lip adhesion (POPLA) compared with previous lip adhesion method: a preliminary study of serial dental casts. Plast Reconstr Surg 103: 1630–1644.

Molsted, K, Dahl, E, Skovgaard, LT, et al. (1993). A multicentre comparison of treatment regimens for unilateral cleft lip and palate using a multiple regression model. Scand J Plast Reconstr Surg Hand Surg 27: 277–284.

Polley, JW, Figueroa, AA (1998). Rigid external distraction: its application in cleft maxillary deformities. Plast Reconstr Surg 102: 1360–1372.

Pruzansky, S (1964). Pre-surgical orthopedics and bone grafting for infants with cleft lip and palate: a dissent. Cleft Palate J 1: 164–182.

Rosenstein, SW, Monroe, CW, Kernahan, DA, et al. (1982). The case for early bone grafting in cleft lip and cleft palate. J Oral Surg 70: 297–309.

Ross, RB, MacNamera, MC (1994). Effect of presurgical infant orthopedics on facial esthetics in complete bilateral cleft lip and palate. Palate Craniofac J 31: 68–73.

Rygh, P, Tindlund, RS (1995). Early considerations in the orthodontic management of skeletodental discrepancies. In: *Facial Clefts and Craniosynostosis. Principles and Management,* edited by TA Turvey, KWL Vig, and RJ Fonseca. Philadelphia: WB Saunders, pp. 234–319.

Santiago, PE, Grayson, BH, Cutting, CB, et al. (1998). Reduced need for alveolar bone grafting by presurgical orthopedics and primary gingivoperiosteoplasty. Cleft Palate Craniofac J 35: 77–80.

Semb, G (1988). Effect of alveolar bone grafting on maxillary growth in unilateral cleft lip and palate patients. Cleft Palate J 25: 288–295.

Semb, G (1991). Analysis of the Oslo Cleft Lip and Palate Archive. Long Term Dentofacial Development. Oslo: Univ. of Oslo. Dissertation.

Severens, JL, Prahl, C, Kuijpers-Jagtman, AM, Prahl-Andersen, B (1998). Short-term cost-effectiveness analysis of presurgical orthpedic treatment in children with complete unilateral cleft lip and palate. Cleft Palate Craniofac J 35: 222–226.

Shaw, WC, Roberts, CT, Semb, G (1995). Evaluating treatment alternatives: measurement and design. In: *Facial Clefts and Cra-*

niosynostosis. Principles and Management, edited by TA Turvey, KWL Vig, and RJ Fonseca. Philadelphia: WB Saunders. pp. 756–766.

Shprintzen, RJ, Siegel-Sadewitz, VL, Amatp, A, Goldberg, RB (1985). Anomalies associated with cleft lip, cleft palate or both. Am J Med Genet 20: 585–595.

Surgeon General's Report (1987). *Children with Special Health Care Needs.* Washington, DC; Government Printing Office.

Tindlund, RS (1989). Orthopaedic protraction of the midface in the deciduous dentition. Results covering 3 years out of treatment. J Craniomaxillofac Surg 17(Suppl 1): 17–19.

Tindlund, RS (1994). Skeletal response to maxillary protraction in patients with cleft lip and palate before age 10 years. Cleft Palate Craniofac J 31: 295–308.

Troxell, J, Fonseca, R, Osbon, D (1982). A retrospective study of alveolar cleft grafting. J Oral Maxillofac Surg 40: 721–725.

Turvey, T, Vig, K, Moriarty, J, Hoke, J (1984). Delayed bone grafting in the cleft maxilla and palate: a retrospective multidisciplinary analysis. Am J Orthod 86: 244–256.

Turvey, TA, Vig, KWL, Fonseca, R (1995). *Facial Clefts and Craniosynostosis.* Philadelphia: WB Saunders.

Vig, KWL (1990). Orthodontic considerations applied to craniofacial dysmorphology. Cleft Palate J 27: 141–145.

Vig, KWL (1992). Timing of alveolar bone grafting: an orthodontist's viewpoint. In: *Problems in Plastic and Reconstructive Surgery,* edited by JA Lehman and D Serafin. Philadelphia: JB Lippincott, pp. 58–72.

Vig, KWL (1999). Alveolar bone grafts: the surgical/orthdontic management of the cleft maxilla. Ann Acad Med Singapore 28: 721–727.

Vig, KWL, Turvey, TA (1985). Orthodontic, surgical interaction in the management of cleft lip and palate. Clin Plast Surg 12: 735–748.

Vig, KWL, Turvey, TA, Fonseca, RJ (1995). Orthodontic and surgical considerations in bone grafting the cleft maxilla and palate. In: *Facial Clefts and Craniosynostosis. Principles and Management,* edited by TA Turvey, KWL Vig, and RJ Fonseca. Philadelphia: WB Saunders.

Washington State Department of Health (1997). *Cleft Lip and Palate: Critical Elements of Care.* Seattle: Division of Family and Community Services, Office for Children with Special Health Care Needs.

Will, LA (2000). Growth and development in patients with untreated clefts. Cleft Palate Craniofac J 37: 523–526.

Winters, JC, Hurwitz, DJ (1995). Presurgical orthopedics in the surgical management of unilateral cleft lip and palate. Plast Reconstr Surg 95: 755–764.

Zins, JE, Whittaker, LA (1979). Membranous vs. endochondral bone autografts: implications for craniofacial reconstruction. Surg Forum 30: 521.

30

Otolaryngologic needs of individuals with oral clefts

PATRICK J. ANTONELLI

Oral clefts can profoundly impact the physiology of the entire upper aerodigestive tract. Although disorders of the upper aerodigestive tract are central to the field of otolaryngology, patients with oral clefts are best managed by a multidisciplinary team. Many of the issues related to the otolaryngologic needs of individuals with oral clefts have been addressed in other chapters (e.g., velopharyngeal insufficiency). Accordingly, this chapter focuses on the ear, nose, and throat issues for which individuals with oral clefts most commonly seek otolaryngologic care (Table 30.1).

EAR

Disorders of the ear are the most common reason that children with cleft palate seek care from an otolaryngologist. Otologic problems in individuals with oral clefts, like those in individuals without clefts, change with age. In early childhood, the primary concerns include acute otitis media, chronic otitis media with effusion, and the cognitive sequelae of hearing loss. With advancing age, otologic concerns shift to the middle ear sequelae of chronic eustachian tube dysfunction and its treatment.

Otitis Media: Classification and Prevalence

Otitis media is defined as any inflammation within the middle ear. The sine qua non of otitis media is effusion within the middle ear space. Further classification is based largely on duration, the nature of the effusion,

and the presence or absence of symptoms (Table 30.2). Though these definitions may seem unambiguous, there are no clear distinctions in clinical practice. Otoscopy is far from 100% accurate (Finitzo et al., 1992; Jensen and Lous, 1999). Otitis media is a dynamic process that may vacillate along a continuum (Paparella et al., 1990). Extrinsic factors may also complicate the distinction between types of otitis media (Kempthorne and Giebink, 1991). For example, a child with persistent otitis media with effusion may become febrile because of a bacterial superinfection in the middle ear. Alternatively, the fever may be due to an unrelated viral illness. These issues must be kept in mind when making therapeutic decisions concerning children with otitis media, particularly children with persistent otitis media with effusion, such as children with cleft palate.

Though clinicians may use many different criteria to diagnose acute otitis media (Hayden, 1981), the criteria proposed by Paradise (1995) have gained the widest acceptance. *Acute otitis media* is generally defined as acute, symptomatic, suppurative middle ear inflammation. Acute otitis media is likely to afflict most children with cleft palate at some point in their early childhood (Skolnik, 1958), but the same is true for children without cleft palate (Teele et al., 1989). Recurrent acute otitis media is only slightly more common in children with cleft palate (Rynnel-Dagoo et al., 1992).

Otitis media with effusion is defined as painless, persistent middle ear effusion. Otitis media with effusion is found in nearly all infants born with cleft palate (Stool and Randall, 1967; Paradise et al., 1969, Dhillon, 1988; Grant et al., 1988). Controlled studies

TABLE 30.1. *Most Common Otolaryngological Issues in Individuals with Oral Clefts*

Ear
    Acute otitis media
    Otitis media with effusion
    Hearing loss and developmental sequelae
    Eustachian tube dysfunction
    Chronic suppurative otitis media
Nose
    Nasal obstruction
    Rhinosinusitis
Throat
    Tonsilitis and tonsillar hypertrophy
    Airway obstruction

have confirmed that otitis media with effusion is far more common in children with cleft palate (Kemaloglu et al., 1999).

Chronic suppurative otitis media is broadly defined by persistent suppuration of the middle ear, manifested by otorrhea through a defect in the tympanic membrane (e.g., a tympanic membrane perforation). Though *persistence* is usually defined as being greater than 6 to 8 weeks, it also implies failed conservative management. Chronic suppurative otitis media is further categorized by the presence or absence of *cholesteatoma* (i.e., the presence of squamous epithelium and accumulation of desquamated skin debris within the middle ear space). The latter classification is of great importance with respect to therapeutic options. Cholesteatoma (Dominguez and Harker, 1988) and tympanic membrane perforation (Gordon et al., 1988) have long been reported to be more common in patients with cleft palate than in those without it (Podoshin et al., 1986; Mawson and Ludman, 1979). This has been substantiated in more rigorous epidemiologic studies (Kemppainen et al., 1999).

Eustachian Tube Dysfunction and the Pathogenesis of Otitis Media

Eustachian tube dysfunction is thought to be central to the pathogenesis of otitis media. The main effect of eustachian tube dysfunction is a gradual absorption of oxygen and carbon dioxide from the middle ear space and the development of negative middle ear pressure (Elner, 1977; Doyle and Seroky, 1994). The negative pressure leads to transudation and accumulation of sterile middle ear effusion (Casselbrandt et al., 1988). This is known as the "hydrops ex vacuo" theory of the pathogenesis of chronic otitis media with effusion.

Otitis media with effusion in individuals with cleft palate is due primarily to eustachian tube dysfunction resulting from tensor veli palatini incompetence (Doyle et al., 1980; Casselbrandt et al., 1988). Although tensor veli palatini dysfunction improves after definitive palatal reconstructive surgery, this may never normalize, and otitis media with effusion remains a common problem after palatal surgery (Matsune et al., 1991; Dhillon, 1988; Tasaka et al., 1990; Rynnel-Dagoo et al., 1992; Robinson et al., 1992; Nunn et al., 1995). This may result from congenital abnormalities of the eustachian tube that are not, and cannot be, addressed by palatoplasty (Yamaguchi et al., 1990; Matsune et al., 1991, 1992; Kemaloglu et al., 1999).

Tubal dysfunction and negative middle ear pressure also predispose to bacterial infection (Meyerhoff et al., 1981). This may lead to recurrent acute otitis media with common upper respiratory pathogens, *Streptococcus pneumoniae*, *Haemophilus influenzae*, and *Moraxella catarrhalis*. Tubal dysfunction is very common in all children (Bluestone and Klein, 1996a) and after viral upper respiratory dysfunction (Buchman et al., 1994). Children with cleft palate, like any other children, are vulnerable to other risk factors for the development of acute otitis media, including day-care attendance, bottle-feeding (vs. breast-feeding), and environmental tobacco smoke exposure. Hence, it can be difficult to isolate the effects of cleft palate from these other factors.

Chronic otitis media with effusion may also be perpetuated, at least in part, by bacterial infection. Though chronic otitis media with effusion (nonsuppurative otitis media) has traditionally been thought of as a sterile process, the same spectrum of bacteria found in acute otitis media may be cultured from the middle ear effusion in up to 30% of cases (Liu et al., 1976; Post et al., 1995). Polymerase chain reaction techniques have

TABLE 30.2. *Classification of Otitis Media*

Class	Duration	Effusion	Symptoms
Acute otitis media	Brief	Suppurative	Pain, fever
Otitis media with effusion	Brief, persistent	Nonsuppurative	Painless
Chronic suppurative otitis media	Persistent	Suppurative	Painless, otorrhea

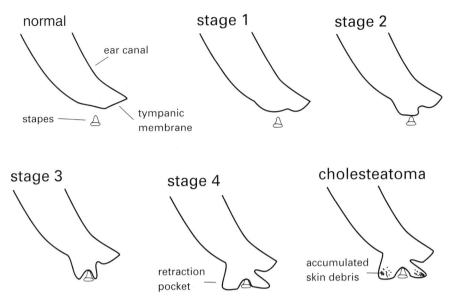

FIG. 30.1. Progression of middle ear atelectasis to cholesteatoma.

suggested that the vast majority of chronic otitis media with effusion cases may yield viable bacteria (Post et al., 1995, 1996; Rayner et al., 1998; Aul et al., 1998). Studies on the role of bacteria in the pathogenesis of chronic otitis media with effusion have not been performed on children with cleft palate.

Persistence of eustachian tube dysfunction after palatoplasty is the primary basis for the development of more serious middle ear pathology in children with cleft palate (Bluestone and Klein, 1996a; Dominguez and Harker, 1988; Goldman et al., 1993; Muntz, 1993). Persistent eustachian tube dysfunction leads to chronic negative middle ear pressure. Chronic negative middle ear pressure leads to inward distention of the tympanic membrane. This may eventually cause irreversible tympanic membrane pathology, such as atelectasis (collapse), perforation, or cholesteatoma (epidermoid cyst) (Bluestone and Klein, 1996a). These conditions are thought to occur along a continuum, and atelectasis is considered a precursor to perforation and cholesteatoma (Fig. 30.1) (Sade and Berco, 1976; Wells and Michaels, 1983; Wolfman and Chole, 1986). If the tympanic membrane ruptures in response to the chronic negative middle ear pressure, a chronic tympanic membrane perforation may result. If the tympanic membrane remains intact, atelectasis will usually develop. Less commonly, atelectasis will progress to cholesteatoma formation.

Atelectasis of the pars tensa (Color Fig. 30.2) is commonly graded using the classification system of Sade and Berco (1976) (Fig. 30.1). Stage 1 involves tympanic membrane retraction toward the promontory with loss of its biconvex contour. Stage 2 involves further retraction of the pars tensa such that the tympanic membrane contacts the incus and/or the stapes. In stage 3, the tympanic membrane contacts the promontory but does not adhere to it. In stage 4, the tympanic membrane adheres to the promontory and ossicular damage is commonly seen. Attic retraction (Color Fig. 30.3) is graded similarly (Tos and Poulson, 1980). This is considered mild (stage 1) when retraction of the pars flaccida is not accompanied by erosion of the scutum (the superomedial tympanic ring). Moderate attic retraction (stage 2) is manifested by slight bone erosion (exposure of malleus neck). Severe retraction (stage 3) involves exposure of the malleus head.

A cholesteatoma (Color Fig. 30.4) results when skin that is sloughed from the atelectatic tympanic membrane begins to accumulate, forming an expansile cyst. Accumulation of debris in the middle ear space, in conjunction with body heat and moisture from the external ear, creates a nidus for chronic suppurative otitis media. Chronic or recurrent purulent drainage usually occurs. In some cases, no drainage may be seen. In most cases without apparent drainage, the drainage will dry over the defect in the tympanic membrane, giving the appearance of cerumen (Color Fig. 30.5).

Tympanic membrane perforation may lead to recurrent or chronic middle ear infection in one of two ways (Bluestone and Klein, 1996a). The defect in the tympanic membrane may allow contamination of the middle ear with water and pathogens from the ear canal.

Such an infection may be seen after an individual with a tympanic membrane perforation has been swimming. Alternatively, the defect in the tympanic membrane may allow reflux of nasopharyngeal secretions.

In contrast to the pathogens isolated from acute otitis media and otitis media with effusion, the bacteria isolated from chronic suppurative otitis media, with or without cholesteatoma, include *Pseudomonas aeruginosa*, anaerobes, Enterobacteriaceae, and *Staphylococcus* species (Kenna and Bluestone, 1986; Papastavros et al., 1986; Harker and Koontz, 1977). Experimental animal studies have indicated that middle ear infection with *P. aeruginosa* can lead to both conditions (Friedmann, 1955a,b; Kenna, 1988; Antonelli et al., 1988, 1992, 1993). In humans, antipseudomonal treatment can eradicate chronic suppurative otitis media without cholesteatoma (Kenna et al., 1986; Fliss et al., 1990). However, chronic suppurative otitis media can be cured with *tympanoplasty* (repair of the tympanic membrane perforation and removal of the cholesteatoma), without the use of antibiotics. Hence, it is unclear whether bacteria are truly pathogenic (i.e., contribute to the development of tympanic membrane perforation or cholesteatoma) or merely colonize the middle ears with tympanic membrane perforations or cholesteatoma.

Hearing Loss and Cognitive Sequelae of Otitis Media

Chronic otitis media with effusion is clinically relatively silent. Few children with chronic otitis media with effusion have symptoms referable to the ear (Paradise et al., 1969). The most common clinical manifestation of chronic otitis media with effusion is conductive hearing loss (Paradise et al., 1969). Hearing loss due to otitis media with effusion averages 25 to 30 dB but may be as high as 50 dB (Cohen and Sade, 1972; Brown et al., 1983; Fria et al., 1985), yet many parents and treating physicians may be unaware that a child has hearing loss due to otitis media with effusion (Rosenfeld et al., 1998; Brody et al., 1999).

Though hearing loss due to otitis media with effusion is considered mild in children with normal inner ear function, children with chronic otitis media with effusion may experience greater problems in speech and language acquisition, cognitive development, and social maturation than children without it (Stewart et al., 1996; Silverman, 1996). Although a great deal of research continues to look for definitive evidence of lasting speech and cognitive sequelae of chronic otitis media with effusion, the data are conflicting or show only mild effects (Hubbard et al., 1985; Schilder et al., 1993; Welsh et al., 1996; Roberts et al., 1998). For example,

Teele and colleagues (1990) found a significant, lasting effect of chronic otitis media with effusion on intelligence quotient, math skills, and verbal language scores; but these findings have not been corroborated in other well-controlled studies (Roberts et al., 1994). Roberts and colleagues (1995, 1998) have found the greatest correlation between chronic otitis media–related hearing loss and the quality of the home and day-care environments. Hence, the impact of hearing loss due to otitis media with effusion remains unclear.

Treatment of Otitis Media with Effusion and Hearing Loss

Because intratemporal or intracranial complications of otitis media are rare (Bluestone and Klein, 1996b) and hearing loss may have a lasting impact on cognitive development, treatment of otitis media, most commonly chronic otitis media with effusion, has been directed at correcting the associated conductive hearing loss.

Speech and cognitive sequelae with much more severe (sensorineural) hearing loss can be minimized or prevented with appropriate early identification and rehabilitation (Yoshinaga-Itano et al., 1998). However, conductive hearing loss due to chronic otitis media with effusion, unlike sensorineural hearing loss, presents unique difficulties, principally as a result of its fluctuating nature. Even relatively brief periods of conductive hearing loss, in both childhood and adulthood, can have lasting effects on central auditory system processing (Gunnarson and Finitzo, 1991; Moore et al., 1999). Treatment for brief or transient conductive hearing loss, with either surgery or amplification, has not been advocated. Central auditory processing difficulties resolve slowly after resolution of bilateral chronic otitis media with effusion (Hall et al., 1995) or unilateral conductive hearing impairment (Hall and Derlacki, 1986; Magliulo et al., 1990; Hall et al., 1990; Hall and Grose, 1993; Snik et al., 1994; Wilmington et al., 1994). Because this has been found in both children and adults, adaptation following treatment is thought to be independent of critical periods for speech and language development (Hall et al., 1990; Ferguson et al., 1998).

Conductive hearing loss may be readily treated either surgically or with amplification. Unfortunately, no studies have compared language and cognitive development in children with chronic otitis media with effusion treated by amplification against those treated surgically.

Amplification has traditionally relied on the use of hearing aids. Fitting young children with hearing aids can be difficult because hearing loss due to chronic oti-

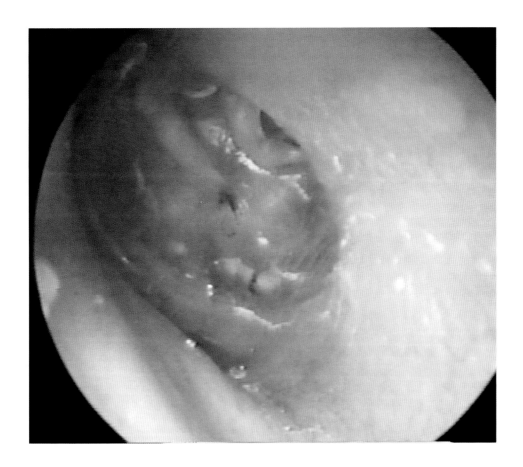

COLOR FIG. 30.2. Stage 4 atelectasis of the tympanic membrane-pars tensa.

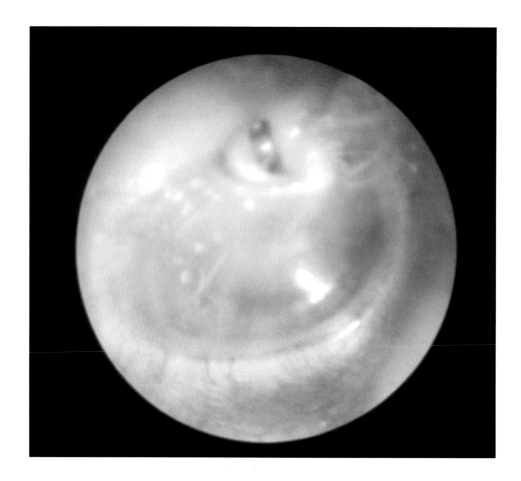

COLOR FIG. 30.3. Stage 2 atelectasis of the tympanic membrane-pars flaccida.

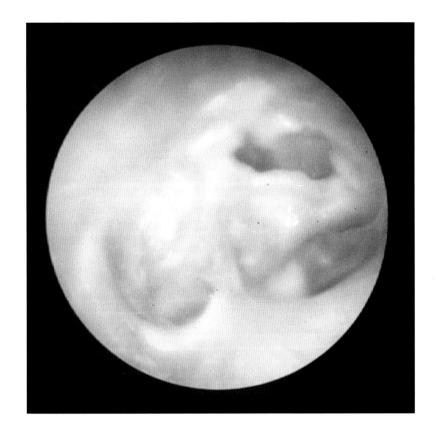

COLOR FIG. 30.4. Cholesteatoma of the left ear. Debris and granulation tissue fill the epitympanic defect.

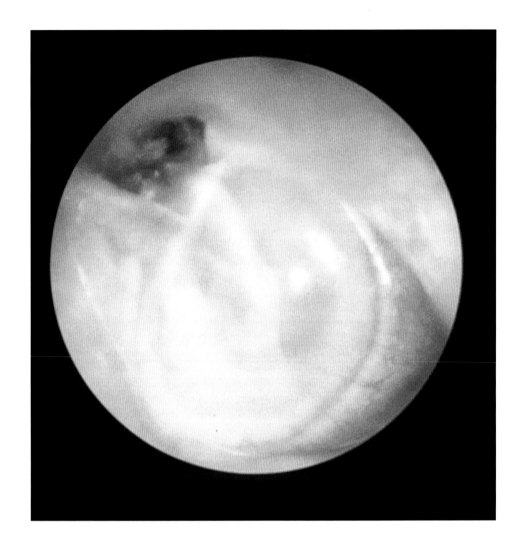

COLOR FIG. 30.5. Cholesteatoma of the right ear obscured by dried drainage that mimics cerumen.

tis media with effusion may fluctuate significantly and young children cannot provide the feedback necessary to readily handle such fluctuations. Although the use of hearing aids for hearing loss due to chronic otitis media with effusion requires frequent audiologic assessment and intervention, they are well tolerated by most children (Updike, 1994; Flanagan et al., 1996; Jardine et al., 1999). Alternative amplification strategies include the use of FM trainers, modification of environmental acoustics, sound-field amplification, and home stimulation language programs (Bergstrom, 1980; Bess et al., 1984; Crandell, 1993).

Surgical treatment of chronic otitis media with effusion involves *myringotomy* (incision through the tympanic membrane) and insertion of a tympanostomy tube through this incision, as described by Armstrong (1954). This bypasses the eustachian tube, allowing ventilation of the middle ear and clearance of middle ear effusion. Clearance of middle ear effusion leads to correction of hearing impairment in the vast majority of children with chronic otitis media with effusion (Fria et al., 1987). The simplicity and prompt auditory benefits of tympanostomy tube placement have led to this procedure becoming the standard of care for chronic otitis media with effusion in the United States (Paradise, 1976; Robinson et al., 1992; Otitis Media Guideline Panel, 1994). The placement of tympanostomy tubes has been cited as the most commonly performed surgical procedure in the United States. Nearly one-third of children less than 2 years old are treated with tympanostomy tubes (Myer and France, 1997). Because chronic otitis media with effusion in children with cleft palate commonly persists for the first few years of life, even after palatoplasty, and tympanostomy tubes commonly extrude in a shorter period of time (Weigel et al., 1989), children with cleft palate who are managed with tympanostomy tubes commonly require multiple tympanostomy tube placement procedures (Muenker, 1980; Robinson et al., 1992; Muntz, 1993). Use of tympanostomy tubes has not been globally adopted as the standard of care. This is likely a function of the limited access to care in developing countries, the expense of surgical intervention, and the potential for sequelae due to tympanostomy tube placement.

A decrease in the incidence of irreversible tympanic membrane conditions (e.g., atelectasis and cholesteatoma) has been perceived by many clinicians. Most have related this decline to an increase in the use of tympanostomy tubes, but Roland et al. (1992) found no correlation between the use of tympanostomy tubes and the incidence of cholesteatoma. On the contrary, a number of studies have implicated tympanostomy tubes in the pathogenesis of middle ear pathology, such

as atelectasis and tympanic membrane perforation (Moller, 1975, 1981; Sade and Berco, 1976; Skinner et al., 1988; Sederberg-Olsen, et al., 1988; Gordon et al., 1988; Le et al., 1991; Robson et al., 1992; Schilder, et al., 1993; Maw and Bawden, 1994). More specifically, the tympanostomy may serve as the nidus for the development of irreversible tympanic membrane pathology, particularly with long-term tube placement (Moller, 1981; Lildholdt, 1983; Gundersen et al., 1984; Mortensen and Lildholdt, 1984; Soderberg et al., 1986; Skinner et al., 1988; Le et al., 1991; Robinson et al., 1992; Robson et al., 1992; Maw and Bawden, 1994; Oluwole and Mills, 1996; Golz et al., 1999a,b). Oluwole and Mills (1996) reported that 70% of tympanic membrane perforations are tube-related. Similar associations have been drawn for cholesteatoma (Golz et al., 1999a).

Adverse middle ear outcomes appear to be more common in children treated with tympanostomy tubes than with myringotomy alone. Compared to treatment with tympanostomy tubes, chronic otitis media with effusion treated by myringotomy alone has been associated with a lower rate of *myringosclerosis* (deposition of hyalinized scar tissue within the lamina propria of the tympanic membrane or submucosally in the middle ear) (Sade and Berco, 1976). Le et al. (1991) found a significantly higher rate of tympanic membrane perforations in ears treated with tympanostomy tubes than with myringotomy alone. Thus, tympanostomy tubes do not protect against long-term adverse middle ear outcomes of eustachian tube dysfunction. Rather, they may increase the risk of their development.

Lildholdt (1983), Skinner and colleagues (1988), and Maw and Bawden (1994) performed long-term, controlled studies on the effects of tympanostomy tubes (with or without concomitant adenoidectomy) for chronic otitis media with effusion in children *without* cleft palate. All enrolled patients had bilateral chronic otitis media with effusion, but tympanostomy tubes were placed in only one ear. These authors assessed the incidence of several forms of tympanic membrane pathology observed in children with chronic otitis media with effusion, including segmental atrophy (loss of the lamina propria, the fibrous, strength layer) of the pars tensa, scarring and thickening of the pars tensa, atelectasis of the pars tensa, attic retraction, myringosclerosis, cholesteatoma, and tympanic membrane perforation. Though ears treated with tubes took less time to resolve the middle ear effusion, other problems were more common in these surgically treated ears. Problems such as myringosclerosis and segmental tympanic membrane atrophy were statistically significantly more common in ears treated with tympanostomy tubes as early as 3 years of age. Skinner et al. (1988) found that less common but more serious problems, such as cholesteatoma, were more common in ears treated with tympanostomy tubes (6.5% vs. 0%), but these differences were not statistically significant. Higher rates of myringosclerosis with the use of tympanostomy tubes have been reported (Sederberg-Olsen et al., 1988; Schilder et al., 1993).

Both Skinner et al. (1988) and Maw and Bawden (1994) treated many of their patients with concomitant adenoidectomy. Adenoidectomy has been shown to significantly impact the resolution of chronic otitis media with effusion and to minimize the recurrence of middle ear effusion, i.e., to minimize the need for repeat tympanostomy tube placement (Gates et al., 1987; Paradise et al., 1990). The benefits of adenoidectomy on chronic otitis media with effusion are greater than those of tympanostomy tubes (Gates et al., 1987; Paradise et al., 1990). The benefit of adenoidectomy is presumably due to its effects on tubal function and nasopharyngeal microflora (Bluestone and Klein, 1996a). Unfortunately, adenoidectomy is relatively contraindicated in children with cleft palate because it places them at an increased risk of velopharyngeal insufficiency (Haapanen et al., 1993). Only a single, small retrospective study has addressed the impact of adenoidectomy on otitis media with effusion in children with cleft palate (Severeid, 1972).

In light of the contraindication for adenoidectomy and the more lasting difficulties with eustachian tube dysfunction in children with cleft palate, it is not surprising that these children undergo more treatment with tympanostomy tubes than children without cleft palate (Muenker, 1980; Robson et al., 1992; Muntz, 1993). As standard tympanostomy tubes extrude or become nonfunctional in 1 to 2 years (Weigel et al., 1989), they are often repeatedly placed in children with cleft palate (Muenker, 1980; Robson et al., 1992). Though longer-acting tympanostomy tubes are available, these are associated with significantly higher rates of serious tympanic membrane pathology, such as cholesteatoma and persistent tympanic membrane perforation (Weigel et al., 1989). Robson et al. (1992) found that children with cleft palate needed an average of 1.66 tympanostomy tubes, despite the use of long-acting tubes. Thus, children with cleft palate and chronic otitis media with effusion are at higher risk than children without cleft palate of experiencing any possible adverse outcomes related to tympanostomy tubes.

To date, only retrospective studies have addressed the long-term middle ear outcomes in children with cleft palate. Gordon et al. (1988) reported that myringosclerosis was significantly more common in the ears of cleft children with chronic otitis media with effusion who had been treated with tympanostomy tubes. Robson et al. (1992) similarly found higher rates of otoscopic abnormalities in the ears of cleft children treated with tympanostomy tubes. Seagle et al. (1998) reported higher rates of otologic and audiologic problems in American children with cleft palate who had been treated with tympanostomy tubes than in Russian children with cleft palate who had not received tympanostomy tubes. Hence, some clinicians have long been advocating more limited use of tympanostomy tubes (Moller, 1981; Gundersen et al., 1984; Robinson et al., 1992; Robson et al., 1992). Use of tympanostomy tubes has been similarly questioned in other craniofacial disorders (e.g., Down syndrome) because of higher rates of such sequelae (Iino et al., 1999). Unfortunately, the long-term value and consequences of tympanostomy tube placement in children with cleft palate and chronic otitis media with effusion are still not clearly understood. This issue has not been formally, prospectively studied in children with cleft palate and chronic otitis media with effusion.

Treatment of Chronic Suppurative Otitis Media

As with chronic otitis media with effusion, chronic otitis media with tympanic membrane perforation or cholesteatoma commonly manifests by hearing loss (Paparella and Schachern, 1984). However, untreated, cholesteatoma and chronic infection can spread into surrounding structures (e.g., the inner ear or cranium) with potentially life-threatening consequences (Sheehy and Brackmann, 1979; Kangsanarak et al., 1993; Burggraff et al., 1995). Simple procedures, such as tympanostomy tube placement, will not correct either of these conditions or their associated hearing loss. Middle ear reconstructive surgery (tympanoplasty with or without mastoidectomy), often requiring multiple procedures, is commonly necessary (Iino et al., 1998; Stangerup et al., 1999; Silvola and Palva, 1999). Although surgical treatment is highly effective for preventing serious intratemporal and intracranial suppurative complications, hearing may remain compromised (Silvola and Palva, 1999). This can have a lifelong impact on quality of life (Mulrow et al., 1990).

Ideally, cholesteatoma should be identified as early as possible, before significant ossicular damage has been incurred and before ossicular removal would be necessary to eradicate the disease. Distinguishing cholesteatoma from end-stage atelectasis can prove challenging. Debris or drainage from a cholesteatoma pocket can look very similar to cerumen (Color Fig. 30.5). Cholesteatoma should be considered if there is any sign or symptom of recurrent or progressive middle ear inflammation (Table 30.3).

TABLE 30.3. *Clinical Findings Consistent with the Diagnosis of Cholesteatoma*

Accumulation of squamous debris within a pars tensa or pars flaccida retraction pocket

Overt chronic purulent drainage from stage 4 atelectasis

Recurrent purulent drainage with the middle ear atelectasis, in the absence of a tympanostomy tube or a perforation

Honey-colored crusting over an advanced retraction pocket, with associated erosion of the bone adjacent to the tympanic membrane

NOSE

The nasal airway is commonly compromised in individuals with oral clefts (Chaudhuri and Bowen-Jones, 1978; Warren et al., 1990; Ishikawa and Amitani, 1994). Nasal airway obstruction is generally not manifest until after cheiloplasty, palatoplasty, or pharyngoplasty (Orr et al., 1987; Josephson et al., 1996; Witt et al., 1996). This can seriously affect spontaneous ventilation in obligate nasal breathers, such as young infants (Sculerati et al., 1994). Older individuals may manifest nasal airway obstruction in more subtle ways, such as obstructive sleep apnea (Nowak and Weider, 1998).

In most cases, the nasal obstruction is ipsilateral to the cleft palate, but both sides may be involved (Sandham and Murray, 1993; Wahlmam et al., 1998; Suzuki et al., 1999; Kunkel et al., 1999). Anatomic deformities include septal deviation (Suzuki et al., 1999), nasal valve stenosis (Wahlmam et al., 1998), posterior choanae (Wahlmam et al., 1998), ectopic teeth (Ranalli et al., 1990; Yeung and Lee, 1996), adenoid hypertrophy (Shapiro, 1982), and skull base encephalocele (Shimizu et al., 1999). Septoplasty and rhinoplasty are often helpful (Lowenthal, 1981), but results may be less than ideal because of midfacial developmental problems (Drake et al., 1993; Mooney et al., 1994; Anastassov et al., 1998).

Adenoid hypertrophy can obstruct the choanae of children with cleft palate. Adenoidectomy is relatively contraindicated in children with cleft palate because of the increased risk for velopharyngeal insufficiency (Pickrell et al., 1976; Croft et al., 1981; Witzel et al., 1986; Haapanen et al., 1993). However, a limited adenoidectomy (i.e., from high within the choanae) may significantly improve the nasal airway with a low rate of velopharyngeal insufficiency in selected patients (Shapiro, 1982; Kakani et al., 2000).

Rhinitis and sinusitis are also relatively common in individuals with cleft palate (Robinson et al., 1982; Ishikawa and Amitani, 1994). These conditions have historically been related to velopharyngeal insufficiency

and reflux of pharyngeal contents into the nasal cavity (Robinson et al., 1982). Stasis of nasal secretions and rhinitis may develop if adenoid tissue or anatomic abnormalities obstruct the choanae. Rhinosinusitis in cleft patients has been attributed to mucociliary dysfunction (Ishikawa et al., 1989). Ishikawa and Amitani (1994) reported rhinosinusitis to be more common both in patients with cleft palate and in congenital (noncleft) velopharyngeal insufficiency relative to normal control subjects. Nasal obstruction and mucociliary dysfunction were significantly more common in cleft palate patients than in congenital velopharyngeal insufficiency subjects or normal controls. Hence, nasal obstruction, mucociliary dysfunction, and velopharyngeal insufficiency may all play a role in the pathogenesis of rhinosinusitis in individuals with cleft palate.

THROAT

Recurrent tonsillitis and sleep apnea secondary to tonsillar hypertrophy are the most common indications for removal of the palatine tonsils in childhood. By virtue of their juxtaposition to the palate, tonsillar pathology can significantly impact palatal function and speech (Finkelstein et al., 1994). Though velopharyngeal insufficiency has been reported to be a complication of palatine tonsillectomy (Haapanen et al., 1994), D'Antonio and colleagues (1996) found no evidence of significant degradation of speech or velopharyngeal function following tonsillectomy in children with cleft palate. A number of reports have documented improvement in palatal function after removal of hypertrophied tonsils (MacKenzie-Stepner et al., 1987; Shprintzen et al., 1987; Kummer et al., 1993).

Palatine tonsillectomy may be necessary to accommodate other cleft palate procedures. Creation of a pharyngeal flap can seriously compromise the airway in the presence of tonsillar hypertrophy (Reath et al., 1987). Though tonsillectomy may be done prior to pharyngoplasty, they may be safely performed simultaneously (Reath et al., 1987; Eufinger and Eggeling, 1994; Eufinger et al., 1994).

Airway obstruction is the most serious of the otolaryngologic conditions involving individuals with oral clefts. Airway obstruction in individuals with cleft lip and palate, as discussed above, is commonly due to nasal abnormalities and adenotonsillar hypertrophy and may be aggravated following palatal or pharyngeal reconstruction. Obstructive sleep apnea may develop later in childhood, well after primary palatoplasty, as adenoid hypertrophy develops (Kiely et al., 1998; Nowak and Weider, 1998). Conservative management, such as continuous positive airway pressure ventilation, may be sufficient (Kiely et al., 1998), but adenotonsillectomy (Shapiro, 1982) or nasal reconstruction may be required (Lowenthal, 1981).

The pharyngeal airway is compromised in individuals with oral clefts (Smahel and Mullerova, 1992). Further compromise by associated anomalies leads to more serious airway compromise (Figueroa et al., 1991). Airway obstruction is of particular concern in patients with hypoplasia of the midface and mandible (Sculerati et al., 1998; Bath and Bull, 1997), as seen with Crouzon's, Treacher Collins, and Apert's syndromes as well as Robin sequence. Conservative measures, such as positioning and continuous positive airway pressure ventilation, may yield an adequate airway, but tracheotomy may be required (Olson et al., 1990; Caouette-Laberge et al., 1994; Lehman et al., 1995; Bath and Bull, 1997; Sculerati et al., 1998).

REFERENCES

Anastassov, GE, Joos, U, Zollner, B (1998). Evaluation of the results of delayed rhinoplasty in cleft lip and palate patients. Functional and aesthetic implications and factors that affect successful nasal repair. Br J Oral Maxillofac Surg 36: 416–424.

Antonelli, PJ, Harada, T, Juhn, SK, Giebink, GS (1988). *Pseudomonas aeruginosa* otitis media in the chinchilla: an animal model of chronic suppurative otitis media [abstract]. Otolaryngol Head Neck Surg 99: 139.

Antonelli, PJ, Juhn, SK, Goycoolea, MV, Giebink, GS (1992). *Pseudomonas* otitis media after eustachian tube obstruction. Otolaryngol Head Neck Surg 107: 511–515.

Antonelli, PJ, Juhn, SK, Goycoolea, MV, Giebink, GS (1993). Middle ear susceptibility to *Pseudomonas* infection during acute otitis media. Ann Otol Rhinol Laryngol 102: 531–536.

Armstrong, BW (1954). A new treatment strategy for chronic secretory otitis media. Arch Otolaryngol 59: 653–654.

Aul, JJ, Anderson, KW, Wadowsky, RM (1998). Comparative evaluation of culture and PCR for the detection and determination of persistence of bacterial strains and DNAs in the *Chinchilla laniger* model of otitis media. Ann Otol Rhinol Laryngol 107: 508–513.

Bath, AP, Bull, PD (1997). Management of upper airway obstruction in Pierre Robin sequence. J Laryngol Otol 111: 1155–1157.

Bergstrom, L (1980). Continuing management of conductive hearing loss during language development. Int J Pediatr Otorhinolaryngol 2: 3–9.

Bess, FH, Sinclair, JS, Riggs, DE (1984). Group amplification in schools for the hearing impaired. Ear Hear 5: 138–144.

Bluestone, CD, Klein, JO (1996a). Otitis media, atelectasis, and eustachian tube dysfunction. In: *Pediatric Otolaryngology*, Vol. 1, edited by CD Bluestone, SE Stool, and MA Kenna. Philadelphia: WB Saunders, pp. 388–582.

Bluestone, CD, Klein, JO (1996b). Intratemporal complications and sequelae of otitis media. In: *Pediatric Otolaryngology*, Vol. 1, edited by CD Bluestone, SE Stool, and MA Kenna. Philadelphia: WB Saunders, pp. 583–635.

Brody, R, Rosenfeld, RM, Goldsmith, AJ, Madell, JR (1999). Parents cannot detect mild hearing loss in children. Otolaryngol Head Neck Surg 121: 681–686.

Brown, DT, Marsh, RR, Potsic, WP (1983). Hearing loss induced by viscous fluids in the middle ear. Int J Pediatr Otorhinolaryngol 5: 39–46.

Buchman, CA, Doyle, WJ, Skoner, D, et al. (1994). Otologic manifestations of experimental rhinovirus infection. Laryngoscope 104: 1295–1299.

Burggraaff, B, Luxford, WM, Doyle, KJ (1995). Neurotologic treatment of acquired cholesteatoma. Am J Otol 16: 480–485.

Caouette-Laberge, L, Bayet, B, Larocque, Y (1994). The Pierre Robin sequence: review of 125 cases and evolution of treatment modalities. Plast Reconstr Surg 93: 934–942.

Casselbrandt, ML, Cantekin, EI, Dirkmaat, DC, et al. (1988). Experimental paralysis of tensor veli palatini muscle. Acta Otolaryngol (Stockh) 106: 178–185.

Chaudhuri, PK, Bowen-Jones, E (1978). An otorhinological study of children with cleft palates. J Laryngol Otol 92: 29–40.

Cohen, D, Sade, J (1972). Hearing in secretory otitis media. Can J Otolaryngol 1: 27–29.

Crandell, CC (1993). Speech recognition in noise by children with minimal degrees of sensorineural hearing loss. Ear Hear 14: 210–216.

Croft, CB, Shprintzen, RJ, Ruben, RJ (1981). Hypernasal speech following adenotonsillectomy. Otolaryngol Head Neck Surg 89: 179–188.

D'Antonio, LL, Snyder, LS, Samadani, S (1996). Tonsillectomy in children with or at risk for velopharyngeal insufficiency: effects on speech. Otolaryngol Head Neck Surg 115: 319–323.

Dhillon, RS (1988). The middle ear in cleft palate children pre- and postpalatal closure. J R Soc Med 81: 710–713.

Dominguez, S, Harker, LA (1988). Incidence of cholesteatoma with cleft palate. Ann Otol Rhinol Laryngol 97: 659–660.

Doyle, WJ, Cantekin, EI, Bluestone, CD (1980). Eustachian tube function in cleft palate children. Ann Otol Rhinol Laryngol Suppl 89: 34–40.

Doyle, WJ, Seroky, JT (1994). Middle ear gas exchange in rhesus monkeys. Ann Otol Rhinol Laryngol 103: 636–645.

Drake, AF, Davis, JU, Warren, DW (1993). Nasal airway size in cleft and noncleft children. Laryngoscope 103: 915–917.

Elner, A (1977). Quantitative studies of gas absorption from the normal middle ear. Acta Otolaryngol (Stockh) 83: 25–28.

Eufinger, H, Eggeling, V (1994). Should velopharyngoplasty and tonsillectomy in the cleft palate child be performed simultaneously? J Oral Maxillofac Surg 52: 927–930.

Eufinger, H, Eggeling, V, Immenkamp, E (1994). Velopharyngoplasty with or without tonsillectomy and/or adenotomy—a retrospective evaluation of speech characteristics in 143 patients. J Craniomaxillofac Surg 22: 37–42.

Ferguson, MO, Cook, RD, Hall, JW 3rd, et al. (1998). Chronic conductive hearing loss in adults: effects on the auditory brainstem response and masking-level difference. Arch Otolaryngol Head Neck Surg 124: 678–685.

Figueroa, AA, Glupker, TJ, Fitz, MG, BeGole, EA (1991). Mandible, tongue, and airway in Pierre Robin sequence: a longitudinal cephalometric study. Cleft Palate Craniofac J 28: 425–434.

Finitzo, T, Friel-Patti, S, Chinn, K, Brown O (1992). Tympanometry and otoscopy prior to myringotomy: issues in diagnosis of otitismedia. Int J Pediatr Otorhinolaryngol 24: 101–110.

Finkelstein, Y, Nachmani, A, Ophir, D (1994). The functional role of the tonsils in speech. Arch Otolaryngol Head Neck Surg 120: 846–851.

Flanagan, PM, Knight, LC, Thomas, A, et al. (1996). Hearing aids and glue ear. Clin Otolaryngol 21: 297–300.

Fliss, DM, Dagan, R, Houri, Z, Leiberman, A (1990). Medical management of chronic suppurative otitis media without cholesteatoma in children. J Pediatr 116: 991–996.

Fria, TJ, Cantekin, EI, Eichler, JA (1985). Hearing acuity of children with otitis media with effusion. Arch Otolaryngol 111: 10–16.

Fria, TJ, Paradise, JL, Sabo, DL, Elster, BA (1987). Conductive hearing loss in infants and young children with cleft palate. J Pediatr 111: 84–87.

Friedmann, I (1955a). The comparative pathology of otitis media—experimental and human, I. Experimental otitis of the guinea pig. J Laryngol Otol 69: 27–50.

Friedmann, I (1955b). The comparative pathology of otitis media—experimental and human. II. The histopathology of experimental otitis of the guinea pig with particular reference to cholesteatoma. J Laryngol Otol 69: 588–601.

Gates, GA, Avery, CA, Prihoda, TJ, Cooper, JC (1987). Effectiveness of adenoidectomy and tympanostomy tubes in the treatment of chronic otitis media with effusion. N Engl J Med 317: 1444–1451.

Goldman, JL, Martinez, SA, Ganzel, TM (1993). Eustachian tube dysfunction and its sequelae in patients with cleft palate. South Med J 86: 1236–1237.

Golz, A, Goldenberg, D, Netzer, A, et al. (1999a). Cholesteatomas associated with ventilation tube insertion. Arch Otolaryngol Head Neck Surg 125: 754–757.

Golz, A, Netzer, A, Joachims, HZ, et al. (1999b). Ventilation tubes and persisting tympanic membrane perforations. Otolaryngol Head Neck Surg 120: 524–527.

Gordon, AS, Jean-Louis, F, Morton, RP (1988). Late ear sequelae in cleft palate patients. Int J Pediatr Otorhinolaryngol 15: 149–156.

Grant, HR, Quiney, RE, Mercer, DM, Lodge, S (1988). Cleft palate and glue ear. Arch Dis Child 63: 176–179.

Gundersen, T, Tonning, FM, Kveberg, KH (1984). Ventilating tubes in the middle ear. Long-term observations. Arch Otolaryngol 110: 783–784.

Gunnarson, AD, Finitzo, T (1991). Conductive hearing loss during infancy: effects on later auditory brain stem electrophysiology. J Speech Hear Res 34: 1207–1215.

Haapanen, ML, Ignatius, J, Rihkanen, H, Ertama, L (1994). Velopharyngeal insufficiency following palatine tonsillectomy. Eur Arch Otorhinolaryngol 251: 186–189.

Haapanen, ML, Veija, M, Pettay, M (1993). Speech outcome in cleft palate patients with simultaneous primary palatal repair and adenoidectomy. Acta Otolaryngol (Stockh) 113: 560–562.

Hall, JW III, Derlacki, EL (1986). Effect of conductive hearing loss and middle ear surgery on binaural hearing. Ann Otol Rhinol Laryngol 95: 525–530.

Hall, JW III, Grose, JH (1993). Short-term and long-term effects on the masking level difference following middle ear surgery. J Am Acad Audiol 4: 307–312.

Hall, JW III, Grose, JH, Pillsbury, HC (1990). Predicting binaural hearing after stapedectomy from presurgery results. Arch Otolaryngol Head Neck Surg 116: 946–950.

Hall, JW III, Grose, JH, Pillsbury, HC (1995). Long-term effects of chronic otitis media on binaural hearing in children. Arch Otolaryngol Head Neck Surg 121: 847–852.

Harker, LA, Koontz, FP (1977). Bacteriology of cholesteatoma: clinical significance. Trans Am Acad Ophthalmol Otolaryngol 84: 683–686.

Hayden, GF (1981). Acute suppurative otitis media in children: diversity of clinical diagnostic criteria. Clin Pediatr 20: 99.

Hubbard, TW, Paradise, JL, McWilliams, BJ, et al. (1985). Consequences of unremitting middle-ear disease in early life. Otologic, audiologic, and developmental findings in children with cleft palate. N Engl J Med 312: 1529–1534.

Iino, Y, Imamura, Y, Harigai, S, Tanaka, Y (1999). Efficacy of tympanostomy tube insertion for otitis media with effusion in children with Down syndrome. Int J Pediatr Otorhinolaryngol 49: 143–149.

Iino, Y, Imamura, Y, Kojima, C, et al. (1998). Risk factors for recurrent and residual cholesteatoma in children determined by second stage operation. Int J Pediatr Otorhinolaryngol 46: 57–65.

Ishikawa, Y, Amitani, R (1994). Nasal and paranasal sinus disease in patients with congenital velopharyngeal insufficiency. Arch Otolaryngol Head Neck Surg 120: 861–865.

Ishikawa, Y, Kawano, M, Honjo, I, Amitani, R (1989). The cause of nasal sinusitis in patients with cleft palate. Arch Otolaryngol Head Neck Surg 115: 442–446.

Jardine, AH, Griffiths, MV, Midgley, E (1999). The acceptance of hearing aids for children with otitis media with effusion. J Laryngol Otol 113: 314–317.

Jensen, PM, Lous, J (1999). Criteria, performance and diagnostic problems in diagnosing acute otitis media. Fam Pract 16: 262–268.

Josephson, GD, Levine, J, Cutting, CB (1996). Septoplasty for obstructive sleep apnea in infants after cleft lip repair. Cleft Palate Craniofac J 33: 473–476.

Kakani, RS, Callan, ND, April, MM (2000). Superior adenoidectomy in children with palatal abnormalities. Ear Nose Throat J 79: 300–305.

Kangsanarak, J, Fooanant, S, Ruckphaopunt, K, et al. (1993). Extracranial and intracranial complications of suppurative otitis media. Report of 102 cases. J Laryngol Otol 107: 999–1004.

Kemaloglu, YK, Kobayashi, T, Nakajima, T (1999). Analysis of the craniofacial skeleton in cleft children with otitis media with effusion. Int J Pediatr Otorhinolaryngol 47: 57–69.

Kemppainen, HO, Puhakka, HJ, Laippala, PJ, et al. (1999). Epidemiology and aetiology of middle ear cholesteatoma. Acta Otolaryngol (Stockh) 119: 568–572.

Kempthorne, J, Giebink, GS (1991). Pediatric approach to the diagnosis and management of otitis media. Otolaryngol Clin North Am 24: 905–929.

Kenna, MA (1988). Chinchilla animal model of chronic suppurative otitis media. Ann Otol Rhinol Laryngol Suppl 97: 19–20.

Kenna, MA, Bluestone, CD (1986). Microbiology of chronic suppurative otitis media in children. Pediatr Infect Dis 5: 223–225.

Kenna, MA, Bluestone, CD, Reilly, JS, Lusk, RP (1986). Medical management of chronic suppurative otitis media without cholesteatoma in children. Laryngoscope 96: 146–151.

Kiely, JL, Deegan, PC, McNicholas, WT (1998). Resolution of obstructive sleep apnoea with growth in the Robin sequence. Eur Respir J 12: 499–501.

Kummer, AW, Billmire, DA, Myer, CM 3rd (1993). Hypertrophic tonsils: the effect on resonance and velopharyngeal closure. Plast Reconstr Surg 91: 608–611.

Kunkel, M, Wahlmann, U, Wagner, W (1999). Acoustic airway profiles in unilateral cleft palate patients. Cleft Palate Craniofac J 36: 434–440.

Le, CT, Freeman, DW, Fireman, BH (1991). Evaluation of ventilating tubes and myringotomy in the treatment of recurrent or persistent otitis media. Pediatr Infect Dis J 10: 2–11.

Lehman, JA, Fishman, JR, Neiman, GS (1995). Treatment of cleft palate associated with Robin sequence: appraisal of risk factors. Cleft Palate Craniofac J 32: 25–29.

Lildholdt, T (1983). Ventilation tubes in secretory otitis media. A randomized, controlled study of the course, the complications, and the sequelae of ventilation tubes. Acta Otolaryngol Suppl 398: 1–28.

Liu, YS, Lang, R, Lim, DJ, Birck, HG (1976). Microorganisms in chronic otitis media with effusion. Ann Otol Rhinol Laryngol Suppl 85: 245–249.

Lowenthal, G (1981). Secondary surgical treatment of intranasal deformities of the unilateral cleft palate nose. Laryngoscope 91: 1641–1646.

MacKenzie-Stepner, K, Witzel, MA, Stringer, DA, Laskin, R (1987). Velopharyngeal insufficiency due to hypertrophic tonsils. A report of two cases. Int J Pediatr Otorhinolaryngol 14: 57–63.

Magliulo, G, Gagliardi, M, Muscatello, M, Natale, A (1990). Masking level difference before and after surgery in unilateral otosclerosis. Br J Audiol 24: 117–121.

Matsune, S, Sando, I, Takahashi, H (1991). Insertion of the tensor veli palatini muscle into the eustachian tube cartilage in cleft palate cases. Ann Otol Rhinol Laryngol 100: 439–446.

Matsune, S, Sando, I, Takahashi, H (1992). Elastin at the hinge portion of the eustachian tube cartilage in specimens from normal subjects and those with cleft palate. Ann Otol Rhinol Laryngol 101: 163–167.

Maw, AR, Bawden, R (1994). Tympanic membrane atrophy, scarring, atelectasis and attic retraction in persistent, untreated otitis media with effusion and following ventilation tube insertion. Int J Pediatr Otorhinolaryngol 30: 189–204.

Mawson, SR, Ludman, H (1979). Diseases of the Ear: A Textbook of Otology, 4th ed. Chicago: Yearbook, pp. 328–330.

Meyerhoff, WL, Giebink, GS, Shea, D (1981). Pneumococcal otitis media following middle ear deflation. Ann Otol Rhinol Laryngol 92: 72–76.

Moller, P (1975). Long-term otologic features of cleft palate patients. Arch Otolaryngol 101: 605–607.

Moller, P (1981). Hearing, middle ear pressure and otopathology in a cleft palate population. Acta Otolaryngol (Stockh) 92: 521–528.

Mooney, MP, Siegel, MI, Kimes, KR, et al. (1994). Anterior paraseptal cartilage development in normal and cleft lip and palate human fetal specimens. Cleft Palate Craniofac J 31: 239–245.

Moore, DR, Hine, JE, Jiang, ZD, et al. (1999). Conductive hearing loss produces a reversible binaural hearing impairment. J Neurosci 19: 8704–8711.

Mortensen, EH, Lildholdt, T (1984). Ventilation tubes and cholesteatoma in children. J Laryngol Otol 98: 27–29.

Muenker, G (1980). Results after treatment of otitis media with effusion. Ann Otol Rhinol Laryngol Suppl 89: 308–311.

Mulrow, CD, Aguilar, C, Endicott, JE, et al. (1990). Quality-of-life changes and hearing impairment. A randomized trial. Ann Intern Med 113: 188–194.

Muntz, HR (1993). An overview of middle ear disease in cleft palate children. Facial Plast Surg 9: 177–180.

Myer, CM 3rd, France, A (1997). Ventilation tube placement in a managed care population. Arch Otolaryngol Head Neck Surg 123: 226–228.

Nowak, KC, Weider, DJ (1998). Pediatric nocturnal enuresis secondary to airway obstruction from cleft palate repair. Clin Pediatr 37: 653–657.

Nunn, DR, Derkay, CS, Darrow, DH, et al. (1995). The effect of very early cleft palate closure on the need for ventilation tubes in the first years of life. Laryngoscope 105: 905–908.

Olson, TS, Kearns, DB, Pransky, SM, Seid, AB (1990). Early home management of patients with Pierre Robin sequence. Int J Pediatr Otorhinolaryngol 20: 45–49.

Oluwole, M, Mills, RP (1996). Tympanic membrane perforations in children. Int J Pediatr Otorhinolaryngol 36: 117–123.

Orr, WC, Levine, NS, Buchanan, RT (1987). Effect of cleft palate repair and pharyngeal flap surgery on upper airway obstruction during sleep. Plast Reconstr Surg 80: 226–232.

Otitis Media Guideline Panel (1994). Managing otitis media with effusion in young children. Pediatrics 94: 766–773.

Paparella, MM, Schachern, PA (1984). Complications and sequelae of otitis media. In: Recent Advances in Otitis Media with Effusion, edited by D Lim. Philadelphia: BC Decker, pp. 316–319.

Paparella, MM, Schachern, PA, Yoon, TH, et al. (1990). Otopathologic correlates of the continuum of otitis media. Ann Otol Rhinol Laryngol Suppl 148: 17–22.

Papastavros, T, Giamarellou, H, Varlejides, S (1986). Role of aerobic and anaerobic microorganisms in chronic suppurative otitis media. Laryngoscope 96: 438–442.

Paradise, JL (1976). Management of middle ear effusions in infants with cleft palate. Ann Otol Rhinol Laryngol Suppl 85: 285–288.

Paradise, JL (1995). Managing otitis media: a time for change. Pediatrics 96: 712–715.

Paradise, JL, Bluestone, CD, Felder, H (1969). The universality of otitis media in 50 infants with cleft palate. Pediatrics 44: 35–42.

Paradise, JL, Bluestone, CD, Rogers, KD, et al. (1990). Efficacy of adenoidectomy for recurrent otitis media in children previously treated with tympanostomy tube placement. JAMA 263: 2066–2073.

Pickrell, KL, Massengill, R, Jr, Quinn, G, et al. (1976). The effect of adenoidectomy on velopharyngeal competence in cleft palate patients. Br J Plast Surg 29: 134–136.

Podoshin, L, Fradis, M, Ben-David, Y, et al. (1986). Cholesteatoma: an epidemiological study among members of kibbutzim in northern Israel. Ann Otol Rhinol Laryngol 95: 365–368.

Post, JC, Aul, JJ, White, GJ, et al. (1996). PCR-based detection of bacterial DNA after antimicrobial treatment is indicative of persistent, viable bacteria in the chinchilla model of otitis media. Am J Otolaryngol 17: 106–111.

Post, JC, Preston, RA, Aul, JJ, et al. (1995). Molecular analysis of bacterial pathogens in otitis media with effusion. JAMA 273: 1598–1604.

Ranalli, DN, McWilliams, BJ, Garrett, WS, Jr (1990). Tooth and foreign object in the nasal fossa of a child with a cleft: case report. Pediatr Dent 12: 183–184.

Rayner, MG, Zhang, Y, Gorry, MC, et al. (1998). Evidence of bacterial metabolic activity in culture-negative otitis media with effusion. JAMA 279: 296–299.

Reath, DB, LaRossa, D, Randall, P (1987). Simultaneous posterior pharyngeal flap and tonsillectomy. Cleft Palate J 24: 250–253.

Roberts, JE, Burchinal, MR, Campbell, F (1994). Otitis media in early childhood and patterns of intellectual development and later academic performance. J Pediatr Psychol 19: 347–367.

Roberts, JE, Burchinal, MR, Clarke-Klein, SM (1995). Otitis media in early childhood and cognitive, academic, and behavior outcomes at 12 years of age. J Pediatr Psychol 20: 645–660.

Roberts, JE, Burchinal, MR, Zeisel, SA, et al. (1998). Otitis media, the caregiving environment, and language and cognitive outcomes at 2 years. Pediatrics 102: 346–354.

Robinson, HE, Zerlin, GK, Passy, V (1982). Maxillary sinus development in patients with cleft palates as compared to those with normal palates. Laryngoscope 92: 183–187.

Robinson, PJ, Lodge, S, Jones, BM, et al. (1992). The effect of palate repair on otitis media with effusion. Plast Reconstr Surg 89: 640–645.

Robson, AK, Blanshard, JD, Jones, K, et al. (1992). A conservative approach to the management of otitis media with effusion in cleft palate children. J Laryngol Otol 106: 788–792.

Roland, NJ, Phillips, DE, Rogers, JH, Singh, SD (1992). The use of ventilation tubes and the incidence of cholesteatoma surgery in the paediatric population of Liverpool. Clin Otolaryngol 17: 437–439.

Rosenfeld, RM, Goldsmith, AJ, Madell, JR (1998). How accurate is parent rating of hearing for children with otitis media? Arch Otolaryngol Head Neck Surg 124: 989–992.

Rynnel-Dagoo, B, Lindberg, K, Bagger-Sjoback, D, Larson, O (1992). Middle ear disease in cleft palate children at three years of age. Int J Pediatr Otorhinolaryngol 23: 201–209.

Sade, J, Berco, E (1976). Atelectasis and secretory otitis media. Ann Otol Rhinol Laryngol Suppl 85: 66–72.

Sandham, A, Murray, JA (1993). Nasal septal deformity in unilateral cleft lip and palate. Cleft Palate Craniofac J 30: 222–226.

Schilder, AG, Van Manen, JG, Zielhuis, GA, et al. (1993). Long-term effects of otitis media with effusion on language, reading and spelling. Clin Otolaryngol 18: 234–241.

Sculerati, N, Gottlieb, MD, Zimbler, MS, et al. (1998). Airway management in children with major craniofacial anomalies. Laryngoscope 108: 1806–1812.

Seagle, MB, Nackashi, JA, Kemker, FJ, et al. (1998). Otologic and audiologic status of Russian children with cleft lip and palate. Cleft Palate Craniofac J 35: 495–499.

Sederberg-Olsen, JF, Sederberg-Olsen, AE, Jensen, AM (1988). Late results of treatment with grommets for middle ear conditions. In: Recent Advances in Otitis Media, edited by DJ Lim. Toronto: BC Decker, pp. 269–271.

Severeid, LR (1972). A longitudinal study of the efficacy of adenoidectomy in children with cleft palate and secretory otitis media. Trans Am Acad Ophthalmol Otolaryngol 76: 1319–1324.

Shapiro, RS (1982). Partial adenoidectomy. Laryngoscope 92: 135–139.

Sheehy, JL, Brackmann, DE (1979). Cholesteatoma surgery: management of the labyrinthine fistula—a report of 97 cases. Laryngoscope 89: 78–87.

Shimizu, T, Kitamura, S, Kinouchi, K, Fukumitsu, K (1999). A rare case of upper airway obstruction in an infant caused by basal encephalocele complicating facial midline deformity. Paediatr Anaesth 9: 73–76.

Shprintzen, RJ, Sher, AE, Croft, CB (1987). Hypernasal speech caused by tonsillar hypertrophy. Int J Pediatr Otorhinolaryngol 14: 45–56.

Silverman, LK (1996). Lost IQ points: the brighter the child, the greater the loss. In: Recent Advances in Otitis Media, edited by DJ Lim, CD Bluestone, M Casselbrant, et al. Hamilton: BC Decker, pp. 342–346.

Silvola, J, Palva, T (1999). Long-term results of pediatric primary one-stage cholesteatoma surgery. Int J Pediatr Otorhinolaryngol 48: 101–107.

Skinner, DW, Lesser, THJ, Richards, SH (1988). A 15 year follow-up of a controlled trial of the use of grommets in glue ear. Clin Otolaryngol 13: 341–346.

Skolnik, EM (1958). Otologic evaluation in cleft palate patients. Laryngoscope 68: 1908–1949.

Smahel, Z, Mullerova, I (1992). Nasopharyngeal characteristics in children with cleft lip and palate. Cleft Palate Craniofac J 29: 282–286.

Snik, FM, Teunissen, B, Cremers, WR (1994). Speech recognition in patients after successful surgery for unilateral congenital ear anomalies. Laryngoscope 104: 1029–1034.

Soderberg, O, Hellstrom, S, Stenfors, L-E (1986). Structural changes in the tympanic membrane after repeated tympanostomy tube insertion. Acta Otolaryngol (Stockh) 102: 382–390.

Stangerup, SE, Drozdziewicz, D, Tos, M (1999). Cholesteatoma in children, predictors and calculation of recurrence rates. Int J Pediatr Otorhinolaryngol 49(Suppl 1): S69–S73.

Stewart, IA, Silva, PA, Williams, S (1996). Relationships of otitis media with effusion in early childhood to educational and behavioral disadvantage during teen years. In: Recent Advances in Otitis Media, edited by DJ Lim, CD Bluestone, M Casselbrant, et al. Hamilton: BC Decker, pp. 337–339.

Stool, SE, Randall, P (1967). Unexpected ear disease in infants with cleft palate. Cleft Palate J 4: 99–103.

Suzuki, H, Yamaguchi, T, Furukawa, M (1999). Rhinologic computed tomographic evaluation in patients with cleft lip and palate. Arch Otolaryngol Head Neck Surg 125: 1000–1004.

Tasaka, Y, Kawano, M, Honjo, I (1990). Eustachian tube function in OME patients with cleft palate. Special reference to the prognosis of otitis media with effusion. Acta Otolaryngol Suppl (Stockh) 471: 5–8.

Teele, DW, Klein, JO, Chase, C, et al. (1990). Otitis media in infancy and intellectual ability, school achievement, speech, and language at age 7 years. Greater Boston Otitis Media Study Group. J Infect Dis 162: 685–694.

Teele, DW, Klein, JO, Rosner, B (1989). Epidemiology of otitis media during the first seven years of life in children in greater Boston: a prospective, cohort study. J Infect Dis 160: 83–94.

Tos, M, Poulsen, G (1980). Attic retractions following secretory otitis. Acta Otolaryngol (Stockh) 89: 479–486.

Updike, CD (1994). Comparison of FM auditory trainers, CROS aids, and personal amplification in unilaterally hearing impaired children. J Am Acad Audiol 5: 204–209.

Wahlmam, U, Kunkel, M, Wagner, W (1998). Preoperative assessment of airway patency in the planning of corrective cleft nose surgery. Mund Kiefer Gesichtschir 2(Suppl 1): S153–S157.

Warren, DW, Hairfield, WM, Dalston, ET (1990). The relationship between nasal airway size and nasal-oral breathing in cleft lip and palate. Cleft Palate J 27: 46–51.

Weigel, MT, Parker, MY, Goldsmith, MM, et al. (1989). A prospective randomized study of four commonly used tympanostomy tubes. Laryngoscope 99: 252–256.

Wells, MD, Michaels, L (1983). Role of retraction pockets in cholesteatoma formation. Clin Otolaryngol 8: 39–45.

Welsh, LW, Welsh, JJ, Healy, MP (1996). Early sound deprivation and long-term hearing. Ann Otol Rhinol Laryngol 105: 877–881.

Wilmington, D, Gray, L, Jahrsdoerfer, R (1994). Binaural processing after corrected congenital unilateral conductive hearing loss. Hear Res 74: 99–114.

Witt, PD, Marsh, JL, Muntz, HR, et al. (1996). Acute obstructive sleep apnea as a complication of sphincter pharyngoplasty. Cleft Palate Craniofac J 33: 183–189.

Witzel, MA, Rich, RH, Margar-Bacal, F, Cox, C (1986). Velopharyngeal insufficiency after adenoidectomy: an 8-year review. Int J Pediatr Otorhinolaryngol 11: 15–20.

Wolfman, DE, Chole, RA (1986). Experimental retraction pocket cholesteatoma. Ann Otol Rhinol Laryngol 95: 639–644.

Yamaguchi, N, Sando, I, Hashida, Y, et al. (1990). Histologic study of eustachian tube cartilage with and without congenital anomalies: a preliminary study. Ann Otol Rhinol Laryngol 99: 984–987.

Yeung, KH, Lee, KH (1996). Intranasal tooth in a patient with a cleft lip and alveolus. Cleft Palate Craniofac J 33: 157–159.

Yoshinaga-Itano, C, Sedey, AL, Coulter, DK, Mehl, AL (1998). Language of early- and later-identified children with hearing loss. Pediatrics 102: 1161–1171.

31

Genetic counseling and interpretation of risk figures

CARMELLA S. STADTER

Genetic counseling, defined as the provision of medical, prognostic, and recurrence risk information about a disorder together with psychosocial support to the family, can be a complex undertaking when dealing with oral clefting. Previous chapters have dealt with medical and prognostic counseling, and this chapter will concentrate on recurrence risk and supportive counseling. Patients and families need to be made aware of their recurrence risks and reproductive options in an easy to understand manner with attention paid to the emotional impact of the information. Counseling an individual with a physical defect of the face, one of the most obvious and public parts of the body, is challenging. As with genetic counseling for any condition, one of the key aspects of supportive counseling for families with oral clefts is listening and allowing them to voice their concerns, frustrations, and joys. As discussed in earlier chapters, cleft lip with or without cleft palate (CL/P) and cleft palate alone (CP) result from distinctly different developmental processes occurring at different gestational ages. While these differences lead to certain counseling issues unique to each condition, there are also a number of important counseling issues shared by both conditions.

RECURRENCE RISKS

A thorough physical examination of the patient and other family members and a careful medical and family history are of utmost importance to the accuracy of recurrence risk counseling. These tools help to establish the etiology of the cleft, whether the cleft is an iso-lated abnormality or part of a multiple malformation syndrome in the patient, and whether there is any familial clustering of oral clefts. Only after establishing the etiology can thorough, accurate, and relevant genetic counseling be provided to the patient and family.

Isolated Oral Clefts

Oral clefts are most often isolated, meaning that they are primary defects with no other associated abnormalities or syndromic features. Among oral clefts, CP is more likely to have associated abnormalities and syndromes than CL/P. Isolated oral clefts have long been assumed to be inherited in a multifactorial manner, meaning that numerous genes in combination with environmental factors contribute to the formation of the cleft. This model assumes a threshold effect in which there is a critical mass of contributory genetic and environmental factors that need to be reached before an oral cleft occurs. Recent studies have questioned the applicability of the multifactorial model to all clefts and have proposed instead a greater degree of heterogeneity than previously thought, with at least some familial oral clefts being the result of the presence of one, or at the most a few, major predisposition genes with incomplete penetrance (Jones, 1993; Carinci et al., 2000). Issues surrounding the genetic mechanisms of isolated oral clefts are explored in much greater detail elsewhere in this book (see Part IV).

While theoretically it is likely that there is heterogeneity among isolated oral clefts, with some families segregating a major predisposition gene with incomplete penetrance, practical genetic counseling for the

TABLE 31.1. *Recurrence Risks for Isolated Oral Clefts*

Affected Family Member	CL/P (%)	CP (%)
1 Sibling	3–7	2–5
2 Siblings	8–14	10–20
1 Parent	2–5	3–7

CL/P, cleft lip with or without palate; CP, cleft palate.
Sources: Lynch and Kimberling (1981), Robinson and Linden (1993), Wyszynski et al. (1996), Harper (1999).

isolated cleft still relies on data of incidence of recurrence within a family compiled over years. If after a thorough evaluation, including a physical examination by an experienced clinical geneticist and a careful family history, the patient is diagnosed with an isolated oral cleft, the family should be provided information on recurrence risks based on empiric data (Table 31.1). In general, the risk increases with the number of affected family members, so it is important to examine other family members for subtle or subclinical oral clefts. Additionally, recurrence risks tend to increase with increasing severity of the oral cleft, so the higher end of the risk figure range may be more appropriate in the case of a bilateral vs. a unilateral oral cleft in the proband (Lynch and Kimberling, 1981; Robinson and Linden, 1993; Wyszynski et al., 1996; Harper, 1999). Bixler (1981) found a much reduced recurrence risk (<1%) when the cleft was sporadic vs. an increased risk (16%) when there was a history of clefting in a first- or second-degree relative.

However, these risks are most appropriately applied to cases of oral clefts in which no, or only an occasional, family member is affected. If the family history shows a number of members affected with oral clefts or other associated abnormalities, then a clefting syndrome or the possibility of mendelian inheritance (e.g., autosomal dominant with decreased penetrance) should be considered. A higher recurrence risk figure based on these findings may be appropriate.

Syndromic Oral Clefts

In approximately 35% to 50% of cases of CP and 7% to 15% of cases of CL/P, other physical abnormalities are seen in the affected individual (Jones, 1993; Robinson and Linden, 1993). The presence of any other birth defect or health concern should prompt an evaluation by a clinical geneticist, looking for evidence of an underlying genetic syndrome. There are well over 200 known syndromes featuring oral clefts, with etiologies including single-gene defects, teratogens, chromosomal abnormalities, and those with uncertain etiology. The more common and relevant of these conditions are dis-

cussed in Part II of this book. However, additional abnormalities that may be seen in a child with a cleft are not automatically assumed to be due to an underlying syndrome. Any associated abnormalities may be due to the same disruptive event as the cleft itself and, therefore, may constitute an association rather than a syndrome.

If a specific syndrome is identified, the recurrence risk is that of the syndrome itself. Of special note are syndromes caused by teratogens, such as fetal alcohol syndrome. The recurrence risk of the syndrome, and thus the oral cleft, should be neglible if the teratogen is removed in future pregnancies. If no specific syndrome is recognized in a child but suspicion of a genetic condition is high based on associated abnormalities, a worst-case scenario recurrence risk of up to 25% for unaffected parents (assuming autosomal recessive inheritance) should be discussed.

Recurrence Risk Reduction

There is a possible decrease in recurrence risks for oral clefts in women taking supplemental folic acid, similar to the situation with open neural tube defects (Hartridge et al., 1999; Mills, 1999). This is most applicable to couples facing the recurrence risk of an isolated cleft. The relationship between folic acid supplementation and oral clefting has not yet been proven and is further discussed in Part III of this book. Alternative reproductive technologies, such as the use of donor egg or sperm, may be options for couples facing a significant recurrence risk of an oral cleft as part of a genetic syndrome. As noted above, for couples facing a recurrence risk based on an oral cleft resulting from a teratogenic exposure, removal of the teratogen, if possible, from the pregnancy environment should remove the risk. Finally, prenatal diagnosis is possible in some cases and can provide parents with valuable information prior to the baby's birth.

Prenatal Diagnosis

Prenatal diagnosis of an oral cleft has been reported using visualization of the fetal facial structures by ultrasound. The accuracy of this diagnosis is highly dependent on many factors, including maternal body habitus, fetal positioning, quality of the ultrasound machine, and skill of the examiner. In general, oral clefts cannot be identified until the second trimester of pregnancy, with CL/P being easier to detect than CP. Use of three-dimensional ultrasound has increased the accuracy of prenatal diagnosis of oral clefts (Jones, 1993; Cockell and Lees, 2000). Prenatal identification of an oral cleft should prompt a careful ultrasound evaluation looking for any associated physical abnormalities that could lead to the diagnosis of a syndrome in a previously low-risk pregnancy. Fetal karyotyping should also be considered, especially in the presence of any additional anomalies.

If the oral cleft in a family is part of a recognized syndrome, prenatal diagnosis for the specific condition may be possible irrespective of the ability to visualize the cleft itself. Known chromosomal abnormalities as well as some single-gene disorders can be diagnosed prenatally by chorionic villus sampling or amniocentesis. Because clinical genetic testing changes so rapidly, the availability of prenatal testing for any given condition should be investigated on a case-by-case basis.

SUPPORTIVE COUNSELING

Emotional support for patients with oral clefts and their families is one of the most important responsibilities of healthcare providers and is ideally provided as a group effort from all members of a craniofacial team, including a genetic counselor. The birth of a child with any type of health problem or physical abnormality can bring on a grieving process in parents. These parents grieve the loss of the "perfect" child they have visualized for 9 months (or longer) while learning to accept the fact that such a rare event as a birth defect has affected their family. As parents go through the stages of grieving, it is important to follow them and make sure they are able to navigate these stages, ideally ending up in acceptance of their child with an oral cleft. Recognition of a family unable to work through these steps and of our limitations in helping them is crucial. A genetic counselor or other craniofacial team member should not hesitate to refer a family to formal therapy if any concerns about their ability to cope arise.

It is also important to remember that each family brings to the counseling session a unique history of experiences that will mold his or her view of the present situation. Often, oral clefts are viewed as merely structural defects that are easily amenable to surgery. Fortunately, this is true for the majority of patients, but it is important not to assume that this is the experience of every patient and family. Is this the first person in the family with an oral cleft, or are there other affected members? Does one of the parents have an oral cleft? Is the oral cleft thought to be isolated in the child, or are there other health concerns and the possibility of a genetic syndrome? Is this a syndrome that has been inherited in the family? Taking the time to listen to a family and learn enough about their experiences to understand their reactions is an invaluable aid in providing useful supportive counseling.

Isolated Oral Clefts

The many medical issues surrounding the birth of a child with an oral cleft can often leave a family feeling overwhelmed. Consultation with a comprehensive craniofacial/oral cleft clinic team can be invaluable to help the parents learn how to manage the medical needs of their child. The type and severity of the oral cleft, especially in terms of its impact on feeding, also greatly affect the amount of support and counseling a family may need. Early contact with a family reassures them that they are not alone and that there are experienced people available to help them care for their child. This "safety net" of healthcare providers will hopefully free parents from some of their worries, allowing them to channel their energies into coping with the emotional aspects of having a child with an oral cleft.

Having other members of the family with oral clefts can be a double-edged sword in regard to how it may impact on a family's reaction. The way in which a family reacts depends greatly on the experience of the other affected family members. If a previous individual with a cleft had a successful repair with few or no complications, this will obviously help allay many of the fears a family may have. However, a previous family member with a poor repair experience may make a family even more frightened of the future. This is especially true of a parent who had a cleft as a child; it is likely that surgical repair was not as good then, so it is not uncommon to encounter a parent with bad memories of the experience. Because the face is the first thing noticed about a person, a less-than-optimal repair can lead to emotional problems, from internal and external sources, especially during adolescence. Envisioning their children going through a similar experience can be very upsetting for parents, and they may be greatly reassured when recent advances in surgical repair are discussed. Finally, the birth of a second child with a cleft forces parents to relive the grieving process and increases their anxiety and risks of having another child with an oral cleft.

Syndromic Oral Clefts

Another important consideration is whether the oral cleft is associated with other health concerns, possibly a recognized syndromic condition. This will have a great impact on how much time and energy the child will spend in hospitals having surgeries and seeing doctors. This will also greatly affect how the parents view their child's oral cleft in that the oral cleft is not the only health problem their child faces. For some families, an oral cleft may be the least of their concerns compared to the other, possibly life-threatening features of the syndrome and severe developmental disabilities. What may have been an emotionally devastating birth defect if isolated may now be viewed as simply a surgically repairable health concern.

The parents of a child with a syndromic oral cleft face all of the emotional issues faced by the family of a child with an isolated oral cleft in addition to those concerning the syndrome. The risk of developmental delay or mental retardation in a child with a syndromic cleft is a significant concern (Kapp-Simon and Krueckeberg, 2000). The presence of mental retardation is one of the most emotionally burdensome aspects of dealing with a syndromic condition. Another consideration is the special instance of a mildly affected parent who is diagnosed with a genetic syndrome after the more severely affected child is born. In this situation, a parent deals with his or her own diagnosis as well as the diagnosis of the child. Thus, families of children with a syndromic oral cleft may warrant closer attention as they cope with the diagnosis of a syndrome as well as the oral cleft and all of the consequences that the diagnosis may hold for the child.

Guilt

Having a child with an oral cleft brings guilt feelings to any parent at having possibly caused the cleft. In the absence of a known teratogen, parents should be reassured that nothing that either of them did before or during the pregnancy caused the oral cleft. Also, no one has any control over the genes they pass on to a child, whether the oral cleft is isolated or part of a recognized syndrome. This becomes an especially emotionally charged issue if one of the parents also has an oral cleft. Again, special attention should be paid to the issue of guilt as it often persists, even when the parents intellectually understand that they had no control over the situation.

For those cases in which the oral cleft is thought to be the result of a teratogen, there will likely always be guilt and remorse on the part of the parents over the use of the medication or drug during pregnancy. If the teratogen, as in the case of antiepileptic medication, carries a definite benefit to the mother despite the risk of oral clefting in the fetus, this benefit and the possible negative ramifications of discontinuing the medication during the pregnancy can be stressed. In cases of teratogens without known benefit, such as alcohol, counseling should stress education of the cause and effect of the teratogen and the benefits of avoiding the exposure in future pregnancies.

Peer Support Groups

Support from healthcare providers can be very valuable to families, especially in the first days and weeks of a child's diagnosis; however, an even more worthwhile source of support is other families of children with an oral cleft. Though we, as healthcare providers, can discuss the medical and psychosocial aspects of having a child with an oral cleft, other families in similar situations are the true experts on the day-to-day realities of raising a child with a cleft. It is also very valuable for children as they grow into adolescence and adulthood to have peers to talk with about problems they face that may be unique to a child with an oral cleft. National support groups geared toward families affected by oral clefting are listed in the Appendix to this book.

These are some of the more important issues that come up when providing genetic counseling for families of a child with an oral cleft. Each family is unique and will teach the healthcare provider a new aspect of coping with a child born with an oral cleft. Our job as providers of genetic counseling is to remain open and to actively listen to families so that we are able to best address their needs with any resources we may have. This is the way in which we continue to learn so that, hopefully, each new family can benefit from our past experience as well as the experiences of previous families.

REFERENCES

Bixler, D (1981). Genetics and clefting. Cleft Palate J *18*: 10–18.

Carinci, F, Pezzetti, F, Scapoli, L, et al. (2000). Genetics of nonsyndromic cleft lip and palate: a review of international studies and data regarding the Italian population. Cleft Palate Craniofac J *37*: 33–40.

Cockell, A, Lees, M (2000). Prenatal diagnosis and management of orofacial clefts. Prenat Diagn *20*: 149–151.

Harper, P (1999). *Practical Genetic Counseling*. Boston: Butterworth-Heineman, pp. 210–212.

Hartridge, T, Illing, H, Sandy, J (1999). The role of folic acid in oral clefting. Br J Orthod *26*: 115–120.

Jones, M (1993). Facial clefting etiology and developmental pathogenesis. Clin Plast Surg *20*: 599–606.

Kapp-Simon, K, Krueckeberg, S (2000). Mental development in infants with cleft lip and/or palate. Cleft Palate Craniofac J *37*: 65–70.

Lynch, H, Kimberling, W (1981). Genetic counseling in cleft lip and cleft palate. Plast Reconstr Surg *68*: 800–815.

Mills, J (1999). Folate and oral clefts: where do we go from here? New directions in oral clefts research. Teratology *60*: 251–252.

Robinson, A, Linden, M (1993). *Clinical Genetics Handbook*. Oxford: Blackwell, pp. 515–521.

Wyszynski, DF, Beaty, TH, Maestri, N (1996). Genetics of nonsyndromic oral clefts revisited. Cleft Palate Craniofac J *33*: 406–417.

32

Psychological care of children with cleft lip and palate in the family

KATHLEEN A. KAPP-SIMON

The birth of a child with a cleft lip with or without palate (CL/P) sets in motion a variety of reactions that have significant consequences for the long-term emotional development of the child within his or her family. Although every family is unique, there is a commonality to the experience of responding to the birth of a child with special medical needs that has been frequently described in terms of shock, sadness, fear, grief, guilt, anger, and other types of psychological distress (Clifford and Crocker, 1971; Spriesterbach, 1973; Drotar et al., 1975; Richman and Harper, 1978; Brantley and Clifford, 1979; Stricker et al., 1979; Barden, 1980; Benson and Gross, 1989; Pillemer and Cook, 1989; Epperson and Meyers, 1990; Speltz et al., 1990; Carreto, 1991; Endriga et al., 1994). Despite the extensive evidence documenting the distress of the initial period following the child's birth, most families cope very well and provide an emotionally healthy environment for their child. However, children live not only in their families but also in society, and there is considerable evidence that individuals with facial differences must negotiate a plethora of personal challenges to self-esteem and social acceptance once they leave the protective environment of the family (Macgregor, 1974, 1979, 1990; Bull and Rumsey, 1988). Nevertheless, most individuals with CL/P are ultimately successful in coping with these difficulties and mature into productive members of society (Strauss, 2001). How families negotiate the risks associated with their child's CL/P while fostering hope and adaptation is the focus of this chapter.

RISK, STRESS, AND COPING

Every family that has a child with CL/P must cope with a significant number of problems and stressors. Some families cope very well, while others do less well. It is critical to identify those factors that are associated with more adaptive outcomes so that practitioners can provide appropriate guidance to families who have a child with CL/P. Eiserman (2001) pointed out that the majority of the research on children with CL/P has focused on factors associated with poor adjustment. In this chapter, we examine that research with the explicit goal of identifying factors that foster adaptation despite the very real difficulties that children and their families face. Wallander and Varni (1992) presented a model on disability, stress, and coping that provides a useful framework for discussing the factors that play an important role in the psychosocial adjustment of children with chronic medical conditions such as CL/P. Within this model, heterogeneous risk factors of the disorder, including medical risks, cognitive risks, functional risks, and psychosocial risks, are identified. The resources that families use to cope with these risks are conceptualized as resistance factors and include contingencies such as the intrinsic characteristics of the child (intrapersonal factors), family mental health, social resources and support (social–ecological factors), and stress processing. The ultimate result of the interplay between risk and resistance factors is the psychosocial adaptation of the affected individual.

RISK FACTORS

Medical Risks

The medical risks associated with different forms of CL/P are varied. A child with an isolated cleft of the soft palate and no known genetic etiology may have some mild feeding problems and require a single surgery to correct the palatal defect, medical management of the ears for otitis media, and monitoring by speech and audiology through early childhood. At the other end of the severity spectrum, a child with a protrusive, complete bilateral CL/P may experience significant feeding problems and require prosthetic management prior to initial lip repair. The severity of the problem may necessitate two surgeries to accomplish initial lip repair, a separate surgery for palatal repair, bone grafting of the alveolar clefts, multiple surgeries to revise the lip and nose at various times throughout childhood and young adolescence, extensive orthodontic treatment with the possibility of orthognathic surgery, ongoing follow-up and surgical interventions by the otolaryngologist, and mildly invasive speech evaluations (e.g., nasopharyngoscopy) and speech therapy. Cleft palate (CP) in the context of Robin sequence may involve other complications, such as airway compromise, that necessitate a tracheotomy in addition to the surgeries to correct the palatal defect. In yet another scenario, a child with CL/P and a genetic deletion, such as a 22q11 disorder, will have the medical risks associated with CL/P as well as the potential of associated problems, including cardiac, neuromotor, seizure or developmental problems. Thus, the specific medical risks associated with a diagnosis of CL/P are heterogeneous. The greater the potential spectrum of medical problems, the greater the potential risk factors for an individual family.

Functional Risks

There are also cognitive risks associated with CL/P. Although the majority of school-aged children with CL/P and CP score in the low-average range of intelligence, verbal IQ is typically lower than nonverbal IQ (Richman and Eliason, 1982). Learning disabilities, particularly in the areas of reading, language, and memory, occur in 30% to 40% of children with CL/P and at significantly higher rates in children with CP (Eliason and Richman, 1990; Broder et al., 1998). There is some evidence that the cognitive problems associated with learning disabilities may present as subtle differences in both verbal and nonverbal developmental progress during infancy and toddlerhood (Kapp-Simon and Krueckeberg, 2000; Speltz et al., 2000). Cognitive problems in more than one-third of children with CL/P represent a significant risk to long-term psychological adaptation. The presence of learning disabilities in so many children with CL/P also confounds studies of psychological adaptation. Children with learning disabilities who do not have CL/P are at risk for behavioral and emotional problems as well as deficits in social skills (Margalit, 1989; McConaughy et al., 1994; Handwerk and Marshall, 1998). Therefore, children with CL/P who also have a learning disability may be dually at risk.

Functional risks associated with CL/P that are separate from cognitive risks generally include speech articulation problems and the possibility of fluctuating conductive hearing loss secondary to otitis media. A significant number of children with a repaired CP require speech therapy to address articulation or language problems (Dalston, 1990; Peterson-Falzone, 1990; Grames et al., 2000). These problems can range from mild to severe. While mild problems may require therapy to correct, they seldom interfere with a child's ability to communicate. However, children whose problems are more severe may have significant difficulty making themselves understood to individuals unfamiliar with their speech patterns. Communication difficulties may alter the way in which family members, teachers, and peers interact with the child. In turn, communication difficulties may have a significant impact on the child's ability to master normal developmental tasks, including personal independence, academic competence, and reciprocal play.

Most children with CP experience multiple episodes of otitis media with effusion, resulting in frequent disruptions of auditory input due to fluctuating mild to moderate conductive hearing loss (Stool, 1990). A number of studies have suggested that these changes in hearing sensitivity may affect the development of language skills and/or reading skills when they occur during the formative years of language learning (Peters et al., 1994; Roberts et al., 1995; Johnson et al., 2000; Kindig and Richards, 2000). While the findings have been inconsistent, the presence of repeated otitis media with effusion with resultant conductive hearing loss is a significant risk factor for children with CL/P.

Psychosocial Risks

Children with CL/P experience a significant number of psychosocial risks, including multiple medical appointments and evaluations, feeding difficulties, repeated surgeries, differences in appearance resulting in possible stigmatization, and the possible need for early intervention programs or special therapies (e.g., speech therapy). Similar to other children, children with CL/P are subject to major life stress, such as the birth of a sibling, a family move, parental divorce, the death of a close relative, or chronic school failure. Likewise, psychosocial stress is part of the daily hassles that all children face, including children with CL/P. These daily hassles can be as mild as being scolded for forgetting homework or more significant, as in peer teasing. Regardless of the severity, however, these daily hassles increase the stress that children feel and contribute to the overall psychosocial risk to which children with CL/P are subjected.

The risks identified above represent areas of potential vulnerability for children with CL/P. The responses to these risks and the methods of coping that develop play a significant role in a child's ability to adapt. A number of researchers have suggested that children with chronic medical conditions are at about twice the risk for problems of maladjustment as their healthy peers (Rutter et al., 1970; Pless and Roghmann, 1971; Wallander et al., 1988). Children with CL/P fall into the same risk rate (Speltz et al., 1997; Kapp-Simon and Dawson, 1998). However, despite the known risks and the increased rate of psychosocial problems for individuals with CL/P, many children are happy and well adjusted and many adults are satisfied with themselves, display good emotional adjustment, and make a significant contribution to society (Strauss, 2001; Eiserman, 2001). What accounts for this differential adaptation? How is it that children faced with a similar set of risks can have such different outcomes?

RESISTANCE FACTORS

Murphy and Moriarty (1976), in their groundbreaking book *Vulnerability, Coping, & Growth: From Infancy to Adolescence*, describe the resilience of a child in the following terms:

> a child is . . . an adapting, plastic individual finding a way to come to terms with changing pressures and opportunities. The latter are experienced individually and selectively as each child's strengths and vulnerabilities make a given situation a source of threat, deprivation, or satisfaction. . . . The adaptational style, then, is a more or less flexible attunement between the range of resources and limitations of the child and the quality of the environmental pressures and opportunities. (p. 166)

As noted earlier, Wallander and Varni (1992) postulate a similar set of resources as moderator variables, which they call "resistance factors." Broadly speaking, they classify these resistance factors as intrapersonal

characteristics, social-ecological characteristics, and the way in which stress is processed by the child and family members.

Intrapersonal Factors

Intrapersonal factors include characteristics intrinsic to the individual, such as temperament, as well as learned characteristics, such as social skills and evaluation of personal competence and self-esteem/self concept. Other factors could also be included under the rubric of intrapersonal factors; however, the current discussion focuses on these three.

Temperament. Temperamental variables are stable characteristics that identify individual differences in children (Thomas and Chess, 1957, 1980; Thomas et al., 1961, 1963). Buss and Plomin (1984) identified three broad constructs that encompass the major dimensions of temperament: *emotionality*, how a child responds to distress, fear, or anger; *activity level*, a child's ability to attend or the degree of cognitive distractibility/persistence present; and *sociability*, a child's tendency to approach or avoid new people or situations. While temperamental characteristics are generally thought to be immutable, in some cases having a genetic basis (Kagan et al., 1987, 1988; Kagan, 1994), they also interact with environmental demands. For example, a child who is inhibited and becomes extremely fearful during medical exams is more likely to react positively if the parent is calm and supportive and the medical staff provides adequate time to become comfortable with the situation than if the adults are quick to make demands and intolerant of the child's justifiable need to acclimate to the exam.

Children with CL/P frequently demonstrate temperamental characteristics consistent with increased anxiety (emotionality), behavioral inhibition (activity level), and social withdrawal (sociability) (Richman, 1976, 1978b, 1998; Richman and Harper, 1978; Richman and Millard, 1997; Kapp-Simon and Dawson, 1998). While it is unlikely that a cautious child will learn to become exuberant or predominantly extroverted, parents and other adults can develop strategies for supporting the inhibited child that foster more adaptive interactions. One basis for that support is encouragement (see Nelsen et al., 1998a, pp. 199–214 for further discussion of this concept). A "slow-to-warm-up child" needs adults to believe that he or she can warm up. When that child is faced with an unfamiliar peer or potentially challenging situation, parents can help if they are able to communicate to their child that they believe the child can be successful. Additional information on responding to temperamental differences in children is provided by Nelsen et al. (1988b).

Social Skills. While temperament is often considered an intrinsic characteristic of individuals, the second intrapersonal characteristic, social skills, includes behaviors that can be taught. Social skills are those behaviors that enhance social interaction. Regardless of temperament, children can learn specific skills that enable them to initiate and maintain social interactions, modulate their emotions, provide social reinforcement to their peers, and solve social problems.

Children with CL/P and other facial differences have been identified as being at risk for difficulties in social relationships. Macgregor (1990) identified social encounters as the most stressful aspect of having a facial disfigurement. In an observational study, Kapp-Simon and McGuire (1997) found that children with craniofacial conditions initiated and received fewer social approaches than their school peers without facial differences and that the strategies that such children used to engage their peers were less effective and more tentative than those used by the comparison group. Macgregor (1990) suggested that the difficulties involved in social encounters occur for individuals with craniofacial conditions because the rituals, typical behaviors, and rules of social conduct are altered when one of the participants is facially disfigured. Difficulties maintaining culturally appropriate interaction sequences are difficult for both the individual with a facial difference and the individual without disfigurement. The nondisfigured participant feels awkward and unsure about how to relate to a person with facial scars. This awkwardness is communicated nonverbally through body movements, postural and facial changes, head positioning, eye movements, gestures, and social distance. Paralinguistic communication, in the tone and pitch of voice, rate of speech, hesitations, and emotional overtones, can also contribute to the discomfort of the situation. In addition, individuals with craniofacial conditions are frequently confronted with impolite stares or intrusive questions. To be successful in this environment, the individual with facial differences must develop coping strategies. However, those strategies that both children and adults report using quite frequently, including feigning unawareness of the other's stares, staring back, making a defiant comment, or withdrawing in hopelessness, are not particularly effective and are more likely to truncate the encounter than to promote interaction.

Learning effective social skills can have lifelong benefits. Research has demonstrated that social deficits can have implications for personal adjustment at later ages (Parker and Asher, 1987). The benefits of positive so-

cial skills have also been demonstrated in studies of adjustment involving children with craniofacial conditions. In longitudinal research, the degree of friendliness displayed by preschool children with craniofacial conditions has been associated with better social adjustment and fewer behavioral problems at school age based on teacher observations (Krueckeberg et al., 1993; Krueckeberg and Kapp-Simon, 1997). In adolescence, parents report that children who have better social skills show fewer emotional or behavioral adjustment problems and are less likely to be socially inhibited or withdrawn (Kapp-Simon et al., 1992).

The social skills needed for effective interaction will vary depending on the age of the child. However, even a preschool child can learn to respond to a question about scarring from the repaired cleft lip in a friendly and effective manner. Parents should be encouraged to provide their children with a vocabulary that they can use to describe the condition, and the children should practice answering questions. Parents can also model appropriate behavior by the way they respond to questions in their child's presence. If families are able to use the same tone of voice and positive emotional energy when talking about their child's cleft as they do when they talk about the child's blue eyes or black curly hair, they will communicate that the cleft is simply another valued part of the child's person. This matter-of-fact approach enables the child to believe that the cleft need not be a source of embarrassment or shame.

As the child matures, more specific skills may be needed. There are a variety of programs geared to the development of social skills for preschool and elementary school students (Cartledge and Milburn, 1980; Coie, 1985; Schneider and Bryne, 1985; Goldstein, 1988; Matson and Ollendick, 1988). Kapp-Simon and Simon (1991) provided a model for social skills training with adolescents who have special needs. For the child with CL/P, specific attention should be paid to skills that encourage good pragmatic communication (eye contact, tone of voice, social distance) as well as specific skills for entering and maintaining conversations, anxiety management, and empathy. The skill of empathy is particularly important for children who are anxious or self-conscious. An empathic response encourages the child to think about the feelings and experiences of the person to whom he or she is speaking rather than to focus on his or her own concerns.

Direct teaching of social skills has been found to be effective. Using a pre-post design, McGuire (1990) evaluated the social skills of 13 children with craniofacial conditions before and after participation in a social skills training group and compared the results with those of seven children who did not participate in the group. The young adolescents who had participated in the social skills group significantly increased the frequency with which they initiated conversations with peers and the frequency with which these contacts became actual conversations. For group participants, these skills increased to be equivalent to the nonclinical group, while they remained unchanged for the comparison subjects with craniofacial conditions.

Robinson et al. (personal communication) also reported increased social competence for participants with craniofacial conditions after a 2-day social skills training workshop sponsored by Changing Faces in England. Only anecdotal reports regarding the improvement in social skills were included in the results; however, reported anxiety decreased significantly after group participation.

Self-Concept. A third intrapersonal consideration that is important when discussing resistance factors is self-concept. According to Kliewer and Sandler (1992), positive self-esteem may enhance an individual's appraisal of a stressor; i.e., a child may view the failure to achieve a particular goal as a challenge to try harder rather than as evidence of a lack of competence. Harter (1985) identified five separate areas of competence believed to be critical to self-evaluation by children and to contribute to overall self-esteem: scholastic achievement, conduct/behavior, physical appearance, athletic achievement, and social acceptance. Harter (1985) described self-esteem as a global judgment that assesses the degree to which the child likes him- or herself, is satisfied with the way he or she is living life, and feels good about him- or herself. Children who believe that they are competent in the classroom, in the orchestra, on the athletic field (regardless of level of play), or in terms of their ability to interact effectively with others are more likely to believe in themselves. Most of their emotional energy can be directed toward continued success in their chosen area. Cleft-related concerns can be relegated to the inconvenience of having to attend medical appointments or to consider surgeries.

SOCIAL–ECOLOGICAL SUPPORT

Children with CL/P receive support from a variety of sources in their environment. To focus on those aspects of the social environment that are common to most children, the following sources of social–ecological support are discussed: family adaptation, financial resources, medical care, and the school environment.

Family Adaptation and Resources

Parental Adjustment. Children with CL/P are born into many different types of family. Prior to the child's birth, some families may be doing well: the marital relationship is stable, and the child is anticipated with eagerness and joy. Other families may be getting along reasonably well: there may be some stresses, possibly mild marital discord, financial problems, or problems with another child. The current pregnancy may be viewed with mixed emotions, though in general the family looks forward to a new addition. A third group of families may not cope particularly well prior to the pregnancy. In some cases, the pregnancy is unplanned; in others, it is planned as a way of "saving the marriage." Marital discord or some other form of significant stress, e.g., job loss or illness of a grandparent, may be present.

The family's level of adaptation, cohesion, and general emotional health will influence its ability to cope with the birth of a child with CL/P (Nash, 1995). For each family, regardless of prior level of functioning, the birth of a child with CL/P marks a time of temporary crisis. Most families anticipate a healthy baby, and the presence of the cleft disrupts their expectations (Endriga and Kapp-Simon, 1999). Clinical experience demonstrates that the family's ability to navigate that crisis will be related to the parents' ability to work through their own emotional responses to this crisis and support each other. Each parent will experience emotional distress, but the two parents may not be at the same stage at similar times. For example, one parent may be dealing with depressed feelings, while the other is angrily searching for something or someone to blame. The ability of the parents to recognize the validity of their own feelings as well of those of their partner, even if they differ from their own, is critical. Acknowledgment of differing emotional responses is the first step toward providing mutual support or, if indicated, seeking outside support to handle intense emotional distress. There is evidence from the broader literature on chronic illness that mothers who experience greater marital satisfaction and broader family and psychosocial support demonstrate healthier mental and physical adjustment (Wallander et al., 1989).

Each parent brings unique abilities to the task of rearing a child with special medical needs. It behooves parents to recognize each other's strengths. For example, one parent may be more competent at negotiating medical terminology and treatment plans, while the other is able to support the child more effectively through an invasive medical procedure. Mutual and respectful acknowledgment of the importance of different types of strength will support the marital relationship and provide the child with optimal care.

Mother–infant attachment may not be affected as negatively as previously thought by the presence of CL/P (Hoeksma and Koomen, 1991; Speltz et al., 1997; Maris et al., 2000). Based on attachment theory, maternal responsiveness is more important than the characteristics of the infant in determining the quality of the mother–infant relationship. The finding that infants with CL/P are as securely attached to their mothers as infants without CL/P is encouraging. These findings suggest that many mothers do overcome the challenges that are a real part of raising a child with CL/P and are able to nurture the infant in an effective and satisfying manner. The characteristics most commonly seen in those mothers whose children were securely attached included belief in their ability to meet their child's needs, satisfaction in their role as parent, and an ability to realistically acknowledge the stress of their current situation (Speltz et al., 1997).

Parents can build on the initial positive attachment that typically develops between mother and infant by ensuring that they have specific parenting skills that enable them to provide emotional support, impart positive discipline, and promote social interaction skills for their child. In at least one study, parents of 2- and 3-year-old children with CL/P reported feeling less competent as parents than other study participants (Speltz et al., 1990), thus highlighting the need for focus on this area. Parents can be encouraged to increase their parenting competence by learning specific parenting skills. This need is supported by research. For example, speaking about the needs for parenting skills, Gottman (1997) states the following:

> In my research, I discovered that love by itself wasn't enough. Very concerned, warm, and involved parents often had attitudes toward their own and their children's emotions that got in the way of them being able to talk to their children when they were sad or afraid or angry. But while love by itself was not enough, channeling that caring into some basic skills that parents practiced as if they were coaching their children in the area of emotion *was* enough. The secret lay in how parents interacted with their children when emotions ran hot. (p. 16)

Gottman outlines a five-step procedure for "emotion coaching," a process of discipline that provides a sound foundation for parenting skills across a large variety of situations. Parents are taught to become aware of their child's emotions, to recognize that times of emotional upset are also moments of potential intimacy with their child, to respond with empathy to their child's distress, to help the child label emotions with words that are appropriate to the age of the child, and to set limits while helping their child solve the problem. Other parenting programs teach similar skills (Gordon, 1970; Nelsen, 1996; Faber and Mazlish, 1998). Consistent use of positive parenting skills will model appropriate social interactions for the child with CL/P and provide the child with the sense of security that comes from knowing that important adults care enough to set reasonable limits.

Social Support. Social and emotional support for parents of children with CL/P is essential, particularly during the first years of the child's life. This support can be provided by extended family, friends, and, for families who choose them, parent-support groups. Many parents seek the help they need, and both Speltz et al. (1990) and Krueckeberg and Kapp-Simon (1993) found that parents of young children with craniofacial conditions did not differ in terms of their social networks or the support they received. This differs from reports by Benson et al. (1991) and Bradbury and Hewison (1994). Benson et al. (1991) found that families of children with craniofacial conditions reported less social support and were less satisfied with their social support networks. Bradbury and Hewison (1994) reported increased parental concern about allowing their infants with visible differences to be seen in public, particularly when their own parents had difficulty adjusting to the child's cleft. Demonstrating the links between various types of resistance factors, Benson et al. (1991) found that parents' satisfaction with social support was related to their child's social competence. Families in which the children with craniofacial conditions displayed more age-appropriate social skill development were likely to have a more extensive social network and experience more satisfaction from those relationships.

Participation in a parent-support group or an online chat room geared to families who have a child with CL/P can be another source of social support for some families. Parents often find it uplifting to speak with another family that has experienced some of the same stages of treatment that they anticipate for their child. As the children mature, they, too, enjoy getting together with others who have had to handle similar peer situations or surgeries. The Cleft Palate Foundation, About Face U.S.A., About Face International, and Wide Smiles provide resources for families looking to make contact with others who have a child with a condition similar to that of their child (see Appendix for Internet addresses).

Financial Resources. Adequate financial resources, including steady employment and medical insurance, are important. The birth of a child with CL/P creates a financial strain for most families (see Waitzman et al., 1994, for an estimate of costs). Even with appropriate medical insurance, there are many needed services that are not adequately covered (Sheils and Wolfe, 1992; Waitzman et al., 1994). Often, tremendous amounts of time need to be devoted to tracking insurance claims, making phone calls, and writing letters regarding denials. With health-maintenance organizations or preferred provider organizations, families struggle to coordinate care and may worry that the practitioners within their provider network do not have sufficient experience in treating CL/P (Fox and McManus, 1998). The financial strain becomes greater as economic need increases because so many of the working poor do not have medical insurance and do not qualify for public assistance.

Especially during the early years of the child's life, multiple medical appointments and surgeries require absences from work. For many families, these absences entail loss of pay or use of vacation time. In either case, family members pay a price to provide appropriate care for their child with CL/P.

In the United States, insurance coverage is generally tied to a parent's job. If that parent loses the job or changes jobs voluntarily, the insurance will no longer be available to the child with CL/P. For some children, care for cleft-related treatment will never again be covered by insurance due to a clause in the family's new insurance excluding preexisting conditions; for others, coverage will be provided only after a waiting period of up to 2 years. Insurance expenses can also create stress for a family when the parent works for a smaller firm, where extraordinary expenses from one member can cause an insurance carrier to drop an account rather than bear the expense of the child with CL/P (see Perrin et al., 1992, for a discussion of healthcare needs for children with chronic illness). Clinical experience demonstrates that families frequently forgo treatment for their child that they feel is less important, such as dental care, speech therapy, or psychological services, when insurance coverage is inadequate. In each case, postponement of, or a decision not to provide, needed care in those areas will increase the child's risk for long-term treatment failure. Provision of these essential services can increase the child's level of invulnerability and thus improve long-term adaptation, the ultimate goal of CL/P-related treatment.

Medical Care

Coordinated, family-centered care is a critical factor in the long-term adaptation of children with CL/P. The American Cleft Palate-Craniofacial Association (ACPA) (1993) provides information on the treatment needs of children with CL/P or other craniofacial conditions. The "Standards of Team Care" (Strauss and ACPA Team Standards Committee, 1998) identifies the makeup of a CL/P or craniofacial team in terms of specialists who should be included on the medical team and the services that should be provided. It is the recommendation of the ACPA that all children with any type of CL/P or craniofacial condition be provided with medical care within the framework of a medical team that meets the standards established through these documents.

Coordinated, multidisciplinary team care for children with CL/P provides many necessary safeguards for the children and their families. The experience of team members with CL/P helps to ease the anxiety that a family with a newborn feels as they realize that the team members understand the condition and can quickly address their initial concerns. Issues such as feeding problems, timing of corrective surgery, and long-term treatment needs can be readily addressed by appropriate team members so that the feelings of crisis are diminished and the family is able to move in the positive direction of intervention. The team is able to provide information about long-term expectations of care that can instill hope, an important ingredient for the success of the child's treatment. Finally, team care allows for coordinated efforts. When indicated, pressure equalizing tubes can be inserted at the time of lip or palate repair, rather than as a separate surgery. Unnecessary secondary surgeries on the palate can be avoided if the speech pathologist is allowed to determine whether speech articulation errors are related to velopharyngeal incompetence or some other cause (Sloan, 2000).

As the child matures, team members work with the family to identify treatment priorities. The family and, when old enough, the child with CL/P are encouraged to voice their concerns. Allowing the child and parents to play a role in the determination of treatment priorities and, when feasible, the timing of interventions empowers the family members. Families do not always make the same decisions that the treatment team members would make under similar circumstances. The role of the team is to present the family with options and then to support the family's decision even when that would not be the decision of the treatment team. This empowerment enables families to be more accepting of the treatment options available as well as the final outcome of the treatment they choose. Satisfaction with treatment outcomes, particularly in terms of appearance, is an important factor. In the study of adolescents with CL/P by Richman et al. (1985), self-reported satisfaction with appearance (not objective ratings of appearance) was associated with level of behavioral inhibition. The greater the level of satisfaction, the less behavioral inhibition observed.

Team care also affords families the opportunities to obtain the psychosocial support they require. Team members generally include a nurse, psychologist, or social worker who is sensitive to the emotional needs of families. These team members specifically assess the strengths of families and work with them to foster the best emotional environment for the child. In addition, psychosocial staff are responsible for assessing the emotional and social adjustment of the child, supporting child and parents, helping to develop parenting skills, providing preparation for invasive medical procedures or surgery, and screening for developmental delay and learning problems (American Cleft Palate-Craniofacial Association, 1993). This type of psychosocial support allows for early identification of areas of concern and development of a treatment plan to address them.

School Support

Children spend a good percentage of their time in school. The school environment is a critical forum in which children are afforded the opportunity for both intellectual and social learning. Children with CL/P face a number of risks within the school environment. Richman (1978a) found that teachers underestimated the intellectual abilities of children with CL/P compared with actual ability, particularly children with more significant scarring. This finding is consistent with other literature that has documented a relationship between cleft-related impairments (e.g., oral–facial differences or speech impairment) and judgments of inferior intellectual functioning (Clifford and Walster, 1973; Shaw and Humphreys, 1982).

Nash (1995) assessed adults with CL/P and found that the vast majority (80.2%, $n = 174$) reported being teased about their cleft when they were children. The finding of increased withdrawal and inhibition at school vs. parental report of the same behaviors at home (Richman, 1976, 1978b) suggests that the stress of social interactions and perhaps competition in the classroom has a negative effect on social adjustment and may even affect achievement. Further support for excessive inhibition of impulse and concern over interpersonal relationships was seen in a study of adolescents using the Minnesota Multiphasic Personality Inventory (Harper and Richman, 1978). In this study, females with CL/P displayed greater dissatisfaction with their life situation, which was interpreted to relate to the greater emphasis on physical appearance in females, particularly during adolescence. Kapp (1979) came to similar conclusions when examining self-concept of adolescents with CL/P.

In addition to the social/emotional concerns that children of school age face, there is the real concern regarding academic difficulties. The rate of learning disabilities for children with CL/P is significantly higher than that of the general population (Broder et al., 1998). As noted previously, these children are doubly at risk and may face social difficulties and assaults on self-esteem from either front.

Despite the risks, the school can become a source of social support for child and family. Teachers can be educated about the multiple risks involved in having CL/P. Education can increase the sensitivity of the teacher to the behavior of all of the children. The goal would be for the teacher to set up a social environment in which each child's uniqueness would be respected and honored. School programs such as the About Face School Program, "Unwrapping the package: dispelling myths about unusual appearances" (About Face, 1996) or "Bully-proof your school" (Short-Camilli et al., 1999) can be used in the classroom to increase the sensitivity of children to the importance of accepting differences in each other. The extent to which the child with a cleft would be singled out during such a discussion is something that should be agreed upon by the parents and teacher in consultation with the child. Families and children differ in their level of comfort in discussing issues related to CL/P in a public forum. However, testimonials that advocate the benefits of such open discussion are certainly found in the parent networks (e.g., Ability Online Support Network, About Face International, About Face U.S.A., Let's Face It, Wide Smiles). Some children enjoy and gain esteem from presenting information about CL/P and their personal history to their classmates using pictures and medical terminology.

Education of the teacher regarding the ways in which teasing occurs in a particular classroom is also critical. Teachers are often unaware of the extent to which a child is victimized because the taunting or bullying takes place out of view and earshot. While the ideal is for a child to address the issues of teasing independently through improved social skills, there are occasions when the adults must take charge to bring about changes in the peer atmosphere (Nash, 1995). When a parent has worked to help the child develop a variety of response strategies to the teasing but the teasing persists, action at the school level is needed. This intervention may require bringing in a counselor or social worker to help the students break the cycle of teasing that has developed (see Wilson, 2001, for information on additional resources that can be used by parents, counselors, or teachers).

The school can also address the special educational needs of those children with CL/P who also have a learning disability. Early memory problems (e.g., rapid naming or verbal memory, such as an inability to label colors, recite the ABCs, or count accurately) may be indicators of potential learning disabilities for many children with CL/P (Buckenburger, 1991; Richman, 2000). Other children, particularly those with CP, may have more pervasive difficulties with language (Richman and Eliason, 1984; Richman et al., 1988; Richman, 1990). Teachers should be made aware of these indicators so that appropriate early intervention can be provided.

Stress Processing

The experience of CL/P clearly increases the number and types of stressors experienced by family and child. Another variable that affects outcome in terms of child adaptation relates to the cognitive appraisal and coping strategies that families adapt in response to those stressors. *Cognitive appraisal* refers to the family's perception of their ability to handle the stresses associated with their child's condition. Four broad areas receive focus: the family's perception of their ability to deal with the child's medical problems and related symptoms, the family's perception of their ability to maintain the child's emotional well-being, the parent's ability to maintain their own emotional well-being, and the parent's ability to maintain the well-being of other children in the family (Sloper, 2000). Coping strategies define the ways in which families respond to stress. A variety of conceptual models have been developed to examine this process. However, Compas et al. (1992) suggest that these models reflect two broad styles of coping: the first focuses on the problem itself, whether that be some aspect of the person, the event, or a combination of the two; and the second focuses on the need to cope with the distressful emotions associated with the event.

There have been no direct studies focusing on stress processing in families whose children have CL/P. Consequently, the information discussed here is drawn from the broader area of research involving children with other types of chronic illness.

Few studies have actually looked at cognitive appraisal as an independent factor associated with adjustment. However, Kazak and Barakat (1997) suggested that perception of illness-related stress is related to adjustment problems. This relationship was empirically demonstrated in the research of Sloper (2000), involving families whose children had been diagnosed with cancer. She found that parents' appraisal of the strain of the illness combined with their confidence in their ability to handle the strain was related to parental distress. Parental confidence in their ability to cope combined with family cohesion were factors associated with less emotional distress for these families.

Positive, problem-focused coping strategies (making a plan and following through with it), as opposed to coping strategies that encompass negative self-criticism, were more effective for mothers in the Sloper (2000) study. Similar findings have been found in other studies where it has been demonstrated that families of children with chronic illness do better when they choose an active, problem-focused coping style (Mullins et al., 1991; Miller et al., 1992a; Thompson et al., 1993; Davis et al., 1998).

Clinical experience provides anecdotal information regarding strategies that families use to help their children cope effectively with CL/P team consultations and surgeries. From an appraisal standpoint, parents acknowledge that cooperating with the various assessments that are part of the team consultation can be stressful for their child. Parents who are effective at supporting their children give the child the message that they believe he or she can cooperate. These parents are able to establish an expectation that the child will talk during the speech exam and will open his or her mouth during the oral exam without making the interaction a power struggle. Some families find success by having their child practice cooperating for the various medical exams using appropriate play medical equipment. The child can be afforded the opportunity to "examine" a parent's or cooperative sibling's mouth and ears as well as "play doctor" with their dolls or stuffed animals. Stressful events, e.g., having blood drawn prior to surgery, can be handled through strategies such as distraction, which encourage the child to think about something else (e.g., count, sing a song, or imagine themselves in a pleasant place) during the stressful procedure or relaxation coupled with positive self-talk (Miller et al., 1992b). The team social worker or psychologist can be accessed by families to help them develop strategies that work most effectively for their child.

Another area of potential stress in families whose children have CL/P is the child's social acceptance, particularly when facial scarring or speech problems are present. Though not specifically assessing cognitive appraisal, the findings of Pope and Ward (1997) on factors associated with peer social competence in preadolescents with craniofacial conditions can be interpreted within this context. They found a relationship between parental worry about their child's social adjustment and the child's social competence. Children whose parents were concerned about them but took active steps to solve the children's social difficulties, such as helping to arrange play dates and encouraging social contact, displayed greater adjustment than children whose parents demonstrated high worry and anxiety about the problem with little or no effective action. In this context, parents or school counselors and social workers can help children develop effective prosocial skills. As described earlier in this chapter, teaching children to approach their peers in a friendly manner, helping them to develop strategies for handling questions about facial scarring or speech difficulties, and teaching them how to respond to bullies are social skills that will facilitate better adjustment.

Enabling families to share their successes can also enhance effective coping. Eiserman (2001) suggests that efforts need to be made to provide families with optimism and models of positive outcome:

> The optimum outcome for families like this was a kind of peace of mind and adaptation that comes when individuals and families accept their circumstances as something: to work with, not against; to help frame their lives, not entirely, but partly; and, which can provide fuel for creating the dreams and hopes they have for themselves and their families. (p 6)

To this end Eiserman (2001) includes a number of vignettes that describe the positive expectations of parents and the adaptive outcomes of adults with the hope of providing models of adaptation for others to emulate.

CONCLUSIONS

In this chapter, I have outlined factors of stress and resistance that interact to moderate adaptation in children with CL/P. Research on children has provided ample evidence of the complicated and multidirectional effects of stress and support on long-term adaptation (Dubois et al., 1992). Children with CL/P face a multitude of challenges specific to the cleft diagnosis, yet they also must cope with the complex set of stresses and challenges to adaptation that are a natural part of childhood. The goal of this chapter was to challenge us to think about interventions and supports that foster optimal development. Children with CL/P have the potential to be significant contributors to society. It behooves us to teach them how to channel the emotional energy required to cope with the variety of challenges inherent in living with CL/P into productive activity. Families should be presented with the expectation that their child with CL/P can cope and actively contribute to society at every stage of development, whether that is in the classroom or in the workforce.

REFERENCES

About Face (1996). *Unwrapping the Package: Dispelling Myths about Unusual Appearances.* Toronto: About Face.

American Cleft Palate-Craniofacial Association (1993). Parameters for evaluation and treatment of patients with cleft lip/palate or other craniofacial anomalies. Cleft Palate Craniofac J *30(Suppl 1):* 4.

Barden, RC (1980). The effects of craniofacial deformity, chronic illness, and physical handicaps on patient and familial adjustment: research and clinical perspectives. In: *Advances in Child Clinical Psychology,* edited by B Lahey and A Kazdin. New York: Plenum, pp. 343–375.

Benson, BA, Gross, AM (1989). The effect of a congenitally handicapped child on the marital dyad: a review of the literature. Clin Psychol Rev *9:* 747–758.

Benson, BA, Gross, AM, Meeser, SC, et al. (1991). Social support networks among families with craniofacial anomalies. Health Psychol *10:* 252–258.

Bradbury, ET, Hewison, J (1994). Early parental adjustment to visible congenital disfigurement. Child Care Health Dev *20:* 251–266.

Brantley, HT, Clifford, E (1979). Cognitive, self-concept, and body image measures of normal, cleft palate, and obese adolescents. Cleft Palate J *16:* 177–182.

Broder, HL, Richman, LC, Matheson, PB (1998). Learning disabilities, school achievement, and grade retention among children with cleft: a two-center study. Cleft Palate Craniofac J *35:* 127–131.

Buckenburger, L (1991). Learning Disabilities in the Cleft Palate Population. Chicago: DePaul Univ. Dissertation.

Bull, R, Rumsey, N (1988). *The Social Psychology of Facial Appearance.* New York: Springer-Verlag.

Buss, AH, Plomin, R (1984). *Early Developing Personality Traits.* Hillsdale, NJ: Lawrence Erlbaum.

Carreto, V (1991). Maternal responses to an infant with cleft lip and palate: a review of the literature. Matern Child Nurs J *10:* 197–205.

Cartledge, G, Milburn, J (eds) (1980). *Teaching Social Skills to Children.* New York: Pergamon.

Clifford, E, Crocker, EC (1971). Maternal responses: the birth of a normal child as compared to the birth of a child with a cleft. Cleft Palate J *8:* 298–306.

Clifford, E, Walster, T (1973). The effect of physical attractiveness on teacher expectation. Sociol Educ *46:* 248–253.

Coie, JD (1985). Fitting social skills intervention to the target group. In: *Issues in Assessment and Intervention,* edited by BH Schneider, KH Rubin, and JE Ledingham. New York: Springer-Verlag, pp. 651–657.

Compas, BE, Worsham, NL, Ey, S (1992). Conceptual and developmental issues in children's coping with stress. In: *Stress and coping in child health,* edited by AM LaGreca, LJ Siegel, JL Wallander, and CE Walker. New York: Guilford Press, pp. 7–24.

Dalston, RM (1990). Communication skills of children with cleft lip and palate: a status report. In: *Multidisciplinary Management of Cleft Lip and Palate,* edited by J Bardach and HL Morris. Philadelphia: Saunders, pp. 746–749.

Davis, CC, Brown, RT, Bakeman, R, Campbell, R (1998). Psychological adaptation and adjustment of mothers of children with congenital heart disease: stress, coping, and family functioning. J Pediatr Psychol *23:* 219–228.

Drotar, D, Baskiewisz, A, Kennell, I, Klaus, M (1975). The adaptation of parents to the birth of an infant with a congenital malformation: a hypothetical model. Pediatrics *56:* 710–717.

DuBois, DL, Felner, RD, Brand, S, et al. (1992). A prospective study of life stress, social support, and adaptation in early adolescence. Child Dev *63:* 542–557.

Eiserman, W (2001). Unique outcomes and positive contributions associated with facial difference: expanding research and practice. Cleft Palate Craniofac J *38:* 236–244.

Eliason, MJ, Richman, LC (1990). Language development in preschoolers with cleft. Dev Neuropsychol *6:* 173–182.

Endriga, M, Kapp-Simon, KA (1999). Psychological issues in craniofacial care: state of the art. Cleft Palate Craniofac J *36:* 3–11.

Endriga, MC, Speltz, ML, Mouradian, W (1994). Change in maternal stress during infancy. *Presented at the annual meeting of the American Cleft Palate-Craniofacial Association, Toronto Canada, April 1994.*

Epperson, MJ, Meyers, BJ (1990). Mother–infant feeding interactions with cleft lip/palate infants: disparity between observations and mother's reports. *Presented at the International Conference on Infant Studies, Montreal, Canada, April 6–8, 1990.*

Faber, A, Mazlish, E (1998). *Siblings Without Rivalry*, exp ed. New York: Avon.

Fox, HB, McManus, MA (1998). Improving state Medicaid contracts and plan practices for children with special needs. In: *The Future of Children: Children and Managed Care*, edited by RE Behrman. David and Lucile Packard Foundation, Los Altos, CA: 8: 105–118.

Goldstein, AP (1988). *The Prepare Curriculum: Teaching Prosocial Competencies.* Champaign, IL: Research Press.

Gordon, T (1970). *P.E.T. Parent Effectiveness Training.* New York: Peter H. Wyden.

Gottman, J (1997). *Raising an Emotionally Intelligent Child.* New York: Fireside.

Grames, LM, Marsh, JL, Pilgram, T, et al. (2000). Speech therapy outcome and duration in children with cleft palate with or without cleft lip. *Presented at the annual meeting of the American Cleft Palate-Craniofacial Association, Atlanta, Georgia, April 12–14, 2000.*

Handwerk, ML, Marshall, RM (1998). Behavioral and emotional problems of students with learning disabilities, serious emotional disturbance, or both conditions. J Learn Disabil *31:* 327–338.

Harper, DC, Richman, LC (1978). Personality profiles of physically impaired adolescents. J Clin Psychol *34:* 636–642.

Harter, S (1985). Processes underlying the construction, maintenance and enhancement of the self-concept in children. In: *Psychological Perspectives on the Self*, Vol. 3, edited by J Suls and A Greenwald. Hillsdale, NJ: Lawrence Erlbaum.

Hoeksma, JB, Koomen, H (1991). *Development of Early Mother–Child Interaction and Attachment.* Amsterdam: Pro Lingua.

Johnson, DL, Swank, PR, Owen, MJ, et al. (2000). Effects of early middle ear effusion on child intelligence at three, five, and seven years of age. Pediatr Psycholog *25:* 5–13.

Kagan, J (1994). On the nature of emotion. In: *The Development of Emotion. Monographs of the Society for Research in Child Development*, Vol. 59, edited by NA Fox. Chicago: U of Chicago, p. 240.

Kagan, J, Resnick, JS, Snidman, J (1987). The physiology and psychology of behavioral inhibition in young children. Child Dev *58:* 1459–1473.

Kagan, J, Resnick, JS, Snidman, J (1988). Biological bases of childhood shyness. Science *240:* 176–171.

Kapp, K (1979). Self-concept of the cleft lip or palate child. Cleft Palate J *16:* 171–176.

Kapp-Simon, KA, Dawson, P (1998). Behavior adjustment and competence of children with craniofacial conditions. *Presented at the annual meeting of the American Cleft Palate-Craniofacial Association, Baltimore, Maryland, April 24, 1998.*

Kapp-Simon, KA, Krueckeberg, SM (2000). Mental development in infants with cleft lip and/or palate. Cleft Palate Craniofac J *37:* 65–70.

Kapp-Simon, KA, McGuire, DE (1997). Observed social interaction patterns in adolescents with and without craniofacial anomalies. Cleft Palate Craniofac J *34:* 380–384.

Kapp-Simon, KA, Simon, DJ (1991). *Meeting the Challenge: A Social Skills Training Program for Adolescents with Special Needs.* Chicago: University of Illinois Press.

Kapp-Simon, KA, Simon, DJ, Kristovich, S (1992). Self-perception, social skills, adjustment, and inhibition in young adolescents with craniofacial anomalies. Cleft Palate Craniofac J *29:* 352–356.

Kazak, AE, Barakat, LP (1997). Parenting stress and quality of life during treatment for childhood leukemia predicts child and parent adjustment after treatment ends. J Pediatr Psychiatry *22:* 749–758.

Kindig, JS, Richards, HC (2000). Otitis media: precursor of delayed reading. J Pediatr Psychol *25:* 15–18.

Kliewer, W, Sandler, IH (1992). Locus of control and self-esteem as moderators of stressor–symptom relations in children and adolescents. J Abnorm Child Psychol *20:* 393–341.

Krueckeberg, SM, Kapp-Simon, KA (1993). Effect of parent factors on social skills of preschool children with craniofacial anomalies. Cleft Palate Craniofac J *30:* 490–496.

Krueckeberg, SM, Kapp-Simon, KA (1997). Longitudinal follow-up of social skillls in children with and without craniofacial anomalies. *Presented at the annual meeting of the American Cleft Palate-Craniofacial Association, New Orleans, Louisiana, April 7–12, 1997.*

Krueckeberg, SM, Kapp-Simon, KA, Ribordy, SC (1993). Social skills of preschoolers with and without craniofacial anomalies. Cleft Palate Craniofac J *30:* 475–481.

Macgregor, FC (1974). *Transformation and Identity: The Face and Plastic Surgery.* New York: Quadrangle.

Macgregor, FC (1979). *After Plastic Surgery: Adaptation and Adjustment.* Brooklyn, NY: Bergin.

Macgregor, FC (1990). Facial disfigurement: problems and management of social interaction and implications for mental health. Aesthetic Plast Surg *14:* 249–257.

Margalit, M (1989). Academic competence and social adjustment of boys with learning disabilities and boys with behavior disorders. J Learn Disabil *22:* 41–45.

Maris, CL, Endriga, MC, Speltz, ML, et al. (2000). Are infants with orofacial clefts at risk for insecure mother–child attachments? Cleft Palate Craniofac J *37:* 257–265.

Matson, JL, Ollendick, TH (1988). *Enhancing Children's Social Skills: Assessment and Training.* New York: Pergamon.

McConaughy, SH, Mattison, RE, Peterson, RL (1994). Behavioral/emotional problems of children with serious emotional disturbances and learning disabilities. School Psychol Rev *23:* 81–98.

McGuire, D (1990). An evaluation of a social skills program for adolescents with facial disfigurement. Chicago: Univ. of Illinois. Dissertation.

Miller, AC, Gordon, RM, Daniele, RJ, Diller, L (1992a). Stress, appraisal, and coping in mothers of disabled and nondisabled children. J Pediatr Psychol *17:* 587–605.

Miller, SM, Sherman, HD, Combs, C, Kruss, T (1992b). Patterns of children's coping with short-term medical and dental stressors: nature implications and future direction. In: *Stress and Coping in Child Health*, edited by AM LaGreca, LJ Siegel, JL Wallander, and CE Walker. New York: Guilford, pp. 157–190.

Mullins, LL, Olson, RA, Reyes, S, et al. (1991). Risk and resistance factors in the adaptation of mothers of children with cystic fibrosis. J Pediatr Psychol *16:* 701–715.

Murphy, LB, Moriarty, AE (1976). *Vulnerability, coping, & growth: From infancy to adolescence.* New Haven, CT: Yale University Press.

Nash, P (1995). *Living with Disfigurement: Psychosocial Implications of Being Born with a Cleft Lip and Palate.* Brookfield, VA: Ashgate.

Nelsen, J (1996). *Positive Discipline*, rev ed. New York: Ballantine.

Nelsen, J, Erwin, C, Duffy, R (1998a). *Positive Discipline: The First Three Years.* Rocklin, CA: Prima.

Nelsen, J, Erwin, C, Duffy, R (1998b). Temperament, what makes your child unique? *Positive Discipline for Preschoolers*, rev 2nd ed. Rocklin, CA: Prima. pp. 75–93.

Parker, JG, Asher, SR (1987). Peer relations and later personal adjustment: are low accepted children at risk? Psychol Bull *102:* 357–389.

Perrin, J, Guyer, B, Lawrence, JM (1992). Health care services for children and adolescents. In: *The Future of Children: US Health Care for Children*, Vol. 2, edited by RE Behrman. David and Lucile Packard Foundation, pp. 58–77.

Peters, SAF, Grievink, EH, van Bon, WHJ, van Schilder, AGM (1994). The effects of early bilateral otitis media with effusion on educational attainment: a prospective cohort study. J Learn Disabil 27: 111–121.

Peterson-Falzone, SJ (1990). A cross-sectional analysis of speech results following palatal closure. In: *Multidisciplinary Management of Cleft Lip and Palate*, edited by J Bardach and HL Morris. Philadelphia: Saunders, pp. 750–757.

Pillemer, FG, Cook, KV (1989). The psychosocial adjustment of pediatric craniofacial patients after surgery. Cleft Palate J 26: 201–208.

Pless, IB, Roghmann, KJ (1971). Chronic illness and its consequences: observations based on three epidemiological surveys. J Pediatr 79: 351–359.

Pope, AW, Ward, J (1997). Factors associated with peer social competence in preadolescents with craniofacial anomalies. J Pediatr Psychol 22: 455–469.

Richman, LC (1976). Behavior and achievement of cleft palate children. Cleft Palate J 13: 4–10.

Richman, LC (1978a). The effects of facial disfigurement on teachers' perception of ability in cleft palate children. Cleft Palate J 15: 155–160.

Richman, LC (1978b). Parents and teachers: differing views of behavior of cleft palate children. Cleft Palate J 15: 360–364.

Richman, LC (1990). Developmental neuropsychological functions of children with cleft at two age levels. *Presented at the annual meeting of the American Cleft Palate-Craniofacial Association, St. Louis, Missouri, April 1990.*

Richman, LC (1998). Fearful shyness versus solitary passivity in socially inhibited children with cleft. *Presented at the annual meeting of the American Cleft Palate-Craniofacial Association, Baltimore, Maryland, April 20–25, 1998.*

Richman, LC (2000). Are reading disabilities of children with cleft related to speech-language variables or to phonemic disassociations? *Presented at the annual meeting of the American Cleft Palate-Craniofacial Association, Atlanta, Georgia, April 12, 2000.*

Richman, LC, Eliason, MJ (1982). Psychological characteristics of children with cleft lip and palate: intellectual, achievement, behavior, and personality. Cleft Palate J 19: 249–257.

Richman, LC, Eliason, MJ (1984). Type of reading disability related to cleft type and neuropsychological patterns. Cleft Palate J 21: 1–6.

Richman, LC, Eliason, MJ, Lindgren, SD (1988). Reading disability in children with clefts. Cleft Palate J 25: 21–25.

Richman, LC, Harper, DC (1978). School adjustment of children with observable disabilities. J Abnorm Child Psychol 6: 11–18.

Richman, LC, Holmes, CS, Eliason, MJ (1985). Adolescents with cleft lip and palate self-perceptions of appearance and behavior related to personality adjustment. Cleft Palate J 22: 93–95.

Richman, LC, Millard, TL (1997). Cleft lip and palate: longitudinal behavior and relationships of cleft conditions to behavior and achievement. J Pediatr Psychol 22: 487–494.

Roberts, JE, Burchinal, MR, Medley, LP, et al. (1995). Otitis media, hearing sensitivity, and maternal responsiveness in relation to language during infancy. J Pediatr 126: 481–489.

Rutter, M, Tizaard, J, Witmore, K (eds) (1970). *Education, Health and Behavior*. London: Longman.

Schneider, BH, Bryne, BH (1985). Children's social skills training: a meta-analysis. In: *Issues in Assessment and Intervention*, edited by BH Schneider, KH Rubin, and JE Ledingham. New York: Springer-Verlag, pp. 175–192.

Shaw, WC, Humphreys, S (1982). Influence of children's dentofacial appearance on teacher expectations. Community Dent Oral Epidemiol 10: 313–319.

Sheils, JF, Wolfe, PR (1992). The role of private health insurance in children's health care. In: *The Future of Children: US Health Care for Children*, Vol. 2, edited by RE Behrman. David and Lucille Packard Foundation, pp. 115–133.

Short-Camilli, C, Garrity, C, Jens, K, et al. (1999). *Bully-Proofing Your School*. Longmont, CO: Sopris West.

Sloan, GM (2000). Posterior pharyngeal flap and sphincter pharyngoplasty: the state of the art. Cleft Palate Craniofac J 37: 112–122.

Sloper, P (2000). Predictors of distress in parents of children with cancer: a prospective study. J Pediatr Psychol 25: 79–91.

Speltz, ML, Armsden, GC, Clarren, SS (1990). Effects of craniofacial birth defects on maternal functioning post infancy. J Pediatr Psychol 15: 177–195.

Speltz, ML, Endriga, MC, Fisher, PA, Mason, CA (1997). Early predictors of attachment in infants with cleft lip and/or palate. Child Dev 68: 12–25.

Speltz, ML, Endriga, MC, Hill, S, et al. (2000). Cognitive and psychomotor development of infants with orofacial clefts. J Pediatr Psychol 25: 185–190.

Spriesterbach, DC (1973). *Psychological Aspects of the Cleft Palate Problem*. Vols 1 and 2. Iowa City: University of Iowa Press.

Strauss, RP, and American Cleft Palate-Craniofacial Association Team Standards Committee (1998). Cleft Palate and Craniofacial Teams in the United States: a national survey of team organization and standards of care. Cleft Palate Craniofac J 35: 473–480.

Strauss, RP (2001). "Only Skin Deep": Health, resilience and craniofacial care. Cleft Palate Craniofac J 38: 226–230.

Stricker, G, Clifford, E, Cohen, LK, et al. (1979). Psychosocial aspects of craniofacial disfigurement. Am J Orthod 76: 410–416.

Stool, SE (1990). Ear disease in children with cleft palate: state of the art. In: *Multidisciplinary Management of Cleft Lip and Palate*, edited by J Bardach, HL Morris, Philadelphia: Saunders, pp. 696–702.

Thomas, A, Birch, HG, Chess, S, Robbins, LC (1961). Individuality in responses of children to similar environmental situations. Am J Psychiatry 117: 798–803.

Thomas, A, Chess, S (1957). An approach to the study of sources of individual differences in child behavior. J Clin Exp Psychopathology Quarterly Rev Psychiatry Neurol 18: 347–356.

Thomas, A, Chess, S (1980). *The Dynamics of Psychological Development*. New York: Brunner/Mazel.

Thomas, A, Chess, S, Birch, HG, et al. (1963). *Behavioral Individuality in Early Childhood*. New York: New York University Press.

Thompson, RJ, Gil, KM, Burbach, DJ, et al. (1993). Psychological adjustment of mothers of children and adolescents with sickle cell disease: the role of stress, coping methods, and family functioning. J Pediatr Psychol 18: 549–559.

Waitzman, NJ, Romano, PS, Scheffler, RM (1994). Estimates of the economic costs of birth defects. Inquiry 33: 188–205.

Wallander, JL, Varni, JW, Babani, L, et al. (1988). Children with chronic physical disorders: Maternal reports of their psychological adjustment. J Pediatr Psychol 12: 197–212.

Wallander, JL, Varni, JW, Babani, L, et al. (1989). J Pediatr Psychol 14: 371–387.

Wallander, JL, Varni, JW (1992). Adjustment in children with chronic physical disorders: programmatic research on a disability-stress-coping model. In: *Stress and Coping in Child Health*, edited by AM LaGreca, LJ Siegel, JL Wallander, CE Walker. New York: Guilford Press, pp. 279–298.

Wilson, B (2001). Resources for people with facial differences. Let's face it. http://www.faceit.org/~letsfaceit.

33

International surgical missions

S. T. LEE

For the foreseeable future, there will always be a need for international surgical missions to deal with the backlog and the increasing number of patients with oral clefts in the world. These volunteer field missions should, however, be only a part of an overall global strategy. Rather, the emphasis should be on genetic and environmental research, to understand the causative factors of oral clefts, which might lead to the development of preventive strategies to reduce incidence.

Based on the current world population and birth statistics (United States Bureau of the Census, www.census.gov/ipc/www/idbnew.html), 132 million babies were born in 2001, out of a global population of 6.2 billion individuals. If the prevalence at birth of cleft lip with or without cleft palate (CL/P) is taken to be 1/500 live births, 264,000 babies were born with oral clefts in 2001. This enormous number illustrates the magnitude of the problem, which needs to be addressed on a global scale. It is likely that the population with oral clefts will increase globally, unless there are dramatic genetic breakthroughs or new preventive strategies that can reduce this ever-increasing number.

Concurrently, there is also the problem of limited global health resources, especially when dealing with a non-life-threatening condition such as cleft lip and palate (CLP). The overwhelming numbers of newborns with oral clefts are found in countries with high birth rates (e.g., China, India, Indonesia, Africa, South America, Southeast Asia) (Lee, 1999b), where there are invariably limited resources for dealing with the problem. This unequal distribution of expertise and resources is a global dilemma. Resource-rich countries have fewer patients, while countries with minimal resources are inundated with more cleft patients than they can handle. Therein lies the challenge of matching the resources/expertise with the CLP population in the world.

PHILOSOPHY OF VOLUNTEER MISSIONS

Traditionally, volunteer surgical missions have been sponsored by religious groups, service clubs, non-government organizations, philanthropic institutions, and altruistic individuals. They are usually motivated by a sense of charity, compassion, and public–spiritedness toward those who belong to the more vulnerable and disadvantaged groups in society.

International cleft missions should mobilize these positive forces and encourage volunteer work as an expression of a concerned and caring society. Voluntary work, as most volunteers on cleft missions have found, is not necessarily a one-way street: the volunteer gives time and expertise and gains much in return from the experience. Interaction with different cultures and different socioeconomic groups can be a very enriching experience, broadening one's outlook of the world community, creating of new bonds, and heightening the sense of personal fulfillment at being able to do something positive, meaningful, and totally voluntary in nature.

GOALS OF INTERNATIONAL MISSIONS

There is a common thread which runs through all of the goals and objectives of international surgical missions. As far as cleft missions are concerned, the "purist" approach is to deal only with oral cleft patients, to the exclusion of any other medical condition.

As far as this author is aware, only a few teams, such as Michael Mars' from the Great Ormond Street Children's Hospital (Mars et al., 1990) and Amado Ruiz-Razura's of Operation San Jose (Ruiz-Razura et al., 2000), conduct their missions in such an exclusive manner. Almost all other missions deal with a high percentage of CLP cases (usually over 80%) and, to a lesser extent, burns, contractures, chronically unhealed wounds from snakebites and other causes, tropical ulcers, and cancrum oris.

Volunteer organizations usually have five main goals, which are humanitarian in nature (for more details, International Medical Corps, 1997; Interplast Australia, 1999; Interplast, Inc., 1998; Operation Smile, 1997):

1. Provision of direct care to cleft patients and those requiring reconstructive and other ancillary services
2. Provision of educational training to the local population of doctors, nurses, and paramedical personnel
3. Provision for more complex cases, who cannot be treated locally, to be brought back to the donor country for treatment
4. Promotion of self-reliance and establishment of local teams capable of continuing the work of volunteer teams
5. Collection of epidemiological and other research data which could give a better insight into the causative factors and result in preventive strategies

PREPARATION FOR A SURGICAL MISSION

The preparation of a surgical mission is as important as the actual execution of the mission itself. The preparatory work may take from 6 months to a year for all of the necessary correspondence and clearance with the relevant medical bodies, ministries, etc. to be completed. Assessment of the needs and the local facilities means that a site usually must be visited by the team leader and key personnel prior to the mission itself.

Embassies in the countries to be visited are usually a repository of relevant information about local health hazards, immunization required for the team, local information on food, accommodation, entry regulations, areas to avoid because of security problems, social taboos, etc. In addition, the ambassador and embassy staff are usually very solicitous and proud of the visiting team and can provide useful contacts with local ministry officials to facilitate the team's movement and activities. Contact with the embassy is to notify the team's visit rather than the actual organization of the mission itself.

Close contact with the main liaison of the host country will need to be maintained. With the availability of the Internet today, communication has become less of a problem. The team composition, the inventory of equipment and supplies, the basic screening of patients before arrival of the team, and the operating schedule for the duration of the mission need to be jointly worked out between the team leader and the liaison beforehand.

As far as the preparation of the team members is concerned, they need to be briefed on the nature of the mission, their individual responsibilities even though they may be volunteers, the local customs and culture, and their role as medical "ambassadors." They need to take the necessary immunization and prophylactic procedures against, e.g., malaria (where chloroquine resistance is a problem, check with World Health Organization and local health authorities on appropriate prophylaxis). Each member of the team should be personally insured against injury as well as covered medicolegally. Either the organization or the institution will need to provide this coverage, and its importance cannot be overemphasized.

RECIPE FOR SUCCESS: THE DOs AND DON'Ts

Guidelines have been drawn up by various volunteer organizations (Lee, 1999a; Reconstructive Surgeons Volunteer Program, 1999; American Cleft Palate Association, 1994) to help those who wish to volunteer their services in developing countries. These guidelines are necessary, to provide a minimum standard of care for cleft patients and to prevent the "downside" of volunteer missions. Much has been written about the unfavorable outcomes of medical missions (Lehman and D'Antonio, 1992), and this disquiet prompted the Reconstructive Surgeons Volunteer Program to organize a symposium entitled "Volunteering Overseas: Avoiding the Downside" in Boston, Massachusetts, in 1998. From these discussions, the following 10 guidelines for the conduct of volunteer surgical missions have been accepted.

Guidelines for Volunteer Medical Missions

1. Go where there is a need and go where you are wanted.
2. The goals should be service, training, education, and, where possible, research.
3. All volunteer missions should liaise closely with the host organization and seek clearance from local government authorities and national organizations.
4. Proper planning and attention to details of the missions will ensure success, e.g., proper timing, cus-

toms and immigration, flight arrangements, and patient screening.

5. Local host participation is important to the success of the mission, e.g., local transport, storage of equipment and supplies, food, and accommodation for team members.

6. Personal health and liability are the individual responsibilities of team members themselves, to avoid sickness during or after the mission. Proper vaccination and prophylactic measures should be undertaken.

7. Sources of funding may be personal donations, industry, philanthropic organizations, private sector, nongovernment organizations, and governments. Recipient countries may contribute toward local transport, food, and accommodation.

8. Team members should be experienced specialists in their own fields, to ensure quality of care. Only senior residents or trainees should be allowed to operate under the supervision of senior team members.

9. Postoperative care and follow-up must be of the highest quality, to avoid complications, especially after the team's departure.

10. Volunteer teams should always avoid self-promoting publicity, especially in the host country. Sensitivities may be aroused by undue and unwanted publicity among the local medical fraternity; but publicity at home, especially after completion of a successful mission, is welcome and good for raising awareness and funds.

In general, volunteers should maintain the highest standards of care. They should work in conjunction with local doctors and transfer skills and knowledge to them so that they can be self-reliant in delivering services after the departure of the team. Technical aid programs to bring doctors, nurses, and paramedical personnel for further training in the donor institutions should be made available. Medical volunteers are ambassadors of care as well as goodwill and should be sensitive to local customs and culture. They should be adaptable to local conditions of medical practice and living. Team members should be chosen for their adaptability as much as their surgical skills.

HOW HOST COUNTRIES CAN ENSURE THE SUCCESS OF A MISSION

The perception by the local professional community of the goals of a volunteer mission is important in determining the level of cooperation. If volunteers are perceived as providing a "superior" service and this is the belief among the local patients, then the local professionals may feel threatened or there may be a "loss of face." It is important to realize that the local professionals may not be able to accept that their skill levels are not equal to the visitors' and that any discussion of sophisticated technology will further enhance feelings of inferiority and animosity. To avoid such negative feelings, active steps should be taken by the volunteer team to dispel such perceptions. The best way to accomplish this is to have the local professionals work alongside the visiting team members from the start.

Host countries can participate actively to ensure the success of missions in several ways.

1. Needs, whether they involve service, training, or equipment and supplies, should be identified as accurately as possible.

2. The patient population needs to be screened so that only those suitable for surgery are presented to the team. Usually, the short duration of the mission precludes dealing with every patient, and there needs to be some prioritization. Investigation and surgery for some complex craniofacial anomalies will need to be done in the donor institution/country.

3. Facilitation of entry and customs requirements as well as local transport and accommodation will allow the volunteer team to settle in and get to work as quickly as possible.

4. Host country and institutions can demonstrate responsibility in the usage of funds and supplies/equipment so that donors can be assured that the donations have reached the people most in need of help.

5. Follow-up of patients after the departure of the volunteer team will need to be carried out by local professionals. Documentation and records are important for subsequent recall of patients who may require staged repair or secondary procedures.

6. To develop the concept of multidisciplinary team care for cleft patients, host countries and institutions should identify suitable individuals for training in orthodontics, speech therapy, pediatric anesthesia, and specialized cleft nursing. They are encouraged to function as a unit and to work with the volunteer team on subsequent visits. If opportunities are available, they should be sent for training in the donor countries/institutions so that eventually a self-reliant and independent CLP team can be created for long-term care of the local cleft population.

FUTURE OF SURGICAL MISSIONS

As Gorney (1987) said: "there is no more undervalued a weapon of foreign policy as reconstructive surgery." When volunteers bring hope to those born with clefts and deformed faces who would otherwise have to face a life as a castaway and shunned by society, they are regarded as angels of hope and humanitarian ambassadors for their countries.

No amount of foreign aid will touch as many lives as those operated on by the volunteer teams or generate the aura of goodwill and understanding between peoples and nations.

However, volunteer missions must be audited for their performance. They must not leave behind a trail of mishaps and complications to sully the reputation of volunteer missions. Untrained personnel and those who do not have the credentials to carry out the surgical procedures in their own countries should not do so in the guise of a "foreign expert" in a developing country. Volunteer missions, after all, are not safaris for hit-and-miss surgeons. They are for the most experienced in the specialty so that spot decisions can be made in the field. There are no intensive care units when something goes amiss, and only experience and clinical judgment of the best course of action will sometimes save the day.

Those who are starting off as volunteers are advised to adhere closely to the guidelines set out by international bodies such as The Reconstructive Surgeons Volunteer Program, The American Cleft Palate Association, and The International Plastic Reconstructive and Aesthetic Society. They should consult veterans of volunteer missions, who will usually have many interesting anecdotes to tell and down-to-earth advice to give. Volunteer missions will continue to be needed until cleft teams are established in all developing countries and the population of individuals with oral clefts stops growing. This will not happen in the foreseeable future, and until it does, volunteerism will provide the avenue for following our humanitarian drive and achieving our hippocratic ideals.

REFERENCES

American Cleft Palate Association (1994). *Cleft and Craniofacial Surgery Services in Developing Nations: Guidelines for Volunteers*, edited by K Stueber and L Wilson.

Gorney, M (1987). Principles of successful medical expeditions to developing nations. In: *A Different Kind of Diplomacy*, edited by JC Fisher and D Armstrong. San Diego: Plastic Surgery Education Foundation, pp. 10–14.

International Medical Corps (1997). *Annual Report 1997*. Los Angeles: International Medical Corps.

Interplast Australia (1999). *Annual Report 1999*. Melbourne: Interplast Australia.

Interplast Inc (1987). *The Story of Interplast—Shared Miracles*. Palo Alto: Interplast.

Lee, ST (1999a). International Plastic Reconstructive and Aesthetic Society, Committee on Projects in Developing Countries. Guidelines for volunteer missions overseas. IPRAS Newsletter.

Lee, ST (1999b). New treatment and research strategies for the improvement of care of cleft lip and palate patients in the new millenium. Ann Acad Med Singapore 28: 760–767.

Lehman, JA, D'Antonio, LL (1992). Volunteer medical missions. Cleft Palate Craniofac J Vol 29, pp. 1–2.

Mars, M, James, DR, Lamabadusuriya, SP (1990). The Sri Lankan Cleft Lip and Palate Project. Cleft Palate J 27: 3–6.

Operation Smile (1997). *Annual Report 1997*. Norfolk, VA: Operation Smile.

Reconstructive Surgeons Volunteer Program (1998). *RSVP Guidelines for Good Guests*. Arlington Heights, IL: Reconstructive Surgeons Volunteer Program.

Ruiz-Razura, A, Cronin, ED, Navavro, CE (2000). Creating long-term benefits in cleft lip and palate volunteer missions. Plast Reconst Surg 105: 195–201.

United States Bureau of the Census. International Data Base. 2001. www.census.gov/ipc/www/idbnew.html.

34

Evidence-based care for children with cleft lip and palate

WILLIAM C. SHAW

GUNVOR SEMB

In the modern age, evidence-based care is considered to be an integration of the best research evidence with clinical expertise and patient values. With respect to therapeutic interventions, the strongest evidence is derived from systematic reviews that provide a synthesis of relevant randomized control trials (Sackett et al., 2000).

For cleft lip and palate care providers, however, there are some challenges ahead. The present scientific basis of the discipline is weak since virtually no elements of treatment have been subjected to the rigors of contemporary clinical trial design (Roberts et al., 1991). Thus, highly complex and varied protocols of care are practised by different teams. Generally speaking, choices regarding surgical technique, timing and sequencing, and ancillary procedures, such as orthopedics, orthodontics, and speech therapy, are arrived at following disappointment in the results of former practices rather than firm evidence that the new protocol has succeeded elsewhere. As a consequence, the unsubstantiated testimony of enthusiasts for a particular treatment has done much to shape current practices. Typically, enthusiastic claims are made for a new type of therapy, the procedure is widely adopted, a flow of favorable clinical reports ensues, little or no positive evidence develops to support the desirability of the procedure, and there is a sharp drop in the number of clinical reports, again without evidence to support the change (Spriestersbach et al., 1973).

JUDGING EVIDENCE OF EFFECTIVENESS

The general rules of health technology assessment are well established and the quality of treatment comparisons conforms to a widely accepted hierarchy, from anecdotal reports to randomized trials and systematic reviews. This hierarchy relates to the degree of effort made to minimize ever-present sources of research bias, "the usual suspects," that readily lead to false conclusions:

1. *Susceptibility bias*. Some patients will inevitably be more susceptible to treatment because their condition is less severe or they inherently possess a better prognosis. Thus, the effectiveness of any technique, applied to a group of cases that are inherently more amenable, will be inflated if compared with another technique applied to a more challenging sample.
2. *Proficiency bias*. In a similar manner, a more skilled surgeon or clinical team can also flatter or inflate the apparent effectiveness of a technique. If operator A is 10% better than operator B and technique X is 5% better than technique Y, a false conclusion will be reached in a comparison of Y performed by A vs. X performed by B.
3. *Follow-up bias*. How confident can the consumer of journal or lecture reports be that the whole story has been given? Can we be sure that follow-up was

as rigorous for the cases that went badly as for those that went well? Without knowing about all of the cases in which the new technique was tried, reliable conclusions cannot be drawn.

4. *Exclusion bias.* In reporting the effectiveness of an intervention, it is often tempting to exclude retrospectively cases where the expected progress was not achieved. Typical grounds for retrospective exclusion might be lack of compliance on the part of the patient or suspicion that an underlying condition (e.g., an ill-defined syndrome) has prevented the intervention from working. Irregular application of the rules of retrospective exclusion clearly can remove any equivalence that comparison groups may have had.

5. *Analysis bias.* Given the virtual absence of agreed rating schemes for outcome evaluation, reporting in the cleft literature is inevitably inconsistent. Without objectivity in appraisal, as achieved with blinded, independent panels, comparisons must be unsure.

6. *Reporting bias.* Clinical researchers, like drug companies, are less likely to report negative findings than positive ones. However, not only are findings more likely to be reported if they are positive, but they are also more readily accepted for publication by journals, more readily accepted for conferences, more often published in English, and more often cited in later publications (Dickersin and Min, 1993; Dickersin et al., 1992; Easterbrook et al., 1991; Egger et al., 1997; Stern and Simes, 1997).

Not surprisingly then, empirical research consistently demonstrates that in studies without randomized control groups an overestimation of effectiveness results (Kunz and Oxman, 1998). Thus, controlled trials of psychiatric interventions found them to be effective only 25% of the time, but in uncontrolled studies of the same medications 75% were positive. Even more dramatically, none of a series of randomized trials of portacaval shunt surgery found clear evidence of benefit, but 75% of uncontrolled studies did. Clearly then, uncontrolled studies, which make up the great majority of the current literature of cleft care, must be appraised with great caution. They should be appreciated for the contributions to knowledge they can make, with recognition of their inherent limitations.

Anecdotal Case Reports

Case reports may signal important new developments in surgical practice, but the evidence they contain for a widespread change in practice remains generally unconvincing in the absence of subsequent confirmatory series.

Case Series

Reports of a series of cases treated by the same method provide more substantial evidence of the merits of a particular technique or program of treatment and a general impression of relative efficacy for the professional community. They are of particular value in demonstrating that new procedures can be reliably performed and can have a low risk of serious morbidity. Rather commonly, however, outcome is measured in the short term and the enthusiasm of the reporters may impair true objectivity. Thus, primary bone grafting, first heralded as an important breakthrough in case series reports, was later shown by randomized control trials to be harmful to facial growth (Rehrmann et al., 1970; Jolleys and Robertson, 1972). However, case series of secondary bone grafting using cancellous iliac crest grafts revealed that one aspect of outcome, the patient's dentition, could be reliably restored beyond previously attainable levels (Boyne and Sands, 1972, 1976; Bergland et al., 1986). The immediacy of these benefits ruled against the need for a randomized trial, though potential growth disturbances still deserved consideration (Semb, 1988). Future trials of bone grafting may, however, still be necessary to examine individual aspects of surgical technique or timing or the suitability of alternative graft materials.

Case series rarely provide evidence of the superiority of one technique over others where a choice of broadly similar methods exists and any improvement may be incremental rather than dramatic. This is a major problem in the evaluation of primary surgical repair since this may be achieved with apparently similar success by methods that differ in technique, timing, and sequence. Meaningful comparison of case series reported in the literature is prohibited by methodological inconsistencies in assessment and by the absence of strict and well-defined entry criteria, such as consecutive cases with an equivalent prognosis.

Uncontrolled Comparison Studies

Opportunities for nonexperimental comparisons of therapies or programs of care can arise in several ways: through coexisting therapies at the same center, through replacement of one therapy with another, or by comparison of treatment centers using different therapies. However, any lack of equivalence between the cases prior to treatment or lack of equivalence in the competence of the clinicians will again undermine the conclusions.

Comparison of Coexisting Therapies.

When using retrospective material such as case notes or clinical databases, checks can be made on the equivalence of the groups, commonly in terms of gender, age, or cleft subtype. Preferably, cases can be matched pairwise on these characteristics. Alternatively, adjustments can be made in the analysis by stratification or the use of multivariate statistical methods. In either case, doubt will remain that important prognostic factors have been masked, for if two or more therapies were being used concurrently within a single center, selective allocation to treatment must be suspected.

Factors that may have influenced clinical decision-making could be unrecorded or unreliably recorded. For example, decisions as to when (at what age) to perform primary surgery may be influenced by unrecorded aspects of the morphology of the cleft, the availability of personnel, the health of the child, or parental attitudes toward the cleft. Should these factors influence outcome, confounding would occur in any study of the effect of age on surgical outcome.

The possibility of confounding in this way is especially likely when treatment was provided 5 or 10 years previously and different staff were involved. Retrospective ascertainment of the details of primary surgery or cleft subtype is difficult, and descriptive terminology may have changed in subtle ways. It may be possible to match or adjust data to remove bias due to gender, age, or cleft subtype; but this gives no guarantee that some other prognostic factor that may affect outcome is not associated with choice of treatment. Also, a critical factor in surgical outcome must be the competence of the surgeon.

Comparison with Historical Controls.

Comparisons with historical controls may arise as natural experiments by changes in therapy within a treatment center. Such research is particularly valuable when durable records (e.g., radiographs, study casts, speech recordings, photographs) are obtained in a standardized way for both subjects treated by a previous method (historical controls) and those treated by the new method, allowing simultaneous unbiased evaluation. Data may already exist on two well-documented treatments used in different time periods.

An alternative circumstance in which such studies arise is where data for a group of patients receiving a standard treatment already exist and can be gathered in a similar way when a new treatment is introduced. This design requires only half the number of patients to be gathered prospectively as a randomized clinical trial and is clearly attractive where recruitment of cases is slow. Furthermore, it has been argued that in circumstances of poor outcome it may be unethical to withhold new treatment in order to create a control group (Gehan, 1984). There are nevertheless several biases and possibilities for confounding that generally favor the newly introduced procedure. In practice, changes in technique at a treatment center often come about as a result of changes in personnel, who may have performed differently with respect to the previous method. This leads to bias due to differences in the skill of personnel associated with either treatment method. For example, a new method of treatment is often tested by an experienced and innovative surgeon, who may be expected to achieve better results than the average surgeon. This clearly introduces the confounding effect of operator skill with treatment. Even where there is stability of staff, bias reflecting gradual changes of ability and technique is highly likely and definition or ascertainment of prognosis may change. New methods may also be initially applied with some selectivity to "suitable" cases as experience is gained. Other aspects of clinical management may have been altered with the intention of improving outcome, creating additional possibilities for bias in favor of the innovative procedure. Multivariate methods have been suggested as a way to adjust for these biases, but serial changes in treatment are likely to take place in parallel, resulting in a strong association between treatment variables. This is one reason why historical control design is generally unsuited to evaluating primary surgery since other changes in the total program of care are likely to have occurred during the extensive recruitment.

Bias favoring the innovative procedure is a major cause for concern with historical control studies as they may either fail to resolve a controversy or create ethical concerns that preclude further, more rigorous comparisons. Favorable outcomes suggested for a new procedure by historical control studies have been disputed by subsequent randomized controlled trials (Pinsky, 1984; Pollock, 1986). Thus, historical control studies could set in motion an unwarranted cycle of change with no benefit to the patient and, consequently, delay the process of development.

The reduction in recruitment time for a historical control study in which data are gathered prospectively on a new method is also less important when evaluating primary surgery due to the extended follow-up required for each case. If, for example, the proposed follow-up of a trial of two methods of primary surgery is 10 years and the recruitment time of patients sufficient for a randomized trial is 4 years, the total duration would be 14 years. The potential saving of time in a partially prospective historical control study would be only 2 years (14%).

Intercenter Comparison. The multicenter approach offers distinct advantages for even the busiest cleft lip and palate treatment centers; the generation of adequate samples within specific cleft subtypes treated by contrasting treatment modalities is extremely difficult. Prospectively planned recall of cases at participating centers allows data on outcome to be collected in a standardized way, and rigorous planning and execution across the centers can ensure consecutive case recruitment and unbiased evaluation (Shaw et al., 1992b).

Provided procedures for entry into the study are equivalent in all participating centers, this strategy is extremely valuable in assessing the outcome of primary surgery together with other major components of the treatment program at respective centers. However, it is difficult, if not impossible, to establish the key beneficial or harmful features of a specific treatment as a general scientific conclusion due to the invariably complex and arbitrary mix of surgical techniques, timing, sequence, ancillary procedures, and surgical personnel (Shaw et al., 1992a). For example, if two centers differ in the use of presurgical orthopedics and types of primary lip and palate surgery, there is no way to determine which of these procedures might be responsible for any difference in outcome between centers, nor would a null result allow the conclusion that individual aspects of the treatment program are equivalent. The method is, therefore, better suited to comparative clinical audit and quality assurance than definitive clinical research. Significant disparities in outcome of the overall treatment process provide a basis for speculating as to the possible cause, and intercenter studies should therefore be highly motivating toward the generation of specific hypotheses for subsequent trials.

An ambitious audit of this kind was conducted in the United Kingdom, to determine the standards of cleft care in the country as a whole, and included a comparison with centers in other European countries (Bearn et al., 2001). Prospectively planned recall of all 5- and 12-year-olds with unilateral cleft lip and palate and standardized recording of a range of outcomes allowed a series of subgroup comparisons as well as comparison with standards elsewhere. The conclusions of this study formed the basis for government recommendations to reconfigure cleft services in the United Kingdom such that care is now concentrated in the hands of a small number of regional specialist centers (Clinical Standards Advisory Group, 1998).

Randomized Controlled Trials

For the comparison of therapies, there is little doubt that the randomized control trial (RCT) is generally the method of choice both scientifically and ethically. Randomization minimizes conscious or unconscious bias in treatment allocation. Prognostic factors, whether known or unknown to the investigator, tend to be balanced between treatment groups. Since patients are followed prospectively according to a clearly defined protocol, missing data are less likely, and the potential loss to follow-up is reduced. If loss does occur, it may be possible to quantify any induced bias, in contrast with retrospective studies, where the researcher may be unaware of patients lost to follow-up, thus introducing bias into the results.

RCTs, however, can also be performed badly. Notably, if the randomization procedure is not strictly applied (i.e., allocation is not fully concealed from the investigators), bias can enter. As with nonrandomized studies, inadequate concealment is associated with higher odds ratios; i.e., an inflated view of effectiveness emerges (Moher et al., 1998).

The ethical issues concerning RCTs in cleft care are interesting (Berkowitz, 1995; Shaw, 1995), particularly the double standards that are applied in clinical experimentation. History tells us that not all surgical innovations are an enduring success. Discredited techniques, though once fashionable, include gastric freezing for bleeding peptic ulcer, carotid body denervation for bronchial asthma, portacaval shunt to prevent esophageal variceal bleeding, nephropexy for viceroptosis, removal of chronically inflamed appendix, and periarterial sympathectomy (Baum, 1981; Salzman, 1985). One dramatic medical example is the prophylactic use of antiarrhythmic drugs during myocardial infarction: at the peak of their use in the late 1980s, it has been estimated that these drugs caused between 20,000 and 70,000 deaths every year in the United States alone, a yearly total of the same order of magnitude as the total number of Americans who died in the Vietnam War (Moore, 1995).

Where the doctor leads, most patients and parents will follow. Such is the desire to shed handicap and stigma. Yet, innovation per se offers no guarantee. Numerous reports show that new treatments are as likely to be worse as they are to be better than existing alternatives (Chalmers, 1997).

What then should be our ethical position? If we wish to test an innovate procedure in an RCT, we must obtain ethical approval from an appropriate body and fully inform each new patient about any uncertainty and risk prior to obtaining signed consent. Ironically, if we wish to test the same innovation on all of our patients, no such rules currently apply (Chalmers and Lindley, 2000). "Ethical codes that seek to protect patients . . . regulate the responsible investigator but not the irresponsible adventurer" (Lantos, 1994). In the United States, the National Commission for the Protection of Human Subjects recommended that "medical committees should be responsible for ensuring that major innovations undergo proper scientific evaluation" and be charged with "determining which new treatments need to be evaluated, the proper method of evaluation and how to limit the use . . . prior to the completion of that evaluation" (Tonelli et al., 1996). As yet, no such body exists in the United States or Europe.

Almost 30 years ago, Spriestersbach and co-workers (1973) identified the need for prospective research to resolve the central problems of cleft management. However, remarkably few RCTs have been performed in cleft lip and palate surgery, despite being the surest means of advancing the discipline in the face of overwhelming uncertainty about the relative efficacy of countless different programs of care around the world. In a review of 25 years of the *Cleft Palate Journal*, only five controlled clinical trials were identified, with only one involving follow-up after surgery of more than 4 years (Roberts et al., 1991).

Robertson and Jolleys conducted two small RCTs of primary surgery in the 1960s. In the first study, a sample was randomized with respect to alveolar bone grafting at the time of primary surgery in infancy (Robertson and Jolleys, 1968). Follow-up revealed a detrimental effect on facial growth in the grafted group (Robertson and Jolleys, 1983). The second study involved two groups of 20 cases, one group having anterior palate closure delayed until age 5 years. No benefit for dentofacial growth was found in delaying hard palate closure (Robertson and Jolleys, 1974). A follow-up study when the children were 11 years of age reached the same conclusion (Robertson and Jolleys, 1990).

In a quasi-RCT on speech outcome, Marsh et al. (1989) alternated (rather than randomized) palate repair with or without intravelar veloplasty in 51 subjects with a broad range of palatal cleft types. Speech evaluations were made at 2-year follow-up. No difference in outcome was detected, but the procedure including intravelar veloplasty required a significantly longer operating time.

Another RCT on speech outcome and maxillary growth in patients with unilateral complete cleft lip and palate operated on at 6 vs. 12 months of age was undertaken in Mexico (Ysunza et al., 1998). The study groups consisted of 41 subjects operated on at 12 months and 35 subjects operated on at 6 months. There was no statistically significant difference in velopha-

ryngeal insufficiency, maxillary arch development, or soft tissue profile as measured on cephalometric radiographs. However, phonological development was significantly better in patients operated at 6 months, and none of the patients in this group developed compensatory articulation. The authors concluded that cleft palate repair performed at 6 months significantly enhances speech outcome and prevents compensatory articulation disorder.

At the Hospital for Research and Rehabilitation of Craniofacial Anomalies, University of São Paulo, Brazil, an RCT comparing velopharyngeal function for speech outcomes in two groups of patients with complete unilateral cleft lip and palate has begun (Williams et al., 1998). The two palatoplasty techniques are the von Langenbeck with intravelar veloplasty and the Furlow procedure. A total of 608 patients will be entered into one of two age categories: patients having surgery before 1 year of age and patients undergoing surgery at approximately 1.5 years of age. This study is designed to determine which of the two surgical procedures is superior at constructing a velum capable of affecting velopharyngeal competence for the development of normal speech.

For patients with velopharyngeal insufficiency, secondary surgery to the pharynx is often recommended. The two most popular techniques are pharyngeal flap and sphincter pharyngoplasty. These techniques are presently being tested in a multisite RCT. Patients are evaluated before and at least twice following surgery by perceptual speech evaluation, video nasopharyngoscopy, nasometry, polysomnographic sleep study, lateral cephalometric radiography, audiometry, and tympanometry. When completed, the study should significantly increase our understanding of both operations and allow an objective comparison between them in terms of speech results, incidence of sleep apnea, other complications, and rate of reoperation, as well as operating time, length of hospital stay, and financial costs (Sloan et al., 1996).

Since 1986, north European teams have been developing a concerted program of multidisciplinary intercenter research on cleft lip and palate, including a comparison of surgical outcome in four Scandinavian centers (Friede et al., 1991; Enemark et al., 1993) and six European centers (Shaw et al., 1992a,b; Mølsted et al., 1992, 1993a,b; Mars et al., 1992; Asher-McDade et al., 1992; Morrant and Shaw, 1996; Grunwell et al., 2000).

Following these collaborations, the limitations of intercenter studies became increasingly obvious to these teams. In particular, it became clear that it would be impossible to separate out the single elements of the package of care provided in the different centers. It was recognized that outcomes of care reflect surgical skill as well as surgical technique and timing and sequence of surgery as well as other auxiliary procedures, such as presurgical orthopedics.

This experience, therefore, provided a compelling stimulus for starting RCTs on primary surgery of clefts. Ten centers are currently participating in a set of three parallel trials, in which teams test their traditional local protocols against a common protocol (Semb and Shaw, 1998). At the time of this writing, almost half of the proposed sample of 450 infants with unilateral cleft lip and palate had been entered.

Randomized trials of nonsurgical intervention have also been completed. These include the use or nonuse of presurgical orthopedics (Prahl et al., 1996), the use or nonuse of arm splints following surgery (Jigjinni et al., 1993), unrestricted sucking after surgery (Lee, 1999), and feeding methods in infancy (Brine et al., 1994; Shaw et al., 1999).

Such efforts demonstrate the feasibility of RCTs in the cleft field and indicate the probable shape of future progress. Thus, trials of sufficient power are likely to be mounted either through collaborations between funding agencies, clinical scientists, and large, possibly developing world centers or through multicenter trials within collaborative groups with strong geographic or cultural links.

MEASURING TREATMENT OUTCOME

The ultimate goal of cleft care is restoration of the patient to a "normal" life, unhindered by handicap or disability. However, the measurement of normalcy is a highly complex proposition, and there is certainly no index at present that would allow sufficiently sensitive comparison between alternative treatment protocols. Clinical trials focus more on "proximate" outcomes. These mainly represent different aspects of anatomical form and function in the parts affected by the clefting process, often reflecting the particular interests of individual disciplines and provider groups. In essence, most measures will be an indication of the degree of handicap that persists despite (or as a result of) treatment, such as shortcomings in speech, hearing, and dentofacial development.

Outcome Measures

Proximate outcome measures must satisfy several criteria. The easiest to meet is that the measurement should be reproducible between and within examiners.

The most suitable statistic for comparing the reproducibility of different measurement scales is the intra-class correlation coefficient, also referred to as the reliability coefficient. In a research setting, a measurement may be broken up into two components: the "true," or error-free, measurement of each case and the error, or "noise," in the measurement that one would wish to minimize. The *intraclass correlation coefficient* is a ratio of the variation of the error-free measurement to the total variation including measurement error. As a ratio, it is dimensionless and, hence, independent of the units of measurement whether they be distances, angles, or scale points in a rating scale. Consequently, it allows cross-comparison of reproducibility between different methods of measurement.

In the unlikely circumstance that a measurement scale is applied without any measurement error, the variation of error-free measurement will equal the total variation. In this case, the intraclass correlation coefficient equals 1. However, a scale containing substantial error will have a much smaller intraclass correlation coefficient. In the worst case, where the measurement error is so great that the scale is unable to distinguish between cases, the intraclass correlation coefficient is equal to 0. At the design stage of a study, poor reproducibility of an outcome measure may be offset by an increase in sample size. The sample size required is increased (relative to that for an entirely reliable scale) by the factor $1/R$, where R is the intraclass correlation coefficient. It is generally estimated using analysis of variance. If the scale used is categorical, the weighted kappa statistic may be used (Cohen, 1968). This is equivalent to the intraclass correlation coefficient if squared weights are used (Fleiss and Cohen, 1973).

Another strategy to improve the reproducibility of a measure is to use the total or mean of a set of measurements from a panel of observers working independently. This also reduces any bias that may related to the idiosyncratic perceptions of a particular observer. It is possible to estimate the reliability of such a pooled value using the Spearman Brown formula (Fleiss, 1986). If R is the intraclass correlation coefficient for a single observer, then the intraclass correlation coefficient for a measurement obtained by totaling the scores of m observers is as follows:

$$R_m = m * \frac{R}{[1 + (m - 1)] * R}$$

More difficult is the requirement of validity that the measure truly represents what it is supposed to represent. For example, do the results of a nasendoscopic examination reflect how well the patient sounds to others? Or does a series of cephalometric measurements actually reflect how well the patient looks to others?

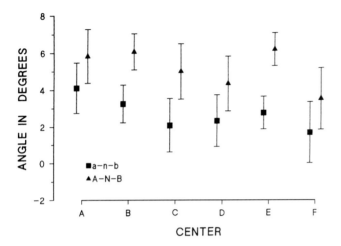

FIG. 34.1. Comparison of maxillo-mandibular profile measurements for unilateral cleft lip and palate. *a-n-b*, hard tissue; *A-N-B*, soft tissue. Data derived from the Eurocleft Study.

External facial appearance is a crucial outcome for patients since this, after all, is what they and society around them actually see. Cephalometric analysis, with its central place in the thinking of orthodontists, is assumed to be an important outcome in its own right, if only as a surrogate measure (Herson, 1989). It is however, an invalid measure of many aspects of external facial appearance.

A particular problem in the study of a congenital condition such as cleft lip and palate arises when outcomes are assessed in childhood, though eventual form and function will not be known until adulthood. This is especially so for aspects of facial growth such as maxillary prominence since this feature deteriorates steadily during growth (Semb, 1991). A useful way to identify potential outcome measures that are valid and predictive is to examine longitudinal archives. The relative prominence of the maxilla in patients with complete clefts is an important outcome for evaluating the success of primary surgery. One common method for doing this is to measure angle a-n-b, the relationship of the anterior outlines of the maxilla and mandible to the fronto-nasal suture. However, identification of point A on the maxillary outline is difficult in early childhood because of the position of the unerupted permanent incisors. In the Eurocleft study (Mølsted et al., 1992), soft tissue analysis at age 10 for unilateral cleft lip and palate was broadly consistent with that derived from hard tissues (Fig. 34.1), and if the soft tissue A-N-B angle could be shown to be adequately predictive, it would be a good alternative. Indeed, it has the further advantages of being measurable on photographs, obviating the need for irradiation and reflecting the actual facial outline observable in everyday life.

TABLE 34.1 *Correlation between Measurement of Maxillo-Mandibular Profile at Age 6 and Subsequently in the Same Cases**

| | Strength of linear relationship with A-N-B at age 6 years (± 1) measured by r^2 (n = 56) | | |
	12 years	15 years	18 years
a-n-b	0.67	0.45	0.27
A-N-B	0.74	0.57	0.46

*Data from the Oslo Archive (Semb, 1991).

Data from the Oslo Archive (Semb, 1991) were examined at a number of age points to assess how well early measurement of the A-N-B angle would predict the situation in adulthood. To assess the strength of any linear predictive relationship, r^2 was calculated between the soft tissue A-N-B angle at age 6 ± 1 year and measurements at a later stage (Table 34.1). Small groups of 20 to 30 unilateral cleft lip and palate patients from Manchester and Oslo were compared in a number of studies at different ages. In Figure 34.2, the average soft tissue A-N-B angle for each center at ages 6, 9, and 12 years is shown. Though the levels of significance for the differences fall just below the 5% level, the differences between each center at different ages are of similar magnitude, reinforcing the predictive worth of the soft tissue A-N-B angle at age 6 ± 1 year.

Measurement Scales

Development of measurement scales that are both reproducible and valid for cleft outcomes is still at an early stage. Preliminary experience comes from comparisons of dentofacial form and relationships in the

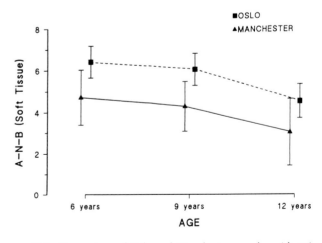

FIG. 34.2. Comparison of Oslo and Manchester samples with unilateral cleft lip and palate for different age groups. Group means with 95% confidence limits.

Eurocleft study using cephalometric analysis for skeletal form (Mølsted et al., 1992), dental arch relationships (Mars et al., 1992), and nasolabial appearance (Asher-McDade et al., 1991, 1992).

Cephalometric measurements, though reproducible, suffer a lack of content validity since they measure three-dimensional structures in a two-dimensional way. Nonetheless, cephalometric relationships can tell a great deal about potential growth inhibition for structures undoubtedly affected by surgical procedures (Semb and Shaw, 1996), and they successfully discriminate between different centers (Mølsted et al., 1992).

To compare dental arch relationships, the Goslon Yardstick, an index designed to systematize subjective perception, was used (Mars et al., 1987). Originally, a large sample of study casts was graded by a panel of orthodontists into a series of five groups containing representative cases ranging from the best (group 1) to the worst (group 5) dental arch relationships. These reference groups were subsequently used to assist in grading new cases. A similar grading system was introduced for use on the study casts of 5-year-old subjects with unilateral cleft lip and palate (Atack et al., 1997). This was extensively used in the recent national enquiry in the United Kingdom described above.

In the Eurocleft study, five observers assessed a sample of 149 study casts using the yardstick and a good level of reliability with an intraclass correlation coefficient of 0.80 was obtained (Table 34.2). The mean of the five measurements was then used as a summary score. Application of the Spearman Brown formula suggests that the reliability of this average score is excellent. From the formula above, the estimated value for the mean of five assessments was 0.95. The mean of the five examiners' scores was sensitive to differences between treatment center (Mars et al., 1992).

In a subsequent study (Morris et al., 1994), an attempt was made to discover whether certain measurements could be made directly without the need of assembling a panel of orthodontists. To relate the subjective assessment of the Goslon Yardstick to objective measurement, overjet, overbite, incisor angulation, and various arch form and crossbite relationships were measured on the same series of study casts using a reflex metrograph. These objective measurements were then used as predictors of the mean Goslon score in a multiple regression analysis. Overjet of the incisor on the unaffected side (all cases were unilateral cleft lip and palate) explained a substantial proportion of the variance ($r^2 = 0.87$). The other measures explained only an additional 3% of the variance.

To compare the nasolabial appearance of patients in the Eurocleft study using photographs, several difficulties were confronted. Technical issues such as film quality, lighting, sharpness of image, facial expression, and background general facial appearance were factors that could influence an observer's opinion. To assess the influence of background appearance, such as hair, eyes, and complexion, a panel of observers was asked to examine independently three frontal views: the nasiolabial area in isolation, the full face, and the surrounding features without the nasolabial part (Asher-McDade et al., 1991). Each view was scored in terms of attractiveness using a visual analogue scale. A strong correlation was found between the full face and surrounding area ($r = 0.53$, $p < 0.001$), indicating that the full face is likely to be influenced by surrounding features.

Consequently, a more valid measure would be based on restricting the areas under consideration to those directly affected by the anomaly and its repair. Thus, the Eurocleft examiners were asked to assess a standardized view of the frontal and lateral views of the nasiolabial area. We considered it important to break down the task into four components: (1) nasal form (frontal view), (2) deviation of the nose from the midline, (3) shape of the vermilion border, and (4) profile including the upper lip. Each observer was asked to score

TABLE 34.2 *Evaluation of Reproducibility for Study Cast (Goslon) and Features of Nasolabial Appearance*[*]

	Goslon	Nasal	Symmetry	Vermilion	Profile	Total
Intraclass correlation coefficient	0.80	0.47	0.36	0.47	0.48	0.49
Lower 95% confidence limit	0.76	0.41	0.30	0.40	0.42	0.43
Sample size	149	115	115	115	115	115
Number of Examiners	*Spearman Brown Estimates of Reliability of Total of Independent Scores*					
3	0.92	0.73	0.62	0.72	0.74	0.75
5	0.95	0.82	0.73	0.81	0.82	0.83
6	0.96	0.84	0.77	0.84	0.85	0.85

[*]All based on six observers except Goslon involving five. Data derived from the Eurocleft study.

each of the components on a 5-point subjective scale, from very good appearance to very poor appearance. A total score was also computed by aggregation of the scores of the four components. The reliability of each component and the total score ranged from 0.47 for nasal form and vermilion border to 0.36 for symmetry (Table 34.2).

We found poor reproducibility compared to that obtained for dental arch relationships, and the reliability of the total score was little better than that for the component scores. In this case, the strategy of splitting the assessment into components appeared to have a limited ability to improve the quality of measurement. Detailed analysis of the data suggested that if one observer scored higher than another for one of the four components, that observer was likely to do so for the other three.

For future work, we will test whether reproducibility is improved by reducing the subjective element, providing reference examples, or "benchmarks" as with the Goslon Yardstick, or by enumeration of specific features for rating. Elsewhere, we have found this to improve reproducibility. For example, rating of dental aesthetics is assisted by providing an illustrated 10-point scale, and orthodontic treatment need on dental health grounds is reproducibly rated when clear diagnostic categories are used (Brook and Shaw, 1989).

Benchmarks must be provided with some caution, however, as the choice of categories for each scale and the subject of each subscale determine the content validity of the total measurement. Thus, there is a danger of imposing the researchers' perceptions of what is important.

An alternative strategy for rating appearance is to rank subjects pairwise against each other. All possible pairs of subjects are compared (Tobiasen, 1989). For each pair, a score of 1 is allocated to the preferred photograph. The score for each case is then its total after comparison with all other cases. One practical difficulty, however, is that the number of comparisons escalates with sample size. The number of possible pairs is equal to $n(n - 1)/2$ for a sample of n cases. Thus, for a sample of 10 subjects, 45 comparisons are needed; for 50 subjects, the number rises to 1225. However, the pairwise technique might be modified by comparing each case against a random or systematic sample of other subjects. For example, the photographs for the complete sample might be arranged in a random sequence and then a score for each case obtained by comparing against the next k subjects. The larger choices for k would improve the reliability of the score for each case but increase the total time to perform the task. A more fundamental limitation is that the scale is meaningful only with regard to the relationship between sub-

jects within the same sample since the comparison is not transferable from one study to another.

The static nature of a still photograph, of course, is a major weakness with respect to validity since the lip in function cannot be judged. Consequently, the use of video recording has been explored (Morrant and Shaw, 1996). An edited sequence for a series of 30 subjects using a number of standardized views of the nasolabial area at rest and function was prepared. A panel of judges then rated the cases using a scoring chart with nine responses for the lip and 10 for the nose.

The nose and lip were assessed separately with eight components and an overall score for lip and nine components and an overall score for the nasal area. For the nasal area, the intraclass correlation coefficient for individual components ranged from 0.40 to 0.27 with 0.52 for the overall score and 0.49 for the sum of the components. For the lip, the intraclass correlation coefficient ranged from 0.39 to 0.10 with 0.28 for the overall score and 0.34 for the sum of components.

While such a dynamic view may be more valid, the interexaminer agreement was generally worse than that achieved from a static image. This may reflect the significantly higher content of information contained in the video format, and by further discussion of the items to be rated and possible provision of improved descriptive categories or illustrated examples, an appearance scale of high validity seems feasible.

TREATMENT COSTS

In most developed countries, the high medical costs of rehabilitating the child with a cleft are borne, or at least supported in part, by the state. Economic pressures around the world now force a re-examination of the true financial costs of treatment, and with declining budgets, clinicians must either be involved in cost control or have arbitrary choices imposed upon them. Surgery is invariably expensive, and successful primary operations that minimize the need for multiple secondary revisions are highly desirable. Furthermore, successful primary repairs are likely to reduce the duration and complexity of ancillary procedures, such as speech therapy, orthodontics, and maxillary osteotomy.

In economic terms, the cheapest care will certainly be that which is provided with a high degree of planning and coordination. Common examples might be combining the placement of drainage tubes with another operation, timing alveolar bone grafting so that natural space closure is facilitated and the duration of subsequent orthodontics is minimized, and recognizing a later need for maxillary osteotomy so that inappropriate early orthodontics is avoided.

BURDEN OF CARE

Since the consequences of an orofacial cleft are apparent through every phase of childhood and adolescence, there is seldom a time when the disciplines involved in care could not recommend some or other intervention. The powerful desire of patients and parents to reach the point where the stigma of clefting will be completely eradicated makes it likely that they will accept most proposals. Most patients and parents will willingly comply with protocols of care recommended by all members of their team, no matter how demanding they may be. They have little choice.

So far, the burden of care has received little attention in cleft care, yet the combined total of operations, other treatment episodes, and review appointments for the first 20 years of life, including all of the disciplines that may be involved, can easily exceed 100. Apart from the pain and suffering and disruption of family life and school attendance, the dependent role in which this places the patient may have an adverse effect on the patient's sense of self-determination or locus of control.

BALANCING OUTCOME, COST, AND BURDEN

Decision analysis (utility theory) is the science of relative utilities or preferences and can be employed to formulate global outcome measures that are more relevant to patients than the short-sighted proximate outcomes that absorb clinicians. Clearly, it behooves the providers of cleft care to seek optimal balance in the development of protocols of care spanning the years from birth to late adolescence.

Undoubtedly, there are intriguing discussions ahead, e.g., the use of early orthopedics and delayed palatal closure. Patients receiving this treatment have to be brought on many additional visits to the treatment center during infancy and childhood and endure the minor risk of impression as well as the greater risk of discomfort associated with the appliances. For the years until the hard palate is closed, they must tolerate a residual cleft or an obturator, while having a clear sense of being an orthodontic patient. How much benefit does this additional treatment have to produce over treatment without early orthopedics to justify its inclusion in care: an average increase in angle s-n-a (maxillary prominence) of 1 degree, a 10% reduction in osteotomy rate in the teens, or a better cosmetic repair of the lip? (If differences do exist, how would they be measured?) Similar questions arise about other elements of care. How often should lip or nasal revision be attempted? When does the law of diminishing re-

turns start to apply? Surgical management of velopharyngeal incompetence is not without some risk, so how bad does the problem have to be to justify the average gain from pharyngoplasty or flap? How much orthodontics should be performed in childhood if the duration and outcome of definitive treatment in the permanent dentition will not be radically altered? These are issues about which patients and parents deserve honest information and the opportunity to have their preferences taken into account.

CONCLUSION

Regrettably, evidence-based care for children with cleft lip and palate is scarcely available. However, there is some evidence that simple treatment protocols that minimize the burden on the child can produce equivalent or better results than complex ones (Shaw et al., 1992a; Shaw, 1997) and no evidence that the opposite is true. Furthermore, centralization of treatment with therapy provided by high-volume operators provides the best setting for good and comprehensive care and at least allows quality assessment within a reasonable period (Shaw et al., 1996).

It has been said that doctors make choices about treatment in three ways: seduction, induction, or deduction. In the seductive method, the clinician simply adopts what he or she has been taught or encouraged to do by teachers or colleagues, i.e., treatment based on faith. The inductive method includes choices based on clinical experience, i.e., on what seems to work or on theories of what ought to work. For example, do extensive muscle repositioning during primary lip repair because this will encourage growth, do minimal tissue mobilization and disturbance during surgery because more surgery means more scar-induced growth disturbance, do not touch the vomer during lip repair because it is a growth center, or do use a vomerine flap because there is no evidence for growth disturbance and it permits good arch development, minimizes fistulae, and provides a good nasal floor for later bone grafting. Finally, there is the deductive, or hypotheticodeductive, method, in which decisions are made on the unbiased evidence of randomized trials. Initiating multicenter collaborations and protocols for these trials is the challenge that must be grasped by today's clinicians who wish to choose the best treatment for their patients. In time, randomized trials will be aggregated in systematic reviews (Chalmers and Altman, 1995), providing as never before a sound evidence base for provision of cleft care.

Following a recent survey of European cleft centers, the register of 201 teams revealed the use of 194 protocols (Shaw et al., 2000). The start of a new millennium appears to be a timely point for concerted action to leave this morass of clinical uncertainty behind. The unfortunate consumers of cleft care certainly deserve better.

REFERENCES

Asher-McDade, C, Brattström, V, Dahl, E, et al. (1992). A six-center international study of treatment outcome in patients with clefts of the lip and palate. Part 4. Assessment of nasolabial appearance. Cleft Palate Craniofac J 29: 409–412.

Asher-McDade, C, Roberts, C, Shaw, WC, Gallagher, C (1991). Development of a method for rating nasolabial appearance in patients with clefts of the lip and palate. Cleft Palate Craniofac J 28: 385–391.

Atack, N, Hathorn, I, Mars, M, Sandy, J (1997). Study models of 5 year old children as predictors of surgical outcome in unilateral cleft lip and palate. Eur J Orthod 19: 165–170.

Baum, M (1981). Scientific empiricism and clinical medicine: a discussion paper. J R Soc Med 74: 504–509.

Bearn, D, Mildinhall, S, Murphy, T, et al. (2001). Cleft lip and palate care in the United Kingdom—The Clinical Standards Advisory Group (CSAG) Study. Part 4: outcome comparisons, training, and conclusions. Cleft Palate Craniofacial J 38: 38–43.

Bergland, O, Semb, G, Åbyholm, FE (1986). Elimination of the residual alveolar cleft by secondary bone grafting and subsequent orthodontic treatment. Cleft Palate J 23: 175–205.

Berkowitz, S (1995). Ethical issues in the case of surgical repair of cleft palate. Cleft Palate Craniofac J 32: 271–276.

Boyne, PJ, Sands, NR (1972). Secondary bone grafting of residual alveolar and palatal clefts. J Oral Surg 30: 87–92.

Boyne, PJ, Sands, NR (1976). Combined orthodontic-surgical management of residual palatoalveolar cleft defects. Am J Orthod 70: 20–37.

Brine, EA, Rickard, KA, Brady, MS, et al. (1994). Effectiveness of two feeding methods in improving energy intake and growth of infants with cleft palate: a randomized study. J Am Diet Assoc 94: 732–738.

Brook, PH, Shaw, WC (1989). The development of an index of orthodontic treatment priority. Eur J Orthod 11: 309–320.

Chalmers, I (1997). What is the prior probability of a proposed new treatment being superior to established treatments. BMJ 314: 74–75.

Chalmers, I, Altman, DC (1995). Systematic Reviews. London: BMJ.

Chalmers, I, Lindley, R (2001). Double standards on informed consent to treatment. In: Informed Consent in Medical Research. Edited by L Doyal and JS Tobias. London: BMJ Publications, Chapter 26.

Clinical Standards Advisory Group (1998). Cleft Lip and/or Palate. London: Department of Health.

Cohen, J (1968). Weighted kappa nominal scale agreement with provision for scaled disagreement or partial credit. Psychol Bull 70: 213–220.

Dickersin, K, Min, YI (1993). NIH clinical trials and publication bias. Online J Curr Clin Trials doc 50.

Dickersin, K, Min, YI, Meinert, CL (1992). Factors influencing publication of research results: follow-up of publications submitted to two institutional review boards. JAMA 267: 374–378.

Easterbrook, PJ, Berlin, JA, Gopalan, R, Matthews, DR (1991). Publication bias in clinical research. Lancet 337: 867–872.

Egger, M, Zellweger-Zahner, T, Schneider, M, et al. (1997). Language bias in randomised controlled trials published in English and German. Lancet 350: 326–329.

Enemark, H, Friede, H, Paulin, G, et al. (1993). Lip and nose morphology in patients with unilateral cleft lip and palate from four Scandinavian centres. Scand J Plast Reconstr Hand Surg 27: 41–47.

Fleiss, JL (1986). Design and Analysis of Clinical Experiment. New York: Wiley.

Fleiss, JL, Cohen, J (1973). The equivalence of weighted kappa and the intra-class correlation coefficient as a measure of reliability. J Educ Psychol Measurement 33: 613–619.

Friede, H, Enemark, H, Semb, G, et al. (1991). Craniofacial and occlusal characteristics in unilateral cleft lip and palate patients from four Scandinavian centres. Scand J Plast Reconstr Hand Surg 25: 269–276.

Gehan, EA (1984). The evaluation of therapies: historical control studies. Stat Med 3: 315–324.

Grunwell, P, Brøndsted, K, Henningsson, G, et al. (2000). A six-centre international study of outcome of treatment in patients with clefts of the lip and palate: the results of a cross-linguistic investigation of cleft palate speech. Scand J Plast Reconstr Hand Surg 34: 219–229.

Herson, J (1989). The use of surrogate endpoints in clinical trials (an introduction to a series of four papers). Stat Med 8: 403–404.

Jigjinni, V, Kangesu, T, Sommerlad, BC (1993). Do babies require arm splints after cleft palate repair. Br J Plast Surg 46: 681–685.

Jolleys, A, Robertson, NR (1972). A study of the effects of early bone grafting in complete clefts of the lip and palate—five year study. Br J Plast Surg 25: 229–237.

Kunz, R, Oxman, AD (1998). The unpredictability paradox: review of empirical comparisons of randomised and nonrandomised clinical trials. BMJ 317: 1185–1190.

Lantos, J (1994). Ethical issues—How can we distinguish clinical research from innovative therapy? Am J Pediatr Hematol Oncol 16: 72–75.

Lee, TK (1999). Effect of unrestricted postoperative sucking following cleft repair on early postoperative course. In: Proceedings of the 4th Asian Pacific Cleft Lip and Palate Conference, Fukuoka, Japan. September 28–30.

Mars, M, Asher-McDade, C, Brattström, V, et al. (1992). A six-center international study of treatment outcome in patients with clefts of the lip and palate. Part 3. Dental arch relationships. Cleft Palate Craniofac J 29: 405–408.

Mars, M, Plint, DA, Houston, WJB, et al. (1987). The Goslon Yardstick: a new system of assessing dental arch relationships in children with unilateral clefts of the lip and palate. Cleft Palate J 24: 314–322.

Marsh, JL, Grames, LM, Holtman, B (1989). Intravelar veloplasty: a prospective study. Cleft Palate J 26: 46–50.

Moher, D, Pham, B, Jones, A, et al. (1998). Does quality of reports of randomised trials affect estimates of intervention efficacy reported in meta-analyses? Lancet 352: 609–613.

Mølsted, K, Asher-McDade, C, Brattström, V, et al. (1992). A six-center international study of treatment outcome in patients with clefts of the lip and palate. Part 2. Craniofacial form and soft tissue profile. Cleft Palate Craniofac J 29: 398–404.

Mølsted, K, Dahl, E, Brattström, V, et al. (1993a). A six-center international study of treatment outcomes in children with clefts of the lip and palate: evaluation of maxillary asymmetry. Cleft Palate Craniofac J 30: 22–28.

Mølsted, K, Dahl, E, Skovgaard, LT, et al. (1993b). A multicenter comparison of treatment regimens for unilateral cleft lip and palate using a multiple regression model. Scand J Plast Reconstr Hand Surg 27: 277–284.

Moore, T (1995). Deadly Medicine. New York: Simon and Schuster.

Morrant, DG, Shaw, WC (1996). Use of standardized video recordings to assess cleft surgery outcome. Cleft Palate Craniofac J *33:* 134–142.

Morris, T, Roberts, C, Shaw, WC (1994). Incisal overjet as an outcome measure in unilateral cleft lip and palate management. Cleft Palate Craniofac J *31:* 142–145.

Pinsky, CM (1984). Experience with historical control studies in cancer immunotherapy. Stat Med *3:* 325–329.

Pollock, AV (1986). Historical evolution: methods, attitudes, goals. In: *Principle and Practice of Research: Strategies for Surgical Investigators,* edited by H Troidl, WO Spitzer, B McPeak, et al. New York: Springer-Verlag, pp. 7–17.

Prahl, C, Kuijpers-Jagtman, AM, Prahl-Andersen, B (1996). *A Study into the Effects of Presurgical Orthopaedic Treatment in Complete Unilateral Cleft Lip and Palate Patients. A Three Center Prospective Clinical Trial in Nijmegen, Amsterdam and Rotterdam. Interim Analysis.* Nijmegen: Academisch Ziekenhuis.

Rehrmann, AH, Koberg, WR, Koch, H (1970). Long-term postoperative results of primary and secondary bone grafting in complete clefts of lip and palate. Cleft Palate J *7:* 206–221.

Roberts, CT, Semb, G, Shaw, WC (1991). Strategies for the advancement of surgical methods in cleft lip and palate. Cleft Palate Craniofac J *28:* 141–149.

Robertson, NR, Jolleys, A (1968). Effects of early bone grafting in complete clefts of lip and palate. Plast Reconstr Surg *42:* 414–421.

Robertson, NR, Jolleys, A (1974). The timing of hard palate repair. Scand J Plast Reconstr Surg *8:* 49–51.

Robertson, NR, Jolleys, A (1983). An 11-year follow-up of the effects of early bone grafting in infants born with complete clefts of the lip and palate. Br J Plast Surg *36:* 438–443.

Robertson, NRE, Jolleys, A (1990). A further look at the effects of delaying repair of the hard palate. In: *Cleft Lip and Palate. Long-term Results and Future Prospects,* edited by AG Huddart and MWJ Ferguson. Manchester: Manchester University Press. Chapter 11, 176–182.

Sackett, DL, Straus, SE, Richardson, WS, et al. (eds) (2000). *Evidence Based Medicine. How to Practice and Teach EBM.* Edinburgh: Churchill Livingstone.

Salzman, EW (1985). Is surgery worthwhile? Arch Surg *120:* 771–776.

Sandy, J, Williams, A, Mildinhall, S, et al. (1998). The Clinical Standards Advisory Group (CSAG) Cleft Lip and Palate Study. Br J Orthod *25:* 21–30.

Semb, G (1988). Effect of alveolar bone grafting on maxillary growth in unilateral cleft lip and palate patients. Cleft Palate J *25:* 288–295.

Semb, G (1991). A study of facial growth in patients with unilateral cleft lip and palate treated by the Oslo CLP team. Cleft Palate J *28:* 1–21.

Semb, G, Shaw, WC (1996). Facial growth in facial clefting disorders. In: *Facial Clefts and Craniosynostosis, Principles and Man-agement,* edited by TA Turvey, KWL Vig, and RJ Fonseca. Philadelphia: Saunders, pp. 28–56.

Semb, G, Shaw, WC (1998). Facial growth after different methods of surgical intervention in patients with cleft lip and palate. Acta Odontol Scand *56:* 352–355.

Shaw, WC (1995). Commentary to "Ethical issues in the case of surgical repair of cleft palate" by S. Berkowitz. Cleft Palate Craniofac J *32:* 277–280.

Shaw, WC (1997). The Eurocleft Study—eight year follow-up. Paper presented at the 8th International Congress on Cleft Palate and Related Craniofacial Anomalies, 7–12 September 1997, Singapore.

Shaw, WC, Asher-McDade, C, Brattström, V, et al. (1992a). A six-center international study of treatment outcome in patients with clefts of the lip and palate. Part 5. General discussion and conclusions. Cleft Palate Craniofac J *29:* 413–418.

Shaw, WC, Bannister, RP, Roberts, CT (1999). Assisted feeding is more reliable for infants with clefts—a randomized trial. Cleft Palate Craniofac J *36:* 262–268.

Shaw, WC, Dahl, E, Asher-McDade, C, et al. (1992b). A six-center international study of treatment outcome in patients with clefts of the lip and palate. Part 1. Principles and study design. Cleft Palate Craniofac J *29:* 393–397.

Shaw, WC, Semb, G, Nelson, PA, et al. (2000). *The Eurocleft Project 1996–2000.* Amsterdam: IOS Press.

Shaw, WC, Williams, AC, Sandy, JR, Devlin, HB (1996). Minimum standards for the management of cleft lip and palate: efforts to close the audit loop. Ann R Coll Surg Engl *78:* 110–114.

Sloan, G, Shaw, WC, Downey, SE (1996). Surgical management of velopharyngeal insufficiency: pharyngeal flap and sphincter pharyngoplasty. In: *Facial Clefts and Craniosynostosis, Principles and Management,* edited by TA Turvey, KWL Vig, and RJ Fonseca. Philadelphia: Saunders, pp. 384–395.

Spriestersbach, DC, Dickson, DR, Fraser, FC, et al. (1973). Clinical research in cleft lip and palate: the state of the art. Cleft Palate J *10:* 113–165.

Stern, JM, Simes, RJ (1997). Publication bias: evidence of delayed publication in a cohort study of clinical research projects. BMJ *315:* 640–645.

Tobiasen, JM (1989). Scaling facial impairment. Cleft Palate J *26:* 249–254.

Tonelli, MB, Benditt, JO, Albert, RK (1996). Lessons from lung volume reduction surgery. Chest *110:* 230–238.

Williams, WN, Seagle, MB, Nackashi, AJ, et al. (1998). A methodology report of a randomized prospective clinical trial to assess velopharyngeal function for speech following palatal surgery. Control Clin Trials *19:* 297–312.

Ysunza, A, Pamplona, MC, Mendoza, M, et al. (1998). Speech outcome and maxillary growth in patients with unilateral complete cleft lip/palate operated on at 6 versus 12 months of age. Plast Reconstr Surg *102:* 675–679.

III

PUBLIC HEALTH ISSUES

35

Prevention of oral clefts through the use of folic acid and multivitamin supplements: evidence and gaps

ANDREW E. CZEIZEL

Oral clefts (OCs) are among the most extensively studied congenital abnormalities (CAs) due to their visibility, which frequently causes serious psychological problems, and their common occurrence (1/500–550 births). CAs including OCs represent a distinct category of disorders because of their early (prenatal) onset without a good chance of spontaneous or medically assisted complete recovery. Thus, prevention of OCs is the optimal solution.

Several maternal and environmental factors have been studied in relation to OCs, and some have possible associations (Wyszynszki and Beaty, 1996). Among maternal factors, epilepsy and/or use of antiepileptic drugs such as phenytoin appear to be important. Many studies have proposed an association between acute viral infections and OCs; however, viruses, medications, hyperthermia, and other related factors are questionable. Drugs such as corticosteroids, ampicillin, metrodinazole, and folate antagonists are potential teratogens in the etiology of OCs as well. Maternal cigarette smoking and alcohol consumption may also have a role as co-teratogens through gene–environment interaction. Pesticides/herbicides, water contaminants, and occupational exposures have been cited as possible causes of OCs, but they probably explain only a small portion of cases. Currently, nutritional factors such as folate deficiency appear to be the most relevant, according to the concept of gene–environment interaction, in the etiology of OCs.

This chapter reviews the primary prevention of OCs through the use of folic acid and multivitamin supplements, with emphasis on our Hungarian studies. "Secondary" prevention of OCs (through the use of high-resolution ultrasound scanning or other diagnostic methods for fetal OCs, followed by elective termination of pregnancy) is not acceptable (the manifestation of OCs in holoprosencephaly or other very severe syndromes may be an exception), and this topic is beyond the scope of this chapter. Possible in utero surgical correction or gene therapy of OCs is premature (Zanjani and Anderson, 1999).

CLASSIFICATION OF ORAL CLEFTS IN HUNGARY

The findings of three Hungarian studies on the primary prevention of OCs will be presented in this chapter, however, before this I summarize our previous Hungarian activities in the research of OCs which explain our classification of OCs. Ascertainment of cases in ad hoc population-based epidemiological studies was based on an active search of all available sources of cases, and on information on the racially homogeneous Hungarian births (Czeizel and Tusnády, 1971, 1972; Czeizel and Nagy, 1986; Czeizel et al., 1986). In addition, the population-based Hungarian Congenital Abnormality Registry, which represents nearly total notification of OC cases thanks to the obligatory reporting system (Czeizel, 1997; Czeizel and Hirschberg, 1997) was used. The classification of OCs and birth prevalences of different OC entities per 1000 total births are shown in Figure 35.1.

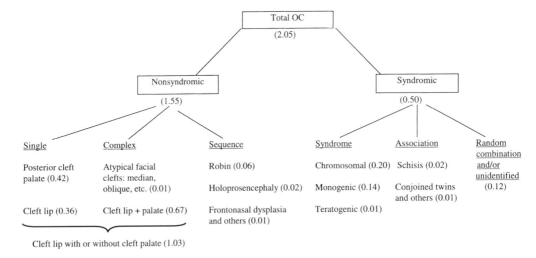

FIG. 35.1. Classification of oral clefts (OCs) and birth prevalences of different OC entities per 1000 total births (in parentheses) in Hungary during the 1980s.

The different origins of posterior cleft palate (CP) and cleft lip with or without cleft palate (CL/P) were shown in the classical work of Fogh-Andersen (1942) and confirmed in our population-based Hungarian epidemiological studies (Table 35.1). Later, it was necessary to differentiate CP and Robin sequence (RS) due to their different origins and clinical manifestations (Table 35.1). A pathogenetic distinction should also be made between isolated, "nonsyndromic" OCs (which are likely due to a localized error of morphogenesis) and multiple, "syndromic" OC (a co-occurrence of two or more different morphogenetic errors in the same person, i.e., OC not part of a sequence) (Czeizel et al., 1988). The difference between nonsyndromic and syndromic CL/P is clearly illustrated by the epidemiological, clinical, and genetic data (Table 35.2). The syndromic CL/P group comprises chromosomal,

mendelian-monogenic, and teratogenic CA-syndromes which include OCs as component element. The origin of nonsyndromic CL/P corresponds to the Gaussian multifactorial threshold model (proportion of heritability $72 \pm 14\%$) (Czeizel and Tusnády, 1984), while that of nonsyndromic CP and RS is also heterogeneous, with a certain proportion of mendelian-monogenic entities (Czeizel and Tusnády, 1972; Czeizel et al., 1986).

The prevalence at birth of OCs in Hungary was 2.05/1000 total births in the 1980s. About three-quarters (1.55/1000, or 76%) were nonsyndromic. The most common categories were CL/P (1.03/1000) and CP (0.42/1000) (Fig. 35.1). These prevalences seem higher than those reported internationally (Tolarova and Cervenka, 1998). This may be due to bias from ascertainment, classification, and certain population characteristics.

TABLE 35.1. *Different Features of Nonsyndromic Cleft Lip with or without Cleft Palate (CL/P), Posterior Cleft Palate (CP), and Robin Sequence (RS) Based on Hungarian Studies (Czeizel and Tusnády, 1971, 1972; Czeizel et al., 1986)*

Type	Critical Period in Postconception (C) Weeks (days) and in Gestational (G) weeks (days)	Localization of CP	Percent Males	Infant Mortality (%)	Familial cluster* (%)		
					CL/P	CP	RS
CL/P (defect of primary palate)	C: 5–7 (35–50) G: 7–9 (49–64)	Most anterior foramen incisivum	65 (male excess)	Low	10.7	0.1	0.0
CP (defect of secondary palate)	C: 8–12 (56–84) G: 10–14 (70–98)	Most posterior foramen incisivum and inverted V	41 (female excess)	Low	0.2	4.7	0.0
RS (early mandibular hypoplasia)	C: 6–9 (42–63) G: 8–11 (56–77)	Inverted U (i.e., rounded shape)	49 (no sex dominance)	High	0.1	0.2	4.5

*Includes first- and second-degree relatives.

TABLE 35.2. *Different Features of Nonsyndromic and Syndromic Cleft Lip with or without Cleft Palate Based on Hungarian Studies (Czeizel and Tusnády, 1971; Czeizel et al., 1988)*

Group	Origin	Right	Left	Both	Percent Males	Birth Weight (g)	Infant Mortality* (%)
		Localization of cleft lip (%)					
Nonsyndromic	Multifactorial	20	60	20	65 (male excess)	3078	4.3
Syndromic	Heterogeneous	33	34	33	51 (no sex dominance)	2675	47.1

*During the study period, between 1962 and 1967, when infant mortality was 3.8% in Hungary.

ANIMAL STUDIES

Treatment of individuals with OCs has improved considerably in recent decades. Nevertheless, the optimal solution is primary prevention. This requires knowledge of causes. The role of dietary deficiencies in the origin of OCs was suggested as early as 1914, when Strauss observed 32 jaguars with CP from one dam by the same sire (Strauss, 1914). When he changed their inadequate diet to fresh meat, no further offspring were born with CP from the same two parents. Pickerill (1914) reported a 99% occurrence of CP in lion cubs born at the zoo. A significant decrease of CP was achieved after the lionesses received a better diet in early pregnancy. In animal studies, the pioneers of teratology (Warkany and Nelson, 1940; Nelson et al., 1952, 1955) induced OCs in more than 90% of rats whose mothers had transitory folic acid deficiency during days 9 through 11 of gestation due to an antimetabolite. Their findings have been confirmed (Lidral et al., 1991). The rate of OCs was reduced in animal experiments by prophylactic vitamins, particularly vitamin B_1 (Schinke et al., 1976; Kreybig, 1981). Bienengräber et al. (1997), however, did not confirm these findings. Peer et al. (1958a) reduced the teratogenic effect of cortisone in mice by administering vitamin B_6, folic acid, or both. In addition, maternal folate supplementation reduced ethanol teratogenicity in CP-susceptible strains of mice (Sakanashi et al., 1996). Finally, folinic acid (the most stable intermediate of folic acid metabolism) reduced the occurrence of OCs in A/WySN mice (Paros and Beck, 1999).

HUMAN STUDIES OF RECURRENCE

The data of previous human intervention studies on the efficacy of vitamins in the reduction of recurrent OCs are summarized in Table 35.3. Conway (1958) used B vitamins together with vitamins A, C, and D. Of 87 women who had already had one child with an OC, 48 received no vitamin supplementation during their 78 subsequent pregnancies and four cases with OC (two CL/P and two CP) were seen among their children. The 39 remaining women were supplemented with the above vitamins during the first trimester of 59 subsequent pregnancies and no recurrent OCs were found ($p = 0.078$). Peer et al. (1958b, 1964) gave 5 mg of folic acid, 10 mg of vitamin B_6, or both to mothers who had previously given birth to children with CL/P at the first suspicion of pregnancy through the fourth month. Of 176 women with this supplementation, four

TABLE 35.3. *Data of Intervention Studies to Check the Efficacy of Vitamins Including Folic Acid in Early Pregnancy for the Reduction of Recurrent Oral Clefts (OC)*

Study	Type*	Sibs (no.)	Recurrent (no.)	OC (%)	Sibs (no.)	Recurrent (no.)	OC (%)
		Supplemented			Unsupplemented		
Conway (1958)	CL/P and CP	59	0	0.0	78	4	5.1
Peer et al. (1958b, 1964)	CL/P	176	4	2.3	418	19	4.5
Briggs (1976)	CL/P	348	11	3.2	417	20	4.8
Tolarova (1982)†	CL/P	84	1	1.2	206	15	7.4
Tolarova (1987)†	CL/P	173	3	1.7	1901	77	4.1
Tolarova and Harris (1995)†	CL/P	214	3	1.4	1901	77	4.1

*CL/P, cleft lip with or without cleft palate; CP, posterior cleft palate.
†There is overlapping in these values due to the cumulative cases.

(2.3%) had children with CL/P compared with 19 of 418 women (4.5%) without vitamin supplementation [relative risk 0.5, 95% confidence interval (CI) 0.2–1.4]. Briggs (1976) supplemented 348 pregnancies of 228 women who had already had a child with CL/P using a multivitamin including 0.5 mg of folic acid, and 11 (3.2%) cases of recurrent CL/P were found. Among the control group of 417 women who also had a CL/P child but did not take supplemental vitamins during their subsequent pregnancies, the recurrent CL/P rate was 4.8% ($p = 0.30$). Tolarova (1982) highlighted the possible primary prevention of CL/P by folic acid and other vitamins in a prospective study of healthy women living mainly in Bohemia who had had one child with unilateral CL/P. These women were encouraged to take three tablets of a multivitamin (Table 35.4) and 10 mg of folic acid per day for at least 3 months before conception and to continue taking these tablets at least until the end of the first trimester of pregnancy. Most of the women also received supplemental iron (75 mg/day of ferrum II fumaricum) and additional vitamin B_6 (1

TABLE 35.4. *Component of Multivitamin Spofavit®
Used in the Studies of Tolarova (1982, 1987) and
Tolarova and Harris (1995) in Addition to
Components of Elevit Pronatal® Used in the
Hungarian Intervention Studies*

Components	Multivitamin (Spofavit®)	Multivitamin (Elevit Pronatal®)
Vitamins		
A	2000 IU	4000 IU*
B_1	1.0 mg	1.6 mg
B_2	1.0 mg	1.8 mg
Nicotinamide	10.0 mg	19.0 mg
B_6	1.0 mg	2.6 mg
B_{12}	—	4.0 mcg
C	50.0 mg	100.0 mg
D_3	100 IU	500 IU
E	2.0 mg	15.0 mg
Calcium pantothenate	1.0 mg	10.0 mg
Biotin	—	0.2 mg
Folic acid	—	0.8 mg
Minerals		
Calcium	—	125.0 mg
Phosphorus	—	125.0 mg
Magnesium	—	100.0 mg
Iron	—	60.0 mg
Trace elements		
Copper	—	1.0 mg
Manganese	—	1.0 mg
Zinc	—	7.5 mg

*Before 1989, 6000 IU.

mg/day). Among 84 pregnancies of 80 fully supplemented women, one (1.2%) recurrence was reported compared with 15 recurrences among 206 pregnancies of 202 women without supplementation (7.4%) ($p = 0.023$). The supplemented and unsupplemented groups also experienced one and six miscarriages, respectively, not included in the data. The frequency of CL/P in the control group, however, was higher than the 4.1% risk for uni- or bilateral CL/P calculated from 2487 sibships in the total Bohemian data set. Tolarova (1987) reported cumulative findings (including data from the 1982 study) that continued to show a significant reduction of recurrent CL/P associated with use of a multivitamin and a very high dose of folic acid supplementation during the periconceptional period. Later, the data set of all subtypes of CL/P, collected from 1970 through 1982, was re-evaluated by Tolarova and Harris (1995). From a group of 2115 women with one previous child with nonsyndromic CL/P, 214 pregnancies were supplemented and three (1.4%) recurrent CL/P cases occurred. However, of 1901 pregnancies without supplementation, 77 (4.1%) ended again with the birth of infants with CL/P ($p = 0.03$). When the supplemented group was divided according to sex and severity, the biggest reduction was found in the group of male probands with unilateral CL (this subgroup had the lowest heritability value and, thus, the largest proportion of environmental factors).

These studies, however, were not randomized, and the possible effect of folic acid could not be distinguished from the possible effect of other vitamins. In addition, both the dose (0.5–10.0 mg) and the design (prospective or retrospective) were different. In general, the observed protective effect did not reach statistical significance (except in the Bohemian data set), but the trend was similar. However, starting vitamins before conception could just as easily be a marker for general health consciousness. Thus, there were two significant goals for further studies. First, it was necessary to organize a double-blind randomized controlled trial (RCT). Second, the reduction of recurrent OCs is important from the aspect of these families, but about 95% of OCs manifested as a *first occurrence*; therefore, the reduction of first occurrences would be of great public health benefit.

THE HUNGARIAN RANDOMIZED CONTROLLED TRIAL

One of the major objectives of the Hungarian RCT of periconceptional folic acid–containing multivitamin supplementation (PFMS) was to evaluate whether multivitamins including 0.8 mg of folic acid can reduce the first occurrence of nonsydromic CL/P and CP. The RCT was based on the periconceptional care program in Hungary (Czeizel et al., 1998; Czeizel, 1999), established in 1984. To be eligible to participate, women planning a pregnancy had to satisfy the following criteria: no infertility, no current pregnancy, and voluntary appearance. Qualified nurses supervised the three steps: checkup of reproductive health, a 3-month preparation period for conception, and better protection of early pregnancy before the usual prenatal care. Supplementation was part of the periconceptional care.

The RCT took place between February 1, 1984, and April 30, 1992. At the first periconceptional care visit, the criteria for eligibility were reviewed. Eligible women were informed about the purpose of the RCT and asked whether they agreed to be randomly assigned to receive a multivitamin pill or a placebo-like trace element pill. The women were then asked to provide written, informed consent and to stop taking any other vitamins. The women entering the RCT were randomly assigned to receive a multivitamin (Elevit Pronatal®; Roche, Switzerland) (Table 35.4) or a trace element supplement as a single tablet each day for at least 1 month before the planned conception. They were asked to record daily their pill taking on a form used to record their basal body temperature and to leave unused tablets in the box. At the second visit, 3 months later, women were supplied with tablets for the next 3 months, advised to attempt conception within this period, and asked to return immediately after the first missed menstrual period. The purpose of the third visit was to confirm pregnancy if a menstrual period had been missed and to supply tablets until the end of the third month of gestation. If a woman did not conceive within this 3-month period, she was given an additional 3-month supply of supplement until the end of 1 year. Compliance in taking the supplement was verified by interview, checking records of basal body temperature, and counting unused tablets. Compliance was categorized as full, partial, or none (Smithells et al., 1980). However, the intention-to-treat analysis was used to evaluate the primary end point of the RCT (Czeizel and Dudás, 1992). Each participant had a certificate with a page including the pregnancy outcome data (date and type of pregnancy outcome, sex, weight, gestational age of singletons or twins, and particularly any defects of the fetuses or newborn infants) filled in by mothers and confirmed by physicians (documented by signature), and women were asked to mail this certificate after the end of pregnancy. When a woman did not mail the certificate, considerable effort was expended to obtain information about her pregnancy outcome. This effort resulted in only 49 of 4753 (1%) confirmed pregnancies with unknown pregnancy outcomes (Czeizel et al.,

1994). Informative offspring (fetuses with prenatally diagnosed conditions aborted after the week 12 of gestation, stillborn fetuses, and liveborn infants) were evaluated with particular attention to the appropriate diagnosis or description of the CA.

The data from the Hungarian RCT showed a significant reduction in the first occurrence of neural tube defects and some other CAs (Czeizel and Dudás, 1992; Czeizel, 1993a, 1996). However, the study did not show a reduction in the occurrence of nonsyndromic CL/P and CP (Table 35.5), though the statistical power of these results was small for these defects (it could detect incidence differences only on the order of 50%).

OTHER HUMAN STUDIES OF OCCURRENCE

Khoury et al. (1989) analyzed the data of the Atlanta Birth Defects Case-Control Study. Mothers who consumed vitamins during pregnancy were at lower risk of having a child with CL/P than mothers who did not take vitamins [odds ratio (OR) 0.74, 95% CI 0.56–0.98], but a statistically significant difference was not found in the CP group (OR 0.93, 95% CI 0.62–1.40). Other studies did not find any association between vitamin use and OCs (Fraser and Warburton, 1964; Saxen, 1975; Hill et al., 1988).

Shaw et al. (1995) investigated whether use of multivitamins containing folic acid from 1 month before through 2 months after conception reduced the risk of OCs in a population-based case-control study in California, 1987–1989. The risk of nonsyndromic CL/P was reduced by half (OR 0.50, 95% CI 0.36–0.68). For CP, this reduction was smaller and not statistically significant (OR 0.73, 95% CI 0.35–1.2). However, the crude ORs for syndromic CL/P (0.61, 95% CI 0.35–1.1) and CP (0.64, 95% CI 0.35–1.2) were also lower, though not significantly. This is surprising because, as mentioned above, syndromic OCs have a different origin. Hayes et al. (1996), in a hospital-based case-control study, compared folic acid supplementation in cases with CL/P ($n = 195$), CP ($n = 108$), and 1167 patient controls with other CAs (e.g., other than OCs, such as neural tube defects and other midline defects). The adjusted relative risks for daily folic acid supplementation during the periconceptional period were 1.32 (95% CI 0.82–2.12) for CL/P and 0.89 (95% CI 0.51–1.58) for CP. However, Werler (1999), from the same research group and using the same approach with "normal" and "affected" controls, found ORs below 1.0 in both CL/P and CP groups regardless of control type. In addition, there was a statistically significant reduction in the occurrence of CP due to multivitamin use after the periconceptional period.

TABLE 35.5. *Results of the Randomized Controlled Trial (RCT) and Two Cohort Controlled Study (TCS)*

Informative Offspring	RCT		TCS	
	Multivitamin	Placebo-like Trace Element	Supplemented	Unsupplemented
Elective termination of pregnancy after fetal diagnosis	3	13	20	8
Stillbirth	11	9	7	8
Live birth	2457	2369	3029	3040
Total	2471	2391	3056	3056
Nonsyndromic OC*				
CL/P	4	3[†]	3[†]	2
Rate per 1000	1.62	1.25	0.98	0.65
CP	0	2	1	1[‡]
Rate per 1000	0.00	0.84	0.33	0.33
Together	4	5	4	3
Rate per 1000	1.62	2.09	1.31	0.98
Syndromic OC				
Chromosomal syndromes	1	2	1	1
Monogenic syndromes	0	0	0	0
Teratogenic syndromes	0	0	0	0
Unidentified syndromes	2	0	0	4
Together	3	2	1	5
Rate per 1000	1.21	0.84	0.33	1.64

*OC, oral cleft; CL/P, cleft lip with or without cleft palate; CP, posterior cleft palate.
[†]Includes one familial case.
[‡]Robin sequence.

In summary, the results of studies using low doses of folic acid (in general, 0.4 mg) are puzzling since they provide different findings despite using similar approaches. Thus, the effects of confounders (such as lifestyle) and other indirect causal factors should not be excluded.

THE HUNGARIAN TWO COHORT CONTROLLED STUDY

The results of previous studies were controversial; nevertheless, the Hungarian RCT was discontinued due to ethical reasons. A two cohort controlled study (TCS) was therefore launched on May 1, 1993, and closed on April 30, 1996 (Czeizel et al., 1999). Cases were recruited from the participants with PFMS of the Hungarian periconceptional care centers after confirmation of pregnancy. They were also supplemented with Elevit Pronatal® (Table 35.4) during the same periconceptional period and using the same criteria of compliance as in the RCT. However, if a woman was pregnant at the start of PFMS, she was excluded from the TCS and referred to regional prenatal care. Matched controls were recruited during *prenatal care*, which is mandatory in Hungary for pregnant women. All pregnant women after the first visit between weeks 8 and 12 of gestation were informed about the purpose of the TCS and invited to take part in the region where cases were recruited. Eligibility of controls was based on three criteria: *(1)* no multivitamin and/or folic acid supplementation in the periconceptional period; *(2)* appropriate matching of age (±1 year), socioeconomic status, and residence of supplemented pregnant women; *(3)* voluntary participation. If unsupplemented pregnant women were eligible for the TCS and agreed to participate, they were asked to sign an informed consent form and to personally deliver or mail their completed pregnancy certificate to the regional prenatal care center after the end of pregnancy. Each supplemented pregnant woman was matched to two unsupplemented pregnant women, the second of whom was enrolled if the first dropped out of the study.

TABLE 35.6. *Data of Liveborn Cases with Nonsyndromic Oral Clefts from the Randomized Controlled Trial (RCT) and the Two Cohort Controlled Study (TCS)*

Study	Group	Birth Year	Gestational Age (weeks)	Birth Weight (g)	Sex	OC	Comment
RCT	PFMS-I	1986	40	3800	M	CL, right + CP	Epicanthal fold
	PFMS-I	1987	39	3000	M	CL, bilateral + CP	—
	PFMS-I	1988	41	4000	M	CL, right + CP	—
	PFMS-II	1988	40	2950	F	CL, bilateral + CP	Mother: epilepsy without anticonvulsant treatment during pregnancy
	PTES-I	1986	37	2450	M	CL, right	Father: CL + CP
	PTES-II	1985	40	3200	M	CL, bilateral + CP	—
	PTES-II	1985	40	3150	M	CL, left	Mild CL: spontaneous closure
	PTES-II	1990	41	3200	F	CP	—
	PTES-III	1987	40	3250	F	CP	—
TCS	PFMS-I	1995	40	5100	M	CL, left + CP	Father: subfertility (AIH)
	PFMS-I	1995	40	4080	M	CP (soft)	—
	PFMS-I	1996	38	3300	M	CL, left + CP	Brother: CL + CP
	PFMS-II	1997	39	3450	F	CL, bilateral + CP	Mother: scoliosis, Father: congenital inguinal hernia Brother (1993): craniostenosis Brother (1995): lethal left heart hypoplasia
	NoS	1995	31	1400	F	CP + mandibular hypoplasia (RS)	Twin A (twin B healthy)
	NoS	1997	39	3600	M	CL, left	Mild CL
	NoS	1998	39	2950	M	CL, bilateral + CP	—

OC, oral cleft; PFMS, periconceptional folic acid–containing multivitamin supplementation; PTES, periconceptional trace element supplementation; NoS, no supplementation; I, fully supplemented; II, partially supplemented; III, unsupplemented; CL, cleft lip; CP, posterior cleft palate; RS, Robin sequence; AIH, artificial insemination by husband.

The data of CAs including OCs were evaluated in 3056 case-control matched pairs. Birth order was lower in the supplemented group (1.2 ± 0.6) due to the larger proportion of women planning first pregnancies compared with the unsupplemented group (1.4 ± 0.7) because primiparous females preferred to take part in periconceptional care. Fetal deaths, infant deaths, and CAs in previous pregnancies were more common among supplemented than unsupplemented women. These differences can be explained by the expected higher medical standard of periconceptional care in couples with previous unsuccessful pregnancy outcomes. Of 172 malformed offspring in the previous pregnancies of supplemented women, six had OCs, while of four previous malformed offspring in the unsupplemented group, none had an OC. In addition, of 3056 case and control mothers, one and none, respectively, had an OC, while of 3056 case and control fathers, three and one, respectively, had OCs. Thus, a higher potential recurrence risk for OCs must be considered in the supplemented group than in the unsupplemented group. All OCs occurred in liveborn infants. The occurrence of CL/P and CP did not show a difference between the supplemented and unsupplemented groups (Table 35.5). One unsupplemented twin infant

had RS, but in general this CA entity is included in the CP group; the other twin was healthy. There was one recurrent case of cleft lip and CP (CLP) in a newborn infant; his brother also had CLP.

The data on all infants with nonsyndromic OCs in the RCT and TCS are shown in Table 35.6. The major methodological factors were similar in the two Hungarian intervention studies (Table 35.7); however, there was a significant difference in design: the RCT was randomized among participants in the coordinating center of periconceptional care, while the TCS was nonrandomized and supplemented women were recruited in all (*n* = 32) periconceptional centers, while unsupplemented controls enrolled in the regional prenatal care clinics. Combination of the data from the RCT and TCS offers an opportunity to estimate the efficacy of PFMS in the reduction of the first occurrence of nonsyndromic CL/P and CP (Table 35.8). (One infant in the trace element group of the RCT who had a father with CLP and one infant and his brothers who had CLP in the supplemented group of the RCT were excluded from the analysis. In addition, ten and one newborn infants with OC who had parents or previous sibs affected with OCs in the supplemented and unsupplemented groups of the TCS, respectively, were also ex-

TABLE 35.7. *Comparison of Major Methodological Factors of the Randomized Controlled Trial (RCT) and the Two Cohort Controlled Study (TCS)*

Method	RCT, 1984–1992	TCS, 1993–1996
Type	Occurrence	Occurrence
Design	Randomized double-blind	Two cohort
Recruitment	Coordinating center of periconceptional care	All centers of periconceptional care and regional prenatal care
Supplementation	Multivitamin: Elevit Pronatal® (incl. 0.8 mg folic acid)	Multivitamin: Elevit Pronatal® (incl. 0.8 mg folic acid)
Time period of supplementation	Periconceptional in both study groups	Periconceptional in supplemented group only
Compliance	Intention-to-treat analysis	Unsupplemented pregnancies excluded
Evaluation	Three time windows: a. Prenatally diagnosed fetal defect b. Birth (still- and liveborn) c. Postnatal development	Three time windows: a. Prenatally diagnosed fetal defect b. Birth (still- and liveborns) c. Postnatal development
End points	Pregnancy outcomes Congenital abnormalities (mainly neural tube defects and OC)	Six major congenital abnormalities* Other congenital abnormalities
Follow-up	Controlled until 1 year of age	Controlled until 1 year of age

*Cardiovascular and urinary tract congenital abnormalities, pyloric stenosis, limb deficiencies, neural tube defect, and oral clefting (OC).

cluded from the denominators due to a 50-fold higher recurrence risk.) There were seven and four CL/P infants in the supplemented and unsupplemented groups, respectively. In addition, there were one and three children with CP in the supplemented and unsupplemented groups, respectively. Crude ORs did not show a difference between the two groups. In addition, there was no significant difference in the first occurrence of nonsyndromic CL/P ($p = 0.47$) and CP ($p = 0.35$) between the supplemented and unsupplemented groups. Thus, the data of 5516 supplemented and 5445 unsupplemented women do not indicate a protective effect of PFMS, including a physiological dose (<1 mg) of folic acid, for nonsyndromic OC.

The so-called syndromic OCs were also evaluated (Table 35.5). There were three and two syndromic OCs in the PFMS and placebo-like trace element groups of the RCT, respectively. One and two fetuses had Edwards' or Patau's syndrome including OCs in the PFMS and placebo-like groups, respectively. Of two unidentified multimalformed cases after PFMS, one newborn was affected with RS (CP + micrognathia) and rib agenesia, while another had bilateral CLP, bilateral congenital structural talipes equinovarus, and spina bifida occulta. There were one and five syndromic OCs in the supplemented and unsupplemented groups of the TCS, respectively. Both chromosomal OCs occurred in Edwards' syndrome. In addition, four unidentified multimalformed infants were found in the unsupplemented group of the TCS: left CLP and polycystic kidney disease type IV causing hydronephrosis (Meckel syndrome?); bilateral CL + ventricular septal defect +

TABLE 35.8. *First Occurrence of Nonsyndromic Cleft Lip with or without Cleft Palate (CL/P) and Posterior Cleft Palate (CP) in the Previous Hungarian Randomized Double-Blind Controlled Trial (RCT) and the Two Cohort Controlled Study (TCS) with (Supplemented) or without (Unsupplemented) Folic Acid–Containing (0.8 mg) Multivitamin during the Periconceptional Period*

Study	Nonsyndromic OC	Supplemented group			Unsupplemented group			OR (95% CI)
		Off.*	No.	Per 1000	Off.*	No.	Per 1000	
RCT	CL/P	2471	4	1.62	2390	2	0.84	1.94 (0.41–9.09)
TCS	CL/P	3045	3	0.99	3055	2	0.65	1.14 (0.20–6.75)
Together	CL/P	5516	7	1.27	5445	4	0.73	1.59 (0.48–5.30)
RCT	CP	2471	0	0.00	2391	2	0.84	0.19 (0.01–4.03)
TCS	CP	3045	1	0.33	3055	1	0.33	1.14 (0.12–10.94)
Together	CP	5516	1	0.18	5445	3	0.55	0.35 (0.05–2.40)

*Off., number of informative offspring evaluated; OC, oral cleft; OR, odds ratio; CI, confidence interval.

cholecyst agenesia + mesenterium commune (one member of a triplet); CP + facial dysmorphism + syndactyly in left hand (II–V fingers) and in right hand (II–IV fingers); RS and bilateral congenital structural talipes equinovarus (the father had micrognathia and high arched palate). The limited number of syndromic OCs does not allow any conclusion; however, these findings do not appear to confirm the observation of Shaw et al. (2000) that women who used PFMS had an elevated risk of delivering a fetus or infant with multiple CAs.

In conclusion, data from the two Hungarian intervention studies do not support a protective effect against nonsyndromic OCs of multivitamins including folic acid (<1 mg).

THE HUNGARIAN CASE-CONTROL SURVEILLANCE OF CONGENITAL ABNORMALITIES

The association between oral supplement use and CA occurrence was also evaluated using a case-control approach in the population-based data from the Hungarian Case-Control Surveillance of Congenital Abnormalities (HCCSCA) between 1980 and 1991 (Czeizel et al., 1996) and between 1980 and 1996 (Czeizel et al., 1999). Cases with nonsyndromic CAs (except for congenital dislocation of the hip, congenital inguinal hernia, and hemangiomas) and multiple CAs reported to the Hungarian Congenital Abnormality Registry in the first 3 months after birth or termination of pregnancy were selected for the HCCSCA. Babies with Down syndrome were used as patient controls. The methods and data set of the above registry have been described elsewhere (Czeizel et al., 2001). Population controls were ascertained from the National Birth Registry of the Central Statistical Office. Two population controls without CAs were matched to every case according to sex, date of birth (within 1 week), and parent's residence (district).

Data on use of vitamins were obtained from three sources. First, a postpaid questionnaire with an explanatory letter and a list of drugs and diseases was mailed to parents immediately after the selection of cases and controls. The questionnaire requested information on drug intake and use of pregnancy supplements, pregnancy complications, and maternal diseases during pregnancy according to gestational month. To standardize the answers, mothers were asked to read a set of lists as a memory aid before they replied. These were lists of medications, including pregnancy supplements such as folic acid, and diseases. The mean return time of completed questionnaires was 1.6 and 3.5 months after birth for the case and population controls,

respectively. Second, mothers were requested to send us the prenatal care logbook and all medical records concerning their diseases during pregnancy and the child's CA. Third, regional nurses were asked to visit and to question nonresponding families in the group of cases. Thus, information was available on 79% (69% from reply, 10% from visit) of cases. The response rate for population controls was 64%, but district nurses did not visit nonresponding population control families because the ethical committee considered this follow-up to be disturbing to the parents of these healthy children. If a case had two population controls, one was randomly excluded. If a case had no population control, another one was selected from the 38,151 population controls on the basis of matching criteria.

Folic acid intake was evaluated according to (1) source of information (maternal self-reported, medically recorded, or both), (2) type of treatment (folic acid alone or folic acid plus other drugs; multivitamins including 0.1–1.0 mg folic acid were excluded due to the small number of pregnant women in the two groups of OC), (3) dose (only one kind of folic acid tablet, 3 mg, was available during the study period, and obstetricians prescribed daily 1–3, but in general 2, tablets, i.e., 6 mg for pregnant women), (4) duration of treatment (after the start of folic acid use, it was generally continued until the end, but at least until the fourth month, of pregnancy), (5) gestational age [calculated from the first day of the last menstrual period, and three time intervals were considered: first month of pregnancy as a continuation of preconceptional treatment; the critical period for primary palatal development, i.e., 49–64 gestational (35–50 postconceptional) days in CL/P, and for secondary palatal development, i.e., 70–98 gestational (56–84 postconceptional) days in CP (Canick, 1954); gestational months after the critical period of orofacial clefts], (6) potential confounding factors (e.g., maternal age, birth order, acute and chronic maternal disorders, and use of other drugs).

At the evaluation of the HCCSCA data set between 1980 and 1996, the study period covered 2,146,574 total births in Hungary; hence, the 38,151 population controls represented 1.8% of Hungarian births. Of 22,834 cases with CA, 1377 and 600 cases with nonsyndromic CL/P and CP, respectively, were evaluated in the case-control matched pair analysis.

Data on maternal age, birth order, pregnancy complications, maternal disorders, and use of other drugs are shown in Table 35.9. Influenza/common cold and epilepsy were more frequent in cases with CL/P or CP compared with their matched controls, while excessive nausea/vomiting was less frequent.

Pregnant women rarely (13.9%–14.8%) used folic acid alone in the two groups. Thus, folic acid alone and

TABLE 35.9. *Some Variables of Total, Cleft Lip with or without Cleft Palate (CL/P), and Posterior Cleft Palate (CP) Cases, in Addition to Comparative Values of Total, Matched CL/P, and CP Controls in the Hungarian Case-Control Surveillance of Congenital Abnormalities between 1980 and 1996*

	Cases						Controls					
	Total (n = 22,834)		CL/P (n = 1377)		CP (n = 600)		Total (n = 38,151)		CL/P (n = 1377)		CP (n = 600)	
Continuous Variables	Mean	SD	Mean	SD	Mean	SD	Mean	S D	Mean	SD	Mean	SD
Maternal age (years)	25.5	5.3	25.7	5.3	26.2	5.5	25.5	5.2	25.7	5.4	25.5	5.2
Birth order	1.9	1.1	1.9	1.1	1.9	1.1	1.7	0.9	1.7	1.1	1.8	1.1
Categorical Variables	No.	%	No.	%	No.	%	No.	%	No.	%	No.	%
Pregnancy complications												
Nausea, vomiting (excessive)	1355	5.8	68	4.9	34	5.7	3042	8.0	99	7.2	59	9.8
Threatened abortion	3430	15.0	204	14.8	91	15.2	6450	16.9	245	17.8	105	17.5
Preeclampsia	656	5.8	68	4.9	34	5.7	1135	3.0	42	3.1	12	2.0
Threatened preterm delivery	2454	10.7	146	10.6	61	10.2	5205	13.6	187	13.6	71	11.8
Anemia	3240	14.2	191	13.9	86	14.3	6365	16 .7	239	17.4	112	18.7
Acute maternal diseases												
Influenza/common cold	4962	21.7	432	31.4	153	25.5	7054	18.5	252	18.3	106	17.7
Respiratory system	2095	9.2	145	10.5	72	12.0	3443	9.0	119	8.6	66	11.0
Urinary tract	1576	6.9	110	8.0	44	7.3	2289	6.0	77	5.6	42	7.0
Genital organs	1633	7.1	118	8.6	33	5.5	2825	7.4	109	7.9	48	8.0
Others	912	4.0	98	7.1	29	4.8	1599	4.2	67	4.9	19	3.2
Chronic maternal diseases												
Epilepsy	55	0.2	8	0.6	5	0.8	61	0.2	3	0.2	0	0.0
Others	3247	14.2	211	15.3	75	12.5	6107	16. 0	226	16.4	87	14.5
Other drugs*												
Acetylsalicylic acid	1001	4.4	72	5.2	30	5.0	1397	3.7	56	4.1	21	3.5
Allylestrenol	3477	15.2	178	12.9	91	15.2	5364	14.1	197	14.3	87	14.5
Aminophenazone	492	2.2	43	3.1	19	3.2	730	1.9	16	1.2	9	1.5
Aminophylline	1369	6.0	91	6.6	46	7.7	2281	6.0	77	5.6	39	6.5
Ampicillin	1616	7.1	121	8.8	47	7.8	2584	6.8	104	7.6	42	7.0
Bromhexine	473	2.1	29	2.1	14	2.3	794	2.1	28	2.0	15	2.5
Cefalexin	261	1.1	18	1.3	10	1.7	368	1.0	16	1.2	10	1.7
Clotrimazole	1636	7.2	117	8.5	34	5.7	3068	8.0	129	9.4	52	8.7
Diazepam	2745	12.0	159	11.5	63	10.5	4125	10.8	155	11.3	47	7.8
Drotaverine	2049	9.0	139	10.1	54	9.0	3482	9.1	132	9.6	54	9.0
Metronidazole	961	4.2	75	5.4	17	2.8	1408	3. 7	45	3.3	21	3.5
Nalidixic acid	242	1.1	13	0.9	4	0.7	377	1.0	17	1.2	7	1.2
Penamecillin	1591	7.0	106	7.7	50	8.3	2239	5 .9	68	4.9	39	6.5
Promethazine	3640	15.9	236	17.1	100	16.7	6020	15.8	205	14.9	106	17.7
Terbutaline	2342	10.3	141	10.2	54	9.0	3996	10.5	145	10.5	63	10.5
Verapamil	341	1.5	12	0.9	7	1.2	501	1. 3	17	1.2	8	1.3

*>1% in the total groups.

with other drugs were evaluated together (Table 35.10) because most other drugs, including other pregnancy supplements (other vitamins, irons, calcium derivatives), had similar occurrence rates in cases and controls. Mothers of newborn infants with CL/P had a significantly *lower* use of folic acid (49.4%) than mothers of matched controls (54.7%). This was the case in the CP group (47.7%) as well compared with their matched controls (55.2%). The proportion of medically recorded folic acid supplementation was similar in the combined control (65.6%) and case (64.2%) groups ($\chi^2 = 5.1$, $p = 0.25$). However, it is worth evaluating

TABLE 35.10. *High-Dose (in General Daily 6 mg) Folic Acid Supplementation in Case-Control Pairs of Nonsyndromic Cleft Lip with or without Cleft Palate (CL/P) and Posterior Cleft Palate (CP) in Addition to Distribution of Gestational Months According to Start of Folic Acid Supplementation and Cumulative Number of Pregnant Women during the Critical Period of CL/P (i.e., 49–64 Gestational Days) and of CP (i.e., 70–98 Gestational Days) and Adjusted Odds Ratio (OR) with 95% Confidence Interval (CI) for Confounding Factors*

Gestational Month	CL/P (n = 1377)					CP (n = 600)				
	Cases		Controls			Cases		Controls		
	No.	%	No.	%	OR (95% CI)	No.	%	No.	%	OR (95% CI)
I	48	3.5	68	4.9	—	12	2.0	20	3.3	—
II	76	5.5	94	6.8	I–II = 0.73 (0.58–0.93)	29	4.8	48	8.0	—
III	239	17.4	246	17.9	II–III = 0.88 (0.74–1.03)	113	18.8	109	18.2	I–III = 0.84 (0.64–1.13)
IV	107	7.8	124	9.0	—	42	7.0	64	10.7	I–IV = 0.72 (0.57–0.90)
V	102	7.4	100	7.3	—	36	6.0	43	7.2	—
VI	41	3.0	59	4.3	—	23	3.8	23	3.8	—
VII	37	2.7	41	3.0	—	24	4.0	14	2.3	—
VIII	25	1.8	16	1.2	—	5	0.8	8	1.3	—
IX	5	0.4	5	0.4	IV–IX = 0.92 (0.81–1.12)	2	0.3	1	0.2	V–IX = 0.99 (0.73–1.38)
Total	680	49.4	753	54.7	I–IX = 0.81 (0.70–0.94)	286	47.7	331	55.2	I–IX = 0.73 (0.60–0.91)
Folic acid alone	191	13.9	204	14.8	I–IX = 0.91 (0.72–1.12)	78	13.0	83	13.9	I–IX = 0.92 (0.73–1.31)

the start of folic acid supplementation according to gestational month (Table 35.10). Folic acid was used only in a small proportion of women in the first month of gestation, which corresponded to the preconceptional supplementation. The increase of folic acid use in the second month of gestation may reflect the early visits to the prenatal care or voluntary folic acid supplementation after the recognition of pregnancy. The maximum rate was seen in the third month of gestation, at the usual time of the first visit to prenatal care. The later start of folic acid supplementation can be explained by a postponed visit to prenatal care or a delay in folic acid use. The major point is the use of folic acid before and during the time of primary and secondary palatal development. Thus, the cumulative number of pregnant women with high-dose folic acid supplementation was calculated during the critical period of CL/P and CP. However, the critical period of primary palatal development (CL/P) includes the last week of the second and the first week of the third gestational months, while secondary palatal development (i.e., CP-forming period) overlaps the last 2 weeks of the third and the first 2 weeks of the fourth gestational months. This explains why there were two estimates for the protective effect of folic acid. (The adjusted OR in case-control pairs was estimated by a conditional logistic regression model for confounding factors.) At the evaluation of primary palatal development, there was a significantly higher rate of supplementation with a high dose (in general, 6 mg/day) of folic acid during the first and second months of gestation in the matched population control group (11.7% vs. 9.0% in the case group), which may indicate a protective effect for CL/P. This was also the case at the evaluation of folic acid supplementation in the first 4 months of gestation (40.2% in matched population controls and 32.6% in cases) in the CP group. There was no difference in the use of folic acid supplementation *after* the critical period of these two kinds of OC between cases and matched population controls (Table 35.10).

The strengths and weaknesses of the HCCSCA have been discussed previously (Czeizel et al., 2001). However, the HCCSCA is the largest case-control data set of its type in the world, and population-based sampling makes risk–benefit assessment possible. A significant reduction was found in the rate of nonsyndromic CL/P and CP due to the pharmacological doses (in general, 6 mg/day) of folic acid supplementation during the critical period of these OC entities in pregnant women. This finding is in agreement with the previously mentioned results of Tolarova (1982, 1987) and Tolarova and Harris (1995) because 10 mg of folic acid was used. The question is whether the reduction of nonsyndromic OCs associated with folic acid supplementation is real or confounded by other factors (e.g., lifestyle). That the effect may be real is supported by the finding that a reduction was seen after the use of folic acid during the critical period of OC development, but not after development of the primary and secondary palate.

Some data of both the TCS and the HCCSCA were published previously (Czeizel et al., 1999); however, the data set of the TCS was complemented by supplemented and unsupplemented pregnant women of three other regional periconceptional care centers, while that of the HCCSCA was modified after the cleaning of multiple CAs and the decision to use one case–one control matched pairs.

In conclusion, folate/folic acid deficiency may play a role in the origin of OCs, and it can be neutralized by supplementation of high-dose folic acid during the critical period of primary and secondary palatal development. According to our study, only high doses (about 6 mg) of folic acid daily during the critical period of OC development reduce the first occurrence of nonsyndromic CL/P and CP. About 30% of first occurrences can be prevented by this method. Our findings agree with the results of Tolarova (1982, 1987), which indicated a reduction of recurrent CL/P after the periconceptional use of 10 mg of folic acid. Thus, the protective effect of folic acid seems to be dose-dependent because only high-dose folic acid supplementation was effective at reducing first and recurrent cases of nonsyndromic CL/P and CP.

BIOLOGICAL PLAUSIBILITY AND PRACTICAL IMPLICATIONS OF THE DOSE-DEPENDENT PROTECTIVE EFFECT OF FOLIC ACID

Berry et al. (1999), in a study in China, showed that the preventive efficacy of folic acid depends on the birth prevalence of neural tube defects. This rule may be valid for nonsyndromic OCs as well. In addition, the population differences in genetic background (ethnicity), lifestyle (e.g., diet), and demographic features (e.g., advanced maternal age) may influence not only on the occurrence of OCs but also on the possible preventive effect of folic acid. These findings demonstrate that here state-of-the-art OC prevention is based mainly on the homogeneous white Hungarian population.

A major proportion of first-occurrence neural tube defects can be prevented by folic acid (Berry et al., 1999) or PFMS (Czeizel and Dudás, 1992). The origins of neural tube defects and OCs may have some similarities. In the early embryo, the neural folds are largely comprised of epithelial cells of the neural plate. After elevation of the neural folds, cells adjacent to the neural plate undergo mesenchymal differentiation and migrate into underlying regions. These neuroepithelial cells, cranial neural crest cells, represent the major cell population that contributes to the formation of, among others, the frontonasal processes and palatal shelves. Thus, closure of the neural tube and development of the face and palate have a common origin, with the same or a similar genetic background (Thorogood and Tickle, 1988). They may share potential candidate genes in folate/folic acid metabolism, providing a plausible biological link between the prevention of neural tube defects and OCs by maternal folate/folic acid supplementation during the critical period for these CAs.

Analysis of the population-based data of multimalformed cases in the Hungarian Congenital Abnormality Registry indicated that the so-called schisis-type CAs, i.e., neural tube defects, OCs, CAs of the midline abdominal region, and diaphragmatic CAs, associated with one another far more frequently than at the expected random combination rates. Their combination with other CAs did not exceed the expected rate. Combinations of two or more schisis-type CAs without other CAs therefore were managed as a provisional entity, named schisis association (Czeizel, 1981) or midline defect (Opitz and Gilbert, 1982). Later, the causal association of schisis-type CAs was confirmed by familial clustering (Fraser et al., 1982). However, there are also differences between these two CA groups; e.g., studies have shown an association between homozygosity for a variant form of the C677T genotype, nor in the methylenetetrahydrofolate reductase (MTHFR) gene and risk of neural tube defects (van der Put et al., 1995; Kirke et al., 1996), while Shaw et al. (1998a, 1999) did not indicate increased risk for CL/P and CP among infants homozygous for the C677T genotype nor an interaction between infant C677T genotype and maternal multivitamin use on the occurrence of these OCs in the United States. However, Wyszynszki and Diehl (2000) reanalyzed the data of Shaw et al. (1999) and concluded that multivitamin supplementation before and during the early weeks of pregnancy may protect against CL/P. Mills et al. (1999) found that the thermolabile variant of MTHFR (TT) was associated with a significantly higher risk for nonsyndromic CP in the Irish population. Thus, ethnic origin may be important. The point is that a multivitamin including a physiological dose of folic acid is appropriate (Czeizel and Dudás, 1992) and that flour-bread fortification with folic acid, vitamin B_6, and vitamin B_{12} (Czeizel and Merhala, 1998) may be effective at reducing neural tube defects but not for OCs because the latter requires a high dose of folic acid.

The available findings about the possible protective effect of folic acid against OCs are conflicting. The data of our Hungarian studies, however, may be appropriate to generate the dose-dependent effect of folic acid hypothesis because this theory is based on the following evidence.

1. It was possible to induce OCs in animal experiments by drastic folate deficiencies (Nelson et al., 1952, 1955), and an association was suggested between antifolate agents and OCs (Hernandes-Dias at al., 2000).

2. There is no evidence of an obvious socioeconomic dependence in the occurrence of nonsyndromic CL/P and CP that may be connected with dietary differences (Czeizel and Tusnády, 1971). Dietary folate intake was not able to reduce the occurrence of OCs (Bower and Stanley, 1992). The usual daily intake of folate is about 0.18 to 0.20 mg, and it is difficult to achieve the necessary two- to threefold increase in folate intake, which would need about 15 servings of broccoli or brussel sprouts. In addition, this dose would not be enough to prevent OCs. Finally, Cuskelly et al. (1996) showed that an extreme increase in consumption of extra folate from natural food is relatively ineffective at increasing folate status.

3. The teratogenic, particularly OC-inducing, effect of anticonvulsant medications, smoking, and alcohol may be related to the reduction of folate that is available to the developing embryo. The teratogenic effect of most anticonvulsants is mediated through folate deficiency (Wegner and Nau, 1992). Smoking can lower serum folate in pregnant women (Houdayer and Bahuau, 1998). Shaw et al. (1996) demonstrated a strong association between periconceptional maternal cigarette smoking, transforming growth factor-α (TGFa) genotype of infants, and risk of OCs. Shaw et al. (1998b) compared infants with the common TGFa genotype whose mothers used PFMS to infants with the A2 genotype (homo- and heterozygous) whose mothers did not use multivitamins and found increased OC risk (for nonsyndromic CL/P, OR = 3.0, 95% CI 1.4–6.6; for syndromic CL/P, OR = 2.4, 95% CI 0.7–11.6; for nonsyndromic CP, OR = 2.6, 95% CI 1.0–7.7; for syndromic CP, OR = 4.2, 95% CI 1.3–16.2; for other known syndromic OCs, OR = 8.1, 95% CI 2.6–27.7). Other candidate genes for nonsyndromic OC and maternal smoking and alcohol consumption were also detected (Romitti et al., 1999). Thus, a gene–environment interaction may play an important role in the origin of OCs.

4. Only the very high dose (6–10 mg) of folic acid reduced both occurrence (Czeizel et al., 1996, 1999) and recurrence (Peer et al., 1964; Tolarova, 1982, 1987; Tolarova and Harris, 1995) of nonsyndromic CL/P and CP in intervention studies.

5. The protective effect of high-dose folic acid is probably different from its reduction of neural tube defects. There is little evidence for a defect in folate metabolism in infants with OCs or their mothers

(Mills, 1999). However, the natural polyglutamate folate and the synthetic monoglutamate folic acid (i.e., two forms of the same vitamin, which is called recently as vitamin B_{11} as a twin to vitamin B_{12}) are pluripotent (Little, 1995). For example, folates also play a role in cell proliferation, and the absence of an adequate level of folates in the embryo leading to less epithelial activity may cause a fusing defect in the craniofacial processes. However, the importance of folic acid/folate in the production of the methyl group needed in the remethylation (i.e., detoxification) of homocysteine should also be considered (Cooper, 1984).

The major question is related to practical use of our knowledge. A higher dose (about 6 mg) of folic acid should be recommended for the reduction of recurrent OCs early during the postconceptional period under medical control (Czeizel et al., 1999). The question is whether it is appropriate to recommend the use of a high dose of folic acid supplementation before conception or after the early diagnosis of pregnancy in all women to reduce the first occurrence of nonsyndromic CL/P and CP. The pharmacological dose of folic acid may have some side effects, e.g., in women with pernicious anemia or epilepsy (Erős et al., 1998). It is reasonable to foresee that, in the future, women will be targeted with high doses of folic acid supplementation based on their genetic composition. Then, primary prevention through pharmacogenetics will be a reality.

REFERENCES

Berry, RJ, Li, Z, Erickson, D, et al. (1999). Prevention of neural-tube defects with folic acid in China. N Engl J Med 341: 1485–1490.

Bienengräber, V, Fanghänel, J, Malek, TA, Kundt, G (1997). Application of thiamine in preventing malformations, specifically cleft alveolus and palate, during the intrauterine development of rats. Cleft Palate Craniofac J 34: 318–324.

Bower, C, Stanley, FJ (1992). Dietary folate and nonneural midline birth defects. No evidence of an association from a case-control study in Western Australia. Am J Med Genet 44: 647–650.

Briggs, RM (1976). Vitamin supplements as a possible factor decreasing the incidence of cleft lip/palate deformities in humans. Clin Plast Surg 3: 647–652.

Canick, ML (1954). Cleft lip and cleft palate. A review of embryology, pathologic anatomy and etiology. Plast Reconstr Surg 14: 30–52.

Conway, H (1958). Effect of supplemental vitamin therapy on the limitation of incidence of cleft lip and cleft palate in humans. Plast Reconstr Surg 22: 450–453.

Cooper, BA (1984). Folate, its metabolism and utilization. Clin Biochem 17: 95–98.

Cuskelly, GJ, McNulty, H, Scott, JM (1996). Effect of increasing dietary folate on red-cell folate: implications for prevention of neural tube defects. Lancet 347: 657–659.

Czeizel, AE (1981). Schisis association. Am J Med Genet 10: 25–35.

Czeizel, AE (1993a). Prevention of congenital abnormalities by periconceptional multivitamin supplementation. BMJ 306: 1645–1648.

Czeizel, AE (1993b). Epidemiological studies of congenital abnormalities in Hungary. Issues Rev Teratol 6: 83–124.

Czeizel, AE (1996). Reduction of urinary tract and cardiovascular defects by periconceptional multivitamin supplementation. Am J Med Genet 62: 179–183.

Czeizel, AE (1997). First 25 years of the Hungarian Congenital Abnormality Registry. Teratology 55: 299–305.

Czeizel, AE (1999). Ten years of experiences in periconceptional care. Eur J Obstet Gynecol Reprod Biol 84: 43–49.

Czeizel, AE, Dobó, M, Dudás, I, et al. (1998). The Hungarian Periconceptional Service as a model for community genetics. Community Genet 1: 252–259.

Czeizel, AE, Dudás, I (1992). Prevention of the first occurrence of neural-tube defects by periconceptional vitamin supplementation. N Engl J Med 327: 1832–1835.

Czeizel, AE, Dudás, I, Métneki, J (1994). Pregnancy outcomes in a randomized controlled trial of periconceptional multivitamin supplementation. Final report. Arch Gynecol Obstet 255: 131–139.

Czeizel, AE, Hirschberg, J (1997). Orofacial clefting in Hungary. Folia Phoniatr Logop 49: 111–116.

Czeizel, AE, Hirschberg, J, Tary, E (1986). Etiological study on the Robin sequence [in Hungarian]. Gyermekgyógyászat 37: 157–171.

Czeizel, AE, Merhala, Z (1998). Bread fortification with folic acid, vitamin B_{12} and vitamin B_6 in Hungary. Lancet 352: 1225.

Czeizel, AE, Nagy, E (1986). Recent aetiological study on facial clefting in Hungary. Acta Paediatr Hung 27: 145–166.

Czeizel, AE, Rockenbauer, M, Siffel, C, Varga, E (2001). Description and mission evaluation of the Hungarian Case-Control Surveillance of Congenital Abnormalities, 1980–1996. Teratology 63: 176–185.

Czeizel, AE, Telegdi, L, Tusnády, G (1988). Multiple Congenital Abnormalities. Budapest: Akadémiai Kiadó.

Czeizel, AE, Tímár, L, Sárközi, E (1999). Dose-dependent effect of folic acid on the prevention of orofacial clefts. Pediatrics 104: e66.

Czeizel, AE, Tóth, M, Rockenbauer, M (1996). Population-based case-control study of folic acid supplementation during pregnancy. Teratology 53: 345–351.

Czeizel, AE, Tusnády, G (1971). An epidemiological study of cleft lip with or without cleft palate and posterior cleft palate in Hungary. Hum Hered 21: 17–38.

Czeizel, AE, Tusnády, G (1972). A family study on cleft lip with or without cleft palate and posterior cleft palate in Hungary. Hum Hered 22: 405–416.

Czeizel, AE, Tusnády, G (1984). Aetiological Studies of Isolated Common Congenital Abnormalities in Hungary. Budapest: Akadémiai Könyvkiadó.

Erős, E, Géher, P, Gömör, B, Czeizel, AE (1998). Epileptogenic activity of folic acid after drug induced SLE. Folic acid and epilepsy. Eur J Obstet Gynecol Reprod Biol 80: 75–78.

Fogh-Andersen, P (1942). Inheritance of Harelip and Cleft Palate. Copenhagen: Arnold Busck.

Fraser, FC, Czeizel, AE, Hanson, C (1982). Increased frequency of neural tube defects in sibs of children with other malformations. Lancet 2: 144–145.

Fraser, FC, Warburton, D (1964). No association of emotional stress or vitamin supplement during pregnancy to cleft lip or palate in man. Plast Reconstr Surg 33: 394–395.

Hayes, C, Werler, MM, Willett, WC, Mitchell, AA (1996). Case-control study of periconceptional folic acid supplementation and oral clefts. Am J Epidemiol 143: 1229–1234.

Hernandes-Dias, S, Werler, MM, Walker, AM, Mitchell, AA (2000). Folic acid antagonists during pregnancy and the risk of birth defects. N Engl J Med *343:* 1608–1614.

Hill, L, Murphy, M, McDowall, M, Paul, AH (1988). Maternal drug histories and congenital malformations: limb reduction defects and oral clefts. J Epidemiol Community Health *42:* 1–7.

Houdayer, CI, Bahuau, M (1998). Orofacial cleft defects: inference from nature and nurture. Ann Genet *41:* 89–117.

Khoury, MJ, Gomez-Farias, M, Mulinare, J (1989). Does maternal cigarette smoking during pregnancy cause cleft lip and palate in offspring? Am J Dis Child *143:* 333–337.

Kirke, PN, Mills, JL, Whitehead, AS (1996). Methylene-tetrahydrofolate reductase mutation and neural tube defects. Lancet *348:* 1037–1038.

Kreybig, TV (1981). Erweiterung der Lippen-Kiefer-Gaumen-spalten-Prävention zur Verkütung anderer Fehlbildungs formen. Munch Med Wochenschr *123:* 1151–1154.

Lidral, AC, Johnston, MC, Switzer, R (1991). The relationship between vitamins and the prevalence of cleft lip in mice [abstract]. J Dent Res *68:* 524.

Little, J (1995). Is folic acid pluripotent? A review of the associations with congenital anomalies, cancer and other diseases. In: *Drugs, diet and disease. Mechanistic Approaches to Cancer*, Vol. 1, edited by DFV Lewis. New York: Ellis Horwood, pp. 259–308.

Mills, JL (1999). Folate and oral clefts: where do we go from here? New Dir Oral Clefts Res *60:* 251–252.

Mills, JL, Kirke, PN, Molloy, AM, et al. (1999). Methylenetetrahydrofolate reductase thermolabile variant and oral clefts. Am J Med Genet *86:* 71–74.

Nelson, MM, Asling, CW, Evans, HM (1952). Production of multiple congenital abnormalities in young by maternal pteroylglutamic acid deficiency during gestation. J Nutr *48:* 61–79.

Nelson, MM, Wright, HV, Asling, CW, Evans, HM (1955). Multiple congenital abnormalities resulting from transitory deficiency of pteroylglutamic acid during gestation in rat. J Nutr *56:* 349–369.

Opitz, JM, Gilbert, EF (1982). CNS anomalies and the midline as a developmental fields. Am J Med Genet *12:* 443–455.

Paros, A, Beck, SL (1999). Folinic acid reduces cleft lip [CL(P)] in A/WySn mice. Teratology *60:* 344–347.

Peer, LA, Bryan, WH, Strean, LP (1958a). Induction of cleft palate in mice by cortisone and its reduction by vitamins. J Int Coll Surg *30:* 249.

Peer, LA, Gordon, HW, Bernhard, WG (1964). Effect of vitamins on human teratology. Plast Reconstr Surg *34:* 358–363.

Peer, LA, Strean, LP, Walker, JC, et al. (1958b). Study of 400 pregnancies with birth of cleft lip-palate infants: protective effect of folic acid and vitamin B$_6$ therapy. Plast Reconstr Surg *22:* 422–429.

Pickerill, HP (1914). The anatomy and physiology of cleft palate and a new method of treatment. In: *Transactions of the 6th International Dental Congress*, London: pp. 453–469.

Romitti, PA, Lidval, AC, Munger, RG, et al. (1999). Candidate genes for nonsyndromic cleft lip and palate and maternal cigarette smoking and alcohol consumption: evaluation of genotype–environment interaction from a population-based case-control study of orofacial clefts. Teratology *59:* 39–50.

Sakanashi, TM, Rogers, JM, Fu, SS, et al. (1996). Influence of maternal folate status on the developmental toxicity of methanol in the CD-1 mouse. Teratology *54:* 198–206.

Saxen, I (1975). Association between oral clefts and drugs taken during pregnancy. Int J Epidemiol *4:* 37–44.

Schinke, G, Sikapa, R, Kreybig, TV (1976). Beeinflussung der Teratogenität von Hydroxamsäuren durch Thiamin (Vitamin B$_1$) bei der Ratte. Z Kinderchir *19:* 333–344.

Shaw, GM, Croen, LA, Todoroff, K, Tolarova, MM (2000). Periconceptional intake of vitamin supplements and risk of multiple congenital anomalies. Am J Med Genet *93:* 188–193.

Shaw, GM, Finnell, RH, Todoroff, K, et al. (1999). Maternal vitamin use, infant C677T mutation in MTHFR and isolated cleft palate risk. Am J Med Genet *85:* 84–85.

Shaw, GM, Lammer, EJ, Wasserman, CR, et al. (1995). Risks of orofacial clefts in children born to women using multivitamins containing folic acid periconceptionally. Lancet *346:* 393–396.

Shaw, GM, Rozen, R, Finnel, RH, et al. (1998a). Infant C677T mutation in MTHFR, maternal periconceptional vitamin use, and cleft lip. Am J Med Genet *80:* 196–198.

Shaw, GM, Wasserman, CR, Lammer, EJ, et al. (1996). Orofacial clefts, parental cigarette smoking and transforming growth factor alpha gene variants. Am J Hum Genet *58:* 551–561.

Shaw, GM, Wasserman, CR, Murray, JC, Lammer, EJ (1998b). Infant's TGF-alpha genotype, orofacial clefts and maternal periconceptional multivitamin use. Cleft Palate Craniofac J *35:* 366–370.

Smithells, RW, Sheppard, S, Schorah, CJ, et al. (1980). Possible prevention of neural tube defects by periconceptional vitamin supplementation. Lancet *1:* 339–340.

Strauss, OA (1914). Predisposing causes of cleft palate and harelip. In: *Transactions of the 6th International Dental Congress*. London: pp. 470–471.

Thorogood, P, Tickle, C (1988). Craniofacial development. Development *103:* 1–257.

Tolarova, M (1982). Periconceptional supplementation with vitamins and folic acid to prevent recurrence of cleft lip. Lancet *1:* 217.

Tolarova, M (1987). Orofacial clefts in Czechoslovakia. Incidence, genetics and prevention of cleft lip and palate over a 19-year period. Scand J Plast Reconstr Surg *21:* 19–25.

Tolarova, M, Harris, T (1995). Reduced recurrence of orofacial clefts after periconceptional supplementation with high dose folic acid and multivitamin. Teratology *51:* 71–78.

Tolarova, MM, Cervenka, J (1998). Classification and birth prevalence of orofacial clefts. Am J Med Genet *75:* 126–137.

Van der Put, NM, Steegers-Theunissen, RP, Frosst, P, et al. (1995). Mutated methylenetetrahydrofolate reductase as a risk factor for spina bifida. Lancet *346:* 1070–1071.

Warkany, J, Nelson, RC (1940). Appearance of skeletal abnormalities in the offspring of rats reared on a deficient diet. Science *92:* 383–384.

Wegner, C, Nau, H (1992). Alteration of embryonic folate metabolism by valproic acid during organogenesis: implications for mechanism of teratogenesis. Neurology *42(Suppl 5):* 17–24.

Werler, MM (1999). Multivitamin supplementation and risk of birth defect. Am J Epidemiol *150:* 675–682.

Wyszynski, DF, Beaty, TH (1996). Review of the role of potential teratogens in the origin of human nonsyndromic oral clefts. Teratology *53:* 309–317.

Wyszynski, DF, Diehl, SR (2000). Infant C677T mutation in MTHFR, maternal periconceptional vitamin use, and risk of nonsyndromic cleft lip. Am J Med Genet *92:* 79–80.

Zanjani, ED, Anderson, WF (1999). Prospects for in utero human gene therapy. Science *285:* 2084–2088.

36

Costs of cleft lip and palate: personal and societal implications

NANCY W. BERK

MARY L. MARAZITA

One of the most common congenital anomalies, cleft lip with or without cleft palate (CL/P) is also one of the most common visible birth defects, occurring in 1 of every 500 to 1000 live births worldwide (Murray, 1995). While the severity of this condition varies, multidisciplinary treatment is often warranted. This may include craniofacial surgery, specialized dental and orthognathic treatment, speech and hearing intervention, and educational, psychological, and social assessment and intervention. The National Institute of Dental and Craniofacial Research (2000) estimates that in the United States the annual health cost for craniofacial anomalies approaches $1 billion and reflects the "comprehensive and time-consuming habilitation required to enable each child born with such birth defects the opportunity to pursue a productive life."

The preceding statement recognizes the inherent right of each individual to pursue a life that is free from the debilitating physical and social effects of a birth defect. The economic cost of CL/P is multidimensional. It is felt by the patient, his or her family, and society. It is highlighted by fiscal burden for the patient and family and can represent lost potential and productivity at the individual, family, and societal levels, which is often forgotten by those focused on dollars, budgets, and reimbursement.

Ideally, this topic should be examined within the rigor of standard health economic paradigms. However, the absence of economic data on clefting prohibits us from assessing the precise fiscal impact of CL/P. The purpose of this chapter then is to elucidate, for the health professional, the myriad costs associated with

this condition and to serve as a springboard for future research that would enable health professionals, including health economists, to better determine the magnitude of these costs. The term *cost* will be used throughout this chapter as a global lay construct reflecting price, loss, and sacrifice. This chapter first addresses the direct financial costs associated with CL/P, with an illustration of early childhood treatment costs in a patient cohort (age 0–6). Next, physical costs are addressed with respect to the morbidity and mortality seen in the CL/P population, including families. Finally, psychosocial costs are reviewed, including those related to health beliefs and behaviors, the impact of facial differences, social competence, and psychosocial interventions.

These categories (financial, physical, and psychosocial) provide a means of conceptualizing the many costs associated with clefting. They are not, however, mutually exclusive. For example, psychosocial costs, such as social anxiety, may influence job opportunities for a patient, in turn impacting his or her income and financial resources. This chapter provides a foundation for understanding these costs and their interrelated nature, as well as the costs associated with the inability or unwillingness to access specialized care.

FINANCIAL COSTS

While there are little data on the medical costs of CL/P, it is well accepted that the medical costs for those with chronic health conditions, including those associated with genetic disorders, exceed costs for those in good health. Variability of medical costs has been associated with disease severity for genetic disorders such as cystic fibrosis, even mild severity being associated with substantial cost (Lieu et al., 1999). In a study of 1993 Medicaid claims data for 310,977 children with one of eight selected chronic conditions, Ireys et al. (1997) found medical care for these children to be 2.5 to 2.0 times more expensive than medical care for children in general. These costs were found to be condition-dependent. While CL/P was not included among these eight conditions, such findings illustrate that medical care costs are burdensome for those with chronic health problems.

While many have acknowledged the overwhelming financial burden associated with CL/P, few have directly assessed the associated financial cost. In perhaps the most frequently cited study of financial cost of CL/P, Waitzman et al. (1994) reviewed the total cost per case based on samples in California, that acknowledging direct and indirect costs. The authors calculated this to range from $29,000 to $246,000. Their conservative estimate of the cost per case, which has been widely quoted in the cleft literature, is $92,000. Waitzman et al. (1994) noted that the "high total cost of cleft lip/palate reflects its high incidence coupled with relatively high frequencies of first-year mortality and activity limitation" (p. 200). This number, while assessing indirect costs, did not include occupational costs to parents or psychosocial costs to the patient, such as pain or anxiety. Thus, this may be an extremely low estimate of the fiscal burden of this birth defect on the patient, family, and society. Direct financial costs include surgeries, dental care, speech and language intervention, audiological assessment, and psychological and educational assessment and intervention. Aspects of the financial impact on the family that are often neglected or unassessed include parking, transportation, and other travel expenses related to patient treatment. Insurance concerns and restrictions, particularly with respect to the identification of CL/P as a pre-existing condition, may impact parental occupational opportunities and advancement (Strauss, 1994).

Also, CL/P is associated with significant costs beyond birth, including nonmedical direct costs such as special education services (Waitzman et al., 1994). For example, children with CL/P are at risk for learning disabilities and other developmental problems (Broder et al., 1998; Kapp-Simon and Krueckeberg, 2000). In comparison to unaffected peers, CL/P children have higher rates of learning disabilities (Richman et al., 1988; Eliason, 1990; Broder et al., 1998). If the educational needs of these at-risk children are routinely assessed and addressed, the financial cost of care rises at the point of

service (e.g., educational testing and intervention can be costly). However, such intervention may prove to defray part of the societal costs and psychosocial impact of CL/P by maximizing educational experiences and promoting the patient's academic success and future occupational opportunities and productivity.

As an illustration of some of the costs associated with cleft lip (CL) and cleft palate (CP), we have summarized the average number of services provided within the University of Pittsburgh Cleft Palate-Craniofacial Center (CPCC), as well as average fees charged, for the first 5 years of life for selected patients from the 1994 birth cohort. Also presented are numbers and fees charged for plastic surgery procedures outside of the CPCC. These numbers do not fully reflect all costs, particularly those associated with dental procedures such as orthodontia and oral surgery. While these specialties are represented within the CPCC, cost assessment and estimates are difficult to track for most patients. Treatments and related billing are often conducted outside of the CPCC by either the affiliated specialty department or specialists. In some cases, patient reluctance to travel long distances for dental procedures has resulted in the seeking of specialty care outside of the team network. This sample may not be representative of all CL/P patients. While the cleft severity of this sample resembles that seen in national birth registry data, socioeconomic status is somewhat lower. This difference would not impact patient treatment needs but could potentially influence parental treatment-seeking behavior. Traditionally, attrition secondary to low socioeconomic status is rare in this group, given the child's obvious medical needs until at least age 6. Nonetheless, these data should be interpreted cautiously with these limitations in mind.

Table 36.1 summarizes the selected patients. Included are patients with nonsyndromic anomalies who were born in 1994, began as patients with the CPCC at birth, and have remained continuously under the care of the CPCC until May of 2000. This cohort was chosen to track patients who had received comprehensive team care at the CPCC rather than patients who may have been seen for isolated visits (e.g., second opin-

TABLE 36.1. *Patients of the University of Pittsburgh Cleft Palate-Craniofacial Center (CPCC) from 1994 Birth Cohort Who Are Currently Active*

	Male	Female	Total
Cleft lip	4	2	6
Cleft lip plus palate	15	6	21
Cleft palate	5	6	11
Total	24	14	38

TABLE 36.2. *Patients from the 1994 Birth Cohort of the University of Pittsburgh Cleft Palate-Craniofacial Center (CPCC) Receiving Services over the First 5 Years of Life*

Diagnosis	CPCC services*			Plastic surgery procedures		
	Minimum	Average	Maximum	Minimum	Average	Maximum
Cleft lip	9	39.7	71	1	1.17	2
Cleft lip plus palate	5	66.0	99	2	3.90	8
Cleft palate	12	41.8	75	0	1.09	3

*Services provided by the CPCC include audiology; speech/language; genetics; pediatrics; ear, nose, and throat consults; dental consults; plastic surgery consults.

ions, lost to follow-up secondary to relocation). As most CL/P children receive care up to age 6 regardless of severity, this cohort enabled us to examine the early financial impact of clefting experienced by nearly all families to some extent. There were 38 such patients, six with CL, 21 with cleft lip with cleft palate (CLP), and 11 with CP. The usual male preponderance was seen for the CL and CLP categories, and the usual slight female preponderance was seen for CP (see Chapter 12 for more details).

Table 36.2 summarizes the total number of services provided by the CPCC over the first 5 years of life for the 1994 birth cohort and the total number of plastic surgery procedures. Presented are the minima, maxima, and averages by cleft type. The specialties providing services within the CPCC include audiology; pediatrics; genetics; ear, nose, and throat (ENT), speech/language, dental (consults), plastic surgery (consults), psychology, and family support. Also summarized is the care received outside of the CPCC and treatment planning after full team staffing of individual cases (see Section II of this book for a full description of multidisciplinary care of CL/P patients; also refer to the American Cleft Palate-Craniofacial Association website www.cleft-line.org). Examples of the plastic surgery procedures provided to this cohort during the first 5 years of life include lip repair, primary nasal reconstruction, poste-

rior and anterior palatal repair, and closure of fistulae (see Chapter 26 for more details on surgery). Not surprisingly, the CLP members of the birth cohort had the highest average number of CPCC services and plastic surgery procedures (about 1.5 times the average for CL or CP individuals and about 4 times the average plastic surgery procedures).

Table 36.3 summarizes the fees billed to these patients. Presented are the minima, maxima, and average fees billed during the first 5 years of life for CPCC services and plastic surgery procedures. These figures represent the fees billed, not those collected. For the purpose of this chapter, billable fees are presented since these are based on the cost of providing the services and, therefore, represent a more accurate reflection of the "costs" of having a cleft than would collections. Again, not surprisingly, CLP individuals have the highest average fees billed over the 5-year period (about 1.5 times the average for CL or CP individuals and about 4 times the average plastic surgery fees).

Table 36.4 presents the categories of service provided by the CPCC for the first 5 years of life. Presented are average numbers of services and average fees billed for each category, by each cleft type. These numbers highlight the direct medical costs faced by those affected by CL/P. However, they capture only a portion of that burden in that costs are often incurred beyond those

TABLE 36.3. *Fees Billed to Patients from the 1994 Birth Cohort of the University of Pittsburgh Cleft Palate-Craniofacial Center (CPCC) for Services over the First 5 Years of Life*

Diagnosis	Fees billed for CPCC services*			Fees billed for plastic surgery procedures*		
	Minimum	Average	Maximum	Minimum	Average	Maximum
Cleft lip	$418.00	$1978.84	$2879.00	$2000.00	$2466.67	$3200.00
Cleft lip plus palate	$125.00	$2591.53	$3940.00	$3700.00	$7738.10	$15,400.00
Cleft palate	$585.00	$1610.09	$2852.00	$2000.00	$2000.00	$4000.00

*These are the fees charged, not necessarily the amount that was collected for the services.

TABLE 36.4. *Categories of Service Provided to Patients of the 1994 Birth Cohort of the University of Pittsburgh Cleft Palate-Craniofacial Center (CPCC) over the First 5 Years of Life*

Category	Cleft lip		Cleft lip with palate		Cleft palate	
	Average No. of Services	Average Fees Billed	Average No. of Services	Average Fees Billed	Average No. of Services	Average Fees Billed
Services provided by the CPCC						
Audiology	12.7	$560.00	17.5	$771.67	12.5	$550.91
Pediatrics/genetics/ ear, nose, throat	7.5	$387.50	12.5	$629.05	8.9	$486.36
Dental consults	4.5	$129.67	9.0	$292.48	1.5	$27.82
Plastic surgery consults	5.8	$285.00	8.9	$454.52	4.9	$242.27
Speech/language	8.5	$216.67	17.1	$443.81	12.9	$302.73
Family support services	0.7	0.0	1.0	0.0	0.9	0.0
Plastic surgery procedures						
Surgery	1.17	$2466.67	3.90	$7738.10	1.09	$2000.00
Total (CPCC + plastic surgery)						
Total	40.87	$4045.51	69.9	$10329.63	42.79	$3610.09

charged by the multidisciplinary center and the surgeon. Likewise, costs extend far beyond the first 5 years of life.

PHYSICAL COSTS

In addition to the financial costs of having an oral cleft are other equally significant costs. There are several morbidity factors associated with having a cleft, as well as increased risk of neonatal mortality. The impact on the family includes problems associated with low birth weight, fetal wastage, and risk of recurrence.

Individual

The two major factors that have been consistently shown to affect the individual with a cleft are associated malformations and neonatal mortality. There is also some evidence that cleft individuals are at risk for low birth weight (Emanuel et al., 1973; Cooper et al., 2000). Table 36.5 presents the percentages of CL, CLP, CL/P, and CP individuals having additional malformations from several large, population-based studies throughout the world. A consistent finding in each of these studies was that the frequency of associated anomalies is higher for CP than for CL/P cases. The percentage of CP individuals having associated anomalies ranges from 15.1% in a large series from Denmark (Christensen, 1999) to 55% in a patient population in California (Jones, 1988). The percentage for CL/P ranges from 6.4% in Denmark (Christensen, 1999) to 29.2% in New York (Druschel et al., 1996). The wide range in the reported percentages from study to study is probably due in part to differences in the definition of associated anomalies, particularly in whether major and minor anomalies are included.

Table 36.6 presents selected population-based studies that tested whether cleft cases had higher neonatal mortality (death during the first year of life) than controls. A consistent finding across these studies was that CL/P and CP individuals with additional associated anomalies were significantly more likely to die during the first year of life than were controls. The results for individuals with isolated CP were also consistent across studies in that they were not more likely to die during the first year of life than controls. However, the results for isolated CL/P were not consistent, with two studies finding a significantly increased risk for cases vs. controls and two studies not finding a statistically significant increased risk.

Furthermore, two studies investigated low birth weight in CL/P and CP individuals vs. controls. Druschel et al. (1996) reported that both isolated CP and CL/P had slightly higher rates of low birth weight [<2500 g, risk ratio = 1.3, 95% confidence interval (CI) 1.0–1.7 for CP; risk ratio = 1.3, 95% CI 1.0–1.5 for CL/P) than did individuals with no anomalies but that CP and CL/P individuals with other anomalies had greatly increased rates of low birth weight (<2500 g, risk ratio = 4.4, 95% C.I. 3.8–5.1 for CP; risk ratio =

TABLE 36.5. *Percentages of Cases Having One or More Other Malformations**

Study Population	CL		CLP		CL/P		CP		Reference
	N	%	N	%	N	%	N	%	
U.S. (Washington), 1956–1965	89	14.6%	161	24.2%	250	20.8%	128	39.8%	Emanuel et al. (1973)
U.S. (California), 1980–1985	—†	—	—	—	259	14.0%	139	55%	Jones (1988)
Saudi Arabia, 1984–1988	68	—	67	—	—	13.4%‡	40	—	Kumar et al. (1991)
The Netherlands, 1981–1988	—	—	—	—	120	23%	48	52%	Cornel et al. (1992)
U.S. (Washington), 1984–1988	—	—	—	—	254	13.4%	130	33.1%	Hujoel et al. (1992)
Italy (Emilia Romagna and northeast), 1981–1989	—	—	—	—	463	23%	303	43%	Milan et al. (1994)
U.S. (New York), 1983–1990	—	—	—	—	1599	29.2%	1187	43.6%	Druschel et al. (1996)
Philippines									
1988–1995 birth records	—	—	—	—	93	20.4%			Murray et al. (1997)
1992–1996 surgical screening	—	—	—	—	1019	6.2%	162	7.4%	
Denmark, 1936–1987	—	—	—	—	4989	6.4%	2301	15.1%	Christensen (1999)

*CL, cleft lip; CLP, cleft lip with cleft palate; CL/P, cleft lip with or without cleft palate; CP, cleft palate.
†No data presented.
‡Presented as the overall proportion of cases with associated malformations; data not presented on each type of cleft.

4.5, 95% CI 3.9–5.2 for CL/P). Menegotto and Salzano (1990) investigated birth weight in isolated CP and CL/P cases vs. controls and found that CP individuals did not have a significantly lower birth weight than controls but that CL/P individuals did ($p < 0.001$).

The associated anomalies, neonatal mortality, and low birth weight have concomitant financial and psychosocial costs. While early mortality may reduce medical costs for families, one might argue that other costs prove to be equally as devastating, particularly from a psychosocial perspective (e.g., psychological trauma, its impact, and subsequent intervention needs). Unfortunately, such costs have been neither well characterized nor well documented in this population.

Family

In addition to the morbidity and neonatal mortality costs to the individual are the costs to the families of affected individuals. In other words, the concomitant costs associated with oral clefting are disproportionately borne by the families in which there is a cleft individual.

First, the risk of having an additional affected family member (recurrence risk) is significantly higher than the population risk of having a cleft for every degree

of relationship (Murray, 1995; Christensen, 1999). Therefore, the financial costs of having an individual with a cleft are magnified within an affected individual's family because there is likely to be an additional affected family member.

Furthermore, that there may be additional noncleft morbidity in families of individuals with a cleft. Although not a consistent finding across all studies, multiple studies have found an increase in fetal mortality in the sibships of cleft individuals (Dronamraju and Bixler, 1984; Menegotto and Salzano, 1990). Also, there may be an increased risk of cancer in the families of cleft individuals. Two genetic loci involved with neoplasms have shown positive linkage or association with nonsyndromic CL/P. Retinoic acid receptor-α (*RARA*, 17q21) has shown positive association with CL/P (see Chapter 20), is involved in the teratogenicity of vitamin A, and is in the same chromosomal region as a major breast cancer gene (*BRCA1*). *BCL3* (19q13) is a proto-oncogene that has shown both positive association and linkage with nonsyndromic CL/P (see Chapter 21). Yang et al. (1994) also showed that there were much higher rates of cancer in the relatives of CL/P probands vs. published population rates. However, this finding was not confirmed by Steinwachs et al. (2000).

TABLE 36.6. *Risks of Dying in the First Year of Life for Cleft Lip with or without Cleft Palate (CL/P) and Cleft Palate (CP)*

Statistically significant increased risk of neonatal death?

Study Population	CL/P		CP		Reference
	Isolated	Multiple Anomalies	Isolated	Multiple Anomalies	
U.S. (Washington, 1956–1965): 251 CL/P, 127 CP vs. overall first-year mortality rate	No, first-year mortality rate = 0.25%	Yes, first-year mortality rate = 4.42%	No, first-year mortality rate = 0.26%	Yes, first-year mortality rate = 4.12%	Emanuel et al. (1973)
Latin America (1967–1981) collaborative study: 741 CL/P, 115 CP vs. matched controls (only isolated cases included)	Yes, *p* value vs. controls <0.001	N/A	No, not significantly different from controls	N/A	Menegotto and Salzano (1991)
U.S. (Washington, 1984–1988): 254 CL/P, 130 CP vs. controls with no anomaly on birth certificate	Yes, odds ratio for dying in first year = 4.6 (95% CI 1.9–11.7)	Yes, odds ratio for dying in first year = 66.6 (95% CI 32.7–135.8)	No, odds ratio for dying in first year = 1.4 (95% CI 0.2–9.1)	Yes, odds ratio for dying in first year = 96.7 (95% CI 61.1–153.0)	Hujoel et al. (1992)
U.S. (New York, 1983–1990): 1599 CL/P, 1187 CP vs. controls with no anomaly	No, risk ratio for dying in first year = 1.4 (95% CI 0.8–2.5)	Yes, risk ratio for dying in first year = 33.8 (95% CI 26.1–43.9)	No, risk ratio for dying in first year = 1.2 (95% CI 0.5–2.7)	Yes, risk ratio for dying in first year = 27.3 (95% CI 20.9–35.7)	Druschel et al. (1996)

As summarized earlier, a high proportion of CL/P and CP individuals have additional associated anomalies (estimates range from 6.4% to 29.2% for CL/P and from 15.1% to 55% for CP). A significant proportion of cleft individuals with associated anomalies have mendelian syndromes with variable expressivity; therefore, some of their relatives may have findings other than a cleft. For example, Stickler's syndrome is the most common syndrome that may include CP; other associated features that may occur alone in carriers of the gene include high myopia and/or detached retina and joint disorders.

In addition to the disproportionate burden borne by families of cleft individuals, those racial and ethnic groups with high birth prevalence of clefts face an increased burden from the costs of clefts secondary to the higher prevalence. As reviewed by Wyszynski et al. (1996), Native Americans have the highest reported birth prevalence of CL/P (3.6/1000 live births), followed by Asians (2.1/1000 in Japanese, 1.3–1.7/1000 in Chinese), Caucasians (1/1000), and individuals of African descent (0.3/1000).

PSYCHOSOCIAL COSTS

Differences can be stigmatizing. For the individual with CL/P, differences often involve varied degrees of facial scarring, dental and orthognathic features such as missing teeth, and speech and language limitations. Syndromic clefts may be associated with a myriad of visible differences, from minor structural ones to major differences in symmetry. The psychosocial implications of CL/P have been acknowledged and examined (Kapp-Simon et al., 1992; Richman and Eliason, 1993), but the costs are rarely assessed. This may be due in part to the lack of available outcome data. Some psychosocial aspects of CL/P (e.g., learning disabilities) have been noted in financial cost studies because of their commonality and the acknowledged fiscal burden. Other aspects that may be more difficult to assess or have more variability among patients and families are reviewed below.

Psychosocial costs often translate into economic costs for the individual, the family, and society. This may occur in a variety of ways. For example, psychosocial factors associated with CL/P may warrant specific treatment that is associated with a financial cost (e.g., psychotherapy). Indirect costs may occur via opportunistic losses related to societal, individual, or familial imposed restrictions or limitations (e.g., vocational obstacles, relationship difficulties). Lack of treatment in any domain has the potential to contribute to psychosocial and financial burdens for the patient and family.

Costs Related to Health Behaviors and Beliefs

Individual. Chronically ill children who undergo frequent invasive medical procedures may be prone to anticipatory anxiety associated with future medical procedures (Jacobsen et al., 1990). Most research in this domain has involved pediatric cancer patients (cf., Redd et al., 1987; Jacobsen et al., 1990; Manne et al., 1992). The impact of early medical experiences on the lives of older CL/P patients has not been comprehensively examined. It is unclear how the early childhood experiences of these patients affect their attitudes toward preventive health behaviors, including medical and dental treatment seeking. However, certain health-related behaviors (e.g., smoking cessation, exercise) can have significant implications in the reduction of costs associated with illness prevention and detection.

Frequent medical appointments, hospitalizations, and associated medical problems (e.g., inner ear pathology) of CL/P children can result in excessive school absences. For some children, these absences may contribute to educational disadvantages. However, there is little research on how these health behaviors and problems impact the future of CL/P individuals from a cost perspective. It has been suggested that the academic performance of CL/P children is negatively influenced by speech, language, and hearing deficits as well as facial differences (Richman and Eliason, 1982). How this directly impacts career development and occupational outcomes is unknown.

Family. The economic burden of CL/P for the family extends beyond the price of surgeries, the cost of orthognathic intervention, or the costs of speech evaluation and treatment. The indirect costs for a parent include such things as lost work hours and opportunities (occupational and social) secondary to the treatment needs of the affected child. While families may be cognizant of these costs, members may also be reluctant to verbalize or elaborate upon these experiences.

Costs Related to Facial Esthetics

The impact of physical appearance, particularly facial attractiveness, on the reactions of others is well documented (cf., Berscheid and Gangestad, 1982; Reis and Hodgins, 1995). Individuals who are perceived by others as attractive are more likely to receive preferential treatment in educational, occupational, legal, and other social settings. Because the majority of research on attractiveness involves unaffected individuals ranging from attractive to unattractive, it cannot be assumed that conclusions based on these studies are generalizable to CL/P populations (Reis and Hodgins, 1995).

Certainly, when excluding the specific visible characteristics of the craniofacial anomaly, CL/P patients, like unaffected individuals, span a range of attractiveness. How the interaction between patient attractiveness and severity of the anomaly influences perceived attractiveness is not known. We are currently examining the contributions of facial attractiveness, severity of the anomaly, and auditory attractiveness in predicting perceived attractiveness.

Individual. Berscheid and Gangestad (1982) noted the following:

> The social psychological effects of physical attractiveness are pervasive, strong, and generally uniform in nature. They are such that the physically attractive, whether male or female, old or young, black or white, or of high or low socioeconomic status, receive preferential social treatment in virtually every social situation examined thus far. (p. 290)

Highly attractive individuals have been found to elicit more favorable social impressions, responses, and interactions (Berscheid et al., 1971; Bull and Rumsey, 1988; Feingold, 1992). Individuals with craniofacial differences are more prone than unaffected individuals to unpleasant social responses from others, particularly strangers (Reis and Hodgins, 1995). Individuals with physical deformities are more prone to being avoided by others who may be uncomfortable with, or insensitive to, the anomaly.

Reactions from others and perceived reactions can influence an individual's behavior. Likewise, differential reactions from others may result in different opportunities and/or needs for individuals with visible differences. These experiential differences may translate to financial costs in areas such as career options and need for psychological intervention. It appears that adjustment in cleft adolescents may be related to an affected individual's self-perception of appearance, given that individuals who perceive themselves to be more attractive or less impaired have higher social competence scores (Tobiasen and Hiebert, 1993).

Teacher expectations are influenced by facial disfigurement (Richman, 1978), children with clefts being more likely to be inaccurately assessed with respect to their intellectual ability than their unaffected peers. While there is no direct evidence that this results in negative educational outcomes for the CL/P child, it does have strong implications with respect to teacher expectations, student advising, student opportunities, and educational/occupational/social outcomes for affected individuals.

Family. For most families, the initial reaction to the birth of a child with a cleft involves some degree of distress. This may be exacerbated by the fact that few children are diagnosed in utero, thus preventing any preparation (Berk et al., 1999). While learning of a birth defect or chronic health condition would normally elicit some level of anxiety, there are no data to suggest that the child's condition and treatment needs interfere with parent–child attachment or normal and positive interactions (Richman and Eliason, 1993). However, studies examining the early interaction of mothers and CL/P infants suggest that their interactions differ from those of unaffected infants and mothers. Specifically, affected infants (infants with CL/P and other craniofacial anomalies) and their mothers are less responsive and active in their interactions with one another (Field, 1995). The implications from this research with respect to long-term adjustment and subsequent costs are unknown.

Costs Related to Social Competence

Children and adults with CL/P are at higher risk for psychosocial adjustment problems in areas related to social competence than unaffected peers (Heller et al., 1981; Richman, 1983, 1998; Tobiasen and Hiebert, 1993; Tobiasen, 1995; Berk et al., 2001). Individuals with oral clefts may be more disadvantaged with respect to social affiliation and adaptation than unaffected adults.

A number of studies have revealed a tendency toward social inhibition and withdrawal in children, adolescents, and adults with oral clefts (Peter et al., 1975; Heller et al., 1981; Richman, 1983, 1997, 1998; Kapp-Simon et al., 1992; Tobiasen and Hiebert, 1993; Tobiasen, 1995; Kapp-Simon and McGuire, 1997). These disaffiliation behaviors associated with social anxiety can impair the development or maintenance of social relationships (Leary and Kowalski, 1995). This may have significant implications, given that social relationships, specifically certain forms of social support, may facilitate psychological adjustment and wellness (Wallston, et al., 1983; Cohen and Hoberman, 1983).

Withdrawal behaviors in children and adolescents with oral clefts may be mediated by other variables, particularly those associated with the severity of the craniofacial anomaly, perceived attractiveness, or perceived importance of facial attractiveness (Richman, 1983; Richman et al., 1985; Tobiasen and Hiebert, 1993).

Costs Related to Psychological Intervention

The need for, and benefits of, psychological intervention with CL/P individuals have been implied and acknowledged (Heller et al., 1985; Kapp-Simon et al., 1992; Kapp-Simon, 1995). In a survey of cleft/craniofacial teams, Broder and Richman (1987) found that 80% of team directors identified mental health intervention as important for their patients. Of interest is that these same directors noted that fewer than 50% of patients received psychological services. It is unclear whether this is a reflection of underutilization, inaccessibility, or selective utilization (e.g., utilization by the most severely impaired).

Psychological intervention can enhance adjustment for individuals with CL/P. For example, Kapp-Simon et al. (1992) found social skills to be one of the best predictors of adjustment in adolescents with craniofacial anomalies. They suggested that social skill training may enhance adjustment in this population. Others have found family support groups, neuropsychological testing, and individual psychotherapy, while not warranted in all cases, to be clinically beneficial for some subsets of patients and families. Despite this general professional consensus, there are no data regarding the utilization of psychological services in this population. The percentage of CL/P individuals and families seeking treatment or evaluation is unclear. Costs for individual psychotherapy, like family therapy, differ significantly across practitioners and geographic areas. Third-party coverage is rarely substantial, rendering some families helpless to pursue a course of action they might otherwise seek. In addition, for some individuals, the stigma of seeking psychological and psychiatric services overrides the distress that warrants it. It is also unclear how many individuals refrain from reporting their utilization of psychological services based on this societal stigma.

CONCLUSION

The area of service utilization and costs in clefting has been explored only minimally. Nonetheless, it is clear that the known direct costs of specialty treatment for individuals with CL/P are significant. For the CL/P patient and family, the overwhelming burden is often the fiscal one, with lifetime costs estimated at approximately $92,000 with a range from $29,000 to $246,000 (Waitzman et al., 1994).

Unfortunately, the unknown costs have the potential to equal or exceed these. The most poorly appreciated costs for the individual with CL/P appear to be the nonfinancial costs that directly and indirectly influence finances and future income. The least appreciated and rarely acknowledged burden involves physical and psychosocial costs to patient, family, and society. Physical costs include inequalities of morbidity and mortality that can be associated with clefts as well as ethnic and racial disparities in cleft prevalence.

Psychosocial costs include those associated with the execution of health behaviors, reactions to facial differences, and disparities in social competence (between affected and unaffected individuals). In addition, the inability to access or the unwillingness to utilize treatment has the potential to result in physical, psychosocial, and financial burden to the patient, the family, and society.

Health professionals must be cognizant of the burden facing the CL/P patient and family. This burden extends beyond direct medical costs and must be acknowledged by patients, families, and those who make decisions related to medical coverage/third-party reimbursement and government assistance. To enhance quality of life and maximize patient potential, we must identify at-risk patients and families and provide them with the strategies, resources, and tools to access intervention and support in all of the aforementioned domains.

REFERENCES

Berk, NW, Cooper, ME, Liu, Y, Marazita, ML (2001). Social anxiety in Chinese adults with oral-facial clefts. Cleft Palate Craniofac J 38: 126–133.

Berk, NW, Marazita, ML, Cooper, ME (1999). Medical genetics on the cleft palate-craniofacial team: understanding parental preference. Cleft Palate Craniofac J 36: 30–35.

Berscheid, E, Dion, KK, Walster, E, Walster, GW (1971). Physical attractiveness and dating choice: a test of the matching hypothesis. J Exp Soc Psychol 7: 173–789.

Berscheid, E, Gangestad, S (1982). The social psychological implications of facial physical attractiveness. Clin Plast Surg 9: 289–296.

Broder, H, Richman, LC (1987). An examination of mental health services for cleft/craniofacial patients. Cleft Palate J 24: 158–162.

Broder, HL, Richman, LC, Matheson, P (1998). Learning disability, school achievement, and grade retention among children with cleft: a two-center study. Cleft Palate Craniofac J 35: 127–131.

Bull, R, Rumsey, N (1988). The Social Psychology of Facial Appearance. New York: Springer-Verlag.

Christensen, K (1999). The 20th century Danish facial cleft population—epidemiological and genetic–epidemiological studies. Cleft Palate Craniofac J 36: 96–104.

Cohen, S, Hoberman, HM (1983). Positive events and social supports as buffers of life change stress. J Appl Soc Psychol 13: 99–125.

Cooper, ME, Stone, RA, Liu, Y, et al. (2000). Descriptive epidemiology of nonsyndromic cleft lip with or without cleft palate in Shanghai, China, from 1980 to 1989. Cleft Palate Craniofac J 37: 274–280.

Cornel, MC, Spreen, JA, Meijer, I, et al. (1992). Some epidemiological data on oral clefts in the northern Netherlands, 1981–1988. J Craniomaxillofac Surg 20: 147–152.

Dronamraju, KR, Bixler, D (1984). Fetal mortality in oral cleft families (V): studies of sporadic vs familial and pure vs syndromic clefts. Clin Genet 25: 314–317.

Druschel, CM, Hughes, JP, Olsen, CL (1996). First year-of-life mortality among infants with oral clefts: New York State, 1983–1990. Cleft Palate Craniofac J 33: 400–405.

Eliason, MJ (1990). Neuropsychological perspectives of cleft lip and palate. In: *Multidisciplinary Management of Cleft and Palate,* edited by J Bardach and HL Morris. Philadelphia: Saunders, pp. 825–831.

Emanuel, I, Culver, BH, Erickson, JD, et al. (1973). The further epidemiological differentiation of cleft lip and palate: a population study of clefts in King County, Washington, 1956–1965. Teratology 7: 271–281.

Feingold, A (1992). Good-looking people are not what we think. Psychol Bull 111: 304–341.

Field, T (1995). Early interaction of infants with craniofacial anomalies. In: *Craniofacial Anomalies. Psychological Perspectives,* edited by RA Eder. New York: Springer-Verlag, pp. 99–110.

Heller, A, Rafman, S, Zvagulis, I, Pless, IB (1985). Birth defects and psychosocial adjustment. American J of Diseases of Children 139: 257–263.

Heller, A, Tidmarsh, W, Pless, IB (1981). The psychosocial functioning of young adults born with cleft lip or palate. Clin Pediatr 20: 459–465.

Hujoel, PP, Bollen, AM, Mueller, BA (1992). First-year mortality among infants with facial clefts. Cleft Palate Craniofac J 29: 451–455.

Ireys, HT, Anderson, GF, Shaffer, TJ, Neff, JM (1997). Expenditures for care of children with chronic illnesses enrolled in the Washington State Medicaid program, fiscal year 1993. Pediatrics 100: 197–204.

Jacobsen, PB, Manne, SL, Gorfinkle, K, et al. (1990). Analysis of child and parent behavior during painful medical procedures. Health Psychol 9: 559–576.

Jones, MC (1988). Etiology of facial clefts: prospective evaluation of 428 patients. Cleft Palate J 25: 16–20.

Kapp-Simon, KA (1995). Psychological interventions for the adolescent with cleft lip and palate. Cleft Palate Craniofac J 32: 104–108.

Kapp-Simon, KA, Krueckeberg, S (2000). Mental development in infants with cleft lip and/or palate. Cleft Palate Craniofac J 37: 65–70.

Kapp-Simon, KA, McGuire, DE (1997). Observed social interaction patterns in adolescents with and without craniofacial conditions. Cleft Palate Craniofac J 34: 380–384.

Kapp-Simon, KA, Simon, DJ, Kristovich, S (1992). Self-perception, social skills, adjustment, and inhibition in young adolescents with craniofacial anomalies. Cleft Palate Craniofac J 29: 352–356.

Kumar, P, Hussain, MT, Cardoso, E, et al. (1991). Facial clefts in Saudi Arabia: an epidemiologic analysis in 179 patients. Plast Reconstr Surg 88: 955–958.

Leary, MR, Kowalski, RM (1995). *Social Anxiety.* New York: Guilford.

Lieu, TA, Ray, GT, Farmer, G, Shay, G (1999). The cost of medical care for patients with cystic fibrosis in a health maintenance organization. Pediatrics 103: e72.

Manne, SL, Bakeman, R, Jacobsen, PB, et al. (1992). Adult–child interaction during invasive medical procedures. Health Psychol 11: 241–249.

Menegotto, BG, Salzano, FM (1990). New study on the relationship between oral clefts and fetal loss. Am J Med Genet 37: 539–542.

Menegotto, BG, Salzano, FM (1991). Epidemiology of oral clefts in a large South American sample. Cleft Palate Craniofac J 28: 373–376.

Milan, M, Astolfi, G, Volpato, S, et al. (1994). 766 cases of oral cleft in Italy. Eur J Epidemiol 10: 317–324.

Murray, JC (1995). Face facts: genes, environment, and clefts. Am J Hum Genet 57: 227–232.

Murray, JC, Daack-Hirsch, S, Buetow, KH, et al. (1997). Clinical and epidemiologic studies of the cleft lip and palate in the Philippines. Cleft Palate Craniofac J 34: 7–10.

National Institute of Dental and Craniofacial Research (2000). www.nidcr.nih.gov, p. 1.

Peter, JP, Chinsky, RR, Fisher, MJ (1975). Sociological aspects of cleft palate adults: IV. Social integration. Cleft Palate J 12: 304–310.

Redd, WH, Jacobsen, PB, Die-Trill, M, et al. (1987). Cognitive/attentional distraction in the control of conditioned nausea in pediatric cancer patients receiving chemotherapy. J Consult Clin Psychol 55: 391–395.

Reis, HT, Hodgins, HS (1995). Reactions to craniofacial disfigurement: lessons from the physical attractiveness and stigma literatures. In: *Craniofacial Anomalies. Psychological Perspectives,* edited by RA Eder. New York: Springer-Verlag, pp. 177–198.

Richman, L (1978). The effects of facial disfigurement on teachers' perception of ability in cleft palate children. Cleft Palate J 15: 155–160.

Richman, L (1998). Fearful shyness versus solitary passivity in socially inhibited children with cleft. *Presented at the annual meeting of the American Cleft Palate-Craniofacial Association, Baltimore, Maryland, April 24, 1998.*

Richman, LC (1983). Self-reported social, speech, and facial concerns and personality adjustment of adolescents with cleft lip and palate. Cleft Palate J 20: 108–112.

Richman, LC (1997). Facial and speech relationships to behavior of children with clefts across three age levels. Cleft Palate Craniofac J 34: 390–395.

Richman, LC, Eliason, M (1982). Psychological characteristics of children with cleft lip and palate: intellectual, achievement, behavioral and personality variables. Cleft Palate J 19: 249–257.

Richman, LC, Eliason, MJ (1993). Psychological characteristics associated with cleft palate. In: *Cleft Palate: Interdisciplinary issues and treatment,* edited by KT Moller and CD Starr. Austin, TX: Pro-Ed, pp. 357–380.

Richman, LC, Eliason, MJ, Lindgren, SD (1988). Reading disability in children with clefts. Cleft Palate J 25: 21–25.

Richman, LC, Holmes, CS, Eliason, MJ (1985). Adolescents with cleft lip and palate: self-perceptions of appearance and behavior related to personality adjustment. Cleft Palate J 22: 93–96.

Steinwachs, EF, Amos, C, Johnston, D, et al. (2000). Nonsyndromic cleft lip and cleft palate is not associated with cancer or other birth defects. Am J Med Genet 90: 17–24.

Strauss, RP (1994). Health policy and craniofacial care: issues in resource allocation. Cleft Palate Craniofac J 31: 78–80.

Tobiasen, JM (1995). Social psychological model of craniofacial anomalies: example of cleft lip and palate. In: *Craniofacial Anomalies. Psychological Perspectives,* edited by RA Eder. New York: Springer-Verlag, pp. 233–257.

Tobiasen, JM, Hiebert, JM (1993). Clefting and psychosocial adjustment: influence of facial aesthetics. Clin Plast Surg 20: 623–631.

Waitzman, NJ, Romano, PS, Scheffler, RM (1994). Estimates of economic costs of birth defects. Inquiry 33: 188–205.

Wallston, BS, Alagna, SW, DeVellis, BM, DeVellis, RF (1983). Social support and physical health. Health Psychol 2: 367–391.

Wyszynski, DF, Beaty, TH, Maestri, NE (1996). Genetics of nonsyndromic oral clefts revisited. Cleft Palate Craniofac J 33: 406–417.

Yang, P, Mitchell, E, Marazita, ML, et al. (1994). Do cancers aggregate in families ascertained through probands with cleft lip and/or cleft palate? Am J Hum Genet 55: A97.

37

Insurance and coverage of care

DAVID A. BILLMIRE

The birth of a child with a cleft or a craniofacial defect can be a traumatic event for a family. Feelings of shock, guilt, and inadequacy are common. Once these fears and concerns are addressed and the parents are assured that the problem is not their fault, the next question they invariably ask is how they will pay for the child's care. This is a legitimate concern, especially in view of the current situation regarding healthcare financing and coverage. With about 13% of children having no healthcare coverage at all, 26% covered mainly by Medicaid (Edmunds and Coye, 1998), and the remaining covered by some form of managed care, the treatment of any complex disorder brings anxiety to the family and treatment team. The concern for the family is whether they can afford the care, and the concern for the team is whether they will be allowed to do what can and should be done. Craniofacial disorders are somewhat unique from a medical perspective. They are rarely fatal, their functional aspects (i.e., speech, hearing, and dental) are easily dismissed by managed care, and they have a strong quality-of-life issue with significant aesthetic overlay. Furthermore, they must be treated over the developmental life of the child, which makes them susceptible to claims of pre-existing conditions, and, most importantly, they occur exclusively in children. Children and their parents lack the financial and political wherewithal to effect significant changes in healthcare (Strauss, 1994). Despite all of this, however, it is rare that a child in the United States with a craniofacial disorder does not receive at least basic care.

HEALTHCARE FUNDING

Healthcare is funded through a number of different sources. There is traditional indemnity insurance based on the fee-for-service concept. There are a whole series of health maintenance organization (HMO)–based and propagated programs using various management concepts, discounted fees, contracted services, panels, etc. Finally, there are the government-based and -administered programs such as Medicare, Medicaid, State Children's Health Insurance Program, Civilian Health and Medical Program Uniformed Service (CHAMPUS), state-based special needs programs, and locally administered indigent care programs. Children are usually covered by, or are eligible for coverage under, one of the above programs.

Indemnity Insurance

Traditional indemnity insurance is becoming less common. It is based on a fee-for-service design, and while it may provide the greatest choice of practitioners, it usually does not cover routine care. Denial of care for lack of "medical necessity" is uncommonly an issue as management is left up to the physician and family. However, dental care, a critical factor in clefts, is not covered and speech coverage may be limited.

Health Maintenance Organizations

For most Americans, the majority of healthcare coverage is provided by some sort of managed care organization. The oldest type of this system of healthcare is the HMO. For a prepaid, fixed fee, the organization will provide comprehensive hospital and outpatient services. Kaiser Permante of California is the prototype of this form of healthcare. The federal government became involved in 1973, when Congress passed the Health Maintenance Organization Act of 1973. This law, as well as subsequent amendments and bills, established the ground rules under which HMOs operate. Currently, the majority of HMOs are federally qualified. By being federally qualified, these organizations may offer their products to Medicare clients. They must provide 10 basic benefits, such as physician services; hospitalization; preventive care; emergency services; diagnostic services; rehabilitation services; up to 2 months of physical, occupational, or speech therapy; drug and substance abuse treatment; and home healthcare. These are basic guidelines and the minimum that can be offered.

To provide services, HMOs can either directly employ providers or contract with independent providers. Patients then choose from among the providers or, in some cases, are assigned to specific offices, depending on location. There are four basic types of HMO model currently in existence. The *staff model* is one in which the HMO directly employs the providers. These providers offer services solely to members of the HMO. In the *group model*, the HMO contracts with a number of groups to provide healthcare services to its subscribers. Usually in this situation, the majority of patients treated by the groups are HMO members. In the *network model*, the HMO contracts widely with a number of groups and practitioners to provide services. The HMO members are only a fraction of the group and practitioners' business. In the *independent practice association model*, the HMO contracts with solo practitioners or associations of providers, which in turn contract with their members to provide the necessary services. Typically, an HMO will actually combine two or more of these models to create a system.

Usually, HMOs provide good basic care, but they may fall short in services to children with special needs (Ireys et al., 1996; Fox et al., 1993; Newacheck et al., 2000). By definition, they deal with a fixed practitioner base and obviously cannot provide comprehensive specialty care in every case. In cleft care, this can be a problem if there is no one in the plan who is experienced in the care of such patients. Providers may be reluctant to refer out of their plan due to the added cost. Cleft care has become the hallmark of team management (Bardach et al., 1984, 1992), but the HMOs, despite their stated commitment to quality and health maintenance, may be against referring to a team for management (Cohen, 1995). Comprehensive care of these disorders may be too expensive for the HMOs bottom line.

Preferred Provider Organizations

A preferred provider organization (PPO) offers a system of coverage by contracting to providers at a discount and then offering these services to employers. Enrollees are encouraged to use preferred providers because of lower co-payments and maximum limits on out-of-pocket costs for network services. Enrollees are allowed to see out-of-network providers but at a higher personal cost. Such organizations have become quite popular as they offer both lower premium costs as well as greater choice of providers. One of the notable differences between HMOs and PPOs is that enrollees may visit specialists without the need of authorization from their primary care physician. Like HMOs, PPOs have several different types. A provider-sponsored organization is established by the providers, employers, and other groups. Traditional indemnity companies often set up their own networks or may, in some cases, lease networks from other insurers (the providers themselves may be unaware of this situation). An exclusive provider organization is a system which in nonemergent care is limited to a fixed panel. It is essentially a form of a point-of-service system, allowing some out-of-network care. Specialty PPOs provide a limited range of benefits such as occupational/physical therapy, speech/language, dental, mental health, and pharmacy services.

Point of Service

Point-of-service systems combine the advantages of HMOs with out-of-network coverage. This is done with economic incentives using a fixed co-payment as opposed to a 20% to 30% co-insurance rate. Services obtained out of network are reimbursed at fee-for-service rates, but there is usually a per-person limit. Point-of-service plans are popular as they allow access to specialists for those who are willing to pay.

In addition to private HMOs, there are both Medicare and Medicaid HMOs. The effect of Medicaid HMOs on children with special healthcare needs is questionable. Many of these children are covered under Title V programs with service coordination as part of their management (Fox et al., 1993).

GOVERNMENT PROGRAMS

State Children's Health Insurance Program and Medicaid

While it is true that millions of children are not covered by health insurance, a significant number are eligible for state and federal programs and would be covered if only the applications were filled out (Summer et al., 1997). Traditional pediatric coverage is usually available through the federal Medicaid program. This program was created in 1965 as Title XIX of the Social Security Act (Edmunds and Coye, 1998). It is a federally mandated program, whose original intent was to provide coverage to children similar to that which Medicare provided to the elderly. Medicaid was initially tied to participation in welfare; however, in the mid-1990s these restrictions were loosened. A phase-in program was initiated so that by the year 2002 all poor children under the age of 19 will be eligible for Medicaid. Unlike Medicare, however, the programs are partially state-managed and -funded. While the federally managed Medicare program has consistent rules and levels of reimbursement nationwide, state-funded Medicaid programs have highly variable coverage and reimbursement rates. The low level and variability of reimbursement can and do restrict the availability of care. The State Children's Health Insurance Program (SCHIP) was established in 1998 by federal law (Balanced Budget Act of 1997) (see Families USA, www.familiesusa.org) to help fill in the gaps in children's healthcare for those not eligible for Medicaid. Coverage is available to families with incomes up to twice the federal poverty level. The combination of Medicaid, SCHIP, and private health insurance should theoretically cover the medical needs of all children.

Title V Programs

As parents of a child with a craniofacial disorder know, treatment needs extend beyond classical medical boundaries, specifically in the areas of speech and dentistry. Although Medicaid does include some dental services, these are areas long neglected by traditional insurance. In 1935, along with establishing the Social Security Act, the U.S. Congress created Women and Children's Health Care, now better known as Title V (National Maternal and Child Health Clearing House www.nmche.org). These programs came under the Maternal and Child Health Bureau of the Department of Health and Human Services (www.mchb.hrsa.gov). These programs, currently refered to as Maternal and Child Health and Children with Special Health Needs programs, exist in every state and territory of the United States. The actual administration and scope of these programs vary from state to state. These are variously known as, e.g., crippled children's programs, special needs programs, or children with medical handicaps programs. They are designed to provide services to children with developmental, congenital, and acquired disorders and diseases. In general, these programs are a stopgap measure. They provide payment and often service coordination when no other source is available. They also provide standards of care, which are followed by the Medicaid programs. The programs are usually need-based, with a sliding scale of reimbursement. These programs help pay for critical dental care, such as restoration, splints, and orthodontics and prosthodontics (crown, bridge, dental prosthesis).

With the recent increase in managed care coverage, they have also been forced into an active advocacy program regarding insurance coverage for children with birth defects. Their budgets are becoming strained by the denial and restriction of services created by managed care. What was once thought of as a stopgap measure is now becoming the primary source of services. Recent expansions and changes in both Medicaid and SCHIP have called into question the existence and function of this critical resource.

Alternative Sources

If the above programs fail, there are still individual state-financed and private sources of care. The Shriners Hospitals for Children (www.shrinershg.org/hospitals/) may offer care. The Choices program (Children Healthcare Options Improved through Collaborative Efforts and Services) links these private endeavors with existing state and federal assistance programs.

THE CONTRACTUAL BASIS OF INSURANCE AND MEDICAL NECESSITY

In any type of private insurance, whether it be traditional indemnity, HMO, or governmental, it is critical for the parent and provider to realize that insurance is contract-based. There are obligations on both the parents' (subscribers') and the insurance companies' parts. These are spelled out in the contract. While it may seem logical that a service be covered, unless it is spelled out in the contract, it is likely to be denied. This also entertains the whole concept of medical necessity (Ireys et al., 1999). Currently, *medical necessity* is the determination of whether a specific service will be provided for a specific situation. The legal authority lies with the managed care organization or the insurance company. Typically, the insurance companies' interpretation of medical necessity is often different from that of the physician and patient. Many current definitions of medical necessity, i.e., a service that will significantly improve health, may work to the detriment of children with special health care needs, who need the services simply to maintain function. In the case of children with craniofacial disorders, medical necessity may be used to deny care based on the definition of improving health. After all, one is only improving appearance, not health. Determination of medical necessity is not easy and must be individualized, taking into account the patient, the disorder, and the family situation. While *rationing* (a deliberate decision to protect resources for the group as a whole at the expense of an individual) is conceptually different from medical necessity, in reality, expense can and will factor into the medical necessity decision-making process. Having explored this issue, it is important to again emphasize that medical plans and insurance are contract-based. If the contract excludes coverage for certain services, e.g., dental, scar revision, or jaw surgery, the determination of medical necessity for these services is not an issue for the provider. In other words, the insurance provider will not argue the medical necessity of the service but simply state that it is not a covered service by contract and, therefore, will not be provided. In situations where services are covered and medical necessity is approved, the insurance company may still stipulate restrictions as to length or extent of care.

In the case of a child with special health care needs, it behooves the parents to look closely at the potential health plan and ask the following questions:

- Will the plan allow my child to go to a center and be team-managed?
- Will it allow my child to seek second opinions?
- What providers are in the plan?
- What ancillary services, i.e., speech, does it provide?
- What are the restrictions and exclusions?
- What defines a pre-existing condition?

Since most plans are presented as group plans, it is difficult, if not impossible, to negotiate any of these points. More latitude may be allowed in employer-sponsored or self-insured types of coverage. In larger companies, one can often discuss these points with the benefits manager. Some HMO plans provide service managers for complex cases. If this situation is available, it is advantageous for the parents to see if this type of service coordination can be applied. This can significantly reduce the paperwork and provide uninterrupted care for the child.

ANCILLARY SERVICES

A child with special health care needs often requires extensive use of services beyond those strictly medical. In many ways, these services are as essential, if not more so, to the child's well-being than those provided by medical professionals. These are the services that allow the child to function in life. As they are not often thought of as medical in nature but their need stems from a medical condition, they are usually covered by medical insurance. In craniofacial disorders, both dental and speech services fall under this umbrella.

Speech

The state and federal governments have passed laws mandating that schools provide services for special-needs children. Of significance to cleft children is that speech therapy is included in this mandate. While theoretically this was a good idea, in reality it has become a treatment nightmare. By mandating school coverage for speech therapy, the government has allowed the insurance companies to abrogate their responsibility for this critical service. A number of problems have ensued. First and foremost, school does not usually start until age 5. During the early critical period of speech development, children are left in a treatment limbo. They often do not get necessary diagnostic and treatment services when indicated. Second, school speech programs are geared toward relatively simple cases, such as articulation disorders. They are usually understaffed, meet infrequently, often group-based rather than individual, and in no way adequate for the complex speech problems associated with clefting and craniofacial disorders.

Insurance companies have, as a result, geared their programs for adults. Speech therapy is often available only to treat loss of an acquired skill, such as loss of speech following a stroke or accident. In children, speech is not yet acquired, so it cannot be lost. Therefore, coverage of speech diagnostic and therapeutic services is often denied (remember that contract). Most HMOs are federally qualified, and one requirement is that they provide a minimum of 60 therapy treatments. Most insurance companies have taken this is as their maximum, not minimum. If one reviews most policies, one will see that the number of 60 sessions of speech or occupational/physical therapy is the maximum. This limitation is problematic not only for acquired disorders but also for the complex issues associated with inherited craniofacial conditions. As most speech problems in these children fall under some form of developmental diagnosis code, they are often automatically denied. Speech and language therapists are forced to become creative in order to come up with codes that will allow them to provide necessary services. Currently, there are a number of state and nationwide initiatives to overcome this glaring shortcoming.

Dental

Dental care, a critical component in the care of these children, has traditionally been almost totally ignored by insurance. In the last few years, there has been a proliferation of both dental insurance and dental HMOs. As with medical insurance, these contracts must be closely evaluated to see exactly what is covered and what the restrictions are. Historically, medical insurance coverage occasionally provided for some of the perioperative services required for bone grafting and orthognathic surgery, such as splints and planning, but this is no longer the case. While Medicaid does provide for basic dental care, the complex issues associated with craniofacial disorders are usually not covered. The Title V programs have become an important funding source for these services. These services, although covered by the special needs programs, are reimbursed at levels significantly below the market rate, and it is often difficult to find practitioners who can afford or are willing to provide the often complex treatment needed. The average wage earner, with or without dental insurance, will usually have to personally bear the cost of the child's special dental care needs.

Secondary Surgery

While basic care can be provided by the programs described above, secondary care is increasingly being denied. The American Society of Plastic Surgeons (www.plasticsurgery.org) in a recent poll of its members discovered that 53.5% of the surgeons surveyed have had at least one pediatric patient partially or totally denied coverage for craniofacial or congenital defects. Even when coverage is available, it is getting harder to obtain approval. One of the most common ploys is that of the pre-existing condition. Combine this with the almost revolving-door change in insurance coverage, and one can see that a child with a birth defect is at great risk for disruption or frank denial of care. The American Medical Association (AMA House of Delegates Policy H-475.992) officially defines *cosmetic surgery* as "being performed to reshape normal structures of the body in order to improve the patient's appearance and self-esteem" and *reconstructive surgery* as "being performed on abnormal structures of the body, caused by congenital defects, developmental abnormalities, trauma, infection, tumors or disease." It is clear that congenital defects and their correction fall under the definition of reconstructive surgery. Despite this, insurance companies continue to deny coverage for any surgery beyond initial repair as "cosmetic." There are even reports of denying repair of isolated clefts of the lip as "cosmetic." When dealing with the insurance company, it is important to never refer to any planned surgery on the child as cosmetic. Once they hear this, it can be impossible to dissuade them from changing their stand. The correct term is *congenital deformity,* and any treatment or surgery that improves the situation is *reconstructive.* Nevertheless, it should be emphasized that insurance is a contract. Often, the company has its own definitions of conditions and terms outlined in the contract, which may not be the commonly accepted and assumed definitions. They can and will define anything in the contract that they choose as cosmetic or a noncovered disorder.

The most common denied procedures are scar revision, nasal surgery, bone grafting and closure of the alveolar cleft, and orthognathic surgery. Virtually all

clefts will require at least one scar revision. Surgery unfortunately does not always come out uniformly. Revisions to both the lip and nose are common. A typical reason for denial is either cosmetic or pre-existing condition, or both. The parents and their surgeon will often have to send documentation, letters, pictures, etc., to get coverage. At times, it will appear to be, or actually will be, a delaying tactic on the part of the insurance company. This may be a standard ploy, and parents should not hesitate to appeal all adverse decisions by the carrier. They should know their rights and read the contract. It is important to emphasize the congenital nature of the child's condition in dealing with the carrier. Bone grafting of the alveolar cleft is often denied as it is thought to be a dental procedure. This can usually be overcome with some education of the medical director of the plan and because of the fact that almost all alveolar clefts are associated with a fistula (a covered medical problem). Orthognathic surgery (surgery to reposition the jaws) was at one time almost universally covered for everyone, congenital defect or not. Insurance plans have drastically limited or eliminated this procedure altogether. Even in circumstances with severe malocclusion secondary to either a congenital condition or trauma, this procedure is denied as cosmetic. Sometimes it can be approved if the condition results in airway obstruction and surgery will improve breathing. This is an instance where patients might be better off with one of the government programs than private insurance. There are standards of cleft care published by the American Cleft Palate-Craniofacial Association (1993), which include the necessary orthognathic surgery. Most Title V special needs programs follow these guidelines. The HMOs, which purport to provide comprehensive care, usually do not follow the guidelines.

LEGISLATION

The increasing denial of secondary, advanced, and in some cases primary treatment of craniofacial disorders has, as one would expect, led to some attempt at correction by legislative means. Nationally and in individual states there are bills being submitted and passed which will mandate coverage of reconstructive surgical procedures for children with congenital, developmental deformities, diseases, or injuries. As of this writing, 13 states have passed such bills and there is a bill in Congress which addresses the issue. One of the problems is that the bill mandates surgery only and does not cover ancillary services for needs such as speech, hearing, dental, or psychological therapies. While superficially this may seem to be a good idea, simply mandating the requirement does not guarantee that reimbursement will be adequate or that anyone will be willing to do the procedure. Coverage of breast reconstruction recently became mandated, but reimbursement levels are now so low that many surgeons either are unwilling to do the procedures or provide only the most basic, simple reconstructions.

The medical insurance business in the United States has undergone rapid and profound changes over the last decade and, unfortunately, shows no sign of stabilizing. Many of the problems that allegedly brought about these changes are still present. The treatment of craniofacial problems by an integrated team method is often pointed to proudly as the first attempt by organized medicine to approach a group of disorders in a "managed" manner. Standards of care have been established, treatment plans created, and critical pathways outlined. Furthermore, this has been done in a national, organized, consensus-based forum with multiple disciplines involved. This is exactly what managed care has asked of us, to justify the treatment of any disease. Yet when presented with these facts and reports, their approach is somewhat disingenuous, hiding behind contractual jargon and denying care. Parents need to carefully review their contracts, voice their concerns to their employers, and become advocates for their children. Insurance companies often are unaware of, ignore, or bend the rules. Parents and providers need to know their rights. Appealing decisions has become almost standard operating procedure. Flagrant violations of coverage can and should be reported to the state insurance commission. The Title V programs (www. mchdata.gov) have become increasingly active in this area as they often bear the financial brunt of these denials. In summary, one has to know one's rights, be an advocate, and be persistent.

REFERENCES

American Cleft Palate-Craniofacial Association (1993). Parameters for the evaluation and treatment of patients with cleft lip/palate or other craniofacial anomalies. Cleft Palate Craniofac J 30: 4.

Bardach, J, Morris, HL, Olin, WH, et al. (1984). Late results of multidisciplinary management of unilateral cleft lip and palate. Ann Plast Surg 12: 235–242.

Bardach, J, Morris, HL, Olin, WH, et al. (1992). Results of multidisciplinary management of bilateral cleft lip and palate at Iowa Cleft Palate Center. Plast Reconstr Surg 89: 419–435.

Borah, GL, Hagberg, N, Jakubiak, C, Temple, J (1993). Reorganization of craniofacial/cleft care delivery: the Massachusetts experience. Cleft Palate Craniofac J 30: 333–336.

Cohen, SR (1995). Managed care. Cleft Palate Craniofac J 32: 178.

Edmunds, M, Coye, MJ (ed) (1998). America's Children: Health Insurance and Access to Care. Institute of Medicine and National Research Council, Committee on Children, Health Insurance and Access to Care. National Academy Press, Washington, D.C.

Fox, HB, Wicks, LB, Newacheck, PW (1993). Health maintenance organizations and children with special health needs. A suitable match? Am J Dis Child 147: 546–552.

Ireys, HT, Wehr, E, Cooke, RE (1999). Defining Medical Necessity: Strategies for Promoting Access to Quality Care for Persons with Developmental Disabilities, Mental Retardation, and Other Special Health Care Needs. Arlington, VA: National Center for Education in Maternal and Child Health.

Ireys, HT, Eichler, RJ (1988). Program priorities of crippled children's agencies: a survey. Public Health Rep 103: 77–83.

Ireys, HT, Grason, HA, Guyer, B (1996). Assuring quality of care for children with special needs in managed care organizations: roles for pediatricians. Pediatrics 98: 178–185.

Ireys, HT, Nelson, RP (1992). New federal policy for children with special health care needs: implications for pediatricians. Pediatrics 90: 321–327.

Kuter, R (1998a). The commercialization of prepaid group health care, part I. N Engl J Med 338: 1558–1563.

Kuter, R (1998b). The commercialization of prepaid group health care, part II. N Engl J Med 338: 1635–1639.

Newacheck, PW, McManus, M, Fox, HB, et al. (2000). Access to health care for children with special health care needs. Pediatrics 105: 760–766.

Salyer, KE (1995). Effects of managed care on the treatment of craniofacial deformities. J Craniofac Surg 6: 4.

Shaw, WC, Devlin, HB, Williams, A (1994). Provision of services for cleft lip and palate in England and Wales. BMJ 309: 1552.

Strauss, RP (1994). Health policy and craniofacial care: issues in resource allocation. Cleft Palate Craniofac J 31: 78–80.

Strauss, RP (1999). The organization and delivery of craniofacial health services: the state of the art. Cleft Palate Craniofac J 36: 189–195.

Summer, L, Parrott, S, Mann, C (1997). Millions of uninsured and underinsured children are eligible for medicaid. Center on Budget and Policy Priorities. Available from http://www.cbpp.org/mcaidprt.htm.

38

Parents' perspective on cleft lip and palate

JANE NICHOLSON

When a child is born with a cleft lip and/or palate (CL/P), it is most often a shock at the time of delivery. An enormous amount of information will have to be absorbed above and beyond that which is needed by all new parents. What follows is a compilation of the collective wisdom of a group of parents whose children were born with a cleft. It is our hope that these insights will make it easier for new parents of such children and those who provide care for them.

One mother of a 22-year-old with a repaired cleft lip and palate (CLP) reflected at the time of his graduation, "I wished I would have known how successful he would be and how well he would do. I wish someone had told me his own wonderful spirit would be the driving force of his success. No one tells you that things will be OK." Parents need to know that their children will do well. The key word should be *encouragement*. The encouragement should start from the very beginning.

For most parents, the birth of a child is a joyful event. After months of anticipation, we look forward to seeing and holding that newborn baby. The pain of childbirth will be over, but there can be a very noticeable difference in the tone of the birthing room when a child is born with CL/P.

There is an awkward moment when the doctor breaks the news: "Your child has a cleft lip and palate." Suddenly, all of the relief and joy that had been anticipated is replaced with fear and confusion. Most people have never seen an unrepaired CL/P, and to see it in the face of one's own child is a shock indeed. Those who find out at the time of an ultrasound scan may be equally anxious.

First and foremost, it is important for the medical personnel to assume a positive attitude. It is human na-ture to imagine the worst when one encounters something new and unexpected. Most parents who have lived with a child with a cleft could tell you that the reality is not as bad as they had expected. At every step along the way, health providers can help the parents by reassuring, giving hope, and providing resources.

From the moment of delivery onward, the tone and demeanor of the doctor and staff should be reassuring. "This is a common birth defect and one that can be repaired. Most children do well." If a pediatrician is not already present, then let the parents know that a pediatrician will take a look at the baby and make sure that otherwise everything is all right.

A subset of babies will need initial help with breathing and stabilization. Let the parents know what is taking place. If the baby needs to be moved to another area, make sure that the parents know what is being done and give timely updates. Reunite the parents and baby as soon as possible. Good communication is paramount.

Parents are worried and may feel that they are drowning and need a lifeline. Since their fears are probably far worse than the reality, the sooner they can get accurate information, the better. Be truthful. If you do not know what you are talking about, then do not offer incorrect information. Tell the parents that you will get them to the people who know about CL/P, and then do it.

Some hospitals will be more prepared than others. In a center where children are routinely seen with this problem, there may already be a team in place. Other hospitals should help the parents with their immediate needs and then connect them with specialists who can help with the baby's care.

First, the parents need some time to be with their baby. Let them hold and cuddle the infant. Meanwhile, a plan needs to be made about who needs to see the child and when this can be done. Once a plan is formulated, give the parents an outline of the game plan about who will see them and when.

Write information down and suggest that the parents do too. Because there is so much information, it helps to have it written down. Small amounts of information accumulate quickly. Most parents find it helpful to have some type of organizing notebook. While providing a notebook from the start is not necessary, it can be suggested. The materials provided can be grouped together in a folder. There can be a section where questions are kept.

Remember that many of these are first-time parents. They have to learn all of the same things as new parents. They have the added insecurity of not knowing what additional problems having a child with a cleft will bring. The severe fatigue and emotional roller coaster of postpartum hormonal changes can affect all new mothers. It can help to let the parents know that these are normal feelings.

It is also completely normal to feel sad, overwhelmed, and upset. One nurse told her patient, "First you have to grieve for the loss of the child that you thought you would have, then you will learn to love the child that you have been given." No one expects to have a child with a birth defect. Consideration should be given to having the parents meet with a social worker or psychologist.

Before parents are sent home from the hospital, they need at least the bare facts about the causes of CL/P. At some point, formal counseling with someone from genetics can be very helpful. However, right away, these parents will be faced with many people who will want to know what happened. It is human nature for parents to assume that they somehow caused or are responsible for the birth defect.

A simple explanation is all that is needed to start. "We do not know what causes cleft lips and palates, but we know that it was nothing that you did or failed to do during the pregnancy. They just happen." Some are the result of a genetic syndrome, but most are the result of multifactorial causes. It can happen to anyone in any family. Fingers should not be pointed at anyone. We do not choose the genes that we pass down to children. Be sure they hear "It is no one's fault." It is worth repeating.

Parents also need some idea about what repairs will be done and what they will entail. The initial repairs are not done for several weeks, so let the parents know that they will have time to absorb the information and learn.

Some hospitals have a plastic surgeon or an oral maxillofacial surgeon who can come and speak with the parents to give them information. Depending on the time of day and the other responsibilities of the surgeon, it may be later in the day or the following day when he or she can meet with the parents. If this is the case, then let the parents know. Sometimes, the parents will need to bring their baby to another hospital or clinic. If this is the case, then arrangements should be made on their behalf to have an appointment in a timely fashion. Then, they should be given up-to-date written materials to review on their own prior to this visit. Make sure that pamphlets are not outdated.

Confidence can be infectious. A positive attitude and confidence on the part of the surgeon make a world of difference to the parents. Parents have noted that it felt reassuring to have the plastic surgeon confidently tell them that this is something that can be fixed.

Before and after pictures are very helpful. Some surgeons have a notebook to share with parents so that they can have an idea of what to expect for their child. Many parents remember only people who did not have the most cosmetic repairs. Times and techniques have changed, and they need to know there are wonderful things that can be done with plastic surgery.

Because the cleft is in the middle of the baby's face, it is an instant point of focus. Help the parents learn that there is much more to their baby, something they will learn over time. Tell them their children are beautiful. Emphasize the positives and point out unique features, e.g., "Look at her beautiful eyes, hair, coloring, etc. . . ." Everyone likes to hear nice things about their child.

FEEDING

The most immediate concern is getting the child to eat. Many children with a cleft will have feeding difficulties. Tell the parents that this is the first challenge and that each baby is unique. There are many ways to help a baby eat, and what works for one may not work for another. Through trial and error the best means of feeding each baby will be determined.

One mother lamented that she was told that "these kids fail to thrive." Another said she was told that her child would have feeding problems but he did not. If only the medical staff had been more positive about it, e.g., "Some children with clefts have problems with feeding, but we will work with you to find out what works best for your child."

Bring in the most qualified person or persons to help. This may include a lactation consultant, a postpartum or newborn nurse, a pediatrician, or a speech–language pathologist. Many different specialty bottles, nipples, and feeding devices are available. Parents should not be sent home until a satisfactory means is found to feed their child.

If a mother has planned to breast-feed, then she should be encouraged but should know that up to 85% of babies may not physically be able to breast-feed. The normal mechanics of breast-feeding include suction from the baby's mouth around the nipple and pushing and squeezing the nipple against the roof of the mouth to release the milk. Suction may not be possible because of the cleft, and a defect in the roof of the mouth may make squeezing the milk out impossible. There are some techniques the mother can use to circumvent these problems, but it most often would take the skill of a lactation consultant to help with this complex process.

Some cannot breast-feed despite their best efforts. Many mothers will feel guilty because they feel like they have failed if they cannot breast-feed. Help the parents find the best way to feed their infant. Tell them that what is important is for this baby to eat and grow. If she wishes to pump and save the breast milk, provide access to a hospital-grade pump. Taking care of any infant is time-consuming and taking care of a baby with a cleft can be exhausting, so any saving of time is appreciated.

CLINIC AND HOSPITAL VISITS

Once the baby goes home, the family starts on a journey of clinic visits and surgeries that may last well into the baby's teens. It is overwhelming at first but becomes routine over time. It is important to get off to the right start and to have each clinic visit be a positive experience.

Sometimes coming to the hospital and clinic setting can be a relief. Out in public, families often have to explain about the child's cleft. It can be tiresome as parents would prefer to talk about the same things as all parents. In the medical community, seeing a child with a cleft is common and a cleft is only one of many different medical conditions. Hence, it gives a chance for the kids just to be kids. Joke and laugh with them. Treat them as if they are special.

One parent, a lawyer, commented that when a client steps into his office that person wants to feel that he or she has his undivided attention and at that moment is the most important person in the world to him. It is no different in the medical office. When parents bring their children to a clinic visit, they know that time is very short and much must be accomplished.

When the children come to clinic visits, recognize them as unique individuals. One parent noted, "It is extremely important to remember each child." Before the child walks into the clinic, always take time to read his or her chart. Review what has happened in the medical course of events. Consider having some place on the chart where unique things about the child can be noted, something like "collects rockets" or "plays soccer." Be sure to use the child's name.

Always introduce yourself and tell the family what your function is that day. Even if the child is familiar to you, it can help to say "I'm Doctor X, the oral surgeon. I saw you last December. Today, I want to take a look at you so we can talk about the next surgeries you may need." Or "I'm Doctor Z, one of the resident doctors who works with Dr. X, I am here to find out how you are doing. I have heard a lot about you. After I am done, I'll come back with Dr. X." Coming to clinic visits can be an anxious time, so it helps to know the game plan.

Language is very powerful. Pick the words and phrases you use carefully. Never talk down to a child. Try to be cognizant of the child's age. Although they may be young, they are likely to be smart and perceptive.

Never talk in front of the child as if he or she is not there. If it is necessary to use medical descriptions and technical terms, then explain them to the child and parents. For example, "I want to describe some things in medical terms to my colleagues so they can learn more about you and about your cleft lip and palate. When we are done, we will make sure that we explain everything to you. Then you can ask questions so that we make sure you understand everything too." Always be cognizant that the parents and child are listening. Take time at the end of the visit to make sure that all questions are answered.

Some families make a special event of the day when their children come to the clinic. Remember that these children have to be pulled out of their normal activities and often miss school. Since it is the nature of children to fit in with their peers, it can be awkward to have attention drawn to them because they have a difference. By making it a family day and a positive experience, some of the discomfort from missing activities may be offset.

SURGERIES

"Giving up my child to the surgeon was one of the hardest parts about having a child with a cleft," lamented one mother. It is indeed one of the hardest times and yet has to be faced repeatedly. There are some things that can make it easier.

Make certain everyone knows what to expect. When is the surgery to take place? What does it entail? How long is it expected to take? Will you let me know how things are going if it takes longer than expected? How long will the child be in the hospital? What does the recovery period involve? Who can we contact if we have questions or problems?

Have a written set of instructions. Be specific and detailed. Most parents are not medically oriented. It is better to write too much than not enough.

Let parents be with the child as much as possible. Many hospitals allow the child to be with a parent right up to the time that the child is being put to sleep. This helps the anxiety of both the parents and the child. Make certain parents are able to be with their child at all times in the hospital, including spending the night.

Over time, parents will realize that their child is much tougher than they thought. It does not hurt to hear this ahead of time. Kids become "old pros" at being tough for surgery, but we need to remember that they are still children.

RESOURCES

Parents universally felt that resources were paramount. Providing access to up-to-date resources is a valuable service of healthcare providers.

One of the most helpful resources is another family with a CL/P child. Most parents say they would be happy to help a new family. They can provide a wealth of information because they have been through the same things themselves. If such a network is not available in your community, consider starting one.

SPEECH

Most children with a cleft will need some degree of speech pathology services throughout their lives, but as with information about feeding problems, do not make blanket negative statements. Not all children will have problems, but those who do will have resources available to them.

As parents, we worry about how our children will communicate. Will they be intelligible? Will people make fun of them? Will they sound funny? We do not want anything to interfere with their independence and self-esteem.

Although speech difficulties are common, it is reassuring to know that there are resources to help. Speech–language pathologists have numerous ways to help children.

Parents should be told that there is teaching and assistance through their intermediate school district. Laws are in place which mandate services to children with special needs. They can be directed to these services by a social worker or a cleft support team. There

are also special funds that can be used to support the medical expenses of these children. Parents should not have to worry needlessly when there is funding available.

CONCLUSION

Parents have a special love for their children. All parents want their children to be happy. We want them to be free to enjoy childhood. We want to nuture their self-esteem, to give them the best chance at future endeavors. We all want to protect our children from harm.

While these are universal parental feelings, those of us who have CL/P children worry even more. In fact, because a child has a facial difference, the parents have a heightened sense of protectiveness for that child. While the children can do very well, it takes a while for the parents to see that. We need all of the support and nurturing we can get from healthcare providers. Help us so that we can launch our children into the world, just like that successful college graduate.

STORIES FROM PARENTS OF CHILDREN WITH ORAL CLEFTS

Karen's Story

My 4-year-old daughter, Ashley, is a bundle of smiles and sensitivity, with golden blonde hair. Although Ashley goes to speech therapy only two evenings per week, every night when I pick her up from day care she meets me with a smile and the same one-word question, "Speech?" Ashley truly enjoys the one-on-one instruction she receives from her speech therapist, Andrea, at the Scottish Rite Clinic in Roseburg, Oregon. Although her one-word question may not say much on its own, Ashley uses her eyes, smiles, and gestures to get her point across.

Ashley's story begins much earlier. Ashley's father was born with bilateral CLP. When I was 19 weeks pregnant, we chose to receive genetic counseling prior to the birth of our child. On January 26, 1996, her father and I unexpectedly learned that our daughter would be born with cleft lip (CL) and most likely cleft palate (CP). I began preparation for my daughter's birth with anticipation, shock, guilt, and fear. I made phone calls to doctors, friends, and national support groups to gather information on how to feed our daughter and what to expect with surgeries. My daughter's first encounter with a speech therapist came about while I was putting everything in place to prepare for her birth. I phoned the Child Development and Rehabilitation

Center in Portland, Oregon. The director of the craniofacial team, a speech–language pathologist, spoke
with me about what to expect after the birth of our
child and the services provided by their team. This pre-
birth instruction and the ongoing instruction and support our family receives from our craniofacial team
have been invaluable. Ashley was born with bilateral
CLP. We met with the craniofacial team, including the
speech therapist, for the first time when Ashley was
only 10 days old. I still remember the speech therapist
telling us that the first sounds to expect from Ashley
would be *M, N, H, W,* and *Y* as these do not require
air pressure to make them. My advice to all members
of a craniofacial team working with a parent who is
dealing with acceptance of a child born with a facial
birth defect is that first impressions are always remembered.

Since Ashley's father had first-hand experience of living with CLP and being a registered nurse myself, I felt
informed of what the future might hold and that we
had a foundation of knowledge and experience. However, but despite any knowledge a person has, there is
always more knowledge to obtain. My advice to all
members of a craniofacial team is to never assume that
parents who are members of the medical field or whom
have a cleft themselves comprehend their child's medical care. When Ashley and I are on the patient side of
medical care, I am her mother and no more. I need
things explained clearly and several times before medical information sinks in. The medical field is always
changing, as does the cleft and the child. Please, start
at ground zero and ask parents questions, reinforce information at follow-up appointments, use verbal communication a parent with no background in the medical field would understand, and allow parents time to
ask questions. There is an obvious and enormous benefit to meeting Ashley's needs through the interdisciplinary approach of the craniofacial team; however,
please know that a day with the craniofacial team can
be overwhelming when I walk away with new information about audiology, dentistry, plastic surgery, genetics, otolaryngology, and speech therapy, new information that changes my daughter's life.

The story continued when Ashley was referred to
early intervention for speech therapy. My advice to
members of a craniofacial team making a referral to an
outside agency is to follow through with families, ensuring that children you referred actually qualified for
services. My daughter was denied speech services at
both 10 and 17 months of age due to the wording of
the eligibility criteria, even though she had a wide CP
at 10 months of age and a large palatal fistula at 17
months of age. "Denied services?" I could not believe
it. Ashley had appropriate receptive and expressive lan-

guage at both assessments; however, impaired articulation by itself was not an eligibility criterion. When
she was 3 years old, I was told that the eligibility criteria had changed. What magically changes when a
child turns 3 years old so that she qualifies for speech
therapy? My advice to members of a craniofacial team
is to advocate for patients to receive speech therapy at
an early age and to be aware of eligibility criteria for
speech therapy in agencies with which you work. It
took my questions, ideas from my public health nurse,
and finally a physician to write a medical referral for
early intervention to qualify her for speech therapy.
Yes, even as a registered nurse, I need to bounce
ideas off of my public health nurse, who helps to case-
manage my daughter's medical care.

Ashley ended up qualifying for speech therapy in July
1998. Her speech therapist at the time worked with
Ashley at day care and sent assignments for me to work
on with Ashley at home. Therapy at her day care was
convenient, but I admit that homework was rarely done
because I had little idea of how much emphasis to put
on sounds and what type of correction I was supposed
to be giving Ashley. Although letters sent home for me
to read were beneficial, they did not help me to work
with my daughter. I was missing out on hearing what
Ashley was able to accomplish with her speech therapist at day care. Ashley's speech difficulties involve a
variety of factors, two of which are difficulty effectively
closing her top and bottom lips together as needed to
make sounds and a large palatal fistula. It was not until July 2000 and after two previous palatal surgeries
that Ashley's fistula was finally closed using a tongue
flap graft. Ashley frequently substitutes sounds she cannot make with alternatives and speaks in sentences with
few words or uses gestures to get her intent across. My
advice to all members of a craniofacial team is to make
sure parents observe every speech therapy session while
children are still young as both the child and the parent are impressionable.

In June 1999, as Ashley turned 3 years old, she was
re-evaluated to determine what services to provide for
the next year. The options included continuing speech
therapy at day care, placing her in Headstart preschool,
or attending the Scottish Rite Clinic. A worry her
speech therapist brought to this meeting was that she
could seldom find a quiet place to work with Ashley
at her day care without interruption from other children or teachers. My concern with placing Ashley in
Headstart was that she would start in the morning at
her regular day care, be transported to and from Headstart, and be returned to her regular day care until the
end of the day. I felt this was too much disruption for
a 3-year-old, who at the time had undergone a total of
eight surgeries and just experienced her parents' di-

vorce. My advice to all members of a cranio-facial team is to listen and help the family to look at all factors influencing the decision. Based on Ashley's needs, the decision was made, and Ashley settled in to the routine of speech therapy at the Scottish Rite Clinic. Ashley has remained there for 2 years now, and we are at present discussing how to transition her speech services to the public school next year for kindergarten. I observe every speech session, twice weekly. Ashley is currently working on the *P, B, T,* and *D* sounds while I sit in an adjoining room behind a one-way mirror. The one-on-one environment provides the attention that both she and I need to learn how to help her speech. Tomorrow, when I pick up Ashley from day care, chances are she will run up to me and say "Speech?" and I will remind her to say, "Mommy, are we going to speech today?" So that is how the story goes . . . at least for now.

Tanya's Story

My name is Tanya, of Troy, Tennessee. My husband John and I had a son, Ty, on January 6, 2000. Ty was born with bilateral complete CLP and no upper gums. My husband was born with unilateral CL; therefore, our chances of having a baby with a cleft were slightly higher. I learned how to feed using nasogastric tubes and syringes and later the Haberman feeders, which we still use today. I stress to parents the need to use the proper feeding methods with your children, feed in the upright position to reduce the risk of ear infections, burp also the same way due to the risk of aspiration, and always wash and sterilize everything that goes into their mouths due to infection. Enroll your child in an Early Interventions Program (they work with children up to 3 years of age and help you find the specialists you need). The Tennessee Infant/Parent Stimulation Program also will work with your child as far as hearing, vision, stimulation, and motor skills to make sure they are progressing as they should for their age. Keep all doctors' appointments, which include plastic surgeons, speech therapists, audiologists, and otolaryngologists among others. After surgery, always follow your doctor's suggestions as far as the feeding regimen and arm restraints. It is important not to affect the surgery site in any way by keeping foreign objects, fingers, and other things out of their mouths. So far, we have had no ear infections, but there is a heart murmur that will close spontaneously; finally, he's gaining weight. Make sure you keep your child's immunizations current. Read any and everything you can find on clefts. Unfortunately, we had no information or local groups here. I have been lucky and found everything on my own with the help of the Internet. There, I found the support of other families just like us, who had tons of information to offer. Check out the Widesmiles web site (www.widesmiles.org). Always remember that craniofacial anomalies can be repaired. Your children can grow up to live normal, happy lives with few or no effects. These children will endure much with the many surgeries that lie ahead, but remember that they are young and can heal more quickly. Through this ordeal, I have learned to appreciate how precious life is and how to be a better parent.

Aggie's Story

At the age of 21, I gave birth to a son with complete CP. When he was 3 months old, he had his first surgery. When he was 1.5 years old, his palate was closed. The surgeons explained to me that this is usually a two-part operation and that they like to close the hard and soft palate at the same time. The chances of it reopening were very high, and they were right: his soft palate reopened, to about the size of a dime. When he was 2 years old, the doctors decided to do some lip revisions and close the soft palate again. This operation was successful, and the soft palate stayed closed. When he was 5 years old, they performed a bone graft, to replace bone that was missing on the upper part of his jaw, where his two splits were. Meanwhile, I had to take him for speech therapy for 2 years, twice a week, to help him learn to speak more clearly. At the age of 15, he had grown enough to do the jaw alignment; they had to take out the upper part of his jaw and bring it forward, using metal plates and screws to hold the jaw correctly in his mouth. At the age of 16, he had surgery to reconstruct his nose and more lip revisions. They made the brim of his nose thinner, tucked his nostrils in a little, and built up the cartilage under his nose. Now, at the age of 17, he will be going for more revisions on his face, to make his lips even on both sides. I was very lucky that he was not born with any other problems but the CP. It was very hard for him growing up and making friends, but now he is older and knows how to handle situations. Being born with CP is very hard, but we all manage.

Lynn's Story

My daughter, Elaine, was born with unilateral CL 2 years ago. It was a surprise to my husband, our doctor, and me. When she was born, the nurses and doctor told us how they see CL often, but no one was able to offer us any factual, useful information.

For 2 months, we felt like the only people with a cleft baby. Then, we moved halfway across the country. Within 2 weeks, we were meeting a world-class plastic surgeon at a highly ranked hospital. She was scheduled for surgery within a month. I was nervous about putting my little darling under anesthesia and about changing the little face with the gap, the face I had loved from the first minute I had seen her, the face we bonded with and the smile that filled our hearts. I asked the cleft case nurse if there was a mother I could talk to who had gone through this surgery recently with her baby.

She called an hour later with the name of Susan G. Her son, Lance, had the same kind of cleft and had his repair the day my daughter was born. The way I looked at it was that Susan's family was 3 months ahead of us, so I could ask any question about what to expect during and after surgery as well as the recovery period. The first time we talked, I was overwhelmed by the emotions I revealed to her and found that we shared the same thoughts about the situation. There are some emotions and questions that constantly weigh your mind down: "What did I do wrong?" "How could I have prevented this?" "Why us?" "What if something goes wrong?" "Do we have to do it, she's so cute now?" To find someone who can say she felt the exact same way is like embracing an old friend you shared your deepest secrets with as a child. Friends and family were very supportive and reassuring but did not truly reassure me. I felt like they were patronizing me. They meant well and really tried, but I just did not feel comforted, until I heard Susan say "She'll be fine, and it will all go well." She said the same thing so many people had said to me, but she had the same true-life experience of the cleft, the feelings of guilt, the success of the repair, and the recovery. It was her comments and assurances that finally reached me.

Susan quickly became a wonderful resource, the most comforting and informative, even better than the literature or the Internet because she was a live person with whom I could interact. The doctor and cleft case nurse could only say so much; this was a routine job for them. They see literally hundreds or even thousands of cases,

many much worse than ours, every year, so I turned to Susan. I asked questions about the surgery, how long was he out, how much pain was he in, how long was he in surgery, how long before his swelling went down, etc. She reassured me by telling me how great and how different he looks. She even sent me pictures of him before and after surgery.

The most amazing thing about Susan and her family was how they opened their lives to us in many ways. They invited us to stay with them the night before the surgery because they lived 20 minutes away from the hospital and we lived 2 hours away. They had never met us, except for the numerous phone calls. They fed us dinner, gave us some snacks to get us through the waiting, and most importantly talked to us late into the night. Once the husbands went to bed, Susan and I stayed up talking until I had to give Elaine her last feeding at 3:45 A.M. The ease with which we talked was distracting enough that the night flew by. We talked about the surgery and about our lives, so we were able to relax and enjoy their hospitality.

The surgery went very well, and Susan was right: she looks like a different baby. We still talk to Susan and her family and, when we go for appointments with the plastic surgeon, we visit them. Recently, Elaine had a lip revision, and once again, I was on the phone with Susan because her son had had the same procedure done a couple of months before. She was available for me, and I have also been there for her; we have a bond now, which will always be there, no matter what.

Because the experience of having another mother to talk to was so rewarding for us, I asked that I be put on a list for any other mother who wants information or just to talk. At Elaine's first postoperative visit, I met Tracey S. and her family. I hope I have given her one-tenth of the support and reassurance I was given.

My daughter's cleft story is nothing extraordinary, unless you count Susan and her family. They were amazing, and they made the difference for us. They opened their home, their hearts, their lives, and their ears to us. For that, we will be eternally grateful.

39

Ethical issues in the care of children with craniofacial conditions

RONALD P. STRAUSS

Ethical issues that arise in the treatment of children with craniofacial anomalies often require health professionals, patients, and families to make difficult decisions. In this chapter, we examine the nature of ethical dilemmas and the principles that may guide ethical decision-making. A number of selected issues that affect craniofacial care are presented, but rather than providing answers to ethical dilemmas, we pose questions that readers can use to examine their own values and principles.

Ethical decisions involve questions of meaning and call for a distinction between what is "right" and what is "wrong." In the conduct of clinical care, judgments about fairness, human duty, and personal morals are ethical decisions. These are not technical questions that are meant for experts in ethics; rather, health professionals regularly make ethical decisions in clinical practice (Beauchamp and Childress, 1994; Jonsen et al., 1992).

Biomedical ethics has received considerable attention because clinical practice involves a professional who is called upon to decide or recommend "what is right" for a patient. Decisions that impact the lives of others, particularly in the context of healthcare, have stimulated substantial public and professional controversy. Biomedical ethical issues that generate public and media attention highlight general social and moral issues. In some regards, ethical issues in craniofacial care are particular cases of social and moral decisions that occur in the conduct of other human matters. For example, issues that relate to the access to costly dental services are merely a subset of the issues that relate to how a society manages access to scarce resources. The eth-

ical discourse will consider how individual benefit and the needs of the society can be fairly balanced. In the conduct of ethical decision-making, it may not be possible to both meet the desires of individuals and satisfy the needs of the society at large; however, both perspectives are recognized, and an equitable resolution is sought.

Health professionals have dealt with ethical decisions for many years and have sought to define guidelines for practice in their written codes of ethics (Beauchamp and Childress, 1994). While these codes provide a statement for a profession, they may not provide guidance to individual health professionals who face an ethical dilemma in their clinical practice. When such quandaries occur, a professional must first identify the ethical issue involved. While this seems simple, the routine of clinical practice may hide an ethical issue or the clinician may not consider the ethical aspects of the management decisions being made. Awareness that an ethical dilemma is present is a first step in making a decision. In some settings, the complexity of ethical problems makes ethics consultation useful. Many medical centers have an ethics committee or a consultant ethicist. Consultation may be informative, but the ultimate responsibility for a decision remains with the health professional, in consultation with the family and patient. Often, an ethics consultation will be used to outline the issues, various possible viewpoints, and the possible courses of action.

The values of health professionals, patients, and families determine their interpretation of ethical principles of autonomy, beneficence, and nonmaleficence. These principles may be complementary or in conflict. *Au-*

tonomy implies the ability of an individual to determine how he or she is to be treated by others. It means that a person can freely define the healthcare treatment, outcomes, and process to be used. Autonomy implies the ability to make reasonable decisions in one's self-interest. *Beneficence* is a principle by which a professional provides what he or she believes is best for another person. In the case of healthcare, a professional will judge what form of treatment is offered in a patient's best interest. Sometimes what the patient (or family) sees as the best course of action may not agree with the professional's vision of what would be in the best interest of the patient. When a patient and a professional hold differing views of the right course of action, who is to judge? Health professionals are often seen as being held to a principle of *nonmaleficence*, or the expectation that they will do everything possible to avoid harm, compared to creating good or well-being. In the surgical care of children with craniofacial anomalies, should the surgeon provide an operation to a patient because the family or patient expresses that wish? Should the surgeon provide the patient only with the treatment options he or she believes are optimal and disregard the other possibilities? Should a surgeon who does not believe that he or she can perform an operation without significant risk of harm refer the patient elsewhere? Issues of autonomy and beneficence arise frequently in communicating surgical treatment plans and in negotiating a course of care.

Another concept that affects clinical decision-making is competence. *Competence* implies the legal ability to make healthcare decisions. Adults are assumed to be competent unless their legal decision-making rights have been granted to others, such as a legal guardian or one with power of attorney. Children are not generally considered competent to make independent decisions without a guardian's involvement. The legal age of competence varies considerably across and within nations; however, some pediatricians and ethicists have used the concept of a *mature minor,* in which an adolescent or child is judged to be developmentally capable of making a decision about his or her own care. On occasion, decision-making authority is granted to a legal minor based on his or her ability and desire to decide. Confidential communications between health professionals and adolescents about birth control, sexually transmitted diseases, and substance use may affect how involved the parent or guardian will be in clinical decision-making about the minor. Individuals who because of limited intellectual capacity or disabilities are unable to engage in the informed consent process may be considered not competent.

The difference between legal age of competence and the mature minor concept highlights the idea that there sometimes is a difference between the law and ethics.

It may be legal to allow parents to decide about a 15-year-old patient's planned craniofacial surgery; however, it may be ethical to empower the teen to actually make the treatment decision. It may be legal for a professional to perform a procedure on a patient, but it may not be ethical for him or her to do so.

Justice is a complex principle that involves three related concepts: treating people fairly, giving people what they deserve, and giving people what they are entitled. These concepts may not be in agreement; however, they are tied to distributive justice or approaches to allocate resources in a society (Churchill, 1987). Issues of justice may be found on the macroallocation level, which examines how goods and services are rightly distributed in the society at large. Microallocation issues may affect how a practitioner decides to allocate attention or time and the conduct of clinical care. In the case of craniofacial surgery, the costly nature of care and the scarcity of trained personnel contribute to this being seen as a scarce resource. Various microallocation approaches may be proposed to decide who gets craniofacial surgical care and who does not. Does the sickest person receive care first? Does the wealthiest or the most valued member of society receive care first? Is care distributed on a first-come, first-served basis or by merit? Who will determine? Elements in microallocation decision-making include *(1)* medical indications (who is most likely to appreciate a medical benefit or who is in greatest need), *(2)* patient preferences (what the patient desires in care), *(3)* quality-of-life aspects (how care or lack of care will affect a patient's ability to experience comfort, security, and function), and *(4)* contextual features such as social, cultural, economic, and legal factors (Jonsen et al., 1992).

It is also important to recall that medical practice deals primarily with the doctor–patient relationship, in which the doctor's primary goal is to meet the needs of a patient. On a public health or policy level, health professions are called upon to protect society and to maxime justice. These goals may differ, especially in organizations where the health professional may be asked to meet patient, societal, and market/organizational goals.

Ethics is not only an abstract endeavor; rather, it illuminates real-life problems and guides decision-making. Examples or cases are often useful in making ethical issues real and allowing for debate and consideration of various options (Strauss, 1995).

GATEKEEPING

In the past, many children with major craniofacial deformities did not survive or had a markedly reduced quality of life. This happened because of limitations in the ability to offer nutrition, surgical care, and post-operative assistance (Scheper-Hughes, 1990). The success of neonatal intensive care units, anesthetic advances, and changes in craniofacial surgery have made it possible to treat many serious defects that may once have been untreatable, even lethal. Medical education socializes health professionals and surgeons to be activist in their responses. They are trained to intervene in deformities and seek to repair or alter disabilities when possible. The decision not to offer care or to withdraw care already started is always difficult and places the health professional in struggle with established healing values. Clinical activism expressed as the desire to fix disabilities orients the professional toward providing craniofacial surgical treatment whenever possible.

The professional's role as a gatekeeper to medical and surgical services is critical as the health professional serves as an agent for the society in making such care decisions. The gatekeeper role involves exerting control over the availability of clinical treatment. Furthermore, the gatekeeper explains care to the parties that pay for treatment. The gatekeeper role for clinicians raises some difficult ethical questions (Strauss, 1983). Health professionals must consider whether infants with major and handicapping craniofacial deformities routinely should be offered treatment in the neonatal intensive care unit. Surgeons may find themselves asking whether severely affected children should always receive craniofacial surgical care. They may search for criteria that might be used to decide when to offer such care. Furthermore, questions may arise about who should make the decision to treat or not to treat. Are decisions best left to the parents, to the surgeons, to the ethics committee, or to multiple parties? Indeed, surgeons will likely ask themselves to what extent should the health professional or surgeon direct the use of scarce and costly resources (Ward, 1995). The role of allocating treatment resources raises many questions of distributive justice. Surgeons must puzzle their role in the healthcare system and consider how many resources can be directed toward any individual child.

Several factors may encourage health professional gatekeepers to be overly activist about providing care or to offer access to surgery even in possibly risky or costly situations. Health professionals may consider themselves charged by the society with the role of normalizing children born with defects. This sense of mission may be enhanced by the desire to perform heroic, novel, and highly technical treatments. The health professional's gatekeeper role may also call upon a clinician to consider quality-of-life factors. Knowledge of the social and psychological implications of major craniofacial deformities may impact clinicians' willingness

to offer treatment: they may be willing to recommend care in the hope that nonbiological benefits may result from appearance or functional change.

The role of health professional gatekeeper often implies an ethical conflict of interest. In many settings, the health professional both controls access to medical services and is financially rewarded for providing care. This is most evident in fee-for-service payment contexts where the health professional is compensated for the amount of treatment provided (Hall, 1992).

Capitation payment mechanisms, in which a health professional is uniformly paid for care of patients enrolled in a plan, tend to diminish overtreatment or excessive treatment. The financial reward system of a capitation plan will not reinforce activism. Some managed care plans limit referrals to specialty services by financially rewarding generalists who deny referrals. This may result in too few referrals for craniofacial surgery, even when care is warranted. Health professional compensation mechanisms exert pressures on clinical decision-making and may place stress on ethical roles. When health professionals and healthcare payers are thoughtful in controlling treatment activism, the gatekeeper role is working well.

INFORMED CONSENT, DISCLOSURE, AND CONFLICT RESOLUTION

Nowhere in healthcare is information more critical than in the seeking of informed consent (Beauchamp and Childress, 1994). Questions of health professional–patient–family communication are central to the informed consent process. Health professionals must consider how much detail should be told to patients or families. Does too much detail about risk scare a patient? What complications does a family need to be informed about prior to surgery? Should potentially lethal complications always be communicated? In seeking informed consent, the health professional must decide how much information is needed and can be understood by a patient or family. While there are many examples of informed consent being conducted so that all possible negative outcomes are listed, this may not be in the best interests of the patient or family. Overly graphic or extreme forms of truth-telling may enhance expectations of postoperative pain or disability.

Informed consent may be particularly challenging when cultural, language, or educational differences exist between the health professional and the family. When communicating across social differences, special attention must be paid to ensuring that information is not only provided but also understood (Kleinman, 1979). Families may not comprehend the language of biomedical thinking and often do not understand statistical risk. Special care may be needed to explain the recurrence risk of an anomaly or the chance of a negative surgical outcome to a patient who does not fully understand the meaning of percentages. Ethicists have sometimes wondered if fully informed consent is ever possible. They have considered whether a surgeon can ever accurately convey the likelihood and quality of postoperative pain to a patient. Can the surgeon really know how or what the patient will feel? The limitations of linguistic ability to describe sensations may be felt by clinicians seeking to be fully informative.

Ethical dilemmas have arisen when patients or families have asked a health professional not to inform them about a specific issue. This may occur when a parent does not want to be told about environmental or genetic causes of an anomaly in their child or in a family that does not wish to learn about the recurrence risk of a condition during genetic counseling. In such cases, the health professional may find it difficult to possess important information that the family seeks to avoid or deny. Issues of privacy and confidentiality have also arisen in the counseling setting. Are both parents always informed of the causes or recurrence risks during counseling? What is the potential family harm in truth-telling? Do all family members have a right to know about etiology, or is there ever a right to privacy, even within a family? At what point does the child or a spouse need to be informed of the likelihood of having future offspring with a genetic defect?

The transfer of information about surgical care may be a concern in the teaching and training hospital setting. Should students and residents make it clear to patients that they are inexperienced and in training? Should it be apparent to families exactly who will be making cuts or suturing their child in the operating room? Does seeking care in an academic health center imply that students and residents will be care providers. Issues of truth-telling, of informed consent and of authority to make healthcare decisions occur on a routine basis in professional practice.

Most health professionals see their principal roles as being within the individual doctor–patient relationship. The health professional is seen as having a powerful personal relationship with a patient and the family. Health professionals are taught to see themselves as advocates for the child patient as well as for the parents. They may have difficulties when the interests of patients and parents do not coincide. For example, in a situation where a child has a serious but partially correctable craniofacial defect that would require risky and costly surgical care and the family expresses a wish to avoid treatment, the clinician may be placed in a difficult position. Is the parental decision in the child's best interest? Whose interests does the health professional serve when there is a determination to make? Legisla-

tive and judicial decisions may become central in guiding such medical decisions and in defining the limits of parental autonomy. The surgeon may ask whether it is his or her role to argue for care when a family is risk-averse. There are many examples of health professionals who have sought court-sanctioned permission to provide care on a minor when the family is unwilling to authorize treatment. On occasion, families with religious beliefs that preclude treatment (i.e., Jehovah's Witnesses and blood transfusion) have been forced by court order to comply with surgical recommendations. Does the reverse occur? Can families force a craniofacial surgeon to provide care that he or she believes is unnecessary or too risky? Courts have not forced unwilling surgeons to provide care; however, one might speculate how often craniofacial surgeons are pressured by parents to operate when the expectation of positive clinical outcomes is minimal.

This discussion of information sharing and potential conflicts might be mistakenly taken to suggest that parents, children, and health professionals are often in a contentious relationship. However, this would be inaccurate since most families and health professionals work harmoniously to achieve common goals that are guided by the child's best interest. Such harmony occurs when there is mutual respect and careful information sharing that avoids persuasive or emotional language.

ALLOCATION OF RESOURCES

In the realm of craniofacial care, ethical dilemmas occur not only in the direct provision of craniofacial health services but also in the decisions that guide the healthcare distribution, organization, and policies.

One must first consider that every society has a means to allocate resources. In the United States, we have long sought to understand the role of the healthcare professional in the allocation of care and the control of cost. It is critical to remember that behind a society's allocation of resources lay values, political forces, and a vision of justice. Decisions about how scarce or limited resources should be distributed reflect a society's perspective on equity and justice (Churchill, 1987).

The definition of what is a "just" system for the distribution of services or products varies across countries and cultures. The choice of an allocation approach will determine who receives services and at what cost. Several individual allocation approaches have been promoted as "just."

The *open-market approach* would have services offered to each person according to ability to pay. This approach expands the variety of services available to the wealthy, while limiting access to less affluent populations. The *merit approach* would distribute services to each person according to their efforts to avoid having need. Under this approach, persons who do not smoke tobacco, who abstain from alcohol consumption, and who maintain a healthy lifestyle might be offered access to health services and those with less merit would not. This approach would deny care to precisely the segment of the population most likely in need of health services. The *social worth approach* would give services to persons according to the degree to which they contribute to the society. More highly valued members of society would have greater access and choice of services. Decisions about the value of an individual to the society are loaded with questions of bias, prejudice, and stigmatization. The social worth system was briefly used to allocate kidney dialysis machines in the 1960s in Seattle; however, the basis for establishing social worth was very controversial. This approach has been effectively employed only during wartime or emergencies. The *rights approach* would see access to services or health care as a right, at least for each individual to have equal access to basic care according to the need for services. Two other schemes have been proposed to allocate resources. One scheme uses chance and would see healthcare given to each according to luck or according to a lottery. Another approach would have scarce resources delivered on a *first-come, first-served* basis, according to place in line. A combination of approaches may be used, e.g., when a basic level of need is first met and then potential recipients enter a lottery.

To understand distributive justice in the United States, one might ponder how this society allocates resources such as food, primary education, secondary education, and luxury cars. It becomes immediately obvious that the United States employs a mixture of the various allocation approaches reviewed.

What forces guide resource allocation to craniofacial care? Several social considerations may influence how resources will be allocated to craniofacial care. Decisions may be made in the context of age, in which there is a competition for resources between younger, less powerful interests and older, growing, and more powerful political segments. Furthermore, the visibility of a clinical condition may be a real factor in resource allocation decisions. Visible defects are more likely to affect voter and legislator emotions. Community awareness and human interest are factors that impact social decisions and draw media attention to an issue. Anticipated voter behaviors are probably the single most useful predictor of legislative decisions.

Decisions about the allocation of funds to craniofacial care will be made in the context of limited resources in societies where demands on the healthcare system exceed the system capacity. Fundamental ethical questions will be raised in these deliberations. Advocates for craniofacial care will need to respond when asked about how to use limited dollars for healthcare: e.g., when dollars are limited, should they be spent on population-based prevention or should they be spent on the treatment of relatively rare but disabling conditions? In considering whether limited resources are best spent on prevention or on treatment, some would state that health and economic resources are most rationally invested in maternal and prenatal healthcare and on established preventive regimes. For example, it could be argued that prevention of fetal alcohol syndrome is preferable to focusing resources on its treatment. However, not all conditions are preventable and some preventive methods or approaches have had greater power than others. In making resource allocation decisions, it will be important to consider the efficacy and cost of preventive initiatives. In the case of major craniofacial deformities, current resources might best be spent on research into the prevention of defects. This might involve developing programs that encourage maternal health and nutrition, genetic counseling, screening, and therapy. However, the major craniofacial disorders are rare and currently often of unknown etiology. Given the paucity of preventive craniofacial research and effort, resources are currently focused on clinical treatment.

Health professionals do not ask questions about social justice when encountered with a specific patient's needs. Few would find it reasonable for a clinician to worry about whether the society's resources are better spent on public health or immunization than on expensive surgical reconstruction. Most citizens would agree that public dollars would be better invested in the realm of prevention, yet when faced with the denial of reconstruction to the individual patient due to limited resources, the decision is often to provide care.

Values on the worth of the individual are strongly held, and rationing of U.S. healthcare has proven to be a difficult prospect, though it happens in a de facto way regularly. When rationing of healthcare occurs, it may be through limited insurance policies, total lack of health insurance coverage, or a scarcity of providers or facilities. The issues arise when payment is not available and when care is very costly. If patients cannot themselves afford care and insurers are unable or unwilling to pay, then the true impact of scarce resources becomes apparent.

Low-income and minority populations do not uniformly have access to high-quality health services in the United States. This is reflected in their relatively lower health status when compared to more affluent or nonminority populations. In a society where marked differences in access to healthcare exist, one must ask whether the ability to pay is the most just mechanism for deciding who is to receive care. In the case of major craniofacial deformities, should ability to pay for expensive services guide their availability? In the case of costly procedures that benefit very few persons, political advocacy seems unlikely to be a large force in guiding insurance coverage. Principles of social justice do come into play when decision-makers consider how much quality of life would decline if care were denied or how much gain could be achieved by funding treatment. These decisions are difficult to make, and cost–benefit thinking may be used in making them.

Some of the most difficult resource distinctions occur around the relative worth of social investments in various diagnoses. Why is a cleft palate repair generally seen as cost-effective, while some question a cloverleaf skull deformity repair? Is it that we expect a better outcome from the cleft lip/palate surgery? Or is it that the frequency of cleft lip/palate demands repair, while the scarcity of major craniofacial syndromes does not? If the society can afford to provide cleft repairs, why then not afford craniofacial repairs? Clearly, questions of the magnitude of cost exist. The costs as calculated cannot be merely the direct costs of several years of surgical care; rather, they must also include the costs of parental work loss, of special education, of rehabilitation services, of mental health assistance, of lost patient productivity, and of mental anguish. These costs are generally not measurable, yet they constitute a real part of the losses and quality of life realized. Cost awareness and the need to control the cost of healthcare have affected the willingness to incur extraordinary medical expenses. Cost–benefit calculations have been applied to treatment decisions, but often these calculations break down when the possible denial of care to a specific child becomes a reality. The cost of correcting major craniofacial conditions may sometimes be extremely high but must be weighed against the social and humanitarian costs of not providing access to care. In the current context of declining health dollars and limited resources, it is predictable that some rationing decisions will be made. The allocation approach to be applied is unclear, but it will determine who will be cared for and who will not.

PRENATAL DIAGNOSIS

Prenatal diagnosis of major craniofacial or genetic conditions is increasingly common (Bosk, 1992; Eng et al., 1997). The use of continuous real-time ultrasound allows for the early visualization of fetal defects. Techniques such as amniocentesis, genetic screening, and risk appraisal may provide the family and health pro-

fessionals with information about a child's craniofacial defect prior to birth (Rothman, 1986). Knowledge of a condition during the prenatal period implies the possibility of choice relative to the birth of a child with a defect.

Knowledge about defects prior to birth has caused medicine to face profound questions about how we as a society will deal with prenatal information about serious craniofacial deformities (Murray and Botkin, 1995; Roberston, 1986). Will there be significant pressure on mothers to abort such fetuses in order to avoid the cost and pain of corrections? Will there be rewards for parents who decide to save the society the cost of treatment? Will we stigmatize and harass parents for seeking to terminate a life, regardless of quality, by abortion (Lapham et al., 1996)?

The realities of the high cost associated with the survival and treatment of children with major craniofacial defects may affect how we perceive a parent decision to abort a fetus with an identified deformity. A decision to bear such a child implies major expenditures for the parents and/or the society.

Social values relative to aesthetic and functional conformity may also be challenged by prenatal diagnosis of defects (Wexler, 1995; Wertz and Fletcher, 1989). Will all deformed infants be aborted? How major a deformity must there be to rationalize an abortion (Blumenfeld et al., 1999; Eiserman and Strauss, 1999)? Will there be less tolerance of different appearance or identity if all those with different identities are aborted or corrected? To what extent does living with a range of appearances and disabilities benefit a society? Some would argue that medicine should exert itself to make children look as normal as possible to meet social expectations. Others would say that instead of changing the child or his or her appearance, the focus should be on changing social values to encourage the acceptance of those who appear different. For the moment, there is little question that those who look different are treated as less than equal and often are stigmatized (Fiedler, 1978).

CONCLUDING COMMENTS

The care of children with craniofacial conditions raises many issues that involve ethical and moral choices. In this chapter, we have examined the principles that support ethical decisions and introduced concepts such as autonomy, beneficence, nonmaleficence, competence, justice, and informed consent. Selected ethical issues were considered, including professional gatekeeper roles, informed consent and truth-telling, allocation of scarce resources, and implications of prenatal diagnosis. These were chosen because they demonstrate the range of ethical dilemmas that arise in craniofacial care. Other issues that might have been examined include the following:

- The relationship between risk to the child and benefit
- Professional-peer relations and quality of care
- Issues in surgical and clinical research
- The neonatal intensive care unit as a locus for ethical decisions
- Quality of life with or without surgery
- The control of sophisticated medical technology and the introduction of new techniques

The ethical dilemmas and issues raised in this chapter stimulate moral and personal questions to which there are rarely easy answers. If the answers were apparent, they would not be ethical dilemmas or quandaries. However, health professionals must be prepared to deal with such questions and must find satisfactory answers to the ethical dilemmas that they encounter in their careers. One would hope that there is willingness to consider the complex issues suggested here and that clinicians and those engaged in healthcare financing and policy making will participate in a lively discussion of the ethics of craniofacial care. Toward that end, each participant in the conversation might pose the following questions:

- What moral issues are involved?
- What varied options are possible?
- What are the ramifications of each of the options?
- Does this decision relate to larger ethical questions?
- Is there a philosophy/value system that guides your ethical actions?

REFERENCES

Beauchamp, T, Childress, J (1994). *Principles of Biomedical Ethics*, 4th ed. New York: Oxford University Press.

Blumenfeld, Z, Blumenfeld, I, Bronshtein, M (1999). The early prenatal diagnosis of cleft lip and the decision-making process. Cleft Palate Craniofac J *36*: 105–107.

Bosk, CL (1992). *All God's Mistakes: Genetic Counseling in a Pediatric Hospital*. Chicago: University of Chicago Press.

Churchill, LR (1987). *Rationing Health Care in America: Perceptions and Principles of Justice*. Notre Dame, IN: University of Notre Dame Press.

Eiserman, W, Strauss, RP (1999). Commentary on early prenatal diagnosis and the decision-making process. Cleft Palate Craniofac J *36*: 542–545.

Eng, C, Schechter, C, Rabinowitz, J, et al. (1997). Prenatal genetic carrier testing using triple disease screening. JAMA *278*: 1268–1272.

Fiedler, L (1978). *Freaks, Myths and Images of the Secret Self*. New York: Simon and Schuster.

Hall, MA (1992). The political economics of health insurance market reform. Health Aff (Millwood) 108–124.

Jonsen, AR, Siegler, M, Winslade, W (1992). *Clinical Ethics: A Practical Approach to Ethical Decisions in Clinical Medicine*, 3rd ed. New York: McGraw-Hill.

Kleinman, A (1979). Sickness as cultural semantics: issues for an anthropological medicine and psychiatry. In: *Toward a New Definition of Health*, edited by P Ahmed and G Coelho. New York: Plenum, pp. 53–65.

Lapham, VE, Kozma, C, Weiss, JO (1996). Genetic discrimination: perspectives of consumers. Science *274*: 621–624.

Murray, TH, Botkin, JR (1995). Genetic testing and screening: ethical issues. In: *Encyclopedia of Bioethics*, rev. ed., Vol. 2, edited by WT Reich. pp. 174–178.

Roberston, JA (1986). Legal issues in prenatal therapy. Clin Obstet Gynecol *29*: 603–611.

Rothman, BK (1986). *The Tentative Pregnancy: Prenatal Diagnosis and the Future of Motherhood*. New York: Viking.

Scheper-Hughes, NM (1990). Difference and danger: the cultural dynamics of childhood stigma, rejection and rescue. Cleft Palate J *27*: 301–307.

Strauss, RP (1983). Ethical and social concerns in facial surgical decision making. Plast Reconstr Surg *72*: 727–730.

Strauss, RP (1995). Experiencing ethical dilemmas: cases of ethical decision-making in the care of children with major craniofacial deformities. Cleft Palate Craniofac J *32(6)*: 494.

Ward, C (1995). Essays on ethics relating to the practice of plastic surgery. In: *British Journal of Plastic Surgery*. Harlow: Churchill Livingstone.

Wertz, DC, Fletcher, JC (eds) (1989). *Ethics and Human Genetics: A Cross Cultural Perspective*. Berlin: Springer-Verlag.

Wexler, A (1995). *Mapping Fate: A Memoir of Family, Risk, and Genetic Research*. New York: Random House.

40

Translating research findings into public health action and policy

RICHARD S. OLNEY

CYNTHIA A. MOORE

Cleft lip and cleft palate are important to public health in terms of birth prevalence, associated disabilities, costs of care, and psychosocial impact. Scientific studies relating to these issues are outlined in other chapters of this book. In this chapter, we focus on the practical application of scientific knowledge by public health providers to prevent and ameliorate birth defects at the community level. Some of the examples in this chapter do not necessarily apply directly to orofacial clefts. However, since these examples of birth defect programs include other malformations of similar public health importance such as neural tube defects, or are programs directed at exposures and outcomes that may also be related to orofacial clefts, they represent model approaches to public health aspects of birth defects that may also apply to cleft lip and cleft palate.

One public health program at the Centers for Disease Control and Prevention (Centers for Disease Control and Prevention, Division of Diabetes Translation, 2001) has defined its role in translating research findings into widespread clinical and public health practice in the following ways:

- Targeting special populations to improve access to affordable, high-quality services
- Supporting extramural prevention programs
- Researching better ways to apply scientific findings
- Strengthening surveillance systems to better define and monitor the burden of disease

This conceptual framework will be used here to discuss areas of public health policy and action that may apply to emerging epidemiologic, genetic, and clinical research findings related to cleft lip and cleft palate.

IMPROVING ACCESS TO AFFORDABLE, HIGH-QUALITY SERVICES

The roles of providers and agencies in the public health aspects of genetic disorders and birth defects include preventing such conditions and developing and instituting measures to prevent suffering and related disabilities when such disorders occur (Khoury et al., 1993). Application of the latter approach, sometimes called tertiary prevention but more accurately known as disability prevention, is an important public health activity for children with orofacial clefts (Pope and Tarlov, 1991). In translating scientific advances into practice, public health agencies and providers become involved with clinical programs to ensure that affected children are identified and linked with specialty care shortly after birth, that the costs of such medical care are covered (often with public funds), and that appropriate interventions are actually provided. Public health agencies and related organizations have been involved with a variety of initiatives to ensure that these goals are addressed (Table 40.1).

As noted in Section II of this book, treatment of affected children has traditionally relied on multidisciplinary teams to address a variety of aspects of long-term care beyond surgical repair and often on cutting-edge advances in clinical practice that may be available only at referral centers in certain geographic areas. These teams have existed for many years (Ely, 1969; Ivy, 1971). However, active involvement of state public health agencies with craniofacial teams has been incomplete. *Healthy People 2010* sets national public health priorities in the United States; in the chapter on

TABLE 40.1. *Public Health Initiatives Relating to Comprehensive Clinical Care for Children with Orofacial Clefts and Other Special Healthcare Needs*

Initiative	Goals Addressed	Agencies/Organizations	Internet Address
National Agenda for Children with Special Health Needs	Access to quality healthcare, provider training, financing issues	Health Resources and Services Administration/Maternal and Child Health Bureau (HRSA/MCHB)	http://www.mchb.hrsa.gov/ html/achieving_ measuringsuccess.html
Healthy People 2010	Early identification and referral, surveillance for interventions	Healthy People Consortium (alliance of more than 350 national membership organizations and 250 state agencies, including the Association of State and Territorial Dental Directors, Centers for Disease Control and Prevention, and HRSA/MCHB)	http://www.health.gov/ healthypeople/document/ html/volume2/ 21oral.htm
Recommended Benchmarks of Health Care Benefits for Newborns, Infants Children	Care from qualified providers; coordination of medical, preventive, and developmental services	Federal Interagency Coordinating Council (multiple agencies including the Social Security Administration and Departments of Education, Health and Human Services, Agriculture, Interior, and Defense)	http://www.fed-icc.org/ policy/hcbench.htm
Medical Home Initiatives for Children with Special Needs	Accessible, continuous, comprehensive, coordinated heath-care services	American Academy of Pediatrics, HRSA/MCHB	http://ww.aap.org/ advocacy/medhome/ ResourcesCenter.htm

oral health, objective 21-15 promotes efforts to increase the number of states that have a system for recording and referring children with orofacial clefts to craniofacial rehabilitative teams (US Department of Health and Human Services, 2000). As a baseline, 23 states surveyed and the District of Columbia had such systems in 1997 (US Department of Health and Human Services, 2000). Objective 21-16 advocates for craniofacial health surveillance systems, one purpose of which is to implement and evaluate interventions. In Britain, a craniofacial surveillance system (currently known as the Craniofacial Anomalies Register) has operated since 1982 (Hammond and Stassen, 1999).

Title V of the Social Security Act mandated comprehensive care by states for children with special needs, and state health departments have set up specific offices and coordinators for these efforts through funding by the federal Maternal and Child Health Bureau (currently part of the Health Resources and Services Administration, HRSA/MCHB) (Walker, 2000). Some of these state programs directly fund healthcare reimbursement for children with orofacial clefts who are seen in multidisciplinary craniofacial clinics. The HRSA/MCHB has also promulgated the National Agenda for Children with Special Health Needs to set specific goals (Table 40.1). Important outcomes of this initiative include adequate insurance coverage for all affected children and ongoing comprehensive care for all children. Another component of the agenda is early screening for special needs; e.g., the HRSA/MCHB (in partnership with the CDC and the federal Office of Special Education and Rehabilitation Services) now funds

universal newborn hearing screening programs in many states, which should lead to interventions earlier in infancy for hearing impairment with or without craniofacial anomalies.

The medical home concept is closely related to comprehensive care initiatives for children with special healthcare needs. The essence of the medical home movement is to ensure continuous, coordinated, and comprehensive care for children with chronic conditions, which is a particular necessity when insurance coverage is provided in a managed care environment requiring a single provider to refer for multidisciplinary care (American Academy of Pediatrics Committee on Children with Disabilities, 1997). The HRSA/MCHB has also funded the American Academy of Pediatrics to establish the National Center of Medical Home Initiatives for Children with Special Needs. The goals of the center are to develop advocacy materials for medical home providers and issue recommendations that benefit children with chronic conditions and to assess outcomes (Table 40.1).

PREVENTION PROGRAMS

Examples of public health prevention programs for birth defects or other reproductive outcomes are listed in Table 40.2. State-sponsored prenatal screening programs, although better established than other prevention programs, primarily involve pregnancies affected with neural tube defects, abdominal wall defects, or multiple congenital anomaly syndromes such as trisomy

TABLE 40.2. *Birth Defect Prevention Programs*

Type of Etiologic Risk Factor	Protective Factor or Cause	Outcome	Public Health Interventions
Nutrition	Folic acid	Neural tube defects	Food fortification, targeted supplementation
Behavioral	Smoking	Low birth weight	Smoking cessation programs
Genetic	Chromosomal abnormalities	Trisomy syndromes	Maternal serum screening programs
Teratogenic drugs	Isotretinoin and thalidomide	Associated multiple congenital anomaly syndromes	Pregnancy Prevention Program (isotretinoin), STEPS program (System for Thalidomide Education and Prescribing Safety)

18 or 21 (Cunningham et al., 1998; Cunningham and Tompkinson, 1999; Kirby, 2000). These public health programs will not be considered in detail here because orofacial clefts are not common features of the currently targeted disorders and a limited number of public health agencies and providers are involved with the programs.

The folic acid story is an example of an evolving prevention program that could also potentially prevent orofacial clefts. The role of nutritional factors in preventing orofacial clefts is reviewed extensively in Section I of this book. In summary, some observational studies have shown risk reduction by folic acid/multivitamins in the occurrence of orofacial clefts, although more research is needed to fully evaluate this hypothesis. Based on strong epidemiologic evidence showing the efficacy of folic acid at reducing the risk for another group of congenital anomalies, neural tube defects, public health approaches to increasing folic acid consumption have proceeded in a variety of ways (Watkins, 1998). The most important interventions have included encouraging supplementation (consumption of multivitamins) and food fortification in the United States. These efforts have occurred through partnerships between such groups as federal and state public health agencies, professional organizations, community service and advocacy organizations such as the March of Dimes, and grass-roots spina bifida associations. Because some folic acid–related interventions will have general effects on public health and are not solely targeted to pregnancies at high risk for neural tube defects, these programs might lower the birth prevalence of orofacial clefts.

Smoking cessation programs are another example of widespread public health efforts aimed at effecting a variety of healthy outcomes that could also potentially lower rates of orofacial clefts, based on the epidemiologic evidence discussed elsewhere in this book. In the 1990s, studies showed that approximately one-quarter of U.S. women of reproductive age smoked, while reported smoking rates during pregnancy were slightly less than 20% (Centers for Disease Control and Prevention, 1994; National Center for Health Statistics, 2000). One of the *Healthy People 2010* objectives (16-17) is to increase the cigarette abstinence rate among pregnant women to 99% (US Department of Health and Human Services, 2000). A meta-analysis of smoking cessation programs targeted specifically toward pregnant women showed them to be effective at reducing smoking rates as well as adverse outcomes clearly linked to perinatal tobacco use: low birth weight and preterm birth (Lumley et al., 2000).

A third type of prevention program is aimed at reducing exposure of pregnant women to teratogenic drugs. Currently known teratogens, such as anticonvulsant medications, have been associated with less than 5% of orofacial clefts (Abrishamchian et al., 1994). However, new gene–drug interactions may yet be identified (see Section I of this book), leading to prevention programs. Isotretinoin embryopathy is one condition that occasionally includes cleft palate in addition to other characteristic craniofacial defects, central nervous system abnormalities, and conotruncal heart defects (Fernhoff and Lammer, 1984). In 1988, the drug manufacturer (Hoffmann–La Roche, Inc., Nutley, New Jersey) together with the Food and Drug Administration (FDA) implemented a Pregnancy Prevention Program in women of childbearing age who were receiving isotretinoin (Mitchell et al., 1995). The pregnancy rate among women enrolled in this program was substantially lower than that in the general population, but this voluntary program enrolled only approximately half of the women taking the drug between 1989 and 1993. Even among the 177,216 women enrolled in the program, 402 pregnancies occurred. In 2000, an advisory committee to the FDA recommended that the isotretinoin program be further strengthened by making registration of female patients and verification of a negative pregnancy test mandatory (Food and Drug Administration, 2000; House Committee on Government Reform, 2000; Meadows, 2001). When the notorious teratogen thalidomide was approved by the FDA for limited use in 1998, the experience of the isotretinoin Pregnancy Prevention Program was considered by the

FDA, CDC, and other public health providers in designing a program for its use (Lary et al., 1999). The System for Thalidomide Education and Prescribing Safety (STEPS) program was developed, which includes not only contraception and pregnancy testing but also mandatory registration of prescribers, pharmacies, and patients; informed consent forms for treatment; and tight controls over prescription and dispensation. Although the success of STEPS has yet to be measured, the designs of both of these pregnancy prevention programs can provide lessons for the use of other known teratogens associated with orofacial clefts such as anticonvulsants or when the use of "new" teratogens is considered in the future.

APPLICATION OF SCIENTIFIC FINDINGS

Applying the results of birth defect–related genetic and epidemiologic discoveries to public health practice is a challenging prospect and has resulted in a spate of research to meet this challenge. Khoury et al. (2000) outlined a framework for this research, which includes four main components:

- Public health assessment
- Evaluation of genetic testing
- Development, implementation, and evaluation of population interventions
- Communication and information dissemination

Public health assessment includes application of surveillance and epidemiologic methods. This topic is discussed in Section I of this book. The second research–related component, evaluation of genetic testing, will become important as new molecular and/or biochemical risk factors for orofacial clefts are discovered. Guidelines for evaluation were promulgated by the Task Force on Genetic Testing (Holtzman and Shapiro, 1998; Holtzman and Watson, 1998). These guidelines include both initial evaluations and studies of the use of these tests in actual clinical and public health practice (postmarketing surveillance). The task force identified three important components in the assessment of genetic tests: analytic validity, clinical validity, and clinical utility. *Analytic validity* refers to the sensitivity, specificity, and predictive values of the test itself with respect to genotype. *Clinical validity* refers to these same parameters with respect to phenotype. *Clinical utility* measures the benefits of interventions that follow genetic testing.

Development, implementation, and evaluation of population interventions refer to the real-world application of basic scientific discoveries. Development of a new prevention program for orofacial clefts might involve principles similar to those that have been applied in neural tube defect prevention programs or novel approaches to behavioral or environmental modification of another type of risk factor. A good example of implementation of a genetic test is a pilot demonstration project of newborn screening for cystic fibrosis in the form of a statewide randomized trial in Wisconsin (Farrell et al., 1997, 2001). Evaluation of interventions refers to studies of their effect on morbidity or mortality; for birth defects, this would include the impact on birth prevalence after a prevention program is implemented. The latter would involve surveillance and birth defect monitoring, as discussed below. Evaluations of orofacial cleft morbidity prevention would involve the application of evidence-based medical care (see Section II of this book).

Communication and information dissemination are major components of birth defect prevention programs. Genetic counselors have developed an entire discipline for the study and practice of communicating information about specific genes involved with cleft lip and cleft palate or other disorders. Initial efforts to evaluate the training of genetic counselors, which occasionally takes place within schools of public health, were sponsored by the Office of Maternal and Child Health (now HRSA/MCHB) (Walker, 1998). Folic acid counseling is already the standard of care for genetic counseling about neural tube defect recurrence, and although prevention of orofacial clefts through multivitamin use needs further study, discussions about vitamins may also be important in genetic counseling about recurrence risks for families of children with orofacial clefts (Harper, 1998; Itikala et al., 2001). Prevention programs involved with modifying environmental risk factors, such as smoking or folic acid intake, rely primarily on changing knowledge, attitudes, and behavior of women of childbearing age. For this reason, public health agencies involved with birth defect prevention have increasingly relied on behavioral scientists and researchers in health communication to develop effective prevention messages. Sometimes this has involved the use of novel techniques, such as analysis of survey databases to identify a target audience, selection of focus groups to define motivational concepts, and testing of these concepts in a controlled setting (Centers for Disease Control and Prevention, 1998; Daniel, 1999).

SURVEILLANCE AND MONITORING SYSTEMS

Section I of this book includes a discussion of epidemiologic issues in birth defect surveillance. Table 40.3 illustrates some uses of birth defect surveillance systems for public health action and policy. Many birth

TABLE 40.3. *Examples of Uses of Birth Defect Surveillance for Public Health Action and Policy*

Public Health Issue	Example	Outcome	Internet Address
Clusters/outbreaks	Chorionic villus sampling associated with limb deficiencies	Quantification of risk for counseling (Centers for Disease Control and Prevention, 1995)	http://www.cdc.gov/mmwr/preview/ mmwrhtml/00038393.htm
Services for children with special heath-care needs	Colorado birth defects monitoring program	Needs assessment, service planning and delivery, family support, case identification (Centers for Disease Control and Prevention, 2000; Montgomery and Miller, 2001)	http://www.cdphe.state.co.us/ dc/CRCSN/crcsn_fact_sheets.htm
Community effectiveness of public health interventions	Agency policies for folic acid daily supplementation and food fortification	Analysis of secular trends in neural tube defects since enactment of recommendations/policies (Rosano et al., 1999)	http://www.icbd.org/collab_99.htm

defect surveillance systems have been established in response to concerns about identifying and controlling teratogens, although methodologic issues have put identification of new teratogens lower on their program agendas (Khoury and Holtzman, 1987). Nevertheless, clusters of birth defects and public concerns about specific environmental exposures frequently surface. Occasionally, high rates of orofacial clefts in specific places and times have prompted investigations. For example, a high orofacial cleft rate of 7/1000 births in the Netherlands in the 1960s led to a study that implicated, but could not prove, local chemical combustion as a risk factor (ten Tusscher et al., 2000). An East German secular trend study showed that local rates of orofacial clefts increased after the Chernobyl reactor accident in 1986, but this type of study also can only suggest and not prove causality for etiologic factors (Zieglowski and Hemprich, 1999).

Registry-based studies can help to quantify risks when clusters have suggested etiologies for certain birth defects, which can ultimately lead to policy recommendations. In the early 1990s a prenatal diagnostic procedure, chorionic villus sampling, was associated with a transverse terminal limb deficiencies based on cluster reports, but early recommendations developed at the National Institutes of Health suggested counseling only about a "possible" risk (Report of National Institute of Child Health and Human Development Workshop on Chorionic Villus Sampling and Limb and Other Defects, 1993). A multistate, registry-based case-control study subsequently showed that an increased risk for limb deficiency after the procedure was statistically significant, but lower than first suggested by the early cluster reports (Centers for Disease Control and Prevention, 1995). The results of this study led to new recommendations by the CDC for counseling that (for the first time) quantified the risk; the CDC risk figures

were subsequently adopted in part by a policy-making committee of the American College of Obstetricians and Gynecologists (American College of Obstetricians and Gynecologists Committee on Genetics, 1996).

Surveillance also has the potential to improve medical care for children with orofacial clefts. One of the uses of birth defect surveillance systems is early identification of children who are eligible for social services and special programs (Lynberg and Edmonds, 1994). In some states and countries, birth defect registries are linked to, or part of, a larger system of early identification and case management for children with special healthcare needs. In a 1999 directory of birth defect surveillance programs, 13 U.S. states listed "service delivery" as one of the uses of their data (Centers for Disease Control and Prevention, 2000; Montgomery and Miller, 2001). In a 1996–1997 survey, eight states responded that they linked their birth defect surveillance systems to their databases of children with special healthcare needs (Kirby, 2000). The challenge for the future of database integration is to increase the number of states performing such activities and to demonstrate to the lawmakers and agencies responsible for funding that they contribute to better outcomes (Walker, 2000).

Finally, birth defect monitoring is important to assess the effects of prevention programs. For example, efforts are under way to judge the effect of folic acid prevention programs on secular trends in neural tube defect rates (Rosano et al., 1999). A similar examination of trends in orofacial cleft rates could also provide epidemiologic evidence about the contribution of folic acid fortification to orofacial cleft prevention (Itikala et al., 2001). Neural tube defect trend studies are confounded by prenatal diagnosis. In studies of birth prevalence rates of clefts over time, as mentioned in Chapter 11 of this book, similar confounding is less likely to occur, even with increasing sophistication of prenatal ultrasound, such as the use of three-dimensional techniques. Anticipating the need for these studies is important for placing methodologically sound surveillance systems that include orofacial clefts in as many geographic areas as possible.

CONCLUDING REMARKS

Last (2001) defined *public health* as a combination of social institutions, practices, and scientific disciplines, the aim of which is to improve community health through collective action. Practical efforts to translate scientific advances related to orofacial clefts into improved community outcomes must proceed on several fronts. These efforts often start with legislative or policy-making initiatives; work through innovative, scientifically based prevention or treatment programs; and end with surveillance and monitoring to evaluate their success or failure. In other areas of maternal and child health, medical therapy and public health practice have had dramatic effects, such as 10-fold to 100-fold decreases in infant and maternal mortality over the last century (Wilcox and Marks, 1994). A prevention achievement of this magnitude for cleft lip and cleft palate would be a more complicated but equally worthy goal.

REFERENCES

Abrishamchian, AR, Khoury, MJ, Calle, EE (1994). The contribution of maternal epilepsy and its treatment to the etiology of oral clefts: a population based case-control study. Genet Epidemiol 11: 343–351.

American Academy of Pediatrics Committee on Children with Disabilities (1997). General principles in the care of children and adolescents with genetic disorders and other chronic health conditions. Pediatrics 99: 643–644.

American College of Obstetricians and Gynecologists Committee on Genetics (1996). ACOG committee opinion. Chorionic villus sampling. Int J Gynaecol Obstet 52: 206–208.

Centers for Disease Control and Prevention (1994). Cigarette smoking among women of reproductive age—United States, 1987–1992. MMWR Morb Mortal Wkly Rep 43: 789–791.

Centers for Disease Control and Prevention (1995). Chorionic villus sampling and amniocentesis: recommendations for prenatal counseling. MMWR Morb Mortal Wkly Rep 44(RR-9): 1–12.

Centers for Disease Control and Prevention (1998). *Preventing Neural Tube Birth Defects: A Prevention Model and Resource Guide.* Atlanta: Centers for Disease Control and Prevention.

Centers for Disease Control and Prevention (2000). State birth defects surveillance programs directory. Teratology 61: 33–85.

Centers for Disease Control and Prevention, Division of Diabetes Translation (2001). *Diabetes: A Serious Public Health Problem. At A Glance. 2001.* Atlanta: Centers for Disease Control and Prevention.

Cunningham, G, Kohatsu, N, Stratton, N, Neutra, R (1998). Meeting the challenge of genetics and public health: state perspectives on program activities. California. Community Genet 1: 98–99.

Cunningham, GC, Tompkinson, DG (1999). Cost and effectiveness of the California triple marker prenatal screening program. Genet Med 1: 199–206.

Daniel, KL (1999). Observations from the CDC: using health communications research to reduce birth defects. J Womens Health 8: 19–22.

Ely, JH (1969). The cleft palate team. Bull N Y State Soc Dent Child 20: 9–10.

Farrell, PM, Kosorok, MR, Laxova, A, et al. (1997). Nutritional benefits of neonatal screening for cystic fibrosis. N Engl J Med 337: 963–969.

Farrell, PM, Kosorok, MR, Rock, MJ, et al. (2001). Early diagnosis of cystic fibrosis through neonatal screening prevents severe malnutrition and improves long-term growth. Pediatrics 107: 1–13.

Fernhoff, PM, Lammer, EJ (1984). Craniofacial features of isotretinoin embryopathy. J Pediatr 105: 595–597.

Food and Drug Administration (2000). Dermatologic and Ophthalmic Drugs Advisory Committee; notice of meeting. Federal Register 65: 45384.

Hammond, M, Stassen, L (1999). Do you care? A national register for cleft lip and palate patients. Br J Orthod 26: 152–157.

Harper, PS (1998). *Practical Genetic Counselling.* Oxford: Butterworth-Heinemann, p. 176.

Holtzman, NA, Shapiro, D (1998). Genetic testing and public policy. BMJ 316: 852–856.

Holtzman, NA, Watson, MS (eds) (1998). *Promoting Safe and Effective Genetic Testing in the United States: Final Report of the Task Force on Genetic Testing.* Baltimore: Johns Hopkins University Press.

House Committee on Government Reform (2000). Accutane: Hearings before the House Committee on Government Reform. 106th Cong., 2nd sess., 5 December 2000, Cong Rec 146, D1195.

Itikala, PR, Watkins, ML, Mulinare, J, Moore, CA, Liu, Y (2001). Maternal multivitamin use and orofacial clefts in offspring. Teratology 63: 79–86.

Ivy, RH (1971). Reminiscences of public health in Pennsylvania: the Cleft Palate Program. Trans Stud Coll Physicians Phila 38: 174–183.

Khoury, MJ, Beaty, TH, Cohen, BH (1993). *Fundamentals of Genetic Epidemiology.* New York: Oxford University Press, pp. 324–325.

Khoury, MJ, Burke, W, Thomson, EJ (2000). Genetics and public health: a framework for the integration of human genetics into public health practice. In: *Genetics and Public Health in the 21st Century,* edited by MJ Khoury, W Burke, and EJ Thomson. New York: Oxford University Press, pp. 3–23.

Khoury, MJ, Holtzman, NA (1987). On the ability of birth defects monitoring to detect new teratogens. Am J Epidemiol 126: 136–143.

Kirby, RS (2000). Analytical resources for assessment of clinical genetics services in public health: current status and future prospects. Teratology 61: 9–16.

Lary, JM, Daniel, KL, Erickson, JD et al. (1999). The return of thalidomide: can birth defects be prevented? Drug Saf 21: 161–169.

Last, JM (2001). *A Dictionary of Epidemiology.* 4th ed. New York: Oxford University Press, p. 145.

Lumley, J, Oliver, S, Waters, E (2000). Interventions for promoting smoking cessation during pregnancy. Cochrane Database Syst Rev: CD001055.

Lynberg, MC, Edmonds, LD (1994). State use of birth defects surveillance. In: *From Data to Action: CDC's Public Health Surveillance for Women, Infants, and Children*, edited by LS Wilcox and JS Marks. Atlanta: Centers for Disease Control and Prevention, pp. 217–229.

Meadows, M (2001). The power of Accutane: the benefits and risks of a breakthrough acne drug. FDA Consum *35:* 18–23.

Mitchell, AA, Van Bennekom, CM, Louik, C (1995). A pregnancy-prevention program in women of childbearing age receiving isotretinoin. N Engl J Med *333:* 101–106.

Montgomery, A, Miller, L (2001). Using the Colorado birth defects monitoring program to connect families with services for children with special needs. Teratology *64:* S42–S46.

National Center for Health Statistics (2000). *Health, United States, 2000.* Hyattsville, MD: US Department of Health and Human Services.

Pope, AM, Tarlov, AR (eds) (1991). *Disability in America.* Washington, DC: National Academy Press.

Report of National Institute of Child Health and Human Development Workshop on Chorionic Villus Sampling and Limb and Other Defects, October 20, 1992 (1993). Am J Obstet Gynecol *169:* 1–6.

Rosano, A, Smithells, D, Cacciani, L, et al. (1999). Time trends in neural tube defects prevalence in relation to preventive strategies: an international study. J Epidemiol Community Health *53:* 630–635.

ten Tusscher, GW, Stam, GA, Koppe, JG (2000). Open chemical combustions resulting in a local increased incidence of orofacial clefts. Chemosphere *40:* 1263–1270.

US Department of Health and Human Services (2000). *Healthy People 2010.* Washington, DC: US Department of Health and Human Services.

Walker, AP (1998). The practice of genetic counseling. In: *A Guide to Genetic Counseling*, edited by DL Baker, JL Schuette, and WR Uhlmann. New York: Wiley-Liss, pp. 1–26.

Walker, DK (2000). Integrating birth defects surveillance in maternal and child health at the state level. Teratology *61:* 4–8.

Watkins, ML (1998). Efficacy of folic acid prophylaxis for the prevention of neural tube defects. Ment Retard Dev Disabil Res Rev *4:* 282–290.

Wilcox, LS, Marks, JS (1994). Overview. In: *From Data to Action: CDC's Public Health Surveillance for Women, Infants, and Children*, edited by LS Wilcox and JS Marks. Atlanta: Centers for Disease Control and Prevention, pp. 9–20.

Zieglowski, V, Hemprich, A (1999). Spaltgeburtenrate der ehemaligen DDR vor und nach dem Reaktorunfall in Tschernobyl. Mund Kiefer Gesichtschir *3:* 195–199.

41

Educating the practitioner and the public

MARILYN C. JONES

Although in the aggregate congenital anomalies affect 3% to 4% of all term infants, individual birth defects are usually infrequent enough that the public, most parents at least at the outset, and many professionals have no experience with the specific problem and consequently no skill sets with which to approach affected individuals. Public education plays a significant role in dispelling myths and raising awareness about the issues faced by people with a variety of medical problems. Moreover, increased public awareness can influence attitudes, perceptions, health policy, and research agendas. Advocacy groups, such as AIDS awareness groups and the Breast Cancer Coalition, have demonstrated the impact of aggressive lobbying and public education campaigns. Concomitant with increased awareness of human immunodeficiency virus-related diseases and breast cancer as important health issues has come increased support for affected individuals and increased funding for research and treatment. Patients have been empowered in treatment decisions, public misperceptions have been dispelled, and professionals have broader knowledge of treatment options. This chapter explores past and current educational efforts with respect to cleft lip and palate.

Over the past 20 years, a number of investigators have surveyed groups of parents, professionals, students, and the general public to define the magnitude of the gaps in knowledge and create solutions. The only published study of public awareness dates from the mid-1980s. Middleton et al. (1986) surveyed 1200 individuals selected at random in six cities across the United States regarding their knowledge about cleft palate. More than half of the respondents had never heard of the condition. Over 60% did not know anyone with a cleft palate. Although 82% knew that clefts could be treated, very few understood how this was accomplished and what outcomes could be expected. Based on the preferences of those surveyed, 10 outreach approaches were suggested, including a media blitz, speakers' bureau, and the development of various written and visual educational materials.

A survey of employees of a Louisiana school district demonstrated that 87% of regular education teachers, 85% of special education teachers, and 31% of speech pathologists had no experience with children with clefts (Mitchell et al., 1984). Similarly, Lass et al. (1973) documented significant deficiencies with respect to clefting in the experience of medical and dental students. The need for in-service education, conferences, and curriculum changes in the training of professionals was emphasized.

The American Cleft Palate-Craniofacial Association (ACPA), the major professional association dedicated to the care of affected individuals, first recognized the need to develop educational materials for families in 1966 (Wells, 1979). From initial outreach efforts to families, ACPA established the American Cleft Palate Foundation, now the Cleft Palate Foundation (CPF), in 1973 in response to the growing need to educate a much broader audience. Yet, 10 years after its establishment, gaps in public and professional knowledge remained enormous as evidenced by the above surveys. In response to growing concerns, the CPF sponsored the development of a series of educational pamphlets for parents and professionals, established a telephone 1-800 hotline for families in crisis, and broadened relations with patient/parent advocacy groups such that information could be broadly disseminated.

Professionals involved in research and treatment wrote books for professionals and parents, contributed chapters to texts, produced videos, lectured at professional meetings and incorporated information on cleft lip and palate into training programs in their respective disciplines (Moller et al., 1990; Vallino and Brown, 1996). Despite concerted efforts, the dissemination of information was limited. Although the ACPA information was readily available, to access it, professionals or parents/patients would have to know of the existence of the organization. Since much of the information was written, a certain level of literacy was required of the consumer. Likewise, outreach to other professional organizations met with modest success since most primary care practitioners, nurses, speech pathologists, and dentists perceive clefts as a small enough component of an individual practice or case load to warrant a concerted educational effort. Conferences on cleft-related issues at specialty continuing education meetings tended to attract the interest of the already informed.

The advent of electronic communication, including the Internet and telecommunication, has changed the rules with respect to patient and practitioner education. The Internet has given both patients and practitioners the tools to access information directly without the filter of professional consultation. Superb educational information from the ACPA, the National Institute for Dental and Craniofacial Research, and various support groups is readily available to anyone with a home computer. Some practitioners and hospitals have discovered that web-based educational pieces are excellent marketing opportunities. Consequently, the distinction between education and advertising is becoming less clear in some circumstances. Both educational and marketing campaigns start with identification of a goal. For individual practitioners and some healthcare institutions, this goal is usually increased patient referrals, although the foundations associated with some hospitals may focus more broadly on a general educational mission. Consequently, the information, no matter how excellent, usually reflects the biases of the sponsoring institution, particularly with respect to treatment. Given the lack of outcome data, there is little solid ground for challenging specific treatment recommendations. For patients, frustration regarding the prior dearth of information may be replaced with confusion generated by the plethora of unfiltered and conflicting information available on the web.

Antismoking efforts have demonstrated that public education campaigns can be successful despite well-funded and organized opposition, particularly when the message is simple (stop smoking) and continually reinforced. The more focused public education campaign of the March of Dimes to encourage women of child-bearing age to increase intake of folic acid in advance of pregnancy to reduce the risk of neural tube defects has met with moderate success, particularly with the health-conscious consumer who assumes an active role in treatment. The effort contributed to the decision of the Food and Drug Administration to supplement grain-based foods with a low level of folic acid. Folate status in women of childbearing age has improved over the last 10 years (MMWR 2000b). Targeted efforts to educate practitioners and patients have met with mixed success, if the isotretinoin (Accutane) experience is examined. Despite an active pregnancy-prevention program sponsored by the manufacturer, roughly 900 exposures to this potent human teratogen occurred among 400,000 voluntary enrollees in the Boston University Accutane Survey (MMWR, 2000a). With all of these efforts, the programs involved have identified a message (stop smoking, take folic acid, do not get pregnant while on isotretinoin), a target audience (the general public, practitioners, and patients), and an outcome measure to document their success (number of smokers, number of neural tube births, and number of pregnancy exposures). With respect to cleft and craniofacial defects, one of the educational messages for patients and practitioners is that treatment of affected individuals requires a multidisciplinary effort. Patients are likely to be best served in centers with broad-based, active teams. However, the Eurocleft Project has demonstrated that team care alone is not enough to predict a successful outcome (Shaw et al., 1992, 2000). Treatment teams in the United States need to develop outcome measures to assure the public that appropriate care is being provided. As the risk factors that predispose to cleft and craniofacial anomalies are conclusively identified, public education programs for prevention need to be implemented using strategies that have been successful for other birth defects.

Several issues could be approached immediately. The first is dissemination of information regarding feeding techniques (including breast-feeding) for affected newborns. The target audience for such information would be parents and primary care providers for delivering mothers and newborns, including obstetricians, pediatricians, family physicians, nurse midwives, nurses, nutritionists, and lactation consultants. The mode of communicating this information to professionals could be in-services (at the local level), conferences (at the regional level), Internet hot-links, and articles in broadly circulated professional journals (at the national and international levels). From the parent standpoint, there is no real substitute for one-on-one instruction from a knowledgeable professional; however, videotapes and pamphlets suffice when the former is not available. A web-based database of the many excellent videotapes available with reviews and information on how to access/purchase them might be helpful.

The second relates to the need for broader acceptance of individuals with facial differences. AboutFace International has developed an excellent teaching module for use in elementary schools called "Unwrapping the Package" (www.aboutfaceinternational.org). Such programs need to be easily accessible to parents, teachers, school counselors, and school nurses, who deal with issues of social acceptance and peer interactions on a daily basis. Videotapes addressing social skills training and how to handle teasing might be highly valuable if they were easily accessible. A web-based, peer-reviewed database of such resources would be very helpful.

Lastly, the ACPA message regarding the need for team care is relevant. Perhaps the most practical way to disseminate this information is to assure that the organization's website is among the first to appear on the list of suggestions generated by the major and commonly used Internet search engines when the words *cleft*, *cleft lip*, *cleft palate*, and *craniofacial* are entered in a search. There is much work to be done.

REFERENCES

Lass, N, Gasperini, R, Overberger, J, Conolly, M (1973). The exposure of medical and dental students to the disorder of cleft palate. Cleft Palate J *10:* 306.

Middleton, GF, Lass, NJ, Starr, P, Pannbacker, M (1986). Survey of public awareness and knowledge of cleft palate. Cleft Palate J *23:* 58–62.

Mitchell, CK, Lott, R, Pannbacker, M (1984). Perceptions about cleft palate held by school personnel: suggestions for in-service training programs. Cleft Palate J *21:* 308–312.

MMWR (2000a). Accutane-exposed pregnancies—California, 1999. MMWR Morb Mortal Wkly Rep *49:* 28–31.

MMWR (2000b). Folate status in women of childbearing age—United States, 1999. MMWR Morb Mortal Wkly Rep *49:* 962–965.

Moller, KT, Starr, CD, Johnson, SA (1990). *A Parent's Guide to Cleft Lip and Palate.* Minneapolis: University of Minnesota Press.

Shaw, B, Semb, G, Nelson, P, et al. (2000). *The Eurocleft Project.* Amsterdam: IOS.

Shaw, WC, Dahl, E, Asher-McDade, C, et al. (1992). A six-center international study of treatment outcome in patients with clefts of the lip and palate: part 5. General discussion and conclusions. Cleft Palate Craniofac J *29:* 413–418.

Vallino, LD, Brown, AS (1996). Assessing third-year medical students' knowledge of and exposure to cleft palate before and after plastic surgery rotation. Ann Plast Surg *36:* 380–387.

Wells, C (1979). The American Cleft Palate Association: its first 36 years. Cleft Palate J *16:* 86.

42

Innovations in international cooperation for patients with cleft lip and palate

NAGATO NATSUME

DAVID S. PRECIOUS

Since World War II, there has been a remarkable increase in international activities concerned with public health, an important example of which is the treatment of patients with cleft lip and palate. Most of this treatment is carried out by volunteers from developed countries, who either belong to or participate with nongovernment organizations (NGOs). The stated goals of these NGOs are to provide free surgery, which would otherwise not be available, to patients who have cleft lip and palate; to train surgeons in developing countries to perform these operations; and to donate equipment, instruments, teaching aids, and the like to regions where there is need.

"SAFARI" SURGERY

It is encouraging to note that today many individuals and NGOs perform charitable operations on patients with cleft lip and palate in developing countries. Several organizations send missions to as many as 20 different countries spanning South America, Africa, Asia, and the Middle East. Emphasis on volunteer treatment in Asia is particularly important given the proportionally higher incidence of cleft lip and palate in that population. Thanks to these contributions, many children have been helped and the skills of local surgeons have improved.

Also encouraging is the greater emphasis some organizations are now placing on local self-sufficiency as a necessary condition for long-term treatment of cleft lip and palate in developing nations. Operation Smile (www.operationsmile.org), for instance, trains local medical providers from the mission site while there and, upon departure, leaves behind necessary medical equipment. In 1999, the organization donated sufficient equipment to supply both an operating room and a recovery room in 18 countries. They have also relied on multimedia as a means to pass on knowledge to local missions by donating instructional videos and video equipment. SmileTrain (www.smiletrain.org) also works toward local self-sufficiency. One means that they employ is to co-sponsor educational scholarships for doctors from developing nations to attend international cleft lip and palate meetings.

Strides toward technological enhancement and genetic research are also commendable expansions in the volunteer medical arena. Initiatives taken by SmileTrain include the use of computer animation in teaching and perfecting surgical techniques for cleft lip and palate and the creation of a web-based patient database. Most organizations currently carrying out volunteer surgery are also researching genetic patterns to help explain the cause of cleft lip and palate.

While the increase in volunteer missions and related medical advances is undoubtedly positive, serious considerations remain. The risk of injury to physicians occurring during the mission, for instance, highlights the need to establish comprehensive insurance policies with coverage extending not only to the particular injury but also, potentially, to the long-term disability suffered by a physician unable to carry out his or her former position upon return home.

By far the most critical area in need of attention relates to patient safety, rights, and quality of care. The current situation is in effect a regulatory void. The conduct of a clinician/surgeon at home is governed by the guidelines and standards of relevant licensing and professional bodies. These organizations are generally responsible not only for establishing the principles and rules dictating standards of care but also for enforcing these with disciplinary action in the event of breaches. While abroad, though, there exists no global body with these responsibilities or powers. Despite its ambitious work on a global scale and universal recognition, some argue that the World Health Organization has been reluctant in adopting treaties and creating guidelines with the authority that it does have (Fidler, 1999).

The result of this void is that there is effectively nothing prohibiting a surgeon, untrained in a particular operation at home, from performing such a procedure voluntarily in a developing nation, yet the risk of harm to the patient is potentially serious. There are few provisions for compensation to the patient in the event that the surgery is carried out improperly. Moreover, there is currently no uniform procedure for ensuring informed consent of mission patients either for the actual surgery or for cooperation in genetic research and analysis. Some have argued that there is no need for such a procedure owing to the already desperate medical situation of both the mission communities generally and the patients in particular. One can also envision, though, how a physician–patient information asymmetry that is even greater abroad than at home and compounded by cultural differences underscores the very need to proceed with surgery only under circumstances where patients' rights and safety are accorded the same respect as at home.

This said, there have been some laudable efforts to address this regulatory void. SmileTrain now requires all healthcare providers performing cleft lip and palate surgery for its organization to meet its Safety and Quality Improvement Protocol. This document specifically addresses the issues of patient safety and adequacy of surgeons' qualifications but remains silent with respect to informed consent. The World Health Organization Human Genetics Program (1997) has published *Proposed International Guidelines on Ethical Issues in Medical Genetics and Genetic Services,* which addresses the issue of genetic research being carried out as part of the surgical mission.

The International Cleft Lip and Palate Foundation (ICPF) has addressed these problems. The following guidelines were adopted as the "Zurich Declaration" at the ICPF Cleft 2000 meeting, with 550 members from 56 countries, held in Zurich, Switzerland, in July 2000.

1. A long-term technology transfer plan is needed for charitable operations. A memorandum of understanding between the local people and/or government and the volunteer mission is necessary when the visiting doctors perform operations, donate equipment, and provide education.
2. Medical humanitarian aid, including cosmetic surgery, should not be profit-motivated. These projects should be carried out in a charitable spirit. Furthermore, these operations should not entail an additional financial burden to the host community.
3. Participants should fully understand the host country's laws, customs, and systems and conduct themselves as guests.
4. These charitable activities should not be religiously or politically motivated.
5. Surgeons should act as teachers, practitioners, and learners.
6. Surgery and other treatment should be performed in collaboration with the local doctors, to allow more effective treatment and technology transfer.
7. We must take responsibility for the patients' convalescence. We should also establish a plan of assistance for the patients' independence.
8. The governing body of the organization should maintain a record of the volunteer participants' professional licenses and personal histories. Measures should be taken to ensure the health and safety of the volunteer participants.
9. A fund should be established for medical accident and/or travel insurance for the staff.
10. An important charity mission goal is establishment of centers of excellence.

These guidelines include important items that individuals and NGOs ought to keep in mind when they undertake aid projects abroad. In subscribing to such guidelines, surgeons volunteering in developing countries would be able to work toward the important goal of a universal standard of care for patients, irrespective of nationality or need.

ASSESSMENT OF QUALITY OF SURGERY

There is a need not only to enhance the research infrastructure but also to meet the challenge of improving quality of services by sharing examples of good practice, recognition and appreciation of common problems, and application of one country's demonstrated success to other countries. This task is all the more difficult in countries where patient follow-up is hindered, and sometimes even prevented, by distance, cost of travel, lack of trained clinicians, and culture.

Attempts to assess outcomes of cleft lip and palate surgery based on pre- and postoperative photographs are limited by the inability to assess dynamic function. Even in developed countries, rigor must be applied in the selection of parameters on which will be based the methodology of outcome studies.

In cleft lip/palate patients, aberrations in craniofacial morphology and growth have often been attributed to the technique and timing of lip and palate surgery (Molsted, 1999). This attribution overlooks the influence of inherent growth tendencies, such as those resulting from variation in cranial base morphology. Cranial base patterns may predispose an individual to certain growth patterns irrespective of the technique and timing of cleft surgery. Thus, when evaluating the results of surgical treatment in CLP patients, cranial base morphology should be included as one influential factor in dental/skeletal relationships. For this reason, one must use caution in interpreting studies based on the examination of dental casts, as is done using the Goslon yardstick (Mars et al., 1987).

In cleft lip and palate, an important (perhaps the most important) event for the patient is what happens on the operating table. The aims of physiological surgery for cleft lip and palate are to restore the best anatomy and physiology of the divided muscles, to recover all normal orofacial functions, not to interfere with the process of maxillary growth, and to ensure good development of the facial skeleton. A priori, seemingly, aesthetics is not the primary concern of this surgery, but in fact, it is the best anatomical and physiological reconstruction of the muscles involved in the cleft that ensures the most beautiful facial aesthetics, both at rest and in function (Delaire, 1978).

Assessment of outcomes of primary and secondary surgery based on functional parameters, such as vestibular oral–nasal fistula, palatal oral–nasal fistula, deviation of the nasal septum to the noncleft side, dental overjet, and coincidence of the maxillary dental midline with that of the mandible (to list a few), offers the advantages not only of simplicity and certainty (there is either a fistula or there is not) but also of providing a means by which the clinician can determine the extent to which the specific goals of surgery were achieved (Precious, 2000). An oral–nasal fistula is not a complication of palatal surgery; rather, it is a failure to achieve the purpose of the surgery. This functional approach to outcomes assessment is seen as one practical innovation by the ICPF.

The way forward is through collaborative research to improve understanding, treatment, and prevention of clefts of the lip and palate. There will never be one best technique or one best protocol. We must broaden our approach so that we respect the patient's right to choose, on the basis of adequate information, from alternate treatment plans that meet professional standards of care. Our duty to secure informed consent is of an even higher order when the patient and the family have little or no information about the proposed surgery.

INTERNATIONAL CHARITY OPERATION NETWORK

When NGO aid activities are undertaken without any criteria such as those outlined in the above-mentioned guidelines, unnecessary confusion can occur in aid-recipient countries. If we share our own information, not only can we avoid such risks but also both the NGO and the local people can make use of that information. With this network system, multiple NGOs can exchange information about their activities through the Internet so that more than two NGOs can cooperate with each other when they undertake activities in the same place or arrange a mutually acceptable schedule of activities to avoid ineffectiveness.

The ICPF has established an incubator program, whereby a meeting of like-minded groups and individuals will be held once every 2 years at the ICPF congress. The incubator program facilitates participation and meeting of NGOs in each country, senders of charity operation missions, and recipients. Accordingly, if there is a certain group which is planning to send a mission and another which is seeking surgeons to perform care, they can talk about their needs face to face at the meeting. It is generally agreed that this will foster the establishment of effective new aid projects.

WORLD GENE BANK

Gene analyses used to improve treatment will become much more important for cleft lip and/or palate treatment in the twenty-first century. However, there are still problems with treatment in developing countries, particularly with regard to psychological support for every patient and family. In the twentieth century, individuals, hospitals, and countries made efforts to solve these problems. What is required in the twenty-first century is that all nations, including developing countries, address these problems.

A prerequisite to progress in the twenty-first century is worldwide establishment of an informed consent system in gene analysis therapies and global registration of patients with rare diseases. Thus, the World Cleft Gene Bank was established to ensure patients' rights in gene analysis therapies and to determine the cause of syntrophus in collaboration with the global community. It is vitally important to determine the causes not only of cleft lip and palate alone but also of all congenital syndromes that affect the maxillofacial region. A registration system for rare diseases is as important as the cause-determination project in the gene analysis therapies. Further, the World Cleft Gene Bank will keep a close watch on patients' rights, especially regarding protection of privacy, which sometimes can be overlooked due to competition among researchers.

INFORMATION EXCHANGE FOR PATIENTS/FAMILIES AND DOCTORS

Since cleft lip/palate rarely results in death or serious disease, administrative bodies tend to be reluctant to take quick measures, but in Japan roughly 30% of mothers who delivered a child with cleft lip and palate said that they had considered committing suicide. Mothers who delivered a child with serious bilateral cleft lip and palate said that they had considered not only committing suicide but also killing their own child. Actually, there is a recorded case of a grandmother who killed her cleft lip and palate grandchild. Why do families think of such dreadful things? The reasons are that cleft lip and palate can cause an unaesthetic facial appearance, speech problems, and disadvantages regarding marriage and other social relationships.

Organizations like the ICPF want patients, their families, and doctors to discuss how they can cope with these difficulties, including prejudice by their neighbors and bullying by classmates. In addition, this same initiative includes preparation of a database compiled by contacting governments, including information about what policies the government has in place to care for cleft lip and palate. This is the challenge of the future.

REFERENCES

Delaire, J (1978). Theoretical principles and technique of functional closure of the lip and nasal aperture. J Maxillofac Surg 6: 109–116.

Fidler, DP (1999). International law and global public health. Kansas Law Rev

Mars, M, Plint, D, Houston, W, et al. (1987). The Goslon yardstick: a new system of assessing dental arch relationships in children with unilateral clefts of the lip and palate. Cleft Palate J 24: 314–322.

Molsted, K (1999). Treatment outcome in cleft lip and palate: issues and perspectives. Crit Rev Oral Biol Med 10: 225–239.

Precious, DS (2000). Unilateral cleft lip and palate. In: Cleft Lip and Palate—A Physiological Approach. Oral and Maxillofacial Clinics of North America. Vol. 12. Philadelphia: Saunders, pp. 399–420.

World Health Organization Human Genetics Program. (0000) Proposed International Guidelines on Ethical Issues in Medical Genetics and Genetic Services. Geneva: World Health Organization.

Appendix
Directory of Internet resources

About Face, a nonprofit international organization dedicated to providing information, emotional support, and educational programs to individuals who have a facial disfigurement and to their families. http://www.aboutface2000.org/

American Cleft Palate-Craniofacial Association, a national organization providing lay and professional services for cleft lip, cleft palate, and other craniofacial deformities. http://www.cleftline.org/

American Society of Plastic Surgeons and Plastic Surgery Educational Foundation, http://www.plastic-surgery.org/

Association of Birth Defect Children, an organization providing information to parents and professionals about all kinds of birth defect, resource, support group, and environmental exposure. http://www.birthdefects.org/

Australasian Cleft Lip and Palate Association (ACLAPA), representing the interests of health professionals involved in the management of cleft lip and palate–related conditions. http://aclapa.thehospital.com/

Birmingham Craniofacial Unit (UK), http://www.craniofacial.org.uk/

Center for Craniofacial Development and Disorders (CCDD), http://omie.med.jhmi.edu/craniofacial/

Center for Craniofacial Disorders, Scottish Rite (Atlanta, GA), http://www.choa.org/

Center for the Evaluation of Risks to Human Reproduction, http://cerhr.niehs.nih.gov/index.html

Children's Craniofacial Association, national nonprofit organization, headquartered in Dallas, Texas, dedicated to improving quality of life for people with facial differences and their families. http://www.ccakids.com/

Cleft Club, a Yahoo club for those who are cleft or who know someone with a cleft lip and/or palate. http://clubs.yahoo.com/clubs/thecleftclub

Cleft Club, for anyone dealing with cleft lip and cleft palate, whether you were born with it, are a parent of a cleft kid, or interested. http://www.cleftclub.barrysworld.net/

Cleft Lip and Palate Association (CLAPA), UK organization offering information and support to anyone with, or affected by, cleft lip or cleft palate. http://www.clapa.cwc.net/

Cleft Lip and Palate Association of Ireland (CLAPAI), http://www.cleft.ie/

Cleft Palate-Craniofacial Center at the University of Pittsburgh School of Dental Medicine, http://www.dental.pitt.edu/cleft_palate/about.html

Cleft Palate Foundation (CPF), a nonprofit organization dedicated to assisting individuals with birth defects of the head and neck and their families. http://www.cleftline.org/cpf/cpffrm.html

Cleft-Talk, online support group for parents and individuals. http://www.widesmiles.org/ct/

COGENE, the Craniofacial and Oral Gene Expression Network. http://hg.wustl.edu/COGENE/

Craniofacial Foundation of America. http://www.erlanger.org/cranio/found1.html

Listing in this directory does not imply either approval or disapproval of the Internet resource on the part of the editor. Descriptions were taken from the websites. All websites were functional as of December 11, 2001.

DHMHD, the Dysmorphic Human–Mouse Homology Database. http://www.hgmp.mrc.ac.uk/DHMHD/dysmorph.html

Embryo images of normal and abnormal development. http://www.med.unc.edu/embryo_images/

FACES, the National Craniofacial Association. http://www.faces-cranio.org/

Florida Cleft Palate Association (FCPA), a well-established statewide association of healthcare specialists and parents who welcome opportunities to help children with a facial difference. http://www.floridacleft.org/

Friendly Faces, providing accurate and abundant information regarding various craniofacial conditions and related subjects. http://www.friendlyfaces.org/

Frontiers in Fetal Health, an informative online journal edited by Dr. Anne Pastuszak. http://www.sickkids.on.ca/FrontiersinFetalHealth/FFHArchives.asp

Genetic Alliance, an international coalition representing more than 300 consumer and health professional organizations with millions of members working together to promote healthy lives for everyone impacted by genetics. http://www.geneticalliance.org/

International Clearinghouse for Birth Defects Monitoring Systems, a nongovernmental organization in official relation with the World Health Organization, representing more than 30 malformation-monitoring programs worldwide. http://www.icbd.org/

International Institute for Birth Defects, research institute providing information on cleft lip and palate with an online registry. http://www.cleft.net/

Interplast, works in partnership with Third-World nations to support the development and growth of high-quality, free reconstructive surgery programs for children and adults with birth defects, burns, and other crippling deformities. http://www.teachsurgery.org/public/interplastcd/start.htm

Let's Face It USA, a nonprofit network that links people with facial disfigurement and all who care for them to resources that can enrich their lives. http://www.faceit.org/

March of Dimes, an organization dedicated to improving the health of babies by preventing birth defects and infant mortality through research, community services, education, and advocacy. http://www.modimes.org/

Mouse Genome Database (MGD), maintained by The Jackson Laboratory. http://www.informatics.jax.org

National Center on Birth Defects and Developmental Disabilities (NCBDDD) at the Centers for Disease Control and Prevention. http://www.cdc.gov/ncbddd/

National Institute of Dental and Craniofacial Research (NIDCR) of the National Institutes of Health. http://www.nidcr.nih.gov/

National Maternal and Child Oral Health Resource Center. http://www.mchoralhealth.org/

National Oral Health Information Clearinghouse, an agency of the National Institute on Dental and Craniofacial Research providing information on oral health needs for patients requiring special care. http://www.nohic.nidcr.nih.gov/

Nemours Foundation, a nonprofit organization devoted to children's health and the largest physician practice delivering subspecialty pediatric care in the United States. http://kidshealth.org/kid/health_problems/birth_defect/cleft_lip__palate.html

Northwestern University Cleft Lip and Palate Institute. http://www.craniofacialinstitute.com/

Online Mendelian Inheritance in Man (OMIM). http://www3.ncbi.nlm.nih.gov/omim/

Operation Smile, a private, not-for-profit, volunteer medical services organization providing reconstructive surgery and related healthcare to indigent children and young adults in developing countries and the United States. http://www.operationsmile.org/

Pierre Robin Network, for families whose children have been diagnosed with Pierre Robin sequence/syndrome. http://www.pierrerobin.org/

POSSUM, a computer-based system that helps clinicians to diagnose syndromes in their patients. http://www.possum.net.au/

Recombinant Inbred Strain Distribution Patterns (SDP), maintained by The Jackson Laboratory. http://www.informatics.jax.org/searches/riset_form.shtml

Smiles, a group of dedicated families who have developed a first-hand understanding of the needs of children with cleft lip, cleft palate, and craniofacial deformities. http://www.cleft.org/

Smile Train, a nonprofit organization that provides free medical training and surgeries for cranifacial defects. http://www.smiletrain.org/

Teratology Society, a multidisciplinary scientific society founded in 1960, the members of which study the causes and biological processes leading to abnormal development and birth defects at the fundamental and clinical levels, and appropriate measures for prevention. http://www.teratology.org

Transgenic/Targeted Mutation Database (TBASE), maintained by The Jackson Laboratory. http://tbase.jax.org

WideSmiles, a nonprofit organization providing resources, support, and information for those affected by cleft lip/palate, the fourth most common birth defect. http://www.widesmiles.org/

Glossary

Admixture: The "flow" of genes from one population into another. African-Americans are an example of an admixed population, resulting from the flow of European genes into African populations.

Allele: One of two or more alternative forms of a given gene.

Alveolar ridge: The bony ridge of the gumline containing the teeth.

Articulation: Movements of the mouth and airway that produce speech.

Association (genetic): The nonrandom occurrence of a disease or trait and a particular allele or genotype.

Bifid uvula: The small, cone-shaped tissue in the middle of the soft palate that is split into two parts.

Birth defect: An abnormality of structure, function, or body metabolism which often results in a physical or mental handicap. It may be inherited (genetic) or environmental.

Candidate gene: A gene whose protein product suggests that it could be involved in the etiology of a particular disease or trait.

Case-control study: A study in which people with a disease (cases) are compared to people without the disease (controls) to see if chemical exposures or other factors were different for the two groups.

Caudal: Denoting a position more toward the cauda, or tail, than some specified point of reference, same as *inferior*.

Chromosomal abnormalities: These can be either structural or numerical. Structural abnormalities include translocations, deletions or insertions, duplications, and amplifications. Numerical abnormalities are either a gain or loss of chromosomes.

Chromosome: Microscopic, rod-like structure in the cell's nucleus that carries genetic material. Threadlike structures in the nucleus of a cell, consisting of a highly compacted stretch of DNA with associated proteins, which are sets of linear DNA from which the genes are arranged. They carry all of the instructions for a species. Chromosomes come in pairs. Human beings have, in normal cells, 46 chromosomes, or 23 pairs of chromosomes (22 pairs of autosomes and two sex chromosomes, X and Y). In each pair, one chromosome, containing one copy of each gene, is inherited from the mother and one from the father.

Columella: The central, lower portion of the nose which divides the nostrils into right and left.

Confidence interval (CI): The range of numerical values in which we can be confident (to a computed probability, such as 90% or 95%) that the population value being estimated will be found. Confidence intervals indicate the strength of evidence; wide CIs indicate less precise estimates of effect. The larger the study's sample size, the larger the number of outcome events and the greater the confidence that the true relative risk reduction is close to the value stated. Thus, the CIs narrow and precision is increased.

Congenital defects: Problems or conditions that are present at birth.

Denasality: The quality of voice that lacks normal nasal resonance for *m, n,* and *ng* ("head cold" sound).

Dental arch: The curved structure formed by the teeth in their normal position.

DNA (deoxyribonucleic acid): The substance of heredity. It is the biochemical molecule of which chromosomes and genes are composed. It is the primary genetic material of all cells that tells the cells what to do and when to do it. It contains all of the information necessary for any organism to develop and function. It is the blueprint for all of the structures and functions of a living being. It holds the coded genetic instructions each person inherits from his or her parents. As a coding sequence, it determines the function of a gene, e.g., the synthesis and amino acid sequence of a protein. It is found in all plant and animal cells and carries the genetic information that cells need to replicate, to produce proteins, and to regulate enzyme production. DNA is a long, two-stranded, intertwined, chain-like molecule held together by weak bonds between base pairs of nucleotides (polysugar and phosphate chemical groups). The chain resembles a ladder twisted into a double helix, spiral shape. The four nucleotides, or chemical building blocks, in DNA contain the following bases: adenine (A), guanine (G), cytosine (C), and thymine (T). In nature, base pairs form only between A and T and between G and C; thus, the base sequence of each single strand can be deduced from that of its partner. Most human DNA is nDNA, which is a huge molecule folded tightly and stored in the nucleus of the cell. mtDNA is a much smaller molecule stored in the mitochondria.

mtDNA: Mitochondrial DNA contain the genes that code for some of the enzymes and some of the necessary molecules needed to make those enzymes of the respiratory chain. Mitochondria are the only part of the body cell with separate and unique DNA. Regardless, most of the mitochondria and the respiratory chain are coded by nDNA. mtDNA is inherited only from the mother.

nDNA: Nuclear DNA. Located in the nucleus of the cell, this DNA contains the blueprints for cells that make up the body.

Ectoderm: From the Greek *ektos* (outside) + *derma* (skin). Most dorsal layer of cells of the early embryo, which gives rise to the epidermis, neural tube, neural crest, etc.

Effectiveness: A measure of the benefit resulting from an intervention for a given health problem under usual conditions of clinical care for a particular group; this form of evaluation considers both the efficacy of an intervention and its acceptance by those to whom it is offered, answering the question "Does the practice do more good than harm to people to whom it is offered?"

Efficacy: A measure of the benefit resulting from an intervention for a given health problem under the ideal conditions of an investigation; it answers the question, "Does the practice do more good than harm to people who fully comply with the recommendations?"

Etiologic heterogeneity: The phenomenon by which a certain phenotype (or clinical feature) can be produced by different mechanisms.

Exposure assessment: A process that estimates the amount of a chemical that enters or comes into contact with people. An exposure assessment also describes the length of time and the nature and size of a population exposed to a chemical.

Follow-up: Observation over a period of time of an individual, group, or initially defined population whose relevant characteristics have been assessed in order to observe changes in health status or health-related variables.

Gene: The fundamental unit of heredity, it is a working subunit of DNA. DNA is a substance that tells cells what to do and when to do it. A gene is the position on a chromosome (strand of DNA) where a specific DNA sequence, or allele, resides in the cells and mitochondria. It is a specific, unique stretch of DNA sequence that codes for a single characteristic or component of physical development and function. It contains the code for a specific product, typically a protein such as an enzyme. Examples: ABO blood group gene, Rh blood group gene. The information in genes is passed from parent to child; e.g., a gene might tell some cells to make the hair red or the eyes brown. Changes in the sequence from one allele to another can be transmitted to the next generation.

Genetic marker: A segment of DNA with an identifiable physical location on a chromosome whose inheritance can be followed, often referred to simply as a marker.

Genome scan: Evaluation of linkage using a panel of several hundred polymorphic markers, distributed across the entire genome.

Genotype: Genetic constitution of an individual, often used to refer to the combination of alleles at any given locus.

Hereditary: Transmitted or capable of being transmitted genetically from parent to offspring.

Heredity: The passing of a trait such as color of the eyes from parent to child. A person "inherits" these traits through the genes.

Hypernasality: Speech that sounds overly nasal, as if the person is talking through his or her nose.

Hyponasality: Denasality, a lack of normal nasal resonance during speech.

Intention-to-treat analysis: A method for data analysis in a randomized clinical trial in which individual outcomes are analyzed according to the group to which the patient was randomized, even if the patient never received the assigned treatment. By simulating practical experience, it provides a better measure of effectiveness (vs. efficacy).

Linkage: The association of genes or markers that lie near each other on a chromosome. Linked genes or markers tend to be inherited together.

Linkage analysis: A method to identify whether or not alleles from two loci segregate together in families.

Linkage disequilibrium: Nonrandom association of alleles at different loci in a population.

Locus (plural, loci): The position that a gene occupies on a chromosome or within a segment of DNA.

Lod score (log of the odds of linkage): A statistical estimate of whether two loci are likely to lie near each other on a chromosome and are therefore likely to be inherited together. A lod score of 3.0 (odds of 1000:1 in favor) or more has been traditionally considered strong evidence in favor of linkage.

Malocclusion: A deviation from normal occlusion, i.e., incorrect positioning of the upper teeth in relation to the lower teeth.

Multidisciplinary team: A group of professionals who work together to plan and carry out treatment for patients with cleft lip, cleft palate, and related disorders. The group usually includes surgeons, dental specialists, speech pathologist, and others who meet regularly to evaluate and discuss the patients under their care.

Nasal emission or nasal escape: An abnormal flow of air through the nose during speech, usually indicative of an incomplete seal between oral and nasal cavities.

Nasal septum: The "wall" that divides the nose into right and left halves. It normally joins the roof of the hard palate like an inverted 7.

Nasopharyngoscope: A lighted telescopic instrument used for examining the passages in the back of the throat, useful in assessing velopharyngeal function.

Nonparametric linkage analysis: A number of statistical methods have been developed that do not require a trait locus model to be specified. The most common approach one will encounter in the literature is the affected sib-pair method. This requires families containing two affected siblings and can be shown to be equivalent to a lod score linkage analysis assuming a completely recessive model for the trait locus.

Occlusion: Relationship between upper and lower teeth when they are in contact, refers to the alignment of teeth as well as the relationship of dental arches.

Odds ratio (synonyms: cross-product ratio, relative odds): A measure of the degree of association, e.g., the odds of exposure among cases compared with the odds of exposure among controls.

p **value (probability value):** The probability that a measure of effect is as extreme as or more extreme than that observed even if no effect exists (i.e., if the null hypothesis is false).

Palatal insufficiency: A lack or shortness of tissue preventing the soft palate from contacting the back of the throat (pharynx).

Polymerase chain reaction (PCR): A molecular biological technique for making, from a very small amount of DNA, an unlimited number of copies of a specific segment of DNA.

Polymorphism: A common variation in the sequence of DNA among individuals.

Population stratification: The existence of two or more subpopulations within a larger population.

Prevalence: The proportion of persons with a particular disease within a given population at a given time.

Prolabium: The central area of the upper lip beneath the center of the nose (columella) and between the philtral columns.

Randomized controlled trial: Study design where treatments, interventions, or enrollment into different study groups are assigned by random allocation rather than by conscious decisions of clinicians or patients. If the sample size is large enough, this study design avoids problems of bias and confounding variables by assuring that both known and unknown determinants of outcome are evenly distributed between treatment and control groups.

Recall bias: Systematic error due to differences in accuracy or completeness of recall to memory of past events or experiences.

Recurrence risk: Probability that a person expresses a disease given the existence of an affected relative (of a given type). For example, the population lifetime risk of developing psoriasis is approximately 2%, but if one has an affected parent or sibling, the recurrence risk is 20%.

Relative risk (RR): the ratio of the probability of developing, in a specified period of time, an outcome among those receiving the treatment of interest or exposed to a risk factor compared with the probability of developing the outcome if the risk factor or intervention is not present.

Restriction fragment length polymorphism (RFLP): Genetic variation at the site where a restriction enzyme cuts a piece of DNA. Such variants affect the size of the resulting fragments.

Risk assessment: A process which estimates the likelihood that people exposed to chemicals have health effects. The four steps of risk assessment are hazard identification (Can this substance damage health?), dose-response assessment (What dose causes what effect?), exposure assessment (How and how much do people contact it?), and risk characterization (combining the other three steps to estimate risk).

Risk management: The process of deciding how to reduce or eliminate possible health effects by considering the risk assessment, engineering factors (Can engineering procedures or equipment do the job, for how long, and how well?) and social, economic, and political concerns.

Route of exposure: The way in which a person may contact a chemical substance. For example, drinking (ingestion) and bathing (skin contact) are two different routes of exposure to contaminants that may be found in water.

Short tandem repeat polymorphism (STRP): DNA sequence variation due to the existence of a variable number of copies of the same base sequence on a chromosome.

Single nucleotide polymorphism (SNP, pronounced "snip"): These are simply point mutations of a sufficiently high frequency to be useful for linkage and association analyses. The nucleotide-wise mutation rate is approximately $10 \exp^{-6}$ and randomly occurs within coding or noncoding regions, so that there is approximately one SNP per 1000 base pairs. Because of this density, SNPs are more useful for fine mapping of trait loci known to be within a certain chromosomal region.

Susceptibility locus: Gene which contributes (or is thought to contribute) to the risk of disease but may be neither a necessary nor a sufficient cause of disease.

Transmission-disequilibrium test (TDT): Tests the transmission ratio of alleles at a marker locus from a heterozygous parent to an affected child. There is distortion of the ratio from the mendelian 50:50 only if the marker locus is linked to the trait locus and exhibits allelic association. If a marker locus is close (tightly linked) to the trait locus, then allelic association may be observed; but association does not automatically imply tight linkage.

Velopharyngeal closure: Closing of the nasal cavity from the oral cavity which directs air used in speech through the mouth rather than the nose. It requires interaction of the muscles in the palate and the back of the throat.

Velopharyngeal incompetence: Inability to achieve adequate velopharyngeal closure despite structures that may appear normal.

Velopharyngeal insufficiency: A structural or functional disorder resulting in the inability to achieve adequate separation of the nasal and oral cavities.

Index